Reader's Digest

Family
Medical
Adviser

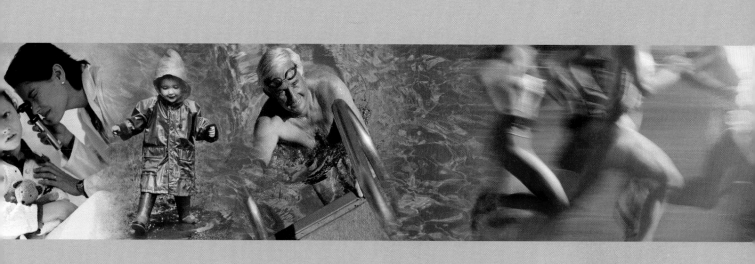

Reader's Digest

Family Medical Adviser

Published by THE READER'S DIGEST ASSOCIATION LIMITED
London • New York • Sydney • Montreal

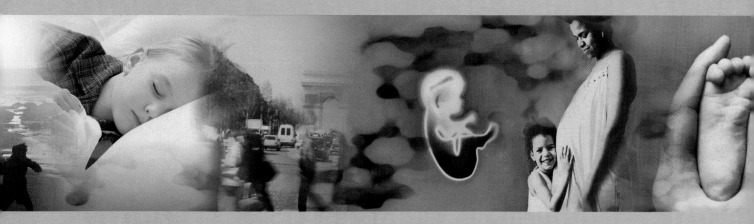

Contributors & consultants

Medical Advisers

Dr Sarah Brewer
MA MB BCHIR

Dr Alex Clarke
DPSYCH MSc BSc (HONS) AFBPsS

Dr John Cormack
BDS MB BS MRCS LRCP

Dr Vincent Forte
BA MB BS MRCGP MSc DA

Dr Judith Hall
BSc PHD MBPS

Dr Jim Lawrie
MB BS FRCGP MA (OXON) MBE

Sheena Meredith
MB BS MRCS (ENG) LRCP (LOND)

Dr Ian Morton
BSc PHD MIBIOL

Dr Melanie Wynne-Jones
MB CHB MRCGP DRCOG

Contributors

Elizabeth Adlam MA
Harriet Ainley BSc
Susan Aldridge MSc PhD
Dr Michael Apple BA
  MBChB MRCGP
Toni Battison RGN RSCN
  PgDip.
Glenda Baum MSc MCSP
  SRP
Nikki Bradford
Dr Sarah Brewer MA MB
  BChir
Jenny Bryan BSc (Hons)
Rita Carter
Dr Alex Clarke DPsych MSc
  BSc (Hons) AFBPsS
Geraldine Cooney BA
Dr John Cormack BDS MB
  BS MRCS LRCP
Dr Christine Fenn BSc
  (Hons) PhD
Dr Vincent Forte BA MB BS
  MRCGP MSc DA
Dr Judith Hall BSc PhD
  MBPS
William Harvey BSc (Hons)
  MCOptom
Caroline Holland BA
John Isitt BA
Dr Gillian Jenkins BM
  DRCOG DFFP BA
Georgina Kenyon BA
Dr Laurence Knott BSc
  (Hons) MB BS
Dr Jim Lawrie MBBS
  FRCGP MA (Oxon)
  MBE

Dr Patricia Macnair MA
  MBChB Dip Aneasth
Oona Mashta BA (Hons)
Sheena Meredith MB BS
  MRCS (Eng) LRCP
  (Lond)
Denise Mortimore BSc
  (Hons) PhD DHD
Dr Ian Morton BSc PhD
  MIBiol
John Newell MA (Camb)
Dr Louise Newson BSc
  (Hons) MB ChB (Hons)
  MRCP MRCGP
Nigel Perryman
Jim Pollard BA MA PCGE
Dr Ann Robinson MBBS
  MRCGP DCH DRCOG
Dr Christina Scott-Moncrieff
  MB ChB FFHom
Helen Spence BA
Dr Jenny Sutcliffe PhD MB
  BS MCSP
Jane Symons
June Thompson RN RM
  RGV
Helen Varley BA
Patsy Wescott BA (Hons)
Ann Whitehead MB BS
  MRCS LRCP MFFP
Dr Melanie Wynne-Jones
  MB ChB MRCGP
  DRCOG

Consultants & Organizations

Alcohol Concern

Alzheimer's Society

Dr Keith Andrews MD FRCP,
The Royal Hospital for
Neuro-disability

Arterial Disease Clinic

Association for Postnatal
Illness

BackCare

Toni Battison RGN RSCN
PgDip

Blood Pressure Association

British Dental Health
Foundation – Dr Nigel L.
Carter BDS LDS (RCS)

British Dyslexia Association

British Lung Foundation

British Red Cross

Cancer Research UK

Dr A Cann, University of
Leicester

CJD Support Network –
Alzheimer's Society

Charles Collins MA ChM
FRCS Ed – Member of
Council for the Royal
College of Surgeons of
England

Dr Carol Cooper MA MB
BChir MRCP

Cystic Fibrosis Trust

Mr R D Daniel BSc (Hons)
FRCS FRCOphth DO

Mr Dai Davies FRCS (plas)

Diabetes UK

Down's Syndrome Association

DrugScope

Eating Disorders Association

The Eyecare Trust

Family Planning Association

Food Standards Agency

Dr Vincent Forte BA MB BS
MRCGP MSc DA

Professor Anthony Frew MA
MD FRCP

Dr Judith Hall BSc PhD MBPS

International Glaucoma
Association

Dr Rod Jaques DRCOG RCGP
Dip. Sports Med. (Dist.)

Dr Laurence Knott BSc (Hons)
MB BS

Dr Richard Long MD FRCP

Dr John Lucocq MB BCh BSc
PhD

Mr W.A. Macleod MBChB
FRCSE

Pamela Mason BSc PhD
MRPharmS

ME Association

Meningitis Research
Foundation

Migraine Action Association

Ian Morton BSc PhD MIBiol

Motor Neurone Disease
Association

Multiple Sclerosis Society

National Asthma Campaign

National Autistic Society

National Blood Service

National Eczema Society

National Hospital for
Neurology and
Neurosurgery

National Kidney Research Fund

National Society for the
Prevention of Cruelty to
Children

Pituitary Foundation

RADAR (The Royal Association
for Disability and
Rehabilitation)

RELATE

Dr Ann Robinson MBBS
MRCGP DCH DRCOG

Royal College of Anaesthetists

Royal College of Speech and
Language Therapists

Royal National Institute for
Deaf People

Royal National Institute of the
Blind

The Society of Chiropodists and
Podiatrists and Emma Supple
FCPodS

SCOPE

Speakability

Penny Stanway MB BS

Terrence Higgins Trust

Dr Mark Westwood MA(Oxon)
MRCP

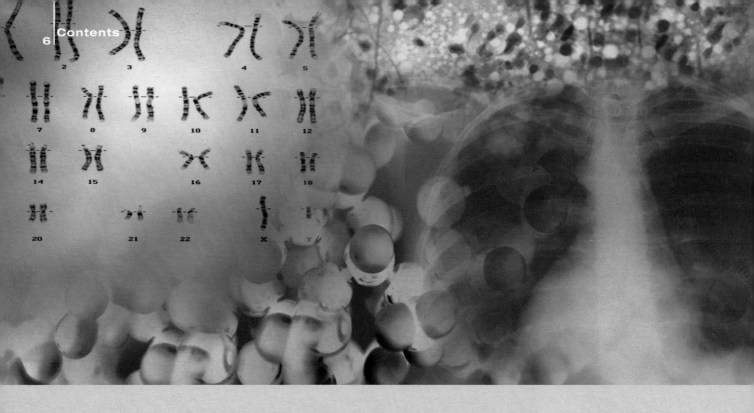

Contents

Important

While the creators of this work have made every effort to be as accurate and up to date as possible, medical and pharmacological knowledge is constantly changing. Readers are recommended to consult a qualified medical specialist for individual advice. The writers, researchers, editors and the publishers of this work cannot be held liable for any errors and omissions, or actions that may be taken as a consequence of information contained within this work.

Your family, your health

We all hope for long life and well-being and, while there can be no guarantee, there is much that we can do to keep ourselves and our families healthy. It helps to know a little about the workings of our bodies and what to do when illness occurs, but caring for your health can be a bewildering business full of difficult choices.

The aim of the *Family Medical Adviser* is to help you to manage your health, and to put you in a position where you can make clear and informed decisions about your treatment and your life.

Symptoms & solutions

You may turn to the book because you have a medical problem and need to know what to do. Knowing how to understand and evaluate symptoms will help you to get the right treatment, at the right time. The *Symptom sorter* is designed to make sense of the most common symptoms and lead you to the likely cause. There's guidance about whether you should seek urgent

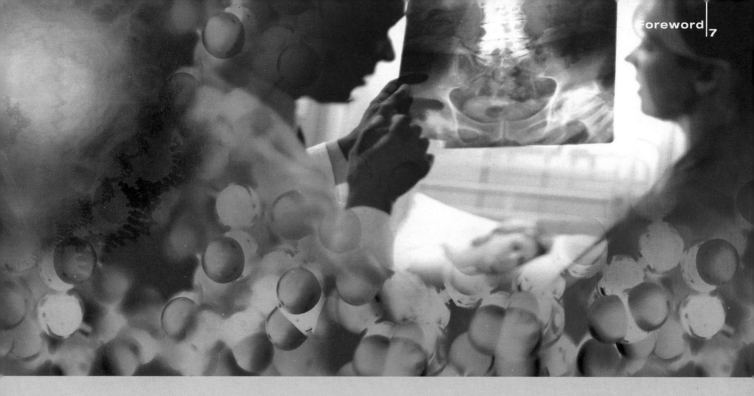

professional advice or make a routine appointment with your GP, and you can turn to the relevant entries in the *A to Z of medicine & health* to find out more.

Health & well-being

Many of the entries in the *A to Z of medicine & health* are descriptions of diseases or definitions of medical terms. To help you to find your way around, each article contains cross references, lists of related topics and words in bold type, which mean that there is a separate entry on that subject.

The information you find will help you to know what questions to ask your doctor and how to interpret the answers. If you are told that you have to undergo a medical procedure – say, a gastroscopy – you'll read about what to expect and how to prepare for it. All the most important conditions and medical issues are discussed at greater length in the special features that appear on coloured pages.

To learn more about the workings of the human body, turn to the *Body systems* pages. Through ground-breaking illustrations and clear explanations, these fascinating layperson's guides reveal the extraordinary complexities of the brain and nervous system *(pages 128–32)*, digestive system *(pages 226–9)*, heart and circulation *(pages 296–302)*, lymphatic system *(pages 380–3)*, muscles *(pages 416–20)*, reproductive *(pages 502–5)* and respiratory systems *(pages 508–11)*, skeleton *(pages 526–9)*, and urinary system *(pages 576–9)*.

If you are prescribed a drug or want to know more about an over-the-counter remedy, look it up in the glossary of *Drugs and their uses*. Using the generic or brand name you can find out how 500 of the most common drugs work and what they treat.

Whatever ailment or treatment you are facing, it is important to remember that you are never alone. The list of 200 *Useful contacts* will put you in touch with research organizations, patient groups and a wealth of information services where you can share experiences, and find help and support.

Your first family reference

A clear and comprehensive 48-page section of *First aid* procedures will equip you to deal calmly and effectively with everything from minor household injuries to major emergencies. Read it now so that you are ready to act whenever your help is needed.

The breadth and authority of this family manual make it an indispensible home reference. With its calm and reassuring tone, clear explanations and helpful illustrations, it will be the first place you turn to for guidance in every medical situation.

Symptom sorter

Symptoms are the sign that something is wrong somewhere in the body or mind. Knowing how to understand and evaluate your symptoms will help you to get the right treatment at the right time.

The Symptom sorter is designed to help you to make sense of the most common symptoms and to guide you to appropriate help. The Quick reference on pages 50 and 51 includes other important symptoms, with advice on the action you should take for each.

How does the Symptom sorter work?

Within each section you will find each symptom discussed briefly in an introduction. The most common causes are then discussed in the column headed Common causes. Next to this you will find information on Action, which tells you what to do and how quickly to do it.

You will also find a list of occasional and rare causes. It is important to be aware of these, but they are much less likely to be the cause of that symptom than the common causes listed. The Symptom sorter is a guide only, not a substitute for actual medical advice or management.

Over-the-counter remedies

For some symptoms the Action column advises using over-the-counter (OTC) remedies – retail products available from pharmacies without a GP's prescription. Always seek the pharmacist's advice when buying any OTC product and read the manufacturer's leaflet for contraindications. Check with your GP if you are in any doubt.

Recommended action

The advice given in the Action column classifies levels of urgency as follows.
- **Dial 999**: in life-threatening emergencies, call an ambulance. Follow the instructions given by the operator and provide information as requested. Remain calm and speak clearly.
- **See GP urgently**: ask for an appointment that same day. If all appointments are already taken for that day, ask to speak to a GP to check how urgently you should be seen. All GPs in the UK provide a 24-hour service for medical emergencies. Outside office hours most surgeries have a recorded instruction on their usual phone number. Alternatively, call NHS Direct (0845 4647); this will put you in contact with an experienced nurse who can advise you further.
- **See GP as soon as possible**: ask for the next available routine appointment.
- **See GP non-urgently**: ask for a routine appointment in the next few weeks or so.
- **Consult a genito-urinary medical clinic, drug and alcohol agency, counselling service**: you can arrange an appointment yourself without being referred by a doctor. To find local branches, consult the telephone directory or phone your local surgery or hospital.

First aid

For emergency treatment refer to the FIRST AID section on pages 590–637.

The symptom sorter is not a tool for self-diagnosis and cannot replace objective professional medical assessment.

Every care has been taken to ensure that the information is up to date and accurate. It is a guide to understanding what symptoms might represent and what appropriate action to take. It has been thoroughly researched and is based on the everyday working experience and knowledge of practising NHS GPs. If you are in any doubt about the importance or urgency of a medical problem, always get advice from your NHS GP's surgery or go to your local hospital casualty department.

Contents

Emergency symptoms

Always consult a doctor urgently if you, or anyone in your care, has any of the following symptoms.

- Sudden, severe, crushing chest pain.
- Severe breathlessness.
- Sudden and lasting confusion or loss of consciousness.
- Severe headache and neck stiffness, particularly if associated with eye pain on looking at a normal-strength light.
- Sudden loss of vision.
- Severe and constant abdominal pain.
- Vomiting blood.
- Jet-black bowel motions.
- Diarrhoea and vomiting lasting more than 24 hours.
- Severe back pain with pain or numbness down both legs and sudden incontinence.

Symptom sorter

Glands, swollen

Swollen glands are enlarged lymph nodes – they swell and become noticeable when they are fighting infection, and may also be sore. The glands most easily felt are under the jaw, all around the neck and in the armpits and groin.

OCCASIONAL CAUSES: glandular fever; cat-scratch fever (common in children); sarcoidosis; German measles (rubella); measles; systemic lupus erythematosis (an inflammatory disease); rheumatoid arthritis; sexually transmitted diseases (eg lymphogranuloma venereum, granuloma inguinale). **RARE CAUSES:** AIDS and AIDS-related complex; tuberculosis; tropical diseases (eg leprosy, filariasis); drug reactions.

COMMON CAUSES	ACTION
General viral infection This is the cause of nine out of ten cases of swollen glands. Enlarged glands may be felt around the body (in the neck, armpits, groin). You may be generally unwell, with a fever.	Rest, drink plenty of non-alcoholic fluids, take paracetamol regularly. If not beginning to improve after five days, call GP for advice.
Localized infection Enlargement of a single group of glands (such as in the neck). Fever and feeling generally unwell; possibly with specific symptoms such as cough or sore throat.	As for General viral infection, above.
Cancer Slowly enlarging, often painless, hard, fixed glands, usually in a single group. Present for six weeks or more.	See GP as soon as possible.
White cell cancers (lymphoma, leukaemia, myeloma) As for Cancer above, but may involve several groups of glands. Night sweats and itching common.	See GP as soon as possible.
Septicaemia (bacterial infection in bloodstream) Several groups of glands are enlarged. Feeling very ill, high fever; possible confusion and delirium.	Urgent GP assessment. A home visit may be necessary if you are confused.

Insomnia

Sleep needs vary with age and according to the individual: infants require at least 16 hours, while adults need 5–8 hours, some 3–4 hours. Insomnia should not be confused with a low requirement for sleep.

OCCASIONAL CAUSES: respiratory problems (eg asthma, chronic obstructive pulmonary disease); inefficient heart pumping (left ventricular failure); overactive thyroid (hyper-thyroidism); benzodiazepine withdrawal; parasomnias (eg nightmares, night terrors, sleepwalking); disruption of biorhythms (eg due to jet lag, shift work). **RARE CAUSES:** malnutrition, low weight; post-traumatic stress disorder; mania; sleep apnoea (cessation of breathing in sleep).

COMMON CAUSES	ACTION
Excess psychological stress You are slow to go off to sleep, may have early morning waking, and feel low or nervous. (Underlying causes include problems with work, relationships or finances.)	See GP as soon as possible.
Clinical depression Early morning waking and low mood, along with low self-esteem, lack of confidence, poor short-term memory, tearfulness, irrational sense of guilt and other symptoms.	See GP as soon as possible.
Chronic excess alcohol Sleep may be totally disrupted. Other signs of alcohol abuse, such as red face and palms, are common.	Seek help from local drugs and alcohol agency.
Hyperstimulation (poor sleeping patterns) You may be wide awake at night and slow to go off, but otherwise well. (Caffeine and nicotine are common underlying causes.)	Change lifestyle to reduce stimulation at night.
Pain of chronic illness Sleep may be totally disrupted. The underlying cause, for example, osteoarthritis, is usually obvious.	See GP as soon as possible to deal with cause.

Memory loss

Memory is classed as short-term (immediate), medium-term (recent) and long-term (remote). For memory loss with acute confusion, see page 50.

OCCASIONAL CAUSES: vitamin B$_1$ (thiamin) deficiency; artery disease; brain tumour. **RARE CAUSES:** subarachnoid haemorrhage (bleeding in brain); some personality disorders; very severe epilepsy; carbon monoxide poisoning; viral encephalitis (inflammation of the brain).

COMMON CAUSES	ACTION
Head injury A head injury can cause all levels of memory loss. If the injury is severe enough to affect the memory, hospitalization is usually needed.	Seek specialist advice from hospital team involved in initial care, or see a GP non-urgently if later.
Dementia, including Alzheimer's disease Gradual onset over a year or two. Short- and medium-term memory affected, long-term memory usually intact. Person usually unaware of problem.	See GP non-urgently for assessment and possible specialist referral.
Stroke Sudden onset. May be associated with collapse, weakness or loss of power of speech.	See GP urgently; a home visit may be necessary.
Depressive illness Gradual onset over two or more weeks, with loss of concentration, constant low mood; loss of appetite, self-esteem; sleep disturbance, fatigue. Usually aware of problem.	See GP as soon as possible for assessment.
Chronic excess alcohol intake Gradual onset. Signs of chronic alcohol excess (eg, lifestyle factors, red face and palms). Person often unaware of problem; invents stories to cover gaps in memory.	See GP as soon as possible. Requires careful assessment.

Muscles, painful

Pain in muscles may be experienced as a short-lived cramp, as a continuous dull ache or as a sharp and severe pain on using the affected muscle. It may be painful to touch as well as to use.

OCCASIONAL CAUSES: peripheral vascular disease (narrowing of blood vessels in legs and arms); diabetic or alcoholic neuropathy (nerve disease); general anaesthesia, side effect of muscle-relaxant drug; underactive thyroid (hypothyroidism); Bornholm disease (devil's grip). **RARE CAUSES:** side effect of drug treatment (eg chemotherapy, cimetidine) or drug withdrawal.

COMMON CAUSES	ACTION
Overuse of muscles, including strain Sudden onset after unusually intense or prolonged activity. Muscle sore to touch and stiff after rest.	Take OTC painkillers, apply heat rubs or take anti-inflammatories. Stay active without straining the affected muscle.
Acute viral illness Sudden onset, with fever and feeling generally unwell. Many muscles are affected, and pain may move from one area to another.	Rest, take non-alcoholic drinks, regular paracetamol or OTC anti-inflammatories. If not settling within five days, call GP for advice.
Depression, ME (myalgic encephalomyelitis)/ chronic fatigue syndrome Vague pains in many different muscles, usually worse after activity. Associated with low mood and tiredness.	See GP non-urgently for assessment.
Inflammatory myopathy (muscle disease) May start suddenly. Marked morning stiffness. Persistent, affecting specific muscles, which may be painful to touch. (Causes include rheumatoid arthritis and scleroderma.)	See GP urgently as some conditions are associated with serious complications if not treated.
Referred joint pain Pain associated with a nearby joint problem and referred (for example, from hip to thigh or shoulder to arm). Made worse if the affected joint is used then rested.	Take OTC painkillers and anti-inflammatories. See GP as soon as possible for assessment.

Numbness and pins and needles

Loss of feeling (numbness) and prickling (pins and needles) in the skin are known medically as paraesthesia. Commonly produced by sitting too long in one position, they may be accompanied by feelings of hot or cold and pain on light touch.

OCCASIONAL CAUSES: multiple sclerosis; spinal cord inflammatory disease (dorsal myelitis); alcoholic polyneuropathy (nerve disease) and vitamin B_1, B_6, and B_{12} deficiency; stroke; injury to peripheral nerve or spinal cord; low blood calcium (hypocalcaemia); kidney failure; low blood sugar (hypoglycaemia); porphyria (an enzyme deficiency); xanthomatosis (fatty deposits affecting nerves); Raynaud's syndrome.
RARE CAUSES: spinal cord tumour; brain trauma, tumour or epilepsy affecting sensory cortex; migraine.

COMMON CAUSES	ACTION
Anxiety with hyperventilation Nervous emotional state, episodes of dizziness, rapid breathing. Often affects hands, feet and area around mouth. In severe hyperventilation, feet and hands may spasm.	To calm symptoms, breathe in and out of a paper bag held loosely over mouth and nose. If not settling, call GP urgently for advice; otherwise see GP non-urgently for help.
Carpal tunnel syndrome (trapped nerve) Pins and needles, pain in hands. Worse at night and after manual work. Finger-thumb grip may be weak.	See GP as soon as possible for assessment.
Sciatica (spinal nerve root compression) Follows severe, sudden lower back pain: numbness and pain spreads from lower back through buttock and down back of leg to side of foot.	See GP urgently or ask for home visit. Try OTC painkillers. If both legs are affected, go straight to casualty: you may need to be hospitalized.
Diabetic neuropathy (nerve disease) Often continuous pins and needles; hot and cold sensations, pain. Affects one or more limbs.	See GP as soon as possible for assessment.
Arthritis in neck (cervical spondylosis) Pain and tingling in back, neck and top of head. Made worse by certain movements.	Take OTC anti-inflammatories or painkillers. If severe, see GP as soon as possible.

Tired all the time

This is the constant feeling of being tired and worn out. Physical and mental activities take more effort, and the ability to keep going is reduced.

OCCASIONAL CAUSES: ME (myalgic encephalitis) or chronic post-viral fatigue syndrome; major organ failure (eg heart, liver, kidney); overactive thyroid (hyperthyroidism); substance misuse; drugs (eg beta-blockers, diuretics).
RARE CAUSES: cancer; tuberculosis or other chronic infection; chronic neurological (nerve) disorders; diabetes mellitus, Addison's disease or other endocrine gland disorders; connective tissue disorders (eg rheumatoid arthritis, polymyalgia rheumatica).

COMMON CAUSES	ACTION
Depressive illness May be worse at some times of the day than others. Associated with tearfulness and loss of confidence, concentration, pleasure, self-esteem. Poor sleep.	If symptoms are present for two weeks or more, see GP as soon as possible. Should respond to treatment.
Stress Tiredness reduces when cause of stress is not present. Identifiable trigger: overwork, young children or boredom.	Try relaxation tapes, yoga, exercise. Take time for self. See GP if this fails.
Anaemia (low red blood cell content) Constant tiredness. Pale lips, tongue and inner eyelids; in extreme cases, shortness of breath on exertion and fainting. Blood loss (eg heavy periods), or lack of iron or B vitamins.	See GP as soon as possible, urgently if extreme symptoms are present.
Acute post-viral fatigue Recent illness. Constant, debilitating fatigue.	Rest, eat well. See GP if symptoms last longer than a month after illness.
Underactive thyroid (hypothyroidism) Gradual onset of constant, debilitating fatigue, associated with coldness and feeling slowed down. Skin may feel dry, hair brittle.	See GP as soon as possible for assessment and possible blood test.

Tremor

Tremor, a repetitive shaking movement of part of the body, is caused by rapid contraction and relaxation of the muscles. It is often noticed in the hands, but can affect any part of the body. It is often embarrassing for the person affected, and can interfere with everyday physical activity.

OCCASIONAL CAUSES: adverse drug reaction; carbon dioxide retention in chronic obstructive pulmonary (lung) disease; multiple sclerosis; chronic liver disease ('liver flap', also called asterixis); any cause of ataxia (clumsy movement), eg tumour, abscess.
RARE CAUSES: hepatic encephalopathy (brain poisoning caused by liver malfunction).

COMMON CAUSES	ACTION
Anxiety Fast, racing heartbeat, palpitations. Nervous emotional state; life stresses likely. Sweaty skin, shaky hands; often breathlessness and pins and needles.	Consider ways to reduce life stress. See GP as soon as possible for confirmation and help.
Thyrotoxicosis (overactive thyroid) Consistently fast heartbeat with missed beats. Gradual, relentless weight loss; feeling hot and dislike of warm environments. Fine tremor of hands.	See GP as soon as possible for assessment.
Drug and alcohol withdrawal Sudden onset with confusion, generalized shaking, fast heartbeat and profuse sweating.	Risk of fits; contact GP urgently. If delirious and confused, dial 999.
Benign essential tremor Usually runs in families. Sufferers notice tremor disappears at rest or on taking alcohol. Otherwise well. Harmless, no known cause.	See GP non-urgently.
Parkinson's disease Tremor worst at rest. Slow movements, shuffling gait, frequent falls and inexpressive, mask-like face.	See GP as soon as possible.

Weight change, excessive

The concept of normal weight is defined by the Body Mass Index (see page 438). Any weight loss or gain that is unexpected and rapid should be investigated.

WEIGHT GAIN
OCCASIONAL CAUSES: liver or kidney failure; drug side affects; hormonal disorders.
RARE CAUSES: anabolic steroid abuse; Cushing's syndrome.

WEIGHT LOSS
OCCASIONAL CAUSES: drug, alcohol or laxative misuse; heart failure; chronic kidney and liver failure; undiagnosed diabetes mellitus; chronic inflammatory conditions; gastro-intestinal disease.
RARE CAUSES: any chronic infection (especially tuberculosis); endocrine disorder; AIDS; malnutrition.

COMMON CAUSES	ACTION
GAIN: Underactive thyroid (hypothyroidism) Gradual onset of constant, debilitating fatigue; feeling cold, slowed down. Skin may feel dry, hair brittle. Fingers and feet may feel swollen.	See GP as soon as possible for assessment and possible blood test.
GAIN: Oedema (tissue swelling) Swelling first of feet, then legs and rest of body. Pressing a finger into the affected part for ten seconds will leave a visible dimple that takes minutes to clear. Many underlying causes including congestive heart failure.	See GP as soon as possible, urgently if short of breath or very ill.
LOSS: Eating disorders (anorexia/bulimia nervosa) **Anorexia**: inappropriate, unshakeable self-image of being overweight; extreme dieting, possibly self-induced vomiting. **Bulimia**: binge-eating alternates with starvation diet, self-induced vomiting common; disordered eating habits.	See GP as soon as possible: these are serious and need expert help. May respond to behavioural treatment; antidepressants can be very helpful.
LOSS: Hyperthyroidism (overactive thyroid) Gradual, relentless weight loss; fast heartbeat with missed beats. Associated with feeling hot and dislike of warm environments; fine tremor of hands.	See GP as soon as possible for assessment.
LOSS: Cancer Rapid weight loss, loss of appetite. Feeling very unwell.	See GP as soon as possible.

Breathlessness, chronic

Breathlessness is the sensation of having to breathe harder than expected for a given level of activity. For example, panting when just walking on level ground, or even having to breathe hard when at rest. It is said to be chronic when it occurs over a long period of time, months or years.

OCCASIONAL CAUSES: bronchiectasis (widening of bronchial air passages); recurrent pulmonary emboli (clots blocking lung arterioles); large hiatus hernia; lung cancer with collapse of part of a lung (lobar collapse); pleural effusion (fluid in lung lining).
RARE CAUSES: pulmonary fibrosis; motor neurone disease; muscular dystrophy.

COMMON CAUSES	ACTION
Obesity Breathlessness occurs in people who are obviously obese. It may be worse when lying down.	Seek dietary advice and ensure clothes are not too tight.
Chronic obstructive pulmonary disease (COPD) Chronic cough and production of phlegm. Nearly always the result of smoking.	Stop smoking. See GP non-urgently for assessment, treatment and possible referral.
Anaemia Pale lips, tongue and insides of eyelids. Increasing fatigue may develop alongside the shortness of breath.	See GP as soon as possible for blood test to confirm the diagnosis and further assessment.
Congestive cardiac failure Always worse on lying down. Ankle swelling, with possible wheezy cough and phlegm.	See GP as soon as possible for assessment and treatment.
Asthma Wheezing and cough brought on by exertion or exposure to allergens such as cats, dogs or pollen.	See GP as soon as possible for assessment and treatment.

Breathlessness, sudden

This is the sudden inability to breathe, or a sudden sensation of not being able to breathe enough for a given level of activity. There is a sense of suffocation or 'hunger for air'. Sudden breathlessness is always a very distressing and frightening experience. Blueish lips (cyanosis) or confusion indicate a severe shortage of oxygen: dial 999 immediately.

OCCASIONAL CAUSES: pneumothorax (air leaking from lung); pulmonary embolism (clot); pleural effusion (fluid in lung lining); severe biochemical imbalance (diabetic ketoacidosis); collapse of part of a lung (lobar collapse) caused by a cancerous tumour.
RARE CAUSES: hypovolaemic shock (lack of blood); obstruction of the windpipe by foreign body.

COMMON CAUSES	ACTION
Acute asthmatic attack Severe difficulty in breathing, with wheezing and drawing in of the skin between the ribs. Inability to speak indicates an extremely severe attack.	Use medication if appropriate. Call GP urgently, or dial 999 if it appears very severe.
Pneumonia Fever, coughing up dirty-looking phlegm, fast breathing rate. Tearing chest pain in deep breathing indicates inflammation of the lung membranes (pleurisy).	Call GP urgently. Continue coughing up of phlegm and keep sitting upright.
Inefficient heart pumping (acute left ventricular failure) Severe shortness of breath on exertion, made worse by lying down. May come on suddenly during the night while asleep; can be the first sign of a heart attack (myocardial infarction).	Sit up in a chair with feet down to relieve the burden on the heart; this could save your life. Dial 999.
Exacerbation of chronic obstructive pulmonary disease (COPD) Long-standing lung disease (such as emphysema); similar features to those of Pneumonia, above.	Call GP urgently.
Hyperventilation (rapid breathing) Overwhelming anxiety. Very fast breathing rate, often associated with 'pins and needles' in fingers, toes and around mouth. Spasm of hands and feet may occur.	Calm symptoms: breathe in and out of a paper bag held over mouth and nose. Call GP urgently for advice.

Chest pain, sudden

Chest pain can take many forms: it may be dull or sharp, aching or stabbing, constant or throbbing, in one place or all over the chest. It may also be referred, felt in another part of the body. For example, heart pain can be felt in the arms, neck and jaw.

OCCASIONAL CAUSES: lung membrane inflammation (pleurisy); peptic ulcer; gallstones; shingles; mastitis (inflammation of the breast).
RARE CAUSES: pulmonary infarct (clot in the lung); inflammation of the heart (eg pericarditis, myocarditis); fractured ribs; dissecting aortic aneurysm (tearing in a swelling of the aorta).

COMMON CAUSES	ACTION
Angina, heart attack (myocardial infarction) Severe, crushing central pain; may be felt in jaw, neck and arms. Nausea; breathlessness; sweaty skin; faintness. Angina is precipitated by exertion and settles with rest. A heart attack may occur at rest and does not settle with rest.	Dial 999 and take half a 300mg aspirin tablet, if not allergic or sensitive to it, to reduce the risk of blood clots (thrombosis).
Reflux oesophagitis (inflammation of the gullet) Anything from mild acid heartburn to symptoms similar to those of Angina, above. Usually acid regurgitation in throat when stooping, lying down and after meals.	If severe, dial 999: requires tests to distinguish it from heart pain. If mild, try OTC antacids or a milky drink.
Anxiety (Da Costa's syndrome) Pain often in one specific point in the chest; related to a stressful event or generally anxious personality.	See GP as soon as possible.
Pulled muscle Usually after physical activity; triggered by certain arm movements. Sore point in affected muscle.	Gentle activity to prevent stiffness. Take OTC anti-inflammatories, painkillers.
Inflammation of the rib cartilage (costochondritis) Often triggered by a general viral illness. Pain on deep breathing in a few points between ribs and breastbone, which are sore to touch.	Take OTC anti-inflammatories, painkillers.

Cough

A cough is a sudden, explosive release of air from the lungs through the mouth. The urge to cough is often a ticklish, irritating sensation, felt in the throat or windpipe. Coughs are often described as productive (with phlegm) or dry (without phlegm). Always see a GP for a cough continuing for six weeks or more. Smoking can be a contributory factor in all of the common causes listed.

OCCASIONAL CAUSES: lung tumour; inefficient heart pumping (left ventricular failure); side effect of ACE inhibitors (high blood pressure drugs); psychological factors.
RARE CAUSES: ear wax or foreign body in ear canal; inhaled foreign body; tuberculosis; cystic fibrosis; cancer of the larynx.

COMMON CAUSES	ACTION
Infection of the upper airways Often follows or accompanies a sore throat or cold. Green or yellow phlegm common in first few days.	Try OTC remedies, steam inhalations. Avoid smoky atmospheres. See GP if not improving after a week.
Chest infection Fever, hot and cold sweats, feeling very unwell; copious yellow, green or brown phlegm that may be bloodstained. In severe cases there may be shortness of breath.	See GP urgently for examination and antibiotic treatment.
Asthma Dry cough, possibly with wheeze, difficulty breathing and chest tightness. Asthma often triggered by emotion, exertion or exposure to allergens such as dogs, cats, pollen.	See GP as soon as possible for examination and treatment.
Nose area inflammations (rhinitis, chronic sinusitis) Stuffy nose with persistent catarrh dripping down back of throat. Sinusitis causes pain over and/or under eyes, and the pain throbs on walking and stooping.	Try OTC remedies. Avoid smoke. See GP if not improving after a week.
Inflammation of the gullet (oesophageal reflux) Acid regurgitation in throat, often on stooping or lying down. Heartburn, often made worse by hot drinks and spicy foods.	Try OTC antacids; avoid trigger foods. See GP if problem continues.

Coughing up blood

Blood can be coughed up from the windpipe or lungs, either on its own or mixed with phlegm. Most of the serious causes listed here are rare; most commonly the blood is from the nose or mouth or caused by a chest infection. But if breathing is difficult phone a GP for urgent advice or dial 999.

OCCASIONAL CAUSES: mitral stenosis (a narrowing of the heart valve opening); bronchiectasis (widening of air passages); polyarteritis nodosa (an inflammation of the artery walls); tuberculosis; tumour of larynx or trachea.
RARE CAUSES: injury-related bruising of the brain (contusion).

COMMON CAUSES	ACTION
Chest infection You will be feeling unwell, have a fever and be coughing up copious yellow, green or brown phlegm. Shortness of breath indicates a severe infection.	Drink plenty of non-alcoholic fluids. See GP urgently or ask for home visit if necessary.
Blood clot on the lung (pulmonary embolism) Sudden shortness of breath and chest pain on deep breathing. May be preceded by calf pain, signifying deep vein thrombosis.	See GP urgently; if breathing is difficult dial 999.
Lung cancer Generally feeling unwell, usually preceded by weight loss, shortness of breath. Rare in non-smokers.	See GP as soon as possible for assessment.
Fluid in the lung (pulmonary oedema) May occur without warning, often while sleeping. Phlegm is pink and frothy. Swollen ankles; severe shortness of breath, made worse by lying down.	Sit in chair with feet down. Dial 999.
Prolonged coughing Coughing is painful. Often linked with a viral infection, (eg a cold), but can occur with any cause of cough (see page 14).	Take frequent sips of cold drinks. Try steam inhalations and humidification.

Palpitations

Palpitations are abnormal-feeling heartbeats, such as fast or irregular ones. They are uncomfortable and often feel like a fluttering in the chest or lower neck. An occasional missed beat (ectopic beat) is normal. Palpitations are more likely to represent a medical problem in people aged over 60 than in younger people.

OCCASIONAL CAUSES: heart disorders (eg mitral valve disease, cardiomyopathy); sick sinus syndrome; electrolyte abnormality (a blood disorder); alcohol abuse; anaemia.
RARE CAUSES: tumour in the chest cavity (a mediastinal tumour); pulmonary embolism (a blood clot in the lung); inflammation of the heart muscle (myocarditis).

COMMON CAUSES	ACTION
Anxiety Fast, racing heartbeat or runs of missed beats lasting seconds or minutes. Nervous emotional state; life stresses likely. Sweaty skin, shaky hands; breathlessness and pins and needles common.	Consider ways to reduce life stress. See GP as soon as possible for confirmation and help.
Missed beats Occasional and infrequent missed beats in an otherwise healthy person. May occur several times a day, but there should not be more than six in one minute.	No action necessary. If there are consistently more than six missed beats per minute, see GP non-urgently.
Overactive thyroid (thyrotoxicosis) Consistently fast heartbeat with missed beats. Gradual, relentless weight loss; feeling hot with dislike of warm environments. Fine tremor of hands.	See GP as soon as possible for assessment.
Heart attack (myocardial infarction) Usually sudden onset of fast and/or irregular heartbeat; with crushing central chest pain that may travel to arms, neck and jaw. Shortness of breath, faintness and nausea.	Dial 999 for ambulance. Take half a 300mg aspirin tablet if not allergic, asthmatic or with stomach problems.
Ischaemic heart disease (blood vessel blockage) Runs of fast and/or irregular heartbeats, brought on by exertion. Often associated with angina (see page 14).	See GP as soon as possible, urgently if this is a new problem and if faint and/or short of breath.

Hair loss

Hair loss may affect just one part of the scalp, appear in patches, or occur in a symmetrical pattern as in male baldness. It is usually painless, unless it is caused by a painful inflammation. Hair loss can affect the whole body.

OCCASIONAL CAUSES: bacterial folliculitis (inflammation of the hair follicles); telogen effluvium (hair falls out suddenly; after a time there is regrowth); endocrine disorders (eg myxoedema, hypopituitarism and hypoparathyroidism); lupus erythematosus (an inflammatory disease); side effect of chemotherapy.
RARE CAUSES: secondary syphilis; trichotillomania (ingrained habit of rubbing, fiddling with or pulling hair out); alopecia totalis (an autoimmune condition).

COMMON CAUSES	ACTION
Male pattern baldness (androgenic alopecia) The scalp is normal. Patchy hair loss works backwards from the forehead, and is more pronounced above the temples. Also thinning crown.	There is no reliably proven treatment for this, although many 'cures' are marketed.
Seborrhoeic dermatitis (fungal infection) Scaly crusts on scalp, often weeping clear fluid. There may be a similar scaly rash on parts of the body.	Control symptoms with OTC antifungal selenium-containing shampoos.
Alopecia areata (bald patches) Patchy hair thinning on a normal scalp. The hairs are tapered, thin towards the ends, like exclamation marks (can be seen under a magnifying glass).	See GP non-urgently for confirmation. Rarely there is an association with uncommon autoimmune diseases.
Allergic dermatitis Patchy hair thinning with a reddened inflamed scalp. There may be similar rashes on the body. Follows use of allergens such as scalp lotion, shampoo.	Avoid allergen if possible. Steroid creams will settle this: see GP non-urgently for advice.
Tinea capitis (fungal infection) Patchy hair thinning, with scaly weeping around areas of scalp. There may be similar ring-shaped areas of skin on the body. 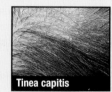 **Tinea capitis**	Use OTC antifungal creams. If you have a cat or dog, get it checked by a vet as it may carry the fungus.

Flat spots

Flat spots are any abnormally coloured, flat areas of skin (macules). They vary from red, white to brown, black and grey. Purple or dark red bruises are called purpura (see page 19). Some red flat spots share causes with erythema (see Red rash, page 22).

OCCASIONAL CAUSES: measles; German measles (rubella); post-inflammatory pigmentation; café-au-lait spots (creamy brown spots); Mongolian spots (brown, slate-grey spots); sensitivity to light as a reaction to certain chemicals; depigmentation (white spots).
RARE CAUSES: infections; Albright's syndrome; neurovascular abnormality; neurofibromatosis (nervous system disorder); pathological freckles.

COMMON CAUSES	ACTION
Allergy or drug reaction Itchy, red, burning spots, often more than 5mm (¼in) in diameter.	See GP urgently if you suspect a drug reaction. If not, try OTC antihistamines.
Flat mole (junctional naevus) Brown spots, often with variable depth of colour; small ones look like freckles. Can be several centimetres (1–2in) in diameter. 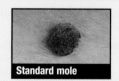 **Standard mole**	No action needed. If it is regularly subjected to damage, changes in size or colour, or becomes lumpy, see GP as soon as possible; this may indicate melanoma.
Non-specific viral rash Red and frequently large area of skin that is painless and does not itch.	No treatment needed unless illness itself requires medical advice.
Chloasma (reaction to sunlight) Mask-like, symmetrical brown area on front of the face. Affects women only, especially those who are pregnant or who take a combined oral contraceptive pill.	No action needed if you are pregnant; if on contraceptive pill, see GP as soon as possible.

Itching

In general, itching is made worse by anything that increases the blood supply to the skin, including alcohol and heat. Calamine lotion, OTC antihistamine tablets or hydrocortisone cream can offer relief. If itching persists for more than a few days, see a GP.

OCCASIONAL CAUSES: ingested allergens such as food (eg strawberries and shellfish) and drugs; jaundice; iron-deficiency anaemia; endocrine disorders (eg diabetes mellitus, hypothyroidism, hyperthyroidism); kidney failure.

RARE CAUSES: psychological factors; diseases of white blood cells (eg leukaemia); itching of unknown cause.

COMMON CAUSES

ACTION

Contact dermatitis
Itchy, inflamed and sometimes weeping skin in one area, where contact with the allergen has been made.

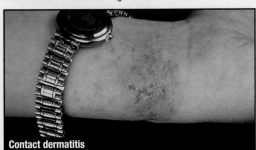
Contact dermatitis

Avoid allergen. Nickel jewellery or jeans studs are common allergens.

Scabies and other skin infestations
Furiously itchy rash, which often spreads from the hands and is worse at night.

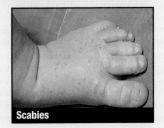
Scabies

Try OTC antiscabies lotion; itching may last up to ten days after end of treatment. Contagious by direct contact only.

Atopic eczema (a skin disease)
Itchy, flaky, inflamed and sometimes weeping skin, often in the bends of the arms and legs.

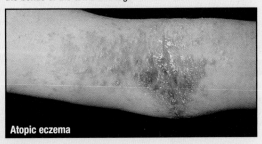
Atopic eczema

Try OTC hydrocortisone cream. See GP if not settling within a week. May need antibiotic cream.

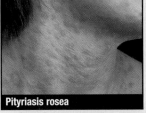
Pityriasis rosea

Pityriasis rosea (skin rash)
Raised, reddened spots 5mm–2cm (¼–¾in) long. Oval patches in characteristic 'Christmas tree' pattern, with long axes pointing the same way. Often starts with one large patch. Takes six weeks to develop and fade.

Try OTC treatments to help symptoms; there is no cure. It is probably caused by a virus, and always goes away on its own.

Psoriasis
Raised, reddened patches from 5mm to many centimetres (¼–2in) in size. Silvery scaling may be seen when scratched.

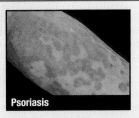
Psoriasis

See GP as soon as possible. There are no effective home treatments.

Blisters

Blisters are categorized into two types according to their size: vesicles are up to 5mm (¼in) in diameter and bullae are more than 5mm (¼in) in diameter. They may be filled with a clear, straw-coloured fluid (lymph) or blood. Blisters may be painless with no unusual sensations or they may be associated with feelings of itching, pain or burning. For blisters filled with pus, see Pus spots, page 21.

OCCASIONAL CAUSES: autoimmune skin disorders (eg pemphigus, pemphigoid); scabies (tiny blisters); dermatitis herpetiformis (a condition that resembles herpes virus infection); bullous impetigo (a skin infection); drug eruption; erythema multiforme (spots are symmetrical with a central blister, like targets).
RARE CAUSES: porphyria (a metabolic disorder); epidermolysis bullosa (a genetic disorder); allergic vasculitis (inflammation of the blood vessels).

COMMON CAUSES	ACTION
Injury Injury usually visible and with obvious cause such as friction, heat, chemical burns or insect bites. Blisters usually more than 5mm (¼in) in diameter. 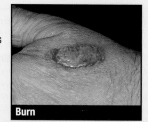 Burn	Do not burst blister; cover with dry plaster. See GP urgently if redness is spreading out from blister and pain increases, since infection is possible.
Cold sore (herpes simplex) Crop of blisters in one area, usually on or around mouth and less than 5mm (¼in) in diameter. Blisters are preceded by skin tingling and pain. 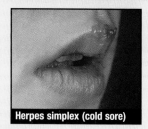 Herpes simplex (cold sore)	Apply OTC antiviral cream as soon as possible. See GP urgently if rash spreads beyond original crop.
Shingles (herpes zoster) Blisters are usually less than 5mm (¼in) in diameter. Always on one side of the body, spreading out in a band around the trunk or down a limb. Pain not helped by OTC painkillers. 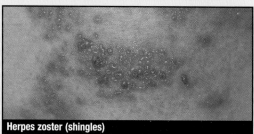 Herpes zoster (shingles)	See GP urgently; antiviral treatment may be needed. It is contagious: avoid contact with adults who have not had chickenpox, especially pregnant women, until the last blister has burst and scabbed over.
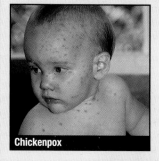 Chickenpox **Childhood viruses** Chickenpox or hand, foot and mouth disease may be the cause. Sufferer may feel mildly ill, as with a cold, before rash appears. Neck glands may be enlarged.	See GP as soon as possible for confirmation. Viral illnesses are contagious: see recommendations for Shingles, above.
Eczema Blisters are often more than 5mm (¼in) in diameter, and may be painful. Commonly on hands, palms or soles of feet. 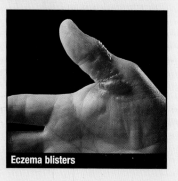 Eczema blisters	See GP as soon as possible, urgently if the skin is very painful – this is unusual and may indicate that the skin is infected or cracked.

Bruising

Bruising is reddish-purple skin discoloration that does not whiten under pressure. The medical name is purpura.

COMMON CAUSES	ACTION
Injury Bruises can be any size, and are usually tender to the touch. The original injury is often minor. 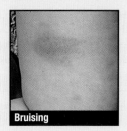 Bruising	No treatment needed, but cold compresses reduce swelling and arnica cream may help to speed up recovery. If repeated bruising appears on areas not subjected to everyday knocks, see a GP as soon as possible.
Senile purpura (age-related bruising) Bruises often appears repeatedly, are widespread and without obvious cause. This is caused by fragile blood vessels in ageing skin.	See GP as soon as possible if there is unexplained bleeding of any sort as well; otherwise no action needed.
Liver disease (especially alcoholic cirrhosis) Widespread bruises of all sizes repeatedly appear. There may be other signs of liver disease or alcohol excess. 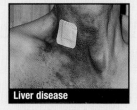 Liver disease	See GP urgently: there may be a blood-clotting problem.
Coughing or vomiting Tiny bruises appear on the face immediately after a violent coughing fit or vomiting, which increases pressure in major blood vessels. Also seen inside lips and eyelids.	No action needed: it looks alarming but is of no importance in itself.
Drug reactions Widespread tiny bruises appear suddenly. They are not painful, but you may feel unwell from some other side effect of the drug (eg steroids, aspirin, warfarin, quinine, thiazides).	See GP as soon as possible; urgently if you are taking warfarin.

OCCASIONAL CAUSES: painful bruising syndrome; connective tissue disorders (eg lupus erythematosis); vasculitis (inflammation of blood vessel walls); platelet (blood) defects; lichen sclerosus et atrophicus (a skin disease).
RARE CAUSES: bone marrow damage (caused by cytotoxic drugs, leukaemia or cancer); inherited blood-clotting disorders (eg haemophilia); infections (eg meningococcal septicaemia); deficiency of vitamin C or K.

Special care: meningitis

Meningitis is an infection of the membranes surrounding the brain and spinal cord (the meninges). Meningitis is very rare, but all parents and carers should know how to recognize it.

The symptoms of meningitis are:
- feeling very unwell, with a fever;
- severe, throbbing headache;
- feeling sick, or vomiting;
- intense dislike of bright light (photophobia), including indoor lighting;
- stiff (not just sore) neck; difficult to turn head;
- floppiness and sleepiness in babies and young children. Older children may be unusually drowsy.

A purplish rash that doesn't fade when pressure is put on the skin is a late and serious sign of the illness. The glass test (see below) can help you to tell whether or not a rash is non-blanching.

All these symptoms can be caused by common illnesses, including migraine and non-serious virus infections. If in doubt phone your GP for advice.

The glass test

Take an ordinary clear glass or plastic tumbler. Place it on the skin next to the spots. Roll it onto the spots, applying firm pressure. Note that the normal skin under the glass goes white as the blood is pushed out of the tiny surface blood vessels.

Meningitis may be indicated if a spot does not fade when the glass is rolled onto it. Call an ambulance if this is the case in an ill child.

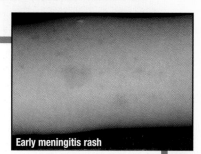
Early meningitis rash

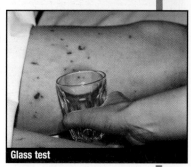
Glass test

Lumps (nodules)

Lumps of more than 5mm (¼in) in diameter, located within or just beneath the skin, are called nodules. Smaller lumps are called papules (see below). Nodules are usually visible, hard, painless and not itchy, depending on the cause.
OCCASIONAL CAUSES: squamous cell carcinoma (skin cancer); kerato-acanthoma (rapidly growing but self-curing skin lump); benign tumour (histiocytoma); gout; lumps on the small joints of fingers, seen in rheumatoid arthritis and osteoarthritis; pyogenic granuloma (a chronic inflammatory lump that bleeds readily) chondro-dermatitis helicis nodularis (inflammation of outer ear).
RARE CAUSES: cancers; uncommon infections (eg leprosy, fish-tank and swimming-pool granuloma): vasculitis (inflammation of the blood vessels).

COMMON CAUSES	ACTION
Xanthoma (fat deposits in the skin) Multiple reddish brown or yellow-whitish lumps, often found around the eyes. 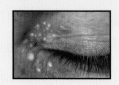	See GP non-urgently: xanthoma may indicate high blood cholesterol level.
Sebaceous cyst (blocked grease gland in skin) Firm or hard lump fixed to the skin, with a central hole or dimple (punctum).	No treatment needed as harmless. See GP non-urgently. Do not squeeze.
Rodent ulcer (basal cell cancer) Reddish-brown lump with rolled-up, pearly edge. The central area often ulcerates. Common in sun exposed areas. 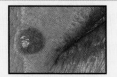	See GP as soon as possible; the lump can be removed by surgery under local anaesthetic. It almost never spreads beyond the area immediately around it.
Viral wart Usually solitary, hard and painless lump on skin surface, but may occur in crops. Common on fingers. On feet viral warts are known as verrucas, and may become painful.	Try OTC remedies. See GP non-urgently if these fail.
Lipoma (benign tumour) Soft, round lump under the skin, can reach 10cm (4in) across.	See GP non-urgently.

Lumps (papules)

Solid, marked skin lumps with a definite circumference, up to 5mm (¼in) in diameter, are called papules. Larger lumps are known as nodules (see above). Papules may be painful or painless, depending on the cause, and may develop into something else.
OCCASIONAL CAUSES: xanthelasma (fat deposits around eyelids); molluscum contagiosum (viral); guttate psoriasis (scaly skin lumps); skin diseases; insect bites.
RARE CAUSES: cancers; acanthosis nigricans (skin thickening associated with stomach cancer); naevoxantho-endothelioma (rounded yellow, firm lumps); pseudoxanthoma elasticum (affects the neck and armpits); tuberous sclerosis (cysts and lumps that calcify and affect different organs).

COMMON CAUSES	ACTION
Blocked sweat gland ducts (milia) Painless crops of solid white spots, often on eyelids or cheeks.	Only treatment is good hygiene. Do not squeeze spots; this causes infection.
Acne (acne vulgaris) Firm, painful lumps that go on to enlarge, develop a yellow head with surrounding inflammation, then burst. May scar on healing.	Practise good hygiene. Contrary to popular belief, a healthier diet will not clear up acne. See GP non-urgently.
Viral wart Usually solitary, hard, painless lump on skin surface, but may occur in crops. Common on fingers. On feet they are called verrucas, and may become painful from pressure of walking.	Try OTC remedies. See GP non-urgently if these fail.
Campbell de Morgan spot (cherry spots or angioma) Bright red round spots, usually on the trunk. They are more common with increasing age.	Completely harmless. Requires no medical treatment.
Skin tag (acrochordon) Finger-like projection of skin. Common in armpits and on neck, and more common with increasing age.	No treatment needed but may become large and uncomfortable. See GP non-urgently if a skin tag is a problem.

Pus spots

Pus spots (pustules) are raised skin lumps that are less than 5mm (¼in) in diameter and filled with pus. They are usually, but not always, caused by infection and can occur anywhere on the body. Avoid squeezing a pus spot, as this can spread infection into surrounding tissues. On and around the nose can be dangerous, as a link exists between the veins here and the large veins around the brain. Although they are very rare, cases of brain infection have been caused this way.

OCCASIONAL CAUSES: inflammation of the sweat gland in the armpits and groin (hidradenitis suppurativa); candidiasis; Staphylococcal (bacterial) infections (eg barber's rash/sycosis barbae); pustular psoriasis; dermatitis herpetiformis (inflamed and infected hair follicles).
RARE CAUSES: jacuzzi folliculitis (inflammation of the hair follicles caused by bacteria in jacuzzis).

COMMON CAUSES

Boil and carbuncle
A boil is a solitary pus spot. A carbuncle has several heads.

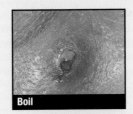
Boil

Impetigo and folliculitis (infections)
Impetigo: crops of golden-yellow pus spots, often on the hands or around the mouth. Common in children.
Folliculitis: often affects regularly shaved areas of body; crops of pustules on hair follicles.

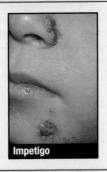
Impetigo

Cold sore (herpes simplex)
Skin tingling and pain precedes crop of blisters, usually less than 5mm (¼in) diameter, in one place.

Acne (acne vulgaris)
Firm, painful lumps which go on to enlarge, develop a yellow head with surrounding inflammation, then burst. May scar on healing.

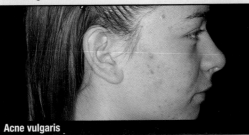
Acne vulgaris

Acne rosacea
Red rash on cheeks, bridge of nose and forehead in 'butterfly' distribution. Pus spots may or may not be present.

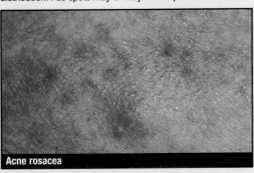
Acne rosacea

ACTION

Cover with dry, non-waterproof dressing. See GP as soon as possible for a carbuncle, or for a boil that has not burst on its own after five days.

Impetigo is highly infectious, so practise good hygiene. See GP urgently to halt infection.

Apply OTC antiviral cream as soon as possible. See GP urgently if rash spreads beyond original crop.

Practise good hygiene. Contrary to popular belief, diet makes no difference. Try OTC remedies; see GP non-urgently if these fail.

See GP as soon as possible.

Red rash

Red rashes are either flushing (see page 51), which disappears in a few minutes, or erythema, which lasts for hours or days. Erythema is caused by relaxation of blood vessels in the skin, which increases the circulation of blood to the skin. Unlike bruising (see page 19), the affected area whitens under pressure. It may be sore, painful or itchy depending on the cause.

OCCASIONAL CAUSES: viral rashes; palmar erythema (red palms); livedo reticularis (a netlike pattern of reddening on the skin); reaction to cold (especially in children); recurrent drug reaction; erythema multiforme (target-like spots).
RARE CAUSES: HIV; erythema nodosum (painful lumps on the shin); sitting in front of the fire for too long (erythema ab igne); Lyme disease (from deer tics).

COMMON CAUSES	ACTION
Cellulitis (skin infection) An area of skin anywhere on the body is red, hot and painful to the touch. You feel unwell, with possible fever.	See GP urgently.
Gout Swollen joint, commonly big toe 'knuckle', top of foot or knee, is extremely painful to touch or move. Skin around the joint is red and hot. In severe cases there may be fever. Gout	See GP urgently.
Burns The skin is very painful to touch and blistering may be present. Heat, contact with a chemical or sunburn may be the cause.	Keep skin cool and dry. Do not use ointments. If burn is large or skin is peeling, go to casualty.
Toxic erythema The skin is not usually painful. Fever and blistering possible. You feel generally unwell. Underlying cause may be a viral infection or drug reaction.	Try OTC antihistamine tablets if itchy. See GP urgently to check if drug reaction, or if very ill with viral infection.
Acne rosacea Rash on cheeks, bridge of nose and forehead in 'butterfly' distribution. Pus spots may be present.	See GP as soon as possible.

Scaly rash and plaque

A scaly rash is a dry, flaky area of skin, nearly always itchy. When it is thickened and raised it is called a plaque. Very serious causes are rare, and most common causes respond well to treatment. Avoid scratching as this will intensify the itching and cause it to spread or become infected. Try OTC antihistamines, hydrocortisone cream or calamine lotion.

OCCASIONAL CAUSES: lichen planus (itchy; usually scaly only on legs); precancerous sun-induced damage (solar keratosis); discoid (disc-shaped) eczema; pityriasis versicolor (skin depigmentation caused by yeast overgrowth); guttate psoriasis (causing scaly lumps).
RARE CAUSES: chronic dermatitis (parapsoriasis).

COMMON CAUSES	ACTION
Psoriasis (chronic skin disease) Raised reddened patches 5mm to many centimetres (¼in or more) in size. Silvery scaling may be seen when scratched.	See GP as soon as possible. There are no effective home treatments.
Atopic eczema and contact dermatitis Itchy, flaky, inflamed and sometimes weeping skin. In atopic eczema it often occurs in the bends of the arms and legs; contact dermatitis often appears on hands.	Try OTC hydrocortisone cream. See GP if not settling within a week. May need antibiotic cream.
Tinea/ringworm (fungal infection) In tinea corporis (ringworm) there is a red ring on the body that slowly expands, leaving a dry, scaly central area. In tinea cruris, there is a red, moist, itchy area in the groin.	Try OTC antifungal cream. See GP if this fails.
Seborrhoeic dermatitis (fungal infection) Scaly crusts on scalp, often weeping clear fluid. There may be a similar scaly rash on other parts of the body.	Control symptoms with OTC antifungal selenium-containing shampoos.
Pityriasis rosea (skin disorder) Patterns of raised, reddened oval spots 5mm–2cm (¼–¾in) long, with lengths of the ovals pointing the same way. Often starts with one large patch, and mostly affects trunk and tops of the arms and legs. Takes six weeks to develop and fade.	Try OTC treatments to help symptoms. There is no known cure but the rash, which is probably caused by a virus, always goes away on its own.

Arm pain

Arm pain can be any sort of pain: dull or sharp, constant or throbbing, aching or shooting, mild or severe, depending on the cause. The same condition, even if serious, can cause a variety of types of pain in different people.

OCCASIONAL CAUSES: inflammation of the gullet (reflux oesophagitis); subacromial bursitis (a form of tissue inflammation); neuritis (nerve inflammation in eg the neck, including post-shingles pain); cervical and thoracic disc prolapse; frozen shoulder.
RARE CAUSES: cancer of the spinal cord and brachial plexus (a network of major nerves); multiple sclerosis.

COMMON CAUSES	ACTION
Tennis elbow (lateral epicondylitis) Pain on bony lump on outer elbow going down back of arm to hand. Gripping and picking things up painful.	Try tennis player's sport support. Rest hand. See GP non-urgently.
Carpal tunnel syndrome (compressed nerve in wrist) Weak grip, tingling in hand especially at night or after using hand for manual task.	Rest hand, and elevate affected arm at night. See GP non-urgently.
Arthritis of the neck (cervical spondylosis) Pain often comes from neck; there may be a grating sensation in the neck.	Try OTC anti-inflammatories or painkillers. See GP non-urgently.
De Quervain's tenosynovitis (tendon inflammation) Pain just above wrist starts after prolonged repetitive actions such as using a screwdriver. Often affects use of thumb.	Prompt treatment with rest and anti-inflammatories important. See GP as soon as possible.
Angina (insufficient oxygen in heart blood) Usually associated with crushing chest pain, cold sweat and shortness of breath. Brought on by physical exertion, cold environment and sometimes large meals.	If severe, with these associations, and lasts more than 15 minutes, call GP urgently or dial 999 for ambulance. If intermittent, see GP as soon as possible.

Foot pain

Foot pain can have any character: it may be dull or sharp, constant or throbbing, aching or shooting, mild or severe, depending on the cause. If there is fever and a feeling of being unwell, infection is likely; see a GP urgently for treatment and to rule out the rare but serious bone infection osteomyelitis.

OCCASIONAL CAUSES: chilblains; Morton's neuroma (a benign tumour); foot bone damage; arthritis (osteo and rheumatoid); Achilles tendonitis/bursitis (inflammations); oedema (fluid accumulation).
RARE CAUSES: march fracture (may be due to a lot of walking); bone infections (eg osteomyelitis, septic arthritis); blockage of the blood vessel (ischaemia).

COMMON CAUSES	ACTION
Gout Sudden onset of pain. The joint, commonly the 'knuckle' of the big toe, is red, hot, and painful to touch or move.	See GP urgently for treatment and blood test to confirm.
Inflamed sole ligaments (plantar fasciitis) Sensation of walking on a pebble in the sole of the foot. Often comes on after an unusual amount of walking.	Try OTC anti-inflammatories and a heel-raise wedge in shoe. If unsuccessful after a month, see GP non-urgently.
Bunion and displacement of big toe (hallux valgus) Tender, bony lump on side of knuckle joint of big toe, which is pointing outwards. **Bunion**	See chiropodist for corrective pads. If unsuccessful and severe, see GP for possible orthopaedic referral/surgery.
Ingrowing toenail, infected Edge of big toe nail is buried in nail fold, which is red, very painful and may leak pus. **Ingrowing toenail**	See GP urgently for antibiotics. When infection is cured, see chiropodist for corrective treatment; if unsuccessful, see GP for minor surgery.
Verruca (foot wart) Gradual onset of pain. Painful flat, warty lump on sole of foot.	Try OTC treatments. See chiropodist to have it filed down regularly.

Calf pain

This is pain in the back of the leg, between the knee and ankle. It may be felt just in the skin, or more deeply, in the muscle of the calf. The type of pain varies and does not usually represent a serious condition.

OCCASIONAL: referred pain from back or knee; alcoholic or diabetic neuropathy (nerve disease); hypocalcaemic cramps (low blood calcium); ruptured Baker's cyst (behind knee); superficial thrombophlebitis (inflammation of the vein wall); deep vein thrombosis (blood clot). **RARE:** motor neurone disease; multiple sclerosis; muscle tension.

COMMON CAUSES	ACTION
Cramp May be brought on by exercise. The calf contracts violently and immediately becomes hard and painful. In elderly people, cramp is often worse at night.	Pull toes towards knee. See GP non-urgently if recurrent: possible blood mineral imbalance/circulatory problem.
Muscle stiffness Both calves sore the day after unaccustomed exercise. Pain reduces once the muscle is used again.	Gradually build up amount of exercise. Keep using legs and pain will settle.
Cellulitis (skin infection) Spreading area of hot, red, swollen skin. May follow a trivial wound or insect bite. Fever and feeling unwell possible.	See GP urgently: requires antibiotic treatment.
Peripheral vascular disease A blood circulation disorder (also called intermittent claudication), this causes cramp in one or both calves after walking. It disappears with rest and recurs after walking the same distance. Sufferers may have noticed cold feet or legs for some time before this starts happening.	See GP as soon as possible for further investigation. If no contra-indications, take half a 300mg aspirin daily to reduce risk of clot. If you smoke, stop.
Muscle injury (for instance, strain) Pain immediately after an injury. May progress to substantial swelling, redness of the calf and disability.	Apply cold compress straightaway to reduce swelling. To prevent disability, important to exercise muscle gently.

Joint pain, multiple

Pain in several joints at once can signify a general infection or disease (more likely in children and young adults), or a widespread inflammatory illness (more likely in people aged 40–60). Osteoarthritis (more common with increasing age) may affect several joints, or just one (see page 26).

OCCASIONAL CAUSES: Reiter's syndrome (an inflammatory disorder); Paget's disease (of the bone); ankylosing spondylitis (an inflammatory disorder); vascular disease (eg giant-cell arteritis, polyarteritis nodosa); malignant tumours (usually secondary); corticosteroid drugs. **RARE CAUSES:** unusual systemic infections that affect the whole body; decompression sickness (the bends).

COMMON CAUSES	ACTION
Rheumatoid arthritis Most common in women aged 20–40. Small joints of the hand, the wrists and ankles usually affected; nearly always affects both sides of body. Possibly generally unwell, with fever.	If the condition has not previously been diagnosed, see GP urgently for treatment and investigation.
Psoriatic joint disorder (arthropathy) Skin psoriasis has usually been present for a time already. Can affect any joint.	See GP as soon as possible; if no contra-indication, take OTC anti-inflammatories.
Viral polyarthritis More common before adulthood. Sudden feeling of being unwell, with a fever, often a few days after the start of a viral illness. Possible rash. Rheumatic fever is rare but has similar symptoms.	Rest and take OTC painkillers or anti-inflammatories; if not better after five days, contact GP for advice.
Systemic inflammatory diseases Usually a sign of some other illness already present, such as bowel problems, skin blisters or rash. Affects any age group. Does not usually improve on its own.	See GP as soon as possible for assessment and treatment.
Osteoarthritis, multiple Morning stiffness and night pain common. Pain improves with activity. Increasingly likely from age 50.	Try OTC anti-inflammatories or painkillers. See GP non-urgently.

Joint pain, single, sudden

A single joint may be painful in an otherwise well person, or it may occur with a pre-existing joint disease. The pain may be dull or sharp, constant or throbbing, aching or shooting, mild or severe, depending on the cause. The most common cause of sudden single joint pain is injury, and the joint most commonly affected is the knee.

OCCASIONAL CAUSES: fracture; blood in the joint (haemarthrosis); inflammation of the kneecap (chondromalacia patellae); anterior (front) knee pain syndromes (eg patellar tendinitis). **RARE CAUSES:** tropical infections; malignant tumours (usually secondary).

COMMON CAUSES	ACTION
Flare-up of osteoarthritis Morning stiffness, swelling, night pain and improvement with activity. Usually a long history of previous problems with the same joint.	Try OTC anti-inflammatories or painkillers; see GP as soon as possible if not better within a week.
Torn ligament Similar to traumatic synovitis (see below), but it is almost impossible to use the joint.	Pain usually requires GP treatment, but worth trying cold compress, OTC anti-inflammatories or painkillers first.
Septic arthritis Severely painful, hot, red, swollen joint that can barely be moved or touched. Fever and general feeling of illness.	See GP urgently or ask for home visit: this emergency needs hospitalization.
Gout Very similar to septic arthritis (see above), but no fever or general feeling of illness. 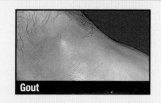 Gout	See GP urgently for diagnosis (blood test) and treatment.
Traumatic synovitis (inflammation) The joint is hot, red and swollen. There is no fever. The inflammation is caused by an injury, which is usually remembered.	Apply cold compress, try OTC painkillers or anti-inflammatories. See GP if not better within a week.

Limping in a child

A limp is an uneven gait. The vast majority of causes in children are not serious and will settle down in time; if it persists beyond a day or two without obvious cause, see a GP, especially if the limping child has a fever.

OCCASIONAL CAUSES: Perthes' disease (hip joint disease, usually in young boys); rheumatic fever; septic arthritis; deviation of the backbone (idiopathic scoliosis); congenital dislocation of the hip. **RARE CAUSES:** bone inflammation (acute osteomyelitis); juvenile rheumatoid arthritis.

COMMON CAUSES	ACTION
Injury, including foreign body in foot There may or may not be obvious signs of injury.	Look at soles of feet for splinters and other objects. If injury obvious, see GP urgently, or go to casualty.
Irritable hip (transient synovitis) Child usually well; problem may start suddenly. The pain may be felt in the knee (referred pain).	See GP as soon as possible.
Acute viral infection, with joint pain Feeling unwell, following a viral infection (such as a cold or sore throat); fever common.	See GP urgently: can mimic rarer, more serious conditions.
Chronic juvenile arthritis Markedly stiff first thing in the morning. Fever possible and several joints likely to be affected.	See GP urgently: can mimic rarer, more serious conditions.
Slipped femoral epiphysis (end of thigh bone) Limp starts suddenly. Most common in boys who are overweight and aged over ten years old.	See GP urgently for assessment.

Nails, abnormal

Many diseases can alter the appearance of the nails, and doctors often start a general examination by looking at the nails. A chiropodist is often the best person to examine an abnormal toenail.

OCCASIONAL CAUSES: horizontal ridging may appear 6–8 weeks after severe illness because of interference with growth; longitudinal ridging (often no known cause); fungal infection of the nail fold (chronic paronychia); dermatitis; clubbing (shape change associated with lung cancer, chronic lung infection, cyanotic heart disease); autoimmune diseases (eg alopecia areata); spoon nails (associated with iron-deficiency anaemia). **RARE CAUSES:** chronic cardiac failure; liver disease; lung tuberculosis; diabetes; rheumatoid arthritis; some cancers; poor circulation.

COMMON CAUSES	ACTION
Injury to nail bed Horizontal ridge on single nail appearing six to eight weeks after an injury such as a hammer blow.	No action needed.
Psoriasis Thickened white nail. Usually associated with a red scaly rash on the body.	Non-urgent GP appointment. Psoriasis needs treatment.
Onychomycosis (fungal infection) Thickened, white and crumbly nail. Can look indistinguishable from psoriasis. Onychomycosis	Non-urgent GP appointment for a lab test on the nail and treatment if positive.
Injury due to biting, hangnail Nails have ragged edges. The adjoining skin is often softened and sore.	Stop biting the nails. Bitter nail paints may help.
Onychogryphosis (thickening of the nails) Usually affects toenails. Gnarled, thick and often long, curly nails.	Seek help from a chiropodist.
White flecks on nails Small white flecks on the nail that move up with the growing nail. 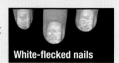 White-flecked nails	No treatment needed. It does not signify calcium deficiency (a common myth); there is no known cause.

Swollen ankles and lower legs

Swollen ankles and lower legs often feel heavy and look puffy. The causes listed here relate to the swelling of the two ankles and lower legs. When just one ankle and lower leg is affected, this is likely to be due to arthritis, varicose veins or injury; very rarely, it results from a tumour in the pelvis pressing on the veins of the leg.

OCCASIONAL CAUSES: severe obesity; pregnancy; abnormal swelling or growth within the pelvis, especially in the ovaries (a pelvic mass); cirrhosis; premenstrual syndrome; anaemia; drug reaction. **RARE CAUSES:** angioneurotic oedema (fluid accumulation).

COMMON CAUSES	ACTION
Congestive heart failure Swelling worsens as the day goes by, often reduced in morning. Associated with shortness of breath on exertion; possible wheezy cough and phlegm.	See GP as soon as possible for assessment and treatment.
Osteoarthritis Morning stiffness, night pain common. Swelling worse when joint pain worse. Increasingly likely from age 50.	Take OTC anti-inflammatories or painkillers. See GP non-urgently.
Kidney disease (nephritis or nephritic syndrome) The hands may also be swollen. Urine may be unusually frothy, bloodstained. You feel generally unwell.	See GP urgently.
Venous insufficiency Common in immobile and elderly people. Swelling often reduced in the morning after lying down at night.	See GP non-urgently for confirmation.
Underactive thyroid (hypothyroidism) Gradual onset, associated with coldness, tiredness and feeling slowed down. Skin may feel dry, hair brittle.	See GP as soon as possible for assessment and possible blood test.

Deafness

Deafness is the complete or partial inability to hear. Before it is diagnosed, deafness in children may cause difficulties at home – parents may think the child is ignoring them – and at school, with poor school performance sometimes being the first sign. More than 3 million adults in the UK have some degree of deafness.

OCCASIONAL CAUSES: fluid in inner ear (Ménière's disease); burst eardrum (barotrauma); nerve disease (viral acoustic neuritis); large nasal polyps or tumour in the nasopharynx (airway behind the nose); drugs (eg streptomycin, gentamycin, or aspirin overdose).
RARE: benign tumour (acoustic neuroma); vitamin B_{12} deficiency; multiple sclerosis.

COMMON CAUSES	ACTION
Ear wax Sense of blockage in the ear, usually painless; possible yellow discharge of liquefied wax. Deafness may be sudden.	Try warm olive oil drops twice daily for a week. If not improving, see your GP or practice nurse.
Middle ear infection (otitis media) Severe, throbbing earache. Sudden relief of pain followed by pus discharge indicates the eardrum has perforated. Deafness sudden.	If not improving within three days, see GP as soon as possible.
Ear canal infection (otitis externa) Severe earache, made worse on pulling outer ear. Common after seaside holidays and in swimmers. Deafness sudden.	See GP as soon as possible for antibiotic/antifungal eardrops. Reduce risk after swimming by washing ears out with boiled, cooled tap water.
Glue ear A common painless childhood problem. Deafness is gradual.	See GP for examination and possible further investigation.
Noise damage to cochlea Onset of deafness very gradual and starts with loss of high-frequency tones. Most common in adults aged over 45.	See GP for examination and possible specialist referral.

Earache

Earache can affect just the inner ear canal or the outer ear (pinna) or both. It can start suddenly or gradually, can be mild or severe, hot, burning, throbbing, stabbing or dull. Referred pain from the throat or upper jaw may be felt in the ear, which shares the same nerve supply.

OCCASIONAL CAUSES: upper jaw joint dysfunction; dental abscess; impacted molar tooth; cranial nerve pain (trigeminal neuralgia); ear canal eczema or seborrhoeic dermatitis.
RARE CAUSES: inflammation behind ear (mastoiditis); arthritis of the neck (cervical spondylosis); benign wax-producing growth (cholesteatoma); cancer; burst eardrum.

COMMON CAUSES	ACTION
Middle ear infection (infective otitis media) Pain does not worsen on pulling external ear; possible ear discharge and fever. Deafness in affected ear.	Take paracetamol, but see GP if not improving after two days, or sooner if discharge appears.
Ear canal infection (infective otitis externa) Pain made worse on pulling external ear; discharge usually present. Possibly some deafness.	See GP as soon as possible for examination and treatment.
Boils of the ear canal and external ear Very painful and made worse by pulling external ear; possible discharge. Boils or acne elsewhere likely.	See GP as soon as possible for examination and antibiotic treatment.
Injury and foreign body (including wax) Deafness, pain on pulling outer ear and possible discharge. Common in toddlers and cotton-bud users.	Do not attempt removal. See GP for removal or referral to specialist.
Throat problems Pain made worse by swallowing. Swelling of glands in neck below jaw. Fever. The cause may be tonsillitis, pharyngitis or an abscess next to a tonsil (quinsy).	See GP for examination and treatment or referral (quinsy requires urgent surgery).

Eyes, red and painful

Eye pain can start suddenly or gradually, can be mild or severe, hot, burning, stabbing or dull and throbbing. All eye pain is serious and needs urgent treatment.
By far the most common cause is infection, as in conjunctivitis; but if only one eye is affected other causes are more likely.

OCCASIONAL CAUSES: other inflammations (eg episcleritis, kerato-conjunctivitis); collagen diseases (eg Reiter's syndrome, systemic lupus erythematosus, ankylosing spondylitis, rheumatoid arthritis); injury such as a bruise or penetrating wound; chemical burns and arc eye, which affects welders; infection of the eyeball capsule (orbital cellulitis).
RARE CAUSES: gout; granulomatous disorders (eg tuberculosis, sarcoidosis, toxoplasmosis); tropical disease (onchocerciasis); malignant tumour in the eye or invasion from tumour directly behind the nose.

COMMON CAUSES	ACTION
Acute conjunctivitis One or both eyes are red and sore, with sticky yellow or green discharge. Blurring of vision temporarily resolved when discharge is wiped away. 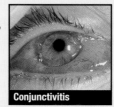 Conjunctivitis	If the eyelids are stuck together, bathe gently with clean, warm water; do not force lids apart. See GP urgently for treatment.
Acute iritis (inflammation of the iris) Vision is blurred. No discharge. Pupil in affected eye does not constrict in light, which hurts the eye.	See GP urgently: requires specialist referral.
Acute glaucoma (high pressure in eye) Blurred vision. The pupil is large and the cornea (the clear part of the front of the eye) may look hazy; eyeball feels hard and is very painful to touch. 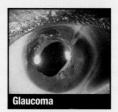 Glaucoma	See GP urgently: requires specialist referral.
Cornea inflammation (keratitis) or corneal ulcer A small grey patch may be seen on the clear part of the cornea (the front of the eye); possible discharge and blurred vision.	See GP urgently: requires specialist referral.
Corneal abrasion or superficial foreign body Impact from a blow or feeling of something getting into the eye is usually remembered. A bruise or foreign body may be visible.	Do not attempt removal. Cover eye and see GP urgently. If high-speed impact from a foreign body (eg a stone) may have occurred, go straight to casualty.

Gums, bleeding

Bleeding gums may be painful or painless depending on the cause. Gum infection is the most common cause, and results from poor dental hygiene. See a dentist first; if there is no dental cause, see a GP non-urgently for investigation.

OCCASIONAL CAUSES: aphthous ulcers; herpes infection of mouth and gums (acute herpetic gingivostomatitis); autoimmune diseases; cancer in the mouth (oral neoplasia); blood abnormalities, especially acute myeloid leukaemia.
RARE CAUSES: malabsorption; scurvy.

COMMON CAUSES	ACTION
Gingivitis (inflammation of the gums) or gum disease The gums are swollen and painful; the breath smells bad.	See dentist as soon as possible.
Pregnancy gingivitis During pregnancy the gums are swollen, but not painful; the breath does not smell bad.	See dentist as soon as possible.
Acute necrotizing ulcerative gingivitis Swollen, painful gums; foul breath; possible fever and feeling generally unwell.	See dentist as soon as possible, or urgently if feeling unwell.
Injury from poorly fitting dentures The cause is usually obvious from looking at the dentures and the sore part of the mouth.	See dentist to check fit of dentures.

Headache

A headache may be dull or sharp, constant or throbbing, aching or shooting, mild or severe. It is usually only a cause for concern if it lasts for several days or more, or is unusually severe. Many people fear it indicates a brain tumour, but this is extremely rare; tension and stress are easily the most common cause.

OCCASIONAL CAUSES: blood sugar deficiency; fatigue or sleep deprivation; nerve pain (eg sphenopalatine, occipital or trigeminal neuralgia); temporal arteritis (inflammation of the artery walls); post-concussional syndrome; drugs (eg nitrates). **RARE CAUSES:** cluster headache; brain tumour; meningitis (see page 19); intracerebral haemorrhage (bleeding into the brain); carbon monoxide poisoning (from a blocked boiler flue).

COMMON CAUSES	ACTION
Anxiety or depression The forehead or back of head may be sore to touch. Often described as feeling like a band around the head.	Take paracetamol for pain. Address causes of tension. If problematic, see GP non-urgently to discuss.
Sinus inflammation (frontal sinusitis) Throbbing pain over eyes made worse by stooping and coughing. Possible fever, green or yellow nasal catarrh.	Try steam inhalations, OTC painkillers, decongestants. If not improving within five days, see GP as soon as possible.
Migraine Severe throbbing headache, usually on one side of the head. Light hurts eyes; nausea, vomiting common. May be preceded by flashing lights or zigzag lines in vision.	Take OTC painkillers; rest in dark room (it often disappears after a sleep). See GP non-urgently if recurrent; if attack very severe and lasting more than six hours, call for home visit.
Arthritis of the neck (cervical spondylosis) Pain is felt from the neck, up the back of the head, and to the top of the scalp; there is often a grating feeling in neck on turning. Common in people aged over 60.	Take OTC painkillers. If home treatment unsuccessful, see GP non-urgently.
Eyestrain Pain usually on one side, over or behind one eye. May happen after prolonged, concentrated reading.	See optician for eye test. Pace periods of reading with rest and looking at distant objects to relax eyes.

Hoarseness

With hoarseness the voice becomes quieter and huskier. It may occur with a sore throat or pain in the windpipe, depending on the cause. In general, slowly increasing and persistent hoarseness is of more concern than sudden hoarseness. See a GP if it lasts two weeks or more. Hoarseness with fever and unusual difficulty in breathing or sensation of swelling in the throat merits an urgent GP appointment.

OCCASIONAL CAUSES: inflammation of the gullet; benign tumours; rheumatoid arthritis of the voicebox; acute epiglottitis (throat inflammation); functional aphonia (loss of voice). **RARE:** cancer of the larynx; chemical or physical damage.

COMMON CAUSES	ACTION
Inflammation of the air passage (acute viral laryngitis) Hoarseness starts suddenly after a sore throat or cold; it is usually painless by then.	Rest voice; it should return within a week. Steam inhalations and soothing drinks may help.
Voice overuse (shouting, screaming) The cause is obvious in an otherwise well person.	As for Inflammation of the air passage, above.
Underactive thyroid (hypothyroidism) Occurs gradually, and is associated with feeling cold, tired and slowed down. Skin may feel dry, hair brittle.	See GP as soon as possible for assessment and possible blood test.
Smoking May follow a sudden excess, for instance, after a party.	As for Inflammation of the air passage, above. Also, stop smoking.
Sinusitis (sinus inflammation) Fever and green or yellow nasal catarrh. Severe, dull pain above and/or below eyes on one or both sides, made worse on stooping.	As for Inflammation of the air passage, above, and use OTC decongestants. If pain not settling within five days, see GP for possible antibiotic treatment.

Neck stiffness, sudden

Neck stiffness is the sensation of tightness and pain in the neck on trying to move the head. Meningitis is a feared cause of neck stiffness but is extremely rare (see page 19). Its symptoms (headache, neck stiffness, dislike of bright light and meningism, see right) occur in any severe general bacterial infection. If in doubt, phone your GP.

OCCASIONAL CAUSES: exacerbation of rheumatoid arthritis; abscess in neck; psychological causes; intracerebral haemorrhage (bleeding into the brain); brain tumour.
RARE CAUSES: inflammation of the brain (meningitis); fracture of a vertebra; bone tumour; uncommon infections (eg tetanus, leptospirosis, psittacosis); brain abscess.

COMMON CAUSES	ACTION
Wry neck (acute torticollis) Often present from waking, or develops after a trivial twisting movement of neck. Turning head to one side is very painful; head often held twisted and to one side.	Take OTC painkillers, gently massage painful muscle. See GP urgently if pain relief is inadequate.
Exacerbation of pre-existing osteoarthritis All neck movements are painful. When the neck is moved a creaking or grating feeling and sound is common.	Take OTC anti-inflammatories or painkillers. See GP as soon as possible if these fail to work.
Viral nose or throat infection Glands in neck enlarged. Feeling unwell with mild fever. General aches and pains common.	Take paracetamol and cool drinks; rest. See GP if not settling within five days.
Whiplash injury Often happens after a road traffic accident. Increasing stiffness and pain over several days following an accident. May be troublesome for months afterwards.	Take OTC anti-inflammatories or painkillers. See GP if not helping. Physiotherapy may be useful.
Meningism Headache, neck stiffness, dislike of bright light. May be caused by infection, eg pneumonia. Severely ill with high fever. Many of the symptoms are the same as for meningitis (see page 19).	See GP urgently; if travel is impossible, ask for a home visit.

Nosebleed

Bleeding from the nose usually settles with simple first aid: sit in a chair with the head slightly forward; firmly pinch the nose between the bony part and the nostrils for ten minutes; do not blow the nose for at least three hours. If bleeding does not stop after an hour, go to casualty for treatment to stop the bleeding.

OCCASIONAL CAUSES: septal granulomas (inflammatory lumps) and perforations; severe liver disease; cancers of nose, sinuses; abnormal anatomy (septal deviation); injury.
RARE CAUSES: thrombocytopaenia (lack of blood-clotting cells); leukaemia; coagulation problems (eg haemophilia, Christmas and von Willebrand's diseases); deficiency of vitamin C or K.

COMMON CAUSES	ACTION
Spontaneous Sudden bleeding with no apparent cause. May be aggravated by nose-picking and sneezing. May recur.	Follow advice in introduction, left. See GP non-urgently if recurrent.
High blood pressure (hypertension); often with artery blockage (atherosclerosis) Nosebleeds come suddenly, with no apparent cause, and tend to be recurrent. Often associated with blockage of the arteries (atherosclerosis).	Follow advice in introduction, left. If you have hypertension, see GP as soon as possible for blood pressure check.
Nasal infection and ulceration Green nasal discharge and crusting usually already present; nose is painful inside.	Follow advice in introduction, left. See GP urgently for assessment.
Drug reactions Sudden bleeding with no apparent cause, and tends to be recurrent. Often associated with unexplained bruising on the body. May be a reaction to warfarin, aspirin or cytotoxic drugs.	Follow advice in introduction, left. See GP urgently for blood test to check blood clotting.
Inflammations of the nose (allergic or atrophic rhinitis) Nosebleeds recurrent, and associated with blocked nose.	Follow advice in introduction, left. See GP non-urgently for assessment.

Symptom sorter

Swallowing, difficulty in

This could be pain on starting to swallow, pain on swallowing, or the sensation of something in the throat when not swallowing. Anyone over the age of 60 complaining of difficulty in swallowing ought to be seen by a GP, especially if the person is unexpectedly losing weight.

OCCASIONAL CAUSES: cancers (eg pharyngeal, bronchial and gastric carcinoma, lymphoma); oesophageal achalasia (muscle abnormality); Plummer-Vinson syndrome (in hiatus hernia); dryness of the mouth (xerostomia). **RARE CAUSES:** skin stiffening caused by scleroderma.

COMMON CAUSES	ACTION
Anxiety (globus hystericus) No difficulty in swallowing solids or liquids, but frequent sensation of something in the throat.	Try to deal with cause of stress. See GP non-urgently for examination and help with anxiety.
Inflammation of the gullet (reflux oesophagitis) Acid regurgitation on stooping and lying down. Heartburn after meals and with hot drinks. Nocturnal cough and foul taste in mouth are common.	Try OTC antacids. If needed, lose weight; wear loose clothing. Stop smoking. See GP non-urgently if this fails.
Narrowing of the bowel (benign peptic stricture) Difficulty in swallowing gradually gets worse. Heartburn and regurgitation of undigested food are possible.	See GP as soon as possible for investigation.
Cancer of the oesophagus, or gullet As for Narrowing of the bowel above, but also with weight loss.	See GP as soon as possible for investigation.
Pharyngeal pouch Intermittent regurgitation of undigested food, hours after a meal. Swelling in neck possible.	See GP non-urgently for specialist referral.

Throat, sore

The pain of a sore throat may be dull or sharp, constant or throbbing, aching or shooting, mild or severe, depending on the cause. Viral infection is the cause in most cases; these will settle with simple home care, eg paracetamol, lozenges and cool drinks or ice cream. In general, if a sore throat is not showing signs of settling within five days, see a GP as soon as possible.

OCCASIONAL CAUSES: thrush (oropharyngeal candidiasis); some forms of nerve pain (eg neuralgia); injury (foreign body or scratch from crispy food); Vincent's angina (ulcerative gingivitis); ulceration.

RARE CAUSES: cardiac angina; oropharyngeal cancer (throat cancer at mouth level); retropharyngeal abscess (abscess in the tissues behind the throat).

COMMON CAUSES	ACTION
Viral pharyngitis (throat inflammation) Often follows a cold. Glands in neck may be enlarged. Feeling unwell with mild fever. General aches and pains common. Throat looks uniformly red but not swollen.	Take paracetamol, anaesthetic lozenges, cool drinks. If not settling in five days, see GP as soon as possible.
Tonsillitis streptococcal pharyngitis ('strep throat') Neck glands enlarged, painful. High fever; red spotty rash on body possible. Pus visible on red, swollen throat. Feeling very ill. Joints may be stiff and sore.	If pus clearly visible, and you are very unwell, see GP urgently.
Glandular fever (Epstein-Barr viral infection) Glands in neck and elsewhere (groins, armpits) swollen; tonsils show white patches. Rash may occur. Extreme tiredness possible for weeks after throat has improved.	See GP as soon as possible to confirm diagnosis (possible blood test) and plan recovery.
Quinsy (peritonsillar abscess) Extreme pain and visible swelling on one side of throat. The uvula, which hangs down at the back of the mouth, is pushed over to one side.	See GP urgently: this requires urgent surgery. If any difficulty in breathing, dial 999 or go straight to casualty.
Gullet inflammation (reflux oesophagitis) Often worse at night; a foul taste is often noted in the morning. Acid heartburn brought on by hot drinks and stooping. Acid may be tasted in the mouth on stooping.	Take OTC antacids. If overweight, lose weight; loosen clothing round waist. If a smoker, stop. See GP non-urgently if problem continues.

Tinnitus

Tinnitus sufferers perceive sounds that are not created outside the body; these may be low- or high-pitched, resembling many different noises.

OCCASIONAL CAUSES: chronic ear infection and glue ear (serous otitis media); a sudden loud noise; head injury; impacted wisdom teeth; drugs (eg aspirin overdose, loop diuretics, aminoglycosides, quinine); high blood pressure (hypertension), blocked arteries (atherosclerosis). **RARE CAUSES:** benign tumour (acoustic neuroma); severe anaemia and renal failure; spasm of the soft palate muscles (palatal myoclonus), arterial bruits (turbulent blood flow and problems affecting the blood flow in the carotid artery); anxiety.

COMMON CAUSES	ACTION
Ear wax Sudden onset of low-pitched noise; may be associated with dizziness and pain in the ear. Otherwise you feel well.	If no pain or previous perforation of eardrum, use OTC wax-removing drops to loosen wax. If this fails, see practice nurse for ear wash-out.
Hearing loss Gradual onset, may be low- or high-pitched noise. Associated with deafness on affected side. There is no dizziness.	See GP non-urgently.
Middle ear inflammation (suppurative otitis media) Sudden onset with severe pain, discharge and deafness on the same side. Fever may be present.	See GP urgently.
Middle ear bone overgrowth (otosclerosis) Very gradual onset with hearing loss in younger people. May be family history of otosclerosis.	See GP non-urgently.
Ménière's disease (inner ear disease) May be present all the time, but is worse at times of flare-ups, when sudden and disabling vertigo and nausea develop. Gradual hearing loss occurs.	See GP non-urgently, or urgently if vertigo is present.

Tongue, painful

Soreness often results when the tongue is accidentally bitten. This is a short-lived problem. For a serious injury to the tongue (which will bleed copiously), go straight to casualty. Longer-term cases should be looked at by a GP or dentist.

OCCASIONAL CAUSES: inflammation of the tongue (glossitis); burning mouth syndrome (psychological cause); fissured tongue (a tongue with cracks on the surface, usually painless); nerve pain (glossopharyngeal neuralgia); lichen planus (an itchy skin disease). **RARE:** cancer of the tongue; drugs (eg mouthwashes, aspirin burns).

COMMON CAUSES	ACTION
Geographic tongue (erythema migrans) Red area with map-like border, slowly changing shape over weeks. It is long-term and gets worse with spicy/bitter foods.	See dentist as soon as possible for assessment.
Thrush (candida infection) Inside of mouth has white patches that scrape off easily. In adults, may be associated with underlying problem, such as diabetes, steroid treatment or taking antibiotics. 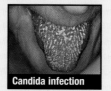 **Candida infection**	See GP as soon as possible for assessment.
Injury May be associated with a jagged tooth edge, the area inside the cheek getting bitten or burnt, or badly fitting dentures.	See dentist as soon as possible for assessment.
Anaemia (deficiency of iron, vitamin B_6 or B_{12}) The lips, tongue and inside of the eyelids may look pale and there may be sores on the corners of the mouth.	See GP as soon as possible for assessment.
Aphthous ulceration The ulcers usually appear in crops, and often recur. 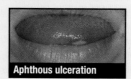 **Aphthous ulceration**	See dentist as soon as possible for assessment.

Abdominal pain: pregnancy

In the later stages of pregnancy, this could be labour. When a period has been missed, severe pain low in one side of the pelvis may represent an ectopic pregnancy (in which the fetus develops outside the uterus). In general, seek medical advice for abdominal pain in pregnancy, or vaginal bleeding with no pain.

OCCASIONAL CAUSES: constipation/irritable bowel syndrome; ectopic pregnancy; appendicitis; red degeneration of fibroid (a fibroid dies and fills with blood); twisting (torsion) and/or rupture of ovarian cyst or tumour. **RARE CAUSES:** twisting (torsion) and/or rupture of the uterus; inflammation of the gall bladder (cholecystitis); liver congestion caused by pre-eclampsia; blood within sheath of rectus muscle.

COMMON CAUSES	ACTION
Strain in symphysis pubis (joint within pubic bone) Severe pain around pubic bone, which is painful to the touch. Worse on standing and walking, relieved by rest.	Rest. Paracetamol is safe to use after the first three months.
Possible miscarriage Brisk vaginal bleeding with crampy, period-like pains. Affects 20–40 per cent of pregnancies in the first three months.	Take urgent GP advice or go straight to casualty.
Labour Very strong cramping pains, becoming longer and more frequent. Some 6 per cent of labours are premature.	Contact midwife, GP or labour ward for confirmation.
Placental abruption Torrential vaginal bleeding in late pregnancy, with severe lower abdominal pain, may indicate that the placenta has become detached from the wall of the uterus.	This is an emergency. Dial 999 and lie down until help arrives.
Kidney infection (pyelonephritis) Fever, frequent passing of small amounts of urine that may be foul and/or bloodstained. Severe, dull pain on one side of the back. More likely after 20 weeks and soon after delivery.	Urgent antibiotic treatment is needed. Contact GP urgently.

Abdominal pain: recurrent, adults

Recurrent pain along with weight loss or red blood in the faeces should prompt making a GP appointment. Jet-black faeces result from bleeding into the stomach; this emergency needs urgent hospital treatment.

OCCASIONAL CAUSES: gallstones; kidney obstruction (hydronephrosis); inflammatory bowel disease; inflammation of the gut (coeliac disease); nerve pain after herpes (post-herpetic neuralgia); spasms in the tubes draining the kidney (ureteric colic). **RARE CAUSES:** chronic pancreatitis (inflammation of the pancreas); subacute (intermittent) obstruction of the bowel (eg adhesions, cancer and diverticulitis); psychological abdominal pain.

COMMON CAUSES	ACTION
Irritable bowel syndrome (IBS) Bloating, crampy, colicky pains, relieved by passing wind or opening the bowels. There is often diarrhoea mixed with pellety faeces and mucus.	Often triggered by stress, so look for and address the cause. Symptoms can be helped by antispasmodics.
Recurrent urinary tract infection Frequent passing of small amounts of urine, often with stinging. Pain is felt low in the pelvis and back, or in one loin if a kidney is affected. Fever may be present.	See GP urgently: swift antibiotic treatment essential. May need later investigation.
Chronic peptic ulcer Continuous gnawing pain felt just under the breastbone. May be relieved by some foods, worsened by others.	Non-urgent GP appointment for investigation and treatment.
Constipation Hard faeces that are difficult to pass. Griping, colicky pain often felt on the left of the abdomen.	Increase fibre and fluid in diet, and level of activity, especially if elderly.
Infection of the alimentary tract (diverticulitis) Severe griping pains all over the abdomen; blood and mucus passed with diarrhoea. Fever.	See GP urgently for antibiotic treatment.

Abdominal pain: recurrent, children

Children may complain frequently of tummy aches, usually a vague and mild pain, felt in varying places in the abdomen. If this recurs over several months, parents should consult a GP. It is very rarely serious (unless it is caused by a urinary infection, which needs vigorous treatment to avoid kidney infection and scarring).

OCCASIONAL CAUSES: protein sensitivity (coeliac disease); parasites in gut; diabetes mellitus; inflamed blood vessels (Henoch-Schönlein purpura); obstruction in the kidney.
RARE CAUSES: sickle-cell disease; tuberculosis; temporal lobe epilepsy.

COMMON CAUSES	ACTION
Recurrent viral illnesses Coincides with a mild, feverish general illness.	Take paracetamol and fluids; rest during illness. Contact GP if significant interference with everyday life.
Abdominal migraine Caused by anxiety, depression or general unhappiness, there is rarely any noticeable illness. Poor school performance is common.	Arrange a non-urgent GP appointment.
Recurrent urinary infections Fever and painful, frequent urination.	Seek urgent GP advice. Needs antibiotics and usually further investigation.
Constipation Colicky or griping pain. May have overflow diarrhoea, when liquid contents of higher bowel bypass hard faeces.	Take plenty of fluids, eat a high-fibre diet, and exercise.
Food allergy Diarrhoea in an otherwise happy, healthy child.	No treatment. Identify and avoid the trigger food.

Abdominal pain: sudden, adults

Sudden, severe and unremitting abdominal pain in adults nearly always warrants an urgent GP examination. It can be felt in any part of the abdomen, or all over, and can have any character. Visit the surgery if possible, or ask for an urgent home visit.

OCCASIONAL CAUSES: gall bladder inflammation (cholecystitis); renal pain or ureteric colic from urinary stone; inflammation of the large intestine (diverticulitis); bowel obstruction (eg adhesions, carcinoma, strangulated hernia, volvulus); kidney infection (pyelonephritis).
RARE CAUSES: Crohn's disease and ulcerative colitis; pancreatitis; hepatitis; blood vessel blockage (bowel ischaemia); dissecting or leaking aortic aneurysm (swelling); ketoacidosis in diabetics.

COMMON CAUSES	ACTION
Peptic ulcer Severe pain just below the solar plexus (breastbone). May be relieved by milky drinks or antacids.	See GP urgently, or ask for home visit.
Acute gastritis (inflammation of the stomach lining) Severe pain just below the solar plexus (breastbone). Vomiting usual.	See GP urgently, or ask for home visit.
Gallbladder or bile duct obstruction (biliary colic) Severe, griping pain just beneath bottom-right ribs. Bowel motions may be pale and urine dark.	See GP urgently, or ask for home visit.
Appendicitis Severe, constant pain in lower-right abdomen, often starting around the navel. Fever usually present. You may feel very ill, and may have vomiting and/or diarrhoea. Symptoms are similar in children.	See GP urgently. Do not eat or drink.
Gastroenteritis (Stomach and intestine inflammation) Colicky pain anywhere in abdomen. Watery diarrhoea and vomiting.	Urgent GP telephone advice needed. Sip clear fluids (water, flat lemonade, diluted squash) even if vomiting.

Abdominal swellings

Most people experience abdominal swelling after certain foods, or too much food; the abdomen returns to normal within a day or two. Progressive swelling needs medical attention, especially if it is associated with weight loss.

OCCASIONAL CAUSES: fluid in the peritoneal cavity (ascites); cancer of the colon (causing partial bowel blockage); ovarian mass (benign cyst or malignant tumours); cancer of the stomach; enlarged liver.
RARE CAUSES: cancer of the pancreas; enlarged spleen (splenomegaly); lymph node swelling around the aorta (para-aortic lymphadnopathy; kidney cysts and cancers.

COMMON CAUSES	ACTION
Pregnancy No periods for three months or more. Nausea and sore breasts may occur several weeks before abdominal swelling is noticed.	Use a home pregnancy test (now as reliable as hospital tests).
Irritable bowel syndrome (IBS) Diarrhoea, slimy or pellety bowel motions, and wind. Frequent changes in size of abdomen. Colicky, griping abdominal pain.	Try a high-fibre diet. Deal with psychological stress (a common cause).
Constipation and wind Overflow diarrhoea, in which liquid contents of the higher bowel bypass hard faeces, may follow a period of constipation.	Try a high-fibre diet and exercise; laxatives may be useful in the short term. In elderly people, see GP if constipation is a new symptom, and laxative treatment fails.
Enlarged bladder (outflow obstruction) Thin, slow stream of urine; dribbling at end of stream.	Seek urgent GP advice. Bladder blockage must be relieved.

Anal pain

With pain, the anal ring of muscle (sphincter) goes into spasm; this can cause constipation, which in turn increases the pain. In general, this symptom needs to be seen by a GP, and promptly if accompanied by weight loss and/or change in frequency and consistency of bowel motions.

OCCASIONAL CAUSES: inflammation of alimentary tract (Crohn's disease); coccygodynia (pain at end of spine); inflammation of the prostate gland (prostatitis); ovarian cyst or tumour.
RARE CAUSES: lesion of the cauda equina (spinal nerve roots); inflammation of the uterus lining (endometriosis); injury.

COMMON CAUSES	ACTION
Anal fissure Pain often starts during a bout of constipation; passing faeces is excruciatingly painful and there is often bleeding.	Use OTC anorectal anaesthetic creams liberally. Try a high-fibre diet to keep faeces soft. If not settling within a few days, see GP.
Thrombosed haemorrhoids and anal haematoma Both thrombosed haemorrhoids and anal haematoma result in a painful, hard lump or lumps on the anus.	As for Anal fissure, above; an ice pack and OTC oral painkillers may be helpful.
Abscess Swelling, bleeding and pus discharge all possible.	See GP urgently; may need surgery.
Muscle spasm (proctalgia fugax) Fleeting, intermittent, severe stabbing pain in rectum. May be associated with anxiety.	See GP non-urgently. Try OTC anorectal anaesthetics and prescribed antispasmodics.
Cancer of the anus and/or rectum Bleeding very likely; you may have a sense of rectal fullness even when no faeces are present.	See GP as soon as possible.

Constipation

Some people naturally open their bowels (defecate) several times a day, others only two or three times a week. Constipation is when defecation is less frequent, or if straining is ever needed. Weight loss and mucus or blood in the bowel motions occurring at the same time as constipation signifies the possibility of a serious problem.

OCCASIONAL CAUSES: dyschezia (ignoring the desire to open bowels long term); chronic laxative use; underactive thyroid (hypothyroidism); cancer of the rectum or colon.
RARE CAUSES: tumours in the pelvis pressing on the colon; intestine inflammation (as in Crohn's disease) with stricture; in infants, Hirschprung's disease (a nerve disorder) and intestinal narrowing.

COMMON CAUSES	ACTION
Low-fibre diet and/or poor fluid intake More likely in people aged over 60, and children who are fussy eaters. Low fruit and vegetable content in diet.	Remedy dietary imbalance and increase daily fluid intake.
Inactivity Very likely in elderly people. Overflow diarrhoea often present: liquid contents of higher bowel bypass hard faeces.	Increase activity. If bedridden, abdominal massage can help.
Irritable bowel syndrome (IBS) Hard, pelletly faeces interspersed with diarrhoea; often with mucus and painful colicky abdominal cramps. Bleeding is never present in IBS alone.	Increase dietary fibre. See GP non-urgently for antispasmodic treatment. Often triggered by stress: identify and remedy cause.
Painful anal conditions Often sudden onset and caused by, for example, anal fissure, haemorrhoids, abscess, florid warts. Attempts to defecate are excruciatingly painful. Blood may be present on paper or in the toilet pan, but not in the faeces.	Use OTC anal anaesthetic ointment and see GP as soon as possible, urgently if fever present (may be an abscess).
Drug treatments More likely in elderly people, and begins soon after starting drug treatment, such as opiates, iron, aluminium hydroxide, trycyclic antidepressants.	See GP for advice on change of treatment if possible.

Diarrhoea

Passing abnormally liquid and frequent faeces is very common; travellers have an increased risk of diarrhoea caused by food poisoning or tropical infection. People who work with food should not return to work until the diarrhoea has cleared and faeces have been tested for disease-causing organisms.

OCCASIONAL CAUSES: lactose intolerance; chronic infection (eg amoebiasis, giardiasis, hookworm, bowel neoplasia); inflammatory bowel disease (eg ulcerative colitis, Crohn's disease); excess alcohol.
RARE CAUSES: laxative misuse; excessive thyroid hormone (thyrotoxicosis); malabsorption (eg coeliac disease); allergy.

COMMON CAUSES	ACTION
Acute gastroenteritis Feeling ill; abdominal cramps and vomiting. Blood in the faeces not uncommon. May be caused by, for example, food poisoning, or infection by rotavirus.	Try OTC antidiarrhoeals/salt-replacement solutions. If fever, continuous pain or vomiting of 24 hours+, see GP urgently or ask for home visit. See GP as soon as possible if diarrhoea lasts 7 days+.
Antibiotic side effect Vomiting may also occur; should settle within a week after antibiotic treatment.	Telephone advice needed from GP about continuing antibiotics. May need a faeces test if it lasts more than a week after end of antibiotics.
Irritable bowel syndrome (IBS) Abdominal cramps, bloating, wind, diarrhoea, pelletly faeces. Blood never present in IBS unless anus is inflamed.	Often stress-related: identify triggering cause. See GP for treatment/advice.
Diverticulitis (infection of the large intestine) Abdominal cramps, bloodstained diarrhoea. Constant pain and fever are serious signs.	Urgent GP appointment needed; request home visit if bedridden.
Overflow in constipation Previous constipation leading up to diarrhoea; abdominal cramps. Especially common in elderly people. Blood never present unless anus is inflamed.	Try OTC laxatives. If unsuccessful or problem recurs, see GP as soon as possible for examination.

Groin swellings

A swelling in the groin is unlikely to need urgent treatment, unless there is severe pain or general unwellness. A lump in the groin of a male with no testicle in the scrotum on that side suggests an undescended testicle; this should be surgically corrected.

OCCASIONAL CAUSES: abscess; cancer that has spread from elsewhere; hydrocele (fluid accumulation) in spermatic cord; low appendix mass; lipoma (a benign fatty tumour).
RARE CAUSES: hip disease; lymphoma (malignant tumour); aneurysm (swelling on the femoral artery); neurofibroma (a benign tumour); undescended testis (especially in infants).

COMMON CAUSES	ACTION
Sebaceous cyst (blocked grease gland in skin) Hard lump within the skin itself. Usually no bigger than 1cm (⅓ in), with a central dimple (punctum).	No immediate treatment needed unless troublesome; infection eventually likely, removal then necessary. See GP non-urgently.
Reactive lymph nodes (reaction to infection) Many lumps, variable in size, can be felt under the skin on either side of groin; these tend to come and go over a few weeks.	No treatment needed. This is simply a sign of a normal immunity, indicating that the lymph nodes are active.
Inguinal groin hernia Soft lump in the groin, appearing or getting bigger on coughing or straining. More common in men. 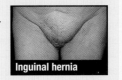 Inguinal hernia	See GP non-urgently, unless it becomes fixed, hard and painful: this may be a strangulated hernia, which is a surgical emergency.
Femoral hernia Similar to inguinal hernia but in the lower groin, and more common in women than men.	See Inguinal hernia, above.
Varicose vein in groin (saphena varix) Looks similar to a hernia but varicose veins are visible lower down the leg. Vibration felt on coughing and straining.	See GP non-urgently for surgical referral.

Rectal bleeding

Bleeding from the anus, on its own, or coating or mixed with bowel motions, is usually a result of constipation: this can cause haemorrhoids (which bleed), or tearing of the lining of the anal canal (anal fissure).

OCCASIONAL CAUSES: benign tumour (villous adenoma); injury; anticoagulant therapy; inflammatory bowel disease; cancer of the colon.
RARE CAUSES: blood clotting disorders; blood vessel blockage in the bowel (bowel ischaemia); abnormal blood vessels in bowel wall (angiodysplasia); telescoping of bowel (intussusception); kidney failure (uraemia).

COMMON CAUSES	ACTION
Haemorrhoids (piles) Blood on paper and sometimes in toilet pan, as well as coating (but not mixed with) faeces. Possible soft and painless, or hard and painful, lumps on anus.	Take OTC haemorrhoidal ointments and laxatives. Have a high-fibre diet. See GP non-urgently for confirmation.
Anal fissure (tear of anal canal lining) Severe, tearing anal pain on passing hard faeces; then pain on passing normal faeces. Blood coating (not mixed with) faeces.	As for Haemorrhoids above, but see GP urgently if pain is severe.
Gastroenteritis (gut infection) Blood mixed with loose or liquid faeces. You may feel unwell; fever is likely if blood present. Colicky abdominal pain and sometimes vomiting.	Take OTC antidiarrhoeals and salt replacement solutions. If constant pain, fever or vomiting for 24 hours+, see GP urgently or ask for home visit.
Diverticulitis (infection of the large intestine) Abdominal cramps and bloodstained diarrhoea. Constant pain and fever are serious signs.	Urgent GP appointment needed; request home visit if bedbound.
Rectal cancer Bleeding, often painless and coating (but not mixed with) faeces. Possible constipation; sense of wanting to open bowels but no motions; mucus or discharge from the rectum.	See GP as soon as possible.

Rectal discharge

Rectal discharge may be identified by a mucus or pus discharge from the anus in the underwear. The main problem may be the resultant itchiness rather than the discharge itself or any dampness. The most common causes are benign, but it is a good idea to see a GP for this symptom to rule out the possibility of cancer.

OCCASIONAL CAUSES: rectal cancer; anal fistula (opening to the skin); benign tumour (villous adenoma); inflammation of the alimentary tract (perianal Crohn's disease); ulcerative colitis is possible.

RARE CAUSES: anal tuberculosis; anal cancer; syphilis; gonorrhoea; AIDS.

COMMON CAUSES	ACTION
Haemorrhoids (piles) Blood on toilet paper, sometimes in toilet pan, and coating (not mixed with) faeces. Soft painless or hard painful lumps may be felt on the anus, or emerge from it while passing faeces, which may be painful.	Take OTC haemorrhoidal ointments and laxatives; try a high-fibre diet. See GP non-urgently for confirmation.
Anal fissure (tear of anal canal lining) Severe tearing anal pain while passing hard faeces. Subsequent pain on passing faeces. Appearance of blood as for Haemorroids, above.	As for Haemorrhoids, above, but see GP urgently if pain severe.
Rectal prolapse Mucus discharge, possibly bloodstained. Rectum protrudes from anus while passing faeces.	See GP as soon as possible.
Rectal inflammation (proctitis) Intense pain in rectum, with mucus discharge, possibly mixed with pus and/or blood.	See GP urgently.
Perianal warts (condylomata acuminata) Cauliflower-like lumps around anus; pus discharge, possibly bloodstained. Passing faeces often painful, hygiene difficult.	Attend genito-urinary medicine clinic as soon as possible.

Vomiting, sudden

Vomiting is often preceded by a feeling of nausea. Blood in the vomit may have a serious cause, and require urgent medical advice. If vomiting is so severe that travel is impossible ask for a home visit. With a vomiting child, go to the surgery with a towel and a bowl or bucket: the wait is likely to be short.

OCCASIONAL CAUSES: low and high blood sugar (hypo- and hyperglycaemia); intestinal obstruction; kidney infection (pyelonephritis); calculus (stone in the ureter).

RARE: peptic ulcer in adults, pyloric stenosis in infants (narrowing of lower outlet from stomach); meningitis (brain inflammation – see page 19); cerebral haemorrhage; bulimia nervosa; severe constipation.

COMMON CAUSES	ACTION
Gastroenteritis (gut infection) Also known as 'food poisoning': feeling ill; abdominal cramps and diarrhoea likely. Blood in the faeces not uncommon.	Take OTC antidiarrhoeals and salt-replacement solutions. If vomiting, fever or continuous pain continues for more than 24 hours, see GP urgently.
Inner ear inflammation (acute viral labyrinthitis) Sudden, severe vomiting and continuous vertigo; associated general viral illness, such as cold. Sensation of sounds in the ears or head (tinnitus) may be present.	See GP urgently; ask for home visit if travel is not possible.
Upper respiratory infection with marked coughing Most common in children, cough, cold or sore throat symptoms are usually present for a day or two before the vomiting, which occurs only with prolonged coughing bouts.	Try OTC decongestants and aromatic oils. Frequent sips of non-milky drinks. See GP urgently if not settled in a day.
Pregnancy Late, missed period. Nausea and sore breasts may occur several weeks before abdominal swelling is noticed.	Consult a home pregnancy test, now as reliable as hospital tests.
Appendicitis and other causes of acute pain Severe, continuous abdominal pain. Possible fever and diarrhoea; you may feel very ill. The abdomen may feel rigid, and movement may be very painful.	See GP urgently.

Breast lumps

A lump that changes in size over time is very unlikely to be cancer. But lumps appearing after the menopause and lumps causing skin dimpling or alterations in breast size or shape, or the direction of the nipple, should always be investigated for the possibility of cancer. Not all lumps require immediate specialist referral, but most GPs now have access to fast-track breast lump clinics.

OCCASIONAL CAUSES:
duct ectasia (dilation); lipoma (a benign tumour); Paget's disease of the nipple; milk-filled cyst (galactocele); multiple cysts.
RARE CAUSES:
tuberculosis; sarcoma; lymphoma; phylloides tumour (benign).

COMMON CAUSES	ACTION
Cancer The lump is hard and irregular, and fixed to surrounding tissues. See introduction for suspicious features.	See GP as soon as possible.
Cyst The lump is smooth and firm, and may change with your menstrual cycle.	See GP as soon as possible.
Abscess Sudden onset of a hot, painful lump with fever and general feeling of illness.	See GP urgently. May need referral to hospital for incision under anaesthetic.
Fibroadenoma (benign lump) Smooth, round, very mobile lump.	See GP as soon as possible for confirmation. Referral may be worthwhile.
Breast tissue change (fibrous dysplasia) Affects both breasts: they feel generally lumpy rather than having individual lumps. May be painful and change with your periods.	See GP routinely for confirmation and treatment.

Breast pain

Breast pain may be dull or sharp, constant or throbbing, aching or shooting, mild or severe, depending on the cause. Like breast lumps, breast pain often raises fear of the possibility of cancer. This is not a common cause, and it is unusual for pain to be the first sign of the disease: a lump would probably have been noticed already. Pain on one side, with a rash on the side of the chest or back (slightly higher than the breast) may be shingles (see page 18).

OCCASIONAL CAUSES:
cancer; onset of puberty; simple cyst; injury; lactation and/or a milk-filled cyst (galactocele).
RARE CAUSES: tuberculosis; (angina); arthritis of the neck (cervical spondylosis); thrombophlebitis (inflammation of the vein); shingles.

COMMON CAUSES	ACTION
Pregnancy One of the earliest signs of pregnancy in a woman who has missed a period. Occurs on both sides. Morning sickness may be present.	If in doubt, get a home pregnancy test (now as accurate as hospital tests). If positive, see GP to discuss.
Menstrual breast pain (cyclical mastalgia) Both breasts become lumpy and tender as the menstrual period becomes due. Can be very sore.	See GP non-urgently to discuss treatment options.
Cracked or inflamed nipple Common in breastfeeding women. May affect one or both nipples or there may be reddening around the nipple on an otherwise normal breast.	Pharmacists and midwives can advise on OTC creams and ointments. Do not stop breastfeeding.
Mastitis (breast infection) One breast is excruciatingly painful and hot. There is reddening of a wedge-shaped area of skin, spreading out from the nipple. Fever is often present. Most common in pregnant or breastfeeding women.	Requires antibiotics. See GP urgently to reduce the risk of abscess formation. Do not stop breastfeeding.
Breast abscess Follows mastitis, sometimes even if treated with antibiotics. Signs as for mastitis, see above, with a hard and very painful lump under the inflamed area.	See GP urgently for hospital referral: requires incision under anaesthetic.

Intercourse, painful in women

Dryness and discharge are just two possible contributory factors to painful intercourse in women. It is a common problem and doctors have much experience in dealing with it; so do not hesitate to seek help.

OCCASIONAL CAUSES: repair of perineum following childbirth; pelvic pain syndrome; fibroids in uterus; retroverted uterus; displaced ovaries (in pouch of Douglas); pelvic adhesions caused by previous surgery or infection; cystitis; urethritis.
RARE CAUSES: large ovarian cyst or tumour; leukoplakia; urethral caruncle (fleshy protrusion); unruptured hymen; anal fissure (tear); thrombosed haemorrhoids (piles filled with clotted blood); perianal abscess.

COMMON CAUSES	ACTION
Vaginismus (spasm and dryness) The vagina is dry on attempting intercourse, and feels tight and too small inside. No pain otherwise; no discharge; normal periods. Psychological cause.	See GP non-urgently to rule out other causes and discuss best approach. Psychosexual therapy can be helpful.
Superficial infection Copious discoloured vaginal discharge that may smell unpleasant. Soreness and itching all the time. Pain from start of penetration. May be caused by bacterial or fungal vaginosis, ulceration or bartholinitis.	See GP urgently for assessment.
Menopausal vaginal dryness (atrophic vaginitis) Gradually increasing difficulty with intercourse. No vaginal discharge. Possible symptoms of menopause, unless already over. Pain from start of penetration.	See GP non-urgently for assessment. If bleeding has occurred, see GP as soon as possible.
Endometriosis (uterus lining tissue at other sites) Heavy, painful periods. Pain on deep intercourse.	See GP as soon as possible for assessment.
Pelvic inflammatory disease (PID) Pain on deep intercourse. Discharge and heavy and painful periods often present.	See GP as soon as possible for assessment.

Pelvic pain, chronic

Pelvic pain is said to be chronic if it has been present for three or more menstrual cycles, either around the time of the periods or throughout the menstrual cycle. The most frequent causes are gynaecological, and a GP might refer you to a gynaecologist.

OCCASIONAL CAUSES: recurrent urinary tract infection; mechanical low back pain (recurrent strain); uterovaginal prolapse; benign tumours (eg ovarian cyst, fibroids); chronic interstitial cystitis.
RARE CAUSES: cancers (eg of the ovary, cervix, bowel); inflammation of alimentary tract (diverticulitis); inflammatory bowel disease; subacute intermittent bowel obstruction; 'forgotten' intrauterine contraceptive device (coil).

COMMON CAUSES	ACTION
Endometriosis (uterus lining tissue at other sites) Often worse around periods, which are often heavy. Painful intercourse.	See GP non-urgently.
Chronic pelvic inflammatory disease (PID) Pain usually throughout the month; may be worse during periods, which are heavy. Difficulty conceiving.	See GP non-urgently.
Pelvic congestion Worse around periods, which are heavier than usual. Usually no problems during the rest of the month.	See GP non-urgently.
Irritable bowel syndrome (IBS) May be worse around periods, which are not heavier than usual. Abdominal bloating, colicky pain, diarrhoea, pellety bowel motions and mucus. Urgent need to open bowels after eating, which often relieves pain.	See GP non-urgently.
Mid-cycle or ovulation pain, period pain Mid-cycle pain is short-lived and felt on one side, occurring 14 days after first day of last period. Period pain is usually just before and in first few days of period.	See GP non-urgently.

Pelvic pain, severe and sudden

Sudden, severe pain felt in the lower abdomen and in the pelvis is mostly felt by women. If the pain is so severe that travel is not possible, ask your GP for a home visit.

OCCASIONAL CAUSES: pelvic abscess; endometriosis (uterus lining tissue at other pelvic sites); pelvic congestion (exacerbation of pelvic pain syndrome); prostatitis (in men); psychosexual factors.
RARE CAUSES: misplaced coil (intrauterine contraceptive device) leading to perforated uterus; referred pain (eg from spinal tumour, bowel spasm); rectal inflammation (proctitis); invasive cancer of ovaries or cervix; degeneration of fibroids.

COMMON CAUSES	ACTION
Acute pelvic inflammatory disease (PID) Pain is constant and severe; it may be felt in the back, and be worse on deep intercourse. Discoloured and/or bloodstained vaginal discharge. Fever; feeling unwell.	See GP urgently for assessment.
Urinary tract infection Low, deep, dull, constant pain, often in the back or higher on one side. Urgent desire to pass urine, but only small quantities passed (with burning pain). Urine may be smelly and/or bloodstained. Fever; feeling unwell.	See GP urgently for assessment.
Miscarriage After a missed period, crampy low pain like a bad period pain. Vaginal bleeding, ranging from a little brown discharge to copious red blood with clots.	Call GP for advice. Wear pad and save any solid material passed.
Ectopic pregnancy (development of fetus outside the uterus) Around two weeks after a missed period, severe crampy or constant pain on one side of the pelvis. Pain is followed by vaginal bleeding, possible serious haemorrhage.	See GP urgently for assessment. If vaginal bleeding has begun, dial 999.

Periods, absent

This refers to periods that have stopped in a previously menstruating woman; periods that never started are referred to as 'delayed puberty' (see page 51). Absent periods are not dangerous, but it is worth seeing a GP to treat the underlying causes.

OCCASIONAL CAUSES: under- or overactive thyroid (hypo- and hyperthyroidism); anorexia nervosa; severe general illness of any kind; excessive exercise or training; adrenal disorders (eg Addison's or Cushing's disease, congenital adrenal hyperplasia).
RARE CAUSES: prolactinoma or other pituitary tumours.

COMMON CAUSES	ACTION
Pregnancy Tender breasts, morning sickness; abdominal swelling after 10–12 weeks.	Try a home pregnancy test, as reliable as hospital tests. See GP if positive.
Physiological factors Causes might include breastfeeding, rapid weight loss or severe emotional stress. Absent periods may be associated with depression.	See GP non-urgently for investigation of weight loss or advice on stress.
Menopause (and premature ovarian failure) Hot flushes, night sweats, and sometimes unpredictable mood swings.	See GP non-urgently for investigation and to discuss available treatments.
Polycystic ovary syndrome (hormonal disorder) Often to some degree overweight, excess body hair and acne.	See GP non-urgently for investigation and possible specialist referral.
Drug treatment Possible milky breast discharge, for example, caused by, phenothiazines, metoclopramide, sodium-valproate, cytotoxics.	See GP non-urgently.

Symptom sorter

Periods, heavy

A period is heavy if bleeding is heavier or longer than the woman thinks it should be. A single heavy period can be caused by emotional upset or excessive exercise, so it is best to wait three cycles to establish a pattern before making a non-urgent GP appointment. (For causes of bleeding outside of periods, see page 51, Vaginal bleeding, irregular.)

OCCASIONAL CAUSES: puberty; menopause; intrauterine contraceptive device (coil); cystic glandular hyperplasia (increased cell production); chronic pelvic inflammatory disease (PID); overactive thyroid (hyperthyroidism). RARE CAUSES: adrenal disorders and excess prolactin; liver disease; dyscrasias (blood abnormalities); endometrial cancer.

COMMON CAUSES	ACTION
Dysfunctional uterine bleeding Periods are heavy but usually painless; the interval between them may be longer than usual. Otherwise you are well.	See GP urgently after three heavy periods.
Cervical or endometrial polyps (benign growths) Heavy periods may be painful; possible bleeding between periods and after intercourse.	See GP urgently after three heavy periods; or sooner if there is bleeding between periods or after intercourse.
Endometriosis (uterus lining tissue at other sites) Heavy periods are generally very painful. Intercourse may be painful; pain in pelvis may persist through the cycle.	See GP urgently after three heavy periods.
Fibroids (benign growths) Heavy periods may be painful. Possible pressure symptoms may be felt: discomfort during intercourse; need to empty bladder frequently and, very occasionally, leg swelling.	See GP urgently after three heavy periods.
Underactive thyroid (hypothyroidism) Heavy, sometimes irregular periods; associated with tiredness, feeling cold and slowed down. Weight gain, dry skin, brittle hair.	See GP urgently after three heavy periods, sooner if associated symptoms have already developed.

Periods, painful

Period pain (dysmenhorroea) is felt in the lower abdomen and back and is not always associated with heavy periods. Half of all the women in the UK have moderately painful periods; and more than ten per cent have severe pain. Painful periods developing later in life are usually treatable.

OCCASIONAL CAUSES: chocolate cyst of ovary (caused by endometriosis); abnormally positioned (retroverted) uterus; inflammation of the cervix (cervicitis); endometrial polyp (benign growth); pelvic pain syndrome. RARE CAUSES: uterine malformation; unbroken hymen; defective development of uterus (hypoplasia); narrowing of the cervix (cervical stenosis); psychological factors.

COMMON CAUSES	ACTION
Primary dysmenorrhoea Pain starts with the first-ever period. Crampy pain is felt in the first few days of the period.	Take OTC painkillers or anti-inflammatories. See GP non-urgently if not settled after first six months, or if especially severe.
Endometriosis (uterus lining tissue at other sites) Pain often not crampy, and may be widespread through lower abdomen. Associated with deep pain on intercourse.	See GP non-urgently for examination and specialist referral for investigations.
Chronic pelvic inflammatory disease (PID) Deep pain felt on intercourse. Pain in pelvis may continue in rest of month. Follows an initial pelvic infection.	See GP non-urgently for examination and possible specialist referral.
Fibroids (benign growths) Progressively more painful periods, sometimes becoming increasingly heavy. Possible pressure symptoms including frequent passing of urine.	See GP non-urgently for examination and investigations.
Intrauterine contraceptive device (coil) Crampy pains felt during periods, which may be heavier than before coil is fitted.	See GP non-urgently to consider coil removal and alternative contraception.

Vaginal discharge

A certain amount of clear mucal discharge from the vagina is normal. Its thickness varies through the menstrual cycle. If it becomes coloured, offensive or excessive, it can be considered abnormal. In all cases, attend a genito-urinary medicine clinic if there is a possibility of a sexually transmitted disease.

OCCASIONAL CAUSES: cervical erosion (ectropion); cervical polyp (a benign growth); lost tampon, or other foreign body; intrauterine contraceptive device (coil); Bartholinitis (inflammation of glands either side of vaginal entrance).
RARE CAUSES: cancer (eg vulval, vaginal, cervical, uterine); benign growth (fibroid).

COMMON CAUSES	ACTION
Excessive normal secretions Clear mucus discharge. May cause external discomfort through continuous dampness. You feel otherwise well.	See GP non-urgently.
Thrush (candida infection) Intense vaginal itching and soreness. There may be pain on passing urine. White, creamy, usually inoffensive discharge.	Take OTC thrush treatment. Your sexual partner, who may have no symptoms, should do the same. See GP if this fails.
Bacterial vaginosis Offensive yellow or greenish discharge. Vagina is usually not sore or itchy.	See GP as soon as possible.
Trichomonal vaginosis Offensive, often fishy-smelling, greyish, frothy discharge. The vagina is sore and itchy.	See GP as soon as possible.
Inflammation of the cervix (cervicitis) Caused by, for example, gonococcus, chlamydia or herpes. The discharge may be yellow or greenish, possibly offensive. Pain on deep intercourse. Vagina may be sore and/or itchy.	Attend genito-urinary medicine clinic as soon as possible. Refrain from sex until treatment is complete.

Vulval irritation

Irritation of the vulva results in itching and soreness. The vulva is made up of the inner and outer lips (labia) of the vagina and the space between them. The causes of vulval irritation may also affect the vagina.

OCCASIONAL CAUSES: inflammation from incontinence (ammoniacal vulvitis); psoriasis; lichen planus (an itchy skin disorder); infestations (eg, scabies, pubic lice); underlying psychosexual problem.
RARE CAUSES: cancer; general disorders causing itching.

COMMON CAUSES	ACTION
Thrush (candida infection) Intense vaginal itching and soreness. Possible pain on passing urine. White, usually inoffensive, creamy discharge.	Take OTC thrush treatment. The same for your sexual partner, who may have no symptoms. See GP if this fails.
Bacterial or trichomonal vaginosis **Bacterial**: offensive yellow or greenish discharge; vagina usually not sore or itchy. **Trichonomal**: offensive, often fishy-smelling, greyish, frothy discharge; vagina is sore and itchy.	See GP as soon as possible or attend a genito-urinary medicine clinic.
Insufficient lubrication during intercourse Sore, possibly itchy vagina. Difficulties with intercourse are usually known already.	Ensure adequate foreplay; use a water-based lubricant gel. See GP non-urgently if problem persists.
Reactions to chemicals Sore, itchy vagina; usually no discharge. Otherwise you feel well. May be caused by bubble baths, feminine-hygiene douches or detergents.	Try OTC hydrocortisone cream; avoid offending product if identified. See GP as soon as possible if not better in five days.
Atrophic vaginitis Around or after the menopause, a sore (not itchy) vagina, with thin, dry and reddened lining of vulva and vagina. No discharge. Difficulties with intercourse.	As for Insufficient lubrication (see above). Discuss hormone replacement therapy (HRT) with GP.

Vulval swellings

A swelling or lump may develop in the vulva (the inner and outer lips of the vagina and the space between them), or originate elsewhere and become displaced into the vulva.

OCCASIONAL CAUSES:
varicose vein; dilated veins (varicocele); benign tumours (eg fibroma, lipoma, hidradenoma); prolapses of the uterus, bladder, rectum or bowel, urethral protuberance/caruncle; cervical polyp (benign growth).
RARE CAUSES: cancer; traumatic haematoma (blood clot in tissue).

COMMON CAUSES	ACTION
Boil Solitary, painful, pus-filled spot, which eventually bursts. It may not heal easily without treatment.	See GP urgently.
Sebaceous cyst (blocked grease gland in skin) Firm or hard lump fixed to the skin, and with a central hole or dimple (punctum).	Do not squeeze the cyst: this could cause painful inflammation. See GP non-urgently. No treatment is needed unless the cyst is causing problems.
Viral warts (condylomata acuminata) Crops of hard whitish or brown lumps appear anywhere on the surface skin of the vulva.	Attend a genito-urinary medicine clinic as soon as possible.
Bartholin's cyst (infected abscess) A painless, firm lump is felt in the lower vulva, under the skin on one side. There is no swelling in the surrounding area.	See GP non-urgently, or urgently if it becomes painful.
Inguinal groin hernia (protrusion) Swelling, usually in one groin, which may extend right into the outer lip (labium major). Increases in size on coughing. More common in smokers, women with chronic cough, and heavy manual workers.	See your GP non-urgently. If the lump cannot be pushed back into the abdomen and it becomes hard and painful, see GP urgently: it may result in possible strangulation of the hernia.

Vulval ulceration and sores

Ulcers and sores are non-healing breaks in a body surface tissue. Consult a doctor about any that appear on the vulva. If there is any possibility of a sexually transmitted disease, attend a genito-urinary medicine clinic.

OCCASIONAL CAUSES:
Bowen's and Paget's diseases; sexually transmitted diseases (eg chancroid, granuloma inguinale, lymphogranuloma venereum); diabetic and mycotic vulvitis (inflammation of the vulva); cancer.
RARE CAUSES: syphilis (primary: chancre; secondary: condylomata lata; tertiary: gumma); Behçet's syndrome; tuberculosis.

COMMON CAUSES	ACTION
Herpes simplex May cause fever and leave you feeling unwell. Crops of blister-like spots develop, becoming pus-filled then painful with scabs. Glands in groin are enlarged. Passing urine can be very painful; catheterization in hospital may be necessary.	Attend a genito-urinary medicine clinic urgently.
Excoriated (badly scratched) thrush (candida infection) Intense vaginal itching and soreness. There may be pain on passing urine. White, creamy discharge.	Take OTC thrush treatment. Your sexual partner should do the same, even if without symptoms. See a GP if this fails.
Abnormal tissue development (vulval dysplasia) Gradual onset of an itchy sore; no accompanying discharge; otherwise you feel well. Most common after the menopause.	See GP as soon as possible.
Squamous cell cancer An itchy, crusty lump gradually enlarges; no discharge.	See GP as soon as possible.
Excoriated (badly scratched) scabies A furiously itchy rash appears, often starting on the hands and spreading. It gets worse at night.	Try OTC antiscabies lotions; itch may last ten days after the treatment ends. It is contagious by direct contact only.

Breast swelling in men

In men, swelling of breast tissue is felt only directly behind the nipple. For causes of lumps in women's breasts, see page 39. The causes are important, so a checkup is advisable.

OCCASIONAL CAUSES: hypothyroidism (underactive thyroid); chronic renal failure and haemodialysis; testicular or adrenal cancer; cryptorchidism, hypogonadism and other causes of impaired testicular function. **RARE CAUSES:** Klinefelter's syndrome (a genetic disorder); acromegaly (a growth hormone disorder).

COMMON CAUSES	ACTION
Puberty Breast swelling often occurs on one side only during puberty. Other causes are very rare at this age.	If it has not settled on its own within three months, see GP non-urgently.
Drugs Both sides swollen; may be feeling generally unwell. Causes include use of spironolactone, cimetidine, digoxin, cyproterone, marijuana.	See GP as soon as possible.
Chronic liver disease Affects both sides. If the cause is alcohol-related, there may be other signs of alcohol excess, for example, red face and palms, weight loss, erratic behaviour and drunkenness.	See GP non-urgently for checkup and advice. Contact local drugs and alcohol agency for long-term help.
Lung cancer Affects both sides. Possible cough, shortness of breath, weight loss, coughing up blood. Rare in non-smokers.	See GP as soon as possible for assessment.
Hyperthyroidism (overactive thyroid) Affects both sides. Feeling unwell, anxious. Possible weight loss, fast pulse, sweaty skin, tremor of hands.	See GP as soon as possible for investigation and treatment.

Impotence

This is failure to achieve a normal erection; either a full erection dwindles before orgasm or it cannot be reached for any length of time. It may have a psychological cause, especially if a good morning erection is regularly achieved. Erections that dwindle after a set period are more likely to have a physical cause.

OCCASIONAL CAUSES: diabetic nerve damage; pelvic or spinal fracture, injury to the penis; post-prostate surgery; anatomical (eg phimosis, tight frenulum); smoking; Peyronie's disease. **RARE CAUSES:** impaired testicular function; spinal cord compression (caused by tumour); blood clot (thrombosis); neurological disorders (eg tabes dorsalis, multiple sclerosis).

COMMON CAUSES	ACTION
Depression or anxiety Low mood, difficulty in sleeping, tearfulness, loss of confidence, all for two weeks or more.	See GP as soon as possible for assessment and treatment.
Excessive alcohol intake Red face and palms. Morning erections infrequent.	Seek help from a local drug and alcohol agency.
Relationship dysfunction Occasional failure to get an erection; good morning erections are usual.	Seek help from a specialist counselling service such as Relate.
Blood vessel problems Erection failure every time. Morning erections infrequent or absent. Cold legs or feet common. Possible causes are arterial insufficiency and excessive venous drainage.	See GP as soon as possible, especially if your legs or feet are cold.
Medication Erection failure every time. Morning erections infrequent or absent. May be caused by, for example, prostate cancer treatments, hypotensives, some antidepressants, spironolactone.	See GP as soon as possible for a review of your medication.

Penile pain

It is important to seek medical advice as soon as possible for penile pain, even if the pain is occasional, and especially if blood is passed painlessly in the urine. If there is no discharge, pain in the penis is unlikely to be caused by a sexually transmitted disease.

OCCASIONAL CAUSES:
herpes simplex; cancer (eg bladder, prostate); injury (eg torn frenulum, zipper injury, urethral injury or foreign body); acute cystitis; anal fissure or inflamed haemorrhoid (pile).

RARE CAUSES: cancer of the penis, rectum and/or anus; Peyronie's disease (pain usually on erection); shingles (herpes zoster).

COMMON CAUSES	ACTION
Balanitis (fungal or bacterial infection of tip of penis) Usually a problem only in uncircumcised men; pus discharge from under the foreskin and painful tip of penis (glans penis). Passing urine may be painful.	See GP urgently.
Prostatic abscess, inflammation (prostatitis) Possible discharge from urethra (opening in end of penis), pain on passing urine. Severe, dull, rectal pain. Fever possible.	See GP urgently.
Urinary stone (calculus) Excruciating pain lasting minutes or hours; may begin on one side of abdomen or back. There may be blood in the urine.	See GP as soon as possible. Sieve urine through a tea strainer to catch stones; retain them to show to your GP.
Inflammation of the urethra (acute urethritis) Continual discharge from urethra with burning pain on passing urine. Fever and joint pains may also occur.	Consult a genito-urinary medicine clinic as soon as possible; until then abstain from all sexual intercourse.
Tight foreskin (phimosis) Difficulty and pain on passing urine through the tight opening in the foreskin, which may balloon during urination. Possible accompanying discharge from under the foreskin.	See GP as soon as possible.

Penile sores and ulceration

Sores and ulcers are non-healing breaks in a body surface tissue. Like penile pain, these symptoms often raise the fear of sexually transmitted disease or cancer. Cancer is a rare cause; sexually transmitted disease is much more likely. If this is a realistic possibility, refrain from all sexual intercourse until seen as soon as possible in a genito-urinary medicine clinic.

OCCASIONAL CAUSES:
shingles (herpes zoster); inflamed glans penis (balanitis circinata caused by Reiter's syndrome); soft sore (chancroid, caused by haemophilus ducreyi); sexually transmitted diseases (eg donovania granulomatis, lymphogranuloma venereum (chlamydial).

RARE CAUSES: primary syphilis (chancre: painful); tertiary syphilis (gumma: painless); penile cancer.

COMMON CAUSES	ACTION
Herpes simplex Crops of blister-like spots that become pus-filled and break down to a painful scab. Glands in groin enlarged. May have fever and be feeling unwell.	Attend a genito-urinary medicine clinic urgently; until then abstain from all sexual intercourse.
Boil/infected sebaceous cyst (blocked grease gland) Solitary, painful pus-filled spot that bursts and may not heal easily without treatment.	See GP urgently.
Warts, condylomata acuminata Crops of hard whitish or brown lumps appear on the surface of the skin, usually at the tip of the penis (glans penis).	Attend a genito-urinary medicine clinic as soon as possible; until then abstain from all sexual intercourse.
Balanitis (fungal or bacterial infection of tip of penis) Usually occurs in uncircumcised men only; pus discharge from under foreskin and painful tip of penis (glans penis). Passing urine may be painful.	See GP urgently.
Injury Injury (eg a zipper injury) is usually obvious. When torn, the frenulum (the bowstring-like thread joining the underside of the penis tip to the penis shaft) often bleeds dramatically.	See GP urgently or go to casualty. To stop any bleeding, apply firm pressure with a clean pad to the bleeding point.

Scrotal swellings

Swellings in the scrotum can affect males of all ages. Testicular cancer is rare, but is most common in the 20–40 age group. All men should practise self-examination of their scrotums at least once a month. See a GP as soon as possible if a lump is discovered.

OCCASIONAL: torsion (twisting) of the testis; infection after surgery or catheterization; haematocele (blood leakage); varicocele (dilated veins); congestive heart failure.
RARE: testicular cancer (seminoma, teratoma).

COMMON CAUSES	ACTION
Inguinal (groin) hernia Swelling usually in one groin and descending towards scrotum; increases in size on coughing. Most common in smokers, men with chronic cough, and heavy manual workers.	See GP non-urgently, more quickly if lump cannot be pushed back into abdomen and is hard and painful.
Sebaceous cyst (blocked grease gland in skin) Firm or hard lump fixed to the skin, with a central hole or dimple (punctum).	Do not squeeze: may make it inflamed. No treatment needed unless causing problems. See GP non-urgently.
Hydrocele (fluid accumulation) Soft, painless swelling around one testicle.	See GP as soon as possible for confirmation.
Epididymal cyst Firm, round swelling at end of one testicle. Usually (but not always) painless.	See GP as soon as possible for confirmation.
Epididymo-orchitis (urinary tract infection) One or both testicles are painful and swollen. You may feel generally unwell, with fever. The infection is sexually transmitted.	See GP urgently.

Testicular pain

When it occurs suddenly, testicular pain is usually excruciating and severe, and is likely to be caused by an urgent problem. A dull, dragging pain suggests a longer-term or less urgent problem. Testicular pain can occur in males of all ages.

OCCASIONAL: varicocele (dilated veins); haematocele (blood-filled swelling); hydrocele (fluid accumulation); injury (fractured testis); undescended or misplaced testis.
RARE: testicular cancer (seminoma, teratoma); syphilis; referred pain from spinal tumours.

COMMON CAUSES	ACTION
Acute orchitis (inflammation of the testes) Both sides affected; testicles painful to touch. Onset over a few hours. Generally feeling unwell, with fever. Glands in armpits, neck, groins may be enlarged and tender. Underlying cause may be mumps or, less commonly, flu or scarlet fever.	Take regular paracetamol. See GP urgently for diagnosis.
Acute epididymo-orchitis (urinary tract infection) Onset over a few hours; usually both testicles painful. Supporting the testicles helps. Fever uncommon; possible discharge, frequent and painful passing of urine. Infection is sexually transmitted.	See GP urgently. Attend genito-urinary medicine clinic if discharge present.
Torsion (twisting) of the testis Sudden onset of disabling, excruciating pain in one testicle which is very painful to touch, and feels hard and high in scrotum. Nausea common. No fever.	See GP urgently or go straight to casualty. Requires operation within four hours of the start of the pain.
Epididymal cyst Firm swelling at end of one testicle, not usually painful to touch. Mild, dull and dragging pain; very gradual onset and may have been present for weeks or longer. Otherwise well.	See GP as soon as possible.
Stone in the ureter (calculus) Sudden, severe pain from one side of back, down through groin and into testicle (referred pain). Pain comes and goes in waves. Blood in urine possible; no fever.	See GP as soon as possible. Sieve urine with tea strainer to catch stones; retain them to show your GP.

Blood in the urine

Blood in the urine always needs to be investigated. It can sometimes be invisible to the eye and may be detected by a routine dipstick test at a medical checkup, or on microscopic examination. Invisible blood in the urine is usually a sign of an underlying problem.

OCCASIONAL CAUSES: jogging and hard exercise; cancer of the kidney; chronic interstitial cystitis; anticoagulant drugs; inflammation of the kidney (eg nephritis, glomerulonephritis). **RARE CAUSES:** renal tuberculosis; polycystic kidney disease; blood diseases (eg haemophilia, sickle-cell disease, thrombocytopaenia; infective endocarditis (heart inflammation); schistosomiasis (tropical disease).

COMMON CAUSES	ACTION
Urinary tract infection Burning, stinging pain on passing urine; frequent passing of small amounts. May have low backache.	Antibiotics are needed: see your GP urgently.
Bladder tumour There may be visible red blood in the urine, and difficulty in emptying the bladder.	See GP as soon as possible; requires specialist referral.
Urinary stones (calculi) in kidney or ureter Excruciating pain on one side of the back, often travelling down to the groin and into the penis, scrotum or vagina.	Call for GP visit for pain relief. Drink plenty of fluids. Later investigation necessary.
Urethritis (inflammation of the urethra) Pus discharge from bladder opening (urethra); stinging, burning pain on passing urine. Underlying cause is often a sexually transmitted disease.	Attend genito-urinary medicine clinic; requires antibiotics and investigation.
Enlarged prostate gland or cancer of prostate Gradual onset of difficulty in starting urination; slow urinary stream, and dribbling afterwards.	See GP non-urgently for examination and further investigation.

Incontinence, urinary

This is the involuntary passage of urine, largely a problem for women. It causes misery through its effect on people's personal hygiene, sexual relationships and ability to go out and about. It is estimated that urinary incontinence affects 15–30 per cent of women of all ages; over 50 per cent of incontinent women never seek help or do so only after many years of misery.

OCCASIONAL CAUSES: excessive urination (polyuria, see page 49); chronic urinary tract infection; interstitial cystitis; bladder stone; surgery or radiotherapy on abdomen and/or pelvis; abnormal opening (fistula), due to surgery or cancer. **RARE CAUSES:** pelvic fracture; congenital abnormalities; nerve damage due to diabetes, syphilis, multiple sclerosis.

COMMON CAUSES	ACTION
Stress incontinence Leakage of small amounts of urine on coughing, straining or lifting. Perhaps caused by sphincter and/or pelvic floor damage through childbirth (often with prolapses).	See GP as soon as possible, or attend a local incontinence clinic.
Surgery to remove prostate gland (prostatectomy) Incontinence after a prostatectomy is usually only temporary.	Seek advice from your GP or hospital team as appropriate.
Urinary tract infections, especially cystitis Low, deep, dull, constant pain; often also felt in the back or higher on one side. Urgent desire to pass urine, but only small quantities are passed. Burning pain on passing urine, which may smell offensive and/or be bloodstained. Fever and feeling unwell.	See GP urgently.
Unstable bladder muscle This may follow, for example, a stroke, dementia or Parkinson's disease. It often disturbs sleep. The urge to pass urine may be so powerful that a toilet is not reached in time.	Restrict fluid intake in evenings. See GP as soon as possible.
Chronic outflow obstruction Gradual slowing of flow, difficulty starting urination, dribbling on stopping. Obstruction may be caused by enlargement of the prostate, narrowing of the urethra or bladder neck.	See GP as soon as possible.

Urination, excessive

Passing increased amounts of urine is nearly always associated with increased thirst.
The medical name is polyuria. (For more frequent passing of normal quantities of urine, see Urinary frequency below. For Urinary retention, see page 50.)

OCCASIONAL CAUSES: relief of chronic urinary obstruction; drugs (eg demeclocycline, lithium carbonate, amphotericin B, gentamicin); low potassium in blood (hypokalaemia); cranial diabetes insipidus; Cushing's syndrome; sickle-cell anaemia; early chronic pyelonephritis (kidney inflammation).
RARE CAUSES: compulsive water-drinking (psychogenic polydipsia).

COMMON CAUSES	ACTION
Diabetes mellitus Continuous, marked thirst. Feeling tired and unwell; weight loss. Abdominal pain and/or vomiting if blood sugar levels very high.	See GP as soon as possible, urgently if you feel unwell. Take fresh urine sample for sugar testing.
Diuretic treatment Symptom usually worse for first few hours after taking treatment. Thirst not usually a problem.	See GP non-urgently if symptom causing major problems.
Excess alcohol intake The need to urinate is increased for several hours during and after excess drinking of alcohol. Dry mouth, hangover later.	Drink plenty of water to replace fluid lost. Avoid alcoholic bingeing.
Chronic kidney failure Often there are no symptoms; possible loss of appetite and weight.	See GP as soon as possible.
High calcium level in blood (hypercalcaemia) May result from, for example, osteoporosis treatment, cancer spread to bones, Paget's disease or hyperparathyroidism. Thirst is continuous. Generally unwell, with muscle cramps or spasms. Possible abdominal pain and vomiting.	See GP urgently or call for a home visit if you are too ill to travel.

Urinary frequency

Urinary frequency is the frequent passing of urine in usually small amounts. If large amounts of urine are passed frequently, this is excessive urination, covered above. (For Urinary retention, see page 50.)

OCCASIONAL CAUSES: inflamed prostate (prostatitis); non-infective interstitial cystitis; urethral syndrome (often after intercourse); stone in the ureter; urethritis (inflammation of the urethra); pyelonephritis (kidney inflammation); thickening and narrowing of the bladder neck (bladder neck hypertrophy); tumour or swelling within the pelvis; habit.
RARE CAUSES: secondary to pelvic inflammation (eg pelvic infection, appendicitis, diverticulitis, adjacent tumour); benign or malignant bladder tumour.

COMMON CAUSES	ACTION
Infective cystitis (bladder infection) Dull, constant pain in stomach, back or kidney area on one side. Urgent desire to pass urine, but little passed, with burning pain. Urine may smell bad and/or be bloodstained.	See GP urgently for assessment.
Bladder stone (calculus) Urinary frequency preceded at some point by excruciating pain that may begin on one side of the abdomen or back. Blood often seen in urine. Frequency intermittent, eased by lying down. Passing urine may be painful or slow.	See GP as soon as possible.
Unstable bladder muscle This may follow, for example, a stroke, dementia, Parkinson's disease. Often disturbs sleep. Urge to pass urine may be so powerful that a toilet is not reached in time.	Restrict fluid intake in evenings. See GP as soon as possible.
Chronic outflow obstruction Gradual slowing of flow, difficulty in starting urination and dribbling on stopping. May be caused by, for example, enlarged prostate or narrowing of bladder neck or urethra.	See GP as soon as possible.
Anxiety Usually long-term, worse with stress and cold weather; fast, racing heartbeat, palpitations, nervous state. Sweaty skin, shaky hands; often breathlessness and pins and needles.	Consider ways to reduce life stress. See GP as soon as possible.

Many other symptoms require medical attention. This quick reference guide helps you to identify some of the most important. The heading indicates what action to take and how urgently to take it.

Emergency: get immediate medical advice/dial 999

Blood in vomit
If blood has been in the stomach for several hours, the vomit looks dark, like coffee grounds. Blood from the stomach passing through the gut turns the faeces jet black and tarry; it is very offensive to smell. Bleeding into the stomach can suddenly get worse. If coughing up blood, see page 15.

Breathing difficulty, sudden and severe in children (stridor)
Anxiety increases the problem, so remain outwardly calm and try to comfort the child while arranging help. In cases of acute airways obstruction by an inhaled foreign body, hold infants upside down and thump the back with the flat of the hand; perform the Heimlich manoeuvre in children too heavy to lift easily (see FIRST AID). Congenital laryngeal paralysis, which is usually detected immediately after birth in hospitals, accounts for one in four infants with stridor; in these cases follow hospital advice. (For shortness of breath in adults, see Breathlessness, chronic and Breathlessness, sudden, both page 13).

Confusion, sudden and severe
Any sudden, severe disorientation or delirium requires urgent hospital investigation to find the cause.

Hallucinations
Hallucinations are defined as the perception of something not actually there. They require urgent medical attention as they may indicate medical conditions such as drug overdose, alcohol withdrawal, acute schizophrenia and other acute psychiatric conditions.

Loss of vision, sudden
It is sensible to go straight to casualty if vision is lost suddenly, especially if the eye is painful (see page 28). For gradual loss of vision, see page 51.

Urinary retention
The severe pain of an enlarged bladder needs urgent relief throught the passing of a tube (catheter) into the bladder, usually through the opening of the urinary tube (urethra). In general, it is quickest and best to attend a casualty department for treatment. For excessive or frequent urination, see page 49.

Urgent but not an emergency: get GP appointment or advice within 24 hours

Ear discharge
This is most commonly caused by an infection requiring antibiotic treatment. For earache, see page 27.

Facial pain
This is often caused by dental problems, including abscesses and jaw joint dysfunction (joint pain, cracking sound on movement). Visit a dentist before seeing a GP.

Facial swelling
See GP urgently or go to casualty if you suspect an allergy (sudden onset); dial 999 if there is difficulty in breathing, or swelling inside the mouth. For swelling, pain and bruising following a blow to the head, go to casualty for X-rays; don't take food or drink until seen. For a dental abscess, see a dentist urgently.

Facial ulcers and blisters
In children, rapidly developing and spreading golden-crusted sores, often around the mouth, may be impetigo. In older people, blisters may indicate shingles (herpes zoster). Both are contagious. For other rashes, blisters and pus spots, see pages 16 to 22.

Fever, prolonged
Seek help for fever of more than three or four days. Mention any recent foreign travel.

Jaundice
Yellow discoloration of the skin and the whites of the eyes caused by deposits of bile pigments. Indicates excessive breakdown of blood cells, a failure of the liver to work properly, or a blockage of the bile ducts.

Jaw, painful and/or swelling
Go to a casualty department for a suspected fracture (inability to open the mouth much). Visit a dentist urgently for dental causes such as: abscess or cyst (severe dull ache and swelling; swollen neck glands and fever); jaw joint dysfunction (pain and possible cracking sound on movement); unerupted teeth; gum swelling.

Loss of consciousness
See GP urgently if also fast or irregular heartbeats and shortness of breath; dial 999 if symptoms are jerkiness of limbs and grunting breathing; this may be epilepsy. For falls with no loss of consciousness, see page 51.

Important but not urgent: get next available GP appointment

Abnormal eating
Although it may be difficult to persuade the person to visit a doctor, it is important to do so before the problem gets out of hand.

Abnormal gait in adults
Make an urgent GP appointment or ask for a home visit if symptoms include disabling vertigo, nausea and vomiting; it may be labyrinthitis, a viral infection. For limping in a child, see page 25.

Excessive body hair
This affects both men and women, but usually refers to excess body hair in a male distribution on a woman (that is, on the face, lower abdomen and upper thighs). There is usually no particular cause. See a GP if it has appeared suddenly; otherwise, see a cosmetician for treatment.

Falls with no loss of consciousness
Such falls are not usually serious, although if a sudden fall accompanies any acute illness, such as a stroke, see GP urgently or ask for home visit. These can be caused by, for example, low blood pressure, poor blood supply to the brain or medication.

Flushing lasting for several minutes
Emotional flushing that lasts seconds, and affects only the face, is normal. If severe or unusually frequent, it can be a sign of an underlying problem; seek a GP's advice.

Faecal incontinence
Most causes are non-urgent: severe haemorrhoids (piles), rectal prolapse, severe constipation or childbirth. Urgent medical attention is required for sudden onset of faecal incontinence with severe back pain and numbness in the back of the thighs; this could indicate a centrally prolapsed lumbar disc. For rectal bleeding and discharge, see pages 37 and 38. For urinary incontinence, see page 48.

Loss of vision, gradual
Emergency or urgent treatment is not needed for most causes, for example, cataracts or long-term damage from diabetes or high blood pressure. But persistent early-morning headaches with double vision may indicate a serious cause. See GP urgently if there is gradual loss of part of the field of vision: this may be creeping inferior retinal detachment, and urgent laser treatment referral may be needed. For sudden loss of vision, see page 50. For painful eyes, see page 28.

Nipple discharge
In general, although infection needs to be dealt with quickly, most causes, such as pregnancy or a reaction to certain drugs, do not need urgent medical attention. An areolar abscess (pus discharge, sometimes bloodstained, from one breast; underlying tissue hot and excruciatingly painful to touch), however, may require immediate surgery, so urgent GP assessment is required. For breast pain and lumps, see page 39.

Nose, blocked
Seek advice from a GP for a blocked nose that is not associated with a simple cold and lasts four weeks or more. For nosebleeds, see page 30.

Puberty, delayed
Delayed puberty is a failure to develop adult sexual characteristics by age 15 in boys, and 14 in girls (or failure to start periods by age 16). Have it investigated by your GP.

Vaginal bleeding, irregular
Menstrual periods are normal vaginal bleeding in women of reproductive age. Any bleeding outside of periods, before puberty or after the menopause is not normal and should be discussed with a GP. If irregular bleeding is associated with discoloured vaginal discharge and pelvic pain, get an urgent GP appointment or go to a genito-urinary medicine clinic; this may be cervicitis (inflammation of the cervix) or a pelvic infection, which need antibiotics. See also Pelvic pain, severe and sudden, page 41.

Vertigo
This symptom manifests itself in the illusion of movement, either of the head or the surroundings; nausea is often present as well. Its causes are quite different from those of dizziness, and although it is not life-threatening, its effects can be disabling and distressing. In cases of severe vertigo where travel is impossible, ask for a home visit. See GP urgently if vertigo appears suddenly and is severe and continuous, as the cause may be viral (for example, a cold or tinnitus). Otitis media (middle ear infection that appears suddenly with severe pain, discharge and deafness on the same side, possible fever and tinnitus) also needs urgent treatment.

Abdominal pain

The abdomen – the lower part of the trunk, running from the diaphragm to the pelvis – contains many of the body's vital organs, including the stomach, kidneys and liver. The abdominal cavity is enclosed at the front by layers of skin and fat and at the back by the spine and lower ribs. The organs in the abdomen are sealed within a smooth, thin membrane called the peritoneum. If this is broken, bacteria can enter the cavity and cause a serious infection (see **Peritonitis**).

TYPES OF ABDOMINAL PAIN

Abdominal pain may be short-lived or chronic (recurring) and felt in various areas. It can take many forms and may be described as griping, gnawing, boring, deep grinding, nagging, bloating, colicky, cramping and stabbing.

▼ **Abdominal pain**
The red areas show the abdominal regions where pain is most often felt. Sudden and sharp pain felt in any of these places is most likely to be digestion-related. Medical advice should always be sought for pain that continues for more than 24 hours.

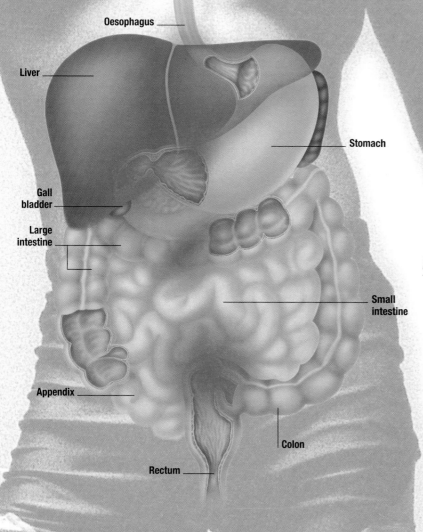

Oesophagus

Liver

Gall bladder

Large intestine

Appendix

Rectum

Stomach

Small intestine

Colon

Because the abdominal cavity contains various body organs and systems, there are many possible causes of abdominal pain. In addition, pain in other areas of the body can suggest a problem in the abdominal area. Pain in the liver, for example, may be felt in the right shoulder. This is known as referred pain.

DIAGNOSIS

To help with diagnosis a doctor may gently investigate tender areas with his or her fingers. He or she may also tap the abdomen; a dull rather than a resonant sound may suggest the presence of fluid or a growth. A stethoscope may be used to listen for abnormal bowel sounds; unusually loud sounds can indicate enteritis (inflammation of the small intestine) or minor digestive problems. The doctor will also take account of any other symptoms, such as swelling, diarrhoea, constipation, abnormal stools, urinary problems, wind, heartburn, vomiting, vaginal bleeding and heavy, painful periods (see also **Symptom sorter**).

CAUSES OF ABDOMINAL PAIN

Abdominal pain may be caused by food poisoning, which may also lead to diarrhoea, vomiting and constipation. Other causes include menstrual problems or pregnancy, hiatus **hernia**, stomach or duodenal **ulcer**, or other damage to the structure of the abdomen. In children, psychological factors, wind, **colic**, appendicitis or inflammation of the lymph glands around the intestines may be responsible. Otherwise, abdominal pain is generally the result of a disorder that affects one of the organs or systems that the abdomen contains.

SEE ALSO *Bladder and disorders; Bowel and disorders; Cancer; Digestive system; Gallbladder and disorders; Kidneys and disorders; Liver and disorders; Pancreas and disorders; Spleen and disorders; Stomach and disorders; Urinary system*

Abscess

An abscess is a collection of pus produced when white blood cells flood into an area of the body, usually to destroy invading bacteria. Abscesses may occur internally – for example, in the teeth, liver, gut, lungs, brain or breast – and may result from conditions such as **appendicitis** or **peritonitis**. A **boil** is a small abscess that forms around a hair follicle in the skin.

SYMPTOMS

- A red, hot, painful swelling.
- Raised temperature and sweating.
- General feeling of illness and loss of appetite.
- Internal abscesses may produce pain or symptoms such as **diarrhoea** or a **cough**.

CAUSES

- Usually bacterial infection, but may be due to irritants entering the tissues.
- Infection is more likely to result if the body defences are weak, as in people with **diabetes** or poor nutrition, or who are suffering from stress.
- Sometimes an abscess is caused by the spread of infection, as in brain abscesses that result from lung, middle ear or sinus infections.

TREATMENT

Small abscesses, such as boils, may be left untreated but larger ones will need treatment to drain the pus.

What you can do

For a small, localized abscess such as a boil:
- apply heat or a magnesium sulphate poultice to encourage the boil to come to a head;
- take paracetamol for pain;
- rest and eat healthily;
- keep flannels separate from those of other household members, and wash carefully before preparing food, to avoid spreading infection.

When to consult a doctor

See your doctor if:
- you develop a fever or **cellulitis**, or begin to feel unwell;
- an external abscess becomes larger than a simple boil, is painful or does not improve;
- the redness spreads to the surrounding skin without the boil coming to a head;
- the boils are recurrent or persistent, or the discharge is continual.

What a doctor may do

Depending on how advanced the abscess is, the doctor may:
- prescribe antibiotics;
- lance the abscess with a sterile needle to allow the pus to drain;
- arrange for you to be admitted to hospital for surgical drainage. Any cavity formed by the abscess will then need to be packed with dressing, to allow it to continue draining and healing. If the cavity is allowed to close up, the abscess may re-form. Swabs will identify any bacteria behind the infection, and you will be screened for undiagnosed diabetes.

Complementary therapies

These are generally no substitutes for the orthodox medical treatment of large abscesses, but complementary treatments may help first aid or prevention.
- **Homeopathy:** try Hepar sulph (Hep.) and Silicea (Sil.) to speed drainage; and Belladonna (Bell.) to cope with throbbing pain.
- **Naturopathy:** a wholefood diet may help to prevent recurrent boils.

COMPLICATIONS

- If an untreated abscess bursts, pus will leak onto the nearest surface. The drained pus from an internal abscess may then collect in a new cavity and form another abscess.
- Infection may spread from an abscess to cause **septicaemia** or may lead to a more extensive infection such as **osteomyelitis, meningitis, encephalitis** or **peritonitis**.
- A brain abscess may be fatal unless it is drained rapidly, or it may leave the person with **epilepsy**.

Acidosis

Acidosis is a condition in which too much acid accumulates in the blood and body fluids. There are various kinds. One of these is ketoacidosis, caused by the body's breaking down muscle and fat and producing ketones. It results from uncontrolled diabetes, alcoholism or extreme diets such as high-protein diets.

SEE ALSO *Alkalosis*

Acne rosacea

Acne rosacea is an inflammatory skin condition that affects around one per cent of the UK population. The majority of sufferers are fair-skinned women aged 35–50.

The causes of acne rosacea are unknown but they are thought to include abnormal sensitivity of blood capillaries and infection of sebaceous (oil) glands with a skin mite, *Demodex folliculorum*. Rosacea tends to recur over a five- to ten-year period, after which it may clear up completely.

SYMPTOMS

There are several ways in which acne rosacea is evident.
- Flushing, especially after drinking alcohol, eating spicy food, consuming hot drinks or entering a warm room.
- Small pimples.
- Fine, dilated skin capillaries (telangiectasia).
- Left untreated, the skin remains permanently red with small, pus-filled blisters called pustules.

TREATMENT

Seek medical advice. Your doctor may prescribe oral antibiotics or metronidazole gel, or refer you to a dermatologist.

Avoid stress, hot liquids, spicy foods, alcohol, vigorous exercise and exposure to sunlight. Avoiding tea, chocolate, cheese, yeast extract, eggs, citrus fruits and wheat may help.

Complementary therapies

- Rosacea may respond to vitamin B complex.
- Natural antiparasitic agents such as tea tree oil applied to the skin may be effective.
- Aloe vera gel helps to reduce inflammation.

Acne vulgaris

Acne vulgaris is an inflammatory skin disease. It affects the sebaceous (oil) glands within the hair follicles on the face, outer ear canal, back, chest and groin. In severe cases, acne may spread as far as the legs. The condition usually starts at puberty and peaks at 17–21.

Four out of five teenagers suffer from acne, which can be an embarrassing condition. One per cent of men and five per cent of women in the UK have problems after the age of 40.

SYMPTOMS
- Greasy skin.
- Spots and pimples on the face, shoulders, back or chest.
- In severe cases, inflamed cysts occur deep in the skin.

CAUSES
Acne is caused by increased activity of the skin's sebaceous glands under the influence of the sex hormones called androgens. Blockage of the duct leading from the sebaceous gland to the skin traps secretions inside to form blackheads. Increased numbers of bacteria on the skin also occur, and can become trapped inside the blocked ducts. Bacterial enzymes break down skin oil to trigger inflammation.

Boys are more prone to acne than girls because they have higher androgen levels, but many girls also suffer, usually in the week before their menstrual period starts.

TREATMENT
Seek help early. Mild acne often responds well to over-the-counter preparations; more severe acne needs prescription drugs. With continuous treatment, nine out of ten people show a 50 per cent improvement within three months and an 80 per cent improvement within six months.

Complementary therapies
Tea tree oil products are often effective.

COMPLICATIONS
Severe acne can leave scars; plastic surgery and other cosmetic treatments may help.

Acoustic neuroma

An acoustic neuroma is a tumour in the hearing (auditory) nerve. Although rare, it accounts for five per cent of all tumours that develop within the skull.

The early symptoms, **dizziness** and tinnitus, do not in themselves suggest serious disease, but seek medical advice if deafness occurs, especially if it is confined to one ear. Diagnosis is by hearing tests and a magnetic resonance imaging (MRI) scan.

SEE ALSO *Ear and problems*

Acrocyanosis

Acrocyanosis makes the hands and feet go cold and blue. Swelling or sweating may also occur, but there is no pain. The condition mainly affects women. The cause is unknown, but cold makes it worse. Sympathectomy (keyhole surgery or injection that severs the nerves which control the arterioles) may relieve symptoms.

Acromegaly

Acromegaly is a chronic metabolic disorder in which too much growth hormone is produced by the **pituitary gland**. The bones of the face, jaw, hands, feet and skull enlarge. It is usually a result of a benign tumour of the pituitary.

Acroparaesthesia

An intense tingling or pricking in the fingers or toes is known as acroparaesthesia. The usual cause is restricted blood supply to the nerves due to resting heavily on a limb during sleep or by a long period of inactivity. Repeated bouts may indicate nerve inflammation or damage.

Acupressure

Acupressure forms part of the system of traditional Chinese medicine. Like **acupuncture**, it is based on the principle that *qi*, or *chi*, meaning 'life force', flows constantly through the body. Any overactivity, blockage or slowing down of *qi* can result in illness. Pressure on certain points (acupoints) on the 12 main energy channels in the body, known as meridians, is thought to regulate the flow of the body's energy, allowing balance to be restored and stimulating the body to heal itself.

The practitioner uses thumb and fingertip pressure to work the appropriate acupoints, rather than the fine needles used acupuncture.

HOW IT CAN HELP
Acupressure is a non-invasive alternative to acupuncture that you can do at home. It is used to treat:
- pain, including chronic back pain, arthritic pain, headaches and migraine;
- gynaecological problems;
- stress and stress-related conditions.

WHAT'S INVOLVED
At your first appointment the practitioner will ask you for a full medical and lifestyle history, and will also take your pulse and inspect your tongue to aid diagnosis.

As well as working on the appropriate acupoints, the practitioner may also show you how to use acupressure as a self-help therapy. The first session will probably last at least an hour; subsequent sessions are likely to take 30–45 minutes.

Acupuncture

Practised in China for more than 2000 years, acupuncture is a form of complementary therapy now offered in NHS pain clinics and recommended by an increasing number of orthodox doctors. It is based on the belief that illness or disease is caused by blockages or imbalances in *qi*, or *chi*, the 'life force' that flows through the body.

Acupuncturists insert fine needles into certain points (called acupoints) on the body's energy channels (meridians) to promote the flow of *qi* and, ultimately, to bring the body back to its natural state of equilibrium.

HOW IT CAN HELP

The effectiveness of acupuncture in the treatment of digestive problems, respiratory disease, pain, neurological disorders, nausea and a range of gynaecological ailments – from premenstrual syndrome to infertility and the menopause – has been officially acknowledged by the World Health Organization. Acupuncture is also often used to treat stress and stress-related conditions.

THE ORTHODOX VIEW

The traditional view among conventional doctors is that acupuncture works by:
■ blocking the body's pain receptors (so that, even though pain signals are still being sent out, the person does not register them);
■ stimulating the nervous system;
■ encouraging the production of endorphins, hormone-like chemicals that enhance mood and are natural painkillers;
■ promoting circulation of the blood.

FINDING A PRACTITIONER

Ask your GP to refer you to an NHS pain clinic, or contact The British Acupuncture Council or The British Medical Acupuncture Society for details of qualified practitioners in your area.

Before arranging treatment, check how long your chosen practitioner trained for, especially if he or she is an orthodox doctor. Some doctors who belong to the British Medical Acupuncture Society are permitted to practise a certain level of acupuncture after a four-day introductory course; other doctors have undergone a three-year training programme. Many non-medical acupuncturists train for at least two or three years, some for five years or more.

WHAT'S INVOLVED

The acupuncturist will ask in detail about your medical history and current symptoms, about any other treatments you are having, your emotional well-being, your lifestyle and your family's medical history. The acupuncturist will take your pulse and inspect your tongue.

After diagnosis, the practitioner will decide what size of needles to use, where to place them and how long to leave them in. Fine stainless-steel needles will then be inserted into the relevant acupoints – usually in a different part of the body from the one that has the problem. The insertion is swift and painless and the most that you should feel is a slight prick to the skin. Tell your practitioner if the needles become uncomfortable during treatment. The needles are left in place for 10–30 minutes before being gently and painlessly withdrawn. Your first session should last up to 1¼ hours and further sessions are likely to be 30–45 minutes long. You may prefer to rest after treatment.

The number of treatments you need depends on the problem. In some cases, one or two sessions may be enough to resolve the problem. In others, you may need several treatments at weekly intervals. Many people also have regular appointments as a preventive measure.

Possible side effects
■ Swelling and discomfort around the site of needle insertion.
■ Brief worsening of symptoms before they begin to subside.
■ If inserted incorrectly, the needles can cause bleeding and even nerve damage. However, this is extremely rare.

Other treatments
Acupuncture treatment may also involve other techniques.
■ Moxibustion – the warming of acupoints with aromatic smoke from a bundle of the dried herb known as moxa (mugwort).
■ Cupping – placing small, bulbous glass cups over acupoints to create a partial vacuum, which then draws blood and *qi* into the area.
■ Electro-acupuncture – connecting the needles to a very small electrical current to increase the stimulation of particular acupoints.
■ **Acupressure** – stimulating the acupoints with finger pressure instead of needles.

HEALTH AND SAFETY

Sterilization of the needles used is crucial to prevent the transmission of infections such as HIV and viral hepatitis. Most acupuncturists use a new packet of needles for each patient. But needles are sometimes sterilized in an autoclave on site, or sent to a local hospital.

SEE ALSO *Chinese herbal medicine*

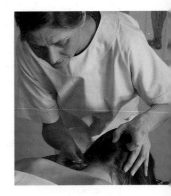

▲ **Painless therapy**
The acupuncturist may gently move the needle by rotating or vibrating it – many people feel no more than a slight tingling or numbness in the area.

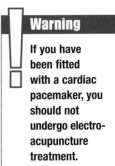

Warning

If you have been fitted with a cardiac pacemaker, you should not undergo electro-acupuncture treatment.

Adenitis

Adenitis is an inflammation of a gland or group of glands. The term is usually used to refer to lymph glands, especially those in the neck, armpit and groin, which are the glands most commonly affected (see **Lymphatic system**). Painful swelling of the glands is often associated with fever and indicates that the body is working to overcome an infection.

Adenoids and problems

The adenoids are the mass of lymphatic tissue at the back of the nasal cavity. The **tonsils**, at the back of the mouth, consist of the same tissue. Both form part of the **lymphatic system**, a network of lymph nodes linked by lymphatic vessels – which defends the body from infection.

Some areas of lymph tissue, such as those in the adenoids and tonsils, are largest during childhood and shrink throughout life.

WHAT CAN GO WRONG
Recurrent infections may lead to enlargement of the adenoids and the tonsils. Enlarged adenoids can block the Eustachian tube that drains the middle ear, resulting in a buildup of thick fluid in the middle ear known as **glue ear**. The fluid interferes with the transmission of sound, causing temporary deafness; in young children, this affects the development of hearing and language skills. The adenoids may also obstruct the flow of air from the nose to the throat, forcing the child to breathe through the mouth. If mouth breathing becomes persistent, the child may develop a nasal voice and a dull facial expression.

Depending on the severity of the symptoms and the age of the patient, a doctor may recommend surgery to remove the adenoids and possibly the tonsils at the same time.

▲ **Shrinking problem**
The adenoids lie at the back of the nose close to where it joins the mouth. Small at birth, they start growing at around 18 months and reach maximum size at about the age of eight.

ADHD

ADHD (attention deficit hyperactivity disorder) is characterized by impulsiveness, inattention and overactivity. ADHD starts in childhood but it is a chronic condition and symptoms may persist into adolescence and adulthood.

In the UK, the disorder is formally diagnosed only when a child is persistently inattentive, impulsive and overactive from an early age, and the main features of the child's behaviour are evident in more than one setting – for example, both at home and in school. The syndrome is present in one to two per cent of schoolchildren in the UK, and is more common in boys. In the USA, the syndrome is diagnosed in three to six per cent of the school-aged population.

SYMPTOMS
A child with ADHD displays the following:
- impulsive and disruptive behaviour;
- impaired attention – inability to concentrate, short attention span;
- hyperactivity – inability to sit still, continual fidgeting and chattering, abundance of energy and need for only a little sleep.

TREATMENT
Although symptoms usually start in the preschool years, there is a wide range of normal behaviour in preschool children, so a definite diagnosis of ADHD may not be made until a child starts school. If you suspect that your child is suffering from ADHD, consult a doctor and talk to your child's teacher.

Before a diagnosis is made, the child will have a full mental health and behavioural assessment by the appropriate specialists.

Once a diagnosis is made, the child will be offered educational support and behavioural therapy such as social skills training.

In some children, symptoms are made more severe by particular foods or food additives, but no single food has been shown to affect all children with ADHD. You may wish to keep a food diary to check if any foods or additives make your child's problems worse.

School-aged children with severe ADHD or those for whom behavioural therapy does not work should be offered additional treatment in the form of a stimulant medication such as Ritalin (methylphenidate hydrochloride) or Dexedrine (dexamphetamine). These drugs are effective in relieving symptoms and may be taken for a number of years. There may be side effects, so drug use should be reviewed.
SEE ALSO *Behaviour problems in children*

Adrenal glands and disorders

The adrenals are a pair of triangular glands located above the kidneys; they are sometimes referred to as the suprarenal glands. They are responsible for producing hormones that help to regulate the body's chemistry and metabolism and enable us to cope with stress. Each gland has two parts, the outer adrenal cortex surrounding the inner core, the adrenal medulla.

THE ADRENAL CORTEX
More than two dozen steroid hormones (corticosteroids) are manufactured by the adrenal cortex. Their production is stimulated

by the adrenocorticotropic hormone (ACTH), produced by the pituitary gland. The release of ACTH is in turn triggered by corticotrophin-releasing hormone (CRH), produced by a part of the brain called the hypothalamus.

The cells of the adrenal cortex are arranged in three layers or zones. The *zona glomerulosa*, the outer layer, produces hormones called mineralocorticoids, which control the body's fluid and mineral balance. The main one is aldosterone, which helps the kidneys to retain sodium (salt) and excrete potassium, thereby helping to regulate blood volume and pressure.

The *zona fasciculata*, the middle layer, produces glucocorticoids, the most important of which is cortisol (hydrocortisone). Cortisol has many functions, but one of the most crucial is helping the body to deal with stress and change. Other functions include:
- helping to control fluid levels in the body;
- helping to maintain blood pressure and cardiovascular function;
- modifying the body's response to inflammation;
- stimulating the liver to raise blood glucose levels and balancing the effects of insulin;
- regulating the metabolism of proteins, carbohydrates and fats.

The *zona reticularis*, the cortex's inner layer, also produces glucocorticoids, together with sex hormones (gonadocorticoids). The main ones are androgens (male sex hormones), although small amounts of oestrogens (female sex hormones) are also produced.

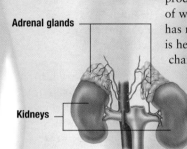

Adrenal glands

Kidneys

▲ **Hormone release**
In males the adrenal glands release sex hormones that promote the development of the testes.

THE ADRENAL MEDULLA
The adrenal medulla consists of a mass of neurons (nerve cells) and is strictly speaking part of the body's autonomic nervous system, which controls involuntary functions such as breathing and heart rate. The medulla secretes two important hormones, adrenaline and noradrenaline, which are involved in activating the body's 'fight or flight' response under stress.

WHAT CAN GO WRONG
Adrenal problems are rare, but may be due to either insufficient production or overproduction of adrenal hormones. Disorders are more likely to affect the cortex than the medulla. Problems with underproduction include Addison's disease. Overproduction disorders include Cushing's syndrome, congenital adrenal hyperplasm and hyperaldosteronism.

Among the most alarming adrenal disorders is Waterhouse–Frederichsen syndrome. In this disorder, fever, bluish discoloration of the skin (cyanosis) due to insufficient oxygen, and bleeding into the skin from the adrenals are caused by severe meningococcal infection. It is fatal if not treated immediately.

Addison's disease
Addison's disease affects four in 100,000 people in the West. In 70 per cent of cases the disease is due to destruction of the adrenal cortex by an **autoimmune disorder** (when the body turns against itself). In the past, tuberculosis (TB) was a major cause, and in the developing world it still is. TB accounts for about one in five cases of Addison's disease in the developed world.

Addison's disease may be caused by problems within the adrenal glands themselves, causing underproduction of adrenal hormones. This is known as primary adrenal insufficiency. It may also be caused by a problem such as a tumour affecting the pituitary gland, which causes failure of ACTH production; this is known as secondary adrenal insufficiency.

Symptoms include weight loss, muscle weakness, fatigue, low blood pressure and an increase in skin pigmentation. Symptoms often appear so gradually that they are missed until a stressful event, infection, trauma or operation triggers acute adrenal failure (Addisonian crisis). This causes severe pains in the abdomen and the back of the legs, confusion and loss of consciousness. If left untreated, it can be fatal.

Cushing's syndrome
Cushing's syndrome is a rare condition that results from overproduction of cortisol or other corticorticoid hormones produced by the adrenal glands. These hormones regulate the use of carbohydrates in the body – an excess upsets the body's regular pattern of converting food into energy.

Symptoms include a rounded 'moon' face, central body fat, muscle wasting, high **blood pressure**, thin skin that bruises easily and reduced resistence to infection. Someone with Cushing's syndrome may also develop glucose intolerance, excessive facial hair, **osteoporosis**, kidney stones, menstrual irregularities or mental health problems such as depression and anxiety.

The disorder may be caused by a problem affecting the adrenals themselves or by excessive secretion of ACTH as a result of a pituitary tumour or, sometimes, by lung or other cancer. It may also be due to overuse of cortisol or other steroid hormones prescribed for the treatment of diseases such as asthma, rheumatoid arthritis, systemic lupus, inflammatory bowel disease and allergies.

Cushing's disease is a type of Cushing's syndrome due to overproduction of ACTH by the pituitary; indeed, 70 per cent of cases of Cushing's syndrome that occur are caused by pituitary problems.

The underlying causes of Cushing's syndrome are better understood now, which could lead

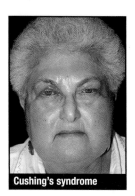
Cushing's syndrome

▲ 'Moon' face
People with Cushing's syndrome, caused by overproduction of corticorticoid hormones, develop a rounded face as part of general weight gain.

to better diagnosis and treatment. Improved methods of measuring the level of ACTH and other hormones are allowing doctors to distinguish between different causes of Cushing's syndrome.

Some research is looking at the origins of the benign pituitary tumours that underlie most cases of Cushing's. The identification of some faulty genes may provide further clues. Other researchers have discovered that retinoic acid, a derivative of vitamin A, can help to inhibit ACTH production in the laboratory.

Congenital adrenal hyperplasia

Congenital adrenal hyperplasia (CAH), also known as adrenogenital syndrome or adrenal virilism, describes a group of rare inherited disorders that affects around one baby in 10,000 worldwide, both boys and girls. It is caused by the lack of an enzyme needed by the adrenal glands to make the hormones cortisol and aldosterone. It results in the overproduction of androgens (male sex hormones).

In male babies there are no obvious symptoms. However, by the age of two or three, a boy with the condition becomes increasingly muscular, the penis enlarges, pubic hair appears and the voice deepens. In female babies, there is masculinization, including an enlarged clitoris. As the girl grows older she develops a deep voice and facial hair, and fails to ovulate and menstruate.

Some forms of CAH can lead to an adrenal crisis in the newborn baby, causing vomiting, dehydration, changes in fluid and mineral balance and disturbances of heart rhythm.

Developments in hormonal and DNA testing could revolutionize detection and diagnosis of congenital adrenal hyperplasia. For example, a heel-prick test can now be carried out on babies in the first week of life that is designed to detect hormonal markers in the blood. This replaces older, slower methods of testing and enables newborn boys who have CAH but exhibit no symptoms to be diagnosed early, thereby avoiding a life-threatening adrenal crisis. Meanwhile, ever more sophisticated gene technology is paving the way for prenatal and neonatal screening.

Hyperaldosteronism

Hyperaldosteronism is caused by excessive production of the hormone aldosterone, which controls the body's water balance. The most commonly known form of the disorder is Conn's syndrome in which, in many cases, the only symptom is raised **blood pressure**, but there may also be excessive thirst and an increased production of urine.

The condition is diagnosed by blood and urine tests. Its underlying cause – which may or may not be a problem affecting the adrenals themselves – needs to be identified and treated.

Tumours affecting the adrenal glands

Occasionally, a benign (non-cancerous) or malignant (cancerous) tumour may develop in the adrenal glands. Some tumours affect production of hormones – causing either underproduction or, more commonly, overproduction – but in many cases hormone production is unaffected. In such cases, they are found only when the person is tested for another illness or condition.

PHAEOCHROMOCYTOMA

A phaeochromocytoma is a rare cancer that often begins inside a group of cells known as chromaffin cells in the adrenal medulla. One of its effects is to cause overproduction of adrenaline and noradrenaline, leading to symptoms of high **blood pressure**, headaches, sweating, pounding of the heart, pain in the chest and a feeling of anxiety. It is sometimes part of a syndrome called multiple endocrine neoplasia (MEN) in which there is thyroid cancer and other hormonal problems.

CANCER OF THE ADRENAL CORTEX

Cancer of the adrenal cortex is a rare form of cancer that can cause either overproduction or underproduction of hormones, leading to a wide range of symptoms including high blood pressure, osteoporosis, diabetes or changes in sexual characteristics such as deepening of the voice, excessive hairiness (hirsutism), swelling of the clitoris or of the breasts. Other symptoms include pain in the abdomen, loss of weight without dieting, and weakness.

NEUROBLASTOMA

A neuroblastoma is a solid tumour affecting nerve tissue that generally begins in the adrenal glands. Children under five are most commonly affected. Symptoms include protruding eyes and dark circles around the eyes.

Agoraphobia

Agoraphobia is a group of **phobias** (intense fears) that includes fear of open spaces, crowded places, being alone, or being anywhere likely to cause sufferers to experience panic.

An estimated 20 per cent of the UK population suffers from some form of it, with more women than men seeking help. It usually starts during the late teenage years or early 20s. You may be more vulnerable to developing agoraphobia if someone in your family has the condition.

SYMPTOMS

The characteristics of agoraphobia include feelings of anxiety and panic such as rapid heartbeat, churning stomach, sweating or a dry mouth, which occur when the sufferer is alone, away from home, in crowds or in public places.

People with agoraphobia avoid situations associated with earlier panic attacks because of their intense fear that the attacks will recur.

TREATMENT

Anyone afflicted by agoraphobia should seek help as early as possible. Join a self-help group for support and to learn coping strategies. Consult a doctor if symptoms worsen or the condition becomes unmanageable.

What a doctor may do

Referral to a psychologist for behaviour therapy or cognitive behaviour therapy may help, as may short course of antidepressants or tranquillizers.

Complementary therapies

The following may help to ease symptoms:
- therapies such as **massage** or aromatherapy;
- **hypnotherapy**.

SEE ALSO *Anxiety; Obsessions and compulsions; Panic attack*

AIDS

AIDS stands for Acquired Immune Deficiency Syndrome, a disease caused by infection with **HIV** (human immunodeficiency virus). The HIV virus can be caught through contact with certain bodily fluids of an infected person.

Saliva, sweat and urine do not contain enough HIV to infect another person. The most common method by which the virus is passed is during sexual intercourse, both heterosexual and homosexual; from mother to baby before or during birth or during breastfeeding; and when injecting drug abusers share needles and other equipment. It is also possible for HIV to be transmitted through organ **transplants**, blood transfusion and the use of blood products; this is rare in the UK because donated blood and tissue are screened for the virus.

SYMPTOMS

When first infected with HIV, some people may notice a brief flu-like illness, but most people are not aware that they have become infected and will have no symptoms for many years. However, once they are infectious, their immune system starts to make antibodies to the virus straight away. When these antibodies are detected by blood testing, people are said to be HIV-positive. Gradually the virus attacks the body's immune system.

The CD4 T-lymphocyte cells in the blood are particularly prone to attack by the HIV virus. These are helper cells that organize the body's response to viral invasion. A normal T-lymphocyte count is 500–1500/ml blood (1fl oz = 28ml).

AIDS has developed once the T-lymphocyte count has dropped below 200/ml and the person is suffering weight loss, diarrhoea, fever, certain types of pneumonia and skin cancer. Damage to the immune system, skin or other defences also makes the person subject to infection with Candida (see **Fungal infections**) or **cytomegalovirus**. People with this test result and the described symptoms are said to have full-blown AIDS.

TREATMENT

If you suspect that you may be infected with the HIV virus, contact your local genito-urinary medicine (GUM) clinic to arrange a test. These are run by your health authority and are usually attached to a general hospital. Many treatments now available can decrease the rate of progress of HIV and alleviate many of the symptoms, but there is as yet no cure for AIDS.

Albinism

Albinism is a condition that prevents the production of the brown pigment melanin, normally found in the skin, hair and eyes. As a result, people with albinism have very pale skin and hair. Their eyes appear pink because of the colour of the blood vessels at the back of the eye, which are normally masked by melanin.

Albinism is fairly common, affecting about one in every 20,000 children born worldwide. It can be a serious health problem in hot countries, where many albinos die of skin cancer in their teens or twenties. They also frequently suffer social ostracism as a consequence of their pale skins. Albinism also occurs in animals.

SYMPTOMS

- Pale skin, white hair and pink eyes.
- Defective eyesight in people with oculo-cutaneous albinism, the commonest form of albinism.
- Susceptibility to sunburn, due to lack of the normal protection provided by melanin.

CAUSES

Albinism is the result of several different genetic mutations, which may be inherited or may occur spontaneously.

COMPLICATIONS

People with albinism have a higher than average risk of developing skin cancers.

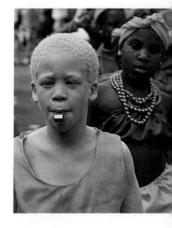

▲ **Skin deep**
In Africa and other parts of the world where most native people have dark skin and hair, albinos can be affected by social discrimination and prejudice.

Alcohol and abuse

Moderate consumption of alcohol promotes relaxation and offers a range of health benefits. But alcohol abuse – when intake rises above moderate levels – presents a severe health risk and can cause great misery.

There are many dangers associated with excessive consumption of alcohol. Some are directly linked to drinking, others are subtle consequences of the damage alcohol can cause. Health risks include the following.

■ Red wine may cause migraine in some susceptible individuals.

■ Alcohol causes weight gain and obesity – it is high in calories with little nutritional value.

■ Nutritional imbalances are caused if drinking interferes with a proper diet.

■ Alcohol can interfere with normal liver function. Cirrhosis of the liver affects one in five heavy drinkers.

■ Alcohol may cause **blood pressure** to rise, which is linked to the risk of coronary artery disease and **stroke**.

■ Alcohol may be dangerous if it is mixed with some medications.

■ Alcohol can provoke melancholy or aggression.

■ Frequent drinkers risk developing problem drinking and alcohol dependence (see below).

■ Pregnant women who drink heavily may cause their baby to be born with **fetal alcohol syndrome**. Consumption of more than 56 units a week in pregnancy can lead to low birth weight, cleft palate and mental retardation.

■ Heavy consumption of alcohol is linked with **infertility**.

■ Excessive drinking leads to increased risk of **cancers** of the mouth, throat, gullet, stomach and liver, and possibly also breast and colon.

In the UK, 65–80 per cent of assault victims needing hospital treatment are intoxicated at the time of injury.

SOCIAL DRINKING OR PROBLEM DRINKING?

There are several warning signs that drinking is getting out of control. You should consider cutting down if you find that you are using alcohol to deal with stress and crises, are organizing your life around the availability of alcohol, developing obsessive attitudes towards alcohol or suffering from frequent hangovers.

Common signs of problem drinking are regular absences from work because of hangovers, family conflicts after drinking, and financial difficulties caused by spending money on drink. Other signs that drinking has become a problem include accidents or injuries due to drinking, forgetting what happened during drinking sessions, and feelings of anger, denial or guilt when others comment on alcohol intake or behaviour.

As well as the potential for causing health problems, financial difficulties, job loss, family breakdown and criminal involvement, about one in 20 of those affected by problem drinking will become alcohol dependent (see below).

Binge drinking

Many people – especially young men, but increasingly young women also – concentrate their drinking into sessions once or twice a week. Such 'binge drinking' is more dangerous to health than drinking the same number of units more evenly spaced throughout the week. Binge drinking may precipitate **gout,** lead to a heart attack, provoke pancreatitis, increase risks of liver damage, and disturb heart rhythm. Binge drinking can also, very rarely, prove fatal (for example, by causing heart failure or by suffocation when people choke on their own vomit). Binge drinking leads to a level of drunkenness that can cause a serious accident.

PROBLEM DRINKING AND CHILDREN

Children of problem drinkers often have difficulty with their self-esteem and are less likely to achieve their potential both in their childhood and later in life. They are more likely than other children to underachieve at school, to have emotional and psychological problems, and to have difficulties making friends. They are also more likely to exhibit antisocial behaviour and to suffer from a psychiatric disorder. As they grow older they have a higher than normal risk of developing alcohol problems of their own, of involvement with recreational and illicit drug-taking and of becoming dependent on either alcohol or drugs.

ALCOHOL DEPENDENCE

A drinking habit that has developed into an addiction is known as alcohol dependence. If the alcohol intake is not maintained, unpleasant withdrawal symptoms result and the person must drink compulsively to avoid them. Withdrawal symptoms include bodily tremors ('the shakes'), anxiety and restlessness, sweating, delusions, hallucinations and delirium.

How alcohol affects the body

Alcohol is absorbed into the bloodstream between 15 and 90 minutes after drinking, depending on the contents of the stomach. On average, it takes one hour per unit for alcohol to be broken down in the liver. The immediate physical effects of alcohol are listed below.

■ Depressed activity of the central nervous system.

■ Faster heart rate.

■ Slower reaction time.

■ Impaired judgment.

■ Reduced coordination.

■ Loss of inhibitions.

As a person gets drunker, effects include:

■ Dehydration.

■ Slurred speech.

■ Clumsiness.

■ Loss of balance.

■ Blurring of vision.

■ Unconsciousness.

The effects of alcohol are greater:

■ For people of small build and low weight.

■ For women – because they metabolize alcohol more slowly than men.

■ For the very young or very old.

■ For some Orientals who metabolize alcohol less readily than Caucasians.

■ When drinking on an empty stomach.

You may still be over the limit for safe driving the morning after late-night heavy drinking.

People with drinking problems that have reached this stage are unlikely to be able to stop drinking unaided, and will need professional help to conquer their addiction. Once this is achieved they will usually have to abstain totally from alcohol for the rest of their lives – there is a high risk of relapse into alcoholism with even 'one little drink'.

RECOGNIZING ALCOHOL DEPENDENCE

Signs of possible addiction to alcohol include waking up feeling shaky and sweaty; needing a drink in the morning; needing to drink more to achieve the same effect; and drinking large quantities without feeling drunk. Many of the indicators of problem drinking may also be signs of developing alcohol dependence.

Alcohol dependence in someone else

Most problem drinkers deny their problem. If you are concerned about someone's drinking, signs include changes in mood and behaviour, memory lapses or confusion about recent conversations and events, unreliability at work or at home, drinking alone or in secret and lying about drinking, neglecting their personal appearance, trembling hands and regular vomiting.

SEEKING PROFESSIONAL HELP

Help with alcohol dependence is available in the UK through the NHS, voluntary organizations and private detoxification and rehabilitation clinics. Most of these organizations will offer support and advice to the family and friends of alcoholics as well as to the problem drinkers themselves. Treatment aims include minimizing the damage that the alcoholic is inflicting on others. If you think you, a friend or a relative may be an alcoholic, consider contacting advice lines and counselling services. You could call your GP, who may refer you to an NHS centre.

TREATMENT OF ALCOHOL DEPENDENCE

The first priority is to get the alcoholic through the symptoms of physical withdrawal when intake is stopped. This process often involves residential treatment.

The next phase is to devise a strategy to help the problem drinker to avoid relapse. Ways of helping a recovering alcoholic to stay off alcohol include counselling, cognitive behaviour therapy, self-help groups such as Alcoholics Anonymous (see box) and aversion therapy.

HOW TO HELP AN ALCOHOLIC

The only person who has control over a problem drinker's drinking is the problem drinker, but you can encourage and support his or her efforts to get better. Discuss the problem when the drinker is sober and focus on the effects the drinking is having on his or her life. Encourage the drinker to take responsibility for his or her behaviour and to seek help from a professional or a support group.

If the problem drinker is your spouse or a close relative, be sure to take care of yourself, maintain separate interests and seek support outside the relationship.

SEE ALSO *Arteries and disorders; Blood and disorders; Heart and circulatory system; Liver and disorders; Pancreas and disorders*

Factfile
Alcoholics Anonymous (AA)

AA is a worldwide network that offers support for maintaining recovery from alcohol dependence.

Its philosophy requires total abstinence from alcohol and the acceptance of the '12 Steps' – a series of slogans and affirmations. These require AA members to acknowledge a 'higher power', admit their problem and discuss it openly at group meetings.

The 12-Step process is not suitable for everyone, but it can be a powerful aid to maintaining abstinence and has been successfully copied by other groups such as Gamblers Anonymous. Support for families is provided through a network called Al-Anon.

Alexander technique

The Alexander technique is a gentle, practical system of exercises designed to help people to develop and maintain good postural habits. Proponents claim that it can alleviate various posture-related health problems.

The Alexander technique is based on the idea that there are correct and incorrect ways of moving, sitting and standing. It was developed in the late 19th century by an Australian actor called Frederick Matthias Alexander after he discovered that changing his posture affected his voice. His techniques, which broadly involve keeping the neck and spine in line, aim to eradicate 'old patterns of misuse' in the body.

WHAT IT IS USED FOR
- Breathing problems.
- Back, neck and joint pain.
- Fatigue, anxiety, stress and headaches.
- To promote self-awareness and confidence.

ORTHODOX VIEW
The Alexander technique is accepted by most doctors. Treatment is available on the NHS in some areas.

FINDING A PRACTITIONER
- Ask a doctor for an NHS referral.
- Contact the Society of Teachers of the Alexander Technique.

WHAT'S INVOLVED
Lessons take place on a one-to-one basis. Alexander technique sessions usually last for 30–40 minutes; most people need 20–30 lessons.

During the lesson, a teacher may ask you to demonstrate sitting, standing and moving, and will show you how to replace any bad habits you may have with better ones. You will be asked to practise between sessions to help you to adapt to new ways of moving.

Alkalosis

Alkalosis is a disturbance in the body's acid/alkali balance that results in the blood and body fluids becoming too alkaline. The acid/alkali balance is regulated by the lungs and the kidneys. There are various types, each with different causes.

Symptoms of alkalosis include confusion, muscle twitches, tremor in the hands, nausea and vomiting, numbness or tingling, and lightheadedness. Treatment for alkalosis consists of correcting the underlying cause, but in severe cases a saline (salt) drip or other treatment may be needed.

SEE ALSO *Acidosis; Adrenal glands and disorders*

Allergic rhinitis

Allergic rhinitis is an inflammation of the moist lining (mucous membrane) of the nose, caused by a reaction to an irritant. This results in attacks of sneezing, nasal discharge or a blocked nose. Excess mucus may also drip into the throat and cause soreness and coughing.

An attack typically lasts for more than an hour. In hay fever (seasonal allergic rhinitis), the problem is limited to a particular time of year; in perennial allergic rhinitis the nasal problems occur throughout the year.

Hay fever

Hay fever is neither caused by hay nor associated with fever. It is the most common of all allergic diseases, affecting 2–10 per cent of people worldwide. Most sufferers will have developed some symptoms by the age of ten. It very rarely starts in people aged over 60.

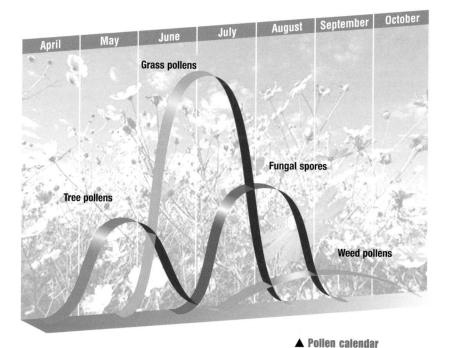

Annual hay fever attacks vary in severity and can recur for 10–15 years, after which they become less troublesome and eventually cease (see also **Hay fever**).

The trigger (allergen) that causes the allergic reaction is pollen from grass, trees, shrubs, weeds or flowers, and spores from moulds and fungi. Pollen counts (the percentage of pollen grains that can be measured in a cubic metre of air) are highest during spring and summer, this is when the plants and grasses that rely on the wind for cross-pollination release their pollen into the air. Twenty per cent of young people in the UK suffer the symptoms of hay fever in the peak months of June and July.

▲ **Pollen calendar**
Sufferers benefit if they keep track of times at which pollen levels put them most at risk of allergic reactions. The graph indicates the months in which the different pollens and spores are most common.

TREATMENT

To reduce exposure to pollen, drive with the car windows closed, keep your bedroom window shut at night, and avoid walking in the countryside, particularly in the late afternoon when pollen falls to ground level.

Over-the-counter antihistamines are the most common treatment for rhinitis. They are effective against sneezing, less so against a runny nose (rhinorrhoea). At one time antihistamines tended to cause drowsiness but modern, non-sedative forms of the drug can be used safely when driving.

Over-the-counter decongestants give relief from nasal discharge and blockage but should only be used for a few days. After longer periods, stopping the drug will cause a rebound swelling of the nasal passages.

Small doses of corticosteroids (prescription drugs administered as a nasal spray or drops) are also an effective treatment for rhinitis. They work especially well when combined with a non-sedative antihistamine. When symptoms are particularly severe and in times of stress a short course of steroids may be justified.

It is also possible for sufferers to receive injections of prepared pollens to desensitize them, but this method is rarely used because it occasionally causes severe allergic reactions and even death in hypersensitive people. If desensitization is considered, skin tests are needed beforehand to decide on the appropriate preparation of pollens.

Perennial allergic rhinitis

Year-round nasal problems are caused by allergens such as house dust mites, feathers and animal fur, or by allergy to certain foods or to drugs such as aspirin. Symptoms are similar to hay fever. Nasal congestion is common and can lead to blockage of the Eustachian tube. This prevents effective drainage of the middle ear and can cause hearing problems, especially in children. The main complications of prolonged allergic rhinitis are sinus infections (**sinusitis**) and growths inside the nose (nasal polyps).

TREATMENT

When specific allergens can be identified, the treatment is broadly the same as for hay fever. Corticosteroid nasal sprays and drops are an effective treatment. Decongestant nose drops or sprays should not be used for more than a few days (as mentioned above).

SEE ALSO *Nose and problems*

Allergies

SEE PAGE 64

Alopecia

Alopecia is the medical word for **baldness**. The most common form is male pattern baldness, or alopecia androgenic, which usually affects older men. The term also refers to hair-loss in which hair follicles stop growing either on a small patch of skin, in one region of the body, or all over the body. In alopecia areata, for example, hair is lost in patches, usually on the scalp.

CAUSES

Apart from male pattern baldness, which is hereditary, the various forms of alopecia are thought to be caused by an overactive immune system attacking the hair follicles. **Stress** plays a major role in triggering hair loss because it reduces blood supply to the scalp; it also seems to increase production of oily secretions by the sebaceous glands connected to each hair follicle.

Occasionally the condition is linked to iron-deficiency **anaemia** or to problems with the **thyroid** gland. Alopecia following illness or pregnancy rarely lasts more than six months.

TREATMENT

There is no effective treatment for male pattern baldness. In alopecia areata, blood tests may show a lack of iron or an inefficient thyroid gland. Most medical treatments such as corticosteroid injections are disappointing.

Complementary and other therapies

■ Homeopathic remedies may help. For alopecia linked with emotional trauma, try a 30c dose of Natrum muriaticum (Nat. mur.) once a week.
■ Massaging the scalp helps to encourage blood flow and to stimulate hair follicles.
■ Cosmetic hair design involves weaving artificial hair fibres into your own hair or onto a fine mesh net to disguise areas of hair loss.

OUTLOOK

Alopecia areata often improves over time. In half of all cases, the follicles start to recover within a year, and the hair grows back. Four out of five sufferers from alopecia areata regrow their hair within five years, but some retain a small bald area.

The condition worsens in around one in ten people. Occasionally, the affected area may grow larger. Rarely, hair loss or general thinning eventually extends all over the scalp to produce alopecia totalis.

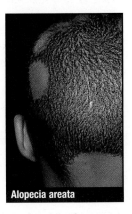

▼ **Irregular hair loss** Hair that comes out in patches could be due to iron deficiency or thyroid problems and should be checked by a doctor.

Alopecia areata

Main types of alopecia

There are various forms of alopecia; hair may be lost from just the scalp or the entire body.

Alopecia androgenic (male pattern baldness) Hair loss occurs over the scalp; the condition mostly affects older men.

Alopecia areata Hair is lost in patches, usually on the scalp.

Alopecia totalis Total loss of scalp hair.

Alopecia universalis Loss of hair over the entire body, including eyebrows and eyelashes.

Allergies

Severe allergic reactions can leave the victim weak and nauseous or gasping for air. Some reactions can even be fatal. People with allergies must learn to identify and avoid the triggers that bring on their attacks.

If you have an allergy, your body is sensitive to – and therefore reacts to – one or more of the many substances to which people are exposed in everyday life. Substances that cause the body to react are called allergens; they include animal hair, pollen, house dust mites and foods such as eggs and shellfish. Allergens may be eaten, inhaled, touched or, in the case of an insect sting, injected under the skin. The allergic reaction often follows quickly.

A wide variety of apparently unrelated ailments – such as **asthma, hay fever, eczema,** contact **dermatitis, nettle rash** (urticaria or hives) – are usually caused by allergies.

When allergens invade the body of an allergic person, the body defends itself by producing antibodies – proteins designed to neutralize the allergens. It is the subsequent reaction between antibody and allergen inside the body that produces the sufferer's allergic ailments.

Some people are allergic to the metallic element nickel, and come out in a rash if they come into contact with it. It is present in some jewellery and coins.

HOW THE BODY RESPONDS TO ALLERGENS

People prone to allergies produce more of a particular type of immunoglobulin, called IgE. IgE forms after the initial contact with an allergen, and becomes attached to cells in the tissues, known as mast cells. When the body encounters the same allergen again it may react with the IgE, causing the mast cells to release a number of chemicals, including histamine. These chemicals cause swelling and inflammation in the surrounding tissues and give rise to various allergic symptoms, depending on which part of the body is affected.

NON-ALLERGIC REACTIONS

Around 10 per cent of hospital patients who are prescribed penicillin show a skin rash, but this is not a true allergy and is not serious; however, 0.1–0.4 per cent of those patients react with severe allergic symptoms including anaphylactic shock (see opposite). A skin test that determines whether or not an individual is sensitive to penicillin is available.

Sometimes allergy-like symptoms are caused by something other than an allergy. For example, histamine can be released in response to an injury, such as a skin graze or damage to the delicate lining of the air passages when certain chemical fumes are inhaled. In these cases, the release of histamine creates allergy-like symptoms although no allergen is involved. Likewise, in susceptible people, allergy-like symptoms can be caused by certain foods that trigger the release of histamine. Other foods can cause similar symptoms because they actually contain histamine (for example, well-ripened cheeses such as mature Brie or fermented foods, especially red wine).

Food intolerance is another reaction that is sometimes confused with food allergy. In food intolerance a number of symptoms, such as headaches, emotional changes, painful joints and muscles, and fluid retention, appear to be caused by eating certain foods.

In such cases there is no hard evidence that the immune system is involved. Doctors do not consider the reaction to be a true allergy, but they find that temporary exclusion of certain foods can relieve symptoms.

TESTING FOR ALLERGIES

Skin and blood tests can help doctors to identify the allergens that may be causing allergic reactions. In a skin-prick test, small amounts of suspected allergens are introduced just under the skin. A weal will develop in the area within a few minutes if the person is allergic to the tested substance. (See **Blood and disorders; Patch test.**)

LIVING WITH ALLERGIES

These strategies will help you to avoid allergic reactions as far as possible while living a full life.
■ Try to identify your allergic triggers. Because these triggers are individual to you, you can minimize the effort needed to avoid allergic attacks if you have a precise idea of what causes your symptoms.
■ Always carry your medication with you, especially if you have asthma, food allergies or are allergic to insect stings.
■ Eat a well-balanced diet, including two to four fruits and three to five vegetables each day.

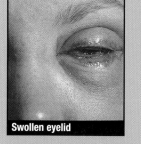

Swollen eyelid

▲ **Allergic reaction**
Swollen eyelids are often a symptom of hay fever. Try not to rub your eyelids. Bathing them in a warm salt solution may help.

ALLERGIES IN CHILDREN

Children have less developed immune systems than adults, which makes them vulnerable to irritants in the environment such as pollen and the droppings of house dust mites. Asthma, eczema and hay fever are the commonest types of allergy in children and may be inherited. As children's immune systems develop, many childhood allergies disappear and most have gone by the time a person reaches adulthood. One common exception is a nut allergy, which usually proves to be a lifelong affliction.

ALLERGY MEDICINES

Several types of conventional medication can be used to relieve allergies; treatment will vary depending on the type and severity of the allergy.

Antihistamine preparations block the action of histamine, while mast-cell stabilizing drugs prevent the release of histamine. Other treaments include corticosteroids, which suppress the allergic reactions, adrenaline injections, which are used for anaphylaxis (see box, below) and desensitization, which involves injecting small doses of the allergen.

COMPLEMENTARY THERAPIES

Many complementary therapists recommend stress management, which can improve the action of the immune system. Changes in diet can also help. **Herbal** or dietary supplements and homeopathic medicines can benefit some allergy sufferers, too. Homeopaths may use remedies made from the allergen that triggers a patient's symptoms, if this is known.

Complementary therapists also use various diagnostic tests: there is little or no scientific support for these tests, but they seem to help some people identify the cause of their allergy. They include pulse tests (checking if the pulse rate is altered by eating a suspect food); the sublingual drop test (which means observing reactions to the application of a suspect substance under the tongue); and an elimination diet (in which the effects of reintroducing suspect foods after they have been excluded are observed).

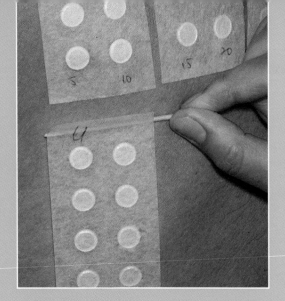

◀ **Patch testing**
Anyone with a contact skin allergy can undergo a test to identify possible allergens. A piece of non-allergenic tape holds samples of the allergens in place for 48 hours, after which the skin is inspected for the redness or swelling that would indicate allergy.

Factfile

Anaphylactic shock

Anaphylactic shock (or anaphylaxis) is an extreme allergic reaction. It can occur within minutes of contact with an allergen or be delayed for several hours. In rare cases it results in death.

Symptoms

■ Itching and swelling around the face and inside the mouth, including the tongue and throat.

■ Difficulty in breathing, together with wheezing, sneezing and a runny nose.

■ Flushed skin and nettle rash (urticaria or hives).

■ Rapid heartbeat and feelings of weakness.

■ Stomach cramps, diarrhoea or nausea.

■ Collapse and loss of consciousness may follow.

What to do if you are at risk

■ If you are at risk of anaphylaxis, carry adrenaline with you at all times and become familiar with how to inject it into your muscles. Label the packs so that someone else can administer the adrenaline in an emergency.

Pre-assembled syringes with adult or child doses are the easiest to cope with.

How to help a victim of anaphylactic shock

■ If the victim has had a previous attack and carries antihistamine medication and an adrenaline injection, these should be given as soon as possible. Adrenaline injections may need to be repeated once or twice at 15-minute intervals. The adrenaline should be injected slowly for anyone with a heart condition, high blood pressure or diabetes.

■ Always send for medical help or an ambulance.

■ Loosen clothing at the neck and around the waist, help the victim to lie down and raise the legs and feet a little if you can. Keep the airway open.

■ If the cause was a bee sting, flick out any remaining sting with your fingernail: avoid squeezing it, because a bee sting contains venom.

■ Anaphylactic shock may develop over the course of a few hours: consult your doctor if the above symptoms occur within a couple of hours of a meal.

Altitude sickness

Altitude sickness, also called mountain sickness, affects people such as climbers and pilots in unpressurized aircraft who are not adapted to living at high altitudes. It can also affect travellers visiting high altitudes.

People are vulnerable to altitude sickness when they ascend rapidly to heights of more than 2400–3000m (8000–10,000ft) above sea level. Air pressure falls with altitude, so at progressively higher altitudes each breath of air contains less oxygen. The levels of oxygen in the blood fall, so that the tissues are deprived of this vital nutrient. To compensate, the heart rate increases, speeding blood flow through the lungs and brain. The lungs can become saturated with water, or fluid may leak into the brain, which can be fatal. Exertion may strain the heart, causing a heart attack.

Gradual ascent is the best way to avoid the problem. Children, elderly people and anyone with lung or heart disease should consult a doctor before travelling to high altitudes.

SYMPTOMS

Symptoms may appear between 8 and 48 hours after rapid ascent to high altitude and include:
- feverishness and severe headache;
- dizziness and unsteadiness;
- nausea and vomiting;
- mental slowness and confusion;
- muscular lethargy and paralysis;
- tightness in the chest and breathlessness;
- loss of appetite and weight;
- insomnia;
- impaired vision and speech;
- euphoria and hallucinations.

TREATMENT

Relatively mild symptoms subside after a few days of rest. People with severe symptoms must descend rapidly to lower altitudes and report to a doctor at once. Breathing in oxygen from a pressurized supply may relieve the effects of fluid in the lungs or brain.

Alzheimer's disease

SEE RIGHT

Amnesia

Amnesia is a loss of memory, either partial or total, caused by disease or injury to the brain, or sometimes by drugs or psychological trauma. In retrograde amnesia, memory about facts or events before the trauma is lost. In

Continued on page 68

Alzheimer's disease

Although Alzheimer's cannot be cured, much can be done to make life easier for people with the condition. Early diagnosis is important.

Alzheimer's disease is the most common cause of **dementia** – a group of symptoms that includes confusion, memory loss, mood changes and speech problems. About 500,000 people in the UK suffer from Alzheimer's, and most are elderly. The condition affects about one in 20 people over the age of 65 and one in five over the age of 80.

A rarer form of Alzheimer's, which tends to run in families, can occur at a much younger age, affecting people in their 30s or 40s. Commoner forms of the disease also appear to have genetic links, but there is no single genetic mutation as occurs with true genetic disorders such as cystic fibrosis.

WHO IS AT RISK?

Research into Alzheimer's disease has identified a 'susceptibility gene' called apolipoprotein E (ApoE). It has been demonstrated that the risk of developing the disease in old age depends at least in part on the configuration of ApoE genes that an individual has inherited.

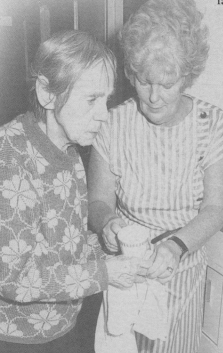

▼ Helping hand
The confusion and disorientation caused by Alzheimer's mean that people with the disease need increasing help with daily activities such as feeding and dressing. In the later stages, full-time residential care becomes necessary.

A wide variety of environmental factors have also been investigated as possible triggers of the disease, especially in genetically susceptible individuals. ApoE plays a role in cholesterol metabolism and heart disease – and people with high cholesterol or high blood pressure, and those who smoke, are all known to have an increased risk of developing Alzheimer's disease. Those who have suffered head or whiplash injuries also seem to be at risk. However, research has failed to support the idea that exposure to aluminium increases the risk of Alzheimer's.

CHARACTERISTICS OF THE DISEASE

Many people complain of poor memory as they grow older, but those with Alzheimer's disease become increasingly forgetful and confused, and this may make them frustrated, angry or frightened. As often happens in elderly people, old memories may remain intact whereas recent events are soon forgotten. People with Alzheimer's also have difficulty finding appropriate words and solving basic problems, and they may show signs of language impairment, such as rambling speech, long pauses and repetition. They are likely to become disorientated and perhaps get lost in familiar places.

As the disease progresses, everyday activities such as dressing, shopping and cooking become increasingly difficult. People with Alzheimer's find it harder and harder to communicate with those around them. They may become depressed and lose interest in the outside world; they are likely to give up interests and hobbies and become indifferent to social conventions and the opinions of others.

Alzheimer's disease is not the only reason why elderly people become confused. Circulatory problems, strokes and the side effects of certain medicines can also cause dementia-like symptoms. It is therefore important to seek medical help for anyone who is becoming confused or forgetful, so that any problems can be swiftly assessed and treated by an expert.

WHAT IS ALZHEIMER'S DISEASE?

First described in 1907 by Alois Alzheimer, a German neurologist, the disease attacks the thinking parts of the brain, including the hippocampus, one of the memory centres. Nerve fibres become tangled (neurofibrillary tangles) and clumps of abnormal protein (neuritic plaques) appear. Cells are destroyed and the brain shrinks. Some of these changes – the shrinkage of brain tissue and enlargement of the fluid-filled ventricles at the centre of the brain – are visible on brain scans. But tangles and plaques are visible under the microscope only when cells from the brain of someone with Alzheimer's is examined after death.

TREATMENT

The nerve damage observed in Alzheimer's disease includes a fall in the nerve transmitter acetylcholine, one of a group of chemicals in the brain that carries messages from one nerve to the next. Drugs currently used to treat the disease are aimed at restoring acetylcholine levels. They include donepezil (brand name Aricept), rivastigmine (Exelon) and galantamine (Reminyl). These drugs, if taken in the early stages of the illness, can slow or halt the deterioration of some patients for several months. They seem to improve the quality of life of people with Alzheimer's disease, enabling them to feel more alert and more willing to take part in social activities.

Complementary treatments such as music therapy and aromatherapy may be helpful to some people.

A POSSIBLE VACCINE

Future treatments are likely to be targeted at two proteins that seem to play key roles in the development of neurofibrillary tangles and neuritic plaques. The first protein, called tau, normally holds nerve fibres together so that they can carry messages efficiently. In Alzheimer's, a chemical change in tau makes it break away from nerve fibres, which then get tangled. Researchers are therefore looking for drugs that can stabilize tau so that nerve fibres stay neat and tidy.

The second protein, called beta amyloid, forms the core of neuritic plaques. Some types of beta amyloid are more harmful than others, and scientists are trying to design drugs that will block production of the harmful varieties.

Trials are also underway to test a vaccine that uses one type of the beta amyloid protein to try to trigger a protective immune response. If this is strong enough, it may help to prevent formation of neuritic plaques.

SEE ALSO *Brain and nervous system*

Guidelines for carers

Carers of people with Alzheimer's can do much to help them to lead lives that are as normal as possible, at least in the disease's early stages.

As a person's mental function deteriorates, full-time residential care is likely to be needed. But thousands of people with early Alzheimer's disease continue to be cared for at home by family and friends. This can be emotionally and physically exhausting for the carers. Availability of support and respite care varies from area to area – local branches of national charities and support groups should be able to advise.

People with Alzheimer's disease often have to make difficult financial and healthcare decisions, and it helps if carers are as honest as possible about what is happening.

There are a number of practical ways to help people with Alzheimer's disease to cope with daily life.

■ Draw up lists of things than need to be done during the day such as washing, getting dressed and preparing food.

■ Label appliances and places where things are kept as a memory aid.

■ Reduce potential hazards – check the safety of cookers and fires, for example.

■ Arrange for home visits by workers from social and other services.

■ Try memory therapy. For example, sit down with the person to look at old photographs and discuss notable family events.

Amnesia continued

anterograde amnesia, memory about events after the trauma is affected. Some people experience both types.

Someone suffering from amnesia caused by a viral infection may find it difficult to identify common objects or remember the meaning of ordinary words.

DURATION

Memory may return within minutes or hours, or more gradually. It may return only when the underlying condition has cleared up. In cases of severe brain injury or progressive diseases, amnesia can worsen or become permanent.

SYMPTOMS

Anterograde amnesia varies from a total lack of recall of events just after an accident to minor difficulty in retaining day-to-day information. It may involve a more serious loss of memory, perhaps leading to permanent disorientation.

Retrograde amnesia may vary from the inability to remember the period just before an accident or the onset of disease to difficulty in remembering minor details. Some affected people are unable to recall anything that has happened in the past 20 years.

CAUSES

Amnesia has many possible causes:
- head injury;
- emotional shock;
- **Alzheimer's disease** and **dementia**;
- **meningitis, encephalitis,** other viral infections;
- brain tumours, brain haemorrhages (see **Brain and nervous system**) and **strokes**;
- heavy drinking or malnourishment.

TREATMENT

If any symptoms of amnesia are noticed after an injury or shock, or if you suffer from repeated bouts of amnesia, seek medical advice.

What a doctor may do

Depending on the suspected source of the amnesia, a doctor may do one of the following.
- Test you for infections or other diseases, and possibly arrange for you to have a brain scan or to see a neurologist or neuropsychologist.
- If the amnesia is due to an emotional shock, refer you for psychiatric help.
- In the case of malnourishment, administer thiamin (vitamin B_1) injections.

Anaemia

Anaemia is a condition in which the quantity of oxygen-carrying haemoglobin in the **blood** is below normal. It is the most widespread of all blood disorders, and can occur in many forms, principally iron-deficiency, megaloblastic, sickle cell, haemolytic and aplastic anaemias.

SYMPTOMS

These symptoms are common to all types of anaemia:
- fatigue and pale skin;
- shortness of breath and palpitations;
- dizziness and disturbed vision;
- headaches and insomnia;
- loss of appetite and indigestion;
- in severe cases, swelling of the ankles;
- in older people, chest pain.

Iron-deficiency anaemia

Iron-deficiency anaemia is the most common form of the disorder. It is caused by a shortage of iron in the blood. This prevents the bone marrow from making enough haemoglobin, the oxygen-carrying pigment in red blood cells – with the result that the body does not get enough oxygen. The condition persists until treated unless the cause is temporary, in which case the body will slowly build up the deficit.

Depending on the cause, the condition could be corrected within three to six weeks of starting treatment. The person may then need to take an iron supplement for six months.

SYMPTOMS

In addition to the symptoms common to all types of anaemia, people with the iron-deficient form suffer from dry, brittle nails and a sore tongue and mouth. In very severe cases, heart failure and **oedema** may occur.

CAUSES
- Loss of blood due to heavy periods (see **Menstruation**).
- Excessive bleeding resulting from an accident or due to surgery.
- A diet deficient in iron.
- **Pregnancy**, which increases the body's need for iron.
- Poor absorption of iron from the diet, usually due to surgical removal of part of the stomach, or to **coeliac disease**.
- Diseases in which there is persistent bleeding, such as **gastritis**, peptic ulcer, bowel disorders including bowel cancer, haemorrhoids (piles) and urinary tract infections.

TREATMENT

Seek medical advice if any of the above symptoms develop.

What a doctor may do
- Carry out tests to measure the level of iron in the blood and the number of red blood cells.
- Investigate any underlying cause of the symptoms, for example, using **endoscopy** or barium X-rays (see **Barium investigations**) to check for digestive tract disorders.
- If the diagnosis is confirmed, prescribe iron-supplement tablets, drugs that control excessive menstrual bleeding or give iron by injection.

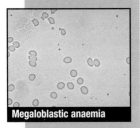

Megaloblastic anaemia

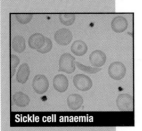

Sickle cell anaemia

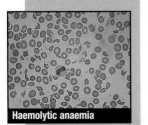

Haemolytic anaemia

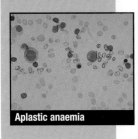

Aplastic anaemia

What you can do

Eat plenty of iron-rich foods such as lean meat, green vegetables, wholemeal bread, pulses, eggs and dried fruits. Avoid drinking tea with meals, since this can inhibit the absorption of iron from food.

Megaloblastic anaemia

This form of the disorder, also known as pernicious anaemia, results from a lack of folic acid or vitamin B_{12}, which prevents the effective production of red blood cells in the bone marrow. The condition persists until treated.

Some surgery is known to cause a deficiency of vitamin B_{12}. Patients who have undergone such surgery can be given injection of vitamin B_{12} to counteract the problems.

With treatment, the outlook for recovery is good, but to prevent recurrence you may need to have B_{12} injections or take folic acid tablets for an indefinite period.

SYMPTOMS

Apart from the symptoms common to all types of anaemia, people with megaloblastic anaemia may have persistent diarrhoea, tingling in the fingers and toes, and a sore tongue. Some may also develop jaundice, which produces a yellowish tinge in the eyes and the skin.

If treatment does not begin within six months of the onset of symptoms, the central nervous system may be irreversibly damaged. Other complications include heart failure, stomach cancer and degeneration of the spinal cord.

CAUSES

- An inability to absorb vitamin B_{12} – often as the result of an **autoimmune disease**. This condition is usually hereditary and is sometimes linked with **diabetes** or **myxoedema**.
- Folic acid deficiency.
- Removal of the small intestine, or the complete removal of the stomach.
  - A vegan diet.
  - Chronic alcohol abuse.
  - Diseases that interfere with the absorption of foods by the body, such as **Crohn's disease** and **coeliac disease**.

TREATMENT

If you develop any of the symptoms described, seek medical advice.

What a doctor may do

- Take a blood sample to assess haemoglobin levels in the blood.
- Refer you to hospital for a bone marrow test.
- Carry out further tests if an underlying cause is suspected.
- Prescribe a course of vitamin B_{12} injections or folic acid tablets.

What you can do

- Eat foods rich in vitamin B_{12}, including meat, poultry, fish, cereals, dairy products and eggs, and foods rich in folic acid, including broccoli, spinach and wholemeal bread.
- During early pregnancy, take a course of folic acid supplements.

Sickle cell anaemia

Sickle cell anaemia is an inherited condition in which the red blood cells contain an abnormal type of haemoglobin. If, because of exertion or respiratory infection, the amount of oxygen in the blood is reduced, the abnormal haemoglobin causes the blood cells to deform into a crescent or sickle shape. These may block blood vessels, reducing blood flow to body tissues, and may be destroyed by the body's immune system. Sickle cell anaemia is found mainly in people of African and Afro-Caribbean descent.

Haemolytic anaemias

Haemolytic anaemias are a group of disorders in which red blood cells are produced at the normal rate but destroyed much faster than usual. The condition may be:

- due to an inherited defect;
- acquired later in life, through an **autoimmune disease**, for example;
- associated with other conditions such as **leukaemia** or **lupus**;
- due to an infectious disease such as **pneumonia** or **malaria**;
- caused by treatment with certain drugs.

TREATMENT

Possible treatments include:

- the removal of the spleen, where many of the red blood cells are destroyed;
- immunosuppressant drugs;
- medication such as antimalarial drugs.

Aplastic anaemia

Aplastic anaemia is a rare type of the disorder in which fewer red blood cells, white blood cells and platelets than normal are produced. It is caused by the bone marrow's inability to produce adequate stem cells. These are the cells that form the basis of all cells in the body. Aplastic anaemia may be the result of a viral infection or an **autoimmune disease,** or it may be a side effect of various drugs or treatment for **cancer** such as **radiotherapy** or anticancer drugs. In many cases no specific cause can be established.

Symptoms can take the form of spontaneous bruising and repeated infections such as sore throats. Treatment may involve a blood transfusion, drugs to stimulate blood cell production, or drugs to suppress the immune system. In severe cases of the disorder, a bone marrow transplant is usually needed.

Anaesthesia and anaesthetics

The development of anaesthetics in the 19th century was a key factor in the advance of modern surgery. Until then, surgery relied on alcohol and narcotics to subdue a patient, often with disastrous results. The drugs used today are easily administered and generally safe.

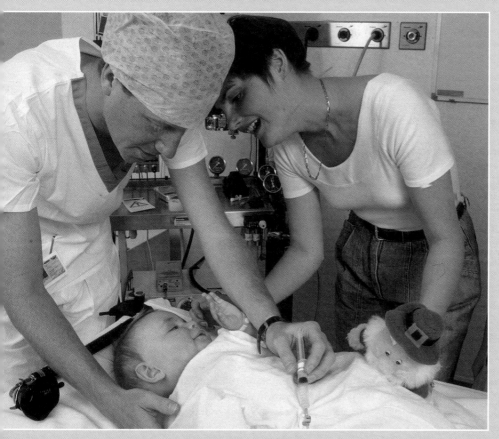

▲ **Parental support**
Parents are encouraged to accompany their children to the anaesthetic room and support them until they are asleep.

Anaesthesia means a loss of sensation. It may occur as the result of a disease, or follow trauma to a nerve. But the word is most often used to mean a loss of sensation induced by drugs. Anaesthesia allows surgical and other procedures to be carried out on patients without pain. There are two types of anaesthesia: general, and local or regional.

GENERAL ANAESTHESIA
In general anaesthesia, an anaesthetist (a doctor with at least six years' specialist training) gives drugs through a vein or by inhalation or, more often, a combination of both. The anaesthetist visits the patient before the operation to assess the individual's needs and answer any questions. Various drugs are used to produce a loss of consciousness and sensation; the anaesthetist chooses the most appropriate combination for the patient and the surgical procedure involved. Patients are advised not to eat or drink for at least six hours before an operation to avoid the risk of vomiting and choking while under general anaesthesia. The anaesthetist monitors the patient throughout the operation, supervises recovery from the anaesthetic and advises on post-operative care, including pain management.

LOCAL ANAESTHESIA
In the case of a local or regional anaesthetic, drugs block all the sensation pathways in one part of the nervous system. This technique is often used in conjunction with general anaesthesia to ensure pain-free recovery. When only a local anaesthetic is used, patients remain conscious during the procedure; they feel no pain, although they may feel pulling or pressure in the area being treated.

Local anaesthetics are introduced directly into the appropriate part of the body or injected around the nerves supplying it. Their effect can be limited to, say, one finger or, in the case of dentistry, to a small part of the mouth. A more specialized technique, known as an epidural, involves injecting an anaesthetic drug into the space around the spinal cord. This blocks off nerves serving the lower part of the body. Epidurals are well established as a form of pain relief during labour.

Local anaesthetic is usually given by injection, but sometimes an ointment, eyedrops, or a spray may be used. Local anaesthesia can also be induced by **acupuncture** and **hypnotherapy**.

RISKS AND COMPLICATIONS
Modern anaesthesia is now very safe, accounting for one death in 250,000. Always tell an anaesthetist if you are taking any medicines or suffer from any medical condition. Sometimes people experience nausea or vomiting after having an anaesthetic, but there are antisickness drugs to counter these after effects.

Anencephaly

Anencephaly is a severe fetal abnormality in which the neural tube (which forms the brain and spinal cord) fails to develop in the womb. It occurs in one in 1000 pregnancies. There is no treatment, and the baby dies at birth or within a few days. The abnormality can be detected by **ultrasound** and amniocentesis tests in early pregnancy.

The cause of anencephaly is unknown, but there is a genetic link. The risk is reduced if a woman who may become pregnant starts taking folic acid supplements from the time she stops using contraception until the end of the 12th week of pregnancy.

A much higher than usual dose of folic acid, taken under medical supervision, can reduce the risk of a baby with anencephaly in women who have a family history of the abnormality.

SEE ALSO *Pregnancy and problems*

Aneurysm

An aneurysm is a swelling that develops in a diseased or weakened artery. It can form anywhere in the body, but most often occurs in the aorta (the main artery of the chest and abdomen). It is more common among people over the age of 55, especially men.

Sometimes aneurysms form in the blood vessels supplying the brain. Usually these are present from birth (congenital aneurysms), but they may form at sites of blood vessel weakness in older people, particularly those with high blood pressure.

Often there is no evidence of a cerebral aneurysm until it ruptures much later in life, causing a subarachnoid haemorrhage. This is a rare cause of sudden, unexpected death in young adults. Survivors may be left with varying degrees of neurological damage.

SYMPTOMS

Many aneurysms have no symptoms and are discovered only through routine examinations and X-rays. Aneurysms in the chest may put pressure on surrounding tissues and interfere with heart function, causing chest or back pain.

CAUSES

The most common cause of an aneurysm is **atheroma** (degenerative

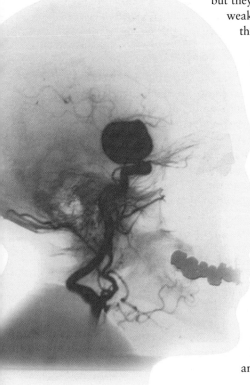

▼ **Brain aneurysm** Injection of a dye into the carotid artery shows the brain's blood vessels on X-ray. Here a brain aneurysm is clearly outlined. The risk of a rupture makes the condition life-threatening.

change) of the wall of the artery, but it is often associated with high blood pressure (hypertension). The cause of congenital aneurysm is unknown.

TREATMENT

If you suspect an aneurysm, seek medical advice urgently. A ruptured aortic aneurysm may cause kidney failure and stroke and can be fatal. Others may remain symptomless for many years, but when they develop, the risk of rupture has to be balanced against any risks of repair by surgery.

What a doctor may do

If there are symptoms, a doctor will investigate further to see whether the aneurysm can be repaired safely by surgery. Doctors may choose not to treat symptomless aneurysms.

Aneurysms over 5cm (2in) wide can be repaired with synthetic tubing to prevent rupturing of the artery.

PREVENTION

The most effective prevention is to adopt a healthy lifestyle with regular exercise. Keep to a healthy weight, do not smoke, and restrict alcohol intake to 21–28 units a week for men and 14–21 units a week for women. Men over 60 with a family history of aortic aneurysm should request ultrasound screening.

Angina pectoris

Angina pectoris is chest pain caused by shortage of oxygen in the heart muscles. By far the most common cause is coronary artery disease that develops in middle age. The arteries that supply the heart become narrowed by deposits (plaques) containing cholesterol, so that blood flow is reduced. Other causative conditions include anaemia, thyroid disease and very fast or slow heart rates.

The condition is aggravated by exertion or stress because these increase demands on the heart. Other triggers include cold weather. It can be relieved by rest or medication.

SYMPTOMS

Angina is marked by a heavy, cramping pain, resembling the effect of a tight band, behind the breastbone. The pain may spread to the neck, jaw or left arm, and occasionally to the right arm. Other symptoms associated with angina include breathlessness, dizziness, sweating, nausea and vomiting.

TREATMENT

If you notice chest pain or severe breathlessness on exertion, consult a doctor. If the pain becomes more frequent, or recurs during minor exertion or when resting, seek medical help urgently. Unstable angina may lead to a heart attack. If an angina attack lasts for more than 15 minutes, call an ambulance.

What a doctor may do

Medication relieves symptoms and reduces the risk of heart attack. In severe cases, coronary artery intervention (**angioplasty** or coronary bypass) may be needed. But in the first instance your doctor may do the following.

■ Examine your heart and chest, and check your blood pressure, pulse, height and weight.

■ Order blood tests for anaemia, diabetes, kidney or liver abnormalities that might affect the severity of angina or the treatment choice.

■ Arrange for a 'fasting' blood test. Restricting to water only for ten hours before the test enables a detailed analysis of cholesterol levels.

■ Arrange an electrocardiogram (ECG or heart tracing) to detect heart damage.

■ Arrange an exercise tolerance (stress) test to show how the heart copes under stress. This is used to confirm the diagnosis.

■ Arrange an ultrasound scan.

■ Book a chest X-ray.

■ Arrange a coronary **angiography**.

■ Order a radio-isotope (thallium) scan of heart function if other tests are not conclusive.

PREVENTION

■ Lose weight.

■ Stop smoking.

■ Drink within safe alcohol limits (14–21 units per week for women, 21–28 for men).

■ Walk briskly for 20 minutes five times weekly (stop or slow down if it brings on symptoms).

■ Adopt a healthier diet.

■ Eat oily fish twice a week.

■ Lower stress levels.

■ Keep blood pressure down to 140/80.

■ In diabetics, good blood sugar control reduces the progression of coronary heart disease.

OUTLOOK

Adopting a healthier lifestyle and appropriate treatment will usually reduce angina symptoms and can also cut the risk of heart attacks, stroke and other circulatory diseases, which are more common in angina sufferers.

SEE ALSO *Arteries and disorders; Heart and circulatory system; Hypertension*

Angiography

Angiography is an X-ray designed to ascertain the shape or direction of an artery. A dye is injected into the artery, and this shows up on the X-ray. It is used to diagnose problems in coronary artery disease and in peripheral artery disease (see **Arteries and disorders**).

The test is painless, once local anaesthetic has been injected to 'freeze' the skin around the artery in the groin or front of the elbow. A long, thin tube (catheter) is inserted into an artery and guided to the correct artery using an X-ray video camera. In coronary angiography, this will be the right or left coronary arteries.

Dye is flushed along the catheter into the artery, and X-ray 'snapshots' are taken immediately; these clearly show any areas of narrowing or blockage.

SEE ALSO *Heart and circulatory system*

Angio-oedema

Angio-oedema is a swelling of the skin and mucous membranes, caused by an excess of histamine released by the body in an allergic reaction. The eyes, face, lips and tongue may swell, restricting breathing. Bee and wasp stings may cause angio-oedema in people sensitive to them. Associated symptoms include headache, painful joints, the sensation of a lump in the throat, wheezing, shortness of breath, vomiting, diarrhoea and abdominal pain.

SEE ALSO *Allergies; Nettle rash*

Angioplasty

Angioplasty is a surgical technique used to widen blood vessels that have been narrowed or blocked as a result of arterial disease of the heart, the limbs or internal organs. In this condition, fatty deposits (atheroma) build up on the artery walls and restrict blood flow. Angioplasty is widely used for dilating the arteries supplying the heart – this is known as a coronary angioplasty.

WHAT'S INVOLVED

'Balloon' angioplasty, the most common technique used in the UK, generally requires overnight admission to hospital. Under local **anaesthetic**, a catheter (a narrow, flexible tube) with a tiny balloon attached to its end is inserted into the artery of the leg. It is guided under **X-ray** control to the narrowed coronary artery and then inflated. This stretches the affected part of the artery, allowing the blood to flow through unrestricted. The balloon is then deflated and the catheter withdrawn.

Angioplasties are successful in most cases, and can be repeated if the artery becomes blocked or narrowed again. Sometimes a synthetic tube or coil known as a stent is inserted into the artery to keep it open; angioplasty can also be used after coronary artery bypass grafts.

OTHER TREATMENTS

Heavily diseased artery sections may not be suitable for balloon angioplasty. Alternative

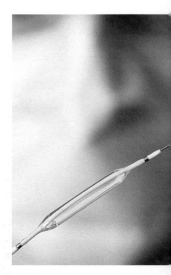

▼ **Balloon therapy**
A surgeon prepares to thread a catheter and balloon into an artery. The 'balloon' is then inflated to widen the narrowed artery.

ways of clearing blocked arteries include using a rotoblator, a revolving burr that drills through the deposits. Sometimes a laser is used to break up the deposits.

SEE ALSO **Arteries and disorders**

Ankle and problems

The ankle is a joint between the uppermost bone in the foot (the talus) and the two bones of the lower leg (the tibia and the fibula), which are bound together by strong ligaments. As it is a hinge joint, the ankle allows movement only in one plane – up and down. Other movements (such as rotation of the ankle) involve bones in the foot itself.

SPRAINED ANKLE

The commonest injury is a sprain of the ligament at its outside edge (the lateral ligament), which results from twisting the ankle. This causes pain, swelling and bruising, which can be severe.

Treat a sprained ankle with rest, by applying an ice pack and compression bandaging, and by elevating it. For more severe sprains, seek medical opinion to rule out a fracture or a torn ligament. A severely sprained ankle may have to be strapped up for two or three weeks.

BROKEN ANKLE

Excessive, violent twisting of the ankle can cause a fracture. Most ankle fractures involve the lower end of the tibia and/or fibula.

If you fall onto your feet from a great height, you may cause a vertical compression injury of the ankle. A combined fracture and dislocation of the ankle is known as a 'Pott's fracture'; this occurs when the lower fibula (and sometimes the tibia as well) fractures and the ligaments tear so that the ankle joint dislocates.

Simple fractures of the ankle are treated by immobilizing the joint in plaster. More severe injuries may require a screw to be surgically inserted into the joint.

SEE ALSO **Arthritis; Bruises; Club foot and hand**

Ankylosing spondylitis

Ankylosing spondylitis is a disease of the joints, mainly affecting the spine. The joints become stiff and inflamed and, if left untreated, may fuse together and become rigid. In the UK about one in 2000 people have the condition, which is most likely to develop in adults between the ages of 20 and 40. Spinal joints are the main ones involved, but in some cases the shoulders, hips and knees may be affected. There is no definite known cause, although there is a genetic link.

SYMPTOMS

Ankylosing spondylitis progresses slowly over many years. Symptoms include:
- repeated attacks of lower back pain in a healthy, fit person aged between 20 and 40;
- early-morning back pain and stiffness, which can move down one or both legs;
- increasing stiffness of the whole spine;
- tenderness over the hip joints;
- limited chest expansion.

TREATMENT

If you suffer from several symptoms, seek medical advice. Also, if there is a family history of the disease, it is advisable to consult your doctor about tests – they can assist in early diagnosis, allowing prompt treatment.

What a doctor may do
- X-ray the lower part of your back and carry out a blood test. If the diagnosis is confirmed, your doctor may refer you to hospital.
- Prescribe painkillers and anti-inflammatory drugs to relieve the symptoms and slow down the progress of the disease.
- Arrange **physiotherapy**, which can help to strengthen spinal muscles, mobilize the joints and stretch ligaments.
- Suggest a hip replacement if hip joints are badly affected.
- Arrange **radiotherapy** occasionally, if pain is severe and uncontrollable.

What you can do
- A daily exercise programme helps to relieve pain and maintain mobility. Swimming is an excellent form of exercise to help to keep the body as supple as possible.
- Lie face down for 20 minutes at the beginning and end of the day.
- Sleep on a firm mattress.
- Keep to a healthy weight.
- Try to maintain good posture (see **Back and back pain**).

Complementary therapies
Hydrotherapy, shiatsu, t'ai chi ch'uan and meditation may all be beneficial. **Acupuncture** may relieve pain.

COMPLICATIONS

Long-term ankylosing spondylitis may cause the spine to become rigid, leading to curvature (kyphosis) which, with neck distortion, can be extremely disabling.

Other potential complications of the disease include ulcerative colitis, Crohn's disease and certain heart defects. Iritis (inflammation of the iris) occurs in 40 per cent of cases.

OUTLOOK

Ankylosing spondylitis may increasingly interfere with work or physical activity.

However, for cases that are treated early with anti-inflammatory drugs and physiotherapy, the outlook is usually good.

Anorexia nervosa

SEE PAGE 75

Anoxia

Anoxia refers to a complete break in oxygen supply to the tissues of an organ even where there is an adequate supply of blood; the term 'hypoxia' means a reduction in oxygen supply to an organ. Despite the difference in meaning, the two words are often used interchangeably to describe a decline in oxygen supply. Some 20 per cent of the body's supply of oxygen is used by the brain. As a result, it is particularly sensitive to anoxia or hypoxia, which can lead to coma or seizures and, if left untreated, death.

CAUSES

The conditions and events that may adversely affect the supply of oxygen to an organ include:
- a heart attack;
- a severe asthma attack;
- an adverse reaction to an anaesthetic;
- inhalation of smoke or carbon monoxide;
- exposure to high altitude;
- strangulation or suffocation;
- poisoning.

TREATMENT

Treatment may include artificial ventilation, oxygen therapy and investigation of any underlying causes.

Antepartum haemorrhage

Antepartum haemorrhage means bleeding from the womb in pregnancy. It may signal a serious problem, so the pregnant woman should seek medical advice promptly if bleeding occurs. Slight spotting around the time of the first missed period is common, but more pronounced bleeding may indicate a complication involving the placenta or a threatened **miscarriage**.
SEE ALSO *Pregnancy and problems*

Anthrax

Anthrax is a disease of farm animals that occasionally spreads to human beings. It may be fatal if left untreated, but is very rare in the UK.
The anthrax bacterium attacks either the skin (cutaneous anthrax) or the lungs (pulmonary anthrax). People may become infected through cuts or sores if handling products from infected animals, or by inhaling large quantities of infected spores. Cutaneous anthrax causes swelling and deep ulcers, but is easily treated in its earliest stages with penicillin. Pulmonary anthrax causes severe breathing problems and pneumonia, and is fatal in most cases.

Anus and problems

The anus is the opening at the lower end of the digestive tract, through which stools (faeces) pass during defecation. It is connected to the rectum by the anal canal, which is about 4cm (1⅜in) long.

Normally, the anus is held closed by two bands of muscle that run around it: the external and internal sphincters. The external sphincter is under voluntary control – it can be relaxed deliberately. The internal one can only be relaxed by the autonomic nervous system, which operates without conscious control.

The lower half of the anal canal has the same number of sensory nerve endings as normal skin; the upper half has no sensory nerve endings and, like the intestines, only responds to increases in tension from the pressure of faeces. For this reason cancer of the lower bowel does not cause pain until it has spread to the lower anal canal.

WHAT CAN GO WRONG?

- The most common problem to affect the anus is **haemorrhoids** – painful swollen veins that may develop either inside or outside the anus.
- Anal fissures are small tears in the lining of the anus, usually caused when a person suffering from **constipation** passes hard stools. Anal fissures are treated with antibiotics and medicated creams.
- Bacteria can invade the tissues of the anal canal to form an anal **abscess**, especially when there is also **Crohn's disease** or a disorder that reduces the efficiency of the immune system. Doctors will drain the abscess.
- Crohn's disease or the presence of an abscess make it likely that an anal fistula will develop. This is a small channel that opens between the rectum and the skin near the anus and is treated with antibiotics and surgery.
- Itching in the anus (*pruritus ani*) can occur for no apparent reason or can be a sign of an infestation by threadworms.
- Very rarely, children are born without an anal opening. The condition, called an imperforate anus, affects one in 5000 births and is corrected by surgery.

Anorexia nervosa

People with anorexia nervosa have an intense fear of putting on weight. The condition can develop when a person focuses on controlling food intake and body shape as a way of coping with painful feelings.

The clearest sign of anorexia is severe weight loss. Sufferers weigh at least 15 per cent less than is usual for their age and height. The condition is more obvious but rarer than **bulimia nervosa**. People can fluctuate between the two conditions. Most sufferers are girls and young women, although men can be affected and even children as young as seven or eight.

People with anorexia restrict the amount they eat and drink not because they are not hungry, but because they cannot allow themselves to satisfy their appetites. They have mixed feelings about 'giving up' their illness because their eating habits have become a way of coping with their emotional problems.

The causes are varied. Some people are more vulnerable due to their genetic make-up or personalities. People with low self-esteem, anxiety or depression may focus on avoiding food to cope with stress or pressure. Traumatic events such as the death of a friend or relative, sexual abuse or divorce can trigger the illness.

HOW OTHERS CAN HELP

The first step is to see a doctor, but it can be hard for people with anorexia to accept that they need help – and they must want to get better before any good can result. Friends and family should try to build a relationship of trust with sufferers without forcing them to get help. The focus should be on emotions rather than on food or weight. It may be useful to suggest that individuals get help to deal with the feelings at the root of the anorexia, rather than the anorexia itself.

A GP can refer someone with anorexia to a specialist in eating disorders. Counselling, psychotherapy or family therapy may address underlying emotional problems, or a psychologist may provide cognitive behaviour therapy. When a person is dangerously underweight, the doctor may advise a spell in a hospital or clinic. Music, dance, drama or art therapy may benefit those who find it hard to express themselves in words. Aromatherapy, **massage** and reflexology can help people to feel more connected with their body.

The Eating Disorders Association provides help and support for people with anorexia, and their family and friends.

LONG-TERM EFFECTS AND RECOVERY

Refusing food over a long period can lead to malnutrition and, sometimes, death. Women can find it difficult to become pregnant and may develop **osteoporosis** (brittle bones). But many of the physical problems associated with anorexia can be reversed once the body is given proper nourishment. Long-term psychological solutions depend on sufferers coming to understand the origins of their eating distress – and finding other ways of coping with their feelings and with stressful situations.

Anorexia affects one in 100 girls and young women in the UK.

Factfile

Signs of anorexia

Many emotional and behavioural changes are linked with anorexia, including:

- an intense fear of gaining weight;
- a belief by sufferers that they are fat when they are underweight;
- mood swings;
- secrecy in regard to food;
- rituals such as cutting food into tiny pieces;

- wearing big, baggy clothes;
- exercising obsessively;
- vomiting or taking laxatives.

Girls and women with anorexia often have irregular then absent periods, while men are likely to suffer a loss of libido. Other physical signs are:

- constipation and abdominal pains;
- downy hair on the body;
- feeling cold, due to poor circulation;
- dry, rough, discoloured skin;
- swollen stomach, face and ankles;
- dizzy spells and fainting;
- restlessness and hyperactivity.

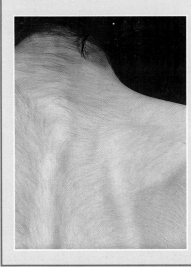

◄ **Keeping warm**
As the body of an anorexic struggles to adapt to decreasing amounts of fat and muscle, it develops a fine covering of hair to help retain body heat.

Anxiety

Anxiety is a normal reaction to **stress**. After a stressful event, the anxiety will usually go away. But anxiety becomes a problem when it persists beyond an event or interferes with your day-to-day life and your relationships.

Anxiety can feed on itself, so that the sufferer worries about feeling anxious which then increases the anxiety. It can lead to **insomnia** or **panic attacks** or may develop into **depression**, an **obsession** or **phobia**.

SYMPTOMS

The symptoms of anxiety can take many forms:
- fearfulness and a pessimistic outlook;
- over-alertness or irritability;
- inability to relax or concentrate;
- tense muscles;
- headaches;
- raised heartbeat, high blood pressure and sweating;
- nausea, sickness or diarrhoea;
- insomnia.

CAUSES

The most common causes of persistent anxiety are stressful life events now or in the past, especially those connected with work, money, relationships, death or divorce.

Another important factor is family history: the way in which your parents cope with pressure and stress can influence the likelihood of your developing an anxiety problem.

Other causes include a poor diet, especially one that includes excess sugar or caffeine, **drug misuse** or the side effects of prescribed drugs.

TREATMENT

Consult a doctor if you are concerned that your anxiety is becoming overwhelming.

What a doctor may do
- Check for any underlying illness.
- Refer you to a counsellor or a psychologist for cognitive behaviour therapy.
- Prescribe tranquillizers or sleeping pills.

What you can do
Reassess your job, ambitions and lifestyle and make changes accordingly. It helps to identify the source of your anxiety – for example, bullying at work.

Complementary and other therapies
- Regular exercise, **massage**, aromatherapy, reflexology or hypnotherapy may help you to relax and sleep better.
- Learn relaxation and breathing techniques from self-help tapes.
- Join a yoga or meditation class.

Aorta and disorders

The aorta is the main artery in the body. It has a thick muscular wall and carries oxygenated blood from the heart to the peripheral arteries to supply the head, trunk, limbs and vital organs.

When oxygenated blood returns from the lungs, it is pumped through the left ventricle and aortic valve into the ascending aorta, where the coronary arteries branch off to supply the heart itself. The aortic valve stops blood from flowing back into the heart when it relaxes.

WHAT CAN GO WRONG

There are a number of conditions and disorders that can develop.

Abnormal development
The aortic valve and the aorta may develop abnormally in the fetus. This can happen in isolation or as part of a syndrome such as **Fallot's tetralogy**. If the aortic valve has two flaps instead of the normal three, it may thicken and stiffen, or it may leak in later life. This makes it harder for the left ventricle to pump blood into the aorta, and can lead to heart failure. In many cases, surgery can correct the condition.

Aortic regurgitation
The aortic valve may leak as a result of damage caused by rheumatic heart disease (see **Rheumatic fever**), heart attack and several other conditions such as rheumatoid arthritis. There can also be a congenital weakness of the valve. Blood ebbs back into the left ventricle from the aorta after each heartbeat, increasing the heart's workload. This can lead to breathlessness or heart failure; treatment with drugs or artificial valve replacement may be needed.

Aortic stenosis
Narrowing of the aortic valve may be caused by rheumatic heart disease, or by hardening caused by calcium deposition, which occurs with ageing. This can cause fainting and breathlessness, and lead to **angina**. An artificial valve replacement is often needed to treat these symptoms, and strenuous activity may be harmful.

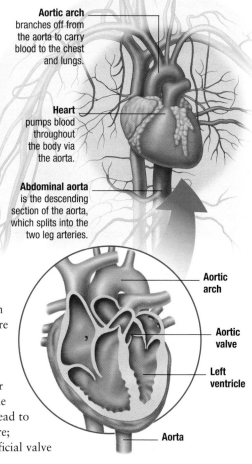

Aorta
The largest artery in the body, the aorta carries blood from the heart to other parts of the body.

Aortic arch branches off from the aorta to carry blood to the chest and lungs.

Heart pumps blood throughout the body via the aorta.

Abdominal aorta is the descending section of the aorta, which splits into the two leg arteries.

Aortic arch

Aortic valve

Left ventricle

Aorta

Coarctation of the aorta

Usually detected in childhood, coarctation of the aorta is a condition in which the aortic arch is abnormally narrowed. It affects one person in 1700, and unless the condition is corrected by surgery, 50 per cent of sufferers will die before the age of 30.

If coarctation is undetected until adulthood, raised blood pressure or premature heart failure may be the first clues to the condition.

Coarctation must be repaired by surgery; the narrowed section is cut out or replaced with an artificial graft, or it may be widened by balloon **angioplasty**. One in ten cases recurs after surgery.

Aortic aneurysm

An aortic aneurysm is a localized swelling caused by weakness in the wall of the abdominal or thoracic aorta. Aneurysms of the abdominal aorta are commonly caused by **atheroma**, a degeneration of the walls of the arteries. Those in the thoracic aorta are more often caused by diseases that affect the wall of the aorta, such as Marfan's syndrome (see below). In both cases, the aneurysm may rupture, leading to internal bleeding.

Marfan's syndrome

Marfan's syndrome is a genetic disorder of connective tissue that produces weakness of the aorta. This leads to dilation of the aorta and results in stretching and leaking of the aortic valve. The wall of the aorta may tear, leading to death in early adulthood, unless the condition is detected by an **ultrasound** picture of the heart and aorta.

SEE ALSO *Heart and circulatory system*

Aphasia

The term 'aphasia' covers a wide range of language impairments caused by damage to the language-processing regions of the brain, usually due to head injury or **stroke**. In 95 per cent of people, the language areas lie in the left cerebral hemisphere. However, in the other five per cent, language is processed in either the right or both left and right sides. The form of aphasia depends on which part of the language area is affected.

There are three common types. Broca's aphasia involves an inability to express language and articulate sentences correctly. Speech tends to be minimal or disjointed, but comprehension is not greatly affected. Wernicke's aphasia involves a difficulty in understanding language, despite the retention of normal intelligence in other ways. Speech is fluent, but the content is garbled or nonsensical.

Anomic aphasia involves a difficulty in retrieving words and using them with good comprehension and grammar.

SEE ALSO *Brain and nervous system; Cerebral haemorrhage; Head and injuries; Stroke*

Apnoea

Apnoea is a pause in breathing during sleep. It lasts between 10 and 30 seconds, and can cause problems both in babies and in adults. There is a possible link between apnoea in babies and cot death (**sudden infant death syndrome**).

In the UK, it affects four per cent of men and two per cent of women in middle age. The symptom, heavy snoring, is caused by the airways closing during sleep. To clear the blockage, the person wakes up (too briefly to remember doing so) 400–500 times a night. Although not in itself fatal, apnoea can cause tiredness and mental health problems. It is associated with increased risk of heart disease. Apnoea can be treated with a breathing aid worn at night.

Appendix and appendicitis

The appendix is a tubular pouch in the large intestine about 9cm (3½in) in length. It has no known function. Appendicitis (inflammation of the appendix) can develop at any time, but is most prevalent in people aged between 8 and 25 years old. It is treated by surgical removal of the appendix, which very rarely has any damaging effect.

Acute appendicitis, which strikes its victims suddenly, is the most common reason for emergency surgery in developing countries.

Chronic (persistent or recurring) appendicitis is far less severe than the acute version of the condition, and may continue for several months before an operation becomes necessary.

SYMPTOMS

There is wide variation in the symptoms of appendicitis, and the condition can easily be confused with many other ailments.

In chronic appendicitis, symptoms may never develop beyond an indeterminate discomfort on the right-hand side of the abdomen. But in about half of all cases of acute appendicitis, the symptoms follow an established pattern.

■ Initially, there is a feeling of discomfort around the navel.

■ Within a few hours, a sharper, more constant pain develops around McBurney's point, which is two-thirds of the way along a line drawn between the navel and the right hip bone. The pain is worse on moving or coughing, and when

pressure is released after the point is pressed.
■ There may be a raised temperature, sickness and vomiting, sometimes accompanied by constipation or diarrhoea.
■ If the appendix is pressing on the ureter, the urine may be bloodstained.

CAUSES
Sometimes the open end of the appendix gets blocked, causing swelling and infection. But the cause of appendicitis is often unknown.

TREATMENT
There are several things you can do before seeking medical help for suspected appendicitis.
■ Lie still, holding a hot-water bottle over the painful area to ease discomfort.
■ Do not eat or drink anything.
■ Do not take painkillers, laxatives or other medication.

When to consult a doctor
If pain has persisted for more than three to four hours, call a doctor. Summon help earlier if the pain grows worse, becomes continuous or keeps you awake during the night.

What a doctor may do
If acute appendicitis is suspected, the doctor will probably send you to hospital immediately for observation or surgery. In some circumstances the doctor may decide to monitor your condition at home.

In cases of acute appendicitis, emergency surgery often proves necessary. Patients are usually discharged from hospital within two to three days after the operation if no subsequent complications occur.

If your condition is chronic rather than acute, surgery may not be necessary for several months.

PREVENTION
Eating a diet high in fibre may help to prevent appendicitis. The condition is less common in countries where a high-fibre diet is the norm.

COMPLICATIONS
■ If treatment is delayed, there is a danger that the inflamed appendix may rupture, spilling its contents into the abdomen and causing the more serious condition of **peritonitis**. This occurs in about 20 per cent of cases.
■ A rupture may form an **abscess**, causing fever and increasing pain in the abdomen.
■ A ruptured appendix can also infect the blood, causing blood poisoning (**septicaemia**).
■ In women, the ovaries and Fallopian tubes may occasionally become infected and blocked, leading to infertility.

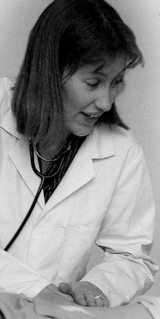

▼ **Telltale touch**
A doctor applies pressure to a patient's abdomen to see if pain in the McBurney's point area worsens after the pressure is released. Such rebound pain is a sign of an inflamed appendix.

Appetite, loss of

The desire to eat is controlled by cells in a part of the brain called the hypothalamus. In a healthy person, these cells integrate information about the fullness of the digestive system, concentrations of nutrients in the blood, the individual's emotional state and whether food is palatable or not. Depending on the balance of these factors, a person may feel full, comfortable (neither hungry nor full), hungry or have no desire for their food.

Social factors also play an important part in determining when people eat food: the internal controls that register when the stomach is full are often overriden.

CAUSES
Sometimes a loss of appetite is nothing to worry about. It may be caused by a slowing of the growth rate in young people, and in women by decreasing oestrogen levels during the menopause or hormone changes during pregnancy. Loss of appetite may also be an adverse reaction to medication – if you think this could apply to you, check with a doctor.

But a seriously diminished appetite can also be an indication of various diseases and conditions, including:
■ a **kidney** disorder;
■ a **liver** disorder;
■ **cancer**;
■ a viral infection such as infectious mononucleosis (see **Glandular fever**);
■ inadequate levels of cortisone hormone (see **Adrenal glands and disorders**);
■ an underactive **thyroid** gland;
■ vitamin deficiency caused by alcohol abuse, or vitamin B_{12} and folic acid deficiency;
■ stomach inflammation (see **Gastritis** and **Stomach and disorders**);
■ irritation or infection of the digestive tract such as that caused by **food poisoning** (see also **Gastroenteritis** and **Digestive system**);
■ a disorder of the red blood cells (see **Anaemia** and **Blood and disorders**);
■ **stress**, **depression** or **anxiety**;
■ an eating disorder.

TREATMENT
If loss of appetite continues for more than a few weeks, seek medical advice for diagnosis and treatment of underlying causes.

What you can do
■ If appetite loss is an acute symptom of food poisoning or of a viral infection lasting only a few days, a diet of plain boiled white rice and plain boiled, cooled water should help.
■ If nausea is one of the acute symptoms, finely grated ginger root (or dried ginger

powder) in hot water may help. Dried
cinnamon in water may also bring relief.
■ For food poisoning with salmonella, cranberry
extract powder dissolved in water helps to
remove the micro-organism from the body.
■ If antibiotics have been prescribed to treat
appetite loss, a course of a probiotic supplement
(containing organisms such as lactobacillus
acidophilus and bifidobacteria) together with
fructo-oligosaccharides (the growth medium for
the probiotic species) can be useful in allowing
repopulation of the gastro-intestinal tract with
'healthy' species of bacteria.

Arm and problems

The arm is made up of three long bones: the
longest, the humerus, is in the upper arm; the
radius and the ulna are in the forearm. The
rounded, upper end of the humerus forms a
joint with the cup of the shoulder blade and it
meets the ulna at the elbow joint. The radius
meets the ulna inside the capsule surrounding
this joint, and both bones connect with the
carpal bones of the wrist joint. The main
muscles of the upper arm are the biceps and
triceps, which raise (flex) and lower (extend)
the forearm. There are two main groups of
muscles in the forearm: the wrist and finger
extensors, which pull the wrist back and extend
the fingers; and the wrist and finger flexors,
which pull the hand down and close the grip.
The muscles move the bones of the arm, wrist
and fingers by means of tendons. Commands
for muscle movements are relayed from the
brain by the median, ulna and radial nerves.

Blood circulates in the arm through the
brachial artery (to the upper arm) and the radial
and ulnar arteries (to the forearm).

WHAT CAN GO WRONG
■ The lower ends of the radius and ulna are the
most commonly fractured bones in the body.
A blow to the ulna nerve at the 'funny bone' –
where the nerve passes over the bottom part of
the humerus at the elbow joint – can cause
intense discomfort but is unlikely to cause a
serious problem.
■ Many common arm problems, such as
arthritis or **RSI** (repetitive strain injury), involve
the joints and muscles. Arthritis and **tendonitis**
can affect the elbow and the structures around
it, while acute frictional tenosynovitis may
cause pain in the tendons of the wrist and
fingers at the lower end of the forearm.
■ An infection can sometimes develop in one
of the arm's bones as a consequence of a
serious fracture or a blood infection
(see **Osteomyelitis**).

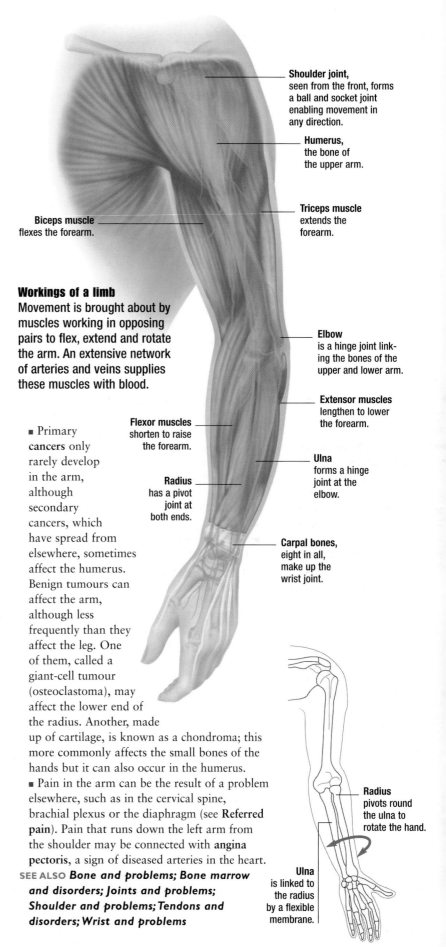

Shoulder joint,
seen from the front, forms
a ball and socket joint
enabling movement in
any direction.

Humerus,
the bone of
the upper arm.

Triceps muscle
extends the
forearm.

Biceps muscle
flexes the forearm.

Elbow
is a hinge joint link-
ing the bones of the
upper and lower arm.

Extensor muscles
lengthen to lower
the forearm.

Ulna
forms a hinge
joint at the
elbow.

Carpal bones,
eight in all,
make up the
wrist joint.

Flexor muscles
shorten to raise
the forearm.

Radius
has a pivot
joint at
both ends.

Radius
pivots round
the ulna to
rotate the hand.

Ulna
is linked to
the radius
by a flexible
membrane.

Workings of a limb
Movement is brought about by
muscles working in opposing
pairs to flex, extend and rotate
the arm. An extensive network
of arteries and veins supplies
these muscles with blood.

■ Primary
cancers only
rarely develop
in the arm,
although
secondary
cancers, which
have spread from
elsewhere, sometimes
affect the humerus.
Benign tumours can
affect the arm,
although less
frequently than they
affect the leg. One
of them, called a
giant-cell tumour
(osteoclastoma), may
affect the lower end of
the radius. Another, made
up of cartilage, is known as a chondroma; this
more commonly affects the small bones of the
hands but it can also occur in the humerus.
■ Pain in the arm can be the result of a problem
elsewhere, such as in the cervical spine,
brachial plexus or the diaphragm (see **Referred
pain**). Pain that runs down the left arm from
the shoulder may be connected with **angina
pectoris**, a sign of diseased arteries in the heart.
SEE ALSO **Bone and problems; Bone marrow
and disorders; Joints and problems;
Shoulder and problems; Tendons and
disorders; Wrist and problems**

Arteries and disorders

As a whole, our arteries constitute a branching system of tubes that carries blood to every tissue in the body. The main arterial 'tree' transports oxygenated blood; the much smaller pulmonary artery picks up blood that has returned to the heart, taking it to the lungs to collect more oxygen.

The **aorta** is the trunk of the arterial tree. Smaller arteries branch off and subdivide until they become arterioles, which are less than 0.1mm in diameter and flow into the blood vessels (capillaries) that supply individual cells. Arterioles receive their own supply of oxygen from the blood they carry; larger arteries are supplied from outside by small arterial 'twigs'.

Muscles in the artery walls contract or relax to control the diameter of the arteries and regulate the blood flow. Sometimes this muscle layer or the artery lining may become stiff or damaged and the arteries may narrow, causing conditions such as aneurysm, arteriosclerosis and arteritis.

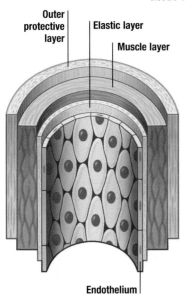

Outer protective layer **Elastic layer** **Muscle layer** **Endothelium**

▲ **Inside a healthy artery**
An artery's inner lining, or endothelium, is enclosed by an elastic layer, a smooth muscle layer (which regulates blood flow) and an outer protective layer.

Arterial aneurysm

Arterial **aneurysm** is a condition in which weakness, then a swelling, develops in an arterial wall. The aorta is most commonly affected, but aneurysms can affect arteries supplying the brain, limbs or internal organs. The main cause is arteriosclerosis, but infection, sudden physical injury, surgery or congenital abnormalities can also trigger an aneurysm.

SYMPTOMS

There may be no symptoms, but seek medical help urgently if you suffer signs of leaking or rupture (bursting) of the artery, such as collapse and shock, or a tearing pain in the chest, abdomen or back. Medical advice should also be sought if you experience:
- painless swelling in the abdomen, neck, arm or leg, which pulses in time to the heartbeat;
- symptoms due to pressure such as abdominal pain, difficulty in swallowing or headaches.

TREATMENT

A leaking aneurysm is a life-threatening condition that requires emergency hospital admission. In less urgent cases, a doctor may arrange tests and set up monitoring procedures.

What a doctor may do
- Check for and, if necessary, treat diabetes, hypertension or raised **cholesterol**.
- Examine the artery by ultrasound, magnetic resonance imaging (MRI) or angiography.

- Monitor the growth of an aneurysm using ultrasound every 6–12 months. Surgery may be needed if an abdominal aortic aneurysm grows larger than 5.5cm (2in) in diameter.
- Advise on changes to a patient's lifestyle that should reduce the risk of further damage.

Surgical options

Surgery can take one of several forms.
- The diseased artery may be bypassed using a section of vein or synthetic tubing.
- A polyester fibre lining tube may be inserted into the artery to provide a new 'inner tube'. In the case of an abdominal aortic aneurysm, a Y-shaped tube is used where the aorta divides into the iliac arteries.
- An endarterectomy may be performed to correct an abdominal aortic aneurysm. This involves reconstruction of the aorto-iliac segment of artery after removal of the diseased section and most of the artery lining.

COMPLICATIONS

The most serious risk posed by an aneurysm is rupture. Sometimes a rupture is incomplete and occurs between the inner and outer layers of the arterial wall. Another possible complication is arterial thrombosis.

PREVENTION

Adopting a healthier lifestyle reduces the chance of further damage (see arteriosclerosis, below).

Abdominal aortic aneurysm affects up to 10,000 people a year in the UK, mostly men over the age of 60. Those at particular risk should have regular ultrasound screening. They include people with a father or brother who has suffered aortic aneurysm, arteriosclerosis, hypertension or ischaemic heart disease.

Arterial thrombosis

Arterial thrombosis is a condition in which an artery becomes blocked, cutting off the blood supply to body organs or tissues. The affected organ or tissue may become damaged or even die. Thrombosis occurs if the blood flows too slowly or clots too easily, and is often the final result of narrowing and hardening of the artery.

Arteriosclerosis

Arteriosclerosis – also known as atherosclerosis – develops over many years. It is a significant cause of heart attacks, strokes and circulatory and memory problems.

As the condition evolves, fatty streaks appear on the artery linings and progress to become fibrous cholesterol-containing plaques (raised circular areas), reducing the diameter of the arteries. The artery walls gradually stiffen – a process called hardening of the arteries – and organs or limbs can become starved of oxygen and other nutrients, leading to permanent

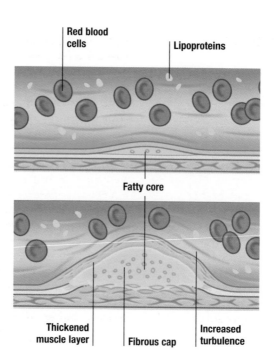

Red blood cells

Lipoproteins

Fatty core

Thickened muscle layer | Fibrous cap | Increased turbulence

► **Narrowing and stiffening**
If an artery's inner wall is damaged, fats, heavy metals, clotting agents and blood cells all stick to the affected area. The immune system tries to heal the wound and to form a cap of fibrous material, or plaque. Buildup of plaque narrows the artery.

damage. Weak points (aneurysms) or blockages (thromboses) may also develop. If the arteries in the neck are arteriosclerotic, the oxygen supply to the brain may be affected, especially when the neck is turned, leading to dizziness.

SYMPTOMS
Arteriosclerosis affects most people by late middle-age, but it has no symptoms until complications such as angina or stroke develop.

TREATMENT
If you consult a doctor about the condition, your **blood pressure** will be checked and the levels of cholesterol and sugar in your blood will be measured. Drugs may be prescribed to reduce blood pressure or levels of cholesterol or blood sugar.

What you can do
Complications associated with arteriosclerosis can be delayed or prevented by making changes to your lifestyle that will reduce health risks. These may include:
■ losing weight and eating a low-fat diet that includes cholesterol-lowering foods;
■ stopping smoking;
■ restricting alcohol consumption to 21–28 units per week for men and 14–21 for women;
■ a brisk 20 minute walk five times a week;
■ lowering stress levels;
■ having regular blood pressure checks.

Complementary therapies
Fenugreek seeds are thought to lower sugar and cholesterol levels, improving circulation.

Arteriovenous fistula

Arteriovenous fistula is a disorder in which an artery drains directly into a vein. The abnormal connection (fistula) causes swollen veins and may deprive the rest of the artery of blood, reducing oxygen supply. If excessive blood is diverted through the fistula, heart failure can develop and the artery may need to be blocked using a tiny coil or plug. It may be congenital or the result of injury or disease.

Arteritis

In arteritis the muscle wall of one or more of the large, mdium or small arteries becomes inflamed, causing narrowing and reduced blood flow. Symptoms include pain and tenderness of the affected skin region – the fingers, for example – or internal organ such as the aorta.

The cause is often unclear, although damage to the artery's own blood supply may be to blame. Arteritis is sometimes linked with diseases such as rheumatoid arthritis or immune system malfunction – in polyarteritis nodosa, for instance. In people with polyarteritis nodosa, the medium-sized arteries become inflamed, reducing blood supply and causing damage to the organs; symptoms include abdominal and testicular pain, chest pain, breathing difficulty or tender lumps under the skin, depending on which organs are affected.

In temporal arteritis, which affects older people, scalp arteries become inflamed, causing headaches and tenderness; this can spread to retinal arteries, causing blindness if not treated.

Treatment of arteritis with anti-inflammatory drugs including steroids is often successful, but lifestyle changes, especially stopping **smoking**, are important in preventing further artery damage. Damaged organs such as the heart or kidney may require additional treatment.

Peripheral arterial disease

In peripheral arterial disease the blood supply to a limb or tissue is reduced or cut off, leading to blood and oxygen shortage (ischaemia). It is commonly caused by a gradual narrowing of the artery. Total blockage may suddenly occur in the form of arterial thrombosis, or a blood clot may break off and travel to block another artery (embolism). Ischaemia may also develop after sudden physical injury, including surgery.

SYMPTOMS
■ A cramp-like pain, which is worse when oxygen demands are high but disappears after rest – for example, in the calf muscles on walking. Pain at rest indicates severe ischaemia.
■ Cold, pale feet or toes that turn blue.
■ Gradual or sudden tissue damage in the legs (leg ulcers, gangrene), heart (angina), brain (stroke) or internal organs.
■ Sudden severe pain in an arm or leg, which turns cold and white.
■ Severe pain in the chest, abdomen or back.

TREATMENT

If you have any of the above symptoms, consult a doctor; if pain is sudden and severe, seek medical advice urgently. If arterial aneurysm, thrombosis, embolism or severe ischaemia is suspected, you will need surgery or treatment to break up clots. In less urgent cases, a doctor may arrange tests and monitoring procedures.

What a doctor may do

■ Check for and, if necessary, treat diabetes, hypertension or raised cholesterol.
■ Measure the arterial pressure in your legs using Doppler ultrasound.
■ Refer you for ultrasound, angiography or magnetic resonance imaging (MRI).
■ Advise you on beneficial lifestyle changes.
■ Prescribe a daily dose of 75mg aspirin.

Surgical options

Surgery may take one of several forms, such as:
■ angioplasty – artery widening or repair;
■ grafting – replacement of diseased section of leg artery with part of another artery or vein;
■ sympathectomy – keyhole surgery or chemical injection that severs the nerves in the back that control leg artery diameter;
■ amputation of foot or leg if gangrene occurs.

COMPLICATIONS

Poor oxygen supply to the legs may lead to leg ulcers. In more serious cases there is a risk of gangrene – and of failure of part or all of a body organ due to lack of oxygen.

PREVENTION

Adopt a healthier lifestyle. Avoid dehydration and prolonged sitting or kneeling, which encourage blood clotting.

Raynaud's syndrome

In Raynaud's syndrome spasm of small arteries, usually in the fingers, produces colour changes – paleness followed by blueness then redness – as well as numbness and sometimes pain.

Raynaud's syndrome may occur as a result of scleroderma, an autoimmune disease causing the skin to thicken, swell and scar on the hands and feet, which become stiff, tight and shiny; ulceration and even gangrene may develop.

Treatment consists of wearing warm or artificially heated gloves and clothing. Drugs such as nifedipine are used to dilate the arterioles. It is important to stop smoking.

Takayasu's disease

Takayasu's disease is a condition of unknown cause in which inflammation and thrombosis in the aorta and other arteries lead to reduced pulses in the limbs, dizziness, raised blood pressure and aortic and other aneurysms. It is also known as 'pulseless disease' and is treated with corticosteroids and arterial surgery.

Arthritis

Eight million people in the UK suffer from some form of arthritis, with pain, stiffness, swelling and loss of mobility in affected joints.

Although arthritis is widespread – about one-fifth of visits to doctors in the UK are arthritis-related – there is an increasingly optimistic outlook for sufferers. Arthritic disease takes many forms, and varies enormously in the severity of its symptoms. But the treatments to alleviate it are becoming ever more effective. For example, lost mobility can now be restored by replacing damaged joints with artificial ones made from alloys of steel and plastics that do not react to the body's tissues or provoke rejection by the immune system.

Shoulders, elbows, hips and knees can all be successfully replaced. Replacement of finger joints in people who were previously unable to open their hands has proved so effective that in some cases, after recovering from surgery, they are able to thread needles.

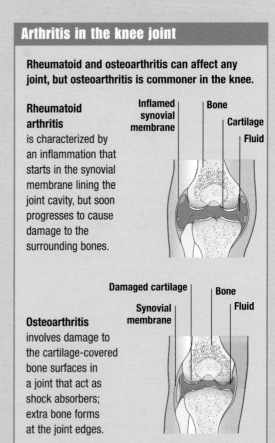

Arthritis in the knee joint

Rheumatoid and osteoarthritis can affect any joint, but osteoarthritis is commoner in the knee.

Rheumatoid arthritis is characterized by an inflammation that starts in the synovial membrane lining the joint cavity, but soon progresses to cause damage to the surrounding bones.

Inflamed synovial membrane — Bone — Cartilage — Fluid

Osteoarthritis involves damage to the cartilage-covered bone surfaces in a joint that act as shock absorbers; extra bone forms at the joint edges.

Damaged cartilage — Bone — Synovial membrane — Fluid

RHEUMATOID AND OSTEOARTHRITIS

Two widespread forms of arthritis, rheumatoid arthritis and osteoarthritis, are chronic disorders that are unlikely to go away once established – as opposed to some other types, such as reactive arthritis, which do not persist and can often go away on their own. Both rheumatoid and osteoarthritis, typically, have 'flare-ups', interrupted by periods of remission that bring spontaneous relief from pain.

Rheumatoid arthritis, which affects about one in 100 people in the UK, is a painful, progressive, inflammatory condition. Joints in the fingers, wrists, knees and shoulders are the most likely to become inflamed. Rheumatoid arthritis can also cause skin lumps (nodules) and damage to the lungs and eyes.

The first signs of the disease are joint pains and stiffness and an under-the-weather feeling, beginning usually between the ages of 30 and 50, although it can strike at any time of life.

Inflammation starts in the lining of the joint (synovium), but it often leads on to damage to the surrounding bones – which is why it is essential to begin treatment early. Treatment focuses on controlling inflammation, alleviating pain and reducing complications. It may involve anti-inflammatory drugs, physiotherapy, exercise and in some cases joint-replacement surgery.

The cause of rheumatoid arthritis is unknown, but it is thought that the body's immune system turns against the tissue and bone in the joint and starts to attack them. As the disease sometimes run in families, it may have a genetic element.

By contrast, osteoarthritis is a degenerative condition with a 'wear-and-tear' element – the protective, shock-absorbing cartilage space between the bones of the joints wears away with age, and new spurs of bone often form at the edges of the joint. Starting from mid-life, osteoarthritis affects mainly the hip, knees, spine and fingers, but can occur in any joint. Abnormal stress, injury to a joint, or obesity, which places extra weight on a joint, may cause the disease to develop.

In more than 50 per cent of osteoarthritis cases, there is remission of pain for many years after an initial painful period.

OTHER FORMS OF ARTHRITIS

There are several other common inflammatory types of the disease, which include:
- reactive arthritis, which can develop after a viral or bacterial infection somewhere else in the body;
- septic arthritis, where there is a viral, bacterial or fungal infection at a joint site;
- gout, where an excess of uric acid leads to inflammation in the toe joint, for example.

▶ Joint distortion
This X-ray of a hand affected by rheumatoid arthritis shows the distortion of the knuckle bones caused by inflammation of the joints.

These varieties of arthritis strike intermittently. Chronic types include connective tissue diseases such as systemic lupus erythematosus, and ankylosing spondylitis, involving inflammation and fusing of the lower vertebrae in the spine.

DIAGNOSING ARTHRITIS

Differing symptoms offer clues for distinguishing between one form of arthritis and another. A general feeling of malaise and severe flare-ups are pointers to rheumatoid arthritis, for example.

If an arthritic condition is suspected, doctors can use X-rays and magnetic resonance imaging (MRI) scans to confirm a diagnosis. Blood tests are carried out to show up a specific condition and to identify or eliminate other diseases.

Management of any chronic arthritic disease is a team job involving GPs, rheumatologists, orthopaedic surgeons, physiotherapists and occupational therapists.

TREATMENT

If you have pain, swelling or stiffness that continues for more than six weeks, consult a doctor and ask to be referred to a rheumatologist.

Most arthritic diseases can be effectively controlled and alleviated by modern treatment. As both severity of symptoms and symptoms themselves vary greatly from person to person, treatment needs to be tailored to each individual.

While the pain of rheumatoid arthritis tends to be worst in the morning, the pain of osteoarthritis gets worse as the day goes on.

Different types of arthritic disease

X-rays and MRI scans can confirm a diagnosis of arthritis. Blood tests are used to identify specific conditions such as rheumatoid arthritis.

DISORDER	DISTINGUISHING FEATURES
Inflammatory types such as rheumatoid arthritis, septic arthritis and gout	The joint lining becomes inflamed. This can damage the surface of the joint and underlying bone
Rheumatoid arthritis	A chronic (recurring) autoimmune disease
Reactive arthritis	Develops after viral or bacterial infection has occurred somewhere else in the body
Septic arthritis	Viral, bacterial or fungal infection at joint site. Treated with intravenous antibiotics
Gout	Excess uric acid causes inflammation in toe joint. An inherited condition that comes and goes
Pseudogout	Calcium crystals form, usually on the knee
Ankylosing spondylitis	Inflammation and fusing of lower vertebrae in spine
Psoriatic arthritis	Associated with psoriasis or colitis
Connective tissue diseases	Include systemic lupus erythematosus
Cervical spondylosis	Spurs of bone form on the neck vertebrae
Polyarteritis nodosa	Rare form of vasculitis, inflammation of medium and small arteries, with impaired circulation. Cause unknown
Osteoarthritis	The cartilage becomes thinner and damaged and extra bone forms at the edges of the joint. Can occur in any joint. Chronic. The immune system is not involved

There are more than 2 million people with osteoarthritis in the UK. More women than men suffer from the disease.

Appropriate drugs and **complementary therapies** combined with **physiotherapy** to help improve movement and instruction on how to protect the joints can often restore sufferers to full lives and minimize their discomfort. If there is severe joint damage and resultant disability, surgery may prove necessary to replace the damaged joint.

Arthritis drugs

A wide range of drugs is used to treat the symptoms and slow progression of the nany forms of arthritic disease.

■ Analgesics such as paracetamol reduce pain.

■ Non-steroidal anti-inflammatory drugs (NSAIDs) reduce swelling and stiffness, and alleviate pain. But they can also irritate the stomach lining so no one should take NSAIDs for more than three days unless under medical supervision. Taking NSAIDs over a long period of time can lead to chronic bleeding ulcers, which can be fatal. About 2000 people die from NSAIDs in the UK every year.

■ Used early in the development of rheumatoid arthritis, some drugs can slow the progression of the condition. Anti-rheumatic drugs such as the immunosuppressant methotrexate and the anti-inflammatory sulfasalazine can be used on a long-term basis. Gold salts, penicillamine and choroquine may work by suppressing the disease process itself.

■ Steroids are powerful anti-inflammatory agents that can be injected or taken in tablet form.

Breakthrough treatments

■ People with rheumatoid arthritis have an excessive amount of the protein TNF (tumour necrosis factor) in their blood and joints. Drugs are available to block the action of TNF, reducing inflammation. Such immunosuppressive drugs are prescribed when standard treatments have not been effective.

■ A new generation of NSAIDs have been developed that have a stronger anti-inflammatory effect than their predecessors, but are less likely to cause intestinal irritation. Hyaluronic acid and derivatives are new non-steroidal drugs that, when injected into the knee joint, temporarily reduce pain and inflammation.

■ Clinical trials are underway to investigate a drug regime that targets the B-cells – the white blood cells that can accidentally make antibodies that destroy healthy tissue.

Complementary therapies

■ The food supplements glucosamine sulphate and fish oil have been proven to have mild anti-inflammatory effects.

■ Warmth may ease pain in osteoarthritic fingers. A cold compress may ease an inflamed joint.

■ For rheumatoid arthritis, try taking two teaspoons of apple cider vinegar in some hot water, twice a day. This can be sweetened with honey to taste, if preferred.

ARTHRITIS IN CHILDREN

One child in 1000 has arthritis. The condition occurs most often at ages 1–4 years, and again at 10–13 years. To counter confusion of names and various presentations of arthritic disease in children, the accepted term in the UK for childhood arthritis is now 'juvenile idiopathic arthritis' ('idiopathic' means 'without clear external cause').

Symptoms are varied and can be confused with other conditions – for example, initially there may be a fever, swollen glands and general aching. Seek out full investigation and careful diagnosis. Treatment involves removal of fluid from the affected joints, drugs such as anti-inflammatories or steroid injections. Regular, gentle exercise often helps to keep joints flexible.

Arthroplasty

An arthroplasty is an operation in which a joint is repaired or replaced to improve its function. One of the most common types of arthroplasty is a hip-joint replacement, in which the hip joint (usually damaged by **arthritis**) is replaced with a new artificial joint.

Asbestosis

Asbestosis is a lung disease caused by inhaling asbestos fibres. It is characterized by scarring of the lung tissue. The main symptoms are shortness of breath, a persistent cough and, less commonly, chest pains. The onset of symptoms can occur between 10 and 40 years after exposure to asbestos. People suffering from asbestosis are more at risk of developing lung cancers and up to 55 times more at risk if they also smoke.

The use of asbestos was regulated in the UK in the early 1970s, but because the symptoms take so many years to develop some 3000 people a year are still dying of asbestosis.

SEE ALSO *Lungs and disorders*

Ascites

Ascites is an abnormal buildup of fluid in the abdominal cavity causing swelling and discomfort. Sufferers may feel short of breath, lose their appetite or regurgitate their food. The most common cause of ascites is cirrhosis of the liver, but other causes include heart failure, kidney disease, pancreatic disease, tuberculosis and some cancers.

To diagnose ascites, a doctor will remove some of the fluid with a needle and send it for analysis or recommend an **ultrasound** scan. Treatment often includes bed rest and a low-salt diet. Diuretics, which make the kidneys excrete more fluid in the urine, can also be used. Ascites sufferers who have liver disease must not drink alcohol.

SEE ALSO *Abdominal pain*

Asperger's syndrome

Asperger's syndrome is a type of **autism** in which social intelligence is severely impaired. People with this condition show normal or even exceptional intelligence in areas that do not involve social interaction. However, they lack 'theory of mind' – the ability to know intuitively what is going on in another person's thoughts – and tend to be very literal-minded. As a result, Asperger's sufferers are very poor at recognizing signs of emotion, which makes them appear insensitive.

In common with other forms of autism, Asperger's syndrome is marked by a rigid adherence to routine and attention to detail. People with Asperger's syndrome are therefore often very good at repetitive tasks requiring high degrees of accuracy.

Aspergillosis

Aspergillosis is an infection of the lungs and airways caused by aspergillus, a fungus that grows on decaying vegetation. While harmless to healthy people, aspergillus may worsen the symptoms of people with **asthma**. It may also lead to inflammation of the lungs and recurrent chest infections.

Aspergillosis can cause a fungus ball to form in people whose lungs have been damaged by tuberculosis, causing them to cough up blood. The disease can be fatal in people with impaired immune systems and those who have undergone transplant operations.

Aspergillosis can be diagnosed by skin or blood tests. It is treated by antifungal drugs and, where appropriate, anti-asthma drugs.

Aspermia

Aspermia, also called azoospermia, is a condition in which the semen contains no sperm. It is generally considered to affect 1 per cent of men in the UK, but research into falling sperm counts suggests the actual rate may be higher.

Aspermia may be genetic in origin or the result of a disease such as cystic fibrosis. In such cases, the condition is rarely treatable. It may be treatable where the cause is a sexually transmitted disease, tuberculosis or the failure of puberty to take place properly. Some cancer treatments may also cause temporary aspermia. In a vasectomy, aspermia is the desired result (see **Sterilization**).

More common is oligospermia, a condition where the ejaculate contains fewer sperm than normal (see **Reproductive system**).

Asthma

Asthma may occur at any age and vary in severity. Some people have infrequent attacks and feel fine in between them; others have to take drugs daily, usually by inhalation, to suppress symptoms.

Asthma attacks can make people feel as if they are suffocating. As they struggle to draw breath through narrowed airways in their lungs, they inhale in short gasps and exhale in long, noisy wheezes. The lower ribcage may contract sharply on inhaled breaths, and the pulse races; in a severe attack, the sufferer's lips may turn blue from loss of oxygen.

Asthma is a condition in which the lining of the airways supplying the lungs swells, restricting air flow and making it hard to breathe. During an attack the airways become narrower; often sticky mucus or phlegm is produced. Sufferers have hypersensitive airways, which are almost always red and slightly inflamed. This means that their lungs are vulnerable to any of a wide range of irritants, including pollen, feathered and furred animals (particularly cats), aspirin and some other drugs, the droppings of house-dust mites, changes in temperature (for example, breathing in very cold air) and cigarette smoke. Some attacks are triggered by non-environmental factors such as respiratory infections, stress, anxiety or exercise.

A GROWING PROBLEM

An estimated 150 million people worldwide suffer from asthma, and every year asthma and other respiratory diseases are becoming more common globally. There are many theories about why the number of asthma cases is rising, but none is free of controversy.

The tendency to develop allergic conditions, such as **hay fever**, allergic asthma and **eczema**, often runs in families. If one or both parents suffer from asthma, hay fever or eczema, the chance of their children developing one of these conditions is higher. Scientists are searching for a genetic link in the hope of developing gene therapy to treat the condition.

Common asthma triggers include viral infections, allergies, irritants and exercise. A third of children who suffer from asthma improve during their teenage years, and have fewer symptoms in adult life.

Among new advances in combating asthma is a preventive injection developed in Switzerland. It is designed to be given every two to four weeks and take the place of existing drug treatments. The drug contains an antibody that can knock out the proteins which trigger allergic asthma attacks.

TREATMENT

Once asthma has been diagnosed, you are likely to be prescribed drugs to prevent or relieve asthma attacks. These are called preventers or relievers (see Drug treatments for asthma, right).

If you continue to have frequent attacks in spite of using an inhaler regularly, the doctor may prescribe additional tablets to be taken orally – for example, a short course of steroid tablets.

Medical terms

The peak-flow meter measures how fast and how hard you can exhale air from your lungs. This is an indication of how well controlled your asthma is – you cannot blow hard when your airways are inflamed. Your peak-flow reading, when compared with levels set by your doctor or with previous readings, can often predict an asthma attack, even a day or two in advance.

Self-help
Action in an attack

The symptoms of asthma are wheezing or whistling in the chest, shortness of breath, a tight feeling in the chest and coughing (dry or with mucus). Consult a doctor if you have any of these symptoms or if your sleep is being disturbed because of breathing difficulties or coughing. If you have an attack, take the following steps:

■ Take two puffs of your reliever inhaler immediately.

■ Try to stay calm and relaxed.

■ Sit in a position you find comfortable.

■ Try to slow your breathing down.

■ Call a doctor or ambulance if the inhaler has no effect after five to ten minutes, and keep using your inhaler every few minutes until help arrives.

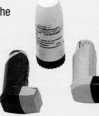

Emergency Symptoms of a severe attack are blue lips, clammy skin, a rapid pulse and gasping for breath. Severe attacks require emergency medical attention.

Drug treatments for asthma

Most people with asthma breathe in the medication they need using an inhaler. Two main types of drugs are taken using inhalers: preventers and relievers.

People use relievers, which usually come in blue inhalers, when they are suffering an asthma attack. Relievers relax the muscles surrounding the airways – the drugs should start to ease your breathing in a few minutes and the relief should last up to four hours. Preventers make the airways less sensitive, reducing the chance of symptoms developing. Preventers should be used every day, usually once in the morning and once in the evening, even if you are feeling well. They generally come in white, brown, orange or red inhalers.

Some people use spacers when taking their asthma medication with inhalers. Spacers are large plastic containers with a mouthpiece at one end and a connection to the inhaler at the other. You can release the medication into the spacer and breathe it in when you are ready or in a number of short breaths rather than one large breath. People who have had to go to the doctor's surgery or hospital accident and emergency department with a severe asthma attack will probably be familiar with the nebuliser – a machine that pumps out a medicated mist that you can breathe in through a mask. At one time the nebuliser was always used to treat severe asthma attacks, but many doctors now report that the latest designs of inhaler and spacer are just as effective as the nebuliser. Nebulisers are still used to treat some elderly or very young people who cannot hold an inhaler.

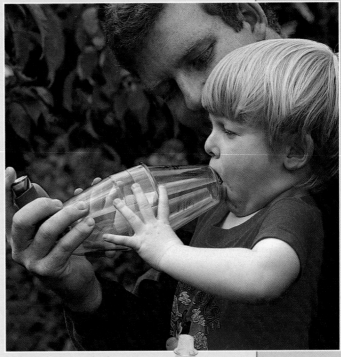

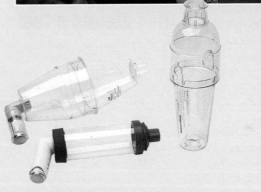

DIETARY SUPPLEMENTS
People with asthma should never stop taking prescribed drugs except on medical advice, but in some cases it may help to take vitamin C supplements as well. Some studies have suggested that a balanced diet with plenty of fruit and vegetables protects against asthma and some other lung diseases. It is also suggested that eating more of certain types of foods and increasing consumption of foods containing vitamin C, magnesium and fish oils (Omega-3 fatty acids) can improve symptoms.

LIVING WITH ASTHMA
The substances that trigger asthma attacks vary from one person to another. If you have asthma, you will be less vulnerable to an attack if you can identify your triggers and avoid them. There are many other ways in which you can make the condition easier to live with.

■ Keep your home clear of dust and pollen.
■ Avoid tobacco smoke.
■ Avoid cats; their fur is highly allergenic.
■ Managing stress and remaining calm helps to reduce the incidence of asthma attacks.
■ Treat colds and flu promptly to reduce the chances of an attack.
■ In winter, wear a scarf over your mouth and nose and breathe through the fabric to warm the cold air.
■ Keep an asthma diary to help you to determine your asthma triggers and control your asthma.
■ Regular exercise, especially swimming, is generally beneficial for people with asthma, but in some people exercise or other exertions can trigger an attack.
■ Some people with asthma find yoga and relaxation techniques beneficial in reducing asthma symptoms.
SEE ALSO ***Respiratory system***

Astigmatism

Astigmatism is an optical defect of the eye that causes sufferers to see objects distorted in size or leaning to one side. This usually occurs because the cornea of one or both eyes is unusually shaped.

Most astigmatism is present from early life; the degree of abnormality usually increases as the eye grows. The condition may also occur as a consequence of injury, certain diseases (especially those of the cornea) or ophthalmic surgery. A swelling in the lid such as a chalazion pressing upon the eye may cause astigmatism; in such cases, the astigmatism resolves once the lesion has been treated. Spectacles or contact lenses can effectively correct the symptoms of astigmatism in the majority of cases.

SEE ALSO **Eye and problems**

Ataxia

Ataxia means loss of physical coordination. It may be caused by a developmental defect such as **cerebral palsy**. Another possible cause is injury to the cerebellum, the part of the brain that controls movement, or to the connections between that area and those that execute movements. An ataxic person retains the power to make normal movements, but is unable to control them. So, for example, an affected person might be able to grip an object firmly but be unable to manipulate it. Dyspraxia is a mild form of the condition, which is manifested as clumsiness or lack of coordination.

SEE ALSO **Brain and nervous system**

Atheroma

In atheroma, deposits of **cholesterol** and blood cells develop on the artery walls. The walls then become hard and rigid and the deposits enlarge into raised circular areas, called plaques. The artery eventually becomes narrowed or blocked. If a crack or fissure forms in a plaque, a blood clot may develop inside the artery. This is an arterial thrombosis, which may break away, leading to **stroke** or **coronary thrombosis.**

Atheroma affects most people by late middle-age, but causes no symptoms until it reaches the stage when the narrowing of an artery interferes with the circulation of the blood. Symptoms then depend on the part of the body affected. Complications such as heart attacks, strokes and circulatory problems can be delayed or prevented by adopting a healthier lifestyle.

SEE ALSO **Arteries and disorders**

Athetosis

Athetosis is the name given to involuntary slow writhing movements. These usually affect the hands and feet, but sometimes involve either one entire side of the body or all of it.

The movements are thought to be reflex actions – alternate grasping and avoidance moves. They occur as a result of damage to, or degeneration of, nerves in the brain that normally prevent them. Such movements tend to increase when the individuals affected are excited or under stress, and to diminish or disappear when they are relaxed or asleep. They may include:
- clenching and unclenching of the fists;
- facial grimaces;
- repeated swallowing;
- hand-wringing;
- writhing of the limbs.

The condition is usually associated with **cerebral palsy**, but drugs used to alleviate the symptoms of **Parkinson's disease** may bring some relief to sufferers.

Athlete's foot

Athlete's foot is a highly contagious **fungal infection** of the foot, which, despite its name, is not confined to athletes.

The infection is caused by a fungus known as *Tinea pedis*, which thrives in moist, warm areas of skin. It is easily spread wherever people walk barefoot – for example, in communal changing areas and showers, and in the bathroom at home. It can also be spread by sharing towels or shoes.

More than 10 per cent of people in the UK are thought to be suffering from athlete's foot at any one time.

SYMPTOMS

The infection most often starts between the little toe and the one next to it, but it can spread around the foot and include the toenails. It is characterized by:
- skin irritation and itching;
- red, raw patches of skin between the toes;
- an unpleasant smell;
- damp and soggy skin that may also crack, flake, bleed and become quite painful.

TREATMENT

The milder, most common form of athlete's foot can easily be treated at home.

What you can do

The important thing is to keep your feet clean: wash them carefully every day and dry them thoroughly after a bath or shower, especially between the toes. In addition:

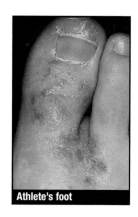

Athlete's foot

▲ **Itchy toes**
Athlete's foot, which usually begins between the toes, is the most common fungal infection of the skin.

■ apply an over-the-counter antifungal cream, spray, liquid or powder to the affected area. Since the fungus burrows deep into the skin, make sure that you continue the treatment for at least ten days after all visible signs of infection have disappeared;

■ wear cotton socks and change them every day, or more frequently if they become damp. Wear open-toed shoes whenever possible;

■ never share towels or shoes; always wear flip-flops in communal changing areas or showers;

■ clean and thoroughly rinse out the bath or shower after use.

When to consult a doctor

Consult a doctor if the infection does not respond to self-help treatment or if it spreads to the nails and other parts of the body. The doctor may prescribe an antifungal cream or, if the infection has spread, an oral medication.

Complementary therapies

Tea tree oil has been shown to be effective in combating athlete's foot. Apply the oil neat to the affected area with a cotton bud, or soak the feet in a basin of water containing a few drops of the oil.

PREVENTION

Maintain good foot hygiene (see What you can do, left) and always wear flip-flops in communal changing rooms and showers.

COMPLICATIONS

If left untreated, athlete's foot can spread to other parts of the body, including the toenails, which turn yellowish brown and become brittle and difficult to cut. If the fungus spreads to the groin, it is known as 'jock itch'.

OUTLOOK

While treatment for athlete's foot is usually effective, reinfection is common, and following preventive measures is recommended.

Atrial fibrillation and flutter

Atrial fibrillation is a condition in which the conduction of electrical impulses through the upper chambers of the heart (the atria) is disordered and chaotic. This leads to an irregular contraction of the lower pumping chambers of the heart (the ventricles). In atrial flutter the atria contract very fast and regularly.

Both conditions reduce the heart's pumping efficiency. They become more common with age, affecting one person in 20 by the age of 75, and may be temporary, lifelong or intermittent.

SYMPTOMS

There may be no symptoms at all or the affected person may experience palpitations, faintness, breathlessness or chest pain.

CAUSES

Atrial fibrillation and flutter often have no obvious cause, and can be brought on by an infection or by excessive alcohol consumption. Disorders that may be the underlying cause include heart disease, respiratory disease, hypertension (high blood pressure) and thyrotoxicosis (see **Thyroid and disorders**).

TREATMENT

Consult a doctor if you have any concerns.

What a doctor may do

Tests, medications and procedures to diagnose and treat the problem may include:

■ blood tests for heart or thyroid disease and for high blood cholesterol levels, which are a major risk factor for heart disease;

■ a chest **X-ray**, electrocardiogram (ECG) or echocardiogram, which involves the use of **ultrasound** to examine the heart;

■ drugs such as digoxin or amiodarone to slow down the heart rate or restore normal heart rhythm or aspirin or anticoagulants to reduce the risk of stroke;

■ cardioversion – a short electric shock treatment, administered under anaesthetic, which may restore normal heart rhythm.

COMPLICATIONS

Atrial fibrillation or flutter may lead to low blood pressure or heart failure. It may also cause strokes from clot formation in the heart.

SEE ALSO *Heart and circulatory system*

Autism

SEE PAGE 90

Autoimmune disease

An autoimmune disease is any disease resulting from a fault in the body's immune system that causes the immune system to attack healthy body tissues.

Some autoimmune diseases seem to occur when cells become altered, perhaps as a result of a **viral infection**, so that the immune system no longer recognizes the cells as part of its own body. Women are generally more likely than men to be affected.

Symptoms and treatment of autoimmune conditions vary according to the particular disease. For example, in the case of rheumatoid arthritis, the joints become extremely painful, stiff and deformed. A wide range of treatments can be prescribed, these include taking anti-inflammatory drugs; the immune system can be suppressed with corticosteroids or the use of still more powerful immunosuppressant drugs.

Autism

Some autistic people are severely disabled, others have above-average intelligence, but all share problems of social interaction and communication, especially when it comes to recognizing and responding to others' emotions.

To varying degrees, autistic people fail to respond to their surroundings or interact with others. There may be hints of the condition from a very early age. A baby may fail to assume the usual anticipatory posture when about to be picked up, for example, and may instead arch away from its mother's grasp and avoid eye contact. If autism is severe, it becomes obvious around the age of two or three, when most children begin to speak. People severely affected by autism do not develop speech and may appear not to understand what is said to them.

Another feature becomes clear around the age of four, when non-autistic children develop the ability to empathize with others by mentally putting themselves in another's place. This social skill never develops in autistic people, although some may learn to understand other people by deduction rather than by intuition. There are several other markers of childhood autism.

- Failure to indulge in 'pretend' play.
- Failure to join in communal games.
- Bizarre and obsessive interests, such as continuously rearranging or spinning objects.
- Preference for sameness – insisting on always taking the same route home or drinking from the same glass, for example.
- Greater interest in objects than people.
- Inability to deceive.
- Inability to understand metaphorical language, resulting in a literal interpretation of everything.

Autism is four times more likely to occur in boys than in girls.

VARIOUS DEGREES OF AUTISM

People who are severely affected by autism may not be able to speak and may appear entirely unresponsive to their surroundings. Some spend almost all their time carrying out a single stereotypical movement such as rocking back and forth or twirling a strand of hair. Others can speak but use words in a very concrete way – for naming objects rather than expressing thoughts. Repetition of words or phrases spoken by another person is common.

Some may have average or above-average intelligence, and may be distinguished only by their social awkwardness; these people have what is known as high-functioning autism. Autism was thought to affect about five children in 10,000, although recent estimates suggest a much higher incidence. However, it is not clear whether these figures signify a sudden increase in the disorder or are simply due to the fact that autism is becoming more widely recognized.

Case study
Understanding an autistic child

An autistic child who does not understand the function of communication becomes frustrated.

Jon, an autistic 12-year-old, loved biscuits. The boy could not speak, so his father taught him to ask for a biscuit by pointing to the tin. Shortly after this, his parents were distressed when Jon's behaviour worsened – several times a day, they found him in the kitchen screaming with anger. Eventually his father discovered what was happening: passing the kitchen window he looked in and saw Jon pointing to the biscuit tin even though he was alone in the room. His father watched as the boy stood there for minute after minute, becoming agitated and then furious. Although Jon had learned that pointing brought him a biscuit, he did not realize that this was because his action communicated a message to another person who then acted on it. Jon had no conception of other people's 'inner worlds' – so, when pointing in the absence of another person failed to get him the goods, he could not understand why his desire was thwarted, and he became angry.

Autistic savants

Some autistic people have astonishing skills in one area, despite having severe problems in everyday functioning.

For example, they may be able to add up huge sums at great speed, memorize telephone directories, or copy a complex image after a single glance.

These skills seem to be executed in an automatic way, without effort or imagination. They may be attributable to malfunction in parts of the brain that normally edit out excessively detailed information.

CAUSES

Autism is a neurodevelopmental disorder – that is, a condition caused by failure of normal brain growth rather than injury or other factors. There is a genetic component: if one child has autism, there is an increased likelihood of two to three per cent that a sibling will be affected. In boys, autistic symptoms may also be a feature of **Fragile X syndrome** – an inherited condition caused by a mutation on the X chromosome of either parent.

Women who contract infections such as rubella or cytomegalovirus during pregnancy have an increased likelihood of delivering an autistic child. The hereditary disorder tuberous sclerosis and the congenital disease **neurofibromatosis** have also been associated with autism, as have infantile conditions such as **febrile convulsions**.

Brain imaging and postmortem studies reveal subtle structural and functional abnormalities in the brains of autistic people, but the cause is not clear. One theory is that autism is caused by dysfunction in the frontal lobes of the brain, where data is combined in a way that makes it meaningful – for example, a house image is linked with its emotional associations to form the concept of 'home'. Autistic people are often unable to make such associations.

Some studies have suggested that the MMR vaccine may trigger the condition in some children, but the available evidence does not support this (see **Immunization**).

TREATMENT

There is no effective treatment for autism, but behavioural problems can be minimized with a consistent routine that increases security.

SEE ALSO *Asperger's syndrome; Brain and nervous system; Disability; Learning difficulties*

Ayurvedic medicine

Ayurvedic medicine has been practised for more than 2000 years on the Indian subcontinent, where it is still widely used. It is based on the idea that people can maintain good health through balancing physical, mental and spiritual energies in the body. This is done through lifestyle, diet and practices such as meditation and yoga.

Ayurvedic practitioners believe that illness occurs when the body gets out of balance. Herbal medicine, massage with therapeutic oils, and purification techniques, such as fasting and enemas, may be used to help to restore the body's equilibrium and bring it back to health.

THE ORTHODOX VIEW

In the West, Ayurvedic practitioners are not usually medical doctors although they may have trained for three or four years. The system tends to be used for chronic conditions such as arthritis, general debilitation, certain women's health problems, asthma and irritable bowel syndrome. Ayurvedic medicine is not widely accepted and is not available on the NHS.

What's involved

Ayurvedic diagnosis is based on the practitioner's assessment of the natural balance of your energies. The practitioner will:
■ question you closely about your lifestyle and diet, and take a full medical history;
■ observe you, taking note of your posture and facial expression;
■ check your pulses, tongue, skin, voice, abdomen, urine, stools and general appearance;
■ recommend changes to your diet and lifestyle;
■ carry out massage, purification techniques and other treatments.

▼ **Herbal healing**
Ayurvedic remedies are often based on herbs and are sold ready-prepared or tailored to the individual.

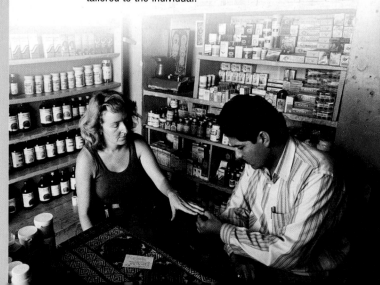

Babies and baby care

Caring for a newborn can be a challenging and even frightening experience, but the exciting developments in the first few months more than make up for the time and effort of early parenthood.

Adjusting to life with your baby is a gradual process that can make some parents feel inadequate at times, but you will gain confidence as your baby grows. In the first days and weeks after birth, regular home visits from a midwife and, later, a health visitor are a valuable source of support. More help and guidance can be found at the local child health clinic.

THE EARLY WEEKS

During the first few days after birth, babies are routinely tested for a metabolic disorder called phenylketonuria, which can cause brain damage if left untreated. The one-off test involves taking a small amount of blood from the baby's heel. Some babies, including those who are particularly heavy or light, are also tested for low blood sugar (hypoglycaemia), which can lead to fits. This test involves taking blood from the heel several times during the first 48 hours.

Several physical changes take place during the first weeks of life. For example, the cord shrivels up and, about ten days after birth, falls off. You will be advised how to keep the cord clean.

Most changes are perfectly normal but can be worrying – for example, blotches, spots or rashes may appear on the baby's skin, but these usually go away without treatment. Jaundice, resulting in yellowish skin, normally clears up after about a week. Do not hesitate to consult your midwife, health visitor or doctor if you have any concerns.

CARING FOR A NEWBORN BABY

Some mothers do not fall in love with their babies instantly. If you feel nothing for your baby at first, don't panic or feel guilty. Just give it time. However, if you feel depressed or are worried that you might harm your baby, it is vital to talk to your midwife, health visitor or doctor. They will help you and offer support, not criticize you.

SLEEPING

Babies vary in the amount of time they sleep. On average, new babies may be awake for eight hours a day, and they usually sleep in stretches of three to five hours. If you put your baby to sleep in the cot while still awake, he or she will learn to fall asleep unaided. Babies who are used to being nursed to sleep may later refuse to settle easily.

Always put your baby to sleep on his or her back instead of on their front or side. This practise has markedly reduced the incidence of cot death (**sudden infant death syndrome**).

CRYING

Babies tend to cry a lot in the early weeks of life because crying is the only way they can make their needs known. Gradually you will learn to distinguish between different cries – hunger, excessive heat or cold, a soiled nappy, loneliness, boredom, tiredness or overstimulation, and **colic**.

The most common reason for crying is hunger, which can be satisfied by a feed – but sometimes the baby cannot be pacified so easily. If the baby feels too hot or cold or is otherwise uncomfortable, being lifted up and comforted may be enough to restore equilibrium. When your baby is crying, follow your instinct and don't worry about 'spoiling' him or her if a cuddle is needed. Rhythmic movement or gentle massage may bring solace. Parents who respond quickly to their babies' cries have been shown to have babies who are more contented and secure.

If you feel your baby cries excessively or often appears to be in pain, seek medical advice.

Factfile
Premature babies

Babies born before the 37th week of pregnancy are described as premature. They are categorized in one of three weight groups:

- 1500–2499g (3lb 5oz–5lb 8oz): low birthweight.

- 1000–1500g (2lb 4oz–3lb 5oz): very low birthweight.

- Below 1000g (2lb 4oz): extremely low birthweight.

Most premature babies are initially cared for in hospital. You may feel helpless, but the hospital staff will be keen for you to visit frequently and to touch, hold and feed your baby. You will be encouraged to breastfeed, if you can, or to feed the baby with expressed breast milk. Breast milk is better-tolerated than formula milk, reduces the risk of infection and contains a host of important factors not found in formula milk.

Before your baby is discharged from hospital, you will be expected to take responsibility for his or her routine care. Your baby's development will be assessed from the expected date of delivery rather than the actual birth date, but immunizations will be given, as usual, at 8, 12 and 16 weeks from the date of birth.

Feeding your baby

Feeds are times to relax with your baby and help you both to learn about each other.

Only breast milk or formula milk made from modified cow's milk should be fed to a baby under one year old. Ordinary cow's milk or other milks such as condensed or goat's milk do not contain the right proportion of nutrients. Soya-milk formula should be used only on the advice of a health professional. A new baby, whether breastfed or bottle-fed, can take about six weeks, sometimes more, to settle into a feeding pattern.

BREASTFEEDING

Breastfeeding brings many benefits to mothers and babies. Not all mothers find it easy, but with calmness and perseverance most challenges can be overcome. Midwives, health visitors and breastfeeding counsellors can give support.

Learning how to 'latch on'

A baby who is not properly attached, or latched on, to the mother's breast will chew or suck on the nipple, which can lead to soreness and other problems. New mothers often need time, patience and practice to get the baby to latch on correctly.

■ Before starting a feed, get into a comfortable position, such as sitting on an upright chair with your feet raised on a cushion. You may need extra pillows to support your back and arms, or to place across your lap for the baby to lie on.

■ If you had stitches after the birth, sitting on a pillow may be more comfortable. If you had a Caesarean, you may want to feed while lying on your side.

■ With the baby's body facing your body, and the baby's head and shoulders at the same level as your nipple, take the baby to your breast (not your breast to the baby) and gently prompt him or her to open the mouth. It may help to support your breast from underneath with your free hand.

■ A properly positioned baby will take in a mouthful of breast, including the nipple and much of the underside of the areola (the dark area surrounding the nipple). You will be able to hear the baby swallowing, and see the ears move.

Breastfeeding challenges

Problems with breastfeeding are not inevitable and can often be prevented by correct positioning and feeding on demand.

The most common challenge is sore nipples, but occasionally other problems such as engorgement (hardening of the breasts), a blocked milk duct or mastitis can arise (see **Breasts and disorders**). In these cases, ask your doctor or health visitor for advice. If breastfeeding is well established and you experience sore nipples or sharp shooting pains in the breast, check your nipples for thrush.

Feeding facts

Breastfeeding, for just a few weeks or even days, is worthwhile for your baby.

How often should I breastfeed?

Feed on demand whenever your baby seems hungry, or feed (or express) when your breasts feel full. In the early days of a baby's life this may mean every two hours. Demand feeding also helps to prevent problems such as engorgement (hardness of the breasts).

How long should I feed for?

Don't limit or time feeds; if you do, your baby may not take in enough high-calorie hindmilk, which satisfies hunger and helps growth (as opposed to the watery foremilk, low in calories and fat, that gives a baby a drink at the start of a feed). Let your baby empty one breast completely before offering the other.

Can I build up my milk supply by offering formula?

On the contrary, the more you breastfeed the more milk your breasts make. If your baby seems hungry soon after feeding, check that he or she is latching on properly and feed more often.

Expressing breast milk

You may need or wish to express breast milk if:
■ your baby is in a special care unit;
■ your breasts are engorged;
■ you are going out for several hours and want someone else to feed your baby;
■ you are returning to work and want to build up a regular store of milk.

Your milk can be expressed straight into a sterile bottle, a sterile plastic container or breast-milk freezer bags. The expressed milk can then be safely stored in a fridge for 24 hours or frozen for up to three months.

You can express milk by hand or with a hand pump, a battery pump or an electric pump. Expressing milk may be hard at first but it gets easier with practice. Before buying a pump, borrow or hire one to make sure that it suits you. To express by hand, support your breast with one hand and stroke downwards from the top of your breast towards the areola with the other hand; squeeze the lower part of your breast with your thumb and

▼ Baby's pause
During a feed you'll notice that your baby takes a short natural break every so often, before starting to 'milk' the breast or suck the bottle's teat more strongly again.

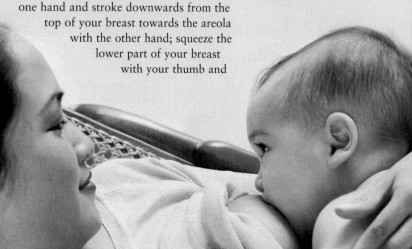

finger, pressing deeply to guide the milk out. Move your fingers and thumb progressively around the outside of your breasts.

BOTTLE-FEEDING FORMULA MILK
Follow the instructions on the packet and use the correct proportion of milk powder to water – otherwise the milk may be too weak or too concentrated. Bottles can be made up and kept in the fridge for 24 hours (discard unused feeds after 24 hours).

Test the temperature of the milk by shaking a couple of drops onto your wrist; it should feel just warm (not hot). Cuddle your baby and support his or her head and back with your arm as you gently insert the teat into the mouth.

After feeding, wash bottles and teats in warm soapy water and place them in a dishwasher – or, if your baby is less than six months old, sterilize them in a chemical solution or an electric steamer.

How much milk?
As a general guide, a baby needs about 150ml milk per kilogram body weight (2½ fl oz per 1lb body weight) per day. An easy way to calculate the correct amount in fluid ounces is to give about half your baby's body weight in pounds for each feed – for example, if your baby weighs 8lb, make up around 4fl oz of milk each feed. He or she will probably take more milk at some feeds and less at others. Never re-use leftover milk.

Feeding problems

Babies always swallow some air when they feed, and many bring up some milk with that air.

Wind If your baby suffers from wind, check that the teat hole in the bottle is not too large or too small. Make sure that the bottle is well tilted when feeding to stop air getting into the feed. Try not to let the baby wait too long for a feed: he or she may swallow air when crying. The best position for burping is over your shoulder – but protect your clothes with a rag.

Possetting Many babies bring back a small amount of milk after a feed; this is called possetting. If the baby is gaining weight, and the vomiting is non-forceful, don't worry. Possetting usually resolves itself once the baby is on solids.

Vomiting If your baby suffers from forceful or projectile vomiting, or appears to be in pain, always contact your doctor.

WEANING
Solid foods can be introduced gradually when your baby is between the ages of four and six months. By six months, a baby needs more iron and other nutrients than milk alone can provide. The aim at this stage is to introduce tastes and get the baby used to a spoon; first foods should be smooth and runny – baby rice or puréed fruit and vegetables, for example. There is no need to add sugar or salt to your baby's foods.

Once the baby is six months old, food should be mashed or minced to give a coarser texture – introducing soft lumps at this age encourages chewing and speech development and helps to avoid fussy eating later. If your baby is drinking less than 600ml (1 pint) of formula milk each day after the age of six months, or you are still breastfeeding, give him or her five drops of combined vitamins A, D and C daily.

Caring for your baby

Your baby relies on you to monitor and meet every need for warmth and comfort.

This small person, who has turned your world upside down, is, for now, completely helpless. But as you and your baby get to know each other, life will become easier and more predictable.

BATHING
You don't need to bath your baby daily. Instead you can 'top and tail' – that is, clean the face, ears, the skin folds of the neck and armpits and nappy area, exposing only the parts you are washing. Always make sure that your baby's skin is quite dry before putting any clothes on. It is easier to dress a baby on a changing table or bed rather than across your knee.

NAPPIES
You can use cloth or disposable nappies, or both. Cloth nappies are cheaper and softer than disposables, and they can be used many times. Disposable nappies are convenient, with no laundering required, but they are expensive, occupy storage space, and are less friendly to the environment than cloth ones.

The number of stools passed varies, and the appearance of a newborn baby's stools changes over a few days from meconium (the first dark green motions) to greenish brown, then yellow. There will probably be more than four stools a day, and two a day by four months. Breastfed babies may have twice as many stools as bottle-fed ones; these are often runny. If stools are hard or look like little pebbles, or none is passed for several days, consult your doctor or health visitor.

Nappy rash
This may appear as a red patch or as open spots, pimples or blisters. A nappy rash that will not heal may be infected with thrush, indicated by whitish spots or patches. To treat or help to prevent a rash, change nappies often, clean the area gently but thoroughly and apply a nappy-rash cream. Expose the baby's skin to the air frequently to aid healing. Avoid plastic pants.

ILLNESSES
Most babies suffer brief and minor illnesses during the first year of life. If your baby has a fever or cold it is not usually necessary to consult a doctor. The following steps will bring relief:
- keep him or her cool (overheating can be dangerous);
- offer extra drinks of breast milk, diluted formula milk or water;
- give the recommended dose of paracetamol syrup for your child's age.

When to consult a doctor

If your baby is ill, you may need to call a doctor to your home urgently. But it is usually better to go to the surgery or to the accident and emergency department of your local hospital, where you are likely to be seen more quickly and the doctor will have more equipment to aid diagnosis. Consult a doctor urgently if your baby has any of the following symptoms:

■ an unexplained rash;

■ keeps crying and cannot be soothed, or has an unusual cry;

■ has cold, clammy skin that is pale and grey;

■ has a temperature over 39°C (102.2°F) with rapid breathing or other signs of illness;

■ passes blood or motions that look like redcurrant jelly;

■ has severe diarrhoea and/or vomiting and is unable to keep fluids down;

■ has a convulsion (fit) or seems floppy;

■ has difficulty in breathing, or turns blue;

■ cannot be woken or is unusually drowsy;

■ is unresponsive or has a vacant expression;

■ has symptoms of **meningitis**. These include fever, vomiting and sensitivity to light.

Complementary therapies

Cranial osteopathy is a therapy offered by some oesteopaths. It involves gentle cranial manipulation and touch to identify and correct disorders throughout the body. It is mostly used to treat babies with feeding difficulties, colic, disturbed sleep and similar problems.

Baby massage is an increasingly popular method of soothing and communicating with babies. Your health visitor can tell you about local classes.

IMMUNIZATION

When children are immunized, they are given a vaccine containing some of the bacteria or viruses that cause a disease. These vaccines do not cause the disease itself but stimulate the body into producing antibodies against it.

During the first year of life, your child can be given vaccines to protect against diphtheria, tetanus, polio, whooping cough (pertussis), *Haemophilus influenzae* type b (Hib) and meningitis C. Some children have adverse reactions to these injections, but serious complications are rare (see **Immunization**).

PHYSICAL AND SOCIAL DEVELOPMENT

In the first year, babies attain an astonishing number of developmental milestones, for example, all babies learn to sit before, months later, they learn to walk. But different children reach these milestones at different times. On average, most babies are sitting by eight months of age, but some may sit as early as five months and others may not sit until ten months.

How to bath a baby

Many babies love bathtime: they relax and enjoy being washed in the soothing warm water.

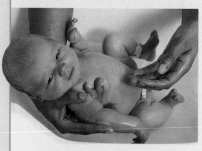

1 Put hot and cold water in the bowl or bath, starting with cold water to avoid scalding. Check the water with the inside of your wrist or your elbow to make sure that it is comfortably warm but not hot.

2 Undress your baby except for the nappy and wrap him or her snugly in a towel, keeping the arms tucked away and leaving the head free.

3 Wash your baby's face with plain warm water and cotton wool. Wash the creases behind the baby's ears and around his or her neck.

4 To wash your baby's hair, tuck his or her body under your arm, supporting the back with your arm and the head with your hand. Hold the baby over the bath, wash and rinse the hair and pat dry.

5 Remove the nappy and clean the baby's bottom. Place your arm behind the baby's back, with your hand firmly holding the baby's arm that is further away from you. With your other hand supporting the legs and buttocks, lower the baby into the bath.

6 Keeping your arm around the head and shoulders, wash the baby's body; sit the baby up and, supporting the chest across your arm, wash the back.

7 Keeping one hand firmly on the baby's shoulder, slide the other hand under the buttocks and lift the baby out of the bath.

8 Dry your baby carefully, especially the skin folds. Rub oil or baby lotion into any dry areas of skin.

! Warning

Never leave young children alone in the bath – even for a moment. They can drown in two inches of water. If you have to go out of the bathroom, wrap your baby up and take him or her with you.

Many physical skills involving hand-eye coordination develop during the first year of life, enabling the baby to use hands and fingers for activities such as grasping and picking up. A baby can hear from birth and reacts differently to different sounds. At first, babies communicate only by crying, but they soon start making the little sounds that are the beginning of speech.

Social and emotional development is equally swift. Most babies return social smiles and responses by the age of six to eight weeks and show likes and dislikes by 24–26 weeks. By the time they reach their first birthday they can understand simple requests. Consult your doctor or health visitor if you are concerned about your baby's development at any stage.

SEE ALSO *Pregnancy and problems*

Back and back pain

The back is a well-designed structure but it is vulnerable to modern living, and back pain is an ever-present fact of life for many people.

The spine is a column of bones that extends from the skull to the pelvis, forming, in profile, a shallow S-shape. It has several functions. It supports the head and allows the body to remain upright, and it provides anchorage points for the ribs, the ligaments and the muscles of the back. This allows very flexible movement of the trunk – forwards, backwards, down to the side and back up, and in a circular movement. The spine also protects the spinal cord (see **Brain and nervous system**) and stores red **bone marrow** to form red blood cells and minerals.

VERTEBRAE AND DISCS

The spine contains 33 bones, or vertebrae. With the exception of the atlas and axis (which are uppermost and act as pivots for the head), all the vertebrae are similar, although they become larger as the spine runs down the body to cope with the increasing weight. Each has five main parts:
- the body or centrum, the main cylinder-shaped part of the vertebra;
- the vertebral arch, the space through which the spinal cord passes down the back;
- two transverse 'processes', bony projections from the body that provide points of contact for ligaments and muscle tendons;
- one spinous process, which can be felt at the back of the spine.

Discs sit between the vertebrae. The discs have a soft, jelly-like centre that is 95 per cent water, and an outer casing made of tough but flexible elastic **cartilage**. They mould themselves into the available space (rather like a balloon full of water) to allow for movement of the spine, and also to act as shock absorbers.

The vertebrae are also linked by facet joints. These bind each set of transverse processes with the ones above and below. Spaces between the vertebrae near the facet joints allow the nerves to enter and leave the spinal cord.

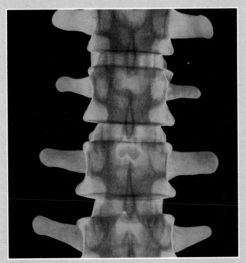

▼ Vertebral structure
Each vertebra consists of a short weight-bearing cylindrical core called the body or centrum. This has bony projections, or processes, to which the muscles and ligaments are attached. Separating the vertebrae are discs encased in cartilage.

CAUSES OF BACK PAIN

Back pain is often the result of lifestyle, ageing or an accident. It can also be caused by conditions that directly affect the spine, including **ankylosing spondylitis, Paget's disease, cancer** and what is popularly known as a slipped disc. It is not in fact the disc that is displaced but the jelly-like centre, which is forced by pressure through a defect in the disc's outer ring and squashed backwards to press on a spinal nerve.

Other conditions may cause pain in the spine even though the spine is not directly affected. These include **influenza**, heart problems, lung problems, kidney problems, an inflamed pancreas or gallbladder, and gynaecological problems. A fractured vertebra or a slipped vertebra (where one vertebra slips out of its position in the spinal column) may be caused by an accident or a fall.

Lifestyle factors
A sedentary lifestyle puts extra pressure on the lumbar spine, especially if you tend to slouch rather than sitting up straight. Pressure in intervertebral discs increases by 50 per cent when you sit with a straight back compared to when you are standing. But when you slouch forward it increases by 150 per cent. Over time, the extra pressure damages the vertebral joints, especially the facet joints, and causes muscular tension, spasms and pain.

People who take excessive exercise or who do a lot of exercise without building up their fitness gradually may suffer soft-tissue damage in their backs. This is because their muscles are not strong enough to cope with the extra demands placed upon them. The muscles may tear or go into spasm, pushing the surfaces of adjacent facet joints down onto each other. The affected joints become inflamed and painful.

Looking after young children involves bending, lifting and stretching, which can lead to back problems if care is not taken. Fashion also takes its toll – wearing high heels increases the pressure on the lower spine. Menstruation can trigger back pain, and a woman's altered posture in late **pregnancy** can result in back pain and **sciatica**.

Osteoarthritis
Osteoarthritis is a common diagnosis of back pain. It is sometimes called spondylosis when it occurs in the spine. As a result of wear and tear,

The cervical spine consists of seven vertebrae, which support the head and neck. The uppermost two are the atlas and axis, which form pivots for the head

Main support
The central structure of the back is the spine. It is held together by joints and ligaments and supported by both large and small muscles.

The thoracic spine serves as attachment points for the ribs and comprises 12 vertebrae

The lumbar spine has five vertebrae that form the lower back

The sacrum has five fused vertebrae, forming a strong joint for the pelvis

The coccyx or tailbone is formed from four vertebrae

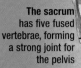

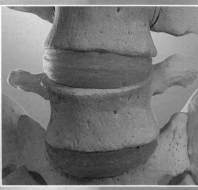

▲ **Vulnerable spot**
Pain often occurs in the lower lumbar region and the sacrum, which links the spine to the pelvic bone.

cartilage in the discs and facet joints starts to harden and turn into bone, and bony spurs grow out from the facet joints. These restrict movement and sometimes even impinge on a nerve. (See **Arthritis**.)

Osteoarthritis is to some extent a natural part of ageing; most people aged over 50 have the condition to some degree, even if they have no symptoms. The condition can develop at any point in the spine, but the lumbar and cervical vertebrae are the most vulnerable to ageing. Other causes include a previous injury, a condition such as ankylosing spondylitis, overuse and poor posture.

Osteoporosis
Osteoporosis is a condition in which the calcium content of bones is reduced, making them thinner, less dense and more likely to fracture. When the vertebrae lose density, they start to crumble, distorting the spinal curves and causing muscle spasms. As the process continues, the vertebrae impact and may trap the spinal nerves, causing considerable pain as well as immobility. (See also **Spine and disorders**.)

TREATMENT FOR BACK PAIN
If you have chronic back pain, the general advice is to carry on as best you can, but to avoid lifting and carrying. According to the Royal College of Physicians, 95 per cent of back pain sufferers do not need bed rest. Contact your doctor if the pain worsens or lasts longer than 48 hours.

If you experience acute, severe back pain or symptoms of sciatica (see Types of back pain, page 98), rest in bed if necessary. If the pain remains after 24 hours, seek medical advice.
What you can do
■ Lay a hot water bottle on the affected area, or use a heat lamp.
  ■ Take over-the-counter medications, such as codeine, paracetamol or ibuprofen – a painkiller and anti-inflammatory – to relieve pain from injury and help the muscles to relax. Or use embrocation creams, which can be rubbed into the skin to relieve stiffness. Hot or cold sprays can be used for the same purpose.
  ■ Arrange for a **massage** to ease muscle tension and spasm.
  ■ Consider using a back brace or belt. These will restrict the small muscle movements and help the muscles to relax.
A corset can be used as a temporary measure only, because long-term use will further weaken the spine's muscular support, making it more vulnerable to stresses.
■ Do graduated exercises to strengthen your back and stomach muscles (see Strengthening your back, page 99).
■ Use relaxation techniques – long-term back pain

Types of back pain

Back problems can have many causes and usually give pain and a degree of immobility. The different types of back pain can be felt in specific places or over wider areas but it is usually possible to establish the nature of the problem from the type of pain and whether it is short or long term.

■ **A sharp, localized pain** that changes with movement is likely to be caused by dysfunction of a facet joint. The pain eases if a movement takes pressure off the joint and worsens and spreads if the pressure is increased.

■ **Chronic back pain** can come and go or it can be felt continuously. It can vary from a dull, muscular ache to a sharp twinge when certain movements are made. Poor posture, weak or imbalanced muscles, soft-tissue damage from unaccustomed exercise, and degenerative conditions such as osteoporosis and osteoarthritis are all possible contributory factors.

■ **General soft-tissue damage** to muscle fibres, tendons and ligaments produces localized acute pain and stiffness that subsides over a few days.

■ **Immobility and severe pain,** and what some sufferers have described as the feeling that the back could 'snap in half', can occur when the back locks in one position. The cause is a dislocation at the facet joints of a vertebra, most often as a result of a sudden movement that involves bending and twisting at the same time.

■ **Muscle spasm** can cause painful hot spots, sometimes called 'trigger points', in the back muscles. These are tender areas that are painful to the touch and can restrict movement. This type of pain occurs after an injury, when the muscle fibres go into spasm to prevent any further damage being done.

■ **General stiffness** in the back, especially first thing in the morning, is often the result of osteoarthritis in people aged over 50, or of ankylosing spondylitis in younger people. But it can also be the consequence of unaccustomed exercise the previous day.

■ **Pain combined with pins and needles**, numbness and muscle weakness can be the result of nerve damage caused by pressure on a nerve or the spinal cord, when it is known as a central spinal stenosis. The pain can also run down the back of the leg and under the foot.

■ **An acute, sharp, burning pain** that is relentless and often immobilizing and debilitating; is usually caused by inflammation of a spinal nerve or pressure on it where it leaves the vertebra.

may be related to stress and other psychological problems, such as **depression**.

When to consult a doctor
■ Get someone to call an ambulance immediately if you suspect that you have hurt your neck or back following an accident or fall. Do not move. Wait for emergency assistance.
■ Go to casualty if your car has been hit from behind while you were sitting in it, even if you feel unhurt – you may have a whiplash injury.
■ Call your doctor if a sudden, immobilizing pain has not improved after 24 hours of bed rest.
■ Call your doctor if a continuous pain has not improved after 48 hours of home treatment.
■ See your doctor if you suspect you may have osteoporosis, you are postmenopausal or have a family history of osteoporosis or have an existing spinal problem.

What a doctor may do
■ Give you a general physical examination, looking particularly at the strength of your muscles and your range of movement.
■ Arrange a bone density scan to rule out osteoporosis.
■ Suggest you wear a corset as a short-term measure – these are available on the NHS.
■ Inject a corticosteroid drug into any painful trigger point.
■ Prescribe **drugs** such as: anti-inflammatories, muscle relaxants, tranquillizers, strong painkillers, steroids or antidepressants, as appropriate.
■ Refer you to a physiotherapist, a muscularskeletal physician or to a surgeon or neurologist.

Physiotherapy
The most common treatment for back pain is **physiotherapy**. Physical methods are either used alone or in conjunction with painkillers. Treatment can include manipulation, exercises, **ultrasound** and hydrotherapy. Physiotherapists also give training on good posture, teach correct lifting techniques and give advice on how to protect your back while performing everyday activities in the home and garden, while travelling and in the office.

Complementary therapies
Increasingly, complementary techniques are being used to treat back pain. These include **osteopathy**, therapeutic **massage**, **chiropractic**, **acupuncture** and the **Alexander technique**. Osteopaths, for example, work on the assumption that many back problems are caused by the displacement of one vertebra in relation to another, and that they can be relieved by identifying the site of the dislocation and applying pressure to reduce it.

Surgery and alternatives
Surgery is used only as a last resort for back problems. There are a variety of options.
■ An injection of a corticosteroid drug and a painkiller into the facet joint to relieve inflammation. This is administered under a local anaesthetic by an anaesthetist.
■ An injection of chymopapain, a chemical derived from the pawpaw fruit, into a prolapsed disc to digest its soft centre. The success rate is 80 per cent, and removes the need for surgery. But the disc remains thin and vulnerable to damage.
■ An emergency operation called a discectomy to remove a prolapsed disc. This will free a trapped nerve when there is a risk of neurological problems affecting other parts of the body.
■ An operation called a spinal fusion to fuse together two or more vertebrae. This can be done using a bone graft from the hip bone or with pins and screws. It will stabilize a slipped vertebra or stop an unnatural spinal curve becoming worse.
■ An operation called a facetectomy to remove

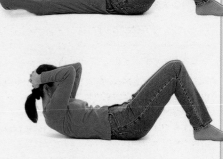

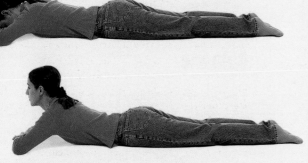

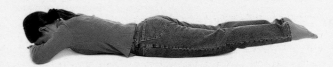

Self-help
Strengthening your back

These simple daily exercises can help strengthen the muscles supporting the spine and reduce the risk of back problems. Do not strain or force the movement, though: stop if you feel discomfort.

2 Turn over onto your back and bend your knees at right angles, with your feet on the floor. Place your hands behind your head and lift your head, shoulders and shoulder blades up off the floor – for safety, do not attempt to sit right up – then lower them slowly and carefully. Repeat five times.

1 Lie on your stomach on the floor with your hands laced under your forehead. Slowly raise your head and shoulders about 20cm (8in) – no more – off the floor, then lower them slowly back to the floor. Repeat five times.

3 With your head on your hands, raise both legs about 15cm (6in) off the floor, then lower slowly. Repeat five times.

bony spurs around a facet joint caused by osteoarthritis. This allows more room for the spinal cord or nerves.

PREVENTING BACK PAIN
In many cases, back problems can be prevented by adopting good posture, using the correct techniques when lifting heavy objects, exercising for strength and flexibility, and taking certain practical measures during everyday life.

The importance of good posture
Bad posture is the most common cause of chronic back pain – and potentially the easiest to avoid.

The back has four natural curves that give it the ability to absorb the stresses of maintaining an upright posture. The sacral and thoracic vertebrae curve backwards (outwards when seen from the side) – they are called primary curves because they are present at birth. The cervical and lumbar vertebrae curve forwards (inwards when seen from the side) and develop shortly after birth as a baby learns to lift the head and sit.

If the back is held either too straight or in an exaggeratedly curved position, the spinal column and its muscles and ligaments are unable to absorb the everyday shocks and stresses of gravity, walking, sitting and weight-bearing, and so become distorted. When the shoulders and upper back become rounded, the unnatural curve is known as a **kyphosis**; the excessive inward curve of a 'hollow back' is called a lumbar lordosis; a sideways curve to the spine is called a scoliosis.

Over time, the muscles and ligaments become either too long or too short and the bones and joints become liable to excessive wear and tear. The result is damage – leading to back pain.

Poor posture quickly becomes a habit, and starts to feel correct even when it is not. Many people find that they need to relearn good postural habits, perhaps with the help of a physiotherapist or an Alexander technique teacher. But you can train yourself to adopt and maintain good posture.

Day-to-day care of your back
Follow these simple rules to minimize the chances of developing problems with your back.
■ Check your posture frequently.
■ Avoid holding any one position for too long.
■ Avoid standing still for long periods – sit or put one foot up on a stool or raised object to reduce the pressure on your back.
■ Ensure that while you are at work any chair that you use regularly protects your back: your feet should touch the ground; the back rest should support your spine; and the chair should be deep enough to support your thighs.
■ If you use a computer, make sure that the screen is at the correct height: you should not have to look down at it.
■ Before embarking on gardening or household chores, warm up with some stretching exercises.
■ Use long-handled tools to take some of the strain out of gardening.
■ Stay fit and keep within the weight limits for your height and age to reduce spinal stress.

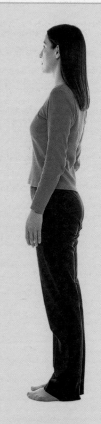

▲ **Natural grace**
If you strive to maintain the correct standing posture at all times, it will eventually become instinctive.

Bacterial infections

Many diseases are caused by bacteria, which are single-cell organisms too small to be seen by the naked eye. Most bacteria are harmless to people and some are beneficial, but others, abundant in the air, soil and water, cause disease by releasing substances that are harmful to human cells.

SYMPTOMS

Bacterial infections can cause:

- skin problems, including rashes;
- breathing problems;
- high temperature or fever;
- stomach pains;
- headaches;
- genito-urinary problems.

COMPLICATIONS

Many bacterial infections can cause further damage to the body and its organs – including **whooping cough, meningitis,** botulism, **tuberculosis, typhoid fever, Legionnaire's disease** and syphilis.

OUTLOOK

Early treatment with antibiotics is often essential for bacterial infections, which may otherwise cause permanent health problems.

Avoiding the spread of infection

Bacterial contamination most commonly occurs through physical contact – from unwashed hands to dirty kitchen utensils.

The simplest, most everyday actions can spread infection.

- Touching or shaking hands with another person.
- Contaminated food infecting the digestive tract.
- Touching food with dirty hands – this will also allow bacteria from the intestine to spread.
- Inhaling droplets breathed, coughed or sneezed out by an infected person – **diphtheria** and **whooping cough** are caught through the lungs in this way.
- Sexual contact. Micro-organisms that enter the genito-urinary system include those causing **sexually transmitted diseases** such as syphilis, pelvic inflammatory disease and gonorrhoea.
- Through hair follicles, cuts and deep wounds.

To prevent infection, you should take the following steps.

- Wash your hands thoroughly and often.
- Store vegetables and meat separately and prepare them on separate chopping boards.
- Cook meat until it is well done.
- Use a handkerchief if coughing or sneezing.
- Wash wounds with antiseptic.
- Get yourself immunized against bacterial diseases such as **tetanus.**

Bad breath

Bad breath, also known as **halitosis,** is unpleasant mouth odour, often caused by poor oral hygiene or, occasionally, stomach problems. If you think that you suffer from bad breath, you should talk to a dentist. If the cause is related to inattentive dental care, you may be advised to see a hygienist.

SEE ALSO *Dentists and dentistry*

Balance

Balance problems may be experienced as toppling or stumbling or, more subtly, by a feeling of unsteadiness, nausea or dizziness. Keeping one's balance depends on a continuous, complex process that involves the eyes, ears, brain and nerves.

Information about body position is fed to the brain in a continuous stream from the eyes, movement sensors in the inner ear, and nerves in the skin, joints and muscles. From this, the brain computes what the body must do to stay 'on course', and transmits instructions back to the limbs. The process involves several areas of the brain, including the cerebellum and the sensory and motor cortices.

ONSET AND DURATION

A balance problem may occur suddenly or over a number of years. Problems with balance are very common in old age, and slow-developing imbalance in later life is unlikely to signify anything sinister – it affects the majority of people over the age of 85. However, any sudden loss of balance should be treated as a medical emergency unless there is an obvious cause such as intoxication. If imbalance develops over several weeks, a doctor should be consulted.

CAUSES

Because it involves so many different parts of the body, the balance system may be disrupted by a very wide range of conditions. It is associated with many different illnesses and can be one of the first signs that a person is tired, intoxicated or very stressed.

Ear disorders

- **Ménière's disease,** an abnormal increase in the pressure in the inner ear.
- **Labyrinthitis,** inner ear inflammation.
- **Otitis media,** inflammation of the middle ear.
- Blocked ears, which may be caused by a buildup of wax.

Nerve disorders

- Inflammation of the nerve fibres, which may be due to viral or bacterial infection.
- Nerve degeneration, which may signify vitamin B deficiency.

- **Multiple sclerosis**, which causes damage to myelin nerve sheaths.

Blood and circulation disorders

- **Anaemia**, which reduces brain oxygen levels.
- Blood poisoning, caused by infections or environmental toxins (see **Septicaemia**).
- Cardiovascular disease, which reduces blood flow to the brain.
- **Hypoglycaemia**, or low blood sugar.
- High or low **blood pressure**.

Brain abnormalities

- A **stroke** that affects the brain's sensory or movement areas.
- A tumour that affects the sensory or movement areas.
- **Motor neurone disease**, which causes death of the brain cells required for movement.

TREATMENT

Treatment will vary, depending on the underlying condition.

SEE ALSO *Blood and disorders; Brain and nervous system; Ear and problems; Heart and circulatory system*

Balanitis

Balanitis is a condition in which both the head of the penis (glans) and the foreskin become inflamed. It can affect men of all ages, and in boys occurs most commonly around the age of three or four years. Unusual among circumcised males (see **Circumcision**), balanitis is best avoided by keeping the penis clean, especially under the foreskin.

Balanitis can develop from infection following damage to the skin surface caused by:

- poor genital hygiene;
- a tight foreskin (phimosis);
- skin disorders such as **Reiter's syndrome**;
- an allergic reaction to a particular soap or washing powder or to the latex or spermicides in condoms;
- sexual activity – although the condition itself is not transmitted sexually, the **candida** fungus can be transmitted and cause localized inflammation.

Most cases clear up without treatment – although you should abstain from sex until the skin has healed. If after a week or two you are still feeling discomfort or are worried that the irritation could be caused by a **sexually transmitted disease**, see a GP or visit your local genito-urinary medicine (GUM) clinic. Antibiotics, antifungals or steroids may be prescribed.

SEE ALSO *Fungal infections; Penis and disorders; Reproductive system*

Baldness

Baldness, also known as androgenic or male pattern baldness, is a common condition that usually poses no health problems. As many as 25 per cent of men in the UK are noticeably balding by the age of 30, and 65 per cent by the age of 60. Baldness can, more rarely, affect women.

SYMPTOMS

In men, the hairline recedes from the front or, less often, from the top of the head; in women, hair tends to thin out all over.

CAUSES

There is a strong hereditary element in baldness, with the biggest influence generally on the mother's side. The trigger, most frequently, is hormonal. Although the mechanism is unclear, testosterone, which increases body hair and reduces scalp hair, is involved.

Other causes can include:

- serious illnesses, infections or fevers;
- **chemotherapy** and **radiotherapy**;
- stress;
- excessive shampooing or blowdrying.

TREATMENT

There is no cure for baldness, but treatments may include:

- hair grafts (the relocation of hairy skin to bald patches), sometimes in tandem with scalp reduction (the removal of bald skin);
- artificial hair fibre implants;
- wigs – provide an effective, short-term solution to, for example, hair loss caused by chemotherapy;
- Minoxidil, which is rubbed on the scalp. This is the only male baldness drug licensed in the UK for sale without a prescription. Research suggests that, after four months' use, it stopped hair loss in about 70 per cent of users and stimulated some growth in half the people who tried it;
- early trials of the drug dutasteride, which breaks down testosterone, look promising.

Anyone considering drug treatments for baldness should first research the latest available products thoroughly with the help of a sympathetic GP or trichologist, a hair specialist.

COMPLICATIONS

- Side effects can arise from any drug treatment.
- **Depression** is a relatively common response to baldness, especially in young men, women and children.

Hair care

You cannot prevent receding hair but you can slow down the process.

- Treat remaining hair gently, especially when it is wet.
- Comb rather than brush your hair.
- To keep hair healthy, ensure your diet contains sufficient protein and iron.
- Wearing your hair short is usually better than trying to disguise a bald patch.

Barber's rash

Known also as folliculitis, barber's rash is an infection of a man's beard area. A similar but usually less serious condition is called razor bumps. Both barber's rash and razor bumps can make shaving difficult and painful.

Barber's rash is caused by infection of the hair follicles by a common skin bacterium, *Staphylococcus aureus*. Infection, and re-infection, often occur through using razors or towels previously used by an infected person.

Razor bumps are caused when facial hair curls and grows back into the skin to cause inflammation. This condition is particularly problematic for men with curly hair.

SYMPTOMS
- In barber's rash, there is itchiness, redness, swelling, multiple small pus-filled blisters and occasionally boils. The condition usually starts on the upper lip, but can spread across the face. It can also occur on the groin and thighs.
- Razor bumps are characterized by redness and inflammation and sometimes by infection.

TREATMENT
- Always use clean towels and razors.
- Wash your face twice daily with hot water and antibacterial soap.
- If you have razor bumps, always shave 'with the grain'. Do not pull your skin taut to get a closer shave.
- Shave less frequently or use an electric razor if it is more comfortable.
- Growing a beard usually solves the problem.
- If your skin is infected and these self-help methods fail to cure the condition, seek medical advice. Your doctor may prescribe an antibiotic cream, a course of antibiotic tablets, or both treatments.

COMPLICATIONS
Scarring can very occasionally result from untreated barber's rash.

Barium investigations

A barium investigation is a diagnostic test used to investigate disorders of the stomach, gullet or bowel. There are three types of barium investigation:
- the barium swallow (used when a doctor wishes to examine the gullet);
- the barium meal (for investigating the stomach and upper intestine);
- the barium enema (used to examine the rectum and lower intestine).

WHAT'S INVOLVED
The first and second types involve drinking a thick, white, often mint-flavoured solution;

in the third the solution is pumped into the rectum. The liquid (a solution of barium sulphate) shows up on **X-rays**: abnormalities of the digestive tract can be seen on X-ray pictures or viewed on an imaging device called a fluoroscope.

For meals and swallows, people are asked to drink up to two cupfuls of the solution and may also be given an injection to paralyse the gut temporarily. The part of the digestive system to be investigated must be empty; for a barium enema, a laxative may first be given to empty the bowel. X-ray pictures will be taken immediately or within 45 minutes depending on where in the gastro-intestinal tract the investigation is centred. Barium investigations cause no discomfort at the time, but patients may find that they have constipation for a day or two afterwards.

Barium meals are not performed as commonly as they once were. Increasingly, medics are using a fibre-optic device called a gastroscope instead. It examines the oesophagus and stomach for any suspected growths and can take tissue samples at the same time.

Since bacteria are the most common cause of stomach **ulcers**, and since barium meals and gastroscopes do not detect bacteria, doctors generally do not use these invasive techniques when first investigating stomach ulcer symptoms.

SEE ALSO *Digestive system; Oesophagus and disorders; Stomach and disorders*

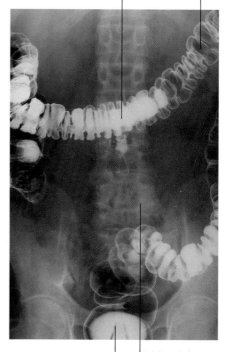

Barium

Large intestine

Spine

Bladder

▲ **Diagnostic meal**
This X-ray image shows part of the large intestine highlighted after a person has taken a barium meal. Medics can use the image to diagnose a digestive complaint.

Bartholin's cyst and abscess

A Bartholin's cyst is a swelling, usually on one side only, of the external female genitals (vulva). The swelling begins as a painless **cyst** but may become infected and enlarged, resulting in a very painful **abscess** that may interfere with sexual intercourse.

It is caused by a blockage in one of the Bartholin lubricating glands, which are positioned at the back of the vulva. It is most common in women of reproductive age.

Any swelling in the vulval area that does not go away after a few days should be medically examined. You may be prescribed a course of antibiotics to treat the condition or referred to a consultant gynaecologist, who will consider surgical removal of the cyst or abscess. To obtain relief yourself at home, try sitting on a cold compress or in a lukewarm bath.

BCG vaccine

The BCG vaccine is administered to provide immunity from **tuberculosis**. Its full name is Bacillus Calmette-Guérin vaccine. The vaccine is produced from live but weakened cattle tuberculosis bacteria, which do not cause the disease in human beings but stimulate the production of specific antibodies. These antibodies react with the human tuberculosis bacteria to give the recipient of the vaccine natural resistance to the disease.

The BCG vaccine is used (following a skin test) for routine vaccination of children, usually between the ages of 10 and 14, and for other people at risk. It is given by injection, generally into the upper arm. Within two to six weeks, a small swelling appears, which heals after six to twelve weeks to leave a small scar.

SEE ALSO *Immunization*

Bedsores

Bedsores are, initially, areas of skin irritation that develop on immobile people confined to bed. They are also known as pressure sores or decubitus ulcers. People at risk include those with a serious debilitating illness, people who have been paralyzed (for example, following a stroke or spinal injury) or those in a coma.

Bedsores result when pressure from the body interferes with the circulation of blood to areas of flesh over bony prominences such as the heels, the base of the spine, the shoulder tips or the elbows. The sores start off as redness on the skin, but these marks become purple before breaking down and ulcerating. Turning the person over at least once every two hours and using rippled bed mattresses, cushions, pillows and sheepskin padding help to prevent bedsores. Treatment may involve the use of antibiotics, ulcer dressings, and surgery to remove dead tissue and apply skin grafts.

SEE ALSO *Skin and disorders*

Bedwetting

Bedwetting (nocturnal enuresis) is defined by doctors as the involuntary wetting of the bed at night by a child over the age of five years.

It is a common problem that can cause considerable distress to both children and their families.

Most children master daytime bladder control between the ages of two and three. Staying dry throughout the night can take longer: up to the age of five bedwetting is considered normal. Before children can stay dry during the night they have to recognize and respond to a full bladder while asleep. This is done either by 'holding on' until morning or by waking up and urinating. Most children who wet the bed grow out of it as they get older.

CAUSES
The reason why some children wet the bed is not fully understood, but factors may include:
■ genes – bedwetting runs in families;
■ sleep disorders;
■ anxiety or psychological problems;
■ a deficiency of a hormone called vasopressin, which reduces secretion of urine when present in the body in normal amounts;
■ developmental immaturity;
■ diabetes or a urinary tract infection.

TREATMENT
Although treatment is not normally given before the age of five years, there are a number of general measures that parents and children can take to cope with bedwetting.
■ Ask your doctor to test your child's urine to exclude any disease.
■ Be reassuring, involve the child in the treatment and give praise for dry nights.
■ Do not restrict your child's fluid intake: the bladder tends to adjust to receiving less fluid and therefore holds less. The Enuresis Resource and Information Centre recommends that children drink around six or seven cups of fluid each day so that their bladders learn to hold a larger capacity. Fizzy drinks and those containing caffeine should be avoided at night, however, because these can act as diuretics and stimulate the kidneys to produce more urine.
■ Try fully wakening your child at a slightly different time each night – this may reduce the number of wet beds.

A doctor or school nurse may suggest other things you can do. For example:
■ star charts – your child is awarded a star on a chart every time he or she stays dry at night;
■ an alarm to wake the child up when urination begins. Alarms can be effective but may take up to 16 weeks to work. For developmental reasons they are recommended by doctors only for children over the age of seven years;
■ medicine, either tablets or a nasal spray, can reduce the amount of urine passed.

SEE ALSO *Urinary system*

Behaviour problems in children

All children have a capacity for mischief, and naughtiness is a perfectly normal way of exploring the limits of acceptable conduct. Such behaviour constitutes a problem only when there is a danger of social or physical damage to a child or others.

Problem behaviour is difficult to define, because what is acceptable in one family may be regarded as outrageous in another. But children are generally reasonable people, and will aim to obey whatever rules parents lay down. Think what might be the cause if a child shows a worrying pattern of behaviour, or if it is getting worse. For example, if a child is persistently aggressive towards a sibling, could it be due to jealousy, boredom, tensions in the family that the child is picking up on, or unrealistic expectations on the part of the parents?

TEMPER TANTRUMS
Most children have uncontrollable fits of anger from time to time, but some are more prone than others to outbursts of kicking, screaming or throwing things. Temper tantrums are usually a passing phase, which begins at about 18 months and can last a year or so. Many parents feel that frustration lies at the root of the 'terrible twos'. Young children have real desires that they cannot quite express, and they are subject to rules and injunctions that they are not equipped to understand. They cannot see, for example, why they can empty a box of toys onto the floor but are not allowed to empty a bag of groceries.

Hard as it may be, ignoring tantrums is a good way of dealing with them. A child is more likely to give up on throwing tantrums if it proves to be an ineffective strategy, so don't use bribes or give in. Once the tantrum is over, make sure that your child knows you still love him or her, but that you dislike the behaviour.

Preventing tantrums
If your child has frequent tantrums, avoid trigger situations. For example, don't press your child to share a treasured toy. Also, decide when it is important to be firm: insist that a child holds your hand in the street, for example, but don't worry about odd socks if your child really wants to wear them.

Unclear rules from adults can be an underlying cause of tantrums, so both parents should try to act consistently. A child may find it confusing if, say, the mother buys sweets at the supermarket but the father won't. Tantrums may also occur if there are too many activities in the day, a child misses a nap, or goes for too long without food. Don't expect too much of your child and allow time for a rest.

BREATH-HOLDING EPISODES
Some children hold their breath when they are crying, feeling upset or in a temper. When this occurs, the child's face turns red, then changes to white or blue. These spells may begin in babies as young as 6 months, peaking between 12 and 18 months, and can continue until the child is 3–3½ years old. In some cases, the child becomes stiff or floppy, and may pass out for a few seconds before starting to breathe again. These episodes are frightening for parents but will not normally harm the child.

Discuss the behaviour with your doctor: as long as your doctor is sure that there is no underlying medical cause of the breathlessness and other symptoms, ignore a child who is having a breath-holding spell. If your child passes out, keep a close watch but move away when he or she starts to regain consciousness.

AGGRESSION
Violent behaviour can be due to something as simple as undeveloped social skills. For example, children aged under two years do not understand the concept of sharing and may become aggressive if they see another child playing with their toys. But a toddler who has started showing signs of aggression needs to know that this behaviour is unacceptable.
- If you see your child about to bite or kick, issue a sharp and unequivocal 'no'.
- Take your child into another room and talk about the behaviour. Even if he or she seems not to understand, the message will sink in over time.
- Consider whether there is a reason for the behaviour, such as a new baby in the family. You may need to make a special effort to prevent older children from feeling neglected when a young baby is demanding much of your attention.
- If children are fighting over toys, distract them with another.
- Take pre-emptive action – for example, put away favourite toys when other children visit.

▼ **Infant rage**
Temper tantrums in public places can be a nightmare for parents, but do stay calm. You may feel embarrassed, but most people will sympathize rather than judge you or your child.

HEADBANGING AND HEAD-ROLLING

It is not unusual for children aged 6–18 months to bang or roll their head in a rhythmical way before going to sleep or if they are tired. Headbanging is alarming for parents, but the habit is harmless and usually resolves itself by the age of four.

Some children bang their heads to attract attention when they are upset. But most have the sense not to bang their heads so hard that they hurt themselves. If necessary, pad the sides of a child's cot, or put padding against a wall. If your child starts to bang the side of the head, check that he or she is not suffering from an ear infection that is causing pain.

Consult a doctor if your child's habit worries you, or if it continues past age four.

JEALOUSY

Many older siblings feel left out when a new baby comes along. It is hard for a first child of any age to let go of exclusive relationships with its parents. But jealousy becomes a problem only if it manifests itself in disruptive reactions such as hitting a new baby, reverting to infantile behaviour or becoming physically destructive.

Try to anticipate jealousy. For instance, move a child out of your bedroom to make way for a new baby before, not after, the baby is born. Think about the cause. Do you always pick up the younger child first? Do you take one's side against another? Children pick up on any hint that a parent's love or attention is being distributed unequally.

The pre-teen years

The pre-teen years are the time when a child's horizons expand beyond the home and the securities of family life.

Behaviour problems can appear suddenly and unexpectedly, and it can come as a shock to parents if a previously well-behaved child becomes aggressive, refuses to go to school or starts to lie or steal. Such behaviour is often a response to some unexpressed unhappiness or anxiety, so any strategy for dealing with problem behaviour must look for these causes as well as deal with their manifestations.

STEALING

If your child is stealing, you need to act quickly. A child who steals from school could end up damaging his or her educational career, and stealing from shops may land an older child in trouble with the police.

Talk to your child to find out the reason for stealing. Some children steal in order to gain the attention that comes with being caught, but the cause is not always psychological: stealing may be done as a silly dare or to gain favour with friends. Bullying can also be at the root of it: bullies sometimes force their victims to steal.

If your child is caught shoplifting, you should insist that he or she goes back to the shop with you to return the item, or that the child pay for it and apologizes to the shopkeeper. Most children will find this experience so mortifying that they will be disinclined to steal again.

Persistent stealing, particularly in children old enough to understand the moral fault involved, usually has some deeper cause. It may need investigation with the help of a psychotherapist, who will help the child to explore the issues behind their behaviour.

LYING

Fantasizing is a normal, and harmless, part of a child's development, but deliberate lying should be discouraged. Children of six or seven inhabit a different moral universe from adults. They believe that the more implausible the lie, the more reprehensible it is – so it is worse to say that you have seen a flying elephant than to claim you did not eat the chocolate in the fridge. Parents should gently make clear the difference between things that are not true because they are stories, and things that are not true because they are deceit.

By the age of seven or eight, children understand that telling lies can have real and unpleasant consequences for other people. But they may still tell lies because they are afraid that they will get into trouble or lose face, or that people won't like

---

Encouraging good behaviour

Parents can help to foster good behaviour in their children with consistent and thoughtful reactions to everyday family issues.

Do

✔ Give your child firm boundaries so that it is clear what you will and will not tolerate.

✔ Be consistent, and if you make a threat carry it out. Parents need to agree on boundaries and sanctions.

✔ Give reasons why you have forbidden something. 'Because I say so' isn't good enough.

✔ Think before you say 'no', then stick to it.

✔ Praise positive behaviour, however infrequent, to raise self-esteem.

✔ Try to spend individual time with each of your children with no interruptions.

✔ Allow your children to bring friends home so that you know who they are spending time with.

Don't

✘ Bribe your child to behave well.

✘ Physically punish your child. Banning television or withdrawing other privileges is more effective.

✘ Apply too much pressure by organizing too many out-of-school activities – children should have time to relax and daydream.

✘ Criticize your child in front of other people.

✘ Try to choose your child's friends.

✘ Give attention only for challenging behaviour.

them if they tell the truth. They generally have a clear intuition that this kind of deception is wrong. Parents can do much by example: displaying a disapproving attitude to dishonesty to underline their child's almost innate sense of right and wrong.

REFUSING TO GO TO SCHOOL

Going to school can be an ordeal for some children and they may refuse to go or pretend to be ill so that they can stay at home. A clear sign of faked illness is when a child complains of stomach aches or headaches on school days, but is fine at weekends.

School phobia may be caused by anxiety at being separated from the parents. This can be caused by the parents' own over-possessive attitude, or it may be that children are worried about what is happening at home while they are at school. Divorce, family illness or bereavement can all cause such anxiety. If one parent dies or leaves the family home, children can worry about the remaining parent. An intimidating teacher or bullying can also be the cause of school phobia. Many children who refuse to go to school are not lazy or disinterested in their own education but, on the contrary, conscientious students who are fearful of failure.

If your child shows signs of school phobia, be firm about the necessity of going to school, and do not give in to faked illness. Discuss your child's attitude towards school with his or her teacher. If necessary, ask for a referral to an educational psychologist.

If the problem seems to be rooted in a situation at the particular school (as would be the case if your child was being bullied) then consider changing schools altogether. Some anxious children do better in smaller schools, where there tends to be more sense of community. Seek recommendations from other parents, phone other schools and ask to visit, and study the reports published by the Office for Standards in Education (OFSTED).

BEATING THE BULLIES

Almost 40 per cent of primary school children say they have been repeatedly bullied, and one in ten say they are both bullies and victims.

Persistent bullying can lead to depression and in extreme circumstances even suicide. Some children who fear bullying play truant rather than go to school.

■ **Signs of bullying** There are many possible signs when a child is being bullied.

▼ **War games** Boys love fighting, and banning rough games is practically impossible. But growing boys do not know their own strength and may need to be told where to draw the line between play-fighting and dangerous aggression.

Obvious clues include a child coming home from school with damaged clothes or property, unexplained bruises or injuries, or changes in behaviour, such as increased timidity or nervousness around certain children. Other signs of bullying may be a child coming home hungry or asking for extra dinner money, developing a reluctance to go to school, or starting to have eating or sleeping problems.

■ **What to do** Make sure your child knows that he or she has your support, and doesn't have to deal with the problem alone. Don't tell him or her to hit back. Encourage your child to tell a teacher and report every act of bullying. Or see the teacher yourself, but make sure you remain calm.

Many children now have mobile phones and bullying by way of phone calls or text messaging is an increasing problem in schools. If your child is a victim of this kind of bullying, tell him or her to write down what the text or caller says and keep a diary of incidents. Consider telling the police as well as a teacher. Making anonymous or abusive phone calls is a criminal offence – contact the charity Bullying Online (www.bullying.co.uk) for further advice.

■ **When your child is the bully** Take time to talk to your child and listen to his or her point of view. Be gentle but make it clear that the bullying has to stop – it can be helpful to ask the child what help he or she needs to stop the behaviour. Try to get to the root of any underlying causes – children may start bullying as a response to unhappiness at home or as an attempt to avoid being bullied themselves.

FIGHTING AND AGGRESSION

Small boys seem to enjoy rough and tumble, and some take longer to grow out of it than others. Such tussles are harmless, even if occasionally they end in tears. As a means of settling disputes, they are probably no worse than the strategy of withholding friendship, which is common practice among girls.

Children of school age should be able to control their anger, and express it verbally, not physically. Aggressive children may be copying violent behaviour experienced in the family: if a parent hits out when angry, the child will see this as acceptable.

Aggression in children can be the result of witnessing violence on television. It may also be due to frustration or unhappiness or a reaction to inconsistent discipline. If a child seems always to be fighting, channel the exuberance into energetic games or sports. Aggressive behaviour can sometimes be countered by giving more praise when due, and by arranging activities that require sharing, cooperation and helpfulness.

SEE ALSO *Psychiatric disorders*

Bell's palsy

Bell's palsy is a form of paralysis that affects the face. It is named after Sir Charles Bell, the who first described it in the 1820s.

SYMPTOMS

Bell's palsy usually occurs on just one side of the face but, very occasionally, both sides may be affected. The paralysis is usually swift: within a few hours the muscles on one side of the face become paralysed and the side of the mouth and lower eyelid droop down. Speech may be slurred and saliva may escape from the affected corner of the mouth. The entire side of the face is flat and expressionless.

CAUSES

Anyone can be affected at any time. The cause is not fully known, but it is believed to be due in most cases to virus-induced inflammation of the nerve that carries signals from the brain to the muscles involved in facial expression.

This nerve (the seventh cranial) is one of the few that emerge directly through small crevices in the skull instead of feeding into the spinal cord. It therefore has to pass through a narrow bony opening; in Bell's palsy it is thought that the inflamed nerve swells and becomes compressed in the channel, and is thus unable to pass signals to the facial muscles.

TREATMENT

If caught early enough, treatment with oral steroids may arrest the condition by reducing inflammation.

OUTLOOK

Most people recover after a few weeks, although sometimes a person is left with a permanent one-sided 'droop', which may benefit from plastic surgery (see **Cosmetic and plastic surgery**). In about one in 20 people, the paralysis remains complete.

Benign tumour

A tumour is an abnormal swelling that results when body cells in an area increase in number at an excessive rate. Benign tumours, such as **cysts**, are usually harmless, although they can cause problems if they grow very large. Unlike cancerous tumours, they do not spread to or invade other tissues in the body (see **Cancer**).

Bilharziasis

Bilharziasis is a widespread disease of the Tropics and is caused by blood parasites. The disease, which is also known as schistosomiasis, is contracted by bathing in water contaminated by worms that harbour the larvae of the parasite. The larvae penetrate the skin and, when mature, settle in the blood vessels of the intestine or bladder. Eggs are released by adult flukes, causing high fever, chills and aches and pains.

In severe cases there may be blood in the urine or faeces, and enlargement of the liver or spleen or both. Diagnosis is made through a blood test and treatment is with anthelmintic drugs that destroy the parasite.

The disease is common in Africa, South America, the Middle East and the Far East.
SEE ALSO *Parasites and parasitic diseases*

Biopsy

In a biopsy a piece of tissue is removed, from the skin or an organ, to be examined more closely. Biopsies may be performed by a GP or at a hospital and are usually used to aid diagnosis. If a woman finds a small lump in her breast, for example, a biopsy may be performed to look for cancerous cells. But biopsies are also performed when cancer is not suspected, for example, to detect such diseases as cirrhosis of the liver, hepatitis and severe anaemia, as well as different types of infection.

WHAT'S INVOLVED

Biopsies are usually performed under local **anaesthetic**. The skin overlying the area is frozen so that it becomes numb, then a needle or knife is used to take a small tissue sample.

Needle biopsy

A fine needle may be used to obtain very small groups of cells or a slightly larger needle used to extract a sliver of tissue. The test should be no more painful than a blood test.

If the biopsy is to be taken from an inaccessible area, such as the lung, **X-rays** are used to ensure that the sample is taken from the correct part.

Incision and excision biopsies

An incision biopsy is a procedure in which part of the abnormal area is removed and taken away for testing; in an excision biopsy, the whole area is removed. Additional equipment may be required by the surgeon so that the sample area can be located properly. For example, an endoscope, a fibre-optic viewing instrument,

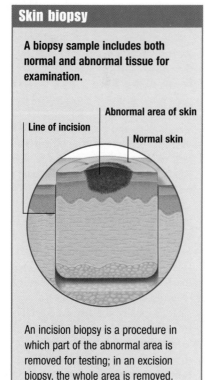

Skin biopsy

A biopsy sample includes both normal and abnormal tissue for examination.

Abnormal area of skin

Line of incision

Normal skin

An incision biopsy is a procedure in which part of the abnormal area is removed for testing; in an excision biopsy, the whole area is removed.

may be used (see **Endoscopy**). In some cases, it may be necessary to use a general anaesthetic during the procedure.

WHAT TO ASK THE DOCTOR

Before the biopsy is performed, ask whether you will have a scar from the procedure. If a larger biopsy is done, a scar may result and stitches will have to be removed; this is usually performed by the practice nurse in a GP surgery.

It is also a good idea to ask why the biopsy is being performed. Often, the doctor will have an idea about what the underlying condition might be.

You should find out if there are likely to be any potential problems caused by the biopsy. After a prostate biopsy test, for example, a little blood loss from the rectum may be experienced. It is also worth checking how long it will take for the results of the biopsy to be returned; this can vary from a few days to a few weeks.

AFTER THE TEST

Once a sample has been taken, it is usually sent to the laboratory so that various tests can be performed on it. A microscope is used to look at the sample in much more detail. Experts use different techniques to analyse the sample to ensure that the correct diagnosis is made, and it may be checked by more than one person.

Sometimes special staining techniques are performed on the tissue to look for certain diseases, and it can take several days for the results to be known.

New molecular biological and genetic techniques are being developed and introduced, which allow more sophisticated tests to be performed. The new techniques also mean that many different tests can be done on smaller pieces of tissue than would have been possible in the past.

After the tests, a written report will be produced and sent to your doctor or specialist, who will discuss the result with you. The result of the biopsy may require a decision about treatment to be made; for example, whether a mastectomy is necessary if breast cancer is diagnosed (see **Breast and disorders**).

Occasionally, the test is inadequate and needs to be repeated. This is usually because the sample taken did not contain enough tissue for the special tests to be performed, or because the sample contained normal rather than diseased tissue. It does not mean that there is a serious problem and you should not be alarmed if a biopsy is repeated. In addition, another biopsy may be carried out at a later stage to assess a person's response to treatment.

Birth and problems

Childbirth is an intensely personal event and every woman's experience of it is different. It is important to weigh up all the issues involved when planning a birth.

What kind of birth you choose will depend on whether there are any medical complications and whether this is your first baby, as well as what kind of pain relief you prefer and whether you want the intimacy of a home birth or the reassurance of being in a large hospital. Discuss the issues with your midwife and birth partner, as well as friends and family who have had babies.

HOSPITAL OR HOME BIRTH?

The majority of women feel more secure giving birth in hospital, where normal pregnancies and uncomplicated births are usually managed by teams of midwives. There is some variation in the facilities offered at different hospitals, but support, advice and pain relief are always available as well as access to medical expertise.

Some mothers prefer to give birth in the familiar surroundings of home, with family and friends present. If there are unexpected complications, however, emergency treatment is delayed. Any woman can request – and insist on – a home birth. If her GP is unwilling to cooperate, the midwife can arrange other medical backup. Factors that make a home birth inadvisable include complications in previous pregnancies, breech presentation, multiple pregnancy and medical problems such as pre-eclampsia (see page 110).

NATURAL AND MANAGED BIRTHS

Natural childbirth aims to deliver the baby with a minimum of medical intervention, managing the birth with breathing and relaxation techniques. Soft lighting and music may be used to create a relaxed atmosphere and the cord is often not cut until it stops pulsating. In a managed hospital birth, on the other hand, labour is actively controlled and the woman is more likely to experience procedures such as induction, the use of forceps and a Caesarean delivery. But there is a growing trend towards less routine use of intervention in hospitals.

Many hospitals ask pregnant women to draw up a birth plan setting out what they would ideally like to happen, and their views on pain relief and intervention. A birth plan is not legally binding but it does provide the person delivering your baby with a clear outline of your wishes.

PAIN RELIEF IN LABOUR

The need for pain relief varies dramatically. It is important to discuss the options beforehand with your doctor, midwife and birth partner.

Natural pain relief

Fear and panic activate hormones that heighten pain, while relaxation techniques and sensory distractions, such as heat and cold or aromatherapy, can help to suppress it. Many antenatal classes teach useful breathing and visualization exercises.

TENS machine

A Transcutaneous Electrical Nerve Stimulation (TENS) machine delivers a small electric current via four electrodes placed at nerve sites on the lower back. Low frequencies release endorphins, the body's natural painkilling opiates, while high frequencies stop pain signals reaching the brain.

Gas and air

A combination of gas (nitrous oxide) and oxygen, delivered via a mask or tube held by the woman to her mouth and nose, numbs the pain centre in the brain. Gas and air takes around 20 seconds to begin working and up to 60 seconds to reach maximum effect, so it is important to start inhaling at the first sign of a contraction.

Pethidine

Pethidine hydrochloride is a pain-relieving drug given via an injection into the thigh or buttock or through a delivery system controlled by the woman. It takes around 20 minutes to work.

Some women find it effective while others say that it makes them feel drowsy while delivering inadequate pain relief. The drug should not be given in the second stage of labour because it suppresses the baby's breathing. Babies born to mothers who have had pethidine are less alert for the first few hours.

Diamorphine

Diamorphine hydrochloride (heroin) has similar benefits and drawbacks to pethidine. Due to its perceived addictive nature, it is not available in all units.

Epidural

Epidural pain relief involves injecting an **anaesthetic** near the spinal nerves to numb the lower body. Some hospitals offer a lower-dose 'mobile epidural', which leaves a degree of muscle strength and sensation in the legs.

If given too early, an epidural increases the likelihood of an assisted delivery with forceps or a ventouse suction device. Follow-up studies show it may also increase the risk of back pain. An epidural is often used in place of a general anaesthetic during a Caesarean.

INTERVENTION IN LABOUR

Many women undergo intervention in labour: in the UK 20 per cent of births are induced, almost 20 per cent are Caesarean deliveries and about 10 per cent are assisted deliveries.

Episiotomy

As the baby's head crowns, it may be necessary to cut the perineum to allow safe delivery of the baby. This is known as an episiotomy, and it may be performed if:
- the perineum is not stretching enough;
- an assisted delivery, using forceps or a ventouse, is required;
- there is a risk of serious tearing.

Medical staff must obtain the woman's consent before performing this procedure. After an injection of anaesthetic, a single cut of around 4cm (1½in) is made. In the United States this is usually a straight line from the vagina towards the anus, but in the United Kingdom the incision is angled to the left. The UK method is harder to repair, but less likely to damage anal muscles.

Dissolving stitches (sutures) are used to repair the cut as quickly as possible after the delivery. Episiotomy increases the risk of discomfort in the postnatal period, and some midwives and doctors believe that small natural tears heal more effectively.

Assisted delivery

Medical staff may decide to assist the delivery if the baby is in distress, the labour is very slow, there is meconium (the baby's first bowel movement) present, or if the mother is too exhausted to push. Forceps or a ventouse are used to hold the baby's head and ease it down the birth canal. An episiotomy may be necessary and pain relief is given.

Caesarean section

A **Caesarean section** is the surgical delivery of a baby through the abdominal wall. It is performed if a vaginal delivery is considered dangerous or

---

Factfile

The baby's position

The contractions of the uterus begin to push the baby out, head first, through the dilated cervix into the vagina or birth canal. The baby shifts its position during labour to ease its passage.

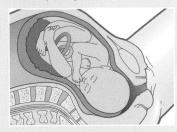

1 The baby has its head lowered onto its chest and usually faces the mother's back as it moves out of the uterus.

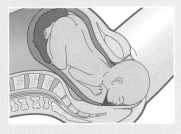

2 Moving down the birth canal, the baby turns according to the shape of the vagina. If the mother is giving birth on her back, the baby usually emerges face down.

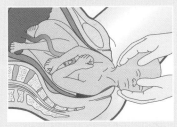

3 Once the baby's head is outside it rotates again, so that the widest shoulder diameter fits the longest diameter of the mother's pelvis. The baby is delivered with its head facing one or other of the mother's thighs.

impossible. An elective Caesarean is one that is planned; a Caesarean carried out in response to a problem arising is called an emergency Caesarean. An epidural or general anaesthetic is given and the baby and placenta are lifted out through a horizontal incision made above the bikini line.

In the 1990s Caesarean rates in the UK climbed dramatically, and around one in five babies are now born in this way. Since a 1993 government report gave the green light for elective Caesareans there has been criticism that some women are now choosing to undergo this surgical procedure in preference to a natural vaginal delivery for the sake of convenience only: women who make an appointment for an elective Caesarean are able to plan for their baby's arrival on a specified date.

MONITORING THE BABY DURING LABOUR

The normal fetal heart rate is 110–160 beats per minute, but this fluctuates with the mother's contractions. Fetal monitoring is used during labour to give warning to midwives and doctors if the baby becomes distressed.

The simplest method of intermittent monitoring of the baby's heartbeat is by using a Pinard stethoscope. This is an earpiece that is placed against the mother's abdomen so the midwife can listen to the baby's heart. An electronic Doppler device, which relies on **ultrasound**, is also used in this way.

Continuous monitoring is advisable if there are complications or a raised risk of fetal distress. If done externally, two straps are placed around the mother's abdomen and connected to an electronic monitor that displays the baby's heart rate and strength, and the timing of contractions. If dilation has begun, a more accurate reading is obtained by attaching a clip to the baby's head.

Some mothers find continuous monitoring intrusive. It also increases the likelihood of intervention because medical staff become aware of problems early on and may be inclined to intervene rather than to wait and see if the problem resolves itself. For this reason the National Institute for Clinical Excellence (NICE) advises that intermittent monitoring is most appropriate for low-risk deliveries.

Induction of labour

Labour may be induced if a woman is two weeks or more overdue to give birth.

Doctors may also decide to induce labour if the baby has stopped growing, the mother has high blood pressure or diabetes, there is not enough amniotic fluid or contractions do not begin within 24–48 hours of the waters rupturing. The Bishop score is used to assess whether an induction is likely to work. This gives a score of zero to three for five factors: the position of the baby and the dilation, consistency, length and position of the cervix. A score of six out of fifteen suggests that induction will succeed.

How is a birth induced?

A synthetic hormone called prostaglandin is administered either orally, vaginally or into the cervical canal itself in order to soften and 'ripen' the cervix. When the cervix begins to dilate, a probe, which looks like a crochet hook, can be used to rupture the waters. If this does not activate regular contractions, an intravenous drip of Syntocinon is given.

WHEN THINGS DON'T GO TO PLAN

The problems that can occur in labour may be a complications of childbirth or the result of a disorder in the pregnancy. The following are common causes of problems in labour.

High blood pressure (hypertension)
One in 20 of the women who experience high **blood pressure** during pregnancy has had long-term hypertension before the pregnancy started. This condition requires careful management because it increases the risk of pre-eclampsia and placental abruption (see below).

Pre-eclampsia
A rise in blood pressure, combined with swollen face, hands, wrists, feet and ankles, and protein in the urine (when there is no urinary tract infection) indicate a pregnancy condition called pre-eclampsia. This usually occurs in the final three months of the pregnancy and is diagnosed when the lower figure in a blood pressure reading rises by 15–20 or goes above 90. Pre-eclampsia is more common in older women and first-time mothers, and is monitored closely since it increases the risk of placental abruption and may develop into eclampsia. Bed rest is advised and a low dose of aspirin may be given.

Eclampsia
Regular antenatal checks mean that pre-eclampsia turns into eclampsia in only one in 2000 pregnancies. This strikes quickly and causes convulsions (fits) and a coma. Apart from the risk of injury and even a heart attack, the mother and her unborn baby may be starved of oxygen. Warning signs include a sharp rise in blood pressure, increased protein in the urine, headache, drowsiness, visual disturbance and nausea. Anticonvulsant drugs are given and a Caesarean is usually performed if the baby isn't yet born.

Gestational diabetes
Pregnancy increases the body's demand for insulin and this activates **diabetes** in two per cent of women. Gestational diabetes is treated by diet or insulin injections. It can accelerate fetal growth, and labour may need to be induced if the baby becomes too large.

Rupture of the amniotic sac
The waters usually break just before, or during, labour, but in one in 14 women this happens too soon. Immediate medical advice is needed as rupture leaves the baby vulnerable to infection and may stimulate contractions. If labour does not begin within 24–48 hours, it is induced.

Premature arrival
A baby born before 37 weeks is pre-term or premature. Babies born after 32 weeks generally do well, but before this may have difficulty breathing. They are at increased risk of jaundice and may have an infection if the early delivery was caused by rupture of the amniotic sac.

Fetal distress

Abnormalities in the heart rate or the presence of fresh meconium are warnings that the baby may not be getting enough oxygen and is in distress. Diagnosis can be confirmed by taking a small blood sample from the scalp. Continued oxygen deprivation causes brain damage, so a decision is usually made to perform a Caesarean or to deliver the baby using forceps or a ventouse.

Breech presentation

One in three babies lie in the womb in a breech (bottom first) position at 30 weeks, but they mostly turn spontaneously and only five per cent remain in it by the due date. It may be possible to turn the baby by manipulating the abdomen in the last few weeks, but this can be uncomfortable and one in ten babies returns to the breech position. Acupuncturists say they can sometimes turn a breech baby by burning moxa, a herb, on certain acupuncture points. Vaginal delivery of a breech baby is possible, but increasing Caesarean rates mean fewer midwives and doctors have experience in delivering breech babies in this way.

Cord prolapse

Occasionally a section of umbilical cord slips out of the uterus in front of the baby. This is more likely to occur in a breech presentation, premature labour or multiple pregnancy.

Prolapse is very dangerous since the cord may be compressed, cutting off the fetal oxygen supply. If this happens, the mother is given oxygen to maximize the baby's supply.

If the prolapse occurs during the first stage of labour, an emergency Caesarean is usually performed. If it happens in the second stage, the baby's position determines whether it will be delivered using forceps or by Caesarean.

Placenta praevia

Placenta praevia, a low-lying placenta, occurs in one in 200 pregnancies and is more common in older mothers. It can cause bleeding and there is an increased risk of haemorrhage. Depending on the position of the placenta, a vaginal delivery may be possible. However, if the placenta is blocking the cervix, a Caesarean is performed.

Placental abruption

In one in 120 pregnancies, the placenta begins to break away from the wall of the uterus before the baby is born. Symptoms include vaginal bleeding, backache and reduced fetal movement. Abruption can cause poor fetal growth and stillbirth, and blood loss in the mother may mean she will need a blood transfusion. The labour may need to be induced or a Caesarean delivery carried out. If placental abruption occurs in the first six months of pregnancy, the death of the fetus is inevitable.

Sudden arrival

If you think the baby is coming too quickly, call the midwife, maternity unit or GP for guidance.

If it appears that the baby may arrive before there is time to reach hospital, call 999 for an ambulance – do not drive yourself. If you are on the way to hospital, the driver should pull over at a safe point, make you comfortable and call 999, giving the exact location and car registration number. If you don't have a mobile phone, flag down another motorist; the mother should never be left alone.

CARE FOR THE NEW BABY

Provided the baby is making some effort to breathe, it is cleaned, weighed and checked for any obvious signs of abnormality. Details of the delivery, time of birth and any drugs given to the mother are recorded, and, in hospital, name bands are placed on the baby's hand and ankle.

Medical staff perform a range of physical checks on newborns, including measuring the skull. The baby's condition is assessed a minute after birth, using the Apgar score so the baby can be given attention if needed. An injection or oral dose of vitamin K may be given. Vitamin K is essential for blood clotting and is given to babies at increased risk of bleeding, such as those born prematurely or with the help of instruments. Many paediatricians believe all babies benefit from vitamin K supplements so some hospitals offer it routinely. The parents are asked for their permission and are given a second oral dose to be administered to their baby four weeks later.

Newborn babies are vulnerable to cold. In the womb they enjoy a constant temperature of 37.7°C (99.9°F), while the average delivery-room temperature is 21°C (69.8°F). Evaporation of amniotic fluid on the baby's skin contributes to heat loss. Because of this, the baby should be dried as quickly as possible and wrapped in a warmed sheet with the head covered.

Most babies breathe within a minute of the birth; if this does not happen the midwife uses suction to clear the airways. A stream of oxygen over the baby's face may prompt a reflex gasp; if this fails, the baby needs assisted ventilation.

CARE FOR THE MOTHER

After the birth a nurse or midwife will take the mother's blood pressure at regular intervals. You will be asked about the amount and consistency of blood loss and have your abdomen palpated – felt firmly – to make sure that your womb is contracting. If you have been given any stitches they will be checked to ensure that they are healing properly. The mother is usually encouraged to put the child to her breast as early as possible, to encourage the early production of milk.

SEE ALSO *Babies and baby care; Postnatal depression; Pregnancy and problems*

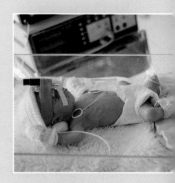

▲ **Early arrival**
In a hospital, medical staff are on hand to provide intensive care for premature babies – particularly those delivered before 32 weeks, who are born significantly under normal weight.

Birthmarks

Birthmarks are areas of discoloured skin that are present at birth or develop in the first few weeks of life. Most birthmarks pose no dangers but can cause the affected person distress, especially if they develop on the face. The most common marks are freckles and moles, caused by abnormal development of skin pigment cells; less common are port-wine stains or strawberry naevi, caused by abnormal dilation of capillaries in the skin.

TREATMENT

Some birthmarks disappear or fade over time without treatment. Others can be disguised with flesh-toned cosmetic creams; colours are available to match most skin tones. Unsightly moles can be removed in the later years of childhood by a plastic surgeon (see also **Cosmetic and plastic surgery**).

Port-wine stains can be treated using an argon **laser**. This emits light absorbed by red pigment, which causes the mark to fade. A patch test is carried out to assess the dose needed and to ensure that there is no scarring. Multiple treatments are needed and there is a 60–80 per cent chance of a 60–80 per cent improvement. The skin may look patchy after treatment, but cosmetic creams can help to disguise this. Seek treatment from a fully trained specialist at an acknowledged centre; ask a GP for advice.

COMPLICATIONS

A strawberry naevus on the face may need early treatment if it interferes with vision, feeding or breathing. Surgery may also be needed if the naevus ulcerates, bleeds or fades leaving an area of slack skin. Those on the lips or the tip of the nose often do not disappear on their own, and are usually treated surgically.

Very rarely, a strawberry naevus causes abnormal blood clotting, resulting in severe haemorrhage (Kasabach-Merritt syndrome); a large, deep naevus may cause **heart failure**. Life-threatening cases can be treated with embolization in which abnormally dilated blood vessels are sealed off.

Facial port-wine stains that develop in skin supplied by a branch of the trigeminal nerve may be associated with abnormalities of blood vessels in the brain coverings (the meninges). This abnormality can lead to **epilepsy** and even a form of **stroke** known as Sturge-Weber syndrome. A port-wine stain that develops on the skin around the eye is associated with an increased risk of **glaucoma**.

Common birthmarks

Birthmarks come in a number of different colours and sizes. Some disappear over time, whereas others require treatment.

▶ **Dark red mark** A port-wine stain is a dark red mark on the skin caused by abnormal dilation of capillaries. Port-wine stains are rare. Most affect the face and neck, which can cause distress in later childhood and adulthood. They are permanent, but can be treated by laser surgery.

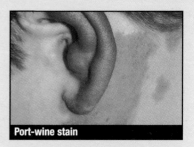
Port-wine stain

◀ **V-shaped patch** As many as 40 per cent of babies have a pinkish-red V-shaped patch on their face, neck or knee, known as a stork mark. Those on the face and knee disappear during the first year of life but those on the nape of the neck are usually permanent.

Stork mark

▶ **Flat or raised skin** Moles may be flat or raised, smooth or hairy areas of skin. Some babies are born with one or more moles. Moles on the face may cause distress and can be removed later in childhood by a plastic surgeon.

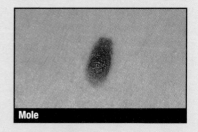
Mole

◀ **Blue-grey spots** Mongolian blue spots appear as a deep, blue-grey discoloration over the lower back; there may be one or several marks. They are caused by the development of pigment cells deep in the skin and are most common in black or Asian babies. The marks usually disappear by the age of seven.

Mongolian blue spot

▶ **Red raised patch** A strawberry naevus is a bright red, raised patch that may appear anywhere on the body during the first four to six weeks after birth. They affect 1 per cent of infants and may grow quite large before starting to fade in the centre. In nine out of ten cases, the strawberry naevus disappears by the age of seven, so these marks are usually best left to fade on their own.

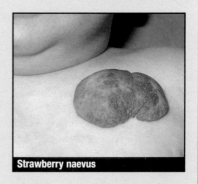
Strawberry naevus

Blackouts

A blackout is the term for any sudden loss of consciousness or vision. It has various causes.

■ **Fainting** – a collapse due to a temporarily insufficient flow of blood to the brain.

■ **Concussion** – disruption of normal brain activity due to an injury to the head.

■ **Seizure** or fit – a sudden surge of electrical activity in the brain. There are many causes, including injury, infection or stroke.

■ Transient ischaemic attacks (**TIA**) – 'mini-strokes' caused by a blood clot or haemorrhage.

■ **Hysterical vision loss** – loss of sight usually due to psychological shock or intense emotion.

Many people experience a blackout at some point. This may be frightening but is not necessarily a sign of disease. However, repeated blackouts should be investigated by a doctor.

Bladder and disorders

The urinary bladder is a hollow, balloon-like, muscular organ that stores urine. No bodily process takes place within the bladder: it does not affect the liquid's concentration nor the balance of its constituents. The bladder is situated behind the pubic bone at the front of the pelvic cavity.

The bladder is highly elastic and can stretch to hold more than 500ml (17fl oz) of fluid. Its size and shape depend on the amount of urine it contains. When empty it is pyramid-shaped with its apex pointing upwards and forward towards the pubic bone. When full, it is egg-shaped and bulges up behind the front abdominal wall, where it may be felt during medical examination if very full.

The neck of the bladder is supported by a sling of muscle known as the pelvic floor. In men, the neck of the bladder is also supported by the prostate gland; this wraps around the urethra (the tube through which urine is emptied) immediately beneath the bladder. In women, the bladder is loosely attached to the cervix and upper vagina, but it is more mobile – one reason why women are prone to stress incontinence (see below).

WHAT CAN GO WRONG?

A number of problems can affect the bladder, of which the most common is an inflammation known as **cystitis**. Most women experience cystitis at least once. Its symptoms are urgent, frequent and uncomfortable urination.

Another common bladder problem is urinary **incontinence**, in which urine leaks from the body involuntarily. This may be due to a weakness of the valve mechanism that keeps the neck of the bladder closed. Such weakness occurs when pressure inside the abdominal cavity temporarily increases – for example, when a person is coughing or sneezing. This is known as stress incontinence.

Other forms of urinary incontinence include urge incontinence, in which an urgent desire to pass urine is accompanied by involuntary contraction of the bladder; total incontinence, due to a complete absence of bladder sphincter activity (for example, in some nervous system disorders such as multiple sclerosis); and overflow incontinence, in which the bladder is always full, due to urinary retention, so that a constant dribbling of overflow urine occurs.

The bladder can also become overactive, causing a frequent and urgent desire to pass urine, with or without urge incontinence. This is thought to happen because the bladder muscle becomes oversensitive and the bladder contracts before it is very full.

Another problem is a bladder calculus. Urine consists of salts dissolved in water, and these salts may crystallize to form a stone called a calculus. A bladder calculus often remains symptomless but can cause discomfort or recurrent urinary tract infections.

Growths may also arise on the bladder lining. These may be benign and produce a wart-like growth known as a bladder polyp, or they may be malignant, causing bladder **cancer**. Bladder tumours may cause no symptoms, or they may produce blood in the urine (haematuria) and recurrent infections. Occasionally, a bladder tumour may obstruct the urethra (causing difficulty passing urine) or a ureter (causing a painful buildup of urine as it travels down towards the bladder from a kidney).

SEE ALSO *Kidneys and disorders; Penis and disorders; Prostate and disorders; Urinary system*

The body has two bladders: the urinary bladder, which stores urine, and the gall bladder, which stores bile.

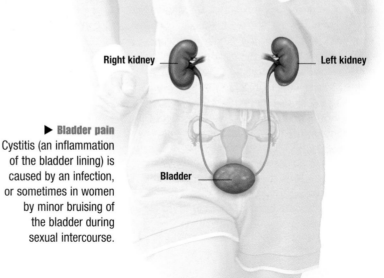

Right kidney — Left kidney

Bladder

▶ **Bladder pain**
Cystitis (an inflammation of the bladder lining) is caused by an infection, or sometimes in women by minor bruising of the bladder during sexual intercourse.

Bleeding

The body's defence system stops minor bleeding in three to ten minutes by forming a clot (see **Blood and disorders; Healing**). Bleeding from an injury to a large vein or artery needs emergency medical treatment as the body cannot cope with major blood loss.

Bleeding without obvious injury may be due to a disease affecting the blood's ability to clot, such as **leukaemia, haemophilia** and abnormal **liver** function – the liver makes the proteins essential to blood clotting. Other common causes are stomach or intestinal **ulcers**.

Minor cases of bleeding cause no symptoms, but continued blood loss of more than 1 litre (around 1¾ pints) leads to low blood pressure, faintness, sweating, rapid pulse, thirst and eventually loss of consciousness.

Bleeding is usually obvious, but sometimes it occurs within the body – for example, after surgery. It is important that patients are monitored after an operation to look for signs of hidden blood loss, such as rapid pulse and falling blood pressure.

SEE ALSO *Arteries and disorders; Blood pressure and problems; FIRST AID; Heart and circulatory system; Liver and disorders*

Blepharitis

Blepharitis is an inflammation of the eyelid margin characterized by redness and crusting of the eyelids and lashes. It is the most common external eye disorder. In more severe cases of blepharitis, the lids may swell and there may be associated **conjunctivitis**. If left untreated over many months, it may lead to eyelash loss and a roughened and irregular lid margin.

Symptoms of blepharitis include itching, a burning sensation, occasional mild pain and crusting of the lids and lashes, particularly upon waking. Its most common causes are seborrhoea (an excess of oily secretions on the skin, causing irritation), dandruff and infection (most commonly by bacteria, but occasionally by other micro-organisms such as the virus **herpes simplex**). In the seborrhoeic form, the lids and lashes are often greasy and matted and the condition responds well to regular bathing of the eyelid margin with a mild baby shampoo or eyelid scrubs, which are available over the counter from a pharmacist. This should be carried out at least twice a day for a fortnight to be effective.

If the condition persists or the symptoms are more severe see a doctor for advice.

SEE ALSO *Eye and problems*

Blindness

In the UK, 25 per cent of people who are registered blind have no perception of light, but most blind people have some degree of vision.

Loss of sight can occur as a result of disease, defect or injury; it may develop gradually or suddenly or be present from birth. Blindness is defined differently from country to country; in the UK, people are said to be blind if they are unable to perform any work for which eyesight is essential. Partial sight has no specific legal definition, but it is a lesser visual disability that can still affect a person's lifestyle or employment. It is not the same as poor vision, which can be corrected with glasses or contact lenses.

CAUSES OF BLINDNESS
Normal vision depends on light passing through the eye and reaching the light receptors in the retina; here, light energy is translated into nerve impulses that are sent to the brain via the optic nerve. Anything that blocks the passage of light or interferes with the nerve impulses can result in blindness.

The major causes of blindness worldwide are: **cataract**, the clouding of the internal focusing lens of the eye; **glaucoma**, nerve damage to the retina and optic nerve caused by high pressure within the eyeball; **trachoma**, a bacterial infection that causes scarring of the cornea and conjunctiva; onchocerciasis, which is a tropical disease of the skin caused by larvae of a parasitic worm; and conditions such as diabetes, which can cause damage to the retina, and dietary deficiency – corneal disease linked to lack of vitamin A, for example, is a major cause of blindness.

BLINDNESS IN THE UK
There are almost 200,000 people registered as blind in the UK and almost 160,000 registered as partially sighted – around 6 in every 10,000. But many blind and partially sighted people are not officially registered, and the actual number is estimated to be just over 1 million. Colour blindness is not really a form of blindness; sufferers, who are usually male, often have good vision but a reduced capacity to perceive various different colours.

Some diseases causing blindness affect different age groups. The majority of blind people are over 65 and have lost their sight as a result of a condition that develops in later life.

Blindness in children

Most conditions that cause blindness in young people are congenital (that is, present from birth). They include disorders of the retina; cataracts; problems caused by infection during **pregnancy** such as rubella or toxoplasmosis; and eye development problems leading to wasting of the optic nerve (optic atrophy). The most common cause of reduced vision in children is amblyopia – or 'lazy eye' – which affects 6 per cent of the population. The condition tends to affect just one eye so is not usually defined as causing blindness or partial sight.

Blindness in adults

The commonest cause of blindness in the adult population is damage to the retina caused by diabetes (diabetic retinopathy). The proportion of people in the UK who develop diabetes is increasing, so the numbers at risk of becoming blind as a result of this condition are rising, too.

There are many other causes of blindness or partial-sightedness in adults. They include **myopia** (short-sightedness), often associated with detachment of the retina. Other conditions include diseases of the retina such as retinitis pigmentosa, which can cause tunnel vision, and diseases associated with the blood vessels such as hypertension (see **Blood pressure and problems**). Inflammatory conditions such as **optic neuritis** (inflammation of the optic nerve) can also cause loss of vision. The eye is such a delicate mechanism that injury can cause serious long-term damage to sight.

Blindness in older age

Most people experience some loss of vision in later life. People who are over 65 are more likely to become blind than those in other age groups. The biggest cause of blindness is age-related **macular degeneration** — the macula is the part of the retina where vision is sharpest. The condition is progressive; eventually a person's vision may deteriorate to the point where they cannot distinguish familiar faces. **Glaucoma** and **cataracts** also commonly affect older people. Age-related cataracts are so common that almost everyone over the age of 65 has some degree of cataract, but vision is not always affected.

COPING WITH BLINDNESS

The level of handicap caused by blindness often depends more on a blind person's attitude than on the degree of sight loss. A well-motivated blind person can often overcome most of the consequences of the disability. Blindness need not affect the person's ability to engage fully in education, a career, family and social life.

But people who have lived most of their life with full vision often find that it takes time to adapt to a sudden reduction in or loss of sight. There are many sources of support for them.

Regular assessment

People adjusting to the loss of sight should keep in regular touch with ophthalmologists and other medical professionals. The management of many of the causes of blindness is continually being improved. A full examination by an optometrist will establish what the best level of achievable vision is at any given stage. The optometrist may recommend magnifiers or low vision aids (LVAs) to help a person to read or watch television. This low-vision assessment is often carried out within a hospital department after referral from a GP. But some optometrists in the community specialize in this area and can also offer the test. Your local health authority should be able to provide information about these services.

Practical support

Social services provide rehabilitation officers who make home visits to people with restricted vision in order to ensure that their living environment is designed to support them. For example, they may make recommendations on how to enhance the contrast of different surfaces and improve lighting in the home. Rehabilitation officers can also provide mobility training and explain other potential sources of practical help. Social workers can offer counselling, including advice and assistance for the family and friends of those who have lost their sight.

For visually impaired people who work, on-the-job assessment of an individual's needs can be carried out. Aids such as portable CCTV systems make it possible for many people with severely impaired vision to read or see a screen well enough to perform many jobs. Children with vision loss may still be able to go to an ordinary school. Education advisers and specialist teachers can design a management plan and provide appropriate LVAs to help a child through school and into higher education.

Charities and self-help groups are often the best sources of information and practical support. They also provide contact with people who have had experience of losing their vision. Among the listed charities and groups, the Royal National Institute for the Blind (RNIB) provides practical support, information about groups within each area and advice on training with techniques such as Braille reading. It lends and sells books and magazines in various formats, including Braille and large-print.

The Guide Dogs for the Blind Association supplies trained dogs for placement with blind people. The dogs make it much easier for blind people to cope with the everyday hazards of urban life, such as crossing roads and negotiating busy public spaces. The association also provides training in using a long cane to aid mobility and reading and writing Braille.

SEE ALSO *Eye and problems*

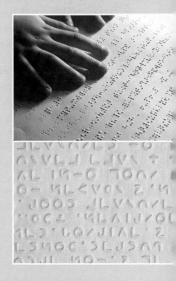

▲ **Feeling the way**
Both Braille (top) and Moon (below) enable people with visual impairments to read and write. Moon is the simpler of the two methods; it has fewer letters that resemble more closely the standard alphabet.

Blind spot

The blind spot is a small area on the retina where the optic nerve is attached. The eye cannot detect images that fall on this spot. But the blind spot is microscopic and the brain compensates for it by 'painting in' the blank area. This subconscious adjustment means that under normal circumstances people remain unaware of the tiny hole at the centre of their vision.

SEE ALSO *Eye and problems*

Blisters

Blisters are collections of fluid beneath unbroken skin. The fluid forms a raised area in which the outer layer of skin (the epidermis) becomes separated from the underlying tissue (the dermis) by straw-coloured fluid (serum) that has leaked from blood vessels. Most occur singly as a result of an injury. Multiple blisters may result from infection or disease. A large fluid-filled blister is known as a bulla, while a small fluid-filled blister is known as a vesicle.

CAUSES

There are many causes of blisters.

■ Injuries, such as burns, sunburn and friction.

■ Infection, for example, **cellulitis**, **impetigo**, **herpes simplex** (cold sores and herpes), **chickenpox**, shingles and molluscum contagiosum.

■ Skin conditions such as **eczema**.

■ Blistering diseases of the skin such as pemphigus vulgaris and **dermatitis** herpetiformis.

An intact blister derived from a non-infectious cause, for example, a burn, helps to protect the underlying tissues from exposure. It also reduces discomfort and the risk of infection. Once burst, exposed nerve endings make a raw blister painful and the blister may also become infected. A blister caused by an infection will be teeming with bacteria or viruses and should also be left intact to reduce the chance of the micro-organisms spreading.

TREATMENT

Do not burst a blister deliberately. If a blister bursts, expose it to the air as much as possible in hygienic surroundings. Cover it with a bandage if there are obvious risks of dirt getting into the wound.

Seek medical advice if a blister becomes infected, with a swollen, tender or red inflamed area spreading around it. You should also consult a doctor if you develop unexplained or widespread blisters: diseases that cause bullae require urgent medical assessment.

SEE ALSO *FIRST AID; Skin and disorders*

Blood and disorders

Every cell in the body is linked by the flow of blood. It acts as both a transport system and a defence mechanism, fighting infection.

There are two types of blood vessel: arteries carry blood from the heart, veins return it to the heart. The average adult has 5 litres (almost 9 pints) of blood circulating through the body. If the circulation stops, death will occur within minutes.

The components of blood

The main components of blood are red blood cells, white blood cells and platelets. These cells float in plasma, a solution that contains important proteins and hormones. Most of the components of blood are manufactured in the bone marrow, from stem cells, and each component has a specific function.

RED BLOOD CELLS

Red blood cells, or erythrocytes, carry oxygen around the body. They contain haemoglobin, a chemical that makes blood red and takes up oxygen from the lungs. When it interacts with oxygen, it forms a compound in the blood called oxyhaemoglobin. As blood passes through the body, this compound is released to help generate energy. Carbon dioxide – a waste product of the chemical reaction that releases this energy – is reabsorbed into the blood and carried back to the lungs, where it is exhaled.

The number of red blood cells in the blood is controlled by a hormone called erythropoietin. When oxygen levels are low, the release of erythropoietin stimulates the formation of more red blood cells in the bone marrow.

WHITE BLOOD CELLS

White blood cells, or leucocytes, are an important part of the body's defence mechanism. There are different types of white blood cells, each with a specific purpose. Lymphocytes, for example, form the antibodies that help the body to fight off infection. Monocytes defend the body against chronic infection, in conditions such as tuberculosis. Neutrophils engulf and digest bacteria and foreign bodies. Other white blood cells contain chemicals such as heparin, which prevents blood coagulation, and histamine, which responds to allergens in conditions such as hay fever and asthma. There is a specialized white blood cell that produces antihistamine, and so controls allergic reactions by inhibiting some of the effects of histamine in the body.

PLATELETS

Platelets help the body to stop bleeding. They are the smallest type of blood cell: there are between 250,000 and 450,000 platelets per cubic millimetre of blood. When a blood vessel is ruptured, the platelets clump together at the site of the injury. They then interact with chemicals in the plasma known as clotting factors. As a result of a series of chemical reactions, the blood is converted from a liquid to a solid state. If the blood lacks any of these clotting factors, as in the condition **haemophilia**, it clots very slowly and the person may experience prolonged bleeding after an injury.

PLASMA

Plasma is the fluid part of blood and carries proteins and nutrients around the body. Plasma proteins include antibodies and fibrinogen, which is involved in blood clotting. Plasma also transports hormones manufactured by various glands in the body, and carries waste products from cells to the liver or kidneys.

Disorders of the blood

The body works to maintain the delicate balance of the different blood components. Various disorders arise when this balance is upset: leukaemia, for example, is a disease that results from the excess production of white blood cells.

DISORDERS OF RED BLOOD CELLS

The most common of all blood disorders is **anaemia**, a reduction in the quantity of haemoglobin in the blood and therefore its capacity to carry oxygen. Its symptoms include tiredness, shortness of breath, headaches, pallor of skin and swelling of ankles in severe cases.

The most frequent cause of anaemia is a deficiency of iron, which is needed for the production of haemoglobin. This is very common in menstruating women, who lose iron when they bleed. It can also occur when the bone marrow lacks Vitamin B_{12} or other substances needed for the formation of blood: it then manufactures fewer red blood cells. A deficiency of folic acid or an inherited defect such as sickle cell anaemia are other causes.

The body can produce too many red blood cells; this condition is called polycythaemia, and is fairly common. It is the body's response to reduced oxygen in the tissues and occurs

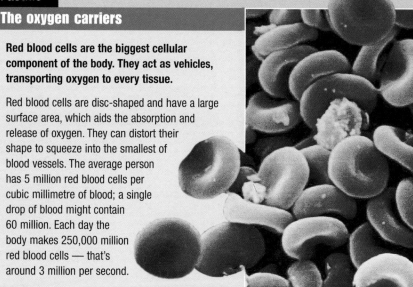

Factfile

The oxygen carriers

Red blood cells are the biggest cellular component of the body. They act as vehicles, transporting oxygen to every tissue.

Red blood cells are disc-shaped and have a large surface area, which aids the absorption and release of oxygen. They can distort their shape to squeeze into the smallest of blood vessels. The average person has 5 million red blood cells per cubic millimetre of blood; a single drop of blood might contain 60 million. Each day the body makes 250,000 million red blood cells — that's around 3 million per second.

naturally in people who live at high altitude. In its early stages, polycythemia produces no symptoms; a flushed face, tiredness, itching and sometimes **gout** can occur later on. Polycythaemia is most likely to affect smokers and people who suffer from chronic lung conditions such as emphysema and chronic bronchitis, which reduce the supply of oxygen to the blood. Red blood cell levels usually return to normal once the underlying condition is treated.

Less commonly, polycythaemia is caused by tumours in the liver or kidneys. A rare cause is an abnormality in red blood cell production in the bone marrow; this is called polycythaemia rubra vera. In this case, a doctor may recommend a bone marrow **biopsy** to aid with diagnosis; treatment may involve removing some blood from the veins every few weeks or the use of radiotherapy or anticancer drug treatment.

DISORDERS OF WHITE BLOOD CELLS

Leukaemia is the name for several cancers in which there is an excess of white blood cells. Leukaemia is quite rare: one in 20,000 people is affected each year in the UK. Leukaemia can be acute, in which there is a rapid onset occurring over a few days or weeks, or chronic, in which abnormalities build up over months or years. Acute leukaemias are more common in children while chronic leukaemias are more likely to arise in adults.

DISORDERS OF PLATELETS

A reduced number of platelets in the blood is a feature of the bleeding disorder thrombocytopenia. The symptoms are easy and spontaneous bleeding, for example, from the gums, and tiny haemorrhages in the skin (called petechiae) that look like purple dots. Thrombocytopenia can follow viral infections or the development of **autoimmune diseases**, as well as a course of certain drugs. The outlook is good once the underlying cause is treated.

Abnormalities in the platelets can also occur as a result of bone marrow disorders. The patient may be referred for a bone marrow **biopsy** to aid diagnosis. If the condition comes on suddenly, other tests may be needed to exclude the possibility of severe infections such as meningococcal **meningitis**.

DISORDERS OF BLOOD PLASMA
Most plasma disorders result from **liver** problems: it is the liver that produces the bulk of the components of plasma. Symptoms of blood plasma disorders include swollen legs, general malaise, poor blood clotting and easy bruising.

Plasma problems are usually detected during investigation of some other disorder such as suspected liver disease.

BLOOD-CLOTTING DISORDERS
The body's blood-clotting mechanism is finely balanced and involves both plasma proteins and the platelets. Abnormality in any one of the factors involved can result in a blood-clotting disorder. The inherited condition **haemophilia**, for example, is caused by a deficiency in the essential clotting factor VIII.

Thrombosis can occur if the blood clots too readily, creating blockages in the arteries. One cause of clotting in the arteries is the buildup of fatty deposits on the blood vessel walls, as occurs in arteriosclerosis. **Deep vein thrombosis** usually occurs as a result of sluggish blood flow; typically circulation may be reduced by the person sitting or lying down for too long, for example, perhaps on a longhaul aircraft flight.

ABNORMAL BLOOD SUGAR LEVELS
Blood sugar is the term used to describe glucose in the blood, a nutrient that provides cells with energy. When sugary and starchy foods are digested, they are converted into glucose which can be stored as glycogen in the liver and muscles for later use.

The level of blood glucose is maintained within narrow limits by various hormones. The predominant hormone is insulin but when too much insulin is produced, **hypoglycaemia** (reduced glucose in the blood) may result, causing temporary symptoms such as cold sweats, irritability and even unconsciousness. When the body fails to produce insulin or fails to respond to it, **hyperglycaemia** (excess glucose in the blood) may result. This is a sign of **diabetes**, typical symptoms of which are excessive thirst and the frequent passing of urine.

BLOOD POISONING
In blood poisoning, also known as **septicaemia**, micro-organisms spread and grow within the bloodstream. The source is often a minor infection such as a skin **boil**, but may also be due to infections in the kidneys, heart, lungs, bowel or brain coverings (meninges). Diabetics are at higher risk of blood poisoning, as are people with lowered immunity – as a result of leukaemia, for example.

Symptoms start with high fever and shivering, then progress to low blood pressure and widespread internal bleeding. The diagnosis involves blood tests to identify the micro-organisms responsible. Treatment requires potent antibiotics, together with an intravenous fluid drip and possibly blood transfusion. Even with prompt, intensive treatment, septicaemia is a highly dangerous illness, and is fatal in 40–55 per cent of cases.

Blood tests
Many specific diseases can be identified through blood tests, which can detect the presence of micro-organisms, antibodies and chemicals (such as glucose) in the blood. The most commonly used blood test is a blood count. This measures the amount of haemoglobin in the blood as well as the number, shape and size of red blood cells, white blood cells and platelets. A blood count aids with the diagnosis of leukaemia, anaemia and thrombocytopenia among other disorders. Blood samples are usually taken from a vein in the arm. Other tests include measuring the time it takes to stop bleeding after a small cut is made to the skin.

Blood transfusion
A blood transfusion usually involves the transfer of blood or certain components of blood from one person into the circulatory system of another person. Blood transfusions are given to patients who have lost a lot of blood after an accident or during surgery, or who have suffered severe internal bleeding. Some conditions such as leukaemia or severe anaemia may also benefit from a blood transfusion. In an exchange transfusion, most of the recipient's blood is replaced: this procedure is used mainly for cases of **haemolytic disease** in newborn babies.

Most blood transfusions involve donated blood; the blood is tested to ensure its compatibility, then stored until required. But it is also possible for people to store their own blood for later use. This process, known as autologous transfusion, is unusual in the UK, but is common in countries where there are doubts about blood safety – especially fears about the transmission of HIV.

It takes two or three sessions to store a substantial quantity of your own blood; for this reason, autologous transfusion is realistic only for non-emergency situations. But a patient's blood is often saved during surgery to be transfused later in the operation if necessary.

Blood transfusions have transformed the outlook for people who have suffered serious injuries and burns. The fact that doctors can now replace or top up a patient's blood makes it possible to perform operations that would otherwise be too risky because of the likelihood of substantial blood loss.

RECEIVING A BLOOD TRANSFUSION

Human blood is not all the same. Before a transfusion is performed, the recipient's blood is crossmatched with the donated blood to ensure that the blood groups are compatible.

Blood is dripped into a large vein, usually in the recipient's arm, via a needle. It takes up to four hours to transfuse a unit of blood, but the process can be done more quickly if needed.

Minor reactions caused by the body's defence system commonly occur after a blood transfusion: these include fever, itching and rashes. More severe reactions are possible if the wrong blood is transfused or if it has not been matched correctly. If this occurs, the recipient's antibodies may destroy the incompatible red blood cells, releasing haemoglobin into the bloodstream. Blood pressure may also fall and the normal blood-clotting mechanism fail, causing extensive internal bleeding; kidney failure may also result.

BLOOD GROUPS

There are four main groups, which cannot always be mixed – a vital consideration when a blood transfusion is necessary. The main blood groups are: A, B, AB and O. Most people of Western origin are either blood group O or A. The definition of the four blood groups is based on the presence or absence of two antigens, A and B. Blood group O contains neither antigen.

As well as this classification, all blood is defined as being Rhesus negative or Rhesus positive, depending on whether or not it contains another group of antigens – the Rhesus factor.

The Rhesus factor

Eighty-five per cent of the population are Rhesus positive; the remainder are Rhesus negative. Although mixing of positive with negative is not desirable, it is possible, but problems may occur if this happens more than once. For example, if a Rhesus negative mother is carrying a Rhesus positive baby, tiny quantities of the baby's Rhesus positive blood can enter the mother's bloodstream. This is usually no problem on the first pregnancy, but the next time the mother carries a Rhesus positive baby her antibodies may enter and destroy the baby's blood. Treatment

Mixing it

The table shows which blood groups can safely be mixed. Forty-six per cent of people of Western origin are blood group O, 42 per cent group A, 9 per cent group B, and 3 per cent group AB.

BLOOD GROUP	CAN DONATE TO	CAN RECEIVE FROM
A	A and AB	A and O
B	B and AB	B and O
AB	AB	A, B, AB and O Universal recipient
O	A, B, AB and O Universal donor	AB and O

involves injecting the mother with antibodies. (See also **Haemolytic disease of the newborn**.)

Matching blood groups

Blood group O is known as the 'universal donor blood' because it can be given in limited quantities to any recipient; blood group AB is called the 'universal recipient' because it can accept limited blood transfusions from any other blood group. But if a transfusion combines other blood groups, there may be serious and even fatal results. Blood in group A contains antibodies, which will react against the antigens of blood group B, for example.

ARTIFICIAL BLOOD PLASMA

The development of a synthetic substitute for blood has been a scientific goal for many years. Although this goal is yet to be reached, substances have been developed that can substitute plasma and therefore restore blood pressure in an emergency.

SEE ALSO *Arteries and disorders; Blood pressure and problems; Capillaries and disorders; Haemorrhage; Heart and circulatory system; Kidneys and disorders; Liver and disorders; Veins and disorders*

Blood pressure and problems

Blood pressure is the pressure created by the flow of blood through the major arteries. Blood pressure is not constant, because blood flows around the body in a series of waves generated by the beating of the heart. With each beat of the heart, there is a point of high pressure and low pressure.

When the heart contracts, the pressure in the arteries reaches its maximum – this is known as systolic blood pressure. The minimum point is reached when the heart relaxes – this is called diastolic pressure. These two points are what is measured when your blood pressure is taken.

There is no such thing as a 'normal' blood pressure, as both the systolic and diastolic pressure vary widely in the population. Your blood pressure can also vary from moment to moment, to cope with the body's hormonal changes. For example, when adrenaline is released into the blood, the pressure rises to send extra blood – and energy – to the muscles.

HOW BLOOD PRESSURE IS MEASURED

Blood pressure is measured using either a mercury or anaeroid sphygmomanometer or a digital monitor; it is a quick and painless procedure. A cuff is placed around the arm and inflated in order to compress the artery. A stethoscope or pressure detector is placed over the artery to gauge the air pressure being exerted. As the pressure falls below systolic blood pressure, the sound of blood pulsing down the artery can be detected; the sound disappears again when the cuff pressure falls to the diastolic blood pressure. Both measurements are recorded.

When blood pressure is tested, both the systolic and diastolic pressure are measured in millimetres of mercury (chemical symbol Hg). Systolic pressure is given first: a reading of 120/80 (an average reading for a fit young person) means a systolic pressure of 120mm Hg and a diastolic pressure of 80mm Hg. A fit middle-aged person might have a reading of 135/90. A reading between 140/90 and 160/110 indicates mild hypertension. Readings above this point indicate severe hypertension. Depending on a person's medical history, a blood pressure reading as low as 95/60 can still be seen as healthy.

Ambulatory blood pressure monitoring

Ambulatory monitoring involves repeated blood pressure checks using a machine that tests blood pressure as the person goes about his or her normal routine. A blood pressure cuff is

Patterns of blood pressure

As we get older our blood pressure has a tendency to rise. The graphs below show the typical patterns for women and men. Age is represented by the numbers along the bottom, while the upper and lower edges of the coloured bands represent systolic and diastolic readings respectively.

Female

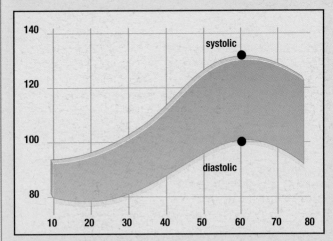

▲ **Rise and fall**
Women's blood pressure tends to peak at the age of 60, at about 130/100.

Male

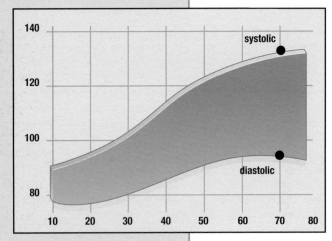

▲ **Sustained risk**
Men's blood pressure rises and remains high, posing risks to health.

worn for 24 hours and inflates automatically, usually every half-hour, including during the night. The person keeps a diary to show what he or she was doing at each point (driving, resting, sleeping and so on). The checks can be helpful to decide if treatment is needed for:

- borderline readings;
- suspected 'white-coat' hypertension – that is, when blood pressure seems to go up in response to being checked in the surgery;
- elderly people or pregnant women;
- suspected night-time hypertension (blood pressure normally falls at night);
- checking whether blood pressure is being over- or undertreated, or when people fail to respond to treatment.

Home monitoring

You can also buy a home blood pressure monitor that can provide extra information, including printouts, to help in diagnosing or treating hypertension. They are prone to error, so choose a brand recommended by your doctor and have it calibrated (for accuracy) regularly. Make sure you follow the manufacturer's instructions. Do not alter your hypertension treatment without asking your doctor's advice.

High blood pressure (hypertension)

Blood pressure naturally increases with age and hypertension often starts in middle-age. More than one-third of adults in the UK are either being treated for high blood pressure or have a blood pressure reading that is greater than 140/90 (a reading that would indicate mild hypertension in middle age). The outward symptoms are difficult to detect: 50 per cent of sufferers are unaware that they have the condition. Because of this, it is usually detected during a routine examination.

Not all the effects of high blood pressure are known, but it can result in damage to the body's vital organs. The heart, brain and kidneys are most at risk: untreated hypertension can lead to heart disease, stroke, dementia or kidney failure. When combined with a high blood **cholesterol** level, high blood pressure will often accelerate the development of arteriosclerosis, a hardening of the arteries. Treatment reduces the risk of heart attack by 20 per cent and of stroke by 40 per cent.

SYMPTOMS

Unless blood pressure is very high, there may be no symptoms of hypertension. When there are symptoms, they may include:

- headaches;
- nosebleeds;
- passing more urine at night;
- symptoms of **angina**, **heart failure**, **stroke** or **oedema** (fluid retention).

Accelerated or malignant hypertension (in which the blood pressure rapidly becomes extremely high), causes severe headaches, visual disturbance, fits and renal failure. Emergency treatment is required.

CAUSES

The causes of hypertension are not fully understood but the vast majority of cases do not occur as a result of an underlying condition. In such cases the condition is called primary or essential hypertension and there are a number of factors associated with it.

There is thought to be a genetic factor, since problems with high blood pressure tend to run in families. Obesity and persistently high alcohol intake are associated with hypertension: avoiding alcohol leads to a prompt fall in blood pressure, and overweight people suffering from hypertension usually show a similar drop, as long as they lose weight gradually. There is also thought to be a link with diet: a diet high in fat and salt may increase the risk of hypertension. Anxiety and stress are also associated with short-term increases in blood pressure.

Five per cent of cases of hypertension are classed as secondary hypertension – they are the result of another disorder. These include:

- **kidney** disease;
- hormonal disorders such as hyperthyroidism, phaeochromocytoma and **Cushing's syndrome**;
- coarctation (narrowing) of the **aorta**;
- pre-eclampsia in **pregnancy**;
- obstructive sleep apnoea.

Some drugs can cause hypertension, including oral contraceptives, steroids, non-steroidal anti-inflammatories, alcohol and some cold remedies.

TREATMENT

Consult a doctor if you develop any of the symptoms described above. You should also have your blood pressure checked regularly – at least once every five years.

What a doctor may do

- Check your blood pressure.
- Arrange ambulatory blood pressure monitoring if your blood pressure varies on different occasions (see page 120).
- Calculate your Body Mass Index (BMI) to determine whether you are in the healthy weight range for your height.
- Check your heartbeat, your abdomen and the functioning of your cardiovascular system (the heart and blood vessels).
- Check for signs of retinopathy, a disorder of the retina often associated with hypertension (see **Eye and problems**).
- Take blood tests to check kidney function, cholesterol levels and glucose levels in the blood.

▲ **Self-testing**
People who have problems with their blood pressure may wish to buy a self-testing kit, like the one shown here, to monitor their condition on a regular basis.

The risks during pregnancy

Three conditions – pregnancy-induced hypertension, pre-eclampsia and eclampsia – can raise the blood pressure of women in pregnancy, in some cases causing serious illness.

Medical researchers do not fully understand why some women develop high blood pressure while pregnant. In most cases the condition causes no serious problems, and the mother's blood pressure returns to its normal level within a week or so of giving birth. But between 5 and 10 per cent of women develop what is known as pre-eclampsia, usually in late pregnancy. Blood pressure starts to rise, and women may experience excessive fluid retention, headaches, visual disturbances, vomiting and upper abdominal pain; a urine test may reveal the presence of harmful proteins.

Pre-eclampsia is usually detected in good time during antenatal checks, but if left untreated it may develop into full-blown eclampsia, in which the woman can suffer seizures and may, in extreme cases, fall into a coma. If pre-eclampsia or eclampsia develop once the fetus is 'viable', labour may be induced or the baby delivered by Caesarean section. In severe cases where the fetus is not yet fully developed, doctors may advise a termination in order to save the mother's life.

Although the exact cause of pre-eclampsia is not known, some women are more at risk: those who are overweight, who have kidney disease, diabetes or pre-existing high blood pressure, and women who are under the age of 19 or over 35.

■ Take additional blood tests to check liver and thyroid function, levels of calcium and protein.
■ Test urine for protein and blood.
■ Arrange an ECG (electrocardiogram) test, chest **X-ray**, echocardiogram (an examination of the heart using **ultrasound**), renal ultrasound or hormone test.

If hypertension is diagnosed, your doctor may:
■ advise changes to your lifestyle, such as taking up exercise or reducing stress;
■ recommend that you follow a healthy balanced diet that is low in fat and salt
■ suggest you lose weight if you are overweight;
■ advise you to reduce your alcohol intake;
■ recommend drug treatment.

Referral to a specialist
You may be referred to a specialist if:
■ tests suggest that you may have an underlying treatable cause for your hypertension (secondary hypertension);
■ you are under 30 years of age;
■ you are pregnant;
■ your blood pressure varies considerably;
■ your blood pressure is difficult to control with drugs;
■ you have severe headaches, visual disturbance or other symptoms of accelerated or malignant hypertension or other complications.

Drug treatment
Different drugs suit different people. Most sufferers are prescribed more than one drug, taking into account:
■ blood pressure level;
■ side effects;

■ co-existing medical problems – target levels are lower for those people who suffer from diabetes or heart disease;
■ risk factors (such as smoking, diabetes or high cholesterol).

Hypertension drugs can take up to four weeks to have full effect: see **Drugs and their uses** for details of the drugs used, how they work and their side effects.

Aspirin is recommended for some people aged over 50 who have controlled hypertension together with diabetes, **angina** or heart disease, or who show evidence of damage to the heart, kidney or retinal arteries, or have a high risk of coronary heart disease. Cholesterol-lowering (statin) therapy is recommended up to the age of 70 for people with a high risk of coronary heart disease due to high blood cholesterol.

Monitoring hypertension
Once hypertension has been diagnosed, your blood pressure and weight should be checked every six months. Your urine should be tested for protein annually.

Certain drugs, including ACE inhibitors, thiazides and angiotensin II receptor antagonists (blockers), may affect blood chemistry and kidney function. These should be checked within two weeks of starting or increasing the dose of these drugs and at regular intervals.

What you can do
Changes to your diet, taking regular exercise, reducing **alcohol** intake and stopping **smoking** can all help to reduce blood pressure. Consult your doctor before starting a new exercise regime or making a drastic change to your diet. Reduce stress levels, which may cause short-term rises in blood pressure. Consider relaxation therapy, yoga or meditation. Keeping a pet or making adjustments to your daily timetable may also help.

Complementary therapies
■ Some people claim that a high potassium intake can help lower blood pressure. Taking potassium supplements is not recommended by most experts, but the following foods are all good sources: bananas, broccoli, potatoes, oranges, melon and pineapple.
■ Avoid ginseng, rosemary, thyme and clary sage as these can raise blood pressure.

COMPLICATIONS
■ Damage to large and small arteries (arteriosclerosis; **atheroma**).
■ Heart strain.
■ **Stroke** or mini-stroke.
■ **Kidney disorders**.
■ Circulatory disorders such as peripheral arterial disease. (See **Arteries and disorders; Heart and circulatory system**.)
■ **Pregnancy** problems (such as pre-eclampsia).

PREVENTION

■ Even if you feel well, you should have your blood pressure checked at least once every five years, and every year if your blood pressure is in the high normal range (above 135/85).

■ Following the lifestyle advice given in Lowering your blood pressure, below) will help to prevent the condition or delay its development. This approach is especially important if you have a family history of raised blood pressure as you may then be particularly at risk of developing problems.

OUTLOOK

Drug treatment is usually effective in keeping hypertension under control. Once drug treatment is started, it is usually necessary for the rest of the person's life.

Low blood pressure (hypotension)

Blood pressure that is lower than normal is not necessarily a problem: some people have naturally low blood pressure. But sudden or prolonged falls can reduce the oxygen supply to the brain and cause episodes of fainting or dizziness.

SYMPTOMS

■ Dizziness or lightheadedness, especially on standing.

■ Blackouts.

■ Fatigue.

CAUSES

■ Getting up after a prolonged period of sitting or lying down.

■ Shock.

■ Pregnancy.

■ Emotion, pain, hunger or prolonged standing, especially when hot.

■ Ageing – automatic reflexes compensate for the natural fall in blood pressure that occurs when we stand up; these work less well as we grow older.

■ Emptying the bladder, especially after getting out of bed.

■ Some forms of heart disease.

■ Overtreatment of hypertension.

■ Some drugs (for example, those taken for **depression** or urinary **incontinence**).

TREATMENT

Treatment for low blood pressure usually involves treating the underlying cause. But in extreme cases, doctors may advise drug treatment to raise the blood pressure.

If you feel dizzy or faint, lie down and raise the feet above the heart. Wearing compression stockings to improve blood return to the heart may help if such spells are frequent. These are not suitable for people with peripheral arterial disease.

SEE ALSO *Arteries and disorders; Blood and disorders; Heart and circulatory system*

Lowering your blood pressure

To lower your blood pressure the British Hypertension Society recommends the following.

■ Keep your Body Mass Index (BMI) below 25; if you are overweight, losing 3kg (6.6lb) can reduce your blood pressure by 7/4 mm Hg.

■ Do not add salt when cooking or at the table, and avoid salty foods such as crisps, salted peanuts and ready-prepared meals.

■ Eat at least two portions of oily fish a week – sardines, mackerel, herring, trout, salmon, pilchards or fresh (but not tinned) tuna. Fish oil capsules are a good alternative; aim for 150–200mg of omega-3 fatty acids daily.

■ Eat a healthy diet – more rice and wholemeal cereals, seven portions of fresh fruit and vegetables daily, and less saturated fat (commonly found in processed foods, animal fats and fats that are solid at room temperature).

■ Take regular exercise – a brisk 20-minute every day should help.

■ Don't smoke.

■ Drink alcohol only within recommended limits – a maximum of 2–3 units a day for women and 3–4 units a day for men (one unit is half a pint of beer or a small glass of wine).

■ Reduce stress – or learn relaxation methods to counteract it.

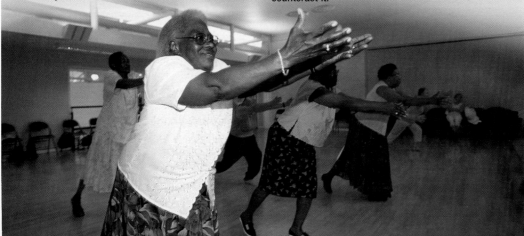

Blue baby

Some babies have a blueish tinge to the skin, which indicates that the infant is not getting enough oxygen. A congenital **heart** defect is the most likely cause.

Lack of oxygen in the blood supply can result from a hole in one of the walls that divide the heart into four separate chambers, or an error in the way that veins and arteries within the heart are connected.

Boil

A boil is a small **abscess** that forms when a hair follicle becomes infected with the common skin bacterium *Staphylococcus aureus*. A collection of boils is known as a **carbuncle**.

Any hair-bearing area of skin can be affected by a boil, but they occur most commonly in places that are prone to friction or where dirt and sweat collect, such as the neck, armpits, groin and buttocks.

A boil first appears as a red, tender lump, which then swells with pus and eventually forms a yellow head before bursting. Any pressure and pain is quickly relieved once the pus comes to the surface.

Recurrent boils may be linked with reduced immunity to infection or with raised blood-glucose levels (see **Diabetes**).

TREATMENT

Boils usually heal quickly, but may need to be treated with antibiotics in the early stages to prevent the infection from spreading, especially if the boil is large or if the person feels unwell. It will also help to apply a hot compress every two hours.

Boils that have come to a head may be treated by lancing under sterile conditions to release the pus and encourage healing. You should never squeeze or burst a boil, since this can cause the infection to spread.

SEE ALSO *Bacterial infections*

Bone and problems

Bones are rigid structures that make up the skeleton and give the body its shape. They are held together with ligaments and meet at the joints. Bones protect the vital organs and act as levers, enabling movement to take place. They also distribute some of the body's essential minerals, in particular, calcium.

Bones have several layers: their spongy interior is surrounded by a hard shell, which in turn is a covered by a thick membrane containing a network of nerves and blood vessels. **Bone marrow** fills the spaces in the spongy bone, and manufactures most of the components of blood.

WHAT CAN GO WRONG

■ The most common problem to affect bone is a **fracture** as a result of a blow or repeated stress. Some conditions make fractures more likely to occur. In older age, **osteoporosis**, which causes bones to become brittle, is often the underlying cause. In young children, frequent fractures may be a result of osteogenesis imperfecta (also known as brittle bone disease).

■ A fracture may cause the bone tissue to die as a result of its blood supply being cut off (avascular necrosis). Also known as ischaemic bone necrosis, it can occur as a result of long-term alcohol abuse or the use of corticosteroids.

■ Osteomalacia is a softening of adult bone, usually caused by an intestinal disease that prevents the absorption of Vitamin D; it is treated with vitamin supplements.

■ **Osteomyelitis** is an infection that causes inflammation in the bone. It usually occurs in newborn babies or young children, and may occur after fractures. Once diagnosed it is treated with antibiotics.

■ Osteosarcoma is a **cancer** that most often affects the ends of long bones. It is the most common form of bone cancer in children. Another form of cancer, called **myelomatosis**, can affect the white blood cells, causing abnormal cells to become lodged in the outer layer of bone and in bone marrow.

■ Fibrous dysplasia is a condition in which the fibrous tissue within bone expands, deforming it and increasing its size. In **Paget's disease**, the outer layer of the bone thickens.

Infected hair follicle

A boil forms when skin bacteria enter a hair follicle and infect it.

As the body fights the bacteria, pus is produced and the boil swells to take on a rounded appearance with a yellow-white tip. The first sign is a painful, itchy lump.

Bacteria enter hair follicle

Sebaceous gland

Hair follicle

A malfunction of the parathyroid glands can cause an excess of parathyroid hormone. This weakens the bones by leaching calcium.

Developmental problems affecting bone include achondroplasia, a hereditary form of dwarfism, and brittle bone disease.

SEE ALSO *Joints and problems; Skeletal system; Spine and disorders*

Bone marrow and disorders

Bone marrow is a soft substance contained within the spongy interior of a bone (see **Bone and problems**). There are two types of marrow: red and yellow. Red marrow manufactures red blood cells, some white blood cells and also the platelets, which play a part in blood clotting. It is found in the bones of the skull, the ribs, the breastbone, the vertebrae and the heads of long bones. Yellow marrow is less active and produces blood cells only when the body is undergoing high physical demand. It is found in the shafts of long bones.

WHAT CAN GO WRONG

The bone marrow may produce insufficient quantities of red blood cells, with serious consequences for all the systems of the body. This occurs in most types of **leukaemia**.

A group of conditions called myeloproliferative disorders cause too many types of blood cells to be produced. These disorders include a type of leukaemia (chronic myeloid leukaemia) and polycythaemia rubra vera, a rare disease, causing the red blood cells to increase to a level that slows the blood flow.

The bone marrow may also be affected by a type of cancer called **myelomatosis**, also known as multiple myeloma. This causes certain cells in the bone marrow (plasma cells) to overproduce one type of antibody at the expense of others, making the person vulnerable to infection.

TREATMENT

Bone marrow disorders are usually treated with drug therapy, **radiotherapy** and **chemotherapy**. A transfusion of red blood cells may also be necessary (see **Blood and disorders**); if treatment is not successful a bone-marrow **transplant** may be performed.

Bornholm disease

Bornholm disease is a viral infection that mainly affects children and young adults. It is also known as epidemic myalgia or devil's grip. Symptoms include a raised temperature, headache and sore throat as well as chest, muscle and stomach pains, made worse by coughing or deep breathing.

The recommended treatment is to rest, drink plenty of fluids, and take painkillers such as paracetamol in the recommended dosage or stronger painkillers prescribed by your doctor. Herbal medicines and homeopathy may help to ease breathing problems, pain and fever. You should contact a doctor if you have severe stomach or chest pain to rule out more serious causes, such as a heart attack or pneumonia.

A full recovery can usually be expected within seven days but, in a few cases, symptoms recur over the following weeks. Complications are rare but the infection may spread to other parts of the body, such as the heart or testicles, or cause a form of **meningitis**.

Bowel and disorders

The bowel is the longest part of the digestive tract. It consists of the small and large intestines and is about 8m (26ft) long. It is the main site in the body for the digestion and absorption of food and water.

The first part of the bowel is the small intestine, which is about 6.5m (21ft) long. Along the internal intestinal wall are finger-like extensions called villi, each about 1mm long (the villi are themselves covered with even smaller microvilli) that increase the surface area of the intestinal wall, which aids the absorption of nutrients.

The small intestine is divided into three parts: the duodenum, where it leaves the stomach; the jejunum, the middle section; and the ileum, which lead into the the large intestine.

The large intestine comprises the colon and rectum. It is shorter, at around 1.5m (5ft), and wider than the small intestine and does not contain villi. Its main function is to absorb water from digested food and turn it into faeces. It starts at a pouch called the caecum, from which the **appendix** protrudes, rises up the right-hand side of the body (the ascending colon) and then across the body (the transverse colon) just below the liver; it then runs down the left side (the descending colon) to terminate at the rectum and anus.

HOW THE BOWEL WORKS

When food enters the small intestine, it is broken down into its component chemicals by enzymes. Bile and pancreatic juices enter the top part of the duodenum through a duct, and other enzymes and mucus are produced by glands in the intestinal walls. The bowel also contains bacteria, which help to break down food as well as manufacturing some types of Vitamin B. The breakdown products are absorbed into the bloodstream through the intestinal wall.

The process is normally so effective that by the time the large intestine starts to fill, the contents consist only of liquid, fibre, some fat, vitamins and mineral salts, bacteria and waste products.

As part of the process of digestion, food is propelled through the bowel by an action called peristalsis. The muscles in the intestinal walls automatically contract and relax in a rhythm – those in front of a portion of digestive material relax, while the ones behind it contract. The result is a rippling, wave-like motion that moves food through the system. Peristalsis takes different forms in different parts of the bowel. In the small intestine, food is moved more slowly and in both directions, mixing it up and allowing more time for digestion. But the muscles of the large intestine contract only a few times a day, usually after meals. This forceful wave of contractions pushes waste products down to the rectum for expulsion during defecation.

Digestive machine
The bowel is a continuous tube about 8m (26ft) long. As food moves slowly through the small and large intestines, nutrients and water are absorbed into the bloodstream through the wall of the intestine. The waste products are then passed out of the body.

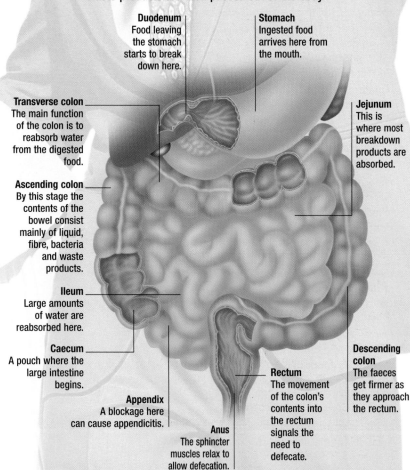

Transverse colon
The main function of the colon is to reabsorb water from the digested food.

Ascending colon
By this stage the contents of the bowel consist mainly of liquid, fibre, bacteria and waste products.

Ileum
Large amounts of water are reabsorbed here.

Caecum
A pouch where the large intestine begins.

Appendix
A blockage here can cause appendicitis.

Duodenum
Food leaving the stomach starts to break down here.

Stomach
Ingested food arrives here from the mouth.

Jejunum
This is where most breakdown products are absorbed.

Rectum
The movement of the colon's contents into the rectum signals the need to defecate.

Anus
The sphincter muscles relax to allow defecation.

Descending colon
The faeces get firmer as they approach the rectum.

BOWEL HABITS
It can take anything from 20 hours to more than 100 hours for food to pass through the digestive tract, and bowel habits vary from person to person. It is considered 'normal' to evacuate your bowels anything from three times a day to three times a week.

A doctor will describe an individual as constipated only if that person's bowel movements are hard, painful to pass or occur less frequently than every two days.

Taking laxatives to increase the frequency of your bowel movements is not advisable because their overuse may damage the intestines. But, if you suffer from persistent constipation, or if your usual bowel habits change and do not return to normal after several days, you should consult a doctor.

WHAT CAN GO WRONG
Problems can occur at any point in the bowel, affecting the absorption of nutrients and the expulsion of waste. Common symptoms of bowel problems are difficulties with defecation, including **constipation, diarrhoea** and **incontinence**. There may also be wind (see **Flatulence**), abnormal or bloody stools and abdominal pain (see **Abdominal pain**).

A number of conditions involve a temporary inflammation of the intestinal wall, generally resulting from bacterial or viral infection. These include **food poisoning, gastroenteritis, ileitis** and **proctitis**.

Coeliac disease
Coeliac disease is an inflammatory condition arising as a result of damage to the small intestine caused by sensitivity to gluten. It adversely affects the absorption of nutrients by the intestines and is one of the main causes of **malabsorption syndrome**.

Crohn's disease
Crohn's disease is a chronic inflammatory disease that usually affects the ileum or the colon. It is also known as inflammatory bowel disease, in which the intestinal wall becomes thickened and ulcerated, sometimes causing an obstruction.

Diverticular disease
Diverticular disease is a condition in which pouch-like protrusions form in the intestinal wall. These may become infected, causing cramps and obstructing the bowel.

Obstruction
The bowel may become partially or completely blocked as a result of impaction of the faeces, or by distortion of the bowel's shape, as in a **hernia**, where a piece of bowel pushes out through the abdominal wall and becomes trapped. Inflammatory disorders may also cause an obstruction.

Irritable bowel syndrome

Irritable bowel syndrome, also called spastic or inactive colon, is one of the most common of all intestinal problems, and probably the least well understood. It is thought to affect between 10 and 12 per cent of adults, and is more prevalent in women.

Irritable bowel syndrome is characterized by bouts of abdominal pain, with diarrhoea or constipation, excessive wind and a feeling that the bowels have not been emptied properly. The cause is not known, although attacks may be associated with stress.

Treatments vary. Some people find that adopting a high-fibre diet is successful; others rely on antidiarrhoeal medicines or antispasmodic drugs; and others recommend psychotherapy or complementary techniques such as hypnosis.

Perforation

The intestinal wall can become perforated as a result of injury or the damage caused by inflammation and ulceration.

A perforated intestine is a medical emergency because the bacteria normally contained within the bowel are a source of infection. Prompt treatment is needed to prevent **peritonitis**, in which infection spreads throughout the abdominal cavity.

Ulcerative colitis

Ulcerative colitis is a chronic inflammatory condition that leads to ulcers forming on the colon and rectum. Like Crohn's disease it is also popularly referred to as inflammatory bowel disease.

Polyps

Small growths called polyps can occur on the lining of the intestines. They are generally harmless, although in large numbers they can cause bleeding and diarrhoea. Suspected polyps should always be investigated, because some types can become cancerous.

Bowel cancer

The bowel may be affected by cancer. Tumours most commonly occur in the lower colon and in the rectum.

Studies comparing different countries suggest that diet has an important part to play in cancer of the bowel. People in Western countries who have low-fibre diets are particularly susceptible.

People who notice a change in their bowel habits – such as constipation or diarrhoea, or the passage of blood, mucus or slime – that persists for more than 14 days are advised to seek medical advice. This applies particularly to people aged 35 or over. But in most cases the changes are likely to stem from a non-malignant bowel condition. **Haemorrhoids** (piles), for example, may cause rectal bleeding.

Other symptoms of bowel cancer include abdominal pain, which may be a generalized ache or localized in the left lower abdomen with feelings of swelling. There may also be anaemia, loss of weight, loss of appetite and a general feeling of ill health.

When to consult a doctor

You should be alert to changes in your bowel movements, and consult a doctor in the following situations.
- If you see blood in your stools.
- If your stools are unusual – tarry, oily, greasy, pale, dark or offensive smelling.
- If an unexplained bout of diarrhoea persists.
- If constipation persists.
- If there is an unexplained change in your bowel habits.
- If you have any acute or persistent abdominal pain or cramps.
- If you have severe wind.
- If fever is associated with these symptoms.

SEE ALSO *Digestive system; Nutritional disorders*

Bradycardia

Bradycardia is an abnormally low heart rate of fewer than 60 beats per minute, which in severe cases can be fewer than 40. The average heart rate for an adult at rest is 72 beats per minute; it is lower during sleep. A fit, active person may have a rate of around 60 and a trained athlete may have a rate that is even lower. But bradycardia can be a symptom of illness and disease as well as a sign of peak fitness.

SYMPTOMS

There may be no symptoms at all or, if any, they are likely to be tiredness, **fainting** and shortness of breath.

CAUSES

Bradycardia may occur during and after fainting. There are several other possible causes:
- heart disease, particularly in elderly people;
- side effects of drugs used to treat heart conditions, high blood pressure, or depression;
- problems such as thyroid or liver disease;
- **hypothermia**;
- brain injury or disease.

TREATMENT

Treatment depends on the cause but may include one or more of the following.
- Stopping or changing any drugs that may be causing the problem.
- Investigation and treatment of any heart, thyroid, liver or brain problem.
- Insertion of an electronic heart **pacemaker** (temporary or permanent).

SEE ALSO *Heart and circulatory system*

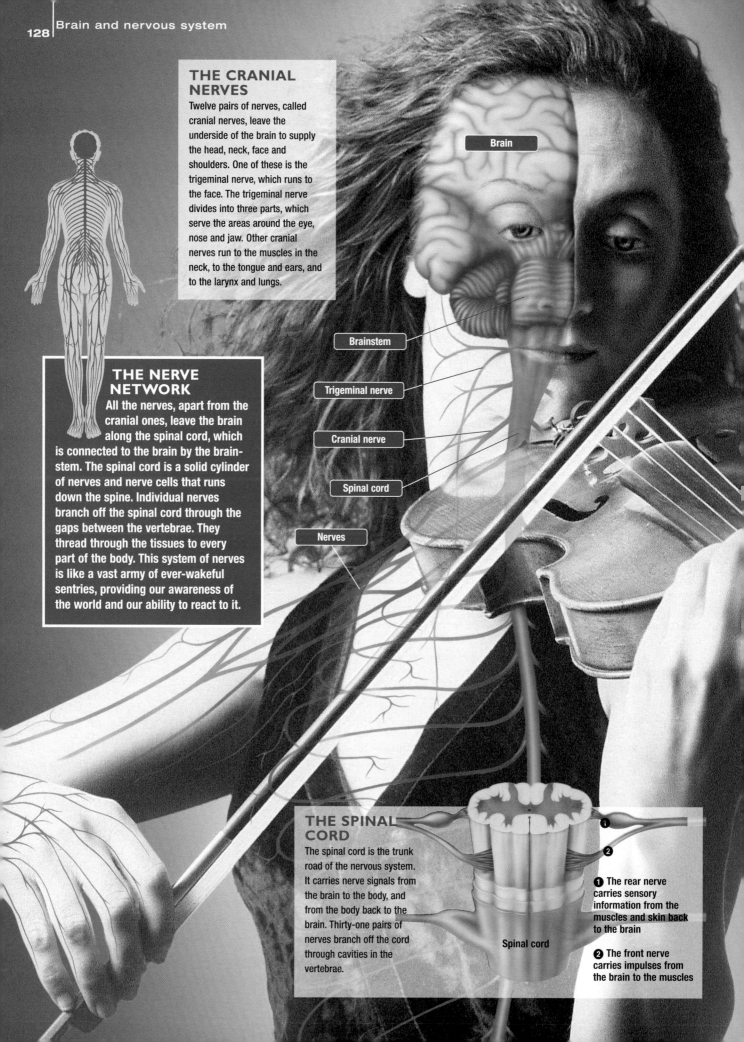

THE CRANIAL NERVES

Twelve pairs of nerves, called cranial nerves, leave the underside of the brain to supply the head, neck, face and shoulders. One of these is the trigeminal nerve, which runs to the face. The trigeminal nerve divides into three parts, which serve the areas around the eye, nose and jaw. Other cranial nerves run to the muscles in the neck, to the tongue and ears, and to the larynx and lungs.

THE NERVE NETWORK

All the nerves, apart from the cranial ones, leave the brain along the spinal cord, which is connected to the brain by the brainstem. The spinal cord is a solid cylinder of nerves and nerve cells that runs down the spine. Individual nerves branch off the spinal cord through the gaps between the vertebrae. They thread through the tissues to every part of the body. This system of nerves is like a vast army of ever-wakeful sentries, providing our awareness of the world and our ability to react to it.

Brain

Brainstem

Trigeminal nerve

Cranial nerve

Spinal cord

Nerves

THE SPINAL CORD

The spinal cord is the trunk road of the nervous system. It carries nerve signals from the brain to the body, and from the body back to the brain. Thirty-one pairs of nerves branch off the cord through cavities in the vertebrae.

Spinal cord

❶ The rear nerve carries sensory information from the muscles and skin back to the brain

❷ The front nerve carries impulses from the brain to the muscles

INSIDE THE BRAIN

The brain's connective tissue consists of glial cells. These supply the nerve cells with nutrients and clear away waste products. There are about 1000 billion glial cells in the brain.

INSIDE A NERVE

Each individual nerve is made up of nerve cells, or neurons, with long branches called axons. Nerve impulses sent from neurons travel along the axons at a rate of 100m (328ft) a second. The axons are encased in a sheath of myelin. If this complex material is damaged, it disrupts the workings of the nerves involved and causes disorders such as multiple sclerosis.

The synaptic bulb is the point where an axon branches off to connect to other neurons.

The fatty myelin sheath insulates the nerve and speeds the transmission of impulses along it.

Neurotransmitters

Axon

Where one axon meets another, neurotransmitter chemicals carry the signal across the intervening space, which is known as the synaptic cleft.

Brain and nervous system

The nervous system consists of the brain and a vast network of nerves through the body. It controls unconscious processes such as breathing as well as complex ones such as playing a violin.

Most nerves have two sets of fibres, sensory and motor, which are like the parallel carriageways on a motorway. Sensory fibres gather information about the outside world and send signals back to the brain; motor fibres then issue instructions to the body to react. So, if sensory fibres detect heat from a flame, the corresponding motor fibres send an urgent message to the muscles to move away.

The conscious mind plays a part in such reactions – you know when you have touched something hot, or that you want to play a note on an instrument. But much of the activity of the nervous system is subconscious. Two groups of nerves – the sympathetic and parasympathetic – regulate heartbeat, sweating and blood pressure, erection and ejaculation. Two other vital elements of the nervous system reside within the brain. The hypothalamus oversees instinctive drives such as hunger and sexual desire; and the limbic system governs still more elemental human impulses such as self-preservation, fear and anger.

The structure and function of the brain

The brain is the command centre of the human body.
It coordinates and controls all the bodily functions.

Anatomists sometimes divide the brain into three main parts: the hindbrain, midbrain and the forebrain. The hindbrain is located at the base of the skull and consists of most of the brainstem and the cerebellum. The brainstem connects with the spinal cord and the brain. All nerve impulses to and from the brain pass through the brainstem. It controls the basic functions that keep us alive, such as heart rate, breathing, blood pressure and swallowing. The cerebellum, which is attached to the brainstem towards the rear of the skull, controls coordination and balanced movement.

The midbrain is the small upper part of the brainstem that connects the hindbrain to the forebrain or cerebrum.

The cerebrum is the largest and most highly developed part of the brain. It comprises two hemispheres that look like the mirror-image halves of a walnut kernel. Its most active parts are located in the highly wrinkled surface layer (the cerebral cortex). The cortex contains the bodies of nerve cells (the grey matter). Beneath this thin layer lie the long axons that connect the cells (the white matter). White matter makes up the bulk of the cerebrum. Nerve impulses are sent by the cells of the grey matter and transmitted via the white matter.

The left and right hemispheres of the cerebrum are bridged by a bundle of nerve fibres (the corpus callosum). Because of the way the nerves are routed, the left side of the brain controls activities on the right side of the body, and the right side of the brain controls those on its left side. The right hemisphere generally controls activities connected to art and the emotions, while the left hemisphere controls language, logic and mathematics.

Our drives and instincts are controlled by the thalamus and hypothalamus in the lower part of the forebrain and by the limbic system (a group of connected structures in different parts of the brain). The thalamus filters nerve impulses as they pass from the brainstem to the cerebrum. The hypothalamus regulates urine production, digestion, thirst, hunger and sexual drive. The limbic system controls emotion and memory.

Factfile

The cerebrum

If you could view the brain through the skull, its most obvious feature would be the grey, wrinkled walnut-like mass of the cerebrum.

The cerebrum divides into two hemispheres, each of which consists of four areas – the frontal (front), temporal (side), parietal (top) and occipital (rear) lobes, which are divided from one another by deep grooves. The frontal lobes control planning and thought processes. The others control our senses – hearing, smell, touch and sight. Also within the cerebrum are the hippocampus and the parahippocampal gyrus. These are elements of the limbic system (see main text). The hippocampus controls recognition and the parahippocampal gyrus regulates memory.

Lying at the centre of the brain are four interconnecting chambers called ventricles, which secrete and store cerebrospinal fluid, a solution of proteins, vitamins and glucose. The fluid flows from the ventricles around the outside of the brain, where it is contained between three layers of a protective membrane called the meninges. Cerebrospinal fluid both nourishes the brain and protects it against shock. The fluid flows down the spinal cord, which it also feeds and cushions against shock. On average the brain weighs 3lb (1.4kg) in a man and 2lb 12oz (1.25kg) in a woman. This difference in weight is related to the difference in body size between the sexes.

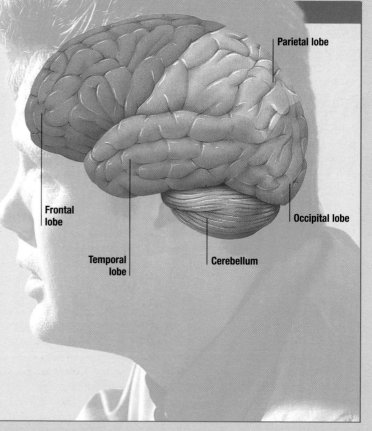

Parietal lobe

Frontal lobe

Temporal lobe

Cerebellum

Occipital lobe

Disorders of the brain

Damage to the brain can be caused both by accidents
and by internal problems such as a stroke or tumour.

Headaches and nausea are two of the most
common symptoms that can affect human beings,
and these usually indicate a minor disorder.
But, occasionally, they can be the first signs
that something is seriously wrong in the brain
or nervous system.

BRAIN INJURY

Head injuries should never be ignored. Anyone
who has hit his or her head in a fall or other
accident should have the injury checked by a
doctor, usually at the nearest general hospital.
Hospital staff will perform **X-rays** or brain scans
to look for skull fractures or signs of bruising,
swelling or bleeding in or around the brain.
Neurological tests check for signs of concussion,
nerve damage or muscle weakness.

Many people with minor head injuries are
treated, then discharged after a short period of
observation. A responsible adult should check
on the person regularly for at least 12–24 hours.
If the person feels worse, becomes drowsy or
unresponsive, or vomits, a doctor or ambulance
should be called and the person should go back
to hospital.

The effects of brain damage after a head injury
depend on which part of the brain has been
injured. Damage to the spinal cord may result
in paralysis and, in general terms, the nearer the
injury is to the brain, the greater the paralysis.

Bleeding in or around the brain may lead to
a blood clot forming between the two outer
membranes around the brain, a subdural
haematoma, or elsewhere in the brain, an
intracerebral haematoma. Haematomas may
be removed surgically if this can be done without
causing further damage.

Intensive rehabilitation at a specialist centre
can improve physical and psychological function
even after a quite severe head injury. Research
is showing that brain and nervous tissues have
much greater powers of renewal and recovery
than previously thought, and improvement may
continue many months after the original injury.

BRAIN TUMOURS

The brain is a common site for tumours that have
spread from other parts of the body – these are
known as secondary tumours. Primary tumours,
those that start in the brain, are rather less
common. Most primary tumours develop in the
glial cells, the supporting tissue of the nervous
system, rather than in the nerve cells themselves.

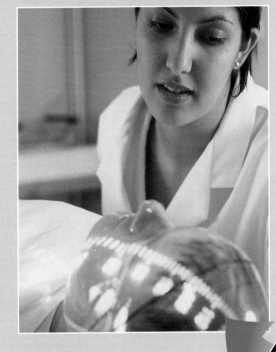

▲ Radiotherapy
A radiographer targets a
brain tumour using laser
crosshairs prior to releasing
radiation on that precise
point to attack the tumour.
The plastic mask on the
patient's head will protect
healthy brain cells from
radiation.

Some brain tumours are benign and do not
spread. These include tumours of the membranes
that cover the brain. But benign brain tumours
can still be dangerous because they can press on
brain tissue as they grow.

Symptoms
In the early stages, headaches, nausea and
vomiting are common symptoms of brain
tumours. They are caused by the pressure of the
growth on nearby tissue. The headache tends to
be worse early in the morning and become better
during the day. Coughing, bending down or hard
physical activity can all make it worse. There may
also be general weakness, visual disturbance,
unsteadiness and personality changes, and it
could trigger **epilepsy**.

Diagnosis
Your doctor will arrange a magnetic resonance
imaging (MRI) brain scan to check for a tumour

Other disorders

The following articles elsewhere in the book give further information on other disorders associated with the brain and nervous system.

Strokes

These arise from blocked or burst blood vessels in the brain, and can lead to partial or complete paralysis, confusion and memory loss, problems with vision or speech.

Alzheimer's disease

This is the most common cause of **dementia**, with symptoms of confusion, memory loss, mood changes and speech problems.

Parkinson's disease

Around one person in 500 develops this disease of the nervous system each year. Its most obvious symptom is tremor.

Schizophrenia

This may be triggered in genetically susceptible individuals by factors such as oxygen deprivation at birth, severe stress, cannabis and LSD.

Multiple sclerosis

Damage to the myelin sheath on neurones leads to disturbed transmission of messages to and from the brain.

Motor neurone disease

The cause of this neurodegenerative condition is unknown. Symptoms include muscle cramps and weakness and gradual loss of movement.

and if necessary, a brain biopsy, in which a small sample of the tumour is taken for examination.

Treatment
Brain tumours are removed surgically if this can be achieved without damaging surrounding brain tissue. Radiotherapy may be used to destroy any cancer cells that are left behind by surgery or, on its own, to treat tumours that are difficult to access for surgery. X-rays can be given from several directions at once, ensuring that a large dose hits the tumour while minimizing exposure to surrounding areas. Anticancer drugs are also used to treat brain tumours.

BRAIN HAEMORRHAGE

The term 'brain haemorrhage' usually means a subarachnoid haemorrhage. This occurs when blood from a burst artery enters the space between the three membranes that protect the brain. It is usually the result of a ruptured aneurysm – a bulge at a weak points in the blood vessel wall, such as a branch-point. If the pressure of blood inside an aneurysm becomes too high, it will burst the blood vessel wall; blood then spreads through and damages the surrounding tissue. Blood can also leak into the space betwen the middle and upper membranes (see Brain injury, page 131)

Symptoms
A sudden, and exceptionally severe headache is the key symptom of a subarachnoid haemorrhage. Some people may also vomit or have a stiff neck. It is essential to seek medical help immediately.

Diagnosis
A subarachnoid haemorrhage can be diagnosed in hospital. Tests include a lumbar puncture in which a sample of cerebrospinal fluid is taken from the spine to check for signs of recent bleeding. An MRI brain scan and an arteriogram, (a test that measures the arterial pulse, see **Arteries and disorders**) is also done to pinpoint the position of the ruptured blood vessel.

Treatment
Treatment of subarachnoid haemorrhage aims to seal off the burst aneurysm and also to prevent spasm in nearby blood vessels, which could starve the brain of oxygen. Sealing off the aneurysm requires surgery. This is usually carried out at a specialist neurosurgical unit.

The drug nimodipine is used to prevent spasm. Treatment is required for about three weeks after the haemorrhage, after which spasm is no longer considered a risk.

BRAIN ABSCESS

An abscess is a collection of pus, usually within a capsule, that forms a cavity within the surrounding tissue. It follows inflammation and damage to tissue caused by a bacterial or other

Endarterectomy

Brain surgeons use specialized technology and highly precise techniques to repair damage and protect the brain's blood supply after a stroke.

After a transient ischaemic attack or stroke, ultrasound tests can show whether there is a blockage in one or both of the carotid arteries that supply the brain with blood. In an endarterectomy operation, a surgeon opens and scrapes clean n artery if it has become blocked by a clot or if the artery wall has degenerated (arteriosclerosis).

Research has shown that people with a block of 70–99 per cent in one or both of these blood vessels will benefit from an operation to clear these blood vessels. A total blockage cannot be cleared because there has to be a trickle of blood getting through for the operation to be worthwhile. Surgery is not recommended for people with blocks of less than 70 per cent because the small risks of surgery start to outweigh the benefits. Surgeons can also operate after an injury, to repair tissue damage and safeguard the blood supply to the brain.

infection. In the brain, an abscess may occur after infection around the outer protective membrane or it may follow chronic ear or sinus infection (sinusitis). The resulting swelling around the abscess can put pressure on nearby brain tissue, causing further damage.

Symptoms
Symptoms may be sudden or develop gradually over a period of about two weeks. They may include any of the following: headache, muscle weakness, seizures, aching or stiffness in the neck, shoulders or back, vomiting, confusion, fever, and problems with speech or vision.

Diagnosis
Neurological tests may suggest the position of the abscess, which can be confirmed with a CT or MRI brain scan. Blood tests should confirm the presence of an infection.

Treatment
A brain abscess needs emergency treatment since it can cause permanent brain damage. Bacterial infections are treated with antibiotics; other antimicrobial therapies may be needed if there is fungal or viral infection. Drugs are also needed to relieve swelling in the brain. If an abscess does not respond to treatment, or pressure in the brain reaches dangerous levels, surgery may be needed to open and drain the abscess or to remove it completely if it is easily accessible.

SEE ALSO *Cerebral thrombosis; Head and head injuries; Learning difficulties; Surgery and surgical techniques*

Breasts and disorders

The primary function of breasts in women is to produce milk to feed a baby. They have little function in men. The female breast consists mostly of milk-producing glands, which are embedded in fat. These glands empty into milk ducts that in turn open out onto the nipple. Each breast has 15–20 sections or lobes. The lobes divide into lobules and each lobule ends in a tiny bulb.

Milk originates in the bulbs and is carried in the milk ducts to openings in the nipple. There are many nerve endings in the nipples, making them sensitive to touch. Men and women can become sexually aroused through touch to the breast area, and many men find female breasts erotic in a sexual context.

Women's breasts vary considerably in shape and size. For most women there are noticeable changes at puberty, during pregnancy and after the menopause. There are also normal tissue changes that occur in response to changing levels of sex hormones during the menstrual cycle. These are called cyclical breast changes, and they can produce swelling, tenderness and pain that fluctuate during the month. Most women also notice changes if they start taking the contraceptive pill or go on **hormone replacement therapy** (HRT).

The most common problems that affect breasts are pain, lumps and nipple discharge.

It is important for women to become aware of the normal condition of their breasts, including the cyclical fluctuations, so that they can promptly notice any abnormal changes such as persistent lumps or swellings. These are unlikely to be cancer (fewer than 20 per cent of breast lumps are cancerous). However, the early diagnosis of breast cancer does improve the outlook and so you should not delay in seeking medical help.

Breast cancer is much less common among men (with approximately 270 men diagnosed in the UK each year), but they also experience breast problems and need to be aware of abnormal changes.

Breast pain

Breast pain is a very common condition: an estimated 70 per cent of women suffer from it at some time during their lives. It is most common among women aged 30–50 and is often accompanied by a general lumpiness of the breast.

There are two types of breast pain: cyclical breast pain, which is worse before a period and better afterwards, and non-cyclical breast pain, which is constant.

SYMPTOMS
- Pain all over the breasts, especially the upper and outer part.
- Nipple tenderness.
- Heavy-feeling breasts.
- In cyclical breast pain, there may be aching down the inner side of the upper arms.
- In non-cyclical breast pain, there may be other symptoms related to the cause of the pain, such as inflammation (see Causes, below).

DURATION
- Any breast pain tends to improve with age.
- For up to 30 per cent of women, cyclical breast pain gets better on its own within three months. But for most affected women, the pain tends to come and go.

CAUSES
- Premenstrual syndrome (see **Menstruation**).
- Hormonal changes, related to oestrogen levels in the body, the effects of **pregnancy**, or taking the contraceptive pill (see **Contraception**) or HRT.
- **Mastitis**, inflammation that usually occurs while breastfeeding (see Breast lumps, opposite).
- Injury, for example, a blow to the breast.
- Breast **cancer** (very rarely a cause).
 Other causes may not be related to the breast, but to other parts of the body.
- Inflammation of the muscles between the ribs (see **Bornholm disease**).
- Inflammation of the ribs.
- Lung disease, such as pneumonia (see **Lungs and disorders**).
- Heart disease, such as angina (see **Heart and circulatory system**).
- Gallstones (see **Gallbladder and disorders**).

TREATMENT
The following measures are sometimes recommended to alleviate breast pain.
What you can do
- Avoid caffeine.
- Consume less salt.
- Take vitamin E or vitamin B_6.
- Wear a bra that gives more support.
- Take an over-the-counter painkiller such as paracetamol.
- Avoid high-impact sports, such as aerobics and jogging, if they make the pain worse.
- Take evening primrose oil (for example, 80mg of Efamast four times daily throughout the month).
- Follow a low-fat diet.
- Keep a symptom diary for three months, charting the days on which you have breast pain and the days of your period. Take note of any other symptoms such as coughing or indigestion (see Symptoms, above). This will allow you and the doctor to decide what type of breast pain you have.

Medical terms

Microcalcifications
Tiny deposits of calcium in the breast, which can show up on a mammogram. Certain patterns of microcalcifications can be a warning sign of breast cancer.

Sclerosing adenosis
A benign breast disease, usually discovered on a mammogram, that involves the excessive growth of tissues in the breast's lobules.

When to consult a doctor

Always consult your doctor if you have any of the following.

- A breast lump (see box on Breast awareness).
- Nipple discharge, especially if bloodstained.
- Persistent or unexplained pain.
- Anxiety about your breast pain.

What a doctor may do

- Ask you about possible causes of the pain.
- Ask you to keep a symptom diary of the pain and your periods, to determine whether you have cyclical or non-cyclical pain.
- Check your breasts for lumps and show you how to check yourself (see box, page 136).
- Refer you to a breast clinic at a hospital within two weeks if you have an undiagnosed lump in your breast.
- Request an **ultrasound scan** if there is generalized lumpiness.
- If you are aged over 35, request a mammogram (a breast X-ray).
- Prescribe hormone treatments, such as danazol or tamoxifen, in severe cases.
- Suggest a change to tibolone if you are having HRT, since this is less likely to cause breast tenderness.

Complementary therapies

Cranial **osteopathy**, a system of gentle manipulation, can alleviate breast tenderness in some women.

COMPLICATIONS

Breast pain can generate a great deal of anxiety, often centred on the fear of breast cancer, although the two are not usually linked.

Breast lumps

Practising breast awareness (see box, page 136) will help you to detect any new lumps in your breasts. If you discover a lump in one breast, check the other breast. If both breasts feel the same, the lumpiness is probably normal. It is best to see a doctor if the lumpiness is new for you, or if it persists after your next period (if you still have periods).

SYMPTOMS

- You may feel a distinct lump or generalized lumpiness.
- Breast tenderness, nipple discharge and other symptoms related to the different causes of breast lumps may also be present.

DURATION

Lumpiness may be a persistent problem from puberty to the menopause although, like breast pain, it tends to improve as you get older.

CAUSES AND TREATMENTS

- **Generalized breast lumpiness** Also known as fibrocystic disease and benign (meaning not cancerous) breast disease. This causes lumpiness around the nipple and the upper

parts of the breasts. It may become a problem in a woman's 30s and 40s, when her breasts gradually change consistency, as milk-producing glands shrink and the proportion of fat in the breast increases. This type of lumpiness disappears after the menopause.

- **Cyclical breast changes** Many women experience breast lumpiness, tenderness and enlargement before and sometimes during their periods. The lumpiness and accompanying symptoms get better when the period ends.
- **Pregnancy** During pregnancy, the milk-producing glands become swollen and the breasts may feel lumpier than usual. In the vast majority of cases, the lumpiness will be related to your pregnancy. It is possible, though very rare, for breast cancer to start when you are pregnant. It is therefore important to see a doctor about any new lumps.
- **Breast swelling in men (gynaecomastia)** A common occurrence in adolescence is a swollen breast in men. It can also be a side effect of drugs, such as cimetidine.
- **Inflammation** Soreness and inflammation of the nipple is common among men and women and is usually due to friction, caused by jogging, for example. Human bites on the breast or nipple, usually as a result of sex games, can become infected and cause a swollen, painful red lump that requires antibiotic treatment.
- **Mastitis** This infection is most often seen in women who are breastfeeding: a duct may become blocked, which causes milk to collect, leading to inflammation and, possibly, infection. The breast appears red and feels warm, tender, and lumpy. In its earlier stages, mastitis can be cured by antibiotics; if a pus-containing **abscess** forms, this will need to be drained or surgically removed.
- **Cysts** These fluid-filled sacs are a common cause of breast lumps in women aged 35–50, and are non-cancerous. They become enlarged, tender and painful just before a period. They vary in size; they can be too small to feel or several centimetres across. **Cysts** show up clearly on an **ultrasound** scan or can be diagnosed by a surgeon inserting a fine needle into the breast to draw off fluid for analysis (a procedure called fine needle aspiration). If there is any doubt about the diagnosis, you will be advised to have the cyst surgically removed.
- **Fibroadenomas** These round, painless, rubbery lumps often move around the breast. They are the commonest cause of breast lumps in young women in their late teens and early 20s. They tend to grow during pregnancy and breastfeeding. They are best diagnosed using mammography or fine needle aspiration (see above and below). Fibroadenomas never

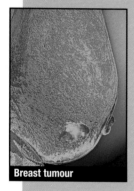

Breast tumour

become cancerous, but your doctor may recommend that you have them removed if there is any doubt about the diagnosis.

■ **Fat necrosis** Painless, round and firm lumps of fatty material may form when a breast is knocked and bruised. These lumps are more common among women with large breasts. The skin around the lump may look bruised and red and you may have noticed the lump soon after being knocked. Fat necrosis can easily be mistaken for cancer, so such lumps are removed as a precaution.

■ **Breast cancer lumps** Breast cancer usually causes a painless lump that most women discover themselves, although it may also be detected during a routine screening mammogram (see opposite). In the UK, mammograms are offered to women every three years between the ages of 50 and 64, and they are available to older women if requested.

Breast cancer

One in 12 women in the UK will develop breast cancer at some stage of her life; breast cancer in men is much rarer. The majority of cases are in women aged over 50 and the incidence rises with age. The earlier the diagnosis and the start of treatment, the better your chances of survival. It is essential to be breast-aware (see box, page 136) and to report to your doctor any lumps or changes in your breasts.

CAUSES

■ **Genetic** About 10 per cent of breast cancer cases in women are caused by an inherited tendency, and most of these are due to an abnormality of one of two genes, BRCA1 or BRCA2. Either parent can pass on these abnormal genes to their children without ever developing the disease themselves.

■ **Age** The risk factor for women developing breast cancer increases with age. There are very few cases in women below the age of 25; after this age, the risk doubles with every ten years of life but the rate of increase lowers after the menopause (see also Hormones, below).

■ **Years of menstrual cycles** Women who start their periods at a young age, have a late menopause and have either not been pregnant or have their first pregnancy at a late age have a slightly increased risk of breast cancer compared to women who have had fewer years of menstrual cycles.

■ **Hormones** Taking the oral contraceptive pill almost certainly does not increase the risk of breast cancer, but using HRT for more than ten years may lead to a small increased risk (2.3 per cent for each year of use). Drugs used in fertility treatments such as IVF may also confer a small increased risk.

Most women have a combination of surgery and radiotherapy to remove cancer in the breast. They may also have chemotherapy, surgical removal of the ovaries and may be given the drug tamoxifen to destroy breast cancer cells within the body and stop the cancer spreading.

■ **Surgery** may be limited to removing just the lump (lumpectomy) or the whole breast (mastectomy). The extent of the operation depends on the state of the disease and the position of the lump. Breast reconstruction can be done at the same time or at a later date. Premenopausal women may be offered surgery to remove the ovaries (oophrectomy) or drugs to induce the menopause, as this is believed to reduce the risk of recurrence.

■ **Radiotherapy** is usually advised for all women after a lumpectomy but is not usually required for women who have a mastectomy.

■ **Chemotherapy** is advised for many women and usually given after surgery to reduce the risk of recurrence. This is known as adjuvant treatment.

■ **Drug treatment** with tamoxifen is effective for all age groups and is now given to most women in a dose of 20mg a day, usually for five years. In premenopausal women, tamoxifen often causes symptoms of the menopause, such as hot flushes.

■ **Geography** Women living in the West have a higher risk of breast cancer than those in the Far East and China. The reason for this is not fully understood but may be due to the relatively low-fat diet of Eastern countries.

■ **Breast disease** Most benign or non-cancerous breast diseases do not increase the risk of breast cancer, but lumps containing cells that show unusual changes may increase the person's risk of breast cancer.

■ **Radiation** Small amounts of radiation such as the level used for a mammogram do not increase the risk of breast cancer, but excessive radiation, especially in teenage girls, may do.

TREATMENT

Consult your doctor as soon as you find a new lump or notice a worrying change in the breast.

What a doctor may do

If you have a lump (or several lumps) in your breast, your doctor might recommend one or more of the following tests.

■ **A mammogram** Breast X-rays, known as mammograms, can be slightly uncomfortable but are a good way of identifying abnormalities in the breast. However, they do not always

If you check your breasts about once a month, preferably after your period, you will become familiar with their normal shape and feel. This will make it easier to identify any changes. Stand in front of a mirror with the light coming from the side; a table or bedside lamp will give a good light.

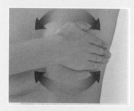

1 To check your breasts, raise your arms above your head and look for any new difference in the shape or size of the breasts. Using the flat of your hand, feel all around the breast.

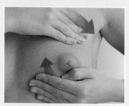

2 Feel all around the breast in concentric circles. Start at the outside and move in towards the nipple. Look for any changes in your nipples or any puckering of the skin. Lie down and feel over the whole breast including the nipple and armpit (some women prefer to do this in the bath using a soapy hand).

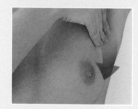

3 Place your fingers high into the armpit feeling downwards towards the breast. Remember to check the other breast.

determine if the abnormality is malignant and further tests are often needed.

■ A breast ultrasound This painless test uses sound waves to produce images of the lump to aid diagnosis (see **Ultrasound**).

■ Fine needle aspiration (FNA) A needle is inserted into your breast lump to extract fluid or a small amount of tissue. The sample is then examined for cancer cells under a microscope.

■ A breast biopsy A sample of tissue is taken out of the breast and examined under a microscope for the purpose of diagnosis.

Complementary therapies

Complementary therapies can have a useful role alongside conventional treatment. Special diets, homeopathy, aromatherapy and reflexology may be offered alongside conventional therapies. It is very important to seek a conventional medical diagnosis of a lump.

COMPLICATIONS

■ The diagnosis can lead to depression, fear and a sense of loss.

■ Surgery can cause wound infection, bleeding and swelling of the arm (lymphoedema).

■ Radiotherapy can cause red, peeling skin and tiredness.

■ Chemotherapy can cause nausea, vomiting and hair loss.

■ Drug treatment can have side effects such as hot flushes, vaginal dryness or weight gain.

PREVENTION

■ Diet A low-fat diet is good for your heart and may prevent other cancers such as bowel cancer. But it is not clear whether it would help to prevent breast cancer.

■ Drug treatment Use of preventive drugs such as tamoxifen for women at increased risk of breast cancer is being investigated. The use of selenium, a trace element in the diet, and retinoids, derived from vitamin A, are also being researched.

■ Surgery Women with a very high risk of developing breast cancer, for example, carriers of abnormal genes predisposing to breast cancer, may choose preventive surgical removal of both breasts and their ovaries.

Nipple discharge

Discharge from the nipple is less common than breast pain or lumpiness but can cause considerable anxiety and distress. It is usually harmless but must be investigated, especially if the discharge is bloodstained and from one breast only. There are several different causes and the treatment will depend on the cause.

CAUSES AND TREATMENTS

■ Pregnancy A straw-coloured liquid often leaks out of one or both breasts during pregnancy. This is harmless.

■ Hormone disturbance Too much prolactin, a hormone that stimulates milk production, or too little thyroid hormone may cause milk to leak out of one or both breasts when you are not pregnant. A blood test can diagnose these conditions. They can be treated with thyroid hormone to compensate for an underactive thyroid, or drugs, such as bromocriptine, that inhibit the release of prolactin.

■ Duct ectasia The milk ducts around the nipple may get wider and shorter as a woman gets older. This is called duct ectasia. It affects 40 per cent of women aged 70 and older and causes a cheesy discharge to leak from the nipple. The nipple may become pulled inwards and look like a horizontal slit, and there may be a hard, doughy lump under the nipple. The doctor may request a mammogram if there is a distinct lump or any blood in the nipple discharge. Duct ectasia persists but does not require treatment unless troublesome. It does not cause any complications.

■ Duct papillomas These are small, harmless growths inside the milk ducts that can cause nipple discharge, which may be bloodstained.

■ Mastitis Infection of the breast can cause pus to leak out of the nipple (see also Breast lumps, page 134).

■ Breast cancer (see Breast cancer, page 135). Cancers that arise inside the milk ducts are called ductal carcinomas. They may cause bloodstained nipple discharge from one breast, a breast lump, or eczema of the nipple. Diagnosis is often made during routine mammography and the cancer may be detected in a precancerous stage, when it is known as ductal carcinoma in situ. Treatment is usually by **mastectomy** (removal of the whole breast) and the outlook is very good for this type of cancer.

Breathing difficulties

In the UK, breathing problems account for more visits to the doctor than any other ailment. Breathing difficulties also account for about 20 per cent of all emergency admissions to hospital.

Breathing problems are linked with swelling or inflammation of the lining of the airways (the bronchi and the bronchioles), which closes up the airways, making it difficult for air to pass through. This can produce a wheezing sound. The passage of air may also be impeded by the production of an excessive amount of mucus or by a blockage caused by inhalation of a foreign object such as a peanut. Other common sources of breathing problems include:
■ damage resulting from an acute infection of the airways and lungs, such as a **cold**, **pneumonia** or **pleurisy**;
■ chronic respiratory conditions, such as asthma or chronic obstructive pulmonary disease (COPD);
■ sleep **apnoea**;
■ smoking;
■ an adverse reaction to drugs (medicinal or recreational);
■ an allergic reaction;
■ **anaphylaxis**;
■ a heart problem.

SYMPTOMS
Breathing problems take several different forms and have a variety of symptoms, ranging from a cough and odd breathing sounds, including wheezing, to being puffed out (fighting for breath, rather than simply feeling breathless after exercise) and pain on trying to breathe. Some people find it hard to breathe when they are lying down.

Symptoms in children
Breathing problems can have rapid and serious effects in young children. Additional symptoms to look out for include:
■ a blueish tinge to the skin, particularly around the mouth;
■ being too breathless to feed;
■ a barking cough;
■ sucking in of the skin around the neck and spaces between their ribs when breathing.

TREATMENT
Treatment will depend on the cause of the breathing difficulty. It may include a course of antibiotics to combat a bacterial infection, giving up smoking, breathing exercises, drugs to counter allergic reactions, oxygen and, in rare cases, surgery.

When to see a doctor
If you are experiencing breathing problems, always err on the side of caution. Seek a doctor's advice if you suffer from any of the following symptoms:
■ shortness of breath without exertion;
■ waking at night feeling breathless;
■ any unexplained shortness of breath;
■ wheezing;
■ chest pain or a feeling of a tight chest;
■ a previously diagnosed breathing problem and you notice your symptoms worsening.

SEE ALSO **Chest pain; Respiratory system; Smoking**

Brittle bones

Brittle bone disease, or osteogenesis imperfecta, is an inherited disorder in which a defect in the production of collagen, a protein, results in bones that are prone to **fractures**.

Many people mistakenly use the term 'brittle bone disease' to refer to **osteoporosis**. But osteoporosis is a condition, rather than a disease – it is a natural part of ageing in which the bones become brittle because more calcium is leached from bone than is absorbed into the structure of the bone.

SEE ALSO **Bone and problems**

Bronchoscopy

A bronchoscopy involves examination of the lungs by means of a flexible instrument with a tiny camera at its end (a bronchoscope). The procedure may be used in the diagnosis of tumours or infections such as tuberculosis, to take a sample of the lung or lung fluid for further investigation, or to remove a foreign object such as a peanut.

The bronchoscope is passed down the patient's nose, past the throat and into the lungs. The examination is a little uncomfortable, so a local anaesthetic is sprayed onto the back of the throat and into the nose. A sedative may be given.

Brucellosis

Brucellosis is a rare bacterial infection caught from farm animals and dairy products. Usually it affects people whose work brings them into contact with cattle, pigs and goats, such as farm workers, abattoir workers or vets. It can also be caught by drinking unpasteurized milk from an infected cow. Brucellosis has an incubation period of 7–21 days.

SYMPTOMS
- Fever in recurring attacks.
- Headache.
- Sweating.
- Joint pains.

CAUSES
Infection with the bacterium *Brucella abortus*.

TREATMENT
- You should contact a doctor if any of the symptoms listed above occur and you are in contact with farm animals.
- A doctor may take blood tests to confirm the diagnosis and prescribe a course of antibiotics or give a course of injections.
- Try to get plenty of rest.

COMPLICATIONS
In rare cases the infection may affect the testes, lungs or heart.

PREVENTION
- Avoid contact with cows when they are calving or have miscarried.
- Do not drink unpasteurized milk.
- Susceptible farm animals should be immunized. Farmers are obliged by law to slaughter affected animals.

OUTLOOK
Health should return to normal within a few weeks if the condition is properly treated. Without treatment, symptoms of infection may recur over many years, with long-term weakness and depression.

SEE ALSO *Bacterial infections*

Bruises

A bruise is a patch of discoloured skin generally caused by an injury. The skin is not broken, but blood leaks out beneath the skin through damaged blood vessels (capillaries). In the course of two to three weeks, the haemoglobin that gives the blood its red colour naturally breaks down, so the bruise changes colour and eventually disappears. Bruising is very common and not usually of any significance, but some people, such as haemophiliacs, are more at risk and may need medical attention.

Bruising may develop at the site of **fractures** and sprained joints (see **Joints and problems**).

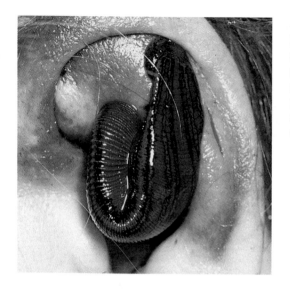

SYMPTOMS
- Localized pain.
- Swelling of the site of injury.
- Discoloration of the skin.

TREATMENT
Home treatment should heal all but the most severe bruises. Treatment in the early stages of the injury will discourage more blood from leaking out of damaged vessels; this will later reduce pain and swelling.

After a period of around 24–48 hours, blood leakage in the bruised area stops and the aim of treatment changes: the goal is now to speed up healing. For this, moist heat – such as that provided by a warm flannel – is best. After a few days, pain and swelling should subside.

When to consult a doctor
- If you cannot use a bruised limb properly.
- If you suffer pain away from the site of the bruise or increasing pain from the bruised area over time.
- If you have a black eye; the force that caused the area to bruise may also have caused a more serious injury, such as damage to the eye itself or a fracture of one of the facial bones.
- If you have received blows to the head, chest or abdomen.
- If swelling remains after a few days.

Complementary therapies
Arnica cream or ointment may help to reduce discomfort and promote healing.

OTHER CAUSES OF BRUISING
Older people may be prone to widespread bruising without apparent cause. This is known as senile purpura, caused by thinning blood vessels.

Repeated bruising, especially after only minor knocks, may indicate an underlying problem:
- vitamin C deficiency;
- bleeding disorders (see **Blood and disorders**; **Haemophilia**);

◀ **Medical leeches**
In some circumstances medical leeches are again being used as a simple and painless method of relieving severe bruising and wounds.

- liver disease (see **Liver and disorders**);
- use of steroid drugs, anticoagulants, non-steroidal anti-inflammatory drugs (NSAIDs) or aspirin.

COMPLICATIONS

Sometimes a large bruise can lead to a **haematoma**. This is common with bruising to the muscle at the front of the thigh. The swelling may need drainage by a doctor.

SEE ALSO *FIRST AID*

BSE

BSE (bovine spongiform encephalitis) is a degenerative disease of the nervous system found in domestic cattle. It is related to similar diseases such as scrapie (which affects sheep) and **CJD** (Creutzfeldt-Jakob disease, found in human beings). These diseases reduce the brain to a spongy consistency, with gaps appearing in the brain tissue. They are believed to be caused by infectious agents called prions, carried in blood and tissue, which destroy brain cells.

When cattle contract BSE, certain parts of their bodies (particularly the brain and spinal cord) harbour large concentrations of prions. Scientists believe that BSE is likely to have been passed from infected cattle to people through foods containing contaminated meat.

Bubonic plague

Bubonic plague is a serious infectious disease caused by the bacterium *Yersinia pestis*. The disease mainly affects rodents but may be transmitted to a human being through the bite of an infected rodent flea. It is now mainly confined to South America, Africa and Southeast Asia. Symptoms include high fever, severe headaches, nausea, vomiting and seizures, as well as painful swellings (buboes) in the armpit, groin or occasionally the neck. These suppurate within one or two weeks, then collapse.

Symptoms start to become evident two to five days after infection. Urgent treatment with antibiotics is essential for recovery. If bubonic plague is left untreated, death is likely within one to two weeks.

Buerger's disease

Buerger's disease is a severe and progressive condition affecting the small **arteries**, mainly in the legs and feet. Caused by smoking and arteriosclerosis, Buerger's disease is seen mainly in cigarette-smoking men under the age of 40. It produces pain in the legs on exercise or even at rest. The feet become cold, discoloured and numb, and the leg veins may become inflamed by thrombophlebitis. Skin ulcers and gangrene may follow, and amputation may be necessary. Stopping smoking is an essential first step. Other measures to alleviate Buerger's disease include regular walking (if possible), losing weight, protecting the skin against heat, cold, infection and injury, wearing well-fitting shoes and taking good care of the feet. Angiography and arterial surgery may be needed.

Bulimia nervosa

People with bulimia have a chaotic eating pattern, with cycles of overeating (bingeing) followed by induced vomiting or the use of laxatives or intensive exercise. Sufferers are obsessed with not gaining weight, their thoughts revolve around food and they have an emotional need to eat that is not satisfied by food alone. The purging episodes are attempts to gain control over the chaotic eating and prevent weight gain.

Bulimia was recognized as a distinct eating disorder only in the 1970s. The incidence of bulimia appears to be increasing rapidly. It is now more common than **anorexia nervosa**, affecting up to ten per cent of young women in the UK. It is less common in men.

The condition is rare before the age of 13 and tends to develop in women in their late teens and early twenties. Bulimic cycles vary: from one purging episode every few months, to several a day.

People can fluctuate between anorexia and bulimia and, without treatment, the problem can persist for many years.

Factfile

Beating bulimia

The first step in conquering bulimia is to see a doctor – but it may not be easy to persuade bulimia sufferers that they have a problem.

- Friends and family members can try to build relationships of trust with sufferers, allowing them to acknowledge their distress without feeling obliged to get help.

- Concentrating on sufferers' emotions may help to take the focus away from food. This can be a difficult step to take without specialist support for family carers.

- A GP should be able to refer someone with bulimia to a specialist in eating disorders. Talking therapies such as psychotherapy, counselling or family therapy may be offered in order to tackle underlying emotional problems. Cognitive behaviour therapy with a psychologist, involving a strict eating plan, can be helpful.

SYMPTOMS

Bulimia is more difficult to spot than anorexia since the person affected often stays within the normal weight range and appears to eat normally. But there are plenty of emotional and behavioural clues to the condition. These include:
- a strong belief that they are fat when in fact they are not;
- an obsession with food and a dread of putting on weight;
- a tendency to disappear immediately after meals (to vomit);
- using laxatives, diuretics or enemas to excess;
- spending large amounts of money on food, or shoplifting for food;
- personality changes and mood swings;
- secrecy and a reluctance to socialize;
- periods of fasting;
- excessive exercising.

There are also some physical signs:
- frequent weight changes;
- sore throat, swollen salivary glands and tooth decay (caused by vomiting);
- poor skin condition;
- in women, irregular periods;
- lethargy and tiredness.

CAUSES

The causes of bulimia are varied. Genetics or traumatic events, such as a bereavement or sexual abuse, may be a factor. Most people with bulimia have low self-esteem or may suffer from **depression**; bingeing may start as a form of comfort eating. When bingeing gets out of control, feelings of guilt and shame lead to vomiting or purging. A vicious circle develops.

TREATMENT

As well as referring people with bulimia to specialists in eating disorders, doctors may prescribe antidepressants and give dietary and nutritional advice.

Nutritional advice may be valuable at some point – when the person is ready to take it – but it should be given in addition to emotional support, not as an alternative to it. It can help the person to address any mineral imbalances, addictions or allergies that may be adding to the disturbed eating pattern.

The Eating Disorders Association offers support for sufferers and their families and friends. Being in touch with an eating disorder support group or helpline can help the person to control the urge to binge.

Complementary therapies

Music, dance, drama or art therapies may help people who find it hard to express emotion in words. **Massage**, reflexology or aromatherapy can help people to feel more connected with their bodies and improve their moods.

COMPLICATIONS

In extreme circumstances, bulimia can cause choking and stomach ruptures. Severe mineral imbalances such as potassium deficiency may affect the internal organs. If laxatives are overused, abdominal pain, damage to bowel muscles and heart failure may result. Rarely, bulimia can be the cause of a fatal heart attack.

OUTLOOK

With help, people can break their bulimic cycle and start to eat normally again. As with all eating disorders, a relapse is likely if the underlying emotional difficulties have not been dealt with.

Bunion

A bunion is a harmless swelling of the joint between the base of the big toe and the first metatarsal bone. A bursa (see **Bursitis**) often develops over the area and the big toe becomes displaced. Bunions are quite common in women aged between 40 and 60.

SYMPTOMS

The joint gradually swells and the skin becomes hard, red and tender. The big toe is then displaced towards the other toes.

CAUSES

The most likely cause is a weakness of the big toe joint or wearing shoes that are too narrow and squeeze the toes together.

TREATMENT

Self-treatment, **chiropody** or surgery will usually dispose of a bunion.
- Wear loose-fitting shoes and protect the bunion with felt pads.
- Regularly soak your feet in a hot foot bath containing grated ginger or Epsom salts.
- If self-treatment fails to ease the discomfort or if the bunion becomes more inflamed and painful over time, seek medical advice.
- A doctor may refer you to a chiropodist for treatment or to hospital for surgery to remove the affected bone at the base of the big toe.

Complementary therapies
- Apply aloe vera gel to inflamed bunions.
- Supplements containing bromelain (an enzyme extracted from pineapple) or devil's claw can help to reduce inflammation and the discomfort of joint pain.

COMPLICATIONS

The base of the big toe can become inflamed and bursitis may develop. Bunions increase the risk of osteoarthritis in the affected joint.

PREVENTION

Ensure that shoes fit well. The feet of children, teenagers and young adults are more easily

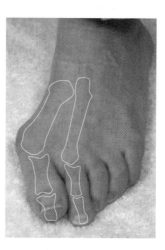

▲ **Tread carefully**
A bunion forms when the foot has been contorted inside an ill-fitting shoe. Here a bunion protrudes from the joint between the big toe and the metatarsal bone.

deformed than adults and are especially at risk of developing bunions from badly fitting shoes. If any swelling or inflammation appears on the big toe joint, protect it with felt pads.

SEE ALSO *Foot and problems*

Burns

A burn is an injury to bodily tissue caused by heat, chemicals or radiation. Burns are common, and range in severity from minor damage to an injury that may be life-threatening.

Burns are classified according to their depth. Burning of the outer layer of skin (the epidermis) is called a first-degree burn. Burning of the epidermis and the underlying layer (the dermis) is called a second-degree burn. Burning of the full thickness of skin and underlying tissues, including nerve endings, is called a third-degree burn. Third-degree burns are painless because they entail damage to the nerve endings, but they are very serious, the most serious of all.

BURN HAZARDS

Burns are extremely common because we use so many devices and substances in our daily lives that pose a danger. Among the causes of burns are:
- dry heat from fire or hot objects;
- moist heat from boiling liquids or steam. Such burns are known as scalds;
- friction;
- chemicals;
- electricity (see **Electrical injuries**);
- radiation from sunlight or nuclear radiation.

SYMPTOMS

The symptoms of burns vary depending on the severity of the injury. They often include:
- pain;
- redness or charring;
- swelling;
- blistering;
- difficulty breathing if the burn or scald is near an airway, or if the cause is smoke inhalation.

A burn is serious if it:
- affects an area greater than the size of a person's hand;
- is painless;
- looks charred, waxy or pale.

WHEN BURNS ARE DANGEROUS

Most victims of severe burns are children or elderly people. Burns that affect more than 15 per cent of the body surface in adults or more than 10 per cent in children pose a risk of serious complications. If more than 30 per cent of the body is burned, the victim may die.

TREATMENT

The faster a burnt area is cooled, the less it will hurt and the fewer complications there will be.

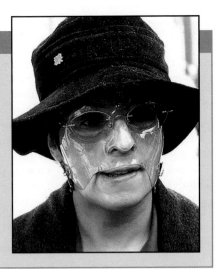

Aids to healing

A mask that follows the contours of the face can be worn to protect new skin.

In the case of severe burns, major reconstructive surgery and skin grafts, a protective mask can be made to fit the individual features of the face. This is worn during the healing process. It aids recovery and the results can be extremely successful.

Immediately flood the burnt area with cold water (or any non-flammable liquid, such as milk): immerse the burnt area or hold it under a cold tap or shower for at least ten minutes.

While doing this, remove rings, watches, boots or other possibly constricting articles near the burn area in case of swelling. Seek urgent medical attention for any serious burn or scald, especially in a child.

Monitor the person's breathing and look for signs of shock. Dress minor burns with a sterile dressing. Polythene bags or cling film make excellent standby burn coverings.

COMPLICATIONS

Severe burns can involve serious complications.
- Fluid loss – due to plasma (see **Blood and disorders**) leaking from damaged vessels.
- Shock – which may require intravenous fluids or transfusion.
- Infection – which may require antibiotics.
- Scarring – third-degree burns may cause skin damage sufficient to require skin grafting.

PREVENTION

The use of a good sunscreen will reduce the risk of sunburn. Always use high-protection sunscreen and reapply it frequently.

Although it is very difficult to make a house completely fire-proof, there are a wide range of precautions that can minimize the dangers.
- Fit a smoke alarm.
- Never leave a hot pan of oil unattended.
- Turn saucepan handles inwards so that children cannot knock or grab them.
- Keep electrical flexes well away from the edge of kitchen worksurfaces.
- Be extremely careful where you put hot drinks when around children.
- Observe safety precautions with open fires, heaters, candles, matches, smoking, fireworks, household chemicals and electricity.

SEE ALSO *FIRST AID*

Bursitis

The bursa is a sac containing lubricating fluid that reduces friction where skin, muscle or tendon moves over bone. In bursitis, the bursa becomes inflamed and excess fluid builds up, interfering with lubrication.

The disorder commonly affects parts of the body where there is particular pressure or friction, such as the kneecap ('housemaid's knee') and the elbow ('student's elbow').

SYMPTOMS

Swelling occurs in the affected area, which may also be tender and hot. The swelling may restrict free movement. It can last for anything from a few days to many months.

TREATMENT

Rest the affected joint as much as possible and take anti-inflammatory painkillers if necessary.

Consult a doctor if the swelling persists for more than two weeks or grows bigger, becomes painful or hot to the touch, or if it interferes with movement.

What a doctor may do

The medical options include:
■ anaesthetizing the affected area and then removing excess fluid by aspiration;
■ injecting hydrocortisone into the emptied sac to reduce the risk of recurrence;
■ prescribing antibiotics if the bursa has become infected;
■ referring the person to a hospital for removal of the bursa under local anaesthetic.

Complementary therapies

Massage the inflamed area with diluted lavender oil. **Acupuncture** can reduce the pain. Apply a compress containing soothing comfrey ointment or slippery elm paste. Some homeopathic remedies can also provide relief.

PREVENTION

Try to avoid prolonged pressure on knees and elbows. Use a rubber mat for kneeling.

Byssinosis

Byssinosis is an occupational disease of the airways caused by breathing in cotton or flax dust. It develops in people who have spent years working with these substances. The exact cause of byssinosis is unknown. Symptoms, which are similar to those of **asthma**, include:
■ chest tightness, a wheeze, and breathlessness;
■ a cough that brings up phlegm.

Smoking aggravates the symptoms. If exposure to the dust is stopped, the symptoms generally disappear. Otherwise, there is a risk of chronic obstructive pulmonary disease.

SEE ALSO *Lungs and disorders*

Callus

A callus, or callosity, is an area of thickened skin that forms on parts of the body where undue pressure or friction is continually exerted. Calluses are most common on the sole of the foot, at the base of the big toe or on the heel. A corn is a type of callus that forms on a toe.

SYMPTOMS

The skin becomes hard, thickened, slightly raised and insensitive.

CAUSES

A callus on the foot may be due to pressure from ill-fitting footwear or from an abnormal gait or abnormality in the foot that causes unequal distribution of weight. A callus on the side of the index finger may result from holding a pencil or pen too tightly. Musicians that play guitar or other stringed instruments often develop calluses on the ends of their fingers as a result of repeatedly holding down or plucking the strings.

TREATMENT

■ A callus on the foot almost always heals when properly fitted shoes are worn.
■ Padding, such as corn plasters, may help to reduce pressure and pain.
■ After soaking the feet, use a skin grater (available from pharmacies) to rub a callus away painlessly.
■ See a doctor if the calluses cause discomfort; the doctor may refer you to a chiropodist or advise you on prevention.
■ If a callus is due to a foot deformity, this may need to be corrected surgically or you may need to have an individually moulded insole made for your shoe.

COMPLICATIONS

A callus can become infected if the skin is cracked. It can then be extremely painful, especially when walking.

PREVENTION

Always wear well-fitting shoes that are wide enough for the foot. This is especially important for children, and shoes should be regularly checked to ensure the correct fit and that there is enough room for growth.

SEE ALSO *Chiropody; Foot and problems*

Cancer

Cancer is a disease that occurs when body cells grow out of control. Many of the 200 different types of cancer can be successfully treated, but medical research continues to seek absolute cures.

Advances in medical knowledge and skill mean that a diagnosis of cancer is no longer an inevitable death sentence. Many people recover completely from their cancer while others can expect a good quality of life for many years. The disease is more likely to occur at a later stage in life – 65 per cent of cancers are diagnosed in people over the age of 65.

WHAT IS CANCER?

A cancer begins when a single cell escapes the normal genetic controls governing cell growth. Exposure to certain chemicals, radiation or a simple mistake in the normal process of cell division can trigger the production of increasing numbers of abnormal cells until a lump or tumour forms, or the number of one type of cell increases dramatically, as in cancers of the blood. This abnormal cell growth is driven by gene damage known as mutations. The rate of growth may be slow; for example, it is estimated that in breast cancer it takes an average of seven years from the first cancer cell to awareness of a lump.

Cancer is a malignant disease that progressively harms the body. There are two principal features in the development of cancer: the spread and invasion of surrounding tissues known as 'local spread', and the invasion of the blood and lymphatic system that carries the cancerous cells to form new tumours in other parts of the body.

Detecting precancerous cells

Precancer is a term used to describe abnormal cells that are more likely to develop into a cancer. It is not inevitable, however, that these cells will become cancerous and they may simply revert back to normal. Precancerous cells may also be called 'premalignant' or, more technically, 'dysplastic'. Screening for precancerous cells, for example, with cervical smear tests, is very important. Detecting precancerous changes allows treatment to be given at the earliest possible stage, minimizing the risk of cancer developing.

WHAT IS A TUMOUR?

Cancers come in all shapes and forms, but generally speaking benign tumours (non-cancerous growths) tend to be smooth, regular lumps and have a clearly defined border or capsule, with a normal blood supply. Malignant tumours, on the other hand, are usually irregular in shape and there may be abnormalities of the blood supply causing the formation of many tiny, fragile blood vessels. The abnormal cells from these tumours penetrate the surrounding tissue.

A primary tumour is the initial cancer. Sometimes it can be difficult to track down the primary cancer. A secondary tumour is a cancer that has spread from the primary site to elsewhere in the body. Secondary tumours are also known as metastases. Widespread secondary cancers are known as carcinomatosis.

DIFFERENT TYPES OF CANCER

There are many types of cancer, and while they may share some features, each is very different in cause, symptoms, treatment and prognosis – essentially, they are individual diseases. Even within a single organ, one of several different types of cancer may develop, depending on which type of cell is involved.

Each type of cancer has its own particular pattern of disease in terms of how fast it grows, how it spreads and how well it responds to treatment. For example, melanomas (pigmented skin cancers) tend to spread through the blood early in their development to distant sites such as the brain or liver. But another type of skin cancer called a basal cell carcinoma very rarely spreads.

HOW COMMON IS CANCER?

Each year in the UK more than a quarter of a million people will receive a diagnosis of cancer. More than one in three will be diagnosed with the disease at some time in their lives and one in four people will die from it.

In adults, the commonest forms are breast cancer (15 per cent of all cancers), lung cancer (15 per cent), bowel cancer (13 per cent) and prostate cancer (8 per cent). The commonest causes of death from cancer are lung cancer (22 per cent of cancer deaths), bowel cancer (11 per cent), breast cancer (9 per cent) and prostate cancer (6 per cent).

Although cancer is mostly a disease of ageing, children do get cancer. The commonest is **leukaemia** (32 per cent of childhood cancers).

Medical terms

Carcinoma Often used as a general word for cancer but refers to one of the commonest types. It develops from cells on the skin surface or cells lining the body's organs, such as the bowel.

Adenocarcinomas are carcinomas that develop from either glandular or secretory cells. Squamous cell carcinomas can develop on the skin and also in the lungs.

Lymphoma Tumours that develop from cells of the lymphatic system.

Sarcoma Cancer that develops from the cells of the connective tissues, such as muscle, bone and cartilage.

Leukaemia Cancer of the cells of the blood system, including the bone marrow.

Staging This is the classification by which doctors judge how far a tumour has spread, in order to plan the most appropriate treatment and estimate prognosis.

Grading Cancers are graded in an attempt to estimate how fast they will grow and how likely they are to spread.

Highly abnormal cells (sometimes called undifferentiated, high-grade or anaplastic) tend to be extremely malignant and therefore have a poorer prognosis.

Cells that appear to be less abnormal (well-differentiated, or low-grade) are less malignant and the prognosis is better.

Cancer: causes and risk factors

Being aware of the causes of cancer can help you to take steps to reduce the risk of disease.

Cancer occurs when the normal control of cell division and reproduction is lost. Damage to a combination of genes known as oncogenes and tumour suppressor genes is responsible for this process. For example, a gene known as *p53* normally plays an important role in preventing cancer by detecting genetic abnormalities within cells and signalling to them to destroy themselves. Damage to genes such as *p53* results in loss of control of cell growth and can lead to cancer.

Many factors can damage the genes and so contribute to cancer, including:

- smoking;
- radiation;
- poor diet;
- infection;
- chemicals;
- inherited gene mutations.

However, the pathway by which most cancers develop is not entirely clear. In most cases, cancer is what doctors call 'multifactorial': that is, several factors add up over time to trigger it. Increasingly, scientists are turning to treatment strategies based on the genetic control of growth, that is, manipulating the mechanism that turns cell growth on and off. Other potential treatments involve mimicking the chemical messages used by cells to control their activity. These are likely to be the cancer treatments of the future.

INHERITED GENETIC CAUSES OF CANCER

Inherited genetic mutations increase the risk of cancer, although other factors, such as exposure to carcinogens, may also be needed for cancer to develop. But in some cases, cancer is caused purely by an inherited genetic fault in the individual. For example, in an inherited condition called Familial Adenomatous Polyposis (FAP), polyps form on the inner surface of the large intestine. Affected people inherit a damaged copy of a gene called APC from their mother or father. Almost inevitably, by the time people with FAP have reached 40 one or more of these polyps has turned into a cancer if left untreated. Breast cancer can also be inherited through a single gene mutation, although in 90 per cent of cases this is not the cause.

CARCINOGENS

A carcinogen is anything that can cause cancer. Many chemicals are carcinogens. Tobacco smoke, for example, contains more than 50 known carcinogens, including benzene, formaldehyde, nitrosamines, radioactive polonium 210 and polynuclear aromatic hydrocarbons.

Some occupations involve exposure to hazards, such as chemicals or radiation, which have been linked to cancers, because the work can bring people who do it into contact with specific carcinogens. Workers in the nuclear power industry, and people working with asbestos or herbicides and insecticides, are examples of people who should always follow existing safety rules to minimize their risk of cancer.

ENVIRONMENTAL AND CHEMICAL EXPOSURE

There are some factors in the environment that may contribute to increased cancer risk. In the workplace, the potential risks should be identified and controlled by employers. At home it may be more difficult to spot the risks. For example, radon, which occurs in some rock formations, is a natural radioactive gas.

Factfile

Cigarettes and cancer

The link between cigarettes and cancer is established beyond doubt.

Tobacco smoke contains dozens of carcinogens that affect not only the smoker but those who breathe the same air, known as passive smoking. Aside from lung cancer, many other types of cancer – including cancer of the mouth, gullet (oesophagus), cervix, and bladder – are also linked to smoking. (See **Smoking**)

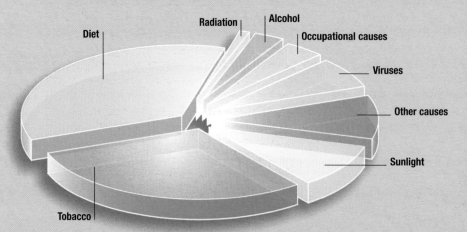

Diet | Radiation | Alcohol | Occupational causes | Viruses | Other causes | Sunlight | Tobacco

◀ **Causes of cancer**
It is estimated that the major causes of cancer are dietary factors (35%) and tobacco (30%). Sunlight accounts for 10% of cancers, viruses 7%, occupational factors 4%, alcohol 3% and radiation 1%.

You can't see it or smell it, and outdoors it rarely accumulates to significant levels. But if levels do build up in a home, the risk of lung cancer is increased. If you are concerned about levels of radon in your area, contact your local authority for advice.

SUNBURN

Exposure to excessive amounts of ultraviolet A and B radiation (UVA and UVB) from sunlight significantly increases the risk of skin cancer, including the most dangerous type, malignant melanoma. Sunburn and tanned skin indicate overexposure to UVA and UVB. Both adults and children should take measures to protect their skin in the sun.

MOLES

Malignant melanomas arise in pigment-containing tissue, usually the skin or eyes, from a mole or pigmented skin lesion. It is important to watch out for changes in moles, in particular, changes in size, shape or colour. These may need medical attention.

Melanomas tend to have an irregular border, an irregular colour (often a mixture of brown, black and even blue), and they can itch, bleed or ooze. Melanomas can appear anywhere on the body, not just at sites of sun exposure.

INFECTION

Certain viral infections may increase the risk of cancer:
■ Human Papilloma Virus, or HPV, is linked to cancer of the cervix;
■ **hepatitis B** increases the risk of liver cancer;
■ HIV increases the risk of tumours, especially Kaposi's sarcoma and lymphoma, possibly due to a secondary viral infection;
■ bladder cancer is more common among those with the tropical disease schistosomiasis.

EARLY WARNING SIGNS OF CANCER

If you notice any of the following symptoms, seek medical advice.
■ Unusual lumps or bumps: especially in the breast, armpit, around the collarbone and neck and in the groin or testis.
■ Changes in the shape or size of a mole or skin lesion.
■ A persistent cough that doesn't settle after a couple of weeks (especially if you smoke).
■ Unexplained loss of weight.
■ An increase or decrease in the number of times you open your bowels each day, especially if you pass blood or mucus with the motions.
■ Intense night sweats.
■ Other unexplained persistent symptoms, including pains, skin discoloration and tiredness.

Cancer: diagnosis and treatment

There are many different symptoms that may indicate cancer, and early detection increases the success of any treatment.

Sometimes a cancer can be immediately identified, but usually tests are needed to confirm the diagnosis. A sample of cells from the cancer will usually be examined under a microscope to look for typical abnormalities. This generally means having a **biopsy,** or small operation, to take some cells from the cancer.

ASSESSING THE CANCER

As well as confirming the diagnosis, it is vital to establish the grade and stage of the cancer (see Medical terms, page 143). In this assessment the cancer will be staged to determine how far the tumour has spread and graded to estimate how fast it is likely to grow.

Several tests, including **X-rays, ultrasound,** CT and magnetic resonance imaging scans, may be needed. Once the stage and grade of the cancer are clear, the most appropriate treatment can start.

TREATMENT

The aim of cancer treatment is to remove all abnormal cells from the body. Each cancer needs a unique approach to its treatment and this is individually planned by an oncologist (a cancer specialist).

Surgery to cut out as much as possible of the cancer is often (but not always) the first step. Some cancers respond particularly well to **chemotherapy** or **radiotherapy.** Other treatments include hormones and vaccines.

If you are prescribed chemotherapy you will be given a combination of drugs by injection or orally, usually as tablets. This continues for a period of days, weeks or months, interspersed with recovery periods. Side effects can include nausea, diarrhoea, fatigue and loss of hair but measures can be taken to reduce this.

Radiotherapy involves the use of carefully targeted high-energy beams of radiation to destroy cancer cells. The treatment is painless but side effects can include redness and irritation of the skin in the area being treated, diarrhoea, nausea, tiredness, cough and shortness of breath.

After an initial course of therapy it may be necessary to continue with long-term drug treatment, known as 'maintenance therapy', to avoid the risk of recurrence.

Factfile

Questions to ask the doctor

Knowing what questions to ask your doctor will help you get the most out of your consultation.

■ What sort of cancer is it?

■ How far has it spread?

■ What is the prognosis for survival?

■ What are the treatments?

■ How likely are these to be successful?

■ What side effects of the treatment can I anticipate?

■ What can I do to improve my chances of recovery?

■ What is the chance of relapse?

■ Is there any risk to other members of my family (possibly from inherited factors)?

In the UK, one in three cancer sufferers is still alive five years or longer after treatment.

PAIN CONTROL

Pain may develop from the cancer itself, from secondary tumours or as a result of cancer treatments. Tiredness, poor sleep and depression can all make pain worse. Be sure to inform your medical team of any new pain you have – there is no reason to suffer unnecessarily.

Painkilling medicines

Almost all cancer pain responds to treatment, although it may take some trial and error to find what works best for each individual. There is a range of painkilling drugs, starting with simple analgesics and working through to more powerful drugs such as morphine.

If you are prescribed morphine it doesn't mean that the cancer has become more serious, simply that it is giving you more pain. Addiction is not an issue – many people use the same dose for months without becoming addicted.

Other pain-control treatments

In addition to drugs, other treatments may be used to control pain, including radiotherapy, nerve blocks, acupuncture, transcutaneous electrical nerve stimulation (TENS), relaxation therapy and hypnotherapy.

CONTROL OF OTHER SYMPTOMS

Other common cancer symptoms, apart from pain, include fatigue, weakness, loss of appetite, weight loss, nausea, bowel upsets, shortness of breath, sleeping problems and depression.

Such symptoms are particularly common in more advanced stages of cancer.

There is always something that can be done, to relieve pain and make the patient more comfortable so don't try to be brave – coping with the symptoms is just as important as treating the cancer.

Cancer in children

Cancer is rare in children. Fewer than one in 600 children aged under 15 years develop cancer. The same sort of treatments are used as for adult cancers (a combination of surgery, chemotherapy, radiotherapy and other treatments), but childhood cancers tend to be more responsive to treatment: ten years after diagnosis, 70 per cent will be cured. This is a great improvement on just 40 years ago, when little more than 20 per cent of child sufferers survived for ten years.

Common childhood cancers include:
- **leukaemia** (about 30 per cent);
- brain tumours (about 25 per cent);
- neuroblastomas, tumours that range from highly malignant to relatively harmless (less than 10 per cent);
- **Hodgkin's** and non-Hodgkin's lymphoma;
- Wilms' tumours, also called nephroblastomas, tumours of the kidneys that can be treated with surgery, chemotherapy and radiotherapy;

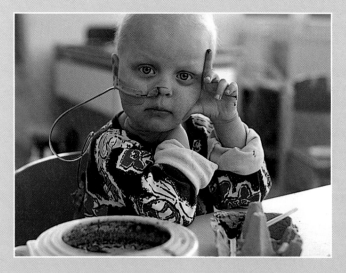

- retinoblastoma (see **Eye and problems**);
- germ cell tumour, mostly found in the testes and ovaries, but may also develop in the chest, abdomen, spine or brain. Most are cured with chemotherapy;
- osteosarcomas, bone cancer, usually affecting the long bones of the leg or arm. They may be highly malignant, but more than half are cured with surgery or chemotherapy.

Helping a child to cope with cancer

Family and friends can be the biggest support when a child has cancer. The following guidelines can help everyone to come to terms with the situation.
- Keep life as normal as possible. Children cope best with a regular routine in familiar surroundings, with the usual family rules. It is natural to want to indulge a child who has been diagnosed with cancer, but maintaining the normal routines and rules of family life ensures that there is less change for the child to deal with.
- Try to keep your own fears contained. It will help a great deal if you can find ways to work through feelings of anger or guilt. Keep some normality in your own life, too.
- Give your child as much chance as possible to talk in case he or she is frightened and needs reassurance about issues such as pain or even dying. Gently try to find ways to help him or her ask questions and get honest answers – this doesn't mean passing on every possible detail. Your child's doctors and nurses will have plenty of experience of dealing with children with cancer and will be able to help you.
- Don't forget the rest of the family. A child with cancer means a family with cancer: no one goes unaffected.
- Keep school and social life going. School and friends are a central part of a child's life and can help them deal with specific issues about their illness. Most hospitals have some special provision for school. Friends should be encouraged to visit as much as possible.

Candida

Candida is an infection of the skin by the yeast-like fungus Candida albicans, which also causes thrush. It can infect all areas of the skin as well as the mucous membranes, but it prefers warm, moist places. It usually occurs in skin folds, such as under women's breasts, in the groin, on the genitals and in the area around the anal orifice. Candida is most likely to affect people with metabolic disorders (such as diabetics), pregnant women, and people who are HIV-positive or who suffer from another type of immunodeficiency.

SYMPTOMS
- Itchy, purple patches on the skin that have a similar appearance to **eczema**.
- A small degree of scaling.
- Blisters resembling spots are often seen around the itchy patches.

CAUSES
A vast number of different micro-organisms, including fungi such as *Candida albicans*, live both on the inside and outside of the human body. Some of these micro-organisms are beneficial and others have no effect until there is either a change in their nature or a decrease in the body's resistance to them. This reaction allows one type of micro-organism to grow excessively, leading to infection.

Infections by *Candida albicans* can be spread by direct contact, sexual contact and, indirectly, via damp towels or flannels.

TREATMENT
- See a doctor for a diagnosis, made on the basis of the skin's appearance or a skin sample.
- Treatment is usually with antifungal cream; the doctor may also prescribe an anti-inflammatory hormone.

Complementary therapies
A homeopath may recommend either Sulphur (Sulphur) or Calcarea carbonica (Calc. carb.).

PREVENTION
- Wash regularly and dry the skin carefully afterwards. Overweight people should be careful to dry all skin folds.
- Wear sandals or leather shoes instead of trainers. Always wear clean socks.
- Wash the hands after touching an infected area and after applying antifungal cream.

COMPLICATIONS
In people with HIV or those taking long-term steroids, the fungus may spread over the entire body, creating a very serious condition called generalized mucocutaneous candidiasis.

OUTLOOK
Like other **fungal infections**, this condition may return if a bodily environment favourable to the spread of the fungus is created once again.

Capillaries and disorders

Capillaries are tiny blood vessels, less than 0.025mm wide. They receive blood from the small arteries and form a network throughout the body, draining back into the system of veins that returns the blood to the heart.

Capillaries deliver oxygen and nutrients via the bloodstream to the tissue fluid that surrounds the body cells; the walls of the capillaries are just a single cell in thickness and so they are permeable, allowing oxygen, water, glucose and other chemicals to pass between the blood and tissue fluid. Capillaries also remove many byproducts of cell metabolism, including carbon dioxide. Other toxins are removed by the lymphatic capillaries, part of the **lymphatic system**.

ADJUSTING TO THE BODY'S NEEDS
Capillaries do not carry blood all the time. They can be rapidly filled or drained according to the need for blood in various organs or areas of the body. For example, most of the capillaries serving the leg muscles will be open when a person is playing football, but closed during sleep. A ring of muscle at the entrance to each capillary controls the blood flow. This allows capillaries to respond quickly to the body's constantly changing needs for blood.
- **During exercise** Lung capillaries lengthen as breathing deepens; this increases their total surface area so that more oxygen can be collected from the lungs. Capillaries in the muscles open to facilitate the delivery of oxygen and glucose. They also carry away waste products such as carbon dioxide and lactic acid, preventing cramp and muscle fatigue.
- **After a meal** Blood is diverted to the gut capillaries to help digestion and transport nutrients to the liver and fat stores. Exercise should be avoided straight after a heavy meal as muscle capillaries will be competing with the digestive system.
- **After injury or during infection** Capillaries deliver more blood to an injured area to promote healing; the skin looks redder, feels warmer and may be swollen or tender.
- **During shock** Shock victims look pale because blood is rerouted from the skin and gut to protect vital organs.
- **In hot or cold environments** When the body is hot, the skin capillaries dilate so heat loss and sweating can increase. When cold, it conserves heat by contracting the skin capillaries.

WHAT CAN GO WRONG
Capillaries are fragile and can be ruptured by an injury or blow to the body tissues. This results in blood cells leaking through the capillary wall, which causes **bruising** or swelling. Ageing,

Healthy resting adults normally extract only a quarter of the available oxygen from capillary blood; a well-trained athlete can triple this during exercise.

vitamin C deficiency and steroid treatment can weaken the tissues that support skin capillaries. This causes more frequent bruising, a condition known as age-related purpura.

Blocked capillaries

- Staying in one position for too long compresses the capillaries, causing localized pain due to lack of oxygen (ischaemia). People with mobility problems should be helped to change their position regularly to avoid this.
- Capillaries in the retina may become blocked as a result of diabetic retinopathy.
- Tissue damage due to blockages in the capillaries may occur in meningococcal septicaemia (see **Meningitis**).

Lung capillaries

Capillaries in the lungs form a network around the air sacs (alveoli), and extract oxygen from the inhaled air.

- Raised pressure in the lung capillaries may force fluid through the capillary walls and 'flood' lung tissues, as in pulmonary **oedema**, causing severe breathlessness.
- The diversion of blood to damaged or non-functioning areas of the lung may prevent lung capillaries from picking up enough oxygen from the air sacs. This occurs in **emphysema** and pulmonary embolism and causes breathlessness. In severe cases the lips and tongue may turn blue.

Kidney capillaries

Kidney capillaries are long and specially adapted to filter blood and regulate the excretion of salt, water and other chemicals. The walls of kidney capillaries may be damaged by infection, **diabetes**, drugs (including painkillers) and diseases such as glomerulonephritis (see **Kidneys and disorders**). If the kidney capillary walls are damaged, fluid, salt and waste products build up in the bloodstream.

Oedema

The levels of fluid in the tissues and blood are roughly constant. But if a capillary is unable to reabsorb sufficient fluid from body tissues, swelling (**oedema**) develops. This usually affects the ankles or legs, but may spread to the abdomen or chest, resulting in breathlessness. Causes include:

- salt or fluid overload, as occurs in kidney, liver and heart failure;
- damage to the capillaries, causing the walls to become more permeable so that excess fluid leaks out;
- excess pressure in the blood flow, which forces too much fluid out of the capillaries, or very low protein levels in the blood (hypoproteinaemia), which allows fluid to leak through the walls and spread into the tissue.

Capillary malformations

- Abnormal dilation of capillaries in the skin may cause **birthmarks** (haemangioma). Some such as a strawberry naevus or stork mark may disappear of their own accord; others, such as port-wine stains may need laser treatment.
- Permanently dilated capillaries in the skin are called telangiectasia. The cause may be genetic or the result of **radiotherapy** or disease. The symptoms are redness and an appearance of broken veins, which may become more prominent after drinking alcohol or coffee. The condition can be treated with laser or light therapy.

SEE ALSO *Arteries and disorders; Heart and circulatory system; Veins and disorders*

▼ Supplying the capillaries
Oxygen-rich blood from the heart travels through the main arteries and then smaller arteries (arterioles) before reaching the capillaries. Because the capillary wall is a single cell in thickness, chemicals and gases can pass in both directions, in and out, with ease.

A process of diffusion

Materials cross the capillary wall by a process called diffusion.

Fat-soluble substances, such as oxygen and carbon dioxide, diffuse far quicker than water-soluble substances because they are better able to penetrate the cell membrane. Ions and many other water-soluble molecules must pass through pores in the membrane. Some molecules, such as proteins, are transported across either through large pores or are carried across by cellular organelles.

The rate of transport

The rate at which molecules are transported across the capillary membrane is not only dependant on the type of molecule but also where the capillaries are in the body.

Fat-soluble substances cross around 100 times faster than water-soluble substances. Different tissues have different pore sizes. The liver, for example, has very big pores, so that even large proteins can readily cross.

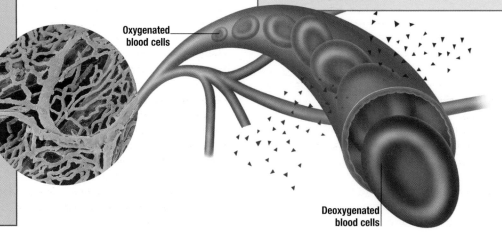

Oxygenated blood cells

Deoxygenated blood cells

Carbon monoxide poisoning

Carbon monoxide is a colourless, odourless gas produced by burning fuel. It is highly poisonous and can kill before anyone is aware of its presence. Anyone can be affected by carbon mononxide poisoning, but children, pregnant women, elderly people and those with heart or lung diseases are the most vulnerable.

When carbon monoxide is breathed in, it binds with haemoglobin (the compound in red blood cells that usually carries oxygen to the tissues) to form the toxic carboxyhaemoglobin. As a result of this, the body becomes starved of oxygen.

A small quantity of carbon monoxide is released whenever a fossil fuel is burnt. Danger arises when levels build up from faults in appliances, cracked or blocked vents, or inadequate ventilation. Modern, well-insulated houses have less natural ventilation than older, more draughty dwellings and in newer homes any buildup of carbon monoxide therefore tends to be more concentrated.

SYMPTOMS
- Flu-like symptoms (headaches, tiredness, dizziness).
- Nausea.
- Irritability.
- Confusion.
- Visual disturbances.
- Breathing difficulties.
- Palpitations.
- Vomiting.
- Fits.
- Paralysis.
- Loss of consciousness.

Acute carbon monoxide poisoning usually causes symptoms after an exposure of three to eight hours. It can kill rapidly, and survivors may be left with long-term brain damage.

Low concentrations of the gas may cause chronic poisoning over time, with low-level symptoms but accumulating neurological damage. Be suspicious if symptoms recur regularly, happen in one part of the house, affect more than one household member or start in winter.

CAUSES
Domestic sources of carbon monoxide include the following.
- Gas or oil boilers and furnaces.
- Water heaters.
- Open fires and wood-burning stoves.
- Charcoal grills and barbecues.
- Gas ranges.
- Fan heaters.
- Gas refrigerators.
- Car exhaust fumes.

TREATMENT
If you suspect carbon monoxide poisoning, turn the appliance off, get out into the fresh air and seek medical attention immediately. Treatment may include oxygen therapy in which the patient is fed pure oxygen through a mask to increase tissue oxygenation, which speeds the elimination of carboxyhaemoglobin. More serious cases may require the patient to be connected to a high-pressure oxygen supply, which pushes oxygen more effectively into the body.

COMPLICATIONS
If rapid treatment is not given, serious complications may arise.
- Coma.
- Brain damage – seizures, impaired memory and intellect, speech disorders, emotional disturbances or balance problems.
- Altered hormone balance and temperature regulation.
- Peripheral nerve damage causing numbness.
- Heart and lung damage.
- Fetal damage.
- Delayed neurological symptoms, months or even years later.

PREVENTION
- Have all heating appliances regularly maintained and chimneys swept annually.
- Never leave a car with its engine running in a garage, especially if the garage is attached to your house.
- Install a carbon monoxide detector that sounds an audible alarm. Place it near bedrooms or living areas but away from open doors, extreme heat or cold.
- Remember that carbon monoxide detectors are not as reliable as smoke alarms; do not use them as a substitute for servicing your appliances.

Carbuncle

A carbuncle is a collection of painful, red **boils**. It is usually caused by the bacterium *Staphylococcus aureus* and can lead to extensive shedding of the surrounding skin. Oral antibiotics are used to treat a carbuncle, and surgery, with a local anaesthetic, is sometimes needed to release trapped pus.

A renal carbuncle is an **abscess** in the outer layer (cortex) of a kidney. This usually results from bloodborne *Staphylococcus* spreading from a boil or carbuncle on the skin.

Symptoms of a renal carbuncle include high, fluctuating fever, and loin pain and tenderness. Treatment is also with antibiotics and surgical drainage.

Cardiac massage

Cardiac massage is an emergency procedure performed when the heart has stopped beating. Forced compression of the heart allows oxygenated blood from the lungs to pump out into the aorta and reach the brain, preventing brain death through lack of oxygen.

In external cardiac massage, crossed hands are placed on the lower breastbone (sternum) and intermittent pressure is applied at a rate of 100 compressions per minute. In internal cardiac massage the chest wall is cut open and the heart is massaged directly with the hand. Internal cardiac massage is performed only rarely, during or after open heart surgery or in cases of extreme emergency.

SEE ALSO *Heart and circulatory system*

Cardiomyopathy

In cardiomyopathy, the heart muscle becomes enlarged or weakened and cannot contract properly, so the pumping action of the heart becomes less efficient. There are two common forms of cardiomyopathy: hypertrophic, causing thickening of the heart muscle, and dilated, in which the heart is enlarged. Symptoms include fainting, palpitations, tiredness, breathlessness and chest pain; arrythmias or **heart failure** can result. Apparently healthy young people may suffer cardiac arrest, especially in the hypertrophic form.

There is a genetic link – 95 per cent of people with hypertrophic cardiomyopathy and 40 per cent of those with the dilated form have relatives with the same condition. Dilated cardiomyopathy can also be a result of **viral infection**, **autoimmune disease**, toxins and metabolic diseases (see **Metabolism and disorders**) or **nutritional disorders**.

The condition can be detected by ECG (electrocardiogram), echocardiogram (using **ultrasound**) and other heart tests. Treatment includes drugs, and in some cases a **pacemaker** may be helpful; in young people a heart **transplant** may be considered. Family members of sufferers may be screened for the condition.

SEE ALSO *Heart and circulatory system*

Carpal tunnel syndrome

Carpal tunnel syndrome is a compression of the median nerve that passes through the carpal tunnel: this is the space in the wrist through which the tendons that flex the fingers also pass. The pressure on the nerve causes pain and the loss of some use of the hand.

Carpal tunnel syndrome is a common condition. More women than men suffer from it. About 50 per cent of cases stem from an existing condition. Left untreated, it grows progressively worse.

SYMPTOMS
- Pain or aching in the hand, especially at night. The discomfort is worse in the thumb, the index finger and the middle finger.
- Numbness, tingling, and pins and needles.
- Weakness in the fingers and thumb.
- In severe cases, pain spreads into the forearm and there may be wasting of the small muscles at the base of the thumb.

CAUSES
- Repetitive use of the wrist.
- Fracture of the wrist.
- **Arthritis**, especially rheumatoid arthritis.
- Underactive thyroid.
- Fluid retention, especially related to pregnancy, periods or the Pill.
- **Diabetes**.

TREATMENT
See a doctor as soon as you notice symptoms.

What a doctor may do
The doctor may tap on the palm side of your wrist over the median nerve; a sharp tingling pain in the wrist confirms the diagnosis. A nerve conduction test may be used to measure the severity of the nerve compression and the doctor may also assess any occupational risk and advise on changes to the way you work.

Your doctor may recommend:
- that you wear a wrist splint at night;
- anti-inflammatory drugs, such as ibuprofen;
- diuretics to reduce fluid retention;
- a steroid injection;
- minor surgery to relieve pressure.

What you can do
- Avoid repetitive actions that may be the cause of the injury.
- Shake your hand and wrist to relieve pressure and hang your arm out of bed at night.
- See a physiotherapist for stretching exercises.

OUTLOOK
Most people make a full recovery.

Median nerve — Carpal tunnel — Ligament

▲ **Occupational hazard**
Repetitive movements involving the wrist can trigger carpal tunnel syndrome. It is particularly likely to affect people who use their fingers a lot, such as computer operators or pianists.

Cartilage

Cartilage is one of the connective tissues of the body, meaning that it serves to hold body structures together. It is a gel made up of water and minerals and bound together by a fibrous mesh. This mesh consists of two proteins, collagen and elastin. Collagen gives cartilage density and strength, while elastin makes it pliable. Cartilage is an important part of the body's joints.

Cartilage turns into bone in a process known as ossification. The skeleton of an embryo is formed of cartilage, which slowly becomes bone.

WHAT CAN GO WRONG

■ Cartilage can degenerate in adulthood, as in the painful condition osteoarthritis. This can occur as a result of wear and tear or as part of the ageing process.

■ Cartilage can be torn as a result of injury. This is most common in the menisci in the knee, but may sometimes occur in one of the rib cartilages. The menisci are especially vulnerable when compression is applied to the knee and it is twisted, as can happen in a sports injury. The menisci tend to degenerate with age and tear much more easily in later life.

Treatment is usually to rest and avoid placing strain or stress on the joint. But in serious cases, **keyhole** surgery may be performed to repair the tear or remove the damaged meniscus completely. It is now possible to culture new cartilage cells in the laboratory. These can then be injected into the joint where they will grow and repair a damaged meniscus.

■ The development of cartilage, and so the growth of bone, can be disrupted by a degeneration of both bone and cartilage. This is known as osteochondritis and incorporates a group of conditions, including Perthes' disease, in which the formation of the bone from cartilage is disrupted. The problem can occur anywhere in the body, but is most common around the knee, elbow, ankle and hip. Inflammation of rib cartilage (**costochondritis**) is a common cause of pain in the chest wall.

■ The knee can be affected by a softening of the articular cartilage beneath the kneecap. This painful condition, called chondromalacia, most often starts in young adults. In severe cases, surgery may be necessary.

■ Cartilage may also be affected by a chondrosarcoma, a form of **cancer**.

SEE ALSO *Bone and disorders; Knee and problems; Skeletal system*

Cataract

A cataract is a painless clouding of the internal focusing lens of the eye. The condition usually progresses gradually and leads to a misting of vision, change in the perception of colours, and short-sightedness.

In developing countries, cataracts still represent a significant cause of **blindness**: 20 million people in the developing world suffer from cataracts.

Most cataracts occur in people over the age of 70. It is usual for both eyes to be affected, often to different degrees. When the affected eye is otherwise healthy, full vision can almost always be restored by surgery.

SYMPTOMS

Initially, as the lens loses its transparency, it may turn yellow. This can give a yellowish tinge to objects and reduce the capacity to recognize blue. As the lens becomes cloudy, sufferers may complain of glare in bright sunlight or of difficulty seeing detail in dimmer light. As the clouding progresses, there is gradual loss of the ability to see detail and contrast, until vision becomes blurred.

The process varies and can occur quickly or over the course of a few years. The extent of the effects upon vision depends upon the area of the lens clouding. Clouding of the centre of the lens (a nuclear cataract) may initially cause a degree of short-sightedness that can be corrected to some extent by wearing spectacles.

If the edge of the lens clouds (a cortical cataract), the effect upon vision may be minimal until eventually the opacity progresses to the centre. This may take some years.

In some rarer cases where the clouding is at the back of the lens (a posterior subcapsular cataract), the effect on vision may be devastating even with minor levels of cloudiness. This is because the clouding is near the point in the eye through which most of the light passes on its way to the retina.

DURATION

Cataracts are permanent once established. But the opaque contents of the lens capsule can be removed to restore vision. The lens capsule remains transparent.

Cataracts that are left alone for many years may eventually cause the capsule to rupture and lead to inflammation within the eye or **glaucoma**. This problem, once common, is now rare due to advances in treatment.

CAUSES

■ The majority of cataracts are a result of the ageing process within the lens.

■ Some cataracts are **congenital** (present at birth). Doctors shine a light into the eyes of

Factfile

Cataract surgery

The surgery to remove a cataract is a procedure normally performed under local anaesthetic.

A small incision is made in the cornea, the transparent covering of the front of the eyeball. An ultrasound probe is inserted through the cut. The probe emits soundwaves that soften the lens tissue; this is then sucked out.

A new artificial lens is then inserted through the cut. The incision is left to heal naturally or can be stitched up.

◀ **Clouded lens**
The cataract can be seen as a milky white circle behind the pupil.

newborn babies to make sure that there is no whitening of the lens.

■ Injury with a blunt object can sometimes result in a cataract. Typically this forms a star-shaped pattern, known as a stellate cataract.

■ Long-term use of some drugs, such as steroids, may lead to cataracts developing.

■ Some diseases increase the risk of cataracts. An example is **diabetes**, which may cause a snowy appearance in the lens or speed up the ageing process that causes cataracts.

TREATMENT

Seek medical help if you have difficulty seeing with either eye. If an optometrist suspects a cataract is the result of a disease or drug, you may be referred to a doctor even if the symptoms are not yet troublesome.

What a doctor or optometrist may do

■ Check your vision with a test chart.

■ Examine your eyes with an ophthalmoscope, a viewing instrument that allows examination of the inside of the eye, or a slit-lamp, an illuminated microscope used to make a detailed examination of the interior structures of the eye.

■ Refer you to an ophthalmologist, a doctor who specializes in eyes.

Treatment is by surgery and involves the removal of the opaque lens material and its replacement by a tiny plastic lens of high optical quality. The decision to treat is usually based upon the extent to which the cataract is affecting your lifestyle.

OUTLOOK

The outlook for treated cases of cataract is excellent: complications are uncommon and good vision is usually restored.

If some clouding recurs after a few months the ophthalmologist can treat the capsule with a laser to leave it permanently clear.

SEE ALSO *Blindness; Eye and problems*

Catarrh

Catarrh is an excessive discharge of mucus (thick phlegm) from the mucous membranes lining the nose, sinuses, throat and air passages. Everyone produces some mucus to protect and lubricate the air passages. Catarrh becomes a problem only when excessive amounts are produced. Causes include infection (such as a cold), **allergy** or an irritant such as smoking or air pollution. Sometimes catarrh can be produced in large quantities even when any obvious irritation has ceased.

Catarrh usually clears up by itself after about three days, but if you have difficulty breathing, a persistent high temperature, facial pain or hearing difficulties you should consult a doctor. Steam inhalation with or without eucalyptus in the water may help, but be careful not to scald your face. There is no clear evidence that complementary treatments are effective against catarrh, although echinacea and high doses of vitamin C – not to be taken by children aged under 12 – may help to combat any infection. Avoid smoking or smoky atmospheres.

Catatonia

Catatonia is a state of stupor in which a person appears unconscious or unaware of his or her surroundings. Muscles may be rigid, and the catatonic person may remain motionless without speaking, then grimace or adopt strange postures. Other features of catatonia may include repeating other people's words or mimicking their movements.

Periods of catatonia may be punctuated by sudden outbursts, periods of excitement or overactivity, panic or hallucinations. Catatonia may be associated with psychiatric disorders such as **schizophrenia** or illnesses such as **encephalitis**.

SEE ALSO *Mental health and problems*

Causalgia

Causalgia is a persistent and severe burning pain that travels along an arm or a leg due to damage to the underlying nerve. It usually follows an injury such as a severe cut or bone fracture. The nerve at the site of the injury continues to send pain signals to the brain even after the injury is healed. The skin over the nerve may become red and tender to the touch, or blue and cold. In some cases, the symptoms may be relieved by surgically severing the affected nerve or other nerves in the vicinity.

SEE ALSO *Brain and nervous system*

Cell and tissue testing

Samples of body cells or tissues can yield a great deal of information about disease processes, and are commonly used to check for signs of cancer. Tests on cells are known as cytology tests; a **biopsy** is a sample of tissue taken from an organ or part of the body. These tests may be performed under local or general **anaesthetic**.

There are three main ways in which cells can be collected. They can be scraped off the body's surface (as in a skin test or **cervical smear**); they can be taken from samples of body products, such as mucus or urine; or fluid can be taken through a syringe, a process known as aspiration cytology.

Biopsy samples may be taken from within the body (by a needle or during an **endoscopy**) either by brushing off and collecting superficial cells or by cutting out a sample. Sometimes cell collections from particular areas are carried out during an **ultrasound** examination; this enables the technician to locate the area for sampling more precisely.

SEE ALSO *Cancer*

Cellulitis

Cellulitis is a spreading bacterial infection of the skin and subcutaneous (under the skin) tissues. It usually affects the lower limbs or face. The condition is particularly common in people with **diabetes** and those with poor circulation in either arteries or veins in the legs. The word is wrongly used in the slimming industry to refer to fatty tissue in buttocks, thighs or arms.

SYMPTOMS
- The person feels ill, hot and shivery.
- The infected area of the skin will become hot, red and tender.
- Blisters may develop if treatment is not started promptly.
- The nearest lymph glands may enlarge and become tender.
- Red lines may be seen along the skin from the area of cellulitis to the lymph glands. These are caused by inflammation of the underlying lymphatic vessels (lymphangitis).
- In one specific form of the condition, **erysipelas**, the inflamed area has a raised edge.

CAUSES
Cellulitis is usually caused by the bacteria *Staphylococcus* or *Streptococcus*, which may enter the body through a cut, scratch, leg ulcer or insect bite, or develop in an area affected by athlete's foot.

TREATMENT
See a doctor as soon as possible if any of the above signs occur.

What a doctor may do
A doctor may:
- prescribe antibiotics and painkillers;
- advise you to keep the area elevated as much as possible to encourage drainage;
- screen you for undiagnosed **diabetes**;
- in more severe cases of cellulitis, admit you to hospital for treatment by intravenous antibiotics. Very occasionally, tissue areas that have died may need to be surgically removed.

Complementary therapies
Tea tree oil is a useful antiseptic for cleansing minor cuts or grazes and can be used as a preventive measure.

COMPLICATIONS
- Blistering and ulceration of the affected part.
- Infection can sometimes spread to the bloodstream causing septicaemia or to the lymph vessels (lymphangitis). If cellulitis occurs on the face, it is possible that the infection may spread to the coverings of the brain (meningitis).

PREVENTION
- Clean dirty cuts and wounds promptly.
- Cover open wounds with a dressing.

OUTLOOK
With prompt treatment, a full recovery is likely and serious complications are rare.

SEE ALSO *Bacterial infections*

Cerebral haemorrhage

Cerebral haemorrhage means bleeding into the brain. This usually occurs following a rupture of a diseased artery, especially in older people with high blood pressure. Less commonly it can be caused by injury, a congenital blood vessel abnormality or illness.

Symptoms of the bleeding can include intense headache, nausea and vomiting, loss of consciousness and other neurological symptoms such as muscle weakness, confusion and speech problems. Bleeding may occur almost anywhere in the brain and the tissue damage that follows can lead to temporary or permanent disability. Large haemorrhages are often fatal within a few days.

Cerebral haemorrhage is a common cause of **stroke**. When the bleeding is into the space below the arachnoid membrane surrounding the brain, it is known as a **subarachnoid haemorrhage**.

SEE ALSO *Brain and nervous system*

Cerebral palsy

People with cerebral palsy lack control over their muscles and movements. Although some sufferers are severely affected, others have a milder form, and the condition need not drastically reduce quality of life.

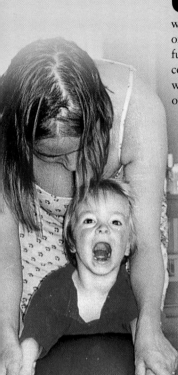

Cerebral palsy is a disability caused by damage to the brain, which can occur during fetal development, birth or soon after. In people with cerebral palsy, part of the brain – usually the one controlling movement and muscles – has not fully developed or does not work normally. The condition can be so mild as to be barely noticeable, with an affected child seeming only slightly clumsy or awkward, or it may be severely disabling. In some children, all four limbs are affected, whereas in others the limbs on one side may be affected. One limb may be shorter or weaker than the other one.

The condition is often – though by no means always – combined with mental disability. About one-third of affected children have low intelligence (an IQ below 70) and another third are slow to learn or have difficulties carrying out complicated mental tasks. Many people with cerebral palsy, including those of normal intelligence, have speech problems or impaired sight or hearing. **Epilepsy** is also associated with the condition.

Diagnosis is usually by assessment of symptoms. Although these are caused by brain injury or dysfunction, the tissue abnormalities are generally too subtle to show up in scans.

CAUSES
Cerebral palsy is due to 'scrambling' of the electrical messages concerned with movement that are transmitted from the brain to the body. It occurs when certain brain cells are damaged, misrouted or killed off by toxins or oxygen starvation.

Researchers have discovered that about one-third of children with cerebral palsy also have a particular tooth abnormality, with patches of thin or missing enamel. The tooth problem develops in the early days of pregnancy, and its association with cerebral palsy suggests that the two conditions may be due to a developmental fault that occurs at this time.

Other cases are associated with maternal illness during pregnancy, and illness or injury to the child shortly after birth.

EARLY SIGNS
The first signs of cerebral palsy usually appear before three years of age. Infants may feel floppy when picked up, or stiff and rigid; in some cases they are floppy at birth but become stiff within about three months. They are usually slow to reach developmental milestones, such as learning to roll over, sit, crawl, smile or walk. They may have unusual posture or favour one side of their body.

MAIN SYMPTOMS
There are three main types of movement disorder: stiff muscles and jerky movements (spastic paralysis), involuntary writhing (athetosis) and loss of physical coordination (ataxia). They may appear singly or in combination.

Jerky movements
With spastic paralysis, walking is invariably difficult because the child's legs press tightly together, producing a characteristic 'scissors' gait. Other signs include:
- persistent twisting of the neck (torticollis);
- involuntary eyelid twitching (blepharospasm);
- muscle spasms that cause grimacing, a 'thick' tongue and difficulty in articulating words (facial dystonia);
- spasm in the jaw muscles (trismus);
- teeth grinding (bruxism).

Involuntary writhing
Athetosis may affect one or all of the limbs or the entire body. These movements may be continuous or intermittent, and tend to be more noticeable when the child is excited or anxious.

Neuromotor therapy

Regular exercise can have a positive effect on children with cerebral palsy.

In neuromotor therapy, the parents of a child with cerebral palsy are taught gentle massage movements to stimulate development of the muscles in the upper body. The therapy is based on the theory that in early life muscles develop in response to stimuli from other parts of the body. As the muscles develop, the skeletal muscles in the child's torso become better balanced leading to improvements in movement and sometimes speech.

Loss of physical coordination

Ataxia commonly occurs in association with spastic paralysis. Actions may be clumsy or uncontrolled. The child may find it hard to manipulate small objects, and when walking may throw the legs out or take uneven steps.

OTHER SYMPTOMS

Parents who are concerned about their child's development should contact their doctor, who can arrange for an assessment at a specialized clinic.

Seizures

Up to half of all children with cerebral palsy have **seizures**, which fall into two main types:

■ Tonic-clonic seizures generally cause patients to cry out and are followed by loss of consciousness, twitching of legs and arms, convulsive body movements and loss of bladder control.

■ Partial seizures may consist of symptoms such as muscle twitches, chewing movements and numbness or tingling, or the individual may hallucinate, stagger, perform automatic movements, or experience impaired consciousness or confusion.

Growth problems

Failure to thrive is common in children with moderate to severe cerebral palsy. It is marked by slowness of growth and development. In babies, this usually takes the form of too little weight gain; in young children, it can appear as abnormal shortness; in teenagers, shortness may be combined with a lack of sexual development. This failure to thrive may be caused by damage to the brain areas that control growth and development.

Impaired vision

■ A condition in which the eyes are not aligned because of differences in the left and right eye muscles (strabismus) is common in children with cerebral palsy. In adults, strabismus causes double vision. Untreated strabismus can lead to very poor vision in one eye and can interfere with certain visual skills, such as judging distances. In some cases, physicians may recommend corrective surgery.

■ Defective vision/blindness in one eye (hemianopia) is common in children whose cerebral palsy affects one side of their body only.

Abnormal sensation and perception

Some children have impaired ability to feel simple sensations such as touch and pain.

TREATMENT

There is as yet no cure for cerebral palsy, but there are therapies that can help to relieve symptoms.

Physiotherapy

Physiotherapy is widely used to increase mobility, and can help to reduce the incidence of spasms.

Speech and language therapy

This might involve learning to control the mouth and throat muscles in order to make speech clearer, or learning to use sign language or a communication aid such as an alphabet board on which words can be spelt out.

Bobath therapy

Children in particular may find this physical therapy beneficial. By learning correct positioning and movement of parts of the body, stiffness can be reduced and muscle control improved; carers can learn to handle and position the child properly.

Conductive therapy

This approach focuses on improving motor skills in conjunction with educational, social and emotional development.

Neuromotor therapy

This therapy aims to restore the capacity of weak and underdeveloped muscles in children with cerebral palsy (see box, left).

Occupational therapy

Children with cerebral palsy can be helped to develop various skills, depending on their mental ability. These may range from dressing and feeding to working with computers.

Recreational therapy

Sports or leisure activities such as swimming, dancing or riding can help coordination and muscle strength and so relieve symptoms.

Botulinum toxin A

Muscle spasms may be relieved by injections of minute quantities of botulinum toxin A, which attaches itself to motor nerves and stops them passing on the deranged signals that cause spastic movements. The injections may be done under local or general anaesthetic, depending on where they are made. Within a few days, the injected muscles relax and remain flaccid for up to four months. After this the nerves come back to life, and physiotherapy is performed to help the affected child direct the muscles in a more functional way.

Surgery

Muscles and tendons that have become permanently contracted through continuous spasm can be lengthened by surgery.

OUTLOOK

Cerebral palsy does not worsen with age, and most people with it can expect a normal lifespan. However, over time the muscle spasms and coordination deficits may create other problems. Single-sided palsy may, for example, cause curvature of the spine or compression of internal organs on one side of the body. An uneven gait places undue stress on certain joints, and this may lead to cartilage degeneration and osteoarthritis. Teeth grinding may wear down the teeth prematurely, which can lead to eating difficulties. Various orthopaedic aids are available, such as built-up shoes, splints and rubber mouth guards, which may help prevent some long-term effects.

SEE ALSO *Brain and nervous system; Disability; Growth and disorders; Learning difficulties*

Cerebral thrombosis

Cerebral thrombosis is an obstruction in one or more of the blood vessels to the brain. A thrombus is a fibrous blood clot that builds up in an artery or vein, usually where the surface is damaged and there are fatty deposits. Most adults have some of this hardening of the arteries (arteriosclerosis), but it is particularly common in those who are overweight, have high levels of **cholesterol** and/or high **blood pressure**.

As the thrombus grows, it reduces the space in the blood vessel, making it increasingly hard for blood to pass through. Eventually, there may be a complete blockage, or part of the thrombus may break off and block a blood vessel elsewhere (thromboembolism). Cerebral thrombosis is a common cause of **stroke**, which occurs in about 100,000 people in the UK each year.

SYMPTOMS

In the early stages, when the blood vessel is starting to become blocked, there may be no symptoms. Once the blood supply to the brain is significantly impaired, symptoms include:

- weakness, numbness, clumsiness or pins and needles on one side of the body, for example in an arm, leg or the face;
- loss of or blurred vision in one or both eyes;
- slurred speech or difficulty in finding words;
- confusion and difficulty concentrating.

These symptoms may last for minutes or hours – see **TIA** (transient ischaemic attack); but if they continue for more than 24 hours they indicate a **stroke**. In either case, seek medical help so that a diagnosis can be made and treatment started.

TREATMENT

Treatment is usually with aspirin and sometimes other anti-clotting agents to prevent further thrombus formation.

Ultrasound scans of the main blood supply to the brain may show narrowing of the carotid arteries. In this case the person may benefit from an operation to scrape out the diseased tissue. People with continuing symptoms of cerebral thrombosis usually benefit from **physiotherapy** and other forms of rehabilitation to help with movement, speech and other problems.

PREVENTION

To reduce your risk of cerebral thrombosis: do not smoke; keep your blood pressure at recommended levels; control your weight; take regular exercise; reduce stress levels; avoid fatty and sweet foods; and eat plenty of fruit and vegetables.

SEE ALSO *Brain and nervous system; Cerebral haemorrhage; Stroke; Subarachnoid haemorrhage*

Cervical smear test

During a cervical smear test, a sample of cells is scraped from the cervix (the neck of the womb), smeared onto a glass slide and preserved with a spray. The smear is then examined under a laboratory microscope for abnormalities. A cervical smear test is an effective way of detecting precancerous cells. There are no symptoms at this stage to suggest anything might be wrong, but any precancerous abnormalites can be detected in a smear sample.

The best time to have a smear test is around two weeks after the first day of your period (mid-cycle). You can have a smear at a GP's surgery, a family planning clinic or an STD (sexually transmitted diseases) clinic.

WHAT'S INVOLVED

A nurse or doctor will perform the procedure; you can request a female doctor or nurse, or ask for a chaperone to be present. You will be asked to lie on your back with your knees bent. A metal speculum is inserted into your vagina and gently opened so that your cervix can be viewed. A sample of cervical cells is scraped off using a wooden or plastic instrument.

AFTER THE TEST

Your smear result will be relayed to you (usually within eight to ten weeks). A smear may be reported as:

- normal (no abnormality seen);
- inadequate (no cells from inside the cervix seen; repeat smear needed);
- showing evidence of the wart virus or other infections;
- indicating severe inflammation, often due to infection;
- showing a precancerous state.

It is important to have regular smear tests (every three to five years) so that any abnormalities can be detected at an early stage. Since most women are now screened regularly, cervical cancer is rarely seen on smears as it is usually picked up at the precancerous stage.

Depending on the results, further tests may be necessary. A smear may need to be repeated after six months or a **colposcopy** may be recommended if precancerous cells are present. This involves the examination of the cervix by means of a viewing instrument; a sample of cells will be taken for further investigation. Precancer is usually treated by a surgical procedure in the abnormal area.

SEE ALSO *Cancer; Cervix and disorders*

UNDER THE MICROSCOPE

The National Cervical Cancer Screening programme picks up thousands of cases of precancerous changes in women.

In this sample from a cervical smear test (top), the cells are of normal size and shape: all clear.

In the abnormal smear (below) the cell nuclei are larger and darker. These changes are known as dyskaryosis and indicate cervical intraepithelial neoplasia (CIN), a precancerous condition that raises the risk of cancer of the cervix.

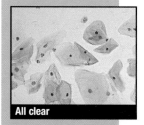

All clear

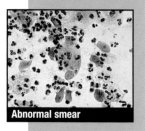

Abnormal smear

Cervix and disorders

The cervix is the neck of the womb (uterus), a short tunnel that leads into the womb from the top of the vagina. It is capable of wide dilation during childbirth, and is lined with mucus. Robust cells, called squamous cells, line the part of the cervix that is in contact with the vagina; more delicate cells line the part that leads into the uterus.

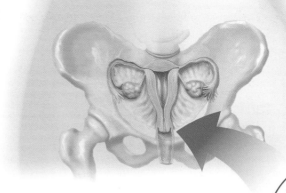

SYMPTOMS

Symptoms of cervical disorders can include:
- abnormal vaginal bleeding, such as bleeding between periods, after sexual intercourse or after the menopause;
- pain during sex;
- vaginal discharge that is bloodstained, foul-smelling or very heavy, or any less obvious change from the woman's normal discharge;
- a lump or ulcer that can be felt during intercourse or on vaginal examination, or can be seen on inspection during a **cervical smear test** or **colposcopy**, the examination of the cervix with a viewing instrument.

TREATMENT

You should see a doctor if you experience any of the symptoms listed above or described in the individual condition entries.

What a doctor may do
- Perform a vaginal examination by inserting a gloved finger into your vagina.
- Perform a speculum examination by inserting a metal instrument into your vagina in order to view your cervix.
- Perform a cervical smear test.
- Refer you to a gynaecologist for further investigations and treatment. This is usually at your local hospital.

Cervical cancer

This potentially preventable **cancer** affects 13 women in 100,000 in the UK. It is most common among women in their early 30s and women over 60.

The disease has a precancerous stage. There are no symptoms of this but the changes in the cells can be detected on a **cervical smear test**. Identifying and treating the precancerous stage can prevent cancer from developing. In the later stages, the disease may cause bleeding after sex or the menopause, or bloodstained vaginal discharge.

DURATION

The disease usually progresses slowly in its precancerous stage. Not all precancerous changes progress to cancer even if left untreated. But once cancer has developed, delay in treatment affects the person's chances of survival.

CAUSES

Cervical cancer has been linked to a virus that is transmitted through sexual intercourse. The human papilloma virus (HPV) is thought to target a number of genes within cells including a tumour suppressor gene called *p53*. Loss of *p53* can lead to a cell becoming cancerous.

The risk of catching the virus may be increased if you:
- have unprotected sex;
- have many sexual partners.

The risk of cervical cancer is also increased in women who smoke.

TREATMENT

There are few symptoms in the early stage of cervical cancer, making regular checks vital.

When to consult a doctor
- If you have any abnormal vaginal bleeding.
- When called for a cervical smear test or follow-up tests.

What a doctor may do

If precancerous changes are detected in a cervical smear test, you will be referred for a **colposcopy**: the cervix will be examined with a viewing instrument and a sample of cells taken for microscopic investigation. If the precancerous changes are confirmed, the abnormal part of the cervix is usually removed. Treatment of cervical cancer depends on the stage of the disease and includes major surgery, followed by **chemotherapy** or **radiotherapy**.

Complementary therapies

Used alongside conventional treatment for cervical cancer, some complementary treatments such as **massage** and aromatherapy may help to improve general well-being.

PREVENTION
- Use condoms during sex to avoid exposing yourself to HPV.
- Have regular cervical smears (at least every three years if HPV has been found).
- Refrain from smoking.
- Consider the sexual health implications of having multiple sexual partners.

OUTLOOK

The earlier cervical cancer is treated, the better the chance of survival. In the first stage of

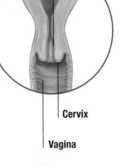

Lining of cervical canal

Cervix

Vagina

▲ **The cervix**
The cervix separates the uterus from the vagina. A narrow canal allows sperm into the uterus and menstrual blood out. During childbirth the cervical canal widens up to 10cm (4in) in diameter.

cervical cancer, in which the disease is confined to the cervix itself, 80 per cent of women live more than five years. Once cancer has spread to distant parts of the body, such as the lungs, only 5 per cent of women live more than five years.

Cervical erosion

This common problem has a misleading name since there is no erosion. Instead, the delicate cells from the inner cervix overgrow onto the outer cervix, in the top of the vagina. The cause is the hormone oestrogen. Women are most likely to develop cervical erosion during pregnancy, when oestrogen levels are high, when using the oral contraceptive pill, or when undertaking a course of **hormone replacement therapy** (HRT) – both HRT and the Pill contain oestrogen.

The symptoms are a clear vaginal discharge, pain during sex, bleeding after sex, and intermittent vaginal bleeding between periods.

TREATMENT

Cervical erosion may disappear without treatment or persist until treated. Treatment involves touching the inflamed area with a silver nitrate stick or using a laser to destroy the affected tissue. The tissue will be replaced over time by normal squamous cells. Erosion needs treatment only if bleeding or discharge occurs.

What you can do

Consider changing your contraception method if you are taking the Pill.

Complementary treatments

Homeopathy can be used to treat vaginal discharge and pain during sex alongside conventional treatment.

COMPLICATIONS

Excessive bleeding may result in **anaemia**.

Cervical polyps

Polyps are non-cancerous (benign) fleshy outgrowths. They can develop from the lining of the cervix (endocervical polyps) or hang down into the cervix from the womb above (uterine polyps). The cause of polyps is unknown and there is no known method of prevention. Symptoms include bleeding after sex, bleeding between periods and abnormal vaginal discharge.

TREATMENT

A doctor may refer you to a gynaecologist for surgical removal. This is a minor operation performed using a hysteroscope, an instrument usually used to examine the uterus.

OUTLOOK

There is no risk of polyps becoming cancerous, but any growths you have may need to be removed to confirm that they are polyps and not cancerous growths.

Cervical warts

Cervical warts are caused by a strain of the human papilloma virus (HPV). Visible, painless warts can appear on the vagina or a sexual partner's penis as well as on the cervix. Other sexually transmitted diseases, such as chlamydia, may be present. Visible warts may disappear without treatment, but the virus may remain present without causing any symptoms or showing any visible signs.

TREATMENT

A doctor will refer you to a gynaecologist or an STD (sexually transmitted diseases) clinic for further investigation and tests. Warts on the cervix can be treated by **cryosurgery**, which involves freezing them with liquid nitrogen, or by laser. Cryosurgery is also used to treat any warts on the vagina.

Complementary therapies

Homeopathic remedies may help if used alongside conventional treatments.

COMPLICATIONS

Increased risk of cervical cancer.

PREVENTION

Practise the same preventive measures as for cervical cancer.

Chlamydia

Chlamydia is a cervical infection caused by the bacterium *Chlamydia trachomatis*, which lives in the cervix and is spread by sexual contact or from mother to baby during birth. Chlamydia is the world's most common sexually transmitted disease. It persists until treated.

In three out of four women, the infection produces no symptoms. Others with chlamydia may have thick yellowish discharge, discomfort passing urine, bleeding after sex, bleeding between periods, pelvic pain or pain during sex.

TREATMENT

When to consult a doctor

If you have any of the symptoms listed above.

What a doctor may do

■ Take swab samples from your vagina and cervix to check for chlamydia and other sexually transmitted diseases or causes of vaginal discharge.

■ Prescribe antibiotic treatment if the infection is diagnosed.

■ Recommend that your partner attends if signs of infection are found.

■ Refer you to a gynaecologist or an STD (sexually transmitted diseases) clinic.

COMPLICATIONS

Untreated chlamydia infection can result in fertility problems (see **Infertility**); the infection may block the Fallopian tubes down which the egg has to travel from the ovaries to mix with the sperm.

Chemotherapy

Strictly speaking, chemotherapy is the treatment of any illness with chemicals. But the term is generally used for a highly effective cancer treatment that kills cancerous cells or interferes with their reproduction.

Chemotherapy is widely used to treat certain cancers. But it is not suitable for all forms of cancer or for all cancer patients. An oncologist (a specialist cancer doctor) will take into account the type and location of the cancer and your age and general health in deciding whether to recommend chemotherapy or other treatments such as surgery or radiotherapy.

Fast-progressing cancers such as Hodgkin's disease and leukaemia tend to respond well to chemotherapy: because the cells are fast-growing, they are quickly affected by the chemotherapy drugs. Chemotherapy is also used for some slower-growing cancers such as those of the ovary, breast or bladder.

The point in your cancer treatment at which chemotherapy is used will also depend on the type, stage and location of a tumour as well as its grade. The grade indicates how closely the cancer cell resembles the normal cell; grade I has the closest resemblance to the normal cell, grade III shows little resemblance. This can help to estimate how aggressive the cancer will be.

Chemotherapy may be used early in treatment to shrink a tumour before surgery or radiotherapy (this is known as neo-adjuvant therapy); straight after surgery to destroy any cancer cells left behind (adjuvant therapy); when cancer has recurred; or to control the symptoms of an advanced cancer (palliative therapy).

Strong drugs are used in chemotherapy, which can have debilitating effects on the rest of the body. Your feelings about whether this treatment is right for you should form part of the decision-making process. In deciding whether or not to have chemotherapy, patients must weigh the side effects against the effectiveness of the treatment in attacking their particular cancer.

WHAT DRUGS ARE USED

Many drugs are used in chemotherapy. Most are poisons that attack cancer cells (cytotoxics), but recent scientific advances are producing new drugs that interfere with the cancer process in other ways. For example, some of these experimental drugs home in on cancer cells by targeting genetic markers and interfering with cell division. Others, called anti-angiogenic drugs, stop the growth of new blood vessels to a cancer.

Most chemotherapy drugs are taken either by mouth or via a tube directly into a large vein in the arm; some can also be taken by injection.

Most currently used cytotoxics affect normal body cells as well as cancerous cells, so they can have unpleasant side effects.

Normal cells tend to recover more quickly than cancerous cells. Chemotherapy is often given in short courses interspersed with several weeks of nontreatment to allow time for normal cells to recover.

EFFECTS ON THE REST OF THE BODY

The side effects of chemotherapy can be very unpleasant and may include intense nausea and sometimes vomiting, a dry mouth, diarrhoea, fatigue, headaches, loss of hair, bone marrow failure with an increased risk of infection, infertility and weight gain.

Everyone reacts differently to chemotherapy. Some people undergo the treatment with few troubles, while others find that the course of chemotherapy causes them even more problems than their tumour did. It is vital to talk to your healthcare team about any problems that you experience since many side effects can be treated.

You may want to take time off work or arrange for help in the home during this period. Take advice from your healthcare team, however, before you make any drastic changes to your normal routine.

Some side effects, such as infertility, make prior planning necessary. Before beginning chemotherapy, women can have sections of their ovaries and eggs stored and men can have sperm set aside for future use.

Treating the side effects

Many of the unwanted effects of chemotherapy can be treated. Options include anti-emetic drugs such as 5HT3 antagonists or steroids such as dexamethasone to treat nausea or vomiting, antidiarrhoeal medicines such as loperamide; constipation treatments such as lactulose; low-dose steroid tablets to maintain your appetite; and growth factors such as G-CSF to boost production of blood cells and fight infection.

Medical terms

Oncologist A doctor who specializes in cancer. He or she may have training in one or more types of the disease.

Induction therapy This is an initial chemotherapy treatment used to reduce the cancer cell count.

Consolidation therapy Treatment that follows immediately after induction therapy to stop a cancer from returning.

Maintenance therapy Longer-term treatment to prevent relapse.

Remission The point when cancer cells can no longer be detected.

Relapse This is the re-occurrence of cancer cells after remission.

Chest pain

The chest (thorax) houses two of the body's vital organs, the heart and lungs, as well as part of the digestive system. Chest problems may involve the circulatory, respiratory or digestive systems, or they may be related to the chest wall – the ribcage, muscles and skin. It can be hard to distinguish chest symptoms: for example, those of heartburn and a heart attack can be similar. Temporary chest pain, lasting a few seconds, is not unusual in healthy people. But if you are worried about any discomfort, it is best to err on the side of caution and consult a doctor.

CAUSES OF CHEST PAIN

Common causes of chest pain include:
- chest infections, including **pneumonia**, **pleurisy** and bronchitis;
- a **heart** attack (also known as acute myocardial infarction or coronary thrombosis);
- **angina pectoris**, due to a failure of the coronary arteries to supply enough blood to the heart;
- **hyperventilation**, also known as overbreathing, in which breathing is unusually deeply and fast;
- **asthma**;
- a collapsed lung (**pneumothorax**);
- fractured or bruised ribs;
- a blood clot in the lungs (pulmonary embolism);
- heartburn;
- hiatus hernia (see **Diaphragm and disorders**);
- **indigestion**, or infection of the **oesophagus**;
- the skin infection shingles;
- infection of the ribs (**costochondritis**).

Chest infections

There are two main types of chest infection: those affecting the upper chest and those affecting the lower chest. Upper chest infections – which include **colds**, flu (**influenza**) and sore throats – are not serious and most people can treat the illness themselves. Lower chest infections, which include pneumonia, pleurisy and **tuberculosis** (TB), are more serious and need medical intervention.

All lower chest infections can cause breathlessness and general pain in the chest. Distinguishing symptoms include:
- in pleurisy, sharp pain, generally on one side, when breathing in (this is known as pleuristic chest pain);
- in pneumonia, pains as in pleurisy, fever, and a cough that produces rust-coloured phlegm (sometimes flecked with blood);
- in TB, fever, cough, loss of appetite over time, tiredness, night sweats, and pus-infected and blood-flecked phlegm.

Most lower chest infections are caused by bacteria, so the main treatment is antibiotics.

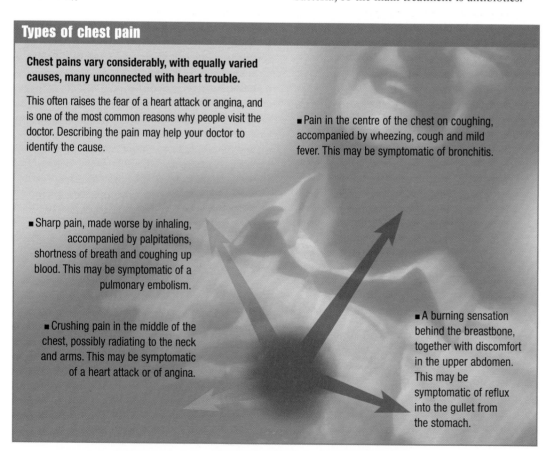

Types of chest pain

Chest pains vary considerably, with equally varied causes, many unconnected with heart trouble.

This often raises the fear of a heart attack or angina, and is one of the most common reasons why people visit the doctor. Describing the pain may help your doctor to identify the cause.

- Pain in the centre of the chest on coughing, accompanied by wheezing, cough and mild fever. This may be symptomatic of bronchitis.

- Sharp pain, made worse by inhaling, accompanied by palpitations, shortness of breath and coughing up blood. This may be symptomatic of a pulmonary embolism.

- Crushing pain in the middle of the chest, possibly radiating to the neck and arms. This may be symptomatic of a heart attack or of angina.

- A burning sensation behind the breastbone, together with discomfort in the upper abdomen. This may be symptomatic of reflux into the gullet from the stomach.

Heart attack and angina

Heart attacks are the biggest killer in the UK – 300,000 people die of them every year. The main risk factors include age, family history, smoking, high **cholesterol**, high **blood pressure** and **diabetes**. Heart attacks are uncommon in men and women under the age of 50, and very rare in healthy men under 30 and in women under 40.

Unlike most other types, chest pain that is due to a heart condition is not affected by breathing in, coughing, eating or drinking. Heart attacks cause a crushing or heavy central chest pain that may spread to the arms or jaw. Other symptoms include breathlessness or sweating. But sometimes a heart attack may cause no symptoms, or pain elsewhere in the chest or in the abdomen. Angina symptoms include breathlessness and a squeezing pain or discomfort behind the breastbone, which normally lasts around two to ten minutes. The symptoms usually disappear if you rest or take medication. Such attacks can often be relieved by drug treatments used either as a spray or tablet put under the tongue (known as a sublingual nitrate). This dilates the arteries, increasing the blood flow to the heart.

Pulmonary embolism

A pulmonary embolism occurs when a blood clot blocks the blood supply to the lungs. This may be caused by part of a larger clot breaking off and travelling through the bloodstream (see **Deep vein thrombosis**). Symptoms develop rapidly and include sharp pain, usually on one side only, when you breathe in (pleuristic chest pain), shortness of breath and coughing up blood. A pulmonary embolism requires urgent medical attention.

Bronchitis and emphysema

Bronchitis and **emphysema** are collectively known as chronic obstructive pulmonary disease (COPD). Both can cause severe shortness of breath and wheezing as well as chest pain. A cough, with or without clear phlegm, is a further symptom of bronchitis. Giving up smoking is very important but only slows the progression of the illness; antibiotics can be used to treat the infections, and steroids and bronchodilators are also used to alleviate symptoms.

Collapsed lung

A collapsed lung may occur spontaneously, be caused by a cracked rib or a chest infection such as pneumonia, or by air getting between the two layers of the pleura (the membrane separating the lung from the chest wall) – a condition known as **pneumothorax**. Symptoms include severe pain on one side of the chest and increasing breathlessness. Seek medical help immediately: serious cases may require urgent hospital treatment; less severe cases generally heal themselves.

Chest injuries

These can be caused by a blow to the chest or a particularly forceful cough. If the pain continues for more than three or four days, see a doctor. Any severe pain should be investigated immediately: one possible cause is a cracked rib, which could protrude into the chest cavity.

Infection of the ribcage

A rare cause of chest pain is an inflammation of the breastbone, known as costochondritis. The pain runs along the edges of the breastbone, but does not cause breathlessness. Painkillers and anti-inflammatories may help.

Heartburn

This term can refer both to indigestion and gastro-oesophageal reflux. Despite the problem's name, it has nothing to do with the heart: the burning pain is caused by stomach acids leaching up into the oesophagus. If you suffer from heartburn, eat little and often, and avoid spicy food. If symptoms persist, seek medical advice: over time heartburn can lead to serious problems.

Hiatus hernia

A hiatus hernia occurs when part of the stomach juts up through the diaphragm into the chest cavity. Pain in the chest, heartburn, belching and difficulty in swallowing may result. Symptoms are alleviated as in heartburn. In severe cases of hiatus hernia, surgery may be necessary.

GENERAL TREATMENT

If you visit your doctor with chest pain, you may be referred to hospital for a chest **X-ray** or an ECG (electrocardiogram). Your treatment will depend on the diagnosis. General treatments include painkillers, which can be bought over the counter. They may help reduce the pain of rib injuries and of infections such as pleurisy. Some painkillers such as ibuprofen may also have anti-inflammatory properties.

Complementary therapies

The following may help some chest problems:
- garlic for heart and circulation problems;
- vitamin C to help boost the immune system;
- echinacea to boost the immune system and help fight a cold. Echinacea should not be taken for more than two consecutive weeks.

Do not stop taking your conventional medication without consulting your doctor.

SEE ALSO *Digestive system; Heart and circulatory system; Lungs and disorders; Respiratory system*

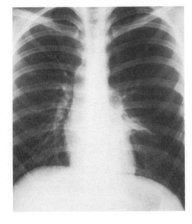

▲ **Chest X-ray**
X-rays give doctors invaluable diagnostic information. This one reveals that a patient's left lung (pictured right) is affected with the condition pneumothorax, in which air enters the pleural cavity, causing the lung to collapse.

Chickenpox

Chickenpox is a highly contagious illness. It is common in children but also affects adults. It usually runs its course without problems and lasts seven to ten days in children. Adults may feel very ill and take longer to recover, however. They are also more likely to suffer complications.

SYMPTOMS

The main symptom is a rash of small red spots that develop into blisters. The number of blisters differs greatly from person to person.
- Before the disease breaks out, the affected person may have a temperature and feel generally unwell. The temperature may last for the duration of the illness.
- The rash usually begins on the body and face and often spreads to the scalp and limbs. It may also spread to the mucous membranes, especially in the mouth and on the genitals.
- The rash is often itchy. The spots develop into blisters in a couple of hours, and the blisters turn into scabs within one to two days.
- New blisters may appear after three to six days.

CAUSES

Chickenpox is caused by the *Varicella-zoster* virus. The viral infection is transferred from one person to another through direct contact with broken chickenpox blisters and through airborne droplets. People with chickenpox should stay at home while infectious to avoid infecting others.

TREATMENT

Treatment focuses on easing symptoms.
- Use camomile lotion to relieve itching.
- Pay attention to personal hygiene and seek cool surroundings – heat and sweat may make the itching worse.
- Avoid scratching the blisters; cut the nails short or wear gloves if necessary.
- See a doctor immediately if you are at risk of developing complications (see below).

People are infectious from about three days before the rash appears. This period continues until all the blisters have formed scabs and new ones have stopped appearing. The incubation period is 10–20 days.

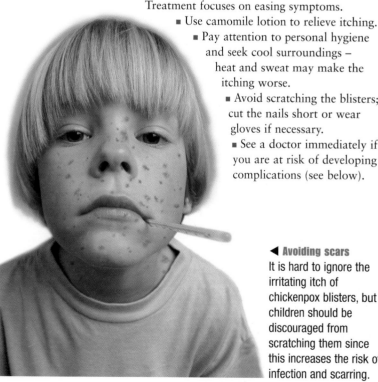

◄ Avoiding scars
It is hard to ignore the irritating itch of chickenpox blisters, but children should be discouraged from scratching them since this increases the risk of infection and scarring.

- A doctor may prescribe antihistamine drugs, which have a heavy sedative effect, to children whose sleep is seriously affected by itching.
- If you have a weak immune system, a doctor may prescribe aciclovir, a medication that works specifically against chickenpox.

COMPLICATIONS

These can be serious. **Pneumonia** may develop. In very rare cases, chickenpox can result in **meningitis** and even inflammation of the heart.

Who is most at risk of complications?
- Pregnant women who have not had chickenpox.
- Anyone with a weak immune system, such as those with leukaemia or HIV.
- Patients taking medication to suppress their immune system, such as long-term oral steroids.

PREVENTION

People who are at particular risk of developing complications and who are exposed to the *Varicella-zoster* virus can be given an injection of *Varicella-zoster* immunoglobin to boost their immunity. Vaccination against chickenpox is also available to those at particular risk.

OUTLOOK

People who have had chickenpox have immunity to the disease for the rest of their life. However, the virus may return later in life in the form of shingles. A person who has shingles can infect others with chickenpox but cannot give shingles to someone else.

Chilblains

Chilblains, medically known as erythema pernio, are itchy purple areas of inflammation that occur on parts of the body exposed to cold for long periods of time. They usually appear a day or two after exposure on fingers, toes and even ears. The inflammation is produced when small blood vessels in the skin go into spasm, thereby reducing the blood supply and causing cell damage. In severe cases, chilblains can develop into painful blisters and may even lead to **gangrene**. After chilblains first occur, the affected area tends to be more sensitive to the effects of cold and so they often recur each year.

Chill

The term 'chill' is used in everyday conversation to describe symptoms of a **fever**. These symptoms include feeling cold, feeling hot and cold alternately (with or without shivering), and a clammy sweat. A raised temperature may be due to viral illnesses such as sore throats, colds, influenza or bacterial infections of the ear, tonsils, upper airways or urinary system.

Certain infections such as abscesses, kidney infections or influenza can be associated with bouts of severe shivering called rigors.

A chill starts suddenly and usually lasts no longer than 48 hours. Elderly people in particular should be careful to keep warm and should attempt to maintain some mobility: there are small but definite risks associated with immobility, such as chest infection or, rarely, **deep vein thrombosis**.

SYMPTOMS

A temperature greater than 40.0°C (104°F) may indicate a chill.

TREATMENT

The treatment for a chill is concerned with tackling the underlying cause.

What you can do

- Drink plenty of water to prevent dehydration.
- Take paracetamol regularly for 48 hours to reduce temperature and relieve symptoms.
- Eat little and often to keep energy levels up.

When to see a doctor

If fever persists for more than 48 hours, or if there are other symptoms such as a rash, severe headache or drowsiness (see **Meningitis**).

Chinese herbal medicine

Chinese herbal medicine uses plants or plant extracts – in the form of pills, teas, ointments, compresses and tinctures – both to prevent and to treat physical, mental and emotional ill health. It is one of the cornerstones of traditional Chinese medicine, a 2000-year-old system that embraces other therapeutic disciplines, including acupuncture and Qigong.

In China herbal remedies form the major part of medical treatments. Some of the plants used, such as peony and forsythia, are familiar to people in the West; many more, such as *Huang bai*, have no direct English translation and would be unfamiliar to most Westerners. The herbs are normally supplied in their raw state and must be soaked in water and boiled for at least 20 minutes; the liquid is then strained and taken while still warm. Chinese herbal teas tend to taste bitter to a Western palate.

The herbs can be taken in many combinations, and a herbalist will make up a recipe that is unique to an individual. In China, people frequently buy herbal remedies over the counter and you can now buy simple remedies without prescription from some health food shops, independent pharmacies and herbal suppliers in the UK. For more serious or chronic conditions, seek the advice of a qualified practitioner. If you have a history of liver disease, such as hepatitis, or if you are pregnant, check with your doctor.

HOW IT CAN HELP

The World Health Organization has published a list of conditions that can benefit from Chinese herbal medicine. It includes arthritis, skin conditions such as eczema and dermatitis, premenstrual syndrome (PMS), hay fever, depression, sciatica, pain, insomnia, diabetes, stroke, potency problems, fertility disorders and cerebral palsy.

HOW IT WORKS

Practitioners of Chinese herbal medicine and other branches of traditional Chinese medicine are governed by five major principles.

- **Holism** This is the concept that the body is a dynamic, integrated whole – which means that something that affects one part will also affect the other parts.
- *Qi* The body is believed to have a 'life force' called *qi* (sometimes written as 'chi'), which should flow smoothly and continuously along interconnected internal pathways called meridians. Practitioners of traditional Chinese medicine believe that illness is the result of this flow becoming diminished, sluggish or blocked.
- **Yin and yang** The body's male or 'yang' energy must balance with its female 'yin' energy. An imbalance between the two can cause physical or emotional problems and illnesses. Pollution, accidents, infection, a bad diet and even the weather are all seen as factors that may create such an imbalance.
- **Organ pairing** Traditional Chinese medicine recognizes 12 organs, and divides them into yin/yang pairs, describing them in terms of the job they do and the way in which they support and interact with each other. Each organ is associated with a complete set of physiological and psychological functions. By contrast, Western medicine describes each organ as a purely physical entity based in a specific place.

The organ pairs are liver–gallbladder, heart–small intestine, spleen–stomach, lung–large intestine, kidney–bladder and triple heater–pericardium. The triple heater does not have a corresponding tissue base and is not recognized in Western medicine.

- **The five elements** The five elements are fire, earth, metal, water and wood. Their qualities are seen as being represented in everything in the universe, including the body's internal organs. In Chinese herbal medicine, herbal remedies are used to balance these five elements within the body. The remedies are classified under the five elements depending on the way they taste (see box, page 164).

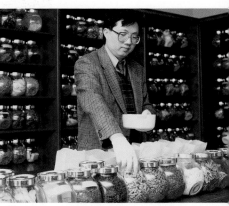

▲ **Chinese herbal pharmacy**
A remedy may contain 20 or more ingredients, carefully mixed by the herbalist, in precise quantities depending on the patient's needs.

How herbs are classified

In Chinese herbal medicine, herbs are classified in the following ways.

- By element. The five herbal elements are sweet (which relates to earth), sour (wood), bitter (fire), pungent (metal) and salty (water).

- As either cold (seen as yin) or hot (yang). For example, *Huang quin* (baical skullcap) is classified as a bitter, cold herb and for that reason is used to treat fevers.

- According to how they operate in certain organs and via particular meridians (see **Acupuncture**).

- By *tendency of action*, whether ascending, descending, floating or sinking. A herb with an ascending (upwards) action, for example, would be used to treat a 'sinking' health problem, such as a bout of diarrhoea.

A practitioner will scrutinize every aspect of your face to assess your state of health. Your eyes are believed to reveal the state of your Shen, the spirit or power behind your personality.

THE ORTHODOX VIEW

There are many published clinical trials that support the effectiveness of Chinese herbal medicine. In 1992 in a trial at Great Ormond Street Hospital for Sick Children in London, 47 children with severe atopic **eczema** – a condition that is hard to treat with conventional medicine – were given Chinese herbal remedies. There was a 60 per cent improvement in four weeks, which increased when the formulae were individually adjusted for those children whom the herbal medicine had not initially helped. Another trial on atopic dermatitis at the Royal Free Hospital in London in 1992 supported these findings.

A study on infertile women at the Qian Fo Shen Hospital in Jinan, China, found that 52 per cent of the women being treated with Chinese herbs became pregnant over the two-year experimental period compared with only 46 per cent of those on fertility drugs.

Studies such as these have brought wider acceptance of Chinese herbal medicine among orthodox doctors. However, its core principles – such as *qi* and yin and yang – are difficult for many to accept. There is also concern about the safety and purity of some of the medicines.

FINDING A PRACTITIONER

- Always consult a practitioner who is fully qualified to practise Chinese herbal medicine. Check that the practitioner is registered with an appropriate professional body.
- For details of local practitioners, contact the Register of Chinese Herbal Practitioners.

WHAT'S INVOLVED

Your first consultation with a Chinese herbal practitioner is likely to take about an hour; the length of subsequent visits will be closer to 30 minutes. Some people begin to feel better after the first session, but you may need to see a practitioner for several months at two- to six-week intervals if you are suffering from a chronic complaint.

A practitioner assesses your health using the 'Four Examinations' of looking, listening and smelling, asking, and touching.

- Looking The practitioner will observe the way that you move as you enter the room, as well as your posture, the colour and tone of your face, your expression and eyes. Your tongue will also be checked, since its colour and coating give important clues about your health.

- Listening and smelling The practitioner also assesses the sound of your voice – a 'laughing' voice, for example, would suggest a fire imbalance, which can relate to heart or circulation problems or to hysteria; your breathing patterns; and the tone of your cough if you have one. He or she will also take note of your body's smell to aid with diagnosis.

- Asking You will be asked questions about yourself and your lifestyle, your sleeping patterns, eating and excretory habits, your medical history and that of your family, and any symptoms and pains.

- Touching The practitioner may gently press your body where you have reported pain, touch your skin if you have a rash, and, most importantly, will check your pulses. There are three pulse points on the radial artery on the inside of each wrist, known as *Chi*, *Guan* and *Cuen*; the practitioner uses them to assess the state of your *qi* and its flow through the organs of the body. There are 28 types of pulse quality, including 'tight, like a lute string', 'choppy' or 'slippery', which help the practitioner to build up a picture of your particular pattern of disharmony.

Once you have been diagnosed, the practitioner will prescribe a remedy. Chinese herbal practitioners have a wide knowledge of the herbs, animal components and minerals that are used to make up individual and standardized formulae. The composition of the remedy may change over the course of your treatment as your body begins to respond. The aim is to reach a point at which your body is in balance and the remedy is no longer needed. The time it takes to reach this point varies.

Possible side effects

Chinese herbs can have powerful actions and side effects can occur, usually in the form of allergic reactions, flu-like symptoms, nausea or diarrhoea. If you experience any of these symptoms, stop taking the remedy straight away and tell your herbalist.

If symptoms persist after you have stopped taking a remedy, seek advice from your GP. Such problems have frequently been linked to poor quality ingredients, or to practitioners who were not properly qualified.

Safety points

- Buy only over-the-counter Chinese herbal remedies that have been standardized and patented for minor ailments. More serious conditions require a full consultation and diagnosis from a qualified practitioner.
- Chinese remedies are individualized and prescribed specifically for you. It is not safe to share remedies.

SEE ALSO *Acupressure; Herbal medicine*

Chiropody

Chiropody is a branch of health care that studies all diseases and developmental and structural problems affecting feet and how we walk. It is also known as podiatry.

In the UK, state-registered chiropodists must complete a three-year degree-level training course approved by the Society of Chiropodists and Podiatrists and the Health Professions Council (HPC). The newly qualified chiropodists can then register with the HPC to gain the letters SRCh, signifying State Registered Chiropodist, after their names.

State-registered chiropodists are fully trained to examine the feet, to diagnose and treat foot problems and to provide treatment and advice in the care of foot-related conditions. They will also give general advice about how to look after your feet – for example, by suggesting what type and style of shoes to wear to avoid developing common problems such as blisters and bunions. Chiropodists may use a range of pharmaceutical preparations, including local anaesthetics, as well as specialized dressings and shoe inserts. They also carry out surgical procedures, such as the removal of ingrowing toenails and the paring away of corns and calluses with a scalpel. Some have additional training in foot surgery and are called podiatric surgeons.

Chiropody is particularly important for people who have reduced sensation in their feet since these people may not realize that they have problems. It is even more crucial for anyone who also has poor circulation to the feet, as occurs in diabetes mellitus or peripheral arterial disease. In extreme cases it is possible that foot infections can lead to **gangrene** if they are not treated promptly.

Chiropody for people with foot problems may be available on the NHS. Many chiropodists also work privately.

SEE ALSO *Ankle and problems; Claw foot; Foot and problems*

▼ **Foot doctor**
Chiropodists can treat varied problems such as athlete's foot, calluses and ingrowing toenails.

Heel pain

Athlete's foot

Bunions

Ingrowing toenail

Calluses

Chiropractic

A chiropractor treats a person by manipulating and adjusting the body's musculo-skeletal system: its bones, joints, ligaments and tendons.

Chiropractors believe that the spine is vitally important for good health because it protects and supports the central nervous system and is the communication highway between the body and the brain.

To function properly, the spine needs to have all its vertebrae correctly lined up in relation to each other. Chiropractic works on the basis that any distortions of the spine affect the way in which other parts of the body function. If one vertebra is out of alignment, for example, it may press against nerves that enter, leave or are integral to the spine, causing inflammation or pinching, as in sciatica. Chiropractors call these misalignments 'subluxations' or 'fixations'.

HOW IT CAN HELP

Chiropractic is usually thought of as a therapy for bad backs, but chiropractors say that they can treat a wider range of health problems. These include pain and disability relating to the musculo-skeletal system, including neck, shoulder and back pain, many types of sports injury and joint problems. Chiropractic is also said to help with indigestion (including colic in babies), constipation, asthma, period pain and headaches.

THE ORTHODOX VIEW

Chiropractic is generally accepted as a valid form of treatment for musculo-skeletal problems. There is a substantial body of research suggesting chiropractic is more effective for acute lower back pain than ordinary physiotherapy as practised in hospitals.

FINDING A PRACTITIONER

■ Chiropractic is only occasionally available on the NHS but most medical insurance companies cover chiropractic treatment if your doctor has recommended it.

■ Contact the General Chiropractic Council for details of professionally qualified chiropractors in your area.

WHAT'S INVOLVED

The number of sessions you need depends on the problem and how long you have had it. It is usual to begin with one to three sessions a week, then to continue with weekly treatments until the condition has cleared or, at least, improved and stabilized. The average number of sessions is two to eight, but you may start to feel better after a single treatment.

A first consultation usually lasts 45 minutes to 1 hour; subsequent appointments last between 15 and 30 minutes. A chiropractor spends most of the first consultation taking a detailed medical history and making a diagnosis. You will be asked about your lifestyle, work, diet, the chairs you use and perhaps the type of bed you sleep in.

The chiropractor will also check your posture as you sit, stand and bend, and will gently manoeuvre you into various positions to check the way that your spine, joints and muscles are working. He or she will also carry out standard tests to check your blood pressure and reflexes, and may also take an X-ray.

A limited amount of therapeutic adjustment may be done during the first session, but treatment usually begins in the second session. The person lies on a special couch to receive gentle physical manipulation. A chiropractor makes well-controlled, precise adjustments to encourage the vertebrae back into their proper positions.

The techniques may include:
■ direct thrusts: precise, rapid, forceful pushes;
■ indirect thrusts: for example, gently stretching a joint over a pad, towel or wedge-shaped block for a few minutes;
■ massage: this may be used to relax a joint or reduce muscle spasm.

Try to rest for an hour after chiropractic treatment, as you may feel tired or disoriented. Around 50 per cent of people who have received treatment feel stiff and sore for a day or two afterwards but this will reduce as treatment progresses.

A gentler form of chiropractic
McTimoney chiropractic is a gentler form of the therapy that is particularly suitable for babies, young children and elderly people.

Practitioners aim to realign the entire body at each session. They manipulate the vertebrae of the spine using only their fingertips – instead of applying ordinary chiropractic's sharp, controlled pushes. They also emphasize the importance of self-help, and will often teach patients a set of simple exercises to carry out on their own at home.

PRECAUTIONS
Chiropractic is not suitable for people with advanced osteoporosis or bleeding problems. Tell the chiropractor if you have any degree of osteoporosis, inflammation, infection, a tumour, circulatory problems (especially an aneurysm) or a recent fracture.

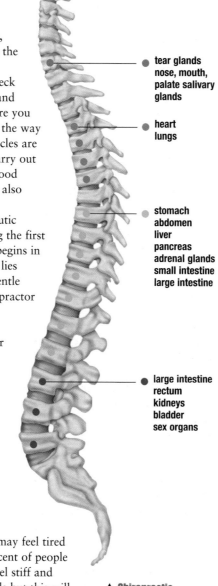

tear glands
nose, mouth,
palate salivary
glands

heart
lungs

stomach
abdomen
liver
pancreas
adrenal glands
small intestine
large intestine

large intestine
rectum
kidneys
bladder
sex organs

▲ **Chiropractic**
Chiropractic works on the premise that misalignments in the spine affect distant parts of the body. A chiropractor will manipulate the vertebra or vertebrae that correspond with the site of a patient's problem. For example, the fifth vertebra corresponds with the mouth and nose.

Chlamydia infections

Chlamydia is a bacterial infection that is passed on through having unprotected sex. It is one of the most common **sexually transmitted diseases** and can affect both men and women. As many as 1 in 14 sexually active young people in the UK have chlamydia at any one time, but all age groups can be infected. If untreated, chlamydia in women can lead to constant pelvic pain, ectopic pregnancies and **infertility**.

SYMPTOMS
About 70 per cent of infected women and 50 per cent of infected men in the UK have no symptoms and are unaware that they have chlamydia. If there are symptoms, they may include:
■ pain when passing urine;
■ a slight vaginal discharge;
■ pain during sex;
■ abdominal pain;
■ pain and cramps in the stomach or lower back;
■ in women, bleeding between periods while taking the contraceptive pill or after sex;
■ in men, a slight discharge from the penis and burning on passing urine.

CHLAMYDIA AND FERTILITY
In women, the bacteria can lie dormant for several months or even years inside the genital tissues before passing through the cervix, or neck of the womb, causing severe, widespread inflammation and pelvic inflammatory disease (PID). This not only causes pain and bleeding, but can also inflame and block the delicate Fallopian tubes with scar tissue. This can lead to an increased risk of an ectopic pregnancy and infertility. In men the infection can spread to the testes, causing inflammation of the tubes surrounding the testes, which can affect movement of sperm. It is thus believed to have long-term effects on male fertility.

DIAGNOSIS
Chlamydia differs from many other infections in that it can be difficult to diagnose. Many doctors advise patients to be tested in a specialist genito-urinary clinic so that a firm diagnosis can be made and treatment with antibiotics given straightaway. An ordinary vaginal swab often fails to pick up chlamydia but newer tests are far better and are claimed to have a 90 per cent success rate.

WHO IS AT RISK?
All sexually active people are at risk, especially those who have had two or more partners in the past year, and also women who have had pelvic inflammatory disease (see **Pelvis and disorders**). Pregnant women, particularly those who are planning to have a termination, and women about to have a coil fitted, are advised to have a test for chlamydia since both

circumstances increase the risk of the infection spreading to the pelvis.

TREATMENT

Chlamydia can be cured when treated early with a course of antibiotics. If a chlamydia infection is detected, recent sexual partners should be tested and treated as well.

Cholecystitis

Cholecystitis is inflammation of the gallbladder. It may be acute or chronic, meaning that it can strike suddenly or be a long-term illness. Acute cholecystitis is usually caused by gallstones (see **Gallbladder and disorders**), but it may rarely be a complication of a tumour. Chronic cholecystitis is caused by a succession of attacks of mild acute cholecystitis, and may result in only moderate symptoms.

Symptoms include nausea, vomiting, mild fever, pain in the upper right abdomen or sometimes in the right shoulder blade that becomes worse on breathing in. Diagnosis is by ultrasound or a **cholecystogram**, and treatment is by antibiotics and, if necessary, surgery to remove the gallbladder (a cholecystectomy).

Cholecystogram

A cholecystogram is an X-ray used to detect gallstones or to check for the presence of a tumour in the **gallbladder**. It is also used to investigate the causes of **cholecystitis** and **liver disorders**. A cholecystogram, also known as an oral cholecystogram (OCG), is normally used when an **ultrasound** scan does not reveal sufficient information.

Cholera

Cholera is an infectious disease caused by a bacterium that undermines the small intestine's capacity to absorb water.

SYMPTOMS
- Stomach pains without feeling sick.
- Mild fever.
- Vomiting.
- In severe cases it produces violent **diarrhoea**.

DURATION

Symptoms occur within a few days: the incubation period is generally less than two days, though it can be as long as five days.

CAUSES

Cholera is caused by ingesting water or food that has been contaminated by cholera-infected faeces. The bacteria can be spread to food if people do not wash their hands thoroughly after using the toilet.

When large numbers of bacteria have passed into the stomach they accumulate and begin to produce toxins that cause the symptoms of the disease. These toxins can affect the cells of the gastro-intestinal tract, causing diarrhoea and rapid fluid loss.

TREATMENT

Treatment is aimed primarily at preventing dehydration. Complementary treatments are not generally deemed appropriate.

What you can do

Consume large quantities of fluid with salt and sugar: for example, add eight teaspoons of sugar and half a teaspoon of salt to one litre of boiled water (water alone is not usually adequately absorbed by the body when a person has cholera).

When to consult your doctor

If you start suffering from severe dehydration – indicated by muscle cramps, a hoarse voice and mental confusion.

What your doctor may do

Replace the lost fluid with a mix of sugar and salts. Severe cases will be treated in hospital, where fluids can be given rapidly via a drip straight into the bloodstream.

COMPLICATIONS

The vast loss of fluid that can occur in a short space of time is particularly dangerous in children, especially in developing countries where they may also be malnourished.

If untreated, the loss of fluid can be fatal within 24 hours.

PREVENTION

Prevention is closely linked to standards of hygiene and the quality of drinking water. If you are concerned about water quality and general hygiene:
- drink only boiled water or use water sterilization tablets;
- boil unpasteurized milk;
- avoid ice cubes;
- refuse food that may not have been hygienically prepared;
- do not eat raw fish and shellfish;
- always peel raw fruit and vegetables before eating them.

OUTLOOK

Mild cases usually recover on their own. Severe untreated cases of cholera have a high mortality rate. If they are treated quickly and properly, patients should make a complete recovery.

Cholesterol

Cholesterol is a soft, waxy, fatty substance found in cells and the bloodstream of human beings and animals. It is not present in plants, and is consequently absent from fruit, vegetables, grains, nuts, pulses and seeds. The main dietary sources of cholesterol for people are:

- meat, particularly liver and other offal;
- poultry;
- fish;
- seafood, such as prawns;
- whole-milk dairy products;
- egg yolks.

THE FUNCTION OF CHOLESTEROL

Cholesterol plays an important role in keeping the body healthy. It forms part of the structure of cell membranes, especially the myelin sheath that insulates nerves (**see Brain and nervous system**), and it is the starting material for the production of the steroid hormones progesterone, cortisol, aldosterone, testosterone, estradiol and calcitriol (see **Endocrine system and disorders**).

In addition, cholesterol is the starting material for the production of bile acids, the most important of which is cholic acid. Problems with the bile can lead to the development of gallstones (see **Gallbladder and disorders**). These usually contain cholesterol, calcium salts from the bile salts and, in some cases, bile pigments.

The body cannot operate without cholesterol, so the liver will manufacture sufficient amounts to serve essential body purposes if the dietary intake of cholesterol is low. The liver can produce as much as 80 per cent of all the body's cholesterol.

CHOLESTEROL AND DISEASE

In addition to its link with gallstones, a high level of cholesterol in the blood (hypercholesterolaemia) is a major risk factor for coronary heart disease, which leads to heart attack. However, some studies show that only around 40 per cent of people with high blood cholesterol levels actually die of heart disease, and experts cannot yet define which people are most at risk. So it is prudent to attempt to normalize blood cholesterol levels by changes in lifestyle and diet.

It is worth noting that a substance called homocysteine in the blood appears to correlate with incidence of heart disease and may be a better indicator of risk than cholesterol.

Research has shown that good intakes of B vitamins, and particularly B_{12} and folic acid, may lower homocysteine levels.

HOW CHOLESTEROL IS TRANSPORTED

Since fats do not mix with water, cholesterol, like other fatty materials, cannot dissolve in the blood. Cholesterol has to be transported to and from the cells by special carriers called lipoproteins, of which there are several kinds. The two main types are low-density lipoprotein (LDL) and high-density lipoprotein (HDL).

Low-density lipoprotein

The principle cholesterol carrier in the blood is low-density lipoprotein. If too much LDL circulates in the blood, it can slowly build up in the walls of the arteries and (together with other substances, such as calcium) can form plaque, a thick, hard deposit that clogs arteries, leading to arteriosclerosis.

If a blood clot (thrombus) forms in the region of a narrowed vessel in a coronary artery, it can block the flow of blood to part of the heart muscle and cause a heart attack. If a clot blocks the flow of blood to part of the brain, the result is a stroke. A high level of LDL cholesterol usually reflects an increased risk of heart disease – which is why LDL is often called 'bad' cholesterol.

High-density lipoprotein

Approximately one-quarter to one-third of blood cholesterol is carried by HDL. This lipoprotein's main function is to carry cholesterol away from the arteries and back to the liver, where any that is surplus to bodily requirements can be passed to the bile and out of the body via the small and large intestines.

HDL also removes excess cholesterol from arteriosclerotic plaques, thereby slowing their growth. HDL cholesterol is often referred to as 'good cholesterol'.

HEALTHY CHOLESTEROL LEVELS

Cholesterol is measured in milligrams per decilitre of blood (mg/dl) and millimoles per litre (mmol/L) – the millimole is a tiny unit used for measuring concentrations of substances such as cholesterol glucose in the blood. An average healthy blood cholesterol level is where total cholesterol is less than 200 mg/dl (around 5 mmol/L) and HDL (high-density lipoprotein) is 40 mg/dl (around 1 mmol/L) or greater.

Nutritionists and medical experts do not encourage people to aim for the lowest blood cholesterol level possible because there is some evidence that low cholesterol levels may be bad for your general health.

Some studies have shown that individuals with the lowest blood cholesterol levels have the highest mortality rate, generally due to cancer

---

Cholesterol health checks

It is possible to buy self-testing kits for measuring your own blood cholesterol, but it is preferable to be tested under medical supervision.

Contact your doctor, who can perform or arrange for a cholesterol check. You should first have the level checked at around the age of 20 and after that every five years – more frequently if you have a family history of heart disease, you have a sedentary lifestyle or you smoke. If the level is too high, your doctor will discuss ways of lowering it that may include dietary and lifestyle improvements.

and conditions unrelated to heart disease. Conversely, studies of people using cholesterol-lowering statin drugs have found no association between lower cholesterol levels and an increase in death from causes other than heart disease.

There is also disagreement among scientists over whether low cholesterol levels increase the risk of depression. Some studies show that low levels of cholesterol are linked with low levels of serotonin (a chemical in the brain); too little serotonin is associated with depression. Expressive angry behaviour, on the other hand, has been linked to high cholesterol levels and heart disease; some experts postulate that anger releases stress hormones that act on fatty tissue and release cholesterol into the bloodstream.

CHOLESTEROL AND DIET

The body – mainly the liver – produces varying amounts of cholesterol (usually around 1000mg per day). Another 500mg can come directly from animal foods.

Generally very little of our blood cholesterol is obtained from dietary sources – you can have high blood cholesterol levels even if you eat a low-cholesterol diet. But there is some evidence that taking care with your diet – in particular, cutting down on saturated fatty acids – can reduce the amount of cholesterol made in the body and so lower blood cholesterol levels in that way.

Nutritionists' advice on diet and cholesterol is as follows.
- Saturated fats and trans fats (fats that are chemically altered by heating, barbecuing and processing) are associated with high blood cholesterol.
- A diet high in polyunsaturated oils can lower cholesterol levels, but it would seem that in this case both LDL and HDL are reduced.
- Using oils high in monounsaturated fatty acids, such as olive oil, on the other hand, appears to reduce LDL cholesterol as well as raising HDL cholesterol.
- Saturated fatty acids are strongly linked with raised cholesterol levels.
- Research into antioxidants (substances that slow down or prevent deterioration caused by oxidation within the body) shows the importance of eating plenty of fruit and vegetables, which are rich in antioxidant nutrients and protect against oxidation of cholesterol particles in the blood.

Reducing blood cholesterol by diet
- Cut down on saturated fatty acids, which are found in dairy foods, oils and margerine spreads, fatty meat products and manufactured bakery products such as cakes, biscuits and pastries. Choose leaner meat and lower-fat dairy products.
- Cut down on fried foods, and ready-made pies, sausage rolls and pasties.
- Increase fibre intake: pectin (from apples and other fruit) helps to prevent excess cholesterol being reabsorbed from the gut.
- Vitamin E inhibits the activity of enzymes involved in making cholesterol within the body. (Consult your doctor before taking vitamin E in supplement form if you suffer from circulatory problems, and especially if taking 'blood-thinning' medication.)
- If you do not eat enough foods containing copper (found in seafood, cherries, cashew nuts), vanadium (black pepper, soya oil, olives) or chromium (whole grains, pulses, liver), or if the combination of foods you eat has a high zinc-to-copper ratio, you may develop high levels of the blood fat triglyceride (hypertriglyceridaemia) and high blood cholesterol. Adjusting your diet to balance the zinc-to-copper ratio and taking supplements of vitamin C and niacin may help reduce levels of blood cholesterol.
- Increase your intake of oily fish: EPA (eicosapentaenoic acid), a polyunsaturated fatty acid found in fish oils, reduces the amount of cholesterol produced by the liver; it also reduces levels of blood triglyceride, another type of blood fat similar to cholesterol.

SEE ALSO *Heart and circulatory system*

Chromosomal disorders

Chromosomal disorders are abnormalities in the number or arrangement of chromosomes in the cells of the human body. Normally, every cell in the human body, with the exceptions of sperm and eggs, has 23 pairs of chromosomes. Sperm and eggs carry single chromosomes instead of pairs, so that when they merge in fertilization the fertilized egg and every cell derived from it receives one member of each pair of chromosomes from the mother and one from the father.

Faults occasionally occur in this pairing off, causing a mutation so that the fetus that grows from the fertilized egg has some kind of chromosomal abnormality.

The best known of these disorders is **Down's syndrome**. Approximately one in 200 children born has a chromosomal disorder and many more fetuses affected are spontaneously aborted. The risk of having a child with a chromosomal abnormality increases as a mother grows older. If she is over 45, the risk of her having a child with Down's syndrome is about one in 40.

SEE ALSO *Turner's syndrome*

A new plant-derived product known as plant stanol ester, present in some margarine-type spreads, has been found to block absorption of cholesterol into the bloodstream, and may therefore reduce the risk of heart disease.

Chronic fatigue syndrome

The overwhelming symptom in chronic fatigue syndrome is long-standing physical and mental exhaustion with no clear cause. Typically, sufferers are tired by even simple everyday tasks such as reading a newspaper or talking to a friend.

There is no diagnostic test for the condition, so it is usually diagnosed by excluding other reasons for the person's symptoms.

Chronic fatigue syndrome may affect people who are very fit, and it is not unusual for the condition to occur in people who have very busy and responsible lifestyles, suggesting that there may be a stress-related trigger to its development. Because of this, the condition has often been trivialized as 'yuppie flu'. But the name is inaccurate since the condition is not confined to youthful high achievers but can affect anyone, including children. Another name for the condition is myalgic encephalomyelitis (ME): myalgic means linked to muscle tenderness and encephalomyelitis is an inflammation in the brain and spinal cord.

SYMPTOMS

The typical symptoms of chronic fatigue syndrome include the following:
- severe fatigue exceeding normal tiredness lasting for six months or more;
- sleep disturbances;
- drowsiness;
- nausea;
- sore throat;
- pain in the muscles/joints, chest pain, headache;
- memory lapses, slips of the tongue.

CAUSES

Doctors are still undecided about the causes of the syndrome. It is likely that there is not a single underlying cause but several, and not all of these will be involved in every person who develops chronic fatigue syndrome. However, the condition that results from these various causes has a pattern of symptoms common in most cases.

WHO IS AT RISK

There are certain factors that appear to increase the risk of chronic fatigue syndrome. These include viral illnesses such as glandular fever or encephalitis, disorders such as depression and recent highly stressful life events such as a bereavement, but chronic fatigue syndrome can sometimes appear without any obvious cause or predisposing factors.

MANAGING CHRONIC FATIGUE SYNDROME

Because there is no clear underlying cause of this condition, there is no obvious medical treatment in the sense of specific medicines that

Therapists and chronic fatigue syndrome

Some experts in chronic fatigue syndrome believe it best to keep the number of clinical investigations of the syndrome to a minimum, but others consider a referral for specialist support to be helpful.

If your GP's diagnosis is that you have chronic fatigue syndrome, you may be offered an appointment with a psychologist at your local hospital. Clinical and health psychologists are experts in behavioural changes. Reducing smoking and alcohol intake, improving your diet, taking plenty of exercise and trying new forms of relaxation are all examples of positive health-related behaviour changes.

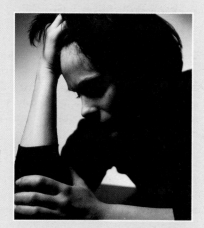

Psychologists working with chronic fatigue syndrome will help you to monitor your behaviour and set yourself realistic goals. Cognitive behaviour therapy may also help you to establish and maintain positive beliefs about the future.

can be used. Instead, health professionals talk of 'managing' the condition and often use the term 'biopsychosocial' for the programme of management. Chronic fatigue syndrome is treated by focusing on the symptoms, investigating the things that are maintaining them, and helping patients to manage these as well as they can. It is important to maintain a daily routine of activity.

For example, most of us respond to fatigue by feeling that we should rest; we may believe that we will delay recovery or even do damage by being active. However, when fatigue is long-lasting, too much rest can produce problems. Loss of muscle tone means even more fatigue when we try to get going again. Therefore the ideal way of managing chronic fatigue syndrome is to put together a programme of graded exercise to increase activity gradually. Built into this programme are periods of planned rest.

Alongside this exercise plan, it is important to ensure that people are eating a balanced diet. Help and advice about healthy eating may also be offered. Therapists call this kind of management 'pacing', and what it really means is making sure that the sufferer balances activity, rest and a carefully balanced diet in an individual treatment plan that gradually increases physical activity and stamina.

Research has shown that the benefits of the graded exercise programme have been a key element in helping people make a successful recovery from chronic fatigue syndrome.

Circumcision

Baby boys used to be circumcised because it was thought more hygienic. In the UK the operation is now most commonly performed as a religious rite, although there are some medical conditions for which it is recommended.

Circumcision in men and boys involves the removal of the foreskin on the penis. The foreskin protects the head (glans) of the penis. Its removal is generally carried out for religious reasons but circumcision may also take place for medical ones.

HOW COMMON IS CIRCUMCISION?

Organizations campaigning against the practice of male circumcision estimate that about one in four males worldwide are circumcised. National rates vary widely from about 80 per cent of males in the USA to 2 per cent in Sweden, where circumcision for non-medical reasons is now illegal. In the UK, infant circumcision of boys for non-medical reasons has not been available on the NHS since 1950; the number of circumcisions for medical reasons fell from 35 per cent of English boys in the 1930s to 6.5 per cent in the 1980s.

Current figures suggest that around 4 per cent of boys in the UK undergo medical circumcision. Some doctors argue that the risks of circumcision far outweigh any possible benefits and that this figure is still too high.

RELIGIOUS CIRCUMCISION

Religious circumcisions are carried out in Jewish, Muslim and African tribal communities. If you are unsure about your religion's reasons for circumcision, your religious leader should be able to explain in detail why the practice is traditionally performed.

MEDICAL REASONS FOR CIRCUMCISION

Medical and physical conditions that may make circumcision necessary include phimosis, in which the foreskin and the glans develop as one, separating only during childhood. The infant foreskin is frequently tight and inelastic. Some doctors may recommend circumcision in these circumstances. Others rightly say that the foreskin usually loosens by the age of three, and that true phimosis, which affects fewer than 1 per cent of boys worldwide, is very rare before the age of five years.

Another possible medical reason for circumcision is recurrent **balanitis**, inflammation of the penis head and/or the foreskin, which can affect men of all ages. Balanitis can develop from infection following damage to the skin surface and is best prevented by keeping the penis clean.

In adults, circumcision may also be offered as a treatment if a tight foreskin is making sex painful. A tight foreskin sometimes afflicts young men in their first few sexual encounters and gradually eases, but for a very few it remains a problem and so treatment is necessary.

Some people claim that circumcision can prevent cancer of the penis, but there is little evidence of this. Circumcision in childhood – but not as an adult – may reduce the risk of penile cancer, but this disease is very rare anyway and the real risk factors are poor personal hygiene and smoking.

Neither does circumcision reduce the risk of **sexually transmitted diseases** (STDs). Some sexually transmitted diseases are more common in uncircumcised men, while others are more common in circumcised men. All men can reduce the risk of an STD by using a condom (see **Contraception**). Two particular concerns for circumcised men are that they are less likely to notice the symptoms of the STD **chlamydia**, so increasing their risk of passing it on, and they appear more likely to develop penile warts.

Circumcision is generally safe. There are serious complications in 2 per cent of medical circumcisions; figures are higher if the surgeon or hygiene practices are below hospital standard. Complications include bleeding, infection, ulceration, and psychological and sexual problems. There are alternative treatments for a tight foreskin, including stretching methods and less invasive surgery. Most doctors will try these before resorting to circumcision.
SEE ALSO **Penis and disorders**

Female circumcision

Around 138 million women worldwide have undergone female circumcision, mainly in Africa.

Female circumcision involves the removal of all or parts of the clitoris and labia; it can be very painful and result in bleeding, infection and long-term physical, sexual and psychological problems. There are no medical reasons for performing a female circumcision, and the procedure is illegal in the UK and many other countries of the world.

There are 3000 cases of female circumcision every year in the UK. The majority – up to 70 per cent – can be reversed to some extent through an operation.

Cirrhosis of the liver

Cirrhosis of the liver is a condition in which fibrous scar tissue replaces normal tissue in the **liver**, impairing its function. The most common cause in the UK is **alcohol** abuse, but **hepatitis** can also be responsible. Alcoholic cirrhosis can develop after about ten years of heavy drinking, although individual susceptibilities vary and women tend to be more vulnerable than men.

The symptoms of cirrhosis include loss of appetite, weight loss and exhaustion. Later, there may be swelling in the abdomen (**ascites**) or legs (**oedema**). Treatment is of the underlying cause, but a liver **transplant** may be necessary in advanced cases.

CJD

CJD (Creutzfeldt-Jakob disease) is a degenerative neurological condition that is invariably fatal. It belongs to a rare group of diseases that invade the brain through an infectious protein known as a prion. Known as a transmissible spongiform encephalopathy, it can be transmitted in certain circumstances, and gives the brain a spongy appearance, with gaps appearing within the brain tissue. Transmissible spongiform encephalopathies can affect both animals and people (see **BSE**).

TYPES AND CAUSES OF CJD

Up to the mid-1990s, three main types of CJD had been recognized: classical, iatrogenic and familial.

■ In classical or sporadic CJD, there is no known source of infection. The condition usually affects people over the age of 50 and is responsible for 85 per cent of all cases.
■ Iatrogenic CJD is a form of the disease that results when the person is contaminated with infected tissue during medical procedures such as treatment with human growth hormone.
■ Familial is an inherited form of CJD.

In 1996, scientists identified a fourth type. This is known as variant CJD (vCJD). This new type was different from classical CJD because it seemed capable of developing in much younger people but did not appear to be inherited or a result of medical procedures.

The cause of vCJD

VCJD is thought to be related to BSE in cattle and is also known as human BSE. Many scientists believe that the prions that eventually produced vCJD came from BSE-infected meat. The strongest, but so far unproven, theory is that infection passed from cattle to people in food, most probably in Mechanically Recovered Meat (MRM). MRM is the meat left on an animal carcass after the prime cuts have been

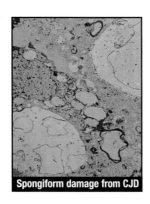

Spongiform damage from CJD

▲ **Damaged tissue**
An autopsy sample of brain tissue affected by CJD shows sponge-like holes in the tissue.

taken: pressure-blasting machines remove it to form a mince-like mixture that some food manufacturers use in cheaper meat products such as economy burgers, sausages and pies.

Until 1995, it was permitted to use animal backbones in MRM production. This posed the risk that recovered meat could have contained potentially infective spinal cord tissue. The brain is also thought to harbour large concentrations of prions and therefore people can acquire the BSE prion through meat that contains pieces of it. There is currently no evidence that muscle, eaten as steak or beef, from BSE-infected cattle poses a risk.

SYMPTOMS

In classical CJD, patients usually suffer from rapidly progressive dementia, with memory loss and confusion. Within weeks, the person may become unsteady on their feet, lacking in coordination and markedly clumsy. Later symptoms can include blurred vision or even blindness, sudden jerky movements and rigidity in the limbs as well as speech or swallowing difficulties. Eventually the person loses the ability to speak or move, and full-time nursing care is needed. Familial CJD has similar symptoms but usually develops over a longer time-span; in those suffering from the iatrogenic form, there may be no symptoms of dementia.

VCJD usually begins with psychiatric or behavioural symptoms such as depression, social withdrawal or anxiety. Sufferers may also develop delusions, paranoia or some hallucinations, and may experience pins and needles or numbness. After some weeks or months, neurological symptoms such as forgetfulness, imbalance, decreasing mobility and clumsiness occur. As the illness progresses, there is an increase of involuntary jerky movements and lack of coordination. This leads to decreasing mobility and an increasing dependence on nursing care.

DURATION

From the onset of symptoms, classical CJD may last for about six months, whereas those with vCJD survive up to 14 months. But there is uncertainty over the incubation period of vCJD. This means that there is no reliable prediction on how many cases could eventually develop. The estimate ranges from only a few hundred to as many as 140,000. By 2001 there had been just over 100 deaths considered to be either definitely or probably caused by vCJD.

HOW CJD IS DIAGNOSED

There is no absolute diagnostic test for any form of CJD that is non-invasive. The only way of definitely confirming a CJD case in human beings is by an autopsy (postmortem). An **EEG** (electroencephalogram) is often used in the diagnosis of classical CJD, which causes changes in the electrical activity of the brain.

In vCJD a brain scan can reveal a characteristic abnormality in an area of the brain called the thalamus. This is not specific to vCJD, but experienced neurologists can exclude other conditions that might produce similar results. A tonsil biopsy may also help to confirm the diagnosis of vCJD; an abnormal protein may be found in the tissue of the tonsil in those suffering with the condition.

TREATMENT

There is no cure for any form of CJD, but scientists are presently trying to develop a vaccine. Some of its symptoms, such as agitation, can be relieved with appropriate medication.

Claudication, intermittent

In claudication the blood supply cannot keep up with increased demand for oxygen and other nutrients from an organ, muscle or tissue, generally when an artery has been damaged. In intermittent claudications the calf and leg are affected, but the pain is similar to that felt in other conditions.

Sufferers develop cramping pain after walking, and may eventually manage to walk only a few metres. Pain is relieved by resting, but recurs on resuming walking. Treatment consists of reducing the factors that cause the condition, graded exercises, medication, or surgery to widen or replace narrowed arteries (see **Angioplasty**).

Claustrophobia

Claustrophobia is the fear of being in an enclosed or confined place from which a quick escape is not possible. Queues or traffic jams can be as frightening for claustrophobics as small rooms or aeroplanes. Claustrophobia may arise from a previous frightening experience, or it may develop for no apparent reason.

There are degrees of claustrophobia. Some people may feel uncomfortable in a crowded train or in a lift but can get on with their lives without too much of a problem. Other people find that their lives are dominated by fear, as they avoid uneasy situations. If this happens to you, see your GP or contact a support group.

Anything that helps you to relax is useful, including self-help tapes or **complementary therapies** that foster relaxation. Your doctor may refer you to a psychologist for behaviour or cognitive therapy or may prescribe a short course of antidepressants or tranquillizers.

SEE ALSO *Anxiety; Panic attack*

Claw foot

Claw foot is a condition in which the tips of the toes are turned under the foot, which is exaggeratedly arched. It is either present from birth or develops as a result of damage to the nerves or blood supply to the foot muscles. **Calluses** and **bunions** form over the prominent bones and pain occurs in the instep. A chiropodist may use a moulded insole to redistribute body weight evenly over the feet. Surgery may involve cutting a tendon beneath the foot in order to flatten it.

Complementary treatments that may help include **chiropractic** and **osteopathy**. Although claw foot is usually a lifelong condition, wearing sensible shoes may ease the pain.

SEE ALSO *Chiropody; Foot and problems*

Claw hand

Claw hand is a condition where the fingers become permanently flexed and contracted, while the joints between the fingers become extended, giving the hand a claw-like appearance with the fingers bent in towards the palm.

It can result from damage to the nerves and muscles that control hand movement, usually through injury to the ulnar and median nerves in the wrist. The condition can also result from a disease of the spinal cord (syringomyelia) and leprosy. Occasionally, the damaged tissue may be repaired by surgery. Symptoms can be helped by wearing splints to straighten the fingers, or surgery to cut tendons in the wrist so that the fingers can be straightened more easily.

SEE ALSO *Dupuytren's contracture*

Cleft palate and hare lip

A cleft palate forms before a baby is born when the halves of the palate, forming the roof of the mouth, fail to join together during the early stages of pregnancy. Similarly, a hare, or cleft, lip occurs when the upper lip does not join together. Clefts vary in their severity, and may involve one or both sides of the lip or the palate.

SYMPTOMS

■ A hare lip can range from a slight notch in the upper lip, to the complete separation in one or both sides of the lip, extending up and into the nose. The upper gum may also be involved.
■ In the case of a cleft palate, there may be a complete opening in the palate or a small hole in the back of the palate. A severe cleft

palate is immediately visible and will be identified at birth but a small opening may not be noticed until a baby starts to feed.

CAUSES

More boys than girls are born with clefts, but in most cases the cause of the condition is unknown. The condition may run in families, and parents with a family history of the condition may be offered genetic counselling prior to attempting to conceive a child. Several studies have linked mothers who smoke during pregnancy to a higher risk of their babies having a cleft palate.

TREATMENT

The usual practice is to repair a hare lip at 6 to 12 weeks, and a cleft palate by 18 months. Further surgery on the original repair is usually required as the child grows. This may take place before the child starts school or during the teenage years. Additional facial surgery may be performed during the late teens to adulthood.

COMPLICATIONS

■ Feeding problems – there is no specific feeding method that is suitable for all infants with clefts and different solutions may need to be tried. Infant nutrition counsellors can provide help.
■ Language and speech difficulties – 50 per cent of children need speech and language therapy and should be routinely checked by a speech therapist.
■ Dental problems – the normal development of the teeth depends largely on the type of cleft.
■ Hearing disorders – middle ear infections and catarrh can be a problem so the hearing should be checked regularly.

■ Psychological and emotional difficulties with regard to appearance – children with clefts can benefit from counselling.

Clubbing of fingers or toes

Clubbing is a thickening of the tissues at the base of the fingernails and toenails. In the early stages, the base of the nail becomes raised, giving the nails an odd, curved appearance. In advanced cases, the end of the finger or toe swells to resemble a club. Clubbing is an important medical sign. Although it may be innocuous and run in families, it is often a sign of an underlying respiratory or heart problem such as **tuberculosis** of the lungs, dilation of airways (bronchiectasis), pus in the chest lining (empyema), disease affecting the small air sacs (fibrosing alveolitis) infection of the heart valves (subacute infective **endocarditis**), congenital heart disease or lung cancer.

SEE ALSO *Heart and circulatory system; Lungs and disorders*

Club foot

Club foot is the deformity of one or both feet at the ankle. It is a congenital disorder – meaning that it is present from birth – and it affects an estimated one in 1000 babies in the UK, more commonly boys than girls. It is usually detected during antenatal scanning.

SYMPTOMS

The heel is drawn up and the sole of the foot is turned inwards so that the foot points downwards and inwards.

CAUSES

Mild cases may result from the baby having too little room to move in the womb, so that a foot is pressed up against the womb wall and normal development is restricted. Club foot can also be an inherited disorder. When this is the case it affects one in 33 babies.

TREATMENT

Club foot is entirely correctable. Splinting or putting the foot in plaster at birth helps to bring it around to the normal position. Exercises help to bring the heel bone down into the heel pad and stretch the inside border of the foot.

Special shoes called Dennis Browne Boots train the feet by using a metal bar to hold them in an overcorrected position.

Surgery may be needed to lengthen the Achilles tendon and release other ligaments and joint capsules at the back and inside border of the foot. Splints are then worn at night only (sometimes up to the age of seven).

Surgical repair

Repairing a hare lip or cleft palate will involve a succession of operations done to match the growth and development of the face.

Initial surgery to treat a hare lip or cleft palate may be carried out when the child is less than 3 months old. By late teens the repair is complete but surgery may leave some scarring, which can be minimized by modern cosmetic surgery techniques as part of the treatment.

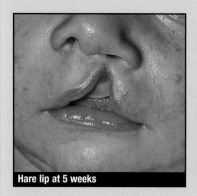
Hare lip at 5 weeks

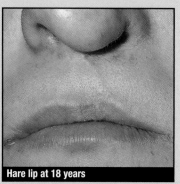
Hare lip at 18 years

Cluster headache

A cluster headache affects one side of the face only, usually around the eye. It may last for anything from 15 minutes to 3 hours, and occur frequently over several days or weeks.

The pain is accompanied by redness and watering of the eye and stuffiness of the nose. The eyelid on the affected side may droop and the pupil may constrict. Cluster headache is treated with anti-migraine drugs.

SEE ALSO *Headache; Migraine*

Coccyx and problems

The coccyx, or tailbone, consists of four fused vertebrae at the base of the spine; it is roughly triangular in shape. The coccyx barely moves in relation to the rest of the spine during standing or walking, but in a sitting position it moves by as much as 22 degrees from the vertical. It is subject to a painful, inflammatory condition known as coccydynia or coccygodynia, which is brought on or aggravated by sitting.

SYMPTOMS
Primary symptoms include:
- deep ache in the coccyx area
- pain and discomfort when sitting;
- pain in the skin tissue covering the coccyx;
- sensitivity to touch around the coccyx.

If the pain persists, secondary symptoms are likely to develop – for example, painful feet from too much standing, exhaustion, lack of sleep, lower back pain as well a general backache and **depression**.

CAUSES
Coccydynia can develop without an identifiable cause, but it is more likely to be the result of a heavy fall onto the coccyx, leading to partial dislocation of a joint in the coccyx, stretched ligaments and muscles around the coccyx, or inflammation of tissues around the coccyx. Other possible causes of coccydynia include childbirth and repetitive strain from cycling or rowing.

TREATMENT
Seek medical advice if symptoms are severe, persistent and interfere with normal activity, and if pain is not relieved by painkillers.

What a doctor may do
The first step is usually to check the coccyx and rectal area to eliminate other conditions, such as abscess or referred pain from a problem elsewhere in the spine. The doctor may then:
- arrange an **X-ray** or magnetic resonance imaging (MRI test) to see if there is a fracture, or a spur of bone on the coccyx;
- administer a local corticosteroid injection to relieve inflammation and pain;
- in cases of unrelenting long-term pain, an operation to remove the coccyx is occasionally necessary; this does not affect mobility.

Complementary therapies
Acupuncture and treatment with a **TENS** machine (a transcutaneous electrical nerve stimulator) may help.

PREVENTION
The following precautions may help to prevent or reduce the severity of coccydynia.
- Avoid long periods of sitting.
- Use a well-padded seat.
- Check your posture – sit correctly.

OUTLOOK
Coccydynia may be short-lived or last for years, and can disappear of its own accord. Most treated cases are completely cured.

SEE ALSO *Back and back pain*

Coeliac disease

Coeliac disease is an inflammatory condition of the small intestine that prevents nutrients in food from being absorbed properly. It is also called gluten-sensitive enteropathy and can cause severe vitamin and mineral deficiencies, leading to further disorders and **malnutrition**.

CAUSES
Coeliac disease results from a hypersensitivity to gluten (a protein in wheat) and similar proteins in rye, barley and oats that lead to inflammation and damage to the lining of the small intestine.

SYMPTOMS
The symptoms of coeliac disease vary widely in severity, tend to develop gradually and may appear at any age.
- Affected babies become miserable and lethargic, with pale, bulky, offensive-smelling stools after gluten is introduced to the diet.
- In adults, there may be tiredness, lethargy and breathlessness with abdominal discomfort, mouth ulcers and **anaemia**.
- In severe cases, there may be serious illness with weight loss, vomiting and diarrhoea.
- Coeliac disease can be associated with an itchy, red skin rash (known as dermatitis herpetiformis).

TREATMENT
A strict gluten-free diet for life is the only treatment. Sufferers cannot eat wheat, rye, barley or oats, or any foods that contain them. A doctor will advise which these are, and may prescribe gluten-free substitutes as well as vitamin and mineral supplements.

Cold, common

The common cold is a contagious viral infection that affects the soft mucous lining of the nose and throat (the upper respiratory tract). For most people colds are a nuisance rather than a health risk, but it is important to be aware that colds can be fatal for babies and elderly people who may develop a serious secondary infection, in particular a chest infection.

More than one hundred different viruses that can cause the common cold have been identified, and most people in the UK can expect to catch between two and four colds each year. A cold usually lasts about a week and is most often contracted during the winter.

Someone with a cold is contagious from the day before the illness breaks out until one to three days after all the symptoms have disappeared. The virus is spread by airborne droplets passed from one person to the next when the sufferer coughs or sneezes. It can also be contracted by someone who has the virus on their hands and then touches their eyes or nose.

SYMPTOMS

The symptoms of a common cold are wide-ranging. They may include:
- a sore throat;
- pain on swallowing;
- sneezing;
- a runny nose;
- a blocked nose;
- earache;
- headache;
- coughing;
- high temperature;
- aching and painful muscles.

TREATMENT

A straightforward common cold causes no serious medical problems and its symptoms will almost always clear up on their own. You need to consult a doctor only if other infections develop or more serious symptoms occur.

There is no effective way of treating a cold. Antibiotics are not appropriate because they are powerless against viruses. But it is possible to relieve some of the misery of a cold's symptoms.

Complementary treatments
- Menthol provides relief from nasal congestion by causing a cool sensation in the nose; it also relieves the symptoms of sore throat and cough by a local anaesthetic action.
- Garlic contains natural antibacterial properties that can help to inhibit infection.
- Zinc medication in the form of cough sweets can coat the common cold viruses, such as the rhinovirus, and prevent them from attaching to the nasal cells.

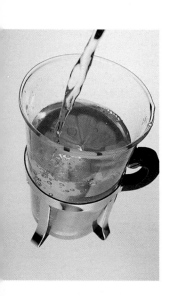

▲ Hot drinks
A steaming medicinal tea or other hot fluid has a soothing effect on sore throats and cough symptoms.

SELF-HELP

Smoking should be avoided because it further irritates the mucous membrane. In order to prevent the spread of infection, always throw away paper tissues after blowing your nose.

PREVENTION

It is practically impossible to avoid catching colds while continuing to lead a normal life, but some precautions are sensible.
- Stay away from people with colds if you can.
- Do not touch your nose or eyes after you have been in physical contact with someone who is suffering from a cold.
- Some scientific studies have shown that taking echinacea may enhance the immune system by stimulating the activity of white blood cells.
- To prevent spreading a cold, wash your hands thoroughly, especially after blowing your nose.
- Keep rooms well ventilated.

COMPLICATIONS

Possible complications of the common cold include inflammation of the eyes, sinusitis, inflammation of the middle ear and tonsillitis. If another germ infects the irritated mucous membrane, it may result in **pneumonia**.

Cold sores

Cold sores are fluid-filled blisters, usually around the mouth but sometimes in the nose, caused by the **herpes simplex** virus HSV-1. Another virus from the same group, HSV-2, usually causes **genital herpes** but there is some crossover between the two types – they can both cause either kind of herpes. The sores are painful and become covered by scabs that fall off after 8–10 days.

The cold sore virus is transmitted by close personal contact such as kissing, and cold sores are infectious until they are completely covered by scabs. The blisters heal without scarring but have a tendency to recur. The virus travels from the skin along nerves to the nerve roots, where it can remain dormant.

A weakening of the body's defences can lead to the virus being reactivated, so people often develop cold sores when they are ill or feeling run down.

SYMPTOMS
- A tingling, itchy sensation is usually felt at the site where the blisters will form.
- Tiny blisters appear, usually on the outer edges of the lips where they join the skin. The blisters become sore and itchy.
- The blisters crust over to form scabs, which last 8–10 days before falling off.
- The problem may recur at any time.

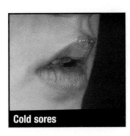

Cold sores

▲ **Cold sores**
Blisters first appear
between one and three
weeks after the virus
has been contracted.

TREATMENT

■ The most successful remedy for cold sores is the drug aciclovir, which prevents the herpes simplex virus from reproducing; to be effective, it must be started as early as possible. Aciclovir is available from pharmacists in the form of a cream (such as Zovirax) for application around the lips and the eyes.

■ If you suffer from severe or recurrent attacks of herpes, consult your doctor, who may prescribe large doses of aciclovir in tablet form.

■ The discomfort of cold sores can be alleviated by simple painkillers such as paracetamol.

■ Apply a lip salve with a high sun protection factor before going out into bright sunlight.

Colic

Colic strictly means any attack of abdominal pain, but the term is generally used to describe bouts of prolonged and unexplained crying in healthy infants in the first few months of life.

Such crying can cause considerable distress to parents when the baby is difficult to console and shows signs of pain and distress. This form of colic – also called infantile colic, three-month colic or evening colic – usually occurs when the baby is between two weeks and four months old. It can happen during the day but is more likely in the evenings.

If you think your baby cries excessively, don't assume that colic is the cause. Crying is a normal feature of infant development. Fussing and crying in the average infant increases from birth to reach about two hours a day at six weeks old, the peak age for crying. Crying then declines until the baby is about four months of age. Infants normally cry much more in the evenings than in the early part of the day, and in the first few hours after they are put to bed.

SYMPTOMS

Colic can be distinguished from ordinary crying by the following symptoms:
■ not relieved by feeding or cuddling;
■ piercing, high-pitched screams;
■ flushing of the face;
■ drawing up of the legs;
■ passing of gas;
■ clenching of the fists.

CAUSES

Although infantile colic has been extensively researched, its causes remain unclear. Results of studies are contradictory. One or more of the following factors may contribute:
■ gastro-intestinal problems such as painful gut contractions caused by an **allergy** to cow's milk;
■ intolerance to lactose, the natural sugar found in cow's milk;
■ excess gas or wind;
■ a behavioural problem resulting from a poor relationship between parent and child;
■ abnormal sensitivity of the child's central nervous system;
■ complications during labour;
■ smoking by one or both parents during and after pregnancy;
■ low birth weight.

TREATMENT

There is no medical consensus on treating infantile colic, but the condition eventually comes to an end of its own accord and seems not to have any long-term adverse effects. Some parents find that colic drops or gripe water can be helpful if their baby suffers from 'wind'; both are available from pharmacists.

Sometimes when a diagnosis of infantile colic is made for an infant who cries a lot and appears to be in pain, an underlying medical problem such as a urinary tract infection can be missed. If your child has a fever, refuses feeds, appears to be in severe pain or has diarrhoea or vomiting, consult your doctor.

What you can do

Many parents feel helpless and guilty when faced with inconsolable crying. A health visitor or doctor may be able to suggest solutions, such as more effective ways of winding your child, or changes to the way you feed your baby or to the baby's routine.

■ Avoid overstimulation. Although rocking may be helpful for some babies, research has found that gently soothing your baby in the cot is more effective than holding and carrying.

■ Give yourself a break. Sometimes you may need to put your crying baby in a safe place, close the door and go into another room for a few minutes to calm yourself down.

■ Do not switch from breastfeeding to bottle-feeding. This may make the colic worse, and breastfeeding is better for your baby.

■ Ask your health visitor to check your breastfeeding technique. Too much foremilk (the watery milk that gives a baby a drink at the start of a feed) may cause colic. Giving only one breast during each feed may help, but remember to express milk from the other breast afterwards so as to avoid discomfort.

■ If you are bottle-feeding, check that the hole in the teat is the correct size. If it is too large, your baby may be gulping down air, which leads to wind. If it is too small, your baby may be having to suck too hard and be taking in air in the process. Ideally, the milk should flow out at a drop a second without the bottle having to be shaken.

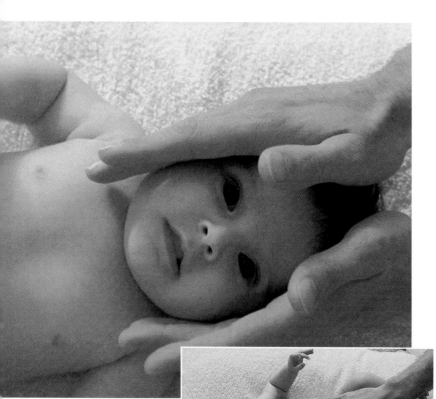

► Healing hands
An osteopath seeks the site of a baby's colic pain (right), and very gently and safely manipulates an infant's skull plates (above). The osteopath believes that the skull plates may have trapped a nerve linked to the digestive system, and so caused the abdominal pain.

■ Try substituting your baby's usual formula for one week with a hypoallergenic formula, to see if this brings any improvement. (Ask your pharmacist or health visitor for up-to-date information on this type of milk.)
■ If breastfeeding, try cutting out spicy or 'windy' foods such as onions, beans and cabbage. Also, try cutting cows' milk from your diet for a week, but get medical supervision to ensure that your diet remains healthy.

Complementary therapies
■ Aromatherapy may help to soothe your baby. Gently massage the baby's tummy with one drop of lavender essential oil in 10ml (2 teaspoons) of carrier oil or add two drops of lavender oil to a warm bath.
■ Try giving your baby a little chamomile, fennel or lemon balm herbal tea, or, if breastfeeding, have some yourself.
■ Try Chamomilla homeopathic remedies.
■ Some parents have found that osteopaths are able to soothe a child with colic (see Osteopathy).

SEE ALSO **Abdominal pain; Babies and baby care; Digestive system**

Colitis, ulcerative

Ulcerative colitis is a chronic inflammation of the colon or rectum, or both, leading to ulceration. The condition affects one in 600 people in the UK, and is most often diagnosed between the ages of 15 and 35 years.

SYMPTOMS
The symptoms are variable, but include diarrhoea in which blood, mucus and sometimes pus is passed, cramping abdominal pains, mild fever and fatigue. In some cases, **anaemia**, eye inflammation, skin disorders and joint pains may occur. The disease involves a variable course of remissions and relapses.

CAUSES
The cause of the condition is unknown, but heredity is thought to play a part. Stress and gastro-intestinal infections may trigger attacks.

TREATMENT
Diagnosis is confirmed by blood tests and a sigmoidoscopy, in which a flexible fibre-optic or video instrument is passed through the anus to view the colon and a small sample of bowel tissue removed for analysis (see **biopsy**). A barium enema may also be used (see **Barium investigations**).

There is no cure for ulcerative colitis, but prescribed anti-inflammatory drugs such as corticosteroids, and antidiarrhoeals can help to alleviate symptoms. Some sufferers find that eliminating cow's milk from their diet improves the condition. Avoiding stress may also help to reduce the number of flare-ups.

OUTLOOK
Although the condition is troublesome from time to time, most people affected by ulcerative colitis are able to lead full lives. However, in around one-third of cases, the colon becomes so damaged that it must be removed by surgery. This is partly because there is a danger that the colon will perforate, and partly because people with long-standing ulcerative colitis are at a higher than normal risk of developing colon cancer.

SEE ALSO **Bowel and disorders; Colostomy**

Collagen diseases

The term 'collagen diseases' covers a group of disorders marked by inflammation in the connective tissues that contain tough, fibrous proteins called collagen. Collagens are found in tissue, including skin, tendons, ligaments, cartilage and bone, and are also distributed in organs. The disorders stem from an immune reaction in the body, which causes inflammation and swelling of various organs and tissues.

Collagen diseases vary widely, and include: systemic **lupus** erythematosus, rheumatoid arthritis and scleroderma, which affects the skin.

Symptoms can include fever, lethargy, joint pain and swelling, skin rashes, fits or convulsions, kidney, heart and lung problems and muscle pain and weakness. Diagnosis is usually confirmed by blood tests, **X-rays** and scans (usually a CT scan or Magnetic resonance imaging/MRI).

A variety of drugs appropriate to the different conditions include painkillers, steroids and other anti-inflammatory drugs. For joint disease **physiotherapy** is helpful and, rarely, surgery is required. In cases of kidney failure, dialysis or transplantation may be necessary.

SEE ALSO *Autoimmune disease*

Colostomy

A colostomy is a surgical operation to create an artificial opening for faeces to leave the body. A cut is made in the abdomen, and connected to another opening in the colon.

A colostomy is often carried out as a temporary measure to allow the bowel to heal after surgery. This type of operation may be necessary to treat conditions such as an obstruction of the bowel, **Hirschsprung's disease**, diverticulitis (see **Diverticular disease**), an imperforate anus or cancer. But, if cancer affects the lower end of the colon or rectum, it may be necessary to remove so much of the bowel that the colostomy must be permanent.

The opening to the abdomen, called a stoma, is about two finger-breadths across, and is connected by seals to a light bag worn outside the body. Faeces pass into the bag, which is then removed and replaced with a new bag.

Specialist stoma nurses teach people with a colostomy bag how to manage the procedure hygienically and efficiently. Although some psychological adjustments may be needed, most people learn to lead normal lives after a colostomy. In time, some people even learn how to make their bowel movements regular.

SEE ALSO *Anus and problems; Bowel and disorders; Ileostomy*

Colour blindness

Colour blindness is the reduced ability to perceive certain colours, usually red or green and, very rarely, blue. Total loss of colour perception is exceedingly rare and usually associated with other eye problems.

People who are colour blind are usually born with the condition. It is caused by a partial or total absence of one or more of the three photo-pigments normally present in the cone receptor cells of the retina. The pigments are sensitive to the three primary colours (red, green and blue), so, if a pigment is missing, the eye cannot detect the colour.

Colour blindness can occasionally result from diseases of the eye or visual system such as cataract, glaucoma, diabetes, optic nerve damage or brain tumour. In such cases, it is known as acquired colour blindness.

Many drugs affect colour perception, such as chloroquine (used to treat arthritis), digoxin (used to treat heart problems) and ethambutol (used to treat tuberculosis).

All children should be screened for colour blindness because it has implications for career choice. Some careers – such as certain jobs within the armed and fire services – require full colour vision; others – such as printing, art teaching and electronics engineering – may be more difficult to do well if you are colour blind. However, most people have no difficulty in living with colour blindness. It does not prevent a person becoming a lorry driver or a bus driver, for example. No link has been shown between defective colour vision and road-traffic accidents. Some colour-blind people even become painters.

CONGENITAL COLOUR BLINDNESS

Red or green colour blindness is usually a congenital condition inherited on the X chromosome. Men have only one X chromosome, and if it is defective colour blindness will be the result. Women, on the other hand, have two X chromosomes. If a woman has one normal and one defective X chromosome, she will not be colour blind since the normal chromosome is dominant. Consequently, colour blindness is much more common among men than it is among women.

Typically, a colour-blind man will pass the defective X chromosome to a daughter, who will act as a carrier but will not herself be colour blind; she will then pass the defect on to a son. In this manner, red or green colour blindness commonly shows up in every other male generation. A woman will be affected only if both parents carry a defective chromosome.

▼ **Three or five?**
People with normal colour vision should read the number 3. Those with red-green deficiencies should read the number 5. People with total colour blindness will not be able to read any numeral.

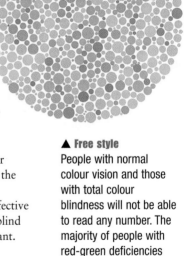

▲ **Free style**
People with normal colour vision and those with total colour blindness will not be able to read any number. The majority of people with red-green deficiencies will read the number 45.

Congenital blue blindness is not linked to the X or Y chromosomes and is much rarer, affecting one in 10,000 people.

SYMPTOMS

■ Often the condition is only detected during an eye examination. Other people may suspect a problem if they notice the sufferer wearing odd-coloured socks or failing to describe coloured objects in the expected manner.

■ People with acquired colour blindness sometimes notice a reduction in the brightness of the colours they see.

TREATMENT

Colour blindness is usually permanent. There is no cure for congenital defects. Some acquired defects may subside to a degree once the underlying disease – for example, optic neuritis – resolves. If you experience a colour defect later in life, consult a doctor; the condition may be a sign of an underlying disease.

What a doctor or optometrist may do

The most common test for colour blindness uses the Ishihara plates (two of which are shown on the previous page). Other tests include:

■ matching similarly coloured dots;

■ ordering variously coloured discs in the sequence requested by the tester;

■ using sequential coloured lights (lantern test).

SEE ALSO *Congenital disorders; Eye and problems*

Colposcopy

Colposcopy is the visual examination of the cervix and upper part of the vagina using a magnifying instrument called a colposcope. It is often carried out after abnormal cells have been detected by a cervical smear test. Its purpose is to detect how much of the cervix is affected and how far any possible cancer has progressed.

Colposcopy is usually performed in a hospital out-patient clinic. A metal speculum is inserted into the vagina, as for a cervical smear, and a powerful magnifying lens is used to view the cervix. A sample of any abnormal-looking area of the cervix is taken to confirm the results of the smear test. The procedure generally involves little or no pain, although a local anaesthetic is sometimes used.

Depending on the results of the colposcopy, the woman may be asked to return for further tests or treatment.

SEE ALSO *Cervix and disorders*

Coma

Damage to the brain or brainstem can cause coma, a state of unconsciousness from which a person cannot be woken.

People in a coma do not respond to external events. They do not move, speak, feel pain or open their eyes. They may not have control of automatic functions such as breathing and heart function and so may may require life support on a ventilator. They have very little brain activity and any responses they do have are very basic reflexes. Such a state of unconsciousness may be caused by an illness such as **stroke, meningitis, diabetes** or **Alzheimer's disease** in its later stages. Coma may occur as a result of a head injury or poisoning by, for example, narcotic drugs or carbon monoxide. Coma may also result where oxygen supply to the brain has been interrupted for several minutes – for example, in a heart attack or as a result of the blocking of the windpipe when a person chokes.

A coma may last for as little as a few hours, and have few long-term consequences, or it may continue for days or weeks. It rarely lasts for more than a month – if a person does not recover or die, he or she usually progresses to the vegetative state.

When coma lasts for longer than a few hours, there is a high chance of very severe brain damage and, even if the person regains consciousness, he or she is likely to suffer some form of permanent after effect such as difficulty with speech, loss of memory or movement impairment.

COMMUNICATING WITH A COMA PATIENT

When the brain is functioning normally, sensory stimulation such as noise, smell or touch sparks off activity in the nervous system and this activity spreads to many areas, including parts of the brain that generate awareness. When someone is in a coma, sensory stimulation may still produce neural activity, even if it does not extend to awareness. This neural activity helps to keep the brain alive – in some people it may make the difference between their falling into a deeper coma or returning to consciousness.

Methods of promoting neural activity include talking gently to the person; playing music at the bedside; wafting strong or familiar smells under the person's nose; massaging, stroking or moving the limbs, and perhaps even stinging or pricking his or her skin; and grasping his or her hands.

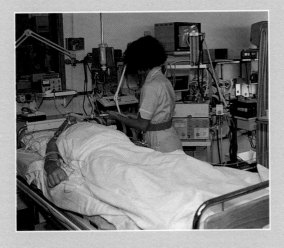

▶ **Coma monitoring**
The condition of a person in a coma is regularly examined for signs of change by a nurse or doctor using intensive care equipment.

COMPLICATIONS OF COMA

People in a coma are kept under close observation in hospital. Their inability to move themselves may cause bedsores to develop, so hospital nurses turn people with coma regularly to prevent this happening.

Patients in coma usually lose the muscle tone in their limbs, but as time passes the limbs become rigid. They can become permanently deformed, unless physiotherapists manipulate the limbs to prevent them 'setting' into an abnormal position.

Inactive people are susceptible to **pneumonia**, and coma patients, whose cough reflex is weak or who have to breath through a breathing tube (tracheostomy tube), are especially vulnerable.

When coma is the result of a head injury, there may be bleeding into the brain, and swelling and congestion of the damaged tissue. An operation may be required to remove the blood clot and decrease pressure in the skull.

Sometimes, the coma state improves but further complications arise such as the development of epilepsy, or bone formation in the muscles.

THE VEGETATIVE STATE

People in coma either die or enter a Vegetative State (VS), in which they have no awareness of their environment but retain the 'lower' brain functions needed for the body to survive. They breathe unaided; their heartbeat, circulation and digestion are normal; and they show a normal sleep/wake cycle. This may be a temporary or permanent state.

A disturbing aspect of VS is that people in this condition often appear to be aware of their surroundings. They might grip an object placed in their hand, or grimace and smile, which can mislead carers into thinking that the person is aware. But the behaviour seen in VS patients is produced reflexively by activity in the brainstem and other 'lower' brain regions and does not signify recovery.

The minimally conscious state
Some patients emerge from the vegetative state into the minimally conscious state, in which their responses to stimuli are above reflex level. For example, they may follow somebody's movements with their eyes or even be able to blink or move their fingers – sometimes on command.

A rehabilitation team experienced in the assessment of profound brain damage should judge the level of a patient's awareness.

OUTLOOK

The outcome for coma and vegetative state patients depends on the cause, location, severity and extent of brain damage, and ranges from total recovery to death. It is difficult to predict what might happen in any individual case.

For those who remain in coma for several weeks and enter into the vegetative state, the outlook is not favourable. Some patients recover, but usually they have some disturbance of memory and some physical disability. Others patients remain severely physically and mentally impaired and a small number remain unconscious. The chances of recovering from a short-lived coma, however, are generally good.

WARDING OFF DIABETIC COMA

Diabetics, especially those treated with insulin, are vulnerable to coma caused by unstable blood levels.

Blood sugar too high
Warning signs include increased thirst and urination, tiredness, breath smelling of nail varnish, and, eventually, unconsciousness.

Seek medical attention immediately as insulin and fluid will be needed. If detected early, increasing the insulin dosage can prevent the condition from worsening and control the diabetes.

Blood sugar too low
Warning signs of low blood sugar levels vary but often include feeling shaky, sweating, tingling lips, paleness, heart pounding, confusion, irritability and faintness leading rapidly to unconsciousness.

If the person is already unconscious seek medical attention urgently. A conscious person should take a sugary drink, followed by a starchy snack, such as a sandwich.

SEE ALSO *Brain and nervous system; Concussion; Head and injuries*

Locked-in syndrome

Some people emerge from coma paralysed and unable to signal their 'return'. Their condition is called locked-in syndrome.

People with locked-in syndrome are often misdiagnosed as being in the vegetative state. They can hear and see, but apart from the ability to look upwards they are totally paralysed. Using the latest technology, such as eye-blink or eyebrow-controlled switches, they can use computers to write out messages, switch on the TV or radio or close the curtains – they can perform any activity controlled by an electricity supply.

Complementary therapies

There are more than 100 different health treatment systems that can be classed as complementary therapies. They all aim to treat the whole person on a mental, emotional and physical level.

Complementary therapies, also widely known as alternative therapies, can be used in conjunction with conventional medicine or, in some cases, in place of it. Many are recognized by the medical establishment and are available on the NHS, while others are on the fringes of credibility. In the 1970s it was regarded as very alternative to see an osteopath for a bad back, but today osteopathy is one of the more widely accepted complementary therapies.

The interest in alternative therapies has increased to such an extent that in some countries there are now more registered complementary therapists than there are GPs. Americans made twice as many visits to complementary practitioners during the 1990s as they did to their family doctors. Around half the population of the USA and Australia and one-third of people in the UK use complementary therapies of some sort.

Research shows that most people who choose to be treated with complementary therapy do so out of frustration with the available orthodox medical treatments, are satisfied with the results, and feel more in control of their illness.

▼ Healing herbs
A vast range of plants is available to both the medical herbalist and the aromatherapist. Leaves, root, bark, seeds, flowers or berries may be used in herbal remedies or massage oils depending on their specific properties.

HOW COMPLEMENTARY THERAPY WORKS

Whether you visit a chiropractor, reflexologist, acupuncturist or any other good complementary therapist, he or she is likely to spend a large part of the consultation listening to what you have to say. The therapist will search for the reason behind your health problem in addition to giving you symptomatic relief for the pain or disorder that brought you to seek help in the first place.

One of the biggest differences between orthodox and complementary therapies is that you and your therapist are seen as partners in your recovery. You are not the passive receiver of medical care, as is often the case in conventional medicine. Imagine that you have arthritis, for example. A GP is likely to prescribe a synthetic drug to soothe the pain and reduce the inflammation, following a short appointment lasting perhaps ten minutes. A complementary practitioner, on the other hand, would usually spend an hour on a first appointment, take a detailed medical history, and would adopt a broader approach both to tackle the arthritis from different angles and to find out what is causing it. A medical herbalist, for example, would treat the pain or inflammation with herbal medication, and provide some soothing herbal poultices for use at home. The herbalist would talk to you about various issues.

■ **What you eat** The herbalist may suggest that you cut out foods that could aggravate your condition, such as red meat. You may also be referred to a nutritionist or clinical ecologist (a medical doctor who has undergone extensive further training in nutrition), who could check whether you have any of the food intolerances that can be linked with arthritis, and advise you on adapting your diet.

■ **Your job and lifestyle** The therapist may be able to help you to identify specific areas where your daily stress load could be reduced, or suggest stress-reducing techniques to suit you. This may help to alleviate certain symptoms of the arthritis and also enhance your overall well-being.

■ **Exercise or movement** The therapist may recommend appropriate gentle exercise, such as swimming, to help you to keep your body moving and prevent stiffness.

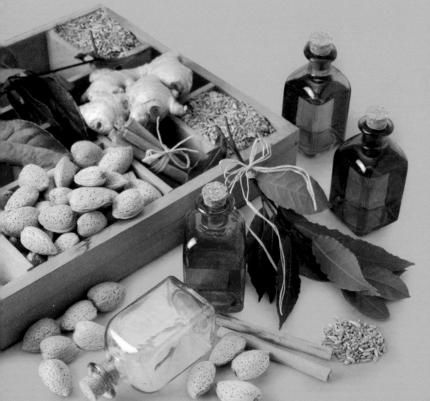

The variety of complementary therapies

So many forms of complementary therapy are available that the choice can be bewildering. The following lists are not all-inclusive but should provide you with a starting point. It is important to be aware that you should always contact your GP or hospital if you have any conditions that require either surgery or an emergency life-saving procedure.

Common complaints

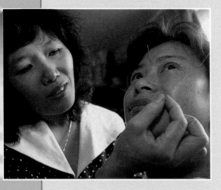

There are some generally useful complementary therapies. These include:

- **acupuncture** – (left) can help to relieve headaches, insomnia and tiredness;
- **Ayurvedic medicine** – has been used to treat eczema, asthma and arthritis;
- **Chinese herbal medicine** – treats eczema, hay fever, asthma, bronchitis and menstrual problems;
- **herbal medicine** – treats many of the same kinds of problems as Chinese herbal medicine;
- **homeopathy** – can be used to treat a wide variety of complaints, including colds, coughs and allergies;
- **naturopathy** – useful in treating arthritis, emphysema, ulcers, allergies, rashes and colds.

Muscular and skeletal problems

Back pain, sciatica, neck pain, joint problems, sports injuries and related problems, such as some headaches, may be treatable by:

- **Alexander technique** – by training the body to adopt the correct posture, all manner of muscular and skeletal problems can be improved. It also helps respiratory and digestive disorders;
- **Bowen technique** – light, precise movements can release tension in the muscles and realign the body, so easing pain and disorders in the muscles, joints and spine;
- **chiropractic** – can relieve pain through joint manipulation. Can be used for slipped discs, sciatica, lumbago and tennis elbow;
- **cranial-sacral therapy** – subtle manipulation of the head can help back and neck pain as well as migraine;
- **Feldenkrais technique** – lessons in the correct movement of the body can help to ease back and neck pain and muscle injuries;
- **massage therapies** – gentle manipulation and deep tissue work can take muscles out of spasm and improve the blood supply, so enhancing the healing process;
- **osteopathy** – treats mechanical problems associated with the spine, joints and muscles. Used for neck and back pain, sports injuries and osteoarthritis;
- **rolfing** – deep tissue massage helps realign the body and so eases pain and tension in the spine and joints.

Stress-related problems

Stress can be linked to a wide range of conditions. Complementary therapists believe that these conditions can often be improved by working to relieve underlying stress:

- **acupuncture** – the purpose is to restore the body to a state of balance, which naturally relieves any stress;
- **aromatherapy** – scented oils and, perhaps, gentle massage relax or stimulate the body and mind;
- **autogenic training** – mental exercises tackle stress through autosuggestion;
- **Bach flower remedies** – aim to release emotional blocks and so enhance a person's sense of well-being;
- **colour therapy** – aims to improve mood and relieve stress through the use of colour;
- **homeopathy** – individualized remedies can treat emotional problems and stress;
- **massage** (above) – relieves stress by inducing a feeling of deep relaxation;

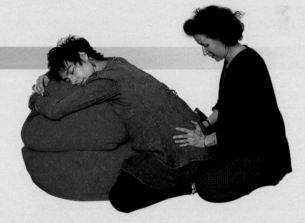

- **reflexology** – massaging certain points on the feet and so rebalancing the body's systems promotes relaxation and relieves stress;
- **reiki** – a Japanese form of healing based on chanelling energy, it usually helps the recipient to feel deeply relaxed;
- **shiatsu** – a firm massage focusing on particular pressure points can improve vitality and release tension and stress;
- **tai chi ch'uan** – this gentle exercise involves graceful flowing movements that can relax the body and mind, so banishing stress. It also enhances the circulation and breathing.

In the UK there are 40,000 registered complementary therapists and 36,000 GPs.

CHOOSING THE RIGHT THERAPY

The range of available therapies can seem bewildering, especially since many of them are said to help with a wide variety of different problems. The table on page 183 provides a rough guide to the complementary therapies that can be used to help common conditions. This should help you get the most out of your sessions.

Some forms of complementary therapy are available on the NHS via GP referral. Most British medical insurance companies will fund treatment by the major complementary therapies if recommended by your GP or a specialist. However, even if the therapy is being paid for by the NHS or a medical insurance company, you may still need to find the therapist yourself.

It is worth taking time to do a little research. Find out more about your condition and read up on the appropriate therapies, so that you can make an informed choice about the right one for you. Many complementary therapists belong to a professional association, which will often provide information about the therapy and its suitability for specific conditions. There are also helplines and support groups for many conditions. These can be a good source of information both about the condition and the treatment options available.

FIND A THERAPIST YOU TRUST

Many people find a therapist through word-of-mouth or by contacting the relevant professional association. Personal recommendation is usually the best indication of a trustworthy therapist, but remember that what suits a friend may not suit you. The Institute of Complementary Medicine can provide contact details for therapists. Talk to the therapist for a few minutes over the phone before you make an appointment. Ask about their qualifications and where they trained, and check these out with the relevant body.

Work with your therapist

Whichever therapy you choose, give it some time to work. You may begin to feel better after the first session, but many therapies take a couple of weeks or longer to take effect. Ask the therapist how long it is likely to be before you see results.

Be an active participant in getting well. Follow any extra dietary or lifestyle advice or relaxation techniques that the therapist gives you. Ask questions about your treatment.

COMBINING ORTHODOX AND COMPLEMENTARY MEDICINE

Many forms of complementary therapy are compatible with orthodox medicine: you do not necessarily have to choose between them. However, you should check with your doctor and the complementary practitioner if you wish to combine treatments.

If you have a chronic health problem such as asthma or arthritis, it may respond best to two or three therapies simultaneously, as well as some sensible self-help measures.

Safety

Complementary therapies generally work more gently and subtly than much of orthodox medicine. The therapist will seek a more complete understanding of the patient as an individual and involve him or her in the treatment. But some treatments can still cause harm if used inappropriately or by a therapist who has not been properly trained. For example, manipulation techniques such as those used in osteopathy and chiropractic can damage nerves and vertebrae, and there is even the risk of a stroke. If acupuncture needles are inserted incorrectly they may cause pain, swelling, bleeding and, very occasionally, nerve damage.

There is no reliable information about the incidence of adverse side effects from most complementary therapies; however, studies suggest complication rates ranging from 3 to 24 per cent.

The orthodox view

The medical profession is increasingly receptive to complementary therapies. There is enthusiasm especially about integrated medicine, combining orthodox and complementary treatments.

■ Ten per cent of GPs now treat their patients with complementary therapies themselves. For example, one in five Scottish GPs has a basic training in homeopathy.

■ Complementary therapies are a growing part of multidisciplinary services in NHS hospitals on palliative-care units, such as pain clinics and cancer units. Acupuncture is now used in most NHS chronic pain services.

■ Four out of ten GP practices in the UK were providing some form of complementary medicine services for their patients in 1995. It is estimated that by 2001 the figure was nearer 50 per cent.

The placebo effect

Many orthodox doctors suggest that much of the success of complementary medical treatments is due to the placebo effect (when a patient feels better after taking a pill just because they expect to), rather than the fact that the therapies genuinely work. Others take the more pragmatic attitude that even if this is true, the reason why a therapy works is less important than the fact that it does so.

SEE ALSO *Acupuncture; Alexander technique; Ayurvedic medicine; Chinese herbal medicine; Chiropractic; Herbal medicine; Homeopathy; Osteopathy*

Concentration, loss of

Concentration is when we focus our attention on one task to the exclusion of others, such as when we write a letter or play the piano. Concentration is thought to be a function of parts of the brain directly behind the forehead. People lose concentration temporarily and variably when they are tired, anxious, emotionally upset or when infections or serious illnesses affect brain function. More specifically, consistent loss of concentration can be a sign of brain disorders such as **dementia**, **depression** or psychosis. Children with **ADHD** are easily distracted and find it very difficult to keep their attention on particular activities (see **Behaviour problems in children**).

SEE ALSO *Alzheimer's disease; Brain and nervous system*

Concussion

Concussion is a brief period of unconsciousness following injury to the head or neck. The most common cause is a blow to the skull, but severe whiplash or shaking may also produce it. Unconsciousness usually lasts for a few seconds and during this time the concussed person may fall over or stagger about looking vacant.

People with concussion lose consciousness because their injury has disrupted electrical activity in the brain. In simple concussion this rights itself quickly, but thinking and sensation may be affected for several minutes, making the person confused and dizzy. If brain activity does not resume, the person goes into a **coma**.

The disruption of normal activity in the brain prevents the memory recording what happened immediately before concussion and as a rule people with concussion do not remember how it happened. It is also quite common to be unable to recall any events in the hour or two before the incident that caused the concussion.

COMPLICATIONS

Most cases of concussion are associated with bleeding in the brain and destruction of some nerve tissue. Bleeding within the brain is potentially dangerous and needs immediate medical attention, so a doctor should always be consulted as soon as possible after concussion.

TREATMENT

If there are no immediate symptoms, the affected person should rest quietly for 24 hours under observation and contact a doctor if the following are experienced:
- vomiting or nausea;
- breathing difficulties;
- visual disturbances.

Any person who may have been concussed and who fails to recover fully in the course of the few days following an incident should visit the doctor again.

What you can do

Everyday activities can be just as dangerous as high-risk ones: you are just as likely to be concussed if you have an accident while cycling without a helmet as you are if you take part in violent or dangerous sports. It is sensible always to protect the head by wearing a suitable helmet or other protective headgear if you take part in any activity where head gear is recommended.

OUTLOOK

A single episode of concussion is unlikely to be harmful but repeated hard blows to the skull, such as a boxer might endure, may lead in the long term to impaired concentration, slow thinking and slurred speech.

SEE ALSO *Brain and nervous system; Head and injuries*

Confusion

Confusion is to some degree a part of normal life – for example, a person who is woken suddenly from a deep sleep remains confused until the brain re-orients itself to the outside environment. But a person who is confused for no obvious reason or continues to suffer confusion for longer than a few seconds needs medical attention. The confusion may be a symptom of dementia, poisoning, stroke, seizure, head injury or **concussion**.

SYMPTOMS

The various symptoms of confusion are not always immediately apparent and may not be noted until a range of symptoms occur simultaneously.
- The confused person's attention meanders or flits from one thing to another.
- When the person is given something on which to focus attention, such as words to read or a simple puzzle to perform, he or she cannot concentrate.
- The person fails to react to significant new features in the environment, such as someone entering the room.
- The person may be unable to follow a train of thought or grasp what is said.
- The person seems to have forgotten how to carry out routine tasks such as using a telephone.
- The person continues or repeats an action long after the original stimulus to act has passed – for example, he or she carries on waving away a fly when the fly is no longer nearby or

continues wiping a misted window when the need to do so has been removed.

■ The person mutters or speaks in nonsensical or disjointed sentences.

Symptoms of confusion often appear in association with other mental dysfunctions such as hallucinations, amnesia, agitation or apathy, weakness, trembling and emotional instability.

CAUSES

Confusion is essentially a dysfunction of attention. The brain areas that control attention are very widely distributed around the brain, so almost anything that interferes with brain function can cause confusion (see **Brain and nervous system**). The condition may come on suddenly (acute confusion) or creep up over a period of weeks (chronic confusion).

Likely causes of acute confusion include:

■ Inflammation of the brain tissue (encephalitis), resulting from a viral or bacterial infection such as flu.

■ Drunkenness.

■ Taking drugs – for example, barbiturates, tranquillizers, antidepressants, antihistamines or narcotics (drugs derived from opium, including painkillers such as codeine and morphine, as well as heroin).

■ Head injury.

■ Stroke.

■ Seizure.

Causes of chronic confusion may be:

■ Dementia.

■ Alcohol dependence.

■ Metabolic disorders – for example, kidney failure, excess blood sugar (**hyperglycaemia**), **acidosis, anaemia** or liver failure.

■ Temporary disruption of the circulation to part of the brain. These mini-strokes or Transient Ischaemic Attack (TIAs) may not be noticed when they first occur.

■ **Schizophrenia.**

■ **Depression.**

It should not be assumed that confusion in an elderly person is an indication of dementia. A doctor should carry out a thorough physical examination to check for other possible causes before making a diagnosis.

TREATMENT

The treatment of confusion depends on the underlying condition. If no obvious cause is found, confusion may be treated with tranquillizers if other symptoms include agitation, or with antidepressants if the confusion is associated with apathy.

SEE ALSO *Alcohol and abuse; Amnesia; Brain and nervous system; Dementia; Encephalitis; Head and injuries; Metabolism and disorders; Schizophrenia; Seizure; Stroke*

Congenital disorders

In the developed world congenital disorders, also known as birth defects, are one of the commonest causes of death in babies.

Most congenital disorders take the form of visible abnormalities that are present from birth. Thousands such disorders are now recognized, including several that are fatal and cause stillbirth. Some spontaneously correct themselves over time.

Congenital defects of the brain and central nervous system and of the heart and blood vessels are the main causes of infant death in developed countries such the USA and the UK. The majority of deaths from such disorders occur in the first year of life, most of them in the first month.

TYPES OF DISORDER

There are three types of congenital disorder. Disorders caused by the defective or abnormal development of an organ or body part are called malformations. They include congenital heart defects, **spina bifida, cerebral palsy** and biochemical disorders such as **cystic fibrosis,** sickle cell **anaemia** and **muscular dystrophy.**

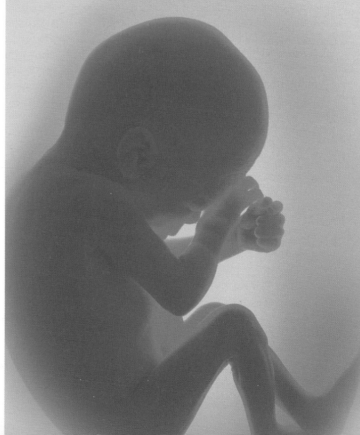

Those caused by damage to a part of a fetus that has previously developed normally are called deformations. An example is club foot.

Those caused by the abnormal development of tissues – which may involve skin, bones, nerves, organs or other tissue – are generally described by doctors as dysplasia.

CAUSES

Congenital disorders may be caused in one of several ways. Some are due to the effects of a mutation (change) in a single dominant gene or in a pair of recessive genes. These mutations may be inherited or may arise spontaneously.

Other disorders are caused by abnormalities involving whole chromosomes or sections of chromosomes (see **Chromosomal disorders**). Some are caused by several genes acting together with an environmental factor.

Some are caused by a fetus being exposed to a teratogen, a chemical or drug that has a harmful effect on fetal development, others by abnormal conditions within the womb – as in the case of club foot, which is caused by a normal foot being crowded during its growth in the womb.

DIAGNOSIS, TREATMENT AND SURVIVAL

Congenital disorders may not be discovered until after a baby is born, although new techniques using ultrasound have made certain abnormalities easier to diagnose antenatally (see page 188). Surgical advances, especially the introduction of cardiopulmonary bypass, have dramatically reduced mortality from congenital heart disorders in the developed world since around 1960.

Babies born with **Down's syndrome** now have a much greater life expectancy than used to be the case. About 90 per cent survive beyond five years of age, although respiratory infections and added complications of congenital heart disorders can still cause early death.

Spina bifida – failure of vertebrae to close during development to protect the spinal cord – is often associated with **hydrocephalus**, swelling of the head due to fluid being unable to drain away from the spaces around the brain. Both conditions can be repaired: by plastic surgery to close the vertebrae and fitting a valve to allow fluid to drain from the brain. **Anencephaly**, the absence of most or all of the brain, is untreatable and always fatal.

THE FUTURE

The rate of serious abnormalities such as Down's syndrome and central nervous system disorders has dropped since 1985 in the developed world. This has been attributed to improved and more accessible screening methods. In addition it is now known that if a woman takes folic acid before conception it reduces the chances of central nervous system defects such as spina bifida.

Research suggests that genetic screening will be developed to detect not only mutations but genetic variations that are partially responsible for characteristics such as intelligence or susceptibility to heart disease or mental illnesses. Doctors are united in opposing the development of screening tests for trivial defects and non-life-threatening characteristics, and would be against offering abortion in cases where these defects have been identified. Strict controls will be needed to prevent the misuse of advances in genetics and screening techniques.

In the long term, cloning techniques may make it possible to add genes to an egg that will benefit not only the person who grows from the egg but also his or her descendants. As such techniques are developed, there is likely to be pressure to use them to try to improve family genes. Most scientists are opposed to such 'germ line gene therapy', but some believe there are circumstances in which it might be justifiable.

Screening for congenital disorders

Screening tests are available that enable the early detection of abnormalities before birth.

Some women are more likely than most to have babies born with congenital abnormalities, and in such cases doctors generally offer tests such as ultrasound scanning (see below), amniocentesis, chorionic villus sampling (CVS) or fetoscopy to check for abnormalities. However, they are unlikely to offer such tests if a woman has indicated that she would not consider having an abortion even if serious genetic abnormalities were identified.

ULTRASOUND

Ultrasound scanning uses beams of high-frequency soundwaves directed into the womb from a probe (the transducer) placed on the abdomen. Some of these waves are reflected in an echo effect: substances such as bone and gas reflect a lot of sound and show up as white in the scan; parts like the placenta, which do not reflect so well, appear grey; the amniotic fluid does not reflect any sound at all so it appears black. By recording the echoes, a detailed picture can be built up of the fetus's position, size and shape and any abnormalities can be identified.

Recent improvements in image sharpness mean that ultrasound scanning can now be used to detect a growing number of congenital disorders.

On average 30 in 1000 babies born worldwide have a congenital disorder.

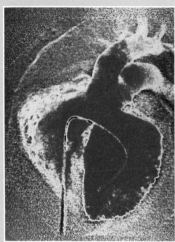

▲ **Heart disease**
A defect called a 'hole in the heart', revealed in this angiogram, causes enlargement of the heart and the pulmonary artery.

Scanning can now be carried out early enough for abortion to be offered if the parents so wish. These include **spina bifida**, **hydrocephalus**, anencephaly, achondroplasia (a growth disorder in which the arm and leg bones fail to grow) and congenital heart abnormalities.

The level of risk
Ultrasound scanning is painless and can be used repeatedly with no health risk to the mother or to the fetus she is carrying.

AMNIOCENTESIS
By performing an amniocentesis a doctor can take fetal cells for chromosomal analysis without disturbing the fetus itself. In an amniocentesis the cells are taken from the amniotic fluid that surrounds the fetus, in which such cells are always present. The chromosomes in the cells can be examined to reveal chromosomal disorders such as Down's syndrome. The amniotic fluid itself can also be analysed to provide evidence that indicates the presence of some other disorders. Higher-than-normal levels of alphafetoprotein, for example, may indicate a fetus affected by spina bifida.

Pregnant women over the age of 38 are normally offered amniocentesis (or chorionic villus sampling, see below) because they have a higher then normal risk of having a baby affected by Down's syndrome. The test may also be offered to women who have already had a child with Down's syndrome or those who have a close relative with the syndrome.

How it is performed
A local anaesthetic is given and then a hollow needle is inserted through the abdominal wall and uterus into the amniotic sac in order to suck out a small fluid sample. The procedure is painless, although the woman may feel a slight pricking. Amniocentesis is usually performed around the 15th–16th week of pregnancy. Throughout the procedure an ultrasound image is generated as a visual guide to the doctor inserting the needle.

The level of risk
Amniocentesis carries a 0.25–0.5 per cent risk of causing a miscarriage, so is used only when the likelihood of having a baby affected by a serious condition outweighs the risk of abortion. The biggest disadvantage of amniocentesis is that it takes place relatively late in pregnancy, and the wait for results is weeks rather than days. The emotional strain of choosing to abort at the fourth or fifth month can be hard to bear.

CHORIONIC VILLUS SAMPLING
Chorionic villus sampling, or CVS, has been developed in recent years to make it possible to sample fetal cells for suspected genetic abnormalities at a much earlier stage of pregnancy than is possible using amniocentesis. Chorionic villus sampling is carried out around the 10th to 12th week of pregnancy.

How it is performed
Using an ultrasound image for guidance, the doctor inserts a fine hollow needle into the uterus

Using ultrasound scanning to detect abnormalities

Women are given a routine ultrasound in about the 12th week of pregnancy to check progress and confirm the forecast delivery date.

Those at risk of having a baby with congenital abnormalities have a second scan in the 16th or 17th week of pregnancy to check for problems. Water-soluble oil is spread over the mother's abdomen so that the scanning head makes good contact with her skin. The handheld transducer is moved over her abdomen and picks up the reflected signal (see main text) before transmitting it to the analyser, which converts the electrical signal into a picture on the screen (right). The scanner produces 30 pictures a second, so radiographer and mother can see the baby moving. The image is recorded on videotape for doctor and nurses to examine later. Modern scans have excellent definition that allows fine detail to be seen. They can be used to examine small parts of the fetus, such as the fingers and toes, for abnormalities.

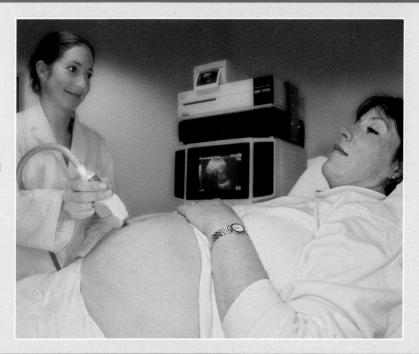

in order to draw off a few cells from the villi at the edge of the placenta. These cells come from the fetus and can be analysed for genetic, chromosomal or biochemical abnormalities. The advantage of chorionic villus sampling over amniocentesis is that it allows earlier and therefore safer abortion.

The level of risk
The test has the disadvantage of a 2 per cent risk of inducing miscarriage – higher than that for amniocentesis. In some teaching hospitals, however, where doctors perform the test several times a day, the risk is far lower.

FETOSCOPY
Fetoscopy is less commonly used than amniocentesis or chorionic villus sampling because it has a much greater risk of causing miscarriage. It is carried out after the 16th week of pregnancy. Fetoscopy is a hi-tech procedure normally only available in larger hospitals.

How it is performed
A thin, flexible hollow tube fitted with a light and a telescopic probe is inserted into the uterus through a small cut through the abdominal wall, made under local anaesthetic. The instrument, called a fetoscope, is used to look at the fetus and to take fetal blood samples from the umbilical cord. Medical staff use ultrasound to guide the fetoscope visually and avoid harming the fetus.

Abnormalities of the face, limbs or body can be viewed, and the fetal blood can be tested for disorders such as thalassaemia or sickle-cell anaemia. A camera is often attached to the instrument to take pictures of the fetus for later use in diagnosis.

The level of risk
Fetoscopy carries a 3–5 per cent chance of miscarriage. It is used only when the mother is at high risk of carrying an abnormal fetus.

GENETIC COUNSELLING
Families with a history of genetic disorders or those who already have a child affected by a genetic disorder may want genetic counselling. This can be arranged through a family doctor. A genetic counsellor can explain how a condition caused by a genetic mutation comes about, and the risks of passing on the condition to another child and to future generations.

Conjunctivitis

Conjunctivitis is a very common disorder of the eye. It involves inflammation of the normally transparent membrane called the conjunctiva that covers the white of the eye and the inner surfaces of the eyelids. The redness is caused by the widening of tiny blood vessels in the membrane, and is usually temporary.

Most cases of conjunctivitis are the result of allergy or infection by bacteria or viruses, or by irritation caused by chemicals, cigarette smoke or contact lenses or, for example, hay fever. Both eyes may be affected, often one after the other.

Acute conjunctivitis lasts for anything from a few days to a few weeks, depending on the cause and whether effective treatment is given. Chronic conjunctivitis lasts for months or years, or may be virtually permanent.

SYMPTOMS
Conjunctivitis causes only slight discomfort or irritation, frequently accompanied by a mild gritty sensation or itching. Sharp pain combined with the feeling that there is a foreign body in the eye is not usually a symptom of conjunctivitis. There are several other signs.
- Pinkness or redness in the membrane covering the white of the eye may be localized or may extend over the whole surface.
- There is commonly a discharge, which may result in blurred vision and cause the eyelids to stick together.
- Occasionally there is a small tender swelling in front of the ear on the same side as the affected eye, and a general feeling of malaise; this is typical of viral conjunctivitis.

TREATMENT
Do not try to treat yourself – it is easy to make the problem worse. Seek medical advice.

What a doctor may do
Sometimes a doctor may refer a person with conjunctivitis to an ophthalmologist, especially if the conjunctivitis is particularly virulent – as, for example, may occur in a newborn infant. Before deciding whether a referral is necessary, the doctor will do some or all of the following.
- Examine the eyes with a hand lens and torch.
- Take a swab of the discharge, if any.
- Check that the vision is unimpaired.
- Carry out tests to eliminate more serious conditions such as acute **glaucoma**, corneal ulcer (see **Cornea and disorders**), a foreign body in the eye, or internal eye inflammation.

Depending on the cause, the doctor may prescribe antibiotics, antiviral drugs, anti-inflammatory drops or antihistamine drops (see **Allergies**). Lubricants or decongestant drops may occasionally be prescribed.

SEE ALSO *Eye and problems*

Constipation

Constipation is a condition in which the bowel is emptied infrequently, the faeces are hard or small, or the elimination of faeces is difficult or painful. It can affect people at any age.

Constipation in babies is hard to diagnose. It may be normal for a baby or young child to defecate only every three or four days; dry, hard stools that are difficult to pass are a more reliable indication. Suspected constipation in infants should be treated by giving them extra bottles of water or diluted fruit drinks.

The tendency to constipation usually persists throughout life unless changes to diet and lifestyle are made. If the constipation has an underlying cause, such as **haemorrhoids**, treating the primary problem may help.

CAUSES

The possible causes of constipation include:
- insufficient intake of dietary fibre;
- inadequate fluid intake;
- old age and consequent reduced mobility;
- drugs, commonly painkillers and antidepressants;
- dehydration and immobility caused by illness;
- medical conditions such as **irritable bowel syndrome**, an underactive thyroid gland (see **Myxoedema**), **multiple sclerosis, stroke, lupus** and **Parkinson's disease**;
- anal fissure – a tear of the skin at the entrance to the back passage, which makes passing faeces very painful (see **Anus and problems**);
- pain caused by **haemorrhoids**;
- the consequences of a surgical operation;
- damage to the colon due to laxative abuse;
- obstruction, narrowing or cancer of the bowel (see **Bowel and disorders**).

TREATMENT

Lifestyle changes are often the most effective way to treat constipation.

What you can do
- Drink more fluids.
- Eat a diet that includes plenty of fibre, bran, bran cereals, wholemeal bread, fresh fruit and vegetables.
- Apply soothing creams or ointments if the passage of faeces is painful.
- Seek advice from your pharmacist on using laxatives and bulking agents – but as a short-term measure only.
- For elderly people, encourage increased mobility and regular trips to the toilet.

When to consult a doctor
Seek medical advice if any of the following circumstances applies.
- The problem persists for over two weeks.
- The problem is severe or is not responding to treatment, and if there is any bleeding from the anus.
- There has been a recent change in bowel habits, particularly if you are over 40.

What a doctor may do
A doctor is likely to advise on increasing fluids, improving diet and incorporating more exercise into the daily routine. Advice may be given on treatment with laxatives and suppositories. In cases where there is a buildup of faeces, an **enema** may be necessary.

A doctor will also investigate and treat any underlying illness. If a problem such as bowel **cancer** is suspected, the patient will be referred to hospital for specialized tests.

Complementary therapies
Herbal medicines and **massage** may help to relieve constipation.

PREVENTION

Adequate fluids and dietary fibre, combined with regular exercise, provide the most effective prevention against constipation.

COMPLICATIONS

Haemorrhoids may result from straining to pass faeces during prolonged constipation.

SEE ALSO *Bowel and disorders*

Contact lenses and problems

Contact lenses are small, shaped lenses that are placed directly onto the front surface of the eye. They are used to correct optical defects such as short-sightedness, long-sightedness, astigmatism and presbyopia (see **Eye and problems**).

Sometimes contact lenses are fitted for therapeutic purposes – for example, to even out distortions of vision caused by an irregular cornea or to protect a severely irritated eye.

Most vision defects are correctable with contact lenses, and the majority of people are able to wear them without too much discomfort – although certain environmental conditions, such as a dusty atmosphere, may increase the likelihood of problems such as chronic eye infection, dry eye or an unstable cornea.

In the case of severely short-sighted people, or where there is a large difference between the lens strength needed to correct each eye, contact lenses may provide a more comfortable and less distorting correction than spectacles.

HOW DO I GET CONTACT LENSES?

Contact lenses may be prescribed only by a registered doctor, optometrist or a dispensing optician with appropriate qualifications.
- At your first appointment you will be given a full eye examination to check the health of your eyes and their suitability for wearing lenses.

■ A trial lens will be inserted to evaluate your response and to establish a good fit. The lens should be comfortable and stable, but not so tight as to restrict tear flow underneath the lens.

■ If you wish to wear lenses full time, you will be advised of a 'building-up' period that will help your eye to adapt to the presence of a lens and to a reduced oxygen supply.

USING CONTACT LENSES

The newer a lens is, and the less it is handled, the lower the risk of infection and the better the quality of image possible through the lens.

Soft lenses are available in a daily disposable form, or may be replaced weekly, fortnightly, monthly or at longer intervals. Rigid lenses tend to require replacement annually. Whatever type of lenses you wear, always keep a spare pair to hand in case of loss or damage.

Storing and cleaning contact lenses

Unless you use daily disposable lenses, you need to establish a routine for cleaning your lenses:

■ never rinse your lenses in tap water;
■ clean them using the recommended solutions;
■ keep the case clean and replace it regularly;
■ for lenses used over longer periods, enzyme tablets may be needed to remove protein.

CONTACT LENSES AND CHILDREN

The high level of care needed to keep lenses clean and safe means that they are not suitable for young children. Older children may wear lenses, but they and their parents need to be aware of the hygienic measures to avoid infections and other problems. Children who wear lenses must have frequent checkups to monitor the health of their eyes.

FOLLOW-UP CARE

■ Eye health and vision should be regularly checked if you wear contact lenses. It is vital to be diligent about attending your aftercare appointments.

■ At each checkup your practitioner will look for changes in the cornea, such as the growth of new blood vessels at the edge of the cornea or localized areas of clouding – these indicate that insufficient oxygen is getting through. You may have to reduce the amount of time you wear lenses or change to a different lens material.

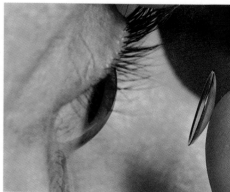

▲ **Inserting a lens**
Place the lens, concave side uppermost, on the inside tip of an index finger. Using a finger from the other hand, gently lift the top eyelid. Looking straight ahead, place the lens on the centre of the eye.

Problems associated with wearing contact lenses

If you wear contact lenses and one or both of your eyes becomes red, blurry or persistently uncomfortable, take out the lenses and seek the advice of your eye-care practitioner. If in doubt, take them out. Never rinse your lenses in tap water – it can cause infection.

SYMPTOM	POSSIBLE CAUSE	ACTION
Discomfort on putting lens in eye.	■ Foreign body in eye. ■ Damaged lens. ■ Corneal abrasion (see **Cornea and disorders**).	■ Remove, rinse and re-insert lens. ■ Replace lens with a new one. ■ Remove lens until eye is better. The eye will usually need a 24-hour break. Ask your practitioner for advice.
Discomfort after wearing lens for a short while.	■ Deposits on lens. ■ Allergic response to lens or to cleaning solution.	■ Remove lenses more frequently for cleaning. Clean them even more carefully. Perhaps try another cleaning solution. ■ Replace lens with a new one.
Discomfort even after removing lens.	■ Possible corneal infection.	■ Seek immediate medical advice.
Discomfort from time to time.	■ Environmental factors such as smoke or dry air. ■ Lens has moved to side of eye.	■ Avoid known irritants, or ask for advice about a lubricant for the eye. ■ Gently lift eyelid and, using other hand, move lens back into position with tip of finger.
Blurred vision.	■ Wearing a right eye lens in a left eye and vice versa. ■ Lens may be scratched or have a deposit on it. ■ Lens does not fit properly.	■ Remove lenses and re-insert them into the correct eye. ■ Replace lens. ■ Change in prescription needed.
Red eye.	■ Infection. ■ Allergic response to solution or lens.	■ Remove lens and seek medical advice. ■ Change solutions or lens material – ask your practitioner for advice – or change to daily disposable lenses.

Contraception

Contraception methods and advice are provided free of charge by the National Health Service and can be obtained from GPs, family planning clinics and many genito-urinary clinics.

The ideal method of contraception does not exist – for most people there is some inconvenience involved. The factors that influence the choice of method include its failure rate, ease of use, side effects, reversibility and the extent of interference with sexual spontaneity. There are also medical factors such as age, history and lifestyle risks, as well as religious beliefs that oppose artificial contraception.

BARRIER METHODS

These form a physical barrier that prevents sperm from reaching an egg. Male and female condoms, the diaphragm and the cervical cap are all barrier methods. Condoms are readily available, simple to use and help to prevent the spread of sexually transmitted infections (STIs) and **HIV**.

Polyurethane male condoms can prevent the loss of sensation sometimes felt with latex ones. The outer ring of female condoms may inhibit foreplay. Diaphragms and caps block or cover the cervix and require specialist fitting and annual checks. Poor-fitting diaphragms may increase the risk of cystitis. Both reduce the risk of cervical cancer and some STIs, but not HIV.

Latex condoms, caps and diaphragms can be damaged by oil-based lubricants and some vaginal medications. If one splits or slips during intercourse, seek emergency contraception.

CHEMICAL METHODS

These are contraceptive products containing chemical substances that kill sperm. They come in the form of pessaries, creams, jellies, foaming tablets, aerosols and vaginal sponges. They can be messy and may rarely cause irritation.

HORMONAL METHODS

Pregnancy can be prevented by altering a woman's hormonal balance. Introducing an increased level of hormones interferes with phases of her menstrual cycle, particularly ovulation.

The Pill

The most commonly used hormonal method is the Pill. There are two types: the combined oral contraceptive (COC) and the progestogen-only pill (POP), which used to be known as the 'mini-pill'. The combined oral contraceptive contains oestrogen and progestogen and prevents ovulation. It is the most commonly used form of contraception among women under 35. It reduces the risk of ovarian and endometrial cancer, but can cause temporary side effects such as weight changes, mood swings and nausea. The pill may also increase blood pressure. Periods on COCs may be shorter and lighter.

The progestogen-only pill thickens cervical mucus to prevent sperm reaching an egg and makes the lining of the uterus unfavourable for implanting an egg. It must be taken at the same time each day. This pill is useful for women who can not take the COC for health reasons such as an increased risk of a blood clot. A doctor should be consulted for further advice.

A woman should use an extra method of contraception if she takes the combined oral contraceptive more than 12 hours late or the progestogen-only pill more than three hours late.

Implants, injections and intrauterine system

These are slow-release methods of delivering progestogen, which work in the same way as the POP and provide contraception for three years. Implants consist of a tiny tube inserted into the

Contraceptive devices: reliability rates

The reliability of contraceptive methods (when they are used correctly) is usually expressed as a percentage of effectiveness.

FEMALE

Female sterilization	over 99%	Female condom	95%
Pill (COC)	over 99%	Diaphragm	92–96%
Implants/injections	over 99%	Cervical cap	92–96%
Pill (POP)	99%	Natural family planning	94%
IUS	98%	Vaginal sponge	90%
IUDs (depending on type)	98%		

MALE

Male sterilization	over 99%	Male condom	98%

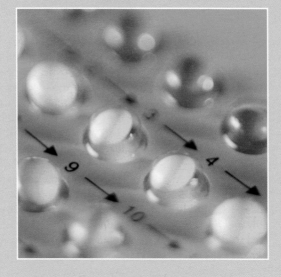

▶ **The Pill**
It is important to take the tablets as directed. Missing a dose, vomiting, diarrhoea and certain antibiotics may lose or reduce protection against pregnancy.

upper arm under local anaesthetic; fertility returns after they are removed.

Injections are given at 8- or 12-week intervals, depending on the type, and cannot be removed once given. Side effects include weight gain, and as with all hormonal methods effectiveness may be reduced by some prescription medicines.

The intrauterine system is a hormonal IUD releasing progestogen. It is an effective method and works for five years. Rarely, there is a risk that the device will perforate the uterus or that the body may expel it.

INTRAUTERINE DEVICES

An intrauterine device (IUD) is a plastic and copper device inserted into the womb via the cervix. It stops sperm from meeting the egg or the egg settling in the lining of the womb. The device works for three to ten years, depending on the type fitted. An IUD does not protect against sexually transmitted infections, so a condom may also have to be used. Disadvantages may include heavier or painful periods and the risk that the device may be spontaneously expelled. There may be slight bleeding between the first two or three periods after it has been fitted. Rarely, IUDs increase the risk of pelvic inflammatory disease and ectopic pregnancy.

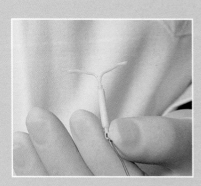

▲ **Intrauterine system (IUS)**
An IUS is fitted in the womb by a trained doctor. It slowly releases the progestogen hormone and works effectively for up to five years.

STERILIZATION

Sterilization is a surgical procedure that may be difficult to reverse and should only be considered if no more children are wanted. In women, the Fallopian tubes, along which the egg travels to the uterus, are cut or blocked by rings or clips. Men have a vasectomy, a minor operation in which the tubes that carry sperm from the testes to the penis are cut.

NATURAL FAMILY PLANNING

Different techniques can be used to predict fertile periods in a woman's cycle, allowing couples to abstain from sex at these times. This may be the only acceptable method for couples who do not want to use 'artificial' contraception. In a 28-day cycle, the fertile time is around 8–9 days.

Pregnancy is unlikely in the early and late phases of the cycle. However, individual cycles vary and sperm can survive for up to seven days, so infertile times can be difficult to predict. Natural family planning can take up to six cycles to learn effectively, and illness, stress and travel may make fertility indicators more difficult to interpret. Natural methods should be taught by a trained Natural Family Planning teacher.

New methods include predictive tests such as Persona, which interpret urine samples, and the temperature method, which relies on the fact that body temperature rises slightly around ovulation.

EMERGENCY CONTRACEPTION

Emergency hormonal contraception (sometimes known as the 'morning-after pill') should be taken within 72 hours of unprotected sex and is available from family planning clinics, NHS walk-in centres and pharmacies. Two pills are taken 12 hours apart. They are more effective the sooner the first pill is taken after sex. The second pill should be taken no later than 16 hours after the first. Hormonal methods work by preventing or delaying ovulation or from preventing implantation of the fertilized egg. A second choice of postcoital contraception is the insertion of an IUD up to five days after unprotected sex. This may stop an egg being fertilized or implanting in your womb and can be used as ongoing method of contraception.

! Warning

■ **Withdrawing the penis before ejaculation is unreliable because of semen leaking before orgasm or during late withdrawal.**

■ **Douching after intercourse is ineffective because sperm penetrate the cervix within 90 seconds of ejaculation.**

■ **Menstruation: it is possible for a woman to conceive during her period.**

■ **Sexual positions and the absence of female orgasm cannot prevent conception.**

■ **If not fully breastfeeding, conception can occur even if periods have not restarted.**

Convulsions

Convulsions are the external physical signs of a **seizure**. People suffering convulsions may fall to the ground and writhe or jerk uncontrollably, or they may tremble all over while remaining standing. They may also lose bladder control and drool at the mouth, their eyes may flicker or roll upwards. They are generally not in control of their bodily actions.

CAUSES

Convulsions are caused by a temporary disturbance in normal brain activity. Neurons in one part of the brain suddenly start to fire (turn on and off) very rapidly and this abnormal activity may spread to the entire brain. The convulsions are the result of the uncontrolled firing of cells in the areas of the brain that produce physical movements. These movements are not under conscious control and a person having convulsions is usually entirely unaware of what is happening.

TREATMENT

Remove anything that could cause injury from around the person who is convulsing – knives, furniture with hard edges and hot drinks, for example. Do not attempt to interfere with people who are suffering convulsions unless they are in immediate danger – if it occurs in the middle of the road, for example.

Biting the tongue is rare, and you do not need to try and wedge anything in the mouth of a convulsing person to prevent it. If you do so, you may cut the mouth and tongue or break the person's teeth while trying to insert the object, or cause them to choke.

If the convulsion continues for more than five minutes, call an ambulance. Otherwise, once the convulsions have stopped, the person should be placed in the recovery position.

Someone coming round from a convulsion will probably be confused and dazed for a few minutes and should be encouraged to lie quietly. The seizure may be followed by intense fatigue, and the person should be allowed to sleep it off as soon as possible.

Convulsions in young children

It can be frightening to witness a child having a convulsion but it is important to keep calm.

Babies and children under five can have fits if the brain becomes inflamed during the feverish stage of an infectious illness. Children suffering convulsions may twitch violently, clench their fists, arch their backs, hold their breath and go very red in the face and neck. Although frightening, isolated fits do not usually have any serious implication for a child's health. At least one in 30 children have them at some time. There is a slightly increased chance of a convulsion in the three months following the MMR (measles, mumps and rubella) vaccination.

If a fit occurs, call an ambulance – a child who has a convulsion should be seen by a doctor as soon as possible. Help the child to cool down by removing clothes and bedding but do not let him or her get cold. Put pillows around the child to stop bangs and bruising. If the child vomits, gently turn his or her head to one side to prevent choking.

Corn

A corn is a thickening of the skin on the toes and feet, usually caused by tight or badly fitted shoes. Soft corns may develop between the toes when they rub together. In hard corns, the skin's outer layer thickens when there is pressure on a bony part of the foot. The corn consists of a central core surrounded by thick layers of skin that become hard and inflexible.

You can buy corn plasters (small rings of sponge) over the counter in chemists. These help to relieve pressure on a corn. A chiropodist or your GP can pare down excess skin using a scalpel. Stubborn corns can be frozen off with liquid nitrogen – a chiropodist or the community nurse at your GP surgery can perform this treatment.

Corns can become infected, especially in diabetics. If you have diabetes and develop corns, have them treated promptly.

SEE ALSO *Chiropody; Foot and problems*

Cornea and disorders

The cornea is a thin transparent area at the front of the eyeball. It acts as the eye's main focusing structure, bending light through the eye's internal lens to a point of focus upon the retina (see diagram, **Eye and problems**).

DISEASES OF THE CORNEA

The cornea's transparency depends upon the collagen fibres in the stroma (see **The layers of the cornea,** right) being separated in a regular way that makes reflected light rays cancel one another out. Swelling of the cornea will disrupt this regular arrangement and make the cornea lose its transparency.

Keratitis

Keratitis is inflammation of the cornea. Contact lens wearers have an increased risk of keratitis: they must stop wearing lenses if keratitis is suspected (see **Contact lenses and problems**). There are four main types of keratitis. All require immediate medical attention.

■ Bacterial keratitis – usually following a wound or weakness that allows bacteria into the otherwise well-protected cornea. A sufferer will often feel severe eye pain, and may have redness in the areas adjacent to the cornea. Bacterial infection can lead to scarring of the cornea within hours. Corneal scarring can make you blind or severely reduce vision.

■ Viral keratitis – often caused by the herpes virus or an adenovirus (see **Viral infections**). A sufferer from viral keratitis will feel eye pain and may also feel unwell, possibly with a sore throat and swollen glands. If you think you may have viral keratitis, avoid using steroid eye drops as they may make the infection worse.

■ Amoebal keratitis – for example, from acanthamoeba found in dirty water in undeveloped countries. The main symptom is severe eye pain.

■ Allergic or non-infective keratitis – symptoms are often mild pain and redness of the eye.

Degenerations of the cornea

The cornea tends to degenerate as you grow older. The most commonly seen degeneration is the buildup of lipid material (see **Cholesterol**) in the periphery of the cornea. It builds up in a ring pattern known as an arcus. The more peripheral the degeneration, the less impact it will have upon your vision.

Abnormal growth

Any of the five major layers of the cornea may grow abnormally, causing the cornea to lose its transparency. Many cases have a hereditary component. Most are painless and progress slowly over years. In keratoconus, for example, the cornea gradually becomes thinner. Some cases eventually require a corneal graft. A cornea from a recently deceased person is sewn into the gap left when a diseased cornea is removed. Because the cornea has no blood vessels in it, rejection is less likely than with other body organs.

OUTLOOK

Diseases of the cornea are often sight-threatening, but technical advances are making **refractive surgery** far more effective. Timed delivery of anti-inflammatory/anti-infective agents is delivering better care of keratitis.

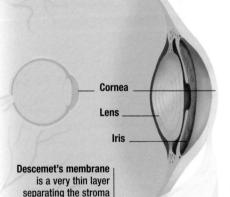

Cornea
Lens
Iris

Descemet's membrane is a very thin layer separating the stroma from the endothelium.

The stroma forms the bulk of the cornea; made up of repeated regular layers of collagen.

Bowman's layer provides a base for the epithelium.

The epithelium protects the exposed surface of the cornea.

The endothelium pumps water out into the anterior chamber of the eye. It is the thin internal lining of the cornea. If the endothelium is damaged, the cornea swells with water and loses its transparency.

The layers of the cornea
The cornea is around 0.55mm ($^2/_{100}$in) thick. It is essentially a modified extension of the skin and consists of five layers. The cornea has very fine nerve fibres, and this makes it highly sensitive to pain. There is no blood supply to the central cornea, which draws nutrition from the eye's aqueous humour.

Coronary angioplasty

A coronary angioplasty is a procedure in which a blockage of one or two coronary arteries is relieved using a balloon catheter (the narrowed artery is expanded by means of a sausage-shaped balloon attached to the tip of a flexible tube) under X-ray control. This procedure cannot be used if there are many areas of narrowing of the arteries.

People are given this procedure when they have **angina** that is not responding to medicine. Half of those who have a coronary angioplasty feel short-term chest pain during the procedure.

In 95 per cent of cases, the operation is a success – the symptoms of angina grow less or disappear altogether for at least two years. Blockage of the coronary arteries recurs after two years in 30 per cent of cases.

SEE ALSO *Angioplasty; Heart and circulatory system*

Coronary artery disease

The left and right coronary arteries supply blood to the heart muscles. The coronary arteries branch off from the aorta (main artery) just after it leaves the heart, and then divide to deliver oxygen to every area of the heart. Coronary artery disease is a condition in which the coronary arteries become narrowed or blocked by fatty or fibrous deposits (atheroma), restricting the supply of oxygen to the heart's muscles. Coronary artery narrowing may produce chest pain (**angina**), especially on exertion. It can also lead to heart failure, although even in severe narrowing there may be no symptoms. Sudden complete blockage of one or more artery branches results in muscle death – a heart attack or **myocardial infarction**.

A tendency to coronary artery disease often runs in families, but it may be brought on by risk factors such as smoking, excess alcohol, raised blood pressure, diabetes, high cholesterol levels, a high-fat diet, or lack of exercise.

SEE ALSO *Heart and circulatory system*

Coronary thrombosis

Coronary thrombosis is a condition in which a branch of the coronary arteries becomes significantly or totally blocked by a blood clot. This cuts off the oxygen supply to part of the heart muscle, leading to permanent damage or even death.

Cosmetic and plastic surgery

Cosmetic surgery is designed to improve appearance – for example, to reshape the nose or flatten the stomach. It is only one element of plastic surgery, which is used largely to reconstruct parts of the body damaged by injuries, growths and defects.

On average plastic surgeons in the UK spend only 15 per cent of their time on cosmetic work. Most of their time is spent on medically necessary plastic surgery.

Plastic surgery encompasses operations to help both patients with congenital or birth deformities and those with acquired deformities resulting from accident, disease or infection. In the first category are people with congenital defects of the breasts, chest, hands and skin, **cleft lip and palate** and other congenital facial deformities (see **Face and problems**) and urogenital defects (see **Urinary system**). In the second are those who have had benign or cancerous growths removed from the breast, head, neck, skin or soft tissue (see **Cancer**), for example, and those who have suffered hand injuries such as **burns** and **scars**.

CLEFT LIP AND PALATE
A child born with a cleft lip (a separation in the upper lip) or cleft palate (a separation in the roof of the mouth) will be offered an operation to close the separation and improve the appearance. He or she may also have difficulty hearing, speaking and eating normally and the operation will only be one part of the package of medical care.

In modifying a cleft lip, a plastic surgeon will normally make a cut on either side of the cleft, turn the cleft's pink outer side inward and draw the muscle and skin on the two sides of the cut and on the lip together. The operation, which leaves a scar that gradually fades, is normally performed when a baby is around 10 weeks old.

In rebuilding a cleft palate the surgeon will normally make a cut either side of the separation and move tissue into the cleft to build the area up. The operation is normally carried out when a child is 9–18 months old.

WOUNDS, GROWTHS AND BLEMISHES
Skin and tissue grafting is used to disguise wounds arising from accidents and to reconstruct areas from which a growth or tumour has been cut. Various procedures carried out under local anaesthetic remove blemishes such as birthmarks and improve the appearance of scars that are red, raised and itchy or keloids – hard raised areas

where an overgrowth of thick tissue develops at the site of a healing scar. For example, laser surgery is used to treat children born with pinkish birthmarks known as port-wine stains. A particular laser light beam that is absorbed by haemoglobin (the red pigment in blood) is used to destroy the abnormal blood vessels in the birthmark. The treatment can lighten the birthmark so effectively that it disappears almost completely. Lasers can also be used to remove skin growths and warts, to blur the edges of a scar, and to improve moles, wrinkles, rough areas and freckles.

RESTORING HAND MOVEMENT
If a person has webbed fingers (syndactyly), the surgeon may be able to make a zigzag cut in the abnormal tissue that joins the fingers, then remove or re-form the tissue there to give a normal hand shape. Surgeons can restore near-normal hand use to children born with more than four fingers on each hand (polydactyly) by removing the extra fingers and rebalancing the hand tendons and joints. Plastic surgeons can also help with developmental hand problems such as **carpal tunnel syndrome** (in which pressure on the nerve in the wrist can cause numbness, aches and problems using the hand), trigger finger and ganglia (see **Hand and problems**) or rebuild a finger or thumb lost in an accident.

In treating carpal tunnel syndrome, for example, the surgeon may cut from the mid-palm to the wrist and remove the tissue that is pressing on the nerve and causing the pain. Keyhole surgery may also be used. Patients wear a splint after the operation to restrict movement.

Skin grafting
Skin grafting is the most widely used form of plastic surgery and is used to cover areas where skin has been lost due to burns, injury or surgery. It is sometimes done using a local anaesthetic, but more complex procedures require a general anaesthetic. The skin is usually taken from some other area of the body (known as the donor site) and stitched to the underlying tissue in the area to be covered (the recipient site).

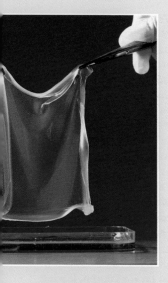

▲ **Laboratory skin**
Human skin grown from living tissues in culture can be used in place of transplanted skin in graft operations.

Patients usually provide their own skin for grafting, but skin from an identical twin has been used. The skin grows back at the donor site, but sometimes the new layer is a slightly lighter colour than the original. Apart from improving appearance, skin grafts to cover large areas of exposed underlying tissue prevent extensive fluid loss and protect wounds from bacterial infection. They can, in some cases, be life-saving.

Skin grafts can be temporary or permanent. Temporary grafts are used in an emergency – when someone has severe burns, for example, surgeons may use skin donated by other people who have died (known as allograft, homograft or cadaver skin) as a temporary cover for the cleaned burn. Alternatively, animal skin (xenograft or heterograft), usually from a pig, may be used. Temporary skin grafts adhere to the wound but are removed when the wound is ready for a permanent graft. In a permanent graft, the patient's own skin is usually used (an autograft).

SKIN GRAFT TECHNIQUES

Various methods of removing and transplanting the skin are used. In pinch grafting, small pieces of skin are placed all over the wound. This technique is very useful where there is poor blood supply or the possibility of infection. In split-thickness grafting, the donor skin is taken from the top layer. This is useful for large areas, but cannot be used for weight-bearing areas or those exposed to friction, such as the hands and feet.

Full-thickness grafting uses all the layers of the skin – being harder-wearing than split-thickness grafting, it can be used for the hands and feet.

In skin flaps, the skin remains attached to the donor site with its blood supply intact. It is not cut loose until the blood supply at the recipient end has fully developed. It is useful for grafts on the face, neck and hands.

Mesh grafting is used when the donor skin is in short supply. Using a meshing machine, small slits are made in the donor material so that it can be expanded like a fish net. Although it means that a larger area can be covered, this method is only used when no other option is suitable because it often leaves small, diamond-shaped scars.

AFTER THE GRAFT

A graft takes about 72 hours to establish its own blood supply. A diet high in protein and carbohydrate will help this process. Infection and trauma may prevent a successful graft, so good nursing is essential, and strict sterile techniques should be used for dressings. Antibiotics may be needed to prevent infection.

Once the wound has healed, regular gentle massage of the scar can help to reduce it. Areas of skin that are usually exposed may need to be protected from sunlight for the first 12 months to prevent excessive formation of pigment.

Someone who has had a skin graft will always have to take care to avoid excessive exposure of the graft to sunlight. Camouflage make-up used in exposed areas may be used to help a person to resume a normal social and working life.

HOW THE GRAFT WILL LOOK

While some grafts may eventually become virtually invisible, others will remain visible, particularly where infection or blood clotting under the graft has complicated recovery. The transplanted skin will retain the characteristics of the donor site. It may therefore not match the colour and texture precisely of the adjacent skin, and may be less or more sensitive than the surrounding skin.

It is thought that scar maturation can be speeded up using silicone gel sheets. These are waterproof flexible sheets that can be applied to soften the scars and reduce inflammation. The degree of improvement depends on the size of the scar, the nature of the skin, and the quality of wound care after the operation. Many patients retain visible marks of surgery at both donor and recipient sites, and it may be a year or more before the final results can be seen.

Scars are always visible to some extent but are most obvious if the excess scar tissue causes the area to be raised. Various techniques can be used to improve scarring. These include laser surgery, in which a high-energy light beam is used to cut away the upper surface of the skin, and dermabrasion, which involves 'sandpapering' the skin using specialist equipment. Dermabrasion is quite painful and it is usually carried out under general anaesthetic.

COMPLICATIONS

Shrinkage or contracture of the graft may occur, with the graft pulling away at the edges. A feeling of tightness or a distorted appearance can result. Grafts do not have sensation and many are less able to withstand damage such as the rubbing of belts and shoes.

Cosmetic surgery

Cosmetic surgery may represent a small proportion of plastic surgeons' work, but its use is growing dramatically in the West. In the USA the number of cosmetic procedures such as liposuction and tummy tucks has risen eightfold since 1990, a rise mirrored in the UK.

THE PURSUIT OF BEAUTY

The practise of cosmetic surgery is increasingly used as a means of remaking the body in the pursuit of ideal beauty.

Tissue expansion

The body can be encouraged to grow the right sort of skin to cover a wound.

Tissue expansion is a skin repair technique that can help to minimize scarring. The surgeon inserts an expander – a device like a balloon – beneath the skin in the area that needs new skin growth. Over a few days the expander is gradually filled with salt water, which stretches the tissue in the area around the recipient site and makes the skin there stretch and grow. The new skin's colour is an almost perfect match for that of the surrounding skin.

Tissue expansion is ideal for repairing the scalp, because the newly grown skin will grow hair in the same way as normal scalp skin – whereas with skin and tissue transplanted from other parts of the body hair growth can be erratic or non-existent.

▼ Laser
A single laser treatment might be enough to remove 'spider veins' on the face. A large, disfiguring birthmark might need ten treatments.

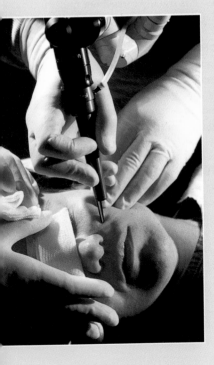

Facelift and forehead lift
Facelifts produce the best results in people whose skin still has some elasticity; they are usually performed, under general anaesthetic, on people in the 40–60 age group.

A common method is to make an incision above the hairline at the temples, following the natural line to the front of the ear, around the earlobe and behind the ear into the scalp. The skin, and sometimes the underlying muscle, is then freed from the underlying bone, stretched tightly and stitched to the solid structures in front of and behind the ear.

In a forehead lift, an incision is made in the hairline or a few centimetres back from the scalp, extending from one side to the other. The skin is then pulled up and tightened, as in a facelift. This can also be carried out with the aid of an **endoscope** and smaller incisions just beyond the hairline, which avoids the need for an ear to ear incision. Sagging eyebrows can also be lifted in this way.

Eyelid reduction
Eyelid reduction, known as a blepharoplasty, is carried out under general anaesthetic. An incision is made, following the natural lines of the upper eyelids, in the creases of the upper lids and just below the lashes in the lower lids, then excess fat, skin or sagging muscle is removed. An incision on the inner surface can be used for some lower-eyelid procedures.

Collagen and botox injections
Animal-collagen injections are commonly given, under local anaesthetic, to smooth out wrinkles and frown lines and to enhance the appearance of the lips. A test dose of collagen is given in the arm first and checked after a month for allergic sensitivity. Collagen breaks down in the body, so the treatment may need repeating. Very fine needles are used, that may leave a small mark for up to a day.

Botox (an abbreviation of botulinum toxin) can be used to treat forehead lines, lines around the nose and mouth, and neck wrinkles. Botox works by paralysing or weakening facial muscles, smoothing out the contours. Re-injection will be needed initially every four to five months to keep the muscles paralysed, then less frequently.

Body sculpturing
Surgery to resculpt the body is increasingly common. Breast enlargement is the most common form of plastic surgery for women in the UK.

Breasts can be reduced surgically or enlarged by the insertion of implants (see **Mammoplasty**). Another form of breast surgery is a mastopexy, in which drooping breasts are improved by removing excess skin from under the breast, remodelling the breast tissue into a tighter cone, and re-siting the nipples at a higher level. Further drooping is possible with ageing and pregnancy, but a good support bra minimizes this possibility.

Another common procedure is the 'tummy tuck' (abdominoplasty). Under general anaesthetic, a long, curved incision is made across the lower part of the abdominal wall at the level of the pubic hair. Excess skin and fat is removed, leaving the belly button in place. A similar procedure called an apronectomy is used for people who have a large fold (or apron) of skin and fat hanging over the pubic area. Most abdominal surgery requires a stay in hospital of 1–3 days.

Liposuction
Liposuction is used to remove fat from certain areas of the body, such as the hips, neck, arms, stomach and thighs. It is usually done under general anaesthetic. A small tube called a cannula, which is attached to a powerful suction machine, is inserted at various points on the body through puncture wounds. It is thought that fat cells do not grow back, so the change in contour is likely to be permanent provided the person does not put on weight. Painful bruising may develop after the operation, and discoloration can last for about a month.

COMPLICATIONS OF PLASTIC SURGERY
If you are treated by a qualified plastic surgeon complications are very unlikely and generally minor. However, they cannot be ruled out entirely and should they occur, a further procedure may be needed. Possible problems include:

- general anaesthetic complications, such as chest infections or vein thrombosis;
- infection of the site of the surgery, leading to delay in healing and increased scarring;
- minor infections. These may need treatment with antibiotics;
- bleeding from a broken blood vessel. The leaking vessel will need to be stitched in cases of severe bleeding;
- blood clots (haematomas) forming beneath the wound. These may be treated with antibiotics or a drainage procedure may be necessary;
- scar problems, such as contraction, widening or thickening of the scar;
- damage to the nerves causing numbness around the scar area.

Costochondritis

Costochondritis is a swelling of the joint between the ribs and breastbone, causing pain in the chest region, especially during coughing or deep breathing. One or more lumps may develop on the wall of the chest. In older people, costochondritis can sometimes be confused with **angina pectoris**.

The cause of costochondritis is unknown. Sometimes the condition resolves without any treatment; more often, the swelling persists, but eventually becomes painless. Painkillers and non-steroid anti-inflammatory drugs (NSAIDs) may be helpful in the interim. Costochondritis is also known as 'Tietze's syndrome'.

Cough

The cough is part of the body's respiratory defence, a forceful blast of air out of the lungs and airways to clear excess mucus or inhaled irritants. Coughs are often a symptom of an underlying disease and can spread infection. Occasionally a violent cough will fracture a rib.

CAUSES

The most common cause of an acute cough (one lasting up to two weeks) is a cold.

Causes of a chronic cough (one lasting more than two weeks) include:
- smoking, which irritates the lungs and airways, causing a constant production of mucus that leads to 'smoker's cough';
- asthma;
- allergic rhinitis;
- sinus problems;
- oesophageal reflux (heartburn);
- bronchitis;
- drugs – in particular ACE inhibitors, which are prescribed for raised blood pressure and heart problems (10 per cent of people using them develop a cough as a side effect).

TREATMENT

Seek medical advice if you have any of the following symptoms (especially if the cough lasts for longer than two weeks):
- thick yellow or greenish phlegm;
- high temperature;
- you are coughing up blood;
- losing weight;
- shortness of breath or wheezing (especially when sleeping or exercising);
- chest pains;
- swelling in the legs.

Treatment depends on the underlying cause and the effect the cough is having on you. Some treatments are designed to stop the cough, others to make it more effective in clearing mucus. If you have a bacterial infection, the doctor is likely to prescribe antibiotics. If you smoke, stop.

Cradle cap

Cradle cap is a condition in which crusty white or greasy brown or yellow scales form on the scalp and sometimes the forehead of a young baby. It is probably caused by overactivity in the baby's sebaceous (oil) glands, and does not usually occur after 12 to 18 months of age.

Cradle cap does not itch or upset a baby, and eventually clears of its own accord. Gentle daily shampooing with a baby shampoo or washing with aqueous cream helps to loosen the scales, as does massaging aqueous cream or warm oil into the scalp.

Sometimes cradle cap spreads to other areas of the body, in which case it is called seborrhoeic eczema or seborrhoeic dermatitis. If this occurs, your doctor may prescribe a mild hydrocortisone cream. Complementary preparations that might help include calendula (marigold) ointment.

Cramp

Cramp is a strong localized contraction of muscle that results in sharp pain and lasts for several minutes. Cramp is common during exercise, but tired and overworked muscles are also susceptible. It may occur where a muscle is held in a certain position – **writer's cramp** is an example – or at night during sleep.

The causes of cramp are not known. One theory is that it is caused by exercise-induced **dehydration** and an imbalance of sodium, potassium, calcium and magnesium, the minerals that help to regulate muscle contraction and relaxation. Another theory is that damage to muscle fibres allows too much calcium to leak into the muscle membranes with the result that the fibres become locked. Cramp occasionally results from a lack of salt.

TREATMENT

For almost immediate relief from pain, stretch the muscle and gently massage the area or ask someone else to do it for you (see right, **Relieving cramps**).

Self-help
Relieving cramps

What you can do to assist someone suffering from cramp depends on where in the body the pain occurs.

- **Lower leg** The sufferer should lie down on his or her back. Take the affected leg and straighten it while pressing down on the knee with your other hand. Hold the foot under the heel and use your other hand to push the toes gently upwards. When the spasm eases, gently massage the affected muscles until the area feels relaxed.

- **Foot** The person with cramp should place the affected foot firmly on the floor. If the toes are in severe spasm, pull the foot upwards slightly to lift the toes off the floor and gently try to straighten them. In cold weather, the sufferer should put on some warm socks.

The following can help to prevent cramps.

- Practise a daily routine of stretching.
- Drink plenty of water before, during and after prolonged exercise. Thirst is a poor indicator of fluid requirements: by the time you are thirsty, you are already dehydrated.
- Herbal remedies such as cramp bark, black haw and valerian may help to prevent cramp. Consult a herbalist for the correct treatment.

When to consult a doctor

Seek medical advice if you experience regular and persistent cramps. These may be caused by poor circulation resulting from other conditions such as **diabetes**. The doctor might carry out tests for diabetes and for cardiovascular and neurological disorders.

SEE ALSO *Muscular system*

Cretinism

Cretinism is a condition caused by a deficiency of iodine due to thyroid dysfunction, usually dating from birth or before. Signs include slow growth and mental development, a large tongue and a hoarse cry. Affected children tend to have coarse facial features and large foreheads. If left untreated, cretinism can cause brain damage leading to permanent mental retardation.

SEE ALSO *Thyroid and disorders*

Crohn's disease

Crohn's disease, also known as regional enteritis, is a chronic inflammatory disease that usually affects the ileum, the lower part of the small intestine (see **Bowel and disorders**). It can, however, involve any part of the digestive tract; in elderly people it often affects the rectum and anus. The intestinal wall thickens in the affected area and **ulcers** form.

Cases of the disease appear to be increasing, especially in children. The condition is most often diagnosed during adolescence and early adulthood, but may appear at any age.

SYMPTOMS

The symptoms are extremely variable, and depend on the area affected and the severity of the condition. Generally, they include:

- diarrhoea, with foul-smelling stools;
- abdominal pain;
- loss of appetite and weight loss;
- fever;
- tiredness;
- anal **abscesses** and sores.

  Additional symptoms may include:
- joint pain;
- mouth ulcers;

Most people who develop Crohn's disease in the UK do so before they reach the age of 30. The peak age is between 14 and 24.

- inflamed eyes;
- painful red lumps on the skin.

TREATMENT

Tests are needed to confirm Crohn's disease and distinguish it from **ulcerative colitis**. They include fibre-optic or video investigations, **barium investigations** and blood tests. Common forms of treatment include:

- anti-inflammatories;
- antibiotics, in the case of abscesses;
- dietary measures – although these vary from person to person, in general, a high-protein, high-calorie, vitamin-rich diet is needed;
- surgery – which may be needed to remove severely affected parts of the bowel;
- stopping smoking, which may help.

PREVENTION

The cause of Crohn's disease is unknown and there are no known preventive measures. The condition has a genetic component.

COMPLICATIONS

The complications of Crohn's disease include intestinal blockage, nutritional deficiencies and an anal fistula – an opening between the anal canal and the surface of the skin that can develop if an abscess in the rectum bursts.

OUTLOOK

Symptom-free periods of remission alternate with relapses, which are more likely to occur at times of emotional stress and after surgery. In some cases, symptoms gradually disappear.

Croup

Croup is an infection of the voice box (larynx), the main airway (trachea) and the bronchi, the two narrow tubes leading from the trachea into the lungs. In the UK, between 80,000 and 100,000 children aged six months to four years suffer from croup each year.

The cause is usually a viral infection. Croup is more common in winter and can be alarming for parents, especially when a child wakes with a distressing, barking cough.

SYMPTOMS

The symptoms of croup include:

- similar symptoms to those of a common **cold**, with a slight fever;
- a hoarse, barking cough;
- noisy breathing.

TREATMENT

Croup should be treated as for a cold.

When to consult a doctor

See a doctor urgently if:

- your child has a high fever;
- there is a marked indrawing of the chest wall with each breath.

Call an ambulance if:

- breathing is rapid and difficult;
- the child is restless and struggling to get air;
- the child turns pale, grey or blueish.

What a doctor may do

- Prescribe steroids, either as a tablet or inhaled mist, to ease breathing.
- Give oxygen, intravenous fluids and plain mist to assist breathing.
- Recommend hospital admission.

What you can do

To relieve the symptoms sit with the child in a bathroom full of steam. Provide plenty of fluids.

COMPLICATIONS

Inflammation and swelling of the narrow airway may result in a life-threatening difficulty in breathing.

OUTLOOK

Croup generally resolves itself without the child becoming severely ill. About 6 per cent of children develop croup repeatedly and suddenly at night without signs of infection. This is known as spasmodic or recurrent croup and often ceases within two hours. The condition is more common in children who suffer from an **allergy**.

Cryosurgery

Cryosurgery is a surgical technique in which liquid nitrogen is used to freeze and hence destroy an unwanted area on the skin such as warts, verrucas and skin blemishes.

Many GPs carry out cryosurgery in their clinics, since it is quick and relatively easy to perform. The area treated may feel sore for a day or two after treatment, and sometimes a blister can form before healing starts.

Depending on the condition, a person may need several cryosurgical sessions, at intervals of three or four weeks.

Cryptorchidism

Cryptorchidism – more commonly known as an undescended testicle – is a condition affecting baby boys in which only one of the two testicles appears in the scrotum. In normal development both testicles descend into the scrotum during the seventh month of pregnancy.

Cryptorchidism affects 3–4 per cent of full-term baby boys worldwide and the risk increases considerably with premature birth.

In most cases, undescended testes drop of their own accord in the first nine months of life; they rarely descend later.

SYMPTOMS

Usually, although not always, the absence of a testicle from the scrotum will be detected at birth or in early infancy. This absence could be caused by:

- the total lack of a testicle;
- a muscle reflex whereby the testicle overreacts to cold or touch and retracts – this is known as a retractile testis and usually corrects itself naturally by puberty;
- the testicle descending to the wrong place, usually into the groin or the base of the penis, a condition known as an ectopic testis;
- the failure of the testicle to descend at all.

CAUSES

In normal development, hormones from the mother and hormones released by the testes cause the spermatic cord to which each testicle is attached to lengthen and the testes to descend into the scrotum. Insufficient hormones or a blockage may prevent this from happening.

TREATMENT

If you are concerned about an undescended testes, see your GP or midwife.

- Hormone injections may be given to stimulate descent. If this does not work, the testicle can be fixed in the right position with a surgical procedure known as an orchidopexy. This should be performed before the child is three.
- Where the other testicle is developing normally, an underdeveloped undescended testicle may be removed. An orchidopexy can also be performed on an ectopic testicle.

OUTLOOK

Cryptorchidism increases the risk of infertility, because the testicle is too hot inside the body. It also increases the risk of testicular cancer.

If the testicle remains undescended into adulthood, the risk of cancer is even higher. Since the testicle is undescended, the cancer is also that much harder to detect. For this reason, an undescended testis in an adult is always completely removed.

SEE ALSO *Testicles and disorders*

Cyanosis

Cyanosis is a blueish discoloration of the skin, lips or tongue that is caused by a lack of oxygen. This is what causes someone to turn 'blue with cold' when low temperatures slow down blood flow. It can indicate more serious problems. For example, fingers that look blue even in warm conditions may be due to a blood circulation problem, while a blueish tongue can be symptomatic of heart disease.

Cyst

A cyst is an abnormal cavity, lined with tissue and filled with fluid. Most cysts are harmless, occuring as lumps anywhere in the body.

COMMON TYPES OF CYST

In general, consult your doctor if you discover any sort of lump. Cysts most often appear on the skin or in the reproductive organs.

Skin

Cysts on the skin, called sebaceous cysts, occur when the grease glands in the skin become blocked. These painless lumps gradually grow bigger, filling with a semi-solid substance. They have to be removed if they become large enough to be a nuisance or risk becoming infected.

Ovaries

Most ovarian cysts are benign (non-cancerous), and many disappear without any treatment. Sometimes, however, a cyst grows very large, and is surgically removed. There are few symptoms associated with ovarian cysts, but they can affect a woman's periods, making them more painful or heavier, or stopping them altogether. A large cyst may also cause pain during intercourse and abdominal discomfort.

Occasionally, ovarian cysts are associated with **endometriosis**. They fill with brown fluid and are known as chocolate cysts.

Testicles

Cysts on the testicles, or epididymal cysts, are common, especially in men over 40. They occur in the epididymis, the tissue around one side and on top of each testicle. They do not need treatment unless they become uncomfortable, when they may be removed surgically.

Cystic fibrosis

▼ **Clearing the way**
Physiotherapy helps to prevent the thick, sticky secretions caused by cystic fibrosis from blocking the airways.

Cystic fibrosis is an inherited genetic disorder. It affects a number of organs in the body, particularly the lungs and pancreas, by clogging them with thick, sticky mucus. There is no cure, but treatment gives children with the disease a higher quality and length of life.

One in 25 people in the UK carries the cystic fibrosis gene, usually without knowing it. If a baby is born with the disease, it means that both parents carry the faulty gene. But even if both parents carry the faulty gene, the child has only a one in four chance of being born with the disease. Gene therapy – in which the correct version of the defective gene is

transported into the lungs – offers hope for the future, but trials are still at an early stage.

SYMPTOMS

Symptoms vary from one person to another, but usually include difficulty with breathing including wheezing and coughing, and susceptibility to chest infections.

A deficiency of the digestive enzymes normally secreted into the gut by the pancreas leads to severe digestive disorders. People with cystic fibrosis are unable to digest fats and proteins properly, so that more undigested food than normal is passed out in unusually bulky stools.

DIAGNOSIS

Cystic fibrosis is not always obvious at birth, but there are early clues to the condition. All affected children overproduce salt in their sweat, so that salt crystals sometimes appear on the skin, which tastes very salty when kissed. Other signs include:

- a persistent cough that worsens with chest infections;
- frequent chest infections;
- stools that are persistently bulky and smell unusually nasty.
- poor weight gain

If a child has some of these symptoms a doctor may recommend that the child's sweat is tested for unusually high levels of salt. Further tests may be needed to confirm diagnosis.

TREATMENT

Depending on symptoms, treatment may involve drugs and **physiotherapy** to clear mucus from the lungs and reduce secretions. A nebulizer may be used to moisten mucus and make it easier to cough. Chest infections need prompt treatment with antibiotics.

Nutrition can be greatly helped by a high-calorie diet and the use of vitamins and enzymes. In very severe cases, a lung transplant may be considered.

LIVING WITH CYSTIC FIBROSIS

Exercise and good nutrition can both do much to help people with cystic fibrosis since a healthy, well-nourished body can deal more effectively with the chest infections and weight loss caused by the disease. An exercise regime devised by a physiotherapist can prevent deterioration of the lungs (see **Physiotherapy**).

Children with cystic fibrosis need to eat more calories and protein than normal to compensate for the loss of fat and protein caused by the disease. For adults with the disease, protein intake should be double the usual recommended amount. Fatty foods, sugary foods, starchy foods, milk and dairy products, and foods rich in vitamins and minerals should also be eaten in abundance.

SEE ALSO *Congenital disorders*

Cystitis

Cystitis is an inflammation or infection of the bladder lining. Cystitis is very common in women, more so than in men because of the difference in anatomy: the urethra (the duct that drains the bladder) is much shorter in women, making it easier for infection to reach the bladder.

SYMPTOMS

The symptoms of cystitis depend on the severity of the infection. In mild cases, only one or two symptoms may occur, but in severe cases a sufferer may develop them all. Symptoms include:
- burning, stinging or discomfort on passing urine (dysuria);
- a need to rush to the toilet;
- passing frequent, small amounts of urine;
- low abdominal pain or tenderness;
- backache;
- unpleasant-smelling, cloudy or bloodstained urine.

An untreated bladder infection can spread upwards to infect the kidneys, resulting in the more serious condition of **pyelonephritis**.

CAUSES

There are two main causes of cystitis:
- infection of the bladder;
- friction or chemical irritation of the urethra (see **Urethritis**).

Infection is usually due to bacteria, such as *Escherichia coli* (*E. coli*), which normally live in the large intestine. Sexual intercourse is one of the commonest triggers of cystitis since it can push bacteria up into the urethra. This is sometimes referred to as 'honeymoon cystitis'.

Irritation of the urethral opening from friction can also cause symptoms of urgency, frequency and discomfort on passing urine.

TREATMENT

Preparations of potassium citrate such as Cystopurin, which make the urine less acid, may be helpful. Cystopurin, taken as an oral powder, is available from pharmacies without a doctor's prescription.

What you can do

As soon as symptoms start, drink a pint of water. Then drink half a pint every twenty minutes for the next three hours if you can. Drinking plenty of water helps to flush out bacteria and to dilute your urine so that it does not sting as much when you urinate.

Unless you suffer from high blood pressure or heart trouble, take a teaspoon of sodium bicarbonate dissolved in water every hour for three hours. This makes the urine less acid, relieves discomfort and helps to stop bacterial growth.

Drinking 300ml (10fl oz) of cranberry juice a day or taking cranberry extracts helps to stop bacteria from sticking to the bladder wall.

When to consult a doctor

Seek medical advice if:
- symptoms last longer than a day or keep recurring;
- you are pregnant;
- your urine is cloudy or stained with blood;
- you develop a fever or uncontrollable shakes.

What a doctor may do

A doctor who suspects a bacterial urinary tract infection may do one or more of the following:
- test your urine using a dipstick test to look for signs of white blood cells, blood, protein and substances produced by bacteria (nitrites);
- send a urine sample to a laboratory to culture and identify any bacteria present, and find out what antibiotics will kill them;
- prescribe antibiotics.

If you suffer from recurrent cystitis, you may be investigated for conditions such as **diabetes**, or anatomical abnormalities of the urinary system using **X-ray**, **ultrasound** or **endoscopy**.

Complementary therapies

Supplements containing natural extracts of the herbs dandelion, bearberry and peppermint can help to prevent recurrent cystitis.

PREVENTION

There are several things you can do to help to prevent recurrent attacks of cystitis.
- When sitting on the toilet, tilt your pelvis up so that your anus is lower than the urethra.
- After passing water, lean forward to squeeze out the last few drops of urine.
- Wipe your bottom from front to back only.
- Wash with warm, unperfumed soapy water after every bowel movement and sexual intercourse.
- Avoid using bubble bath, vaginal deodorants, perfumed soap and talcum powder.
- Drink 2 litres (3.5 pints) of fluid daily.

SEE ALSO *Urinary system*

Cytomegalovirus infection

Cytomegalovirus is a common viral infection belonging to the **herpes** family. It usually remains symptomless or causes a mild flu-like illness. It is passed on by close personal contact with an infected person, via sexual intercourse or blood transfusion. The virus can also pass through the placenta and in rare cases can affect the unborn child. Although the symptoms of cytomegalovirus are milder than those of a common cold, infection may be serious in people suffering from reduced immunity.

Dandruff

Dandruff is a common condition in which there is excessive flakiness of the skin on the scalp but no redness or inflammation.

If the scales causing the flakiness are greasy, stick to the scalp and cause severe irritation, the problem may be a form of **eczema** called seborrhoeic dermatitis. In this case, itchy, flaking skin may also appear on the eyebrows, the beard, on the chest or back and in the creases of the arms and legs.

SYMPTOMS

Dandruff is a harmless condition but it can be itchy or irritating. The white flakes of skin it causes to be shed into the hair and then onto collars and shoulders of clothes can cause self-consciousness and embarrassment.

Dandruff may be more pronounced in people suffering from chronic illnesses, including **AIDS**.

CAUSES

The condition is thought to be linked to an overproduction of yeasts (*Pityrosporum ovale*) that normally live on the human skin.

TREATMENT

Dandruff can be cured quickly and easily by the repeated application of an antidandruff shampoo containing an antifungal agent such as ketoconazole. Regular hair brushing removes dead skin and promotes circulation in the scalp. It is advisable to restrict your intake of sugar which increases the productions of yeast.

When to consult a doctor

Seek medical advice if:
- scratching leads to a scalp infection;
- the dandruff does not respond to several weeks of home treatment;
- your scalp is uncomfortably irritated despite home treatment.

What a doctor may do

- Check that the dandruff is not caused by infection or a skin disorder, such as eczema or **psoriasis**.
- Give further advice on how to treat the dandruff.
- Possibly prescribe antifungal or steroid preparations.

Complementary therapies

- Scalp massage may help to improve circulation.
- Aromatherapy oils such as tea tree can be diluted in a carrier oil and applied overnight.
- Homeopathic remedies may help. Which remedy depends on specific symptoms: some of the most common include graphites, sepia and sulphur.

COMPLICATIONS

Scratching may cause the scalp to bleed or become infected.

Deafness

Deafness is defined as the partial or total loss of hearing in one or both ears. It can be caused by a mechanical problem that blocks the conduction of sound in the ear canal or the middle ear. This is called conductive deafness. Damage to the inner ear, auditory nerve or auditory nerve pathways in the brain, on the other hand, is defined as sensorineural deafness. The two types of deafness can be distinguished by comparing how well a person hears sounds conducted by air with how well a person hears sounds conducted through the bones (see **Diagnosis**).

CONDUCTIVE DEAFNESS

Problems with the conduction of sound from the external ear to the inner ear can be traced to several sites. It can originate in the external ear canal, where it can be caused by:
- a buildup of wax;
- a benign outgrowth of cartilage from a bone (meatal exostoses);
- a buildup of skin cells, often seen mixed with wax, in the ear canal (epithelial debris);

Loss of hearing
The problems that cause hearing loss can be very varied and originate in different parts of the ear.

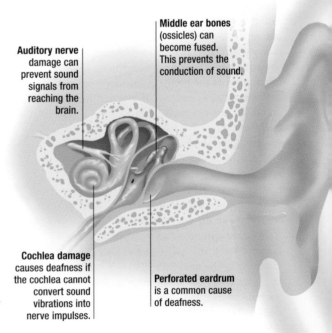

Auditory nerve damage can prevent sound signals from reaching the brain.

Middle ear bones (ossicles) can become fused. This prevents the conduction of sound.

Cochlea damage causes deafness if the cochlea cannot convert sound vibrations into nerve impulses.

Perforated eardrum is a common cause of deafness.

- a developmental abnormality, such that the ear canal has not developed (congenital atresia).

In the middle ear, deafness can be caused by:
- perforation of the ear drum (the tympanic membrane);
- fluid in the ear (glue ear) or inflammation in the middle ear (otitis media);
- otosclerosis, a condition in which the small bones that conduct sound in the middle ear (the ossicles) become fused together;
- damage or trauma to the eardrum or the ossicles, caused by direct force or sudden explosive noises.

In general, conductive deafness responds to treatment and hearing may be recoverable.

SENSORINEURAL DEAFNESS

Sensorineural deafness, also called perceptive deafness, can be of two types: sensory, when the inner ear is affected, and neural, when the auditory nerve or its pathways in the brain are affected.

Causes of sensory hearing loss

- Age: the gradual and progressive loss of hearing that is common with advancing age, also known as presbyacusis.
- Noise damage: prolonged exposure to loud noises causes hearing loss at certain frequencies, particularly those of the human voice.
- Congenital defects, such as the damage caused to the inner ear when a pregnant mother contracts German measles (rubella).
- Ménière's disease (endolymphatic hydrops), a condition caused by a buildup of fluid in the inner ear, resulting in deafness, buzzing in the ear (tinnitus) and vertigo.
- Fractured base of skull, generally caused by a blow to the face or head.

Causes of neural hearing loss

- Brain tumours, causing damage to nearby nerves and the brainstem – the point where the brain meets the spinal cord.
- Infections, particularly in childhood, when the auditory nerve can be damaged by mumps, German measles (rubella), meningitis or inner ear infections.
- Auditory nerve pathways in the brain can be damaged by diseases that destroy the nerve covering such as **multiple sclerosis**.
- Acoustic neuroma, a tumour of the part of the auditory nerve that lies in the inner ear.

In general, sensorineural deafness is hard to treat, and it is very rare for an affected person to recover any hearing.

DIAGNOSIS

A doctor will look in your ears and may use a tuning fork held near your ear and then against your head to establish whether hearing loss is due to conductive defects or sensorineural problems.

A precise diagnosis

As well as audiometry, there are several other tests available, which may be used for a precise diagnosis of hearing problems.

TEST	PROCEDURE
Tympanometry	This tests if the middle ear is working properly. A device blows tiny amounts of air into the ear canal, and measures sound reflected back by the eardrum.
Auditory brain stem response	This test distinguishes between sensory and neural hearing loss by measuring how the nerve impulses in the brain respond to sound.
Electrocochleography	This measures the activity of the cochlea and the auditory nerve and is used in young children with profound hearing loss.
Oto-acoustic emissions	This test measures the 'echo' produced by the cochlea in response to sound. It shows if the cochlea is working properly and is used as a screening test for newborn babies.

For a full assessment of your hearing your GP may refer you to the hospital ear, nose and throat (ENT) clinic or audiology department for an audiometry test. The patient sits in a soundproof room, and is asked to indicate when they hear sounds emitted at specific pitches and volumes from an electronic device called an audiometer.

Hearing by air conduction is tested by asking the patient to listen to the sounds through headphones, so that sound has to travel through the air to reach the eardrum. The faintest sound that can be heard is recorded, to discover whether the ear is less sensitive than it should be. Any hearing

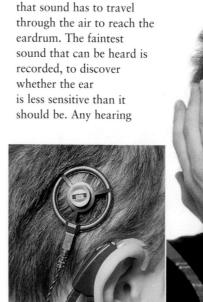

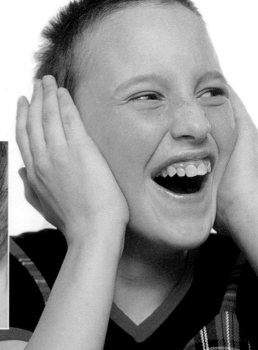

▼ **Loud and clear**
This young girl, who has just received a cochlear implant, is hearing for the first time in her life. She may need time to adjust to hearing the different sounds around her.

loss indicates a problem in the auditory pathway. This could be in the ear canal, the middle ear, the inner ear, the auditory nerve or the auditory nerve pathways in the brain.

Hearing by bone conduction is tested by placing a vibrating pad against the head behind the ear and delivering the sounds from the audiometer by vibration. The vibrations spread through the bone to the cochlea in the inner ear. Specialized hair cells in the cochlea convert vibrations into nerve impulses that travel along the auditory nerve to the brain.

If hearing by air conduction is reduced, but hearing by bone conduction is normal, then there is a conductive hearing loss. If the hearing is reduced by both bone and air conduction then there is a sensorineural hearing loss.

TREATMENT

The treatment of deafness depends on the cause. The most common cause of conductive deafness is wax or skin debris in the external ear canal. Olive oil or sodium bicarbonate eardrops can be used to soften the wax. Sometimes this is sufficient to clear the problem. The skin grows outwards from the eardrum and will carry wax and debris out of the ear canal as long as it is soft enough. If the wax remains in the ear it can be removed by gentle syringing with warm water. This must be carried out by a doctor.

To treat conductive deafness caused by fluid in the middle ear, an ear, nose and throat (ENT) surgeon uses an operating microscope that cuts through the eardrum and sucks out the fluid. A small tube called a grommet may be placed through the eardrum to allow the fluid to drain. The grommet is eventually pushed out as the eardrum heals. Surgery is also effective for conductive deafness caused by **otosclerosis**.

COMPENSATING FOR HEARING LOSS

For many people with deafness there is no cure. Treatment involves compensating for the hearing loss as much as possible. Lipreading, hearing aids and sign language can all help greatly with communication. For some people, a cochlear implant can greatly improve hearing.

Lipreading and sign language

Many local authorities in the UK provide classes to learn, or to learn to teach, lipreading or sign language. Those whose hearing is badly affected, or who are likely to become deaf, should consider attending such classes.

Hearing aids

Sound amplification with a hearing aid will help people with either conductive or sensorineural hearing loss, particularly if they have trouble hearing the sound frequencies of normal speech. The initial experience may be disappointing for some people but hearing improves as they become accustomed to the device, so it is worth persevering with a new aid for a least two months. Modern hearing aids have proved especially helpful in teaching deaf children.

Cochlear implants

A person who is profoundly deaf and cannot hear sounds even with a hearing aid may benefit from a cochlear implant. This can give a sensation of hearing to severely or profoundly deaf adults and children. A cochlear implant is an electronic device made up of external and

Types of hearing aids

Some aids are worn on the body, others in or behind the ear, and they vary greatly in quality and cost. The NHS is beginning to supply digital aids, which generally provide a much better sound quality than analogue aids.

▶ In-the-ear aids
These aids fit entirely into the ear and have an easy-to-use volume control. They are suitable for people with mild to moderate deafness.

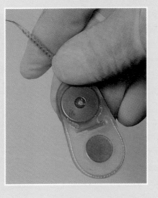

▶ Remote-control aids
The aid (right) fits in the outer ear, while a remote control device allows the wearer to tune to particular frequencies, cutting down, for example, on background noise.

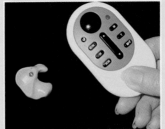

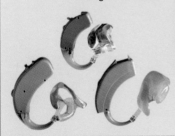

◀ Behind-the-ear aids
These widely used aids are available on the NHS or privately, and are suitable for various degrees of hearing loss. The expensive privately bought aids are more effective.

◀ Cochlear implant
Profoundly deaf people may be able to have a cochlear implant. A small receiver is implanted under the skin on the scalp; this transmits sound impulses via a processor, which the user wears externally. Implants are expensive, but the NHS may pay the costs in some cases.

internal parts. The external part is worn like a hearing aid, either on the head or clipped to clothes. This contains a sound processor that translates sounds into signals which are sent to the internal part surgically implanted in the ear. Electrodes fitted inside the cochlea, in the inner ear, transmit the electrical signals from the sound processor to the hearing (auditory) nerve. These signals are then recognized as sounds by the brain.

A cochlear implant can help deaf people to hear sounds such as doorbells, telephones and alarms. It helps some people with lipreading and allows people to use the telephone. It is more likely to be effective in someone whose hearing loss is recent or who was successfully using a hearing aid before the implant.

Decompression sickness

Decompression sickness is a condition that occurs during a rapid decrease in atmospheric pressure – for example, when divers surface too quickly. As they surface, water pressure falls and the body tissues release gases such as nitrogen and oxygen, disolved in the body fluids during the descent. During a slow ascent they are expelled through breathing; but if a diver's speed exceeds the rate at which nitrogen can be carried to the lungs and exhaled, bubbles may form in the tissues. These may block blood vessels, causing pain, especially in the joints. Bubbles may lodge in the lungs, the ear, the spinal cord and the brain, affecting breathing and nerve function and possibly causing paralysis and death.

Decompression sickness is also called caisson disease because it affects construction workers in caissons (watertight containers used to carry out construction work under water).

SYMPTOMS

These may appear up to 24 hours after a dive.
- Itching and mottled skin.
- Severe pains around shoulder and knee joints.
- Breathlessness or chest pain.
- Pins and needles or numbness.
- Visual disturbances.
- Dizziness, staggering and weakness.
- Nausea, vomiting.
- Severe headache.

Treatment involves sitting in a hyperbaric (decompression) chamber while air pressure is first increased to the level to which the sufferer was exposed, then reduced at a safe rate to sea-level pressure. Divers can prevent decompression sickness by using the correct air mixture, and surfacing at the rate recommended in a reliable manual for the duration and depth of the dive.

Deep vein thrombosis

Deep vein thrombosis (DVT) is a condition in which the blood clots in a deep vein, causing a blockage, usually in the leg or pelvis. Part of the blood clot may detach and travel to the lungs, resulting in a life-threatening pulmonary embolism.

CAUSES

Deep vein thrombosis occurs when blood is more prone to clotting, due to:
- thrombotic blood disorders;
- raised oestrogen levels (during pregnancy, or when taking the contraceptive pill or hormone replacement therapy);
- dehydration;
- immobilization during prolonged bed rest, air travel or after an operation.

DVT may also be triggered by vein damage caused by thrombophlebitis.

SYMPTOMS

Deep vein thrombosis may have no visible signs, but it usually produces deep, boring pain, tenderness, warmth, swelling and redness. Walking may be painful if the calf is affected.

Diagnosis is confirmed using various methods: a blood test; an ultrasound to show blood flow; or venography, in which dye is injected into a vein and tracked using X-rays (similar to angiography). More than one test for blood disorders and underlying causes may be needed.

A blocked vein may lead to dilated skin veins, and long-term swelling (oedema). A firm elastic stocking is a helpful preventative measure but may not be suitable for people with peripheral arterial disease.

TREATMENT

Treatment consists of injections of an anticoagulant drug such as heparin, to thin the blood, followed by anticoagulant tablets such as warfarin. Treatment lasts for at least three months, depending on the cause of the DVT and the likelihood of recurrence. Women should not take oestrogens again. A chest X-ray and ECG are required to exclude the presence of a pulmonary embolism.

Air travellers should avoid dehydration, move the legs frequently, and take medical advice about aspirin and compression stockings.

Degenerative diseases

Dramatic increases in life expectancy over the past 50 years mean that a growing number of people are suffering from age-related degenerative problems, ranging from arthritis to Alzheimer's disease.

egenerative disease is a term used by doctors to describe any progressive breakdown in the structure or working of a body organ or system. The breakdown may be due to ageing, have a genetic or environmental cause, or result from wear and tear – repeated physical strain, for example. Strictly, the term excludes damage caused by injury or cancer, but it is often broadly interpreted. As life expectancy in the developed world increases with each new generation – more than 1600 people now reach the age of 100 each year in the UK, compared with 200 each year around 50 years ago – so does the number of people with degenerative diseases.

The most common types of degenerative diesease are cardiovascular disease, **arthritis**, **osteoporosis** and **Alzheimer's disease** (see also **Heart and circulatory system**).

One in three people in the UK over the age of 80 are disabled by a degenerative disease.

Diseases not linked to age

Some degenerative diseases are not confined to old age. For example, muscular dystrophy, a severe muscle-wasting disease, affects infants and children as well as adults.

Motor neurone disease – a group of degenerative disorders that affect nerves in the upper or lower parts of the body – often strike in middle age; symptoms may include difficulty in swallowing, limb or facial weakness, slurred speech, muscle cramps, impaired mobility and, in the later stages, respiratory problems. Other degenerative disorders not strongly linked to old age are **multiple sclerosis**, **Huntingdon's disease** and **CJD**. The cause is often unknown, although genetic factors may be involved. CJD, which usually affects young people, is believed to be caused by eating the meat of cattle affected by BSE.

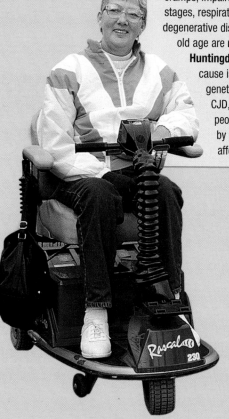

◄ **On the move again**
Some people whose walking ability has been severely impaired by a degenerative disease can regain a measure of independence with a pavement buggy or similar mobility aid.

PROTECTING YOURSELF AGAINST DEGENERATIVE DISEASES

Although degenerative diseases are closely associated with age, they are not an inevitable consequence of it. Many conditions are now being linked to chronic infections, toxins and immune system disorders that – if recognized early enough – can be treated before they start to cause damage.

For example, eating sensibly can protect your heart and perhaps prevent late-onset diabetes. A diet high in antioxidants and low in saturated fats can arrest, and perhaps reverse, the gradual clogging of arteries that limits the supply of blood and strains the heart. A diet low in refined sugar may prevent the exhaustion of insulin-producing cells that leads to late-onset diabetes, which in turn can cause degeneration of the kidneys and eyes.

Osteoarthritis – the erosion of bone in joints – can be caused either by physical wear and tear or by untreated rheumatoid arthritis, a chronic disorder that eats away the protective cartilage, leaving the bones exposed. Wear and tear may be minimized by avoiding the sort of physical exercise that stresses the joints, while rheumatoid arthritis can be treated with anti-inflammatory drugs.

Osteoporosis – the weakening of bone mass – can be limited by weight-bearing exercise that encourages new bone growth. Even the brain degeneration that causes dementias such as Alzheimer's disease may be limited by ensuring that the brain is kept active.

Degenerative diseases tend to be progressive, but there are few symptoms that cannot be relieved by good medical care.

SEE ALSO *Brain and nervous system*

Dehydration

Dehydration is a condition resulting from loss or lack of water in body tissues. Excessive water loss is frequently combined with a loss of sodium and potassium, which may cause body organs to malfunction.

Dehydration is a consequence of inadequate water intake or water loss through diarrhoea, vomiting or excessive sweating during a fever. It may also be caused by uncontrolled **diabetes** or some types of kidney failure.

Babies dehydrate much faster than adults because any substantial water loss represents a higher percentage of their bodies' water content.

If you fear that a baby in your care may be dehydrated, gently pinch the skin on the baby's forearm and pull it up, then release. If the skin at once resumes its normal appearance, the baby is probably not dehydrated, but if the skin remains puckered, seek medical advice urgently.

SYMPTOMS

Typical symptoms of dehydration include:
- concentrated (dark-coloured) urine;
- dry skin and mouth;
- swollen tongue;
- rapid pulse and rapid breathing;
- cold feet and hands;
- loss of skin elasticity;
- in severe cases, lightheadedness, irritability, confusion and loss of consciousness.

TREATMENT

It is necessary to rehydrate the body with rehydration fluids as quickly as possible.

What you can do
- Drink rehydration fluids. These contain essential salts and glucose and can be bought in pharmacies in powder or tablet form to dissolve in water. Sports drinks are not advised.
- Prepare a home-made rehydration drink by mixing one teaspoon of table salt with eight teaspoons of sugar in one litre of tap water.

When to consult a doctor
Consult a doctor immediately if a baby shows any symptoms of dehydration, or if an adult shows severe signs.

Severe dehydration requires hospitalization so that fluids can be replaced through a drip.

COMPLICATIONS

If dehydration is untreated, blood pressure will fall to dangerously low levels, causing shock and damage to the kidneys, liver and brain.

PREVENTION

Drink plenty of water, especially during hot weather, before and after strenuous exercise and during a fever. Drink rehydration fluids when suffering from diarrhoea or vomiting.

OUTLOOK

Recovery is good if fluids are replaced quickly.

Delirium

A delirious person is confused, disoriented and agitated, and is likely to suffer hallucinations or delusions. In delirium tremens – a symptom of withdrawal from chronic alcoholism – a person has the symptoms of delirium and may also shake uncontrollably.

SYMPTOMS

People who are delirious typically mutter or shout incoherently, and may be convinced that other people are out to harm them.

CAUSES

Delirium may be caused by anything that disturbs the normal functioning of the brain. This includes head injury, brain inflammation from infectious illness, drug abuse and adverse reaction to medicinal drugs. It is commonly seen after surgery (especially in children and elderly people), as a reaction to anaesthesia.

TREATMENT

Treatment depends on the cause. If delirium occurs after a head injury or as a reaction to a drug, the affected person should be seen urgently by a doctor. If the delirium is linked with fever, the person should be soothed, kept cool and watched carefully, in consultation with a doctor. If a delirious person lapses suddenly into unconsciousness, or starts convulsing, a doctor should be called.

A person suffering from delirium should be encouraged to lie down in a fairly light, cool room (darkness increases the likelihood of hallucination). Other people can help by providing soothing talk aimed at calming and allaying fear, and gentle distraction during periods of lucidity.

Delirium tremens

Delirium tremens is a type of delirium linked almost exclusively with a sudden withdrawal from alcohol after very heavy (and usually long-term) over-consumption

The condition comes on hours or days after the person has stopped drinking, and its start is marked by irritability, restlessness, lack of concentration and insomnia or disturbed sleep with nightmares. There is a characteristic shaking (tremor), most noticeable in the hands but sometimes extending to the entire body. About one in four people with delirium tremens has a seizure.

Delirium tremens usually lasts for several days, during which time the affected person shows increasing distress and confusion. He or she may experience terrifying hallucinations – of foul smells, threatening voices and the sensation of being pushed or hit. Sometimes the affected person sweats profusely and becomes dehydrated. Recovery is usually quite sudden, but in about one in 10 cases the person dies from physical disorders caused by long-term abuse of alcohol.

A person suffering from delirium tremens should be taken to hospital, where doctors may prescribe sedative drugs and vitamin B injections.

Delusions

Delusions are mistaken or false beliefs that cannot be altered by rational argument. People who are mentally ill may have a false belief that they are all-powerful or that they are victims of persecution or an external force that is taking over their bodies or minds. Some people who believe that their body has changed in some way react by trying to do harm to themselves.

Delusions are a common feature of mental distress, particularly **paranoia** and **dementia**, and may be a symptom of **schizophrenia** or **manic depression**.

TREATMENT

Trying to empathize with the feelings of fear, confusion and isolation experienced by the person suffering from delusions may help to alleviate the problem; trying to reason with the person about the delusions does not. A doctor may prescribe drug treatment – generally tranquillizers.

SEE ALSO *Mental health and problems; Psychosis*

Dementia

Dementia is a gradual, long-term deterioration of a person's ability to think clearly and to remember everyday events. Eventually it leaves the person unable to live independently.

The most common form of dementia is **Alzheimer's disease** but other causes include **Huntingdon's disease**, impaired blood supply to the brain, **CJD** and **AIDS**. Dementia may also be caused by drug or alcohol abuse.

Although dementia most commonly affects people later in life, it is not the same as poor memory or forgetfulness, which some people complain of as they grow older.

SYMPTOMS

In the early stages, people affected by dementia may become confused and forgetful and find it difficult to make decisions.

As the disease progresses, the affected person can develop feelings of anxiety, fear and aggression. Delusions and paranoia are common – for example, patients may believe that their relatives are stealing from them or trying to harm them.

In the later stages, people with dementia may lose long-term memory and fail to recognize even their close family members.

TREATMENT

Treatment of dementia is geared to enabling people with the condition to lead lives that are as near normal as possible for as long as possible. It may include practical assistance

In the UK, dementia affects one in ten people over the age of 65 and one in five over the age of 80.

in the home, such as the provision of meals or help with personal and domestic hygiene, as well as emotional support for both the person with dementia and that person's carers.

When Alzheimer's disease is in its early stages, drugs may help to preserve the affected person's mental faculties for several months and may also alleviate symptoms such as aggression, irritability, restlessness and depression.

Residential care is likely to be needed in the later stages of dementia.

Complementary therapies

Complementary therapies cannot provide a cure for dementia but relaxation techniques and aromatherapy may be soothing.

Some essential oils such as rosemary, herbs such as gingko biloba, and the nutrient lecithin – which occurs naturally in egg yolks and is also available as a supplement – peanuts and green leafy vegetables, may help to improve the powers of memory.

COMPLICATIONS

As dementia progresses, an affected person will no longer be able to manage his or her own affairs. It is important to seek legal advice before major problems arise.

PREVENTION

Dementia related to poor blood supply to the brain may be prevented by reducing risk factors such as smoking and high blood pressure. But, since the causes of most forms of dementia are not fully understood, there are limited opportunities for prevention.

OUTLOOK

Dementia usually becomes progressively worse until death occurs, often from respiratory infection or other chronic illness. But the person's emotional health and general well-being can be improved by sensitive care and good support services.

SEE ALSO *Alzheimer's disease; Brain and nervous system; Huntington's disease*

Dentists and dentistry

Regular visits to your dentist from an early age will help to maintain healthy teeth and gums. A dentist will also check for problems involving the tongue or soft tissues of the mouth and provide advice on how to prevent disease.

Dental checks every six months used to be standard, but the recommended interval between visits now varies, depending on the state of your teeth and the advice of your dentist. Most dentists advocate preventive care to keep treatments to a minimum. Patients are shown how to care for their teeth and given oral health advice to help to keep their mouth free from disease. As well as attending checkups, consult a dentist if you suffer from toothache, chip or lose a tooth, or have problems with dentures. Your dentist can also advise on how to deal with bad breath and jaw problems. Anaesthetics and new techniques have taken much of the pain out of dentistry, and a focus on prevention means that drastic treatments have become rarer.

FINDING THE RIGHT DENTIST

Before registering with a dentist, decide exactly what kind of service you want.
■ NHS treatment provides routine care at fixed prices. But it is not always easy to find an NHS dentist, and not all treatments are covered.
■ Private care offers longer sessions with a dentist and a greater choice of treatment options, but it is usually more expensive than NHS care.
■ Some practices provide both NHS and private treatment and allow you to choose between them depending on your treatment needs.

You may also want to consider registering with one of the following types of dental practice:
■ a practice with a hygienist who will advise on brushing and flossing to improve preventive care;
■ a family practice geared to treating children;
■ a practice with expertise in treating nervous patients that offers sedation;
■ a practice that has late or unusual opening hours to fit in with your working life;
■ a practice that provides cosmetic dentistry treatments such as bleaching;
■ a practice that offers a dental scheme whereby you pay a set amount annually for dentistry.

NHS Direct can provide details of NHS dentists in your area, many of whom offer private care.

THE DENTAL CHECKUP

After enquiring about any problems since your last visit, the dentist will examine your mouth under a bright light, often using a mirror and a probe. The dentist will check that any new teeth such as wisdom teeth are emerging correctly and will look for any signs of decay or gum or mouth disease. Water and air from a syringe may be used to clean off any debris; air blown onto the teeth may also indicate any sensitivity. After every dental session, the tray of instruments used is sterilized and the gloves are thrown away.

The dentist works with a nurse, who will use a suction device to remove excess saliva from your mouth, prepare instruments and fill in records.

If your last dental checkup was some time ago, X-rays may be taken to see whether there are any hidden problems such as decay between your teeth or problems in the roots. Bite-wing X-ray films are placed between your teeth, one for each side, and an X-ray machine placed by your cheek. Panoramic X-rays, or OPG (orthopantomograph) machines, may be used to provide an image of the whole jaw as well as sectional images of teeth, roots and sinuses. Some practices have intra-oral cameras linked to a monitor so that the dentist can use images of the patient's mouth to explain problems and treatment options.

If you require treatment, you will usually need to make another appointment. If you are unclear about what is being recommended, ask for a treatment plan and an estimate of the cost.

Your dentist or a hygienist may also scale and polish your teeth to remove plaque and calculus. Plaque is a sticky film containing bacteria that can build up in the mouth; the bacteria can produce acids that attack the teeth, penetrating the enamel and causing decay. Calculus is plaque that has hardened on the teeth.

HAVING A TOOTH EXTRACTED

If you are having a tooth extracted, eat before you go to the dentist – you will not be able to eat for some hours afterwards. Your blood sugar level can drop after an extraction, making you feel faint or weak. If this happens, have a drink

---

Avoiding tooth problems

To maintain good oral health, take your dentist's advice:

■ brush twice a day with a toothpaste containing fluoride;

■ avoid sugary snacks and drinks;

■ have regular dental checkups;

■ chew sugar-free gum

■ don't smoke;

■ limit fizzy or acidic drinks.

of squash or juice to restore your blood glucose levels. Avoid drinking anything very hot or cold, and do not touch the area where the tooth has been extracted or you may hinder the healing process. Wrap a clean handkerchief around cotton wool, lay it across the socket and bite onto it to stop any bleeding. Go back to the dentist if this fails to stop the bleeding.

REPLACING MISSING TEETH
If one or two teeth are extracted or lost, they may be replaced with a bridge whereby an artificial tooth is attached to adjoining teeth. Crowns are made to fit the natural teeth either side of the gap. They are fixed onto the plate and cemented over the natural teeth. Several treatment sessions may be needed to have a bridge fitted. Dentures may be used where more than two teeth are lost (see page 214).

A permanent dental implant can be used to replace one or more missing teeth. A hole is drilled in the jaw and a small titanium rod inserted, usually under local anaesthetic. The screw is left to heal for several months before an artificial tooth is placed over the top although, increasingly, teeth are being placed on the implants immediately. Implants can be an alternative to dentures, but inserting them can be a long and expensive process.

MAJOR DENTAL TREATMENT
If decay invades the pulp of the tooth, after an abscess has caused infection there, root canal treatment may be necessary. In this procedure, the remaining pulp and nerve are removed, the roots and abscess are drained, and antiseptic is used to sterilize the cavity. The root canals are shaped with a series of files and the roots and interior of the tooth are then filled; in some cases the tooth is covered with a crown to strengthen it. The procedure may require several sessions.

If root canal treatment does not successfully remove all the infected pulp from a tooth, an apicectomy may be necessary. This is a surgical procedure in which an incision is made in the gum and the end of the root is cleaned and trimmed. This is usually carried out in the practice under a local anaesthetic.

Difficult extractions – such as removing a wisdom tooth that has become stuck (impacted) because of lack of space in the mouth – are usually done in the practice under a general anaesthetic. Antibiotics may be prescribed for any infection.

NUMBING THE PAIN
Most dental treatments are carried out under local anaesthetic. An anaesthetic such as Lignocaine is injected into the gum near the tooth to be treated. An anaesthetic gel can be applied before the injection to numb the area and reduce discomfort. Injections are a very effective way of numbing the nerves in the mouth so that no pain is experienced during treatment. But people who are very anxious about treatment can have it carried out under sedation. This usually takes the form of inhaling gas and air (nitrous oxide and oxygen), but a sedative can also be injected into a vein. Not all dental practices have the facilities to offer sedation.

Some dentists offer relaxation techniques, including hypnotherapy, which can induce a state of altered consciousness to make the patient relaxed and immune to discomfort.

DENTAL SPECIALISTS
Most dental care and treatment is carried out by general dental practitioners in their surgeries, but complex work may require specialist treatment. Dental specialists include:
■ endodontists, who specialize in root canal treatment and apicetomies;
■ orthodontists, who deal with irregularities and overcrowding of teeth and correction of the bite;
■ periodontists, who treat advanced gum disease;
■ oral surgeons, who carry out extractions, jaw surgery and may insert implants;
■ restorative dentists, who provide crowns, bridges and fillings;
■ prosthodontists, who specialize in dentures.

ORTHODONTICS
Orthodontic treatment is used to straighten or realign crooked or crowded teeth, but it is not simply a cosmetic procedure – it prevents decay by enabling the teeth to be cleaned properly. Orthodontics can also improve your bite in cases where teeth do not meet correctly – a bad bite makes it harder to chew food thoroughly and strains the jaw muscles. Most orthodontic patients are children or teenagers, but adults can also benefit.

Simple treatment may require the person to wear a removable brace that exerts gentle sustained pressure to move the teeth into the correct position.

A fixed brace is necessary for more complex treatment, and some patients need to wear additional headgear at night, to increase the pressure. This process usually takes a minimum of between 18 months and two years, with visits to the dentist every four to six weeks. Once the teeth are in the correct position, a retainer may have to be worn for a further six months to maintain the position of the teeth.

Orthodontic work on children's teeth may be available on the NHS; some adults may also be entitled to NHS treatment. Private orthodontists offer tooth-coloured brackets, which make the brace less visible.

Only healthy teeth are regarded as suitable for orthodontic treatment, and while wearing braces it is important to clean your teeth properly.

ROUTINE AND COSMETIC TREATMENT

Almost everyone has at least one filling at some point in their lives. Fillings are used to replace a decayed area of a tooth and to prevent the decay from spreading. The decayed area is removed, usually by drilling. Other methods include air abrasion, which is precise and virtually pain-free, or use of laser or a gel such as carisolv, that dissolves soft tissue. But these methods may not be suitable and are not widely available.

Chipped or cracked teeth can be repaired. A tooth may be given a replacement surface in the form of thin porcelain veneer. This is often used to improve the appearance of teeth that are irregular or stained. Discoloured teeth can also be lightened with hydrogen peroxide (bleach).

A protective cover, or crown, can be fitted over a tooth that is broken down through decay, badly discoloured or misshapen. Crowns are made of porcelain or porcelain bonded to metal. The tooth is ground down and shaped into a peg. An impression of the peg is made and a temporary cover is fitted while the crown is made in a laboratory to the dentist's prescription. The crown, which should match the shade of existing teeth, is cemented into place. Fitting a crown may require two or three appointments. Teeth may need to be extracted if they are badly decayed or loosened due to gum disease. Extractions can also be performed to make room in the mouth for orthodontic work. They are usually done in the dentist's surgery under a local anaesthetic, but more complex procedures may need to be carried out in hospital.

TREATMENT FOR GUM DISEASE

Gum problems are usually treated by a dentist. Inflammation of the gums, or gingivitis, is very common and is caused by bacteria in plaque. The dentist or a hygienist will use a scaler to remove plaque and calculus from the teeth and advise you on preventive care.

Gingivitis can develop into periodontal disease, which causes the gums to recede followed by eventual tooth loosening and loss. Treatment can involve root planing, a special cleaning of the roots of the teeth, antibiotics, mouthwashes, or surgery to remove the diseased area of the gum. A periodontist may be consulted about how to prevent periodontal disease.

Gum disease can be prevented by careful home care including brushing and flossing, as well as having regular visits to your dentist or hygienist.

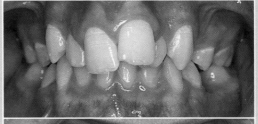

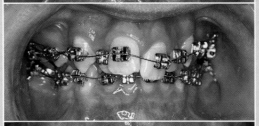

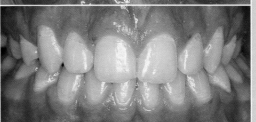

◀ **Crooked correction**
In cases where teeth need radical realignment, a fixed brace is used. The first step is to fix a small bracket to each tooth.

◀ **Straightening up**
The brackets are joined by a flexible wire, which allows the teeth to be guided accurately and gently into place.

◀ **Raising a smile**
Even though the process may take several months or more to complete, the end result should be a straight set of teeth set off by a radiant smile.

TREATMENT FOR JAW PROBLEMS

Aches around the face and head may be caused by the teeth meeting incorrectly and abnormal clenching or grinding; a dentist can treat this problem or give you advice about how to deal with it. If you grind your teeth at night, you may wake up with a dull headache. A dentist may advise wearing a special mouthguard at night or may refer you to an orthodontist to correct your bite.

TREATMENT WITHIN THE NHS

Fees for specific dental health treatments within the NHS are set by the Department of Health, limited by a maximum amount payable for any course of treatment. The patient pays the dentist 80 per cent of the cost of the treatment and the remainder is paid to the dentist by the NHS. The dentist will need to obtain official approval for any course of dental work costing more than the set maximum.

Children and young adults under the age of 18, expectant mothers, mothers of children under 12 months and some benefit claimants are exempt from fees. There are restrictions on the types of treatment you can have on the NHS – for example, you may be offered only amalgam fillings in certain teeth.

By law, Primary Care Trusts must ensure that there is enough NHS dental provision in the area, and some provide dental centres staffed by salaried dentists. These clinics deal mostly with patients who are in pain and need emergency treatment care.

If you lose a tooth, a dentist may be able to re-implant it. Placing the tooth in milk improves the chances of saving it.

PRIVATE TREATMENT

Private patients pay for all their dental treatment and the cost varies greatly between practices. If you are considering private treatment, it is advisable to follow up recommendations and visit several practices before choosing one. Some dentists provide both NHS and private care. Certain dentists belong to a national payment plan scheme such as Denplan or Cigna; others have their own plan.

DENTAL STANDARDS

There are more than 30,000 dentists and some 12,000 dental practices in the UK. All practising dentists are obliged to register with the General Dental Council (GDC) and to conform to the council's ethical code. Those who fail to do so and whose practice or behaviour falls below acceptable standards may be struck off.

HOMEOPATHIC DENTISTRY

Complementary therapies such as homeopathy cannot offer an alternative to dental treatment but can provide a useful adjunct to it. Some dentists are trained in homeopathy and may offer remedies such as arnica to reduce swelling and pain after extractions. Few homeopathic dentists use mercury in their fillings.

DENTISTRY FOR CHILDREN

It is never too early to start instilling healthy practices and teaching children to look after their teeth. Introduce your baby to a trainer mug for drinking as soon as you can; sucking on a bottle should be discouraged as soon as an infant is old enough to drink from a mug or glass. Infants should never be allowed to go to sleep with a bottle in their mouth, especially one that contains sweet drinks.

When children are very small, plaque can be removed from their teeth with a cotton bud. Later on, this may be replaced by a child's toothbrush and toothpaste, which has a lower level of fluoride than ordinary toothpaste.

Parents should oversee a child's toothbrushing until the child is about seven years old. Before this age, it is advisable to make sure that the child does not use too much toothpaste as this may cause mottling of the teeth (fluorosis). A pea-sized smear of toothpaste is recommended.

Children can start visiting the dentist when their first teeth appear, and all children should have seen a dentist by the time they are two years old. Regular checkups help to ensure that the teeth are coming through correctly and allow the child to get used to seeing a dentist.

Practices specializing in children's dentistry help make visits enjoyable; for example, stickers may be given to reward children for good behaviour.

As your child's permanent teeth appear, plastic sealants may be recommended to protect the biting surface of the first molars. These teeth have tiny cracks (fissures) between them that are particularly susceptible to decay. However, covering the cracks with sealant helps to keep decay at bay. The process is pain-free and is recommended when the permanent molars have just come through, between the ages of six and thirteen.

When children need fillings in their first teeth, the dentist may insert glass ionomers, which leach fluoride into the teeth to strengthen them. Baby teeth provide the spaces for the second teeth to grow into, so it is worth taking care of them. If a child loses some first teeth, the permanent teeth may be overcrowded when they come through and extractions may be necessary. Children's teeth may become discoloured from toothpaste or antibiotics, particularly tetracycline. White filling material or veneers can be used to conceal small stains when the child is older.

SEE ALSO *Gums and gum disease; Halitosis; Teeth and problems*

Dentures

Dentures can be fitted to replace missing teeth. They may be partial, replacing one or more teeth, or complete, replacing all teeth in both jaws. Unlike crowns and bridges, dentures are removable.

Dentures are artificial teeth attached to a plastic or metal plate that rests on the ridges of the gums or clasps onto any natural teeth. Suction and muscle control keep them in place; lower dentures have no suction and tend to move more.

Dentures are made specially for each individual, but they often become uncomfortable or loose because the gums and supporting bones shrink after natural teeth have been extracted; the shrinkage occurs rapidly for the first six months, then more slowly.

An annual checkup will allow early detection of any problems such as mouth cancer. All dentures should be checked if they become uncomfortable.

Dentures should be removed at night and left in a denture cleaner. If they are left in place, the roof of the mouth becomes soft and spongy and a yeast infection may develop. Denture wearers should brush their gums and palate twice a day to keep them healthy. Some wearers use dental fixative to keep dentures in place but this is not recommended for regular use; your dentist can adjust your dentures to make a better fit if they have become loose and are uncomfortable

Ill-fitting dentures may make the mouth sag at the corners, causing a buildup of saliva, which can lead to infection. The wearer may stop eating foods that need chewing, and there is a danger of serious weight loss and health problems linked with poor diet, such as vitamin deficiency. Another unpleasant side effect is mouth ulcers.

As people age, the soft tissue of the mouth thins and dentures can become painful, rubbing the inside of the mouth. A dry mouth – a common side effect of some medications such as antidepressants and of some cancer treatments – exacerbates the problem, and may also cause your dentures to fit less well.

Depression

Depression is a common illness that affects most people at some point in their lives. When it grips someone, activities that were previously fulfilling seem to become a waste of time.

In its mildest form, depression means feeling miserable and dissatisfied. If you have mild depression, you can carry on with a normal life, but everything seems more of a struggle. Severe depression can stop you living your life the way you want to. You may feel helpless and even suicidal. When negative thoughts dominate a person's life and continue for a long time, the depression is described as 'clinical'.

More women than men experience depression – in the UK, one in six women and one in nine men seeks medical help for depression. Depression is common in older people, but it can be mistaken for an early sign of dementia or overlooked as 'just getting old'. Children and young people can also get depressed.

COMMON CAUSES

The causes of depression are many and various. You may know why you are depressed – it may be a natural reaction to something happening in your life, such as divorce – or there may be no apparent cause. Depression sometimes runs in families, but how much this is due to genetics and how much to environment or upbringing is not clear. Negative life experiences are more likely to lead to depression if your feelings about the negative event are not expressed or explored.

Common causes of depression include recent life events, such as a bereavement; financial or relationship problems; **disability**; childhood experiences that have affected the way you feel about yourself and the world; and traumatic experiences such as a physical attack. Other possible triggers of depression are recent life changes, such as moving house or having a baby. Poor diet, lack of exercise and physical illness sometimes lie behind bouts of depression.

SYMPTOMS

Depression affects different people in different ways and there is a wide range of emotional and physical symptoms. These include sadness, low mood, constant irritability, seeing the worst in everything, feeling worthless, guilty and despairing, and losing interest in things you used to enjoy such as reading, sport, social activities, music or sex. Depressed people are also often preoccupied with thoughts of death or suicide.

▼ **A common affliction**
Depression is nothing to be ashamed of – one person in 20 in the UK is seeking help for the condition at any given time.

Other symptoms include eating problems – for example, having no appetite and losing weight, or overeating and gaining weight – and sleep problems such as waking early, having difficulty getting to sleep, or being unable to get up.

Depression may be an underlying cause if you have serious problems involving concentration, thinking or making decisions, or if you feel agitated, anxious and unable to relax (see **Anxiety**). Likewise, if you feel tired all the time or as though you have no energy, or if you suffer from headaches, aches and digestive pain, depression may be at the root of your problems.

How to help someone who is suicidal

If someone you are close to seems suicidal, talk about their feelings and draw up a personal support list together. Include names, phone numbers and addresses of people, helplines, organizations or professionals. Persuade him or her to keep the list by the phone and to call someone when suicidal feelings arise.

If you think someone is in real danger of suicide or has an acute mental health problem and will not seek help, you can contact social services. It may be possible to arrange for that person to be encouraged to accept treatment.

If you are the parent of an adolescent who seems suicidal, encourage him or her to talk to you about their worries. Do your best to help your child to find ways to solve the problems.

On a practical note, keep only small amounts of drugs such as paracetamol, and lock away all medicines. Keep strong alcohol locked away, too. These measures can help to prevent an angry or impulsive suicide attempt. If family problems are distressing your child, ask your GP to refer you for family therapy.

> For many people, a combination of talking treatments and antidepressants is the best way of coping with depression.

Postnatal depression

Many women feel exhausted, helpless or even frightened for several days or weeks after giving birth. In a few mothers, this reaction is stronger and longer-lasting, and may develop into a mental disorder known as postnatal depression.

Women with postnatal depression may suffer mood swings and feel angry and rejecting of their baby and of their partner. They often feel anxious and have panic attacks. Some also have physical symptoms such as digestive problems and stomach or chest pains.

Try to make time for yourself – a night out or even just a visit to the salon for a haircut may help you to move on from the depression. If you can, take daily exercise – it helps to ease tension. Make sure you eat regularly, because you may feel worse if you go for long periods without food. Most women have good spells when post-natal depression eases and bad ones when it is worse, and the proportion of good spells gradually increases.

TREATMENT

It can be very difficult to seek help when you feel depressed and listless, but deciding to do something about your depression is the first step to putting things right. See a doctor if you have had five or more of the symptoms described above for at least two weeks.

The sooner you obtain treatment for severe depression, the sooner you will start to get better. If you feel unable to help yourself, or feel desperate or suicidal, see a doctor, telephone the Samaritans or tell someone you trust.

A doctor may talk to you about your feelings and symptoms and may also want to talk to family members or a close friend. The doctor will also want to eliminate physical causes. Depression may be a symptom of an underlying condition, or may even be a side effect of medication.

The doctor will discuss options for treatment, or possible combinations of treatments, and may prescribe antidepressants or other drugs. You may be referred to another practitioner for talking therapies such as counselling, cognitive behaviour therapy or psychotherapy.

If you are severely depressed, you may be admitted to the psychiatric ward of a hospital.

Depression may disappear without treatment, especially if it is a normal reaction to a life event. But if it persists it can disrupt your life and relationships. Your treatment should depend on the severity of the depression, how long you have had it and how much it is disrupting your life.

Medication

Antidepressant drugs are the most common drug treatment for depression. They do not cure depression but can reduce the symptoms and

---

Offering help and support

Anyone at risk of suicide needs someone to talk to. If a suicidal person confides in you, try not to feel overwhelmed by the responsibility.

Do

- ✔ Listen, and encourage the person to talk about his or her feelings.
- ✔ Talk openly about suicide – this does not make it more likely to happen.
- ✔ Take talk of or threats of suicide seriously.
- ✔ Give the person a list of contacts to call when feeling suicidal.

Don't

- ✗ Try to 'jolly them out of it', or dismiss the person's feelings of hopelessness.
- ✗ Let the person think that suicide is the only option: show him or her that there is help and support available.
- ✗ Ignore what lies underneath the suicidal feelings.
- ✗ Neglect yourself – make sure you get support and advice.

help you through a crisis to the point where you can help yourself. Antidepressants aim to restore chemicals in the brain to a healthy level. This involves increasing levels of noradrenaline and seratonin, two chemicals in the brain that affect mood. Antidepressants fall into three main groups: tricyclics, monoamine oxidase inhibitors (MAOIs) and seratonin-specific reuptake inhibitors (SSRIs).

Antidepressants do not offer instant relief – they often take between two and four weeks to have an effect. They do not work for everyone, and can cause unpleasant side effects. Tricyclics can cause drowsiness, blurred vision, a dry mouth and constipation. MAOIs can interact with other drugs and foods containing tyramine (such as cheese), causing a sudden rise in blood pressure. SSRIs may cause agitation and nausea.

Electroconvulsive therapy (ECT)
Electroconvulsive therapy may be given to severely depressed people when antidepressant drugs have failed to work. The depressed person is put to sleep with an anaesthetic, then a small electric current is passed through the brain. The electric shock gives the brain a seizure. This stimulates the release of the neurotransmitter chemicals that carry messages between brain cells, which appears to improve the mood of the depressed individual.

ECT is a controversial treatment that can have side effects such as short-term memory loss. Doctors will recommend it only as a last resort.

Talking therapies
Therapies such as counselling, cognitive behaviour therapy and psychotherapy can help people who want to explore and understand themselves and their depression. These talking therapies can be beneficial used alongside antidepressants or instead of them.

Counselling examines your feelings at the time of the depression and can help you to adjust to life events, illnesses or losses. Cognitive behaviour therapy aims to encourage you to replace negative thought patterns with positive ones. Psychotherapy helps you to find and explore the root causes of your depression.

Some people find it unhelpful to focus on their problems. What seems to matter most in talking therapies is the relationship between individual and therapist. Continue treatment only if you feel comfortable with the counseller or therapist.

Talking therapies are available within the NHS in some areas, both in GPs' surgeries, mental healthcare clinics and in hospitals. Many voluntary organizations and self-help groups offer counselling and support at low cost or free of charge or you may choose to consult a fee-charging therapist privately.

Staying well

There are many things that you can do to help you to stay well once your depression has lifted.

■ Join a support group to meet others who suffer from depression. It can alleviate feelings of isolation and helplessness.

■ Look after yourself physically and reduce the stress in your life. Take regular exercise, eat well and practise relaxation techniques.

■ You may need to stay on medication or persist with talking therapy for a time to avoid a relapse.

■ Know your triggers. Be aware of the kinds of things that make you depressed and avoid them if possible.

■ Notice early-warning signs. You may be able to avoid a crisis and get help quickly. It helps if people around you are aware of these signs, too.

What you can do
There are no instant solutions to depression. What you can do for yourself depends on how low you are feeling. You may feel paralysed and unable to act. If so, you may need professional help or drugs to get you to a point where you can take action to help yourself. Depression feeds on itself – you get depressed, then you become more depressed about being depressed. If you can break the cycle of negative thoughts, you can begin to break the hold that depression has on you. Joining a support group can help to ease isolation and boost self-esteem.

Complementary therapies
Many people find complementary therapies useful for emotional problems. Therapies that can be helpful for depression include aromatherapy, **massage, acupuncture** and meditation. Many therapies and treatments can be used alongside orthodox medical treatment, but always consult your GP first.

OUTLOOK
Depression can be treated, and most people recover from it, whatever the cause. You may have to try several treatments before finding the treatment or combination of treatments that is best for you.

LIVING WITH A DEPRESSED PERSON
If relatives or friends are depressed, show that you care by listening sympathetically and being affectionate. Encourage them to talk about how they feel and help them to decide what they can do to deal with the depression. Get some support for yourself – from other family members, depression support groups or carers' groups.

SEE ALSO *Chronic fatigue syndrome; Insomnia; Manic depression; Postnatal depression; Seasonal affective disorder*

Dermatitis

Dermatitis, or eczema, is an inflammatory skin condition. The term 'contact dermatitis' refers to two types of eczema – irritant and allergic. Irritant eczema is triggered by substances that directly damage the skin, while allergic eczema occurs when someone becomes sensitized to something in the environment. Atopic eczema (atopic dermatitis) is a pink scaly rash that is very itchy. It may appear only on wrists and ankles, knee and elbow creases, or it can be much more extensive. There are a number of other types (see box below).

SYMPTOMS

Symptoms of dermatitis vary from mild to severe and can include:
- a patch of dry, scaly, thickened skin;
- redness;
- itching;
- blisters;
- weeping sores that may become infected;
- crusting
- severe inflammation with blisters on hands and feet (pompholyx, see box below).

TREATMENT

Treatment for dermatitis depends on the cause.
- Avoid contact with the substance that triggers the reaction.
- Regularly apply emollients, non-cosmetic moisturizers available from pharmacies and on prescription. A twice daily application of steroid cream may be prescribed, the strength of which depends on the body part affected and the age of the person concerned. Hydrocortisone cream is available from pharmacies without a prescription.

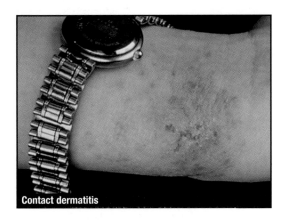

Contact dermatitis

▲ **Contact dermatitis** People who are allergic to the nickel used in some metal watchstraps develop a painful dermatitis rash on their wrist.

- Occasionally, in cases of severe dermatitis, an oral corticosteroid may be prescribed.
- Antihistamines, which can help to reduce itching and swelling, may be prescribed.
- In the case of pompholyx, patch-testing for specific common allergies may be carried out. One in ten people shows a consistent positive result, allowing easy resolution of the problem.

Complementary therapies

Aloe vera and evening primose may be helpful.

COMPLICATIONS

Chronic actinic dermatitis can spread to cause redness over the whole body (erythroderma). This can result in serious loss of body heat and fluids, and in extreme cases heart failure.

PREVENTION

To prevent dermatitis, avoid known allergens and use emollients and soap substitutes daily.

The types and causes of dermatitis

Most types of dermatitis are triggered by contact with an external irritant, but allergy to gluten and the presence of particular antibodies in the blood are among the internal causes.

Allergic contact dermatitis A reaction that occurs in people allergic to substances such as nickel. An estimated one in four people in the UK is affected by nickel-induced contact dermatitis. Common irritants include perfume, chromium and some plants, especially cacti and varieties of the primula family.

Irritant dermatitis This may occur in anyone whose skin comes into contact with chemical irritants such as acids, alkalis, solvents and detergents.

Chronic actinic dermatitis A relatively rare form of allergy to sunlight. Severe cases can also be triggered by exposure to artificial lighting.

Pompholyx Blisters form on the hands and feet in this acute form of dermatitis. It may be caused by wearing powdered natural rubber latex gloves. Using powder-free, non-latex gloves usually solves the problem.

Dermatitis herpetiformis This is an itching, blistering, symmetrical rash that usually appears on the knees, elbows, buttocks or shoulders, and is associated with sensitivity to gluten, which is found in bread and other grain products. Sufferers are advised to adopt a gluten-free diet.

Atopic dermatitis Also known as eczema, atopic dermatitis is an inherited tendency that affects people with a family history of disorders such as asthma, eczema and hay fever. It causes very dry, intensely itchy skin and in severe cases eruptions and crusting of the skin. Atopic dermatitis is associated with the presence of certain antibodies in the blood.

Detached retina

The retina is the light-sensitive membrane at the back of the eye. When it becomes partially separated from its underlying bed, the condition is called a detached retina. It usually occurs because a hole or tear in the retina has allowed fluid to accumulate behind it, and the pressure of the fluid forces the retina away from its bed.

SYMPTOMS

Symptoms include seeing:
- unusual flashing lights;
- a shower of dark floating spots;
- a large floating ring;
- a black curtain with a sharp, curved edge that appears to move inwards from the periphery of vision, obscuring all vision beyond its edge.

If you have the condition and it is not treated, you will lose all useful vision in the affected eye. The more quickly you have an eye operation, the better the prognosis.

CAUSES

The development of a detached retina is often preceded by degenerative changes in the retina that result in holes or tears. The main causes are:
- severe short-sightedness (myopia);
- a penetrating injury to the eyeball;
- abnormalities in the eye's vitreous humour, the transparent, jelly-like substance contained in the vitreous cavity behind the eye's lens;
- a tumour in the eye;
- **eclampsia** (convulsions in pregnancy);
- diabetic retinopathy (see **Diabetes**).

In some cases, eye injury that results in a detached retina can be caused by a heavy blow to the head.

TREATMENT

Treatment usually involves an operation to seal off holes in the retina. This may be carried out using a freezing probe or a laser.

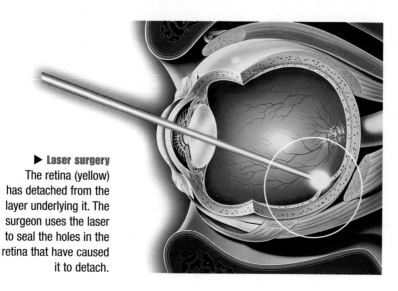

▶ Laser surgery
The retina (yellow) has detached from the layer underlying it. The surgeon uses the laser to seal the holes in the retina that have caused it to detach.

PREVENTION

Anyone at risk should have regular eye examinations with an optometrist.

OUTLOOK

With effective surgery, the recovery prospects are excellent.

SEE ALSO *Eye and problems*

Detoxification

Detoxification is the removal or neutralization of toxic or poisonous substances from the body. This is a natural function carried out by the liver to counteract the effects of potentially harmful substances – including drugs and alcohol. The term is also used to mean a process of withdrawal from alcohol or drugs under medical supervision. Its meaning has further expanded from there to include various minimal dietary regimes used in complementary medicine and nutritional therapy and aimed at cleansing the body internally.

Medically supervised detoxification is used for drug addiction where unpleasant symptoms of withdrawal such as **delirium** are likely to occur once drug intake is stopped. It is used particularly for addiction to alcohol – the process is colloquially known as 'drying out'.
- The supervised detoxification process usually involves a stay as an in-patient at a psychiatric hospital or special treatment unit.
- The body is weaned off the substance in a controlled environment in which the addicted person is isolated from any temptations to relapse, and doctors can help to control distressing symptoms.
- Once the substance has been removed from the body, longer-term treatment and counselling will usually be needed to ensure continued abstinence.

SEE ALSO *Alcohol and abuse; Drugs, misuse of; Liver and disorders*

Diabetes

Diabetes is the name given to two metabolic disorders, the most common form is diabetes mellitus. Diabetes insipidus is much rarer but both are characterized by excessive thirst and increased urination.

In the UK, around 1.4 million people are known to have diabetes mellitus, and it is thought at least a million more people have the condition without being aware of it. This is because the most common form of the condition (known as Type 2 diabetes) may produce only mild symptoms, so it can easily be overlooked.

Diabetes mellitus

Diabetes mellitus is the most common disorder affecting the glands of the **endocrine system**. It is caused by a shortage or lack of the hormone insulin produced by the pancreas. The body uses insulin to absorb glucose into cells, and a deficiency leads to abnormally high levels of glucose in the blood and the urine. This causes problems and defects in various parts of the body. There are two main types of diabetes mellitus: Type 1 and Type 2.

■ **Type 1** This is also known as insulin-dependent or juvenile diabetes. In most cases it first appears under the age of 40, and it is commonly discovered in teenagers. The onset is usually sudden – the production of insulin completely halts due to the destruction of pancreatic cells.

■ **Type 2** Non insulin-dependent diabetes is also known as late-onset diabetes as it commonly affects people over the age of 40. It occurs when the insulin produced is not sufficient for the body's needs. The body may be insulin-resistant, in which case the cells are unable to respond to normal levels of insulin. At first the pancreas tries to right the situation by producing more insulin, but it is unable to keep this up over time, and eventually it is unable to release enough to keep the blood glucose levels stable.

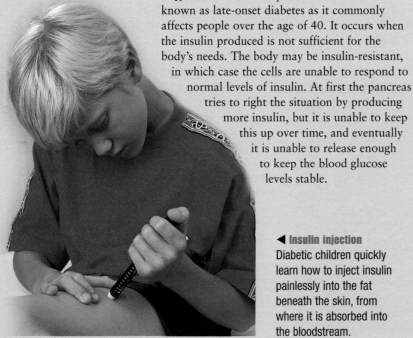

◄ Insulin injection
Diabetic children quickly learn how to inject insulin painlessly into the fat beneath the skin, from where it is absorbed into the bloodstream.

CAUSES AND RISK FACTORS

Genes play a part in both types of diabetes mellitus, but environmental factors are thought to be the triggers. Of the people who inherit the genes for Type 1 diabetes, only a small proportion actually develop the condition. Many people newly diagnosed with Type 1 diabetes have antibodies to a protein found in cow's milk, leading some researchers to suggest that feeding babies with formula milk may trigger the immune system to destroy pancreatic cells. It is more commonly thought that Type 1 diabetes occurs as a result of a viral infection that damages the pancreas.

Type 2 is by far the most common form of diabetes mellitus. Risk factors include a family history of diabetes, increasing age and being of Asian or Afro-Caribbean origin. Being overweight, particularly if you store fat around the waist, is another risk factor as **obesity** is known to increase insulin resistance. Weight loss and keeping active reduce insulin resistance.

Globally, the number of people who have this form of diabetes is rising. This is attributed to the fact that people in the developed world are increasingly inactive and overweight.

SYMPTOMS

The following symptoms are associated with uncontrolled Type 1 and Type 2 diabetes due to excessive levels of glucose in the blood (**hyperglycaemia**). People with Type 2 diabetes may experience only some of the symptoms, or only in a mild form, leading many to be unaware that they have the condition. The symptoms include increased urination (polyuria), excessive thirst (polydipsia), fatigue, unexplained weight loss, genital itching or thrush, blurred vision and tingling in the hands and feet.

DIAGNOSIS AND MANAGEMENT

Diabetes is diagnosed by a blood test to check for glucose. A urine sample may be taken and a glucose-tolerance test may also be performed. Type 1 diabetes is more easily identified than Type 2, which may go undetected for between nine and twelve years.

People with Type 1 diabetes always need to inject insulin because their body is unable to make the hormone. They inject up to five times a day, depending on their lifestyle. They also need to follow a balanced diet to ensure that their blood sugar levels are stable and do not fluctuate too widely.

Initially, people with Type 2 diabetes are often able to control their symptoms with regular injections of insulin. Diet, regular exercise, weight loss (if necessary) and oral medication to help the body utilize insulin more efficiently all play a part in managing the condition. As the condition progresses, people may have to rely on insulin injections to balance their blood sugar. Possible future alternatives to injected insulin include nasal and oral sprays, patches, tablets and inhalers.

COMPLICATIONS AND OUTLOOK

Most people with diabetes lead a healthy life. However, there is a risk of serious complications if the condition is not tightly controlled. A short-term risk in Type 1 diabetes is ketoacidotic coma.

Diet and exercise to control diabetes

People with diabetes should pay careful attention to diet and activity levels.

The diet should be the same as is recommended for general health, with plenty of fresh fruit and vegetables, wholegrain cereals and pulses, some low-fat protein, less saturated fat (choose poly-unsaturated and monounsaturated varieties), and a minimum of fatty, sugary foods and salt. Eating regularly helps to maintain stable blood glucose levels, and regular exercise is important for managing the diabetes. It can also help to control blood glucose and blood pressure, strengthen the heart and lungs and aid weight control.

This is the result of the body breaking down fat and muscle to create energy normally provided by glucose.

Both types of diabetes can lead to complications from the effects of persistently raised levels of blood glucose on the body's blood vessels and nerves. These include coronary heart disease, **stroke** and kidney disease, as well as nerve damage and lack of blood supply to the feet, which in severe cases can result in amputation. Diabetic retinopathy, a disease of the retina, can lead to **blindness**. It is the most common cause of blindness in people aged 20–65 in the UK.

Pregnancy and diabetes

Gestational diabetes mellitus (GDM) affects a small number of pregnant women. It usually develops during the second or third trimester as a result of the body's failure to produce enough insulin to meet the extra demands of pregnancy. Although blood glucose levels usually return to normal after delivery, women who have had GDM have a higher risk of developing Type 2 diabetes in later life.

Pregnant women with diabetes must control their blood glucose level prior to conception and throughout pregnancy to avoid the risk of complications. Too much glucose in the bloodstream increases the risk of malformation. In addition, the baby may grow too big and need to be delivered by Caesarean section.

Diabetes insipidus

Diabetes insipidus is a completely separate disorder from diabetes mellitus. The similar names derive from the fact that excessive urination is a symptom of both (diabetes means overflow). Thirst is the other main symptom. In diabetes insipidus these symptoms are caused by an imbalance of antidiuretic hormone (ADH), or vasopressin, which is stored in the pituitary gland and maintains the fluid balance within the body.

There are four types. Neurogenic diabetes insipidus is caused by a deficiency of ADH, while the nephrogenic form is caused by an inability of the kidneys to respond to ADH. The third type, gestagenic, appears during pregnancy and the fourth, called dipsogenic, is caused by abnormal thirst and excessive intake of fluids.

The treatment depends on the cause. In some types, a synthetic form of ADH is taken in a nasal spray or tablet. For sufferers of the dipsogenic form of the disease, the only treatment is limitation of fluid intake with, occasionally, a small dose of synthetic ADH at night.

In the UK, diabetes mellitus is up to five times more common among people of Afro-Caribbean and Asian origin than it is among the European population.

Dialysis

Dialysis is a medical procedure that artificially cleans the blood of people whose kidneys have stopped functioning. Normally, the kidneys filter poisonous waste products such as urea, together with excess salts, minerals and water from the blood to form urine. The urine is then excreted from the body. When the kidneys fail, these waste products accumulate in the blood and, if not treated, this can be fatal.

Kidney failure usually develops slowly, and in its early stages can be treated with drugs and by controlling your diet and daily liquid intake. You may be prescribed drugs to to control blood pressure and balance blood acidity. A dietician may advise you to reduce your salt intake or to eat fewer protein-rich foods such as fish, meat, cheese, milk and eggs. People in the early stages of kidney failure are advised to drink around 3 litres (5 pints) of liquid daily.

Dialysis is given in severe cases of kidney failure, either until the kidneys recover or until a donor kidney becomes available for transplantation.

HOW DIALYSIS WORKS

Dialysis works by passing the patient's blood over one side of a semi-porous membrane while the other side of the membrane is washed with a purifying solution known as dialysate. The pores in the membrane allow the molecules of waste products into the dialysate while holding back the larger blood cells and proteins. The dialysate and waste products are then drained and discarded.

There are two main types of dialysis: peritoneal dialysis and haemodialysis (see box). For the first type, a catheter must be inserted through the abdominal wall into your abdominal cavity. This is done in a short operation in hospital under general anaesthetic. You will usually be allowed to return home within two days of the operation. Around two weeks later you will begin a week-long training programme in how to perform peritoneal dialysis..

Most patients undergoing haemodialysis have a short operation to have a sterile, closeable opening (fistula) made in their arm through which a good flow of blood can exit to the dialysis machine. The operation is performed in hospital under local or general anaesthetic. Dialysis centres in hospitals are staffed by specialist nurses, and which type of dialysis is used depends on their assessment of your condition. The nurses may visit you at home to explain the practicalities of your treatment and how to fit it into your routine with the least disruption. Family members and close friends can attend these sessions with you if you wish.

Peritoneal dialysis

Once you have learned how to do it, peritoneal dialysis can usually be self administered and carried out at home or during breaks at work.

Continuous ambulatory peritoneal dialysis (CAPD) uses the membrane that surrounds the abdominal organs (the peritoneum) to filter blood, the task usually carried out by the kidneys.

A catheter is passed through an opening in the abdominal wall. Three or four times a day, a bag of dialysate is attached to the catheter by means of a plastic tube. It is then held aloft so that the fluid can run into the abdominal cavity.

The emptied bag is detached, and waste products and excess water in the blood are left to pass across the membrane and into the dialysate fluid.

After 3–4 hours, the fluid containing these toxins is drained back into the bag and discarded. The process lasts 30–40 minutes.

A variant of this process is called automated peritoneal dialysis (APD). It is done at night over 8–9 hours; most people learn to sleep while their blood is being filtered.

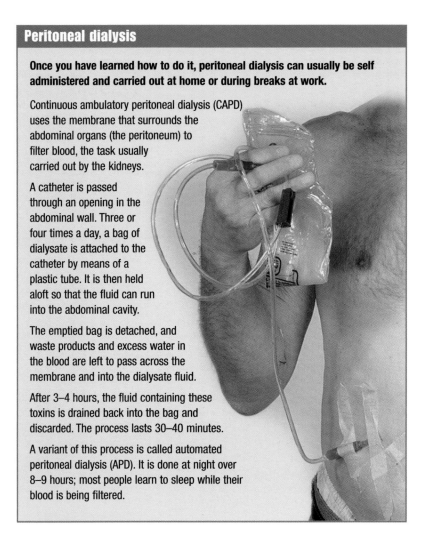

LIVING WITH DIALYSIS

Beginning dialysis treatment does not mean you have to give up your usual occupation. Nurses and doctors encourage dialysis patients to continue their normal activities as before and many employers will agree to adjust your schedule so that you can perform CAPD (continuous ambulatory peritoneal dialysis) or attend a dialysis centre for haemodialysis. However, heavy physical labour is not advised and some people with very demanding jobs – such as building labourers or packers – may need to leave the job on medical grounds.

You should be able to continue driving, although doctors will advise you not to drive immediately after haemodialysis during the first two months of treatment. The medical team will encourage you to exercise and maintain fitness for the general benefit of your health but contact sports such as football or rugby are not recommended for dialysis patients with a fistula because of the risk of damaging it. If you smoke, you will be strongly advised to stop because of the damage the habit does to your lungs and heart.

Haemodialysis

Haemodialysis treatment requires the patient to be connected to a dialysis machine.

It is usually carried out in a dialysis centre, but some people treat themselves at home.

In haemodialysis, an artificial membrane made of cellulose is used to cleanse the blood. An initial operation is necessary to make an opening in the arm, giving access to the vein. During haemodialysis, blood flows from the vein, via tubing, into one side of the artificial membrane, which is attached to a machine.

Dialysate fluid flows into the other side of the membrane. Toxins and excess water from the blood can then pass across the membrane into the dialysate fluid. Once the blood has been filtered, it is returned to the body. The dialysate fluid is discarded.

The whole process takes about 3–4 hours. It usually needs to be done three times a week.

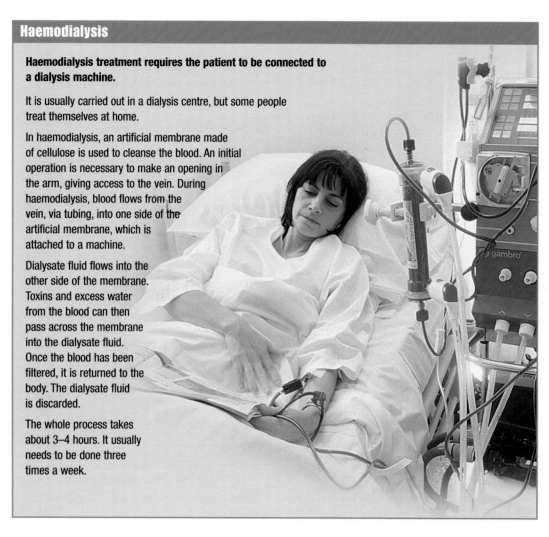

The role of diet

If you are undergoing haemodialysis, you will be on the kidney machine for an average of 12 hours a week. For the rest of the time your kidneys will not be efficiently filtering waste products from your blood. You need to follow a limited diet to control production of waste and fluid. You can eat normal amounts of protein, but must restrict potassium (found in chocolate, fruit and potatoes) and salt. You will be prescribed drugs to prevent excretion of phophates (phosphate binders). The amount of liquid you can drink depends on the amount of urine you produce each day – this varies between individuals and may change after you start treatment. During your training period on the treatment your urine production will be monitored. You will then be given a liquid allowance – 500ml (⅘ pint) daily plus a volume equal to the amount of urine produced.

If you are undergoing peritoneal dialysis, you must be careful to eat enough protein, as each time you drain the dialysate you lose protein. Eat plenty of high-protein foods such as chicken, eggs and fish. There are no limits on potassium-rich foods, and there is usually no need for phosphate binders. You will be given a daily liquid limit. Too much liquid necessitates a stronger mixture of dialysate, which damages the peritoneum over time. Dialysis patients are allowed to drink alcohol in moderation, but it must be counted as part of your diet and fluid allowance.

OUTLOOK

Your kidney function may improve, but if it does not you will have to continue dialysis for life unless you have a kidney transplant. Your medical team will discuss with you whether you are suitable for a transplant. This is usually considered the best option because it can restore your health to its level before you developed kidney disease. The general health of long-term dialysis patients will be closely monitored. Long-term haemodialysis can lead to high blood pressure (hypertension), anaemia and cardiovascular problems. Some people taking peritoneal dialysis in the long term develop an inflamed peritoneum (peritonitis).

SEE ALSO *Blood and disorders; Kidneys and disorders; Transplants*

In the UK over 180,000 people of all ages are affected by kidney disease. Each year almost 6,000 people are newly diagnosed.

Diaphragm and disorders

The purpose of the diaphragm is to work the lungs in the breathing process. As the diaphragm contracts, its shape becomes flatter increasing the volume of the chest cavity. Atmospheric pressure then forces air into the lungs, which expand to fill the space. The diaphragm then relaxes and pushes upwards, deflating the lungs and causing the person to breathe out.

WHAT CAN GO WRONG

Problems arise when the stomach or other abdominal organs push up through the abdomen.

Hiatus hernia

When part of the stomach juts up through the diaphragm into the chest cavity, the condition is known as a hiatus hernia. The cause is not known, but risk factors seem to be increasing age, obesity and smoking, all of which may weaken the diaphragm.

Often a hiatus hernia has no symptoms. Where there are symptoms, these include:
- chest pain;
- **heartburn;**
- difficulty in swallowing;
- belching.

You may be able to reduce heartburn by losing weight if you are overweight, refraining from large meals and spicy foods, eating at least 2–3 hours before lying down and not wearing tight clothes.

Treatments are given to reduce stomach acidity and to strengthen the opening from the stomach. Surgery may be necessary if symptoms persist or if complications such as gastro-oesophageal reflux occur. In gastro-oesophageal reflux, the contents of the stomach pass back into the oesophagus.

Diaphragmatic hernia

In some babies the diaphragm does not form properly, with the result that one of the abdominal organs pushes up into the chest cavity. This generally leads to a collapsed lung. Symptoms include:
- severe breathing difficulties;
- skin turning blueish;
- pauses in breathing.

If your child has any of these symptoms, seek urgent medical advice.

Paralysis of the diaphragm

This condition most commonly affects babies, particularly those born in the breech position or with the aid of instruments. If the muscles of the diaphragm weaken, the contents of the abdomen push up into the chest cavity. Breathing capacity, especially when lying down, can be significantly reduced. A typical symptom is night-time breathlessness.

SEE ALSO *Chest pain; Respiratory system*

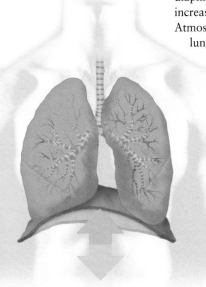

▲ **Flexible muscle**
The diaphragm is attached to the lower ribs at the sides and to the breastbone and backbone at the front and back. When it relaxes it forms a dome shape, forcing air out of the lungs. When it contracts , it flattens out and moves downwards, causing the lungs to fill with air.

Diarrhoea

Diarrhoea is the frequent passage of loose, watery stools, often with explosive bowel movements. It is a common symptom of a wide range of conditions. Travellers' diarrhoea is one of the commonest illnesses experienced in tropical or subtropical countries (see **Travel and tropical disease**).

Diarrhoea can be very serious in babies and in elderly people because of the associated dangers of **dehydration**. It kills more than 3 million children each year, mainly in developing countries.

SYMPTOMS
- Frequent, loose, watery bowel movements.
- Abdominal pain (sometimes).
- Fever (sometimes).
- Nausea and vomiting (sometimes).
- Loss of appetite (sometimes).
- Dehydration – signs that a person is dehydrated include concentrated dark urine, dry skin and mouth, loss of skin elasticity, sunken eyes and, in severe cases, lightheadedness or confusion.

DURATION
- Acute diarrhoea comes on suddenly and lasts from a few hours to two or three days.
- Chronic diarrhoea can last for more than three weeks and may recur.

CAUSES
Diarrhoea is a symptom of many illnesses.
- Bacterial and viral infections that irritate the intestinal lining, with the result that more fluid passes from the blood into the intestines.
- Food that is contaminated, usually by *Staphylococcus* bacteria (see **Food poisoning**).
- A food allergy, such as hypersensitivity to gluten in wheat, or lactose or glucose intolerance (see **Coeliac disease; Allergies**).
- Anxiety and **stress**.
- A reaction to certain **drugs** such as antibiotics, some antacids, and blood pressure and arthritis medications.
- The abuse of laxatives.
- More rarely, **dysentery** or **typhoid fever**.
- Chronic and debilitating diarrhoea may be caused by intestinal disorders such as **Crohn's disease** and **colitis**.

TREATMENT
You can usually treat diarrhoea at home using over-the-counter medicines.

How to deal with diarrhoea in babies and toddlers

Diarrhoea in babies is normally caused by a viral infection. Other causes include lactose intolerance and coeliac disease (gluten-sensitive enteropathy).

- Check there is nothing irritating in your child's diet – or yours if you are breastfeeding.

- Give plenty of fluids but do not give solid food.

- Give oral rehydration sachets, available from the chemist, dissolved in water that has been boiled.

- Gradually re-introduce solid foods for toddlers when the diarrhoea stops.

- Wash your hands thoroughly after handling or changing your child.

Call a doctor

- If there are signs of dehydration.

- If your child is vomiting, feels pain, is not gaining weight or has blood in his or her stools.

- If your child has a high fever or is floppy.

What a doctor may do

- Prescribe a special baby milk containing no sugars.

- Refer the child to a paediatrician.

What you can do

- Rest, take 3–4 litres (5–7 pints) of fluids a day and avoid food, especially dairy products.
- Buy oral rehydration sachets from your pharmacist. Alternatively, make up a solution of 4 level teaspoons of sugar and ½ a level teaspoon of salt dissolved in 1 litre (1.75 pints) of clean water.
- Take over-the-counter antidiarrhoeal medicines unless you have blood or pus in your motions.

When to consult a doctor

Go to your doctor if:
- diarrhoea lasts more than 24 hours in a baby or in frail or elderly people;
- there is blood or pus in your motions;
- symptoms are severe and persist for longer than three days;
- others are simultaneously affected;
- you have returned recently from abroad;
- there are signs of dehydration.

What a doctor may do
- Prescribe oral rehydration salts.
- Prescribe an antidiarrhoeal drug, such as loperamide.
- Arrange for testing of the faeces.

Complementary therapies
Relaxation techniques and meditation may be helpful if diarrhoea is stress-related.

PREVENTION
Follow good hygiene practices. Wash your hands thoroughly after using the lavatory and make sure children do the same.

COMPLICATIONS
Dehydration can be life-threatening, especially in babies or elderly people.

OUTLOOK
Most people recover from an acute attack within a few days with no side effects.

Diathermy

Diathermy is the use of a high-frequency electrical current to generate heat within the body to treat certain conditions. The current passes between the electrodes which are placed on the skin. To treat rheumatic conditions and sciatica, diathermy skin pads are used. These direct a diffuse heat inward to body tissues – stimulating blood flow and promoting healing. Powerful currents concentrated at a point with a diathermy needle or knife can be used to destroy tumours, warts, ulcers and polyps.

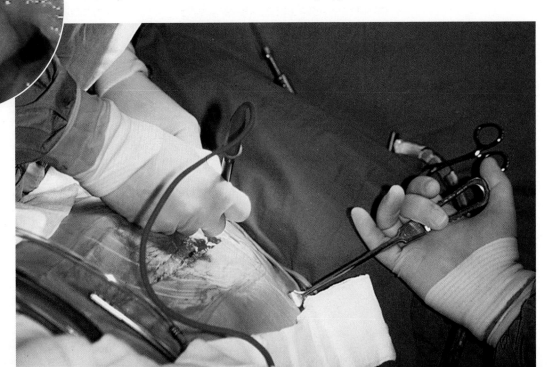

▲ **Diathermy**
The intense heat generated by a diathermy needle can be used to stop bleeding during conventional surgery or bloodlessly to destroy an ulcer (right). The electricity used in diathermy runs at 10 to 25,000 million oscillations per second.

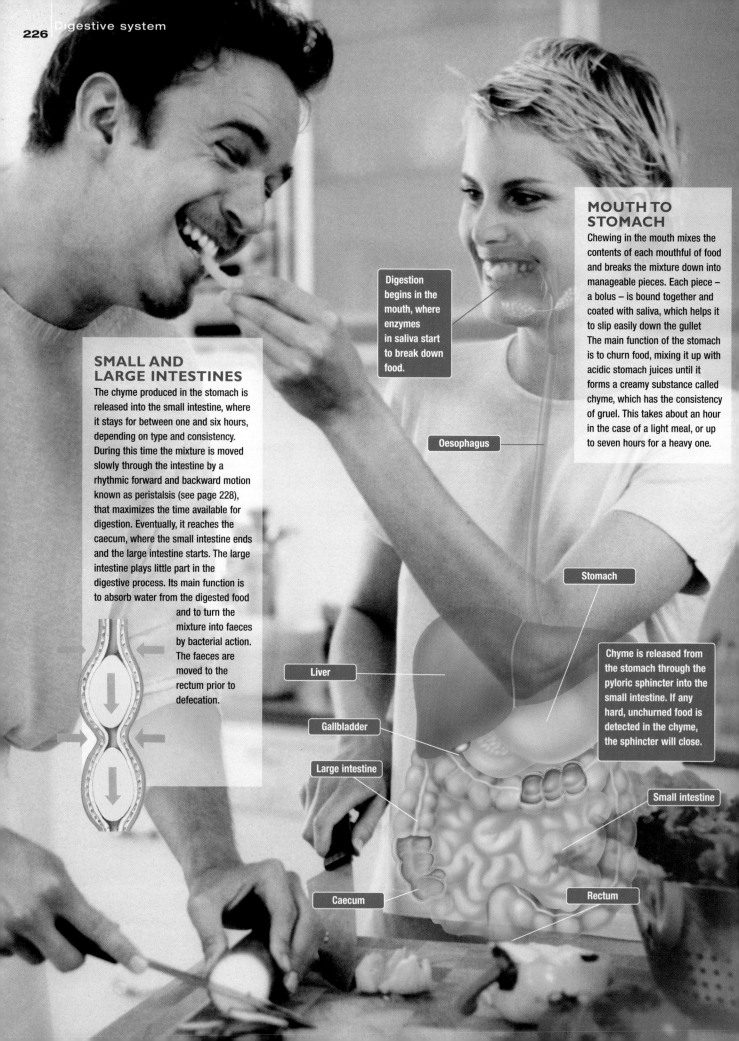

MOUTH TO STOMACH

Chewing in the mouth mixes the contents of each mouthful of food and breaks the mixture down into manageable pieces. Each piece – a bolus – is bound together and coated with saliva, which helps it to slip easily down the gullet The main function of the stomach is to churn food, mixing it up with acidic stomach juices until it forms a creamy substance called chyme, which has the consistency of gruel. This takes about an hour in the case of a light meal, or up to seven hours for a heavy one.

Digestion begins in the mouth, where enzymes in saliva start to break down food.

Oesophagus

SMALL AND LARGE INTESTINES

The chyme produced in the stomach is released into the small intestine, where it stays for between one and six hours, depending on type and consistency. During this time the mixture is moved slowly through the intestine by a rhythmic forward and backward motion known as peristalsis (see page 228), that maximizes the time available for digestion. Eventually, it reaches the caecum, where the small intestine ends and the large intestine starts. The large intestine plays little part in the digestive process. Its main function is to absorb water from the digested food and to turn the mixture into faeces by bacterial action. The faeces are moved to the rectum prior to defecation.

Stomach

Chyme is released from the stomach through the pyloric sphincter into the small intestine. If any hard, unchurned food is detected in the chyme, the sphincter will close.

Liver

Small intestine

Gallbladder

Large intestine

Caecum

Rectum

Digestive system

The digestive system consists of a 6.5m (21ft) tube called the digestive tract, which runs from mouth to anus, together with the pancreas, liver and gallbladder. Problems can affect any part of the system.

In the digestive tract, food is broken down so that the sugars, fats, proteins, minerals, vitamins and water that it contains may be absorbed into the blood and used to fuel the body. People usually think of digestion as taking place in the stomach. But in fact it occurs mainly in the intestines, where most of the nutrients are absorbed. The enormous surface area of the lining of the small intestine, together with the thinness of the lining, and the closeness of the interior blood and lymph vessels to it, make absorption possible.

The motion that passes out at the anus consists of the unuseable elements of food – mainly cellulose – and the bacteria that aid the breakdown of food in the intestines. However, even though some elements of food do not nourish the body they do play an important part in digestion. The roughage, or fibre, in food helps to carry away wastes and may even help to protect against diverticular disease and cancer of the colon and rectum.

THE DIGESTIVE TRACT

Food may take many hours to pass along the convoluted, looping and twisting tube of the digestive tract from the mouth to the anus via the oesophagus, the stomach and the small and large intestines. The muscular walls of the tube contract rhythmically to propel the food along, while a series of valves normally prevent digested or semi-digested food from passing in the wrong direction, back up the tract to the mouth.

Blood carried by arteries to the intestines flows through capillaries in the villi, where it picks up absorbed nutrients. The nutrient-rich blood is then delivered by veins to the liver for further digestion. Lymph vessels transport digested fats from the villi into the bloodstream.

SPECIALIZED LINING

The stomach is lined with glands that secrete the gastric juices involved in the digestion of food (see page 387). The glands open into the main stomach cavity through gastric pits, which are visible in this micrographic image as dark holes. The lining of the small intestine contains numerous fingerlike projections called villi. These are made up of cells that are specialized for absorbing nutrients.

How the body regulates digestion

Unconscious processes govern our appetite and the breaking down of nutrients in the food we eat.

Your appetite for food is a biological response. The hypothalamus, one of the parts of your brain that governs unconscious responses, monitors the levels of glucose circulating in your blood. When levels of blood glucose fall, the hypothalamus sends messages both to the higher centres of your brain in the cerebrum , which makes you think consciously of the need for food, and to your digestive system, preparing it for action. (see **Brain and nervous system**).

Normally, you then find and eat some food, your blood glucose levels rise and the situation is stabilized. However, if you don't eat anything the signals from the hypothalamus become stronger. Your stomach starts to rumble and your appetite slowly starts to turn to hunger. As this grows sharper, you may feel hunger contractions, in which the muscles of your stomach wall contract forcefully for several minutes, causing you quite considerable discomfort.

HOW FOOD MOVES THROUGH THE SYSTEM

Rhythmic muscular movements, known as peristalsis, move the products of digestion through the digestive tract. The muscles in the walls of the digestive tract contract and relax in a rhythm which is controlled by the autonomic (unconscious) nervous system. The muscles in front of a parcel of food relax, while the ones behind it contract – and the result is a rippling, wave-like motion that moves food through the system. Food in the stomach is churned back and forth by three layers of muscle, so that it is thoroughly mixed. In the small intestine, food is moved more slowly and in both directions so that more time is allowed for digestion and absorption of nutrients. The muscles of the large intestine contract only a few times a day, usually after a meal. This is a forceful wave of contractions that pushes waste products down to the rectum so that they can be expelled when we defecate.

Factfile

Digestive enzymes and bacteria

Enzymes present in the small intestine break down large, complex molecules of food into simpler molecules that are small enough to pass through the intestinal wall into the blood.

Intestinal enzymes help to break down sugars from carbohydrate into glucose, the simplest form of sugar, and proteins into amino acids, their most basic chemical form. They also help to split fats into their constituent fatty acids. Helpful bacteria, called probiotics, live in the digestive tract and play a vital role in breaking down the chemicals there.

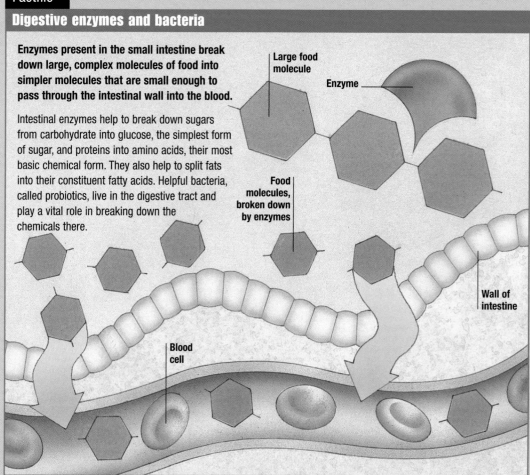

Large food molecule

Enzyme

Food molecules, broken down by enzymes

Wall of intestine

Blood cell

What can go wrong

Damage to the liver, pancreas, or intestinal lining can cause painful disruptions of digestion and, ultimately, nutritional problems.

The most common cause of disruption to digestion and the absorption of nutrients is damage to the lining of the intestine or another part of the digestive tract.

Gastroenteritis is inflammation of the lining of the stomach and intestines. It leads to vomiting and diarrhoea, usually with abdominal cramps and colicky pains, a slightly raised temperature and perspiration. Traces of blood are sometimes found in vomit or stools. It is caused by bacterial or virus infection, usually from half-cooked or reheated food.

Gastritis is irritation of the stomach lining. It may be either acute (caused by something a person has eaten or drunk) or chronic (long-term and not linked to a specific incident). It also causes pain in the upper abdomen, nausea, vomiting and diarrhoea.

Ileitis, also known as **Crohn's disease**, is inflammation of the lower part of the small intestine. The cause is not known. Parts of the intestinal wall thicken and infection or ulcers may develop. It causes chronic diarrhoea, which is associated with poor appetite, fever, weight loss and abdominal pain. Sometimes ileitis may be mistaken for acute **appendicitis**.

Colitis is long-term inflammation of the colon (large intestine), which causes ulcers to form. It can cause frequent bloody diarrhoea, with fever, poor appetite, loss of weight and anaemia.

PROBLEMS WITH DIGESTIVE ENZYMES

Less common causes of digestive problems are metabolic disorders, in which there is a deficiency of one or more of the digestive enzymes. In addition, any problem that affects the pancreas, such as cancer or chronic inflammation, is likely to disrupt the supply of pancreatic enzymes to the small intestine and disturb the process of digestion there. Secretions from the pancreas are released in response to a hormone that starts to circulate when food is detected in the first part of the small intestine (the duodenum).

Similarly, diseases that affect the gallbladder or the liver will disrupt the supply of bile and so affect the body's ability to digest fats. Bile, which is produced in the liver and stored in the gallbladder, contains complex chemicals called bile salts, which help to break down fats into their constituents. Bile production is stimulated by a hormone whose release is triggered by the presence of fatty foods in the duodenum.

PHYSICAL PROBLEMS

Physical problems such as the twisting or displacement of the intestines also disrupt the digestive process. In a hiatus **hernia**, the stomach bulges through the diaphragm at the weakest point where the oesophagus passes through. The hernia is not visible and often symptomless – symptoms where present are those of indigestion (see below).

An **intussusception** is a twisted intestine, in which part of the intestine pushes inside the length of intestine next to it, like a glove finger turning inside itself. It is most common in babies under 12 months, and affects boys more than girls, causing severe pain, vomiting and passing of blood and mucus from the rectum. In adults it is far less common and occurs where there is a polyp or cancer within the bowel. Other physical problems that obstruct the bowel, such as impacted faeces and tumours, can also cause serious digestive problems. (see **Colorectal cancer**)

SYMPTOMS OF DIGESTIVE PROBLEMS

The general symptoms of mild digestive disorders are familiar to us all – **abdominal pain,** loss of appetite, **heartburn, indigestion, diarrhoea, constipation, nausea,** vomiting and flatulence. More serious ones include blood in the vomit or stools, weight loss and yellow skin or eyes.

See your doctor if there is a large amount of blood in vomit or motions, if you or a person for whom you are caring suffers prolonged or severe vomiting with abdominal pain or diarrhoea or if you notice a rapid deterioration in a baby or elderly person who is vomiting or has diarrhoea.

Dealing with indigestion

Doctors define indigestion as discomfort in the upper middle part of the abdomen, sometimes speading up behind the breastbone. It is associated with nausea and belching wind, which may bring acid up to the mouth. If you have these or similar symptoms, work out which foods make the pain worse and avoid them. Alcohol can provoke digestive problems and should never be taken to excess. Stress can make indigestion worse, as can eating irregularly and smoking. If you suffer from indigestion, do not take aspirin or any drug containing it, unless instructed to do so by your doctor – aspirin irritates the stomach. Always tell your doctor if the symptoms of your indigestion grow worse or change in nature.

SEE ALSO ***Bowel and disorders***

OTHER DISORDERS

Coeliac disease
This is a disorder in which an intolerance to gluten – a protein found in barley, rye and wheat – makes people unable to absorb essential nutrients from the intestines.

Diabetes
In this condition, the body cannot make full use of sugar and starches from the diet, because the pancreas is not producing enough of the hormone insulin. Sugar accumulates in the blood and tissues, causing defects in various parts of the body.

Diverticular disease
Diverticula are pouches that form in the mucous lining of the large intestine. They contain no muscle, so cannot be emptied by muscular contraction and may become infected.

Diphtheria

Diphtheria is a highly contagious bacterial infection that generally affects the throat but may also affect other mucous membranes and the skin. The bacteria release a toxin into the bloodstream; this toxin can obstruct the airways and damage the heart and nervous system. The infection is rare in most Western countries due to an effective vaccination programme.

SYMPTOMS
These can take the form of:
- sore throat;
- mild fever;
- tiredness;
- coughing and breathing difficulties;
- crusty scabs on the skin;
- enlarged lymph nodes in the neck;
- irregular heartbeat.

DURATION
The disease breaks out two to five days after infection. The affected person may be infectious for four weeks, sometimes longer.

CAUSES
The bacterium *Corynebacterium diphtheriae* is spread by coughs and sneezes. It can also be caught by touching people who have acquired immunity to the illness and may have no symptoms, but who harbour the organisms in their nose or skin (carriers).

TREATMENT
Early treatment is always required, so seek urgent medical advice at the earliest opportunity.

What a doctor may do
- Admit you to hospital.
- Prescribe **antibiotics** and diphtheria antitoxin.
- Treat complications as they arise.

Complementary therapies
Herbal remedies, including echinacea, may be used alongside orthodox medical treatment.

PREVENTION
The infection is best prevented by vaccination in childhood and boosters to maintain immunity.

COMPLICATIONS
The toxin produced by the diphtheria bacterium can cause asphyxiation and damage to the heart muscles or nervous system, resulting in heart failure or paralysis.

OUTLOOK
Diphtheria is potentially fatal, but most people recover fully with urgent medical treatment.

SEE ALSO *Bacterial infections*

Disability

Globally, almost one person in five has some kind of disability, ranging from mild impairments to severely disabling conditions.

Three-quarters of people affected by disability are mildly disabled: they are unable to do all the things they would like to do. One quarter are severely disabled, in that they cannot carry out the everyday activities associated with their age group, such as playing (in the case of children), going to work, or being able to look after themselves without assistance.

DEFINING DISABILITY
The term disability is used both as a general description and as a legal definition. There is an important difference between people with a temporary disability and those officially assessed and recognized as disabled. The latter are eligible to receive state benefits, which may include financial assistance with housing, nursing care, domestic help, physical aids such as wheelchairs, and concessions such as free parking.

Temporary incapacity due to acute illness does not usually qualify as disability, but repetitive functional impairment due to relapsing conditions such as **multiple sclerosis** or rheumatoid arthritis may do so. Certain disabilities may not be recognized as official disabilities. For example, the ten most common causes of disability in the developed world, as listed by the World Health Organization (see box, page 231), include alcohol abuse, depression and obsessive-compulsive disorders, but few people with these conditions are in receipt of disability benefits.

Disability may be primarily physical, marked by an inability to:
- sit, stand, or walk for long enough to allow the person to fulfil their daily tasks;
- lift or carry a weight;
- coordinate movements, such as manipulating objects by hand;
- remain alert for long periods without severe fatigue;
- breathe, eat and attend to bodily needs unaided;
- operate in a normal environment (for example, at normal temperature or both in and outside a building);
- see and hear well enough to function normally.

Or it may be primarily mental, marked by an inability to:
- understand, carry out or remember instructions;

Leading causes of disability in the developed world

Disability can have many causes and occur at any stage of life. It results in the inability to function normally because of physical or mental impairment.

■ **Depression** is the most common cause of disability worldwide, and affects between 13 and 15 per cent of the population. The condition is often overlooked because the symptoms are largely hidden.

■ **Alcohol abuse** affects about 10 per cent of people. This condition is rarely recognized as a disability.

■ **Osteoarthritis** affects 6 per cent of people. It is a progressive erosion of the bones in joints, preventing normal movement and causing chronic pain.

■ **Dementia** and other degenerative brain diseases, including Alzheimer's and Parkinson's diseases, affect about 5 per cent of people.

■ **Schizophrenia** affects 4 per cent of people. It is a brain disorder which, left untreated, causes apathy, paranoia, hallucinations and delusions.

■ **Manic depression** (bipolar disorder), a condition in which the affected person swings between depression and mania, affects 3.5 per cent of people.

■ **Cerebrovascular disease** (which affects the brain and its membranes) is a cause of disability in 3.2 per cent of people. It can take the form of a **stroke** or brain haemorrhage, and frequently causes brain damage.

■ **Diabetes**, mainly type 2, affects 3.1 per cent of people. Left untreated, this condition causes visual impairment and kidney disease.

■ **Obsessions and compulsions** affect 3.1 per cent of people. Sufferers cannot function normally because they are restricted by obsessive thoughts or compulsions to carry out repetitive actions.

■ **Drug abuse** is the cause of disability in 2.9 per cent of people. The adverse effects of drug abuse may cause permanent mental and physical incapacity.

■ communicate through speech and the written word;
■ maintain the appropriate mood in a changing situation;
■ attend to relevant stimuli;
■ maintain a grasp of reality free of hallucinations and delusions.

Many disabilities are the result of a combination of physical and mental factors caused by a primary brain disorder such as **cerebral palsy** or **Parkinson's disease**.

CHILDHOOD DISABILITY

About half a million children in the UK are clearly disabled, and many more have mental or physical impairments that may or may not be recognized as a disability. The most common types of recognized disability are listed below.

■ Inherited disorders – **Huntington's disease** and Duchenne **muscular dystrophy**, for example.
■ Developmental abnormalities – including **autism**, cerebral palsy and **growth disorders**.
■ Disease-related disabilities – such as those caused by **polio** and bacterial **meningitis**.
■ Accidental disabilities – for example, severe head injury and damaged or amputated limbs.

The importance of early intervention

Children are in some ways more liable to disability because their brains and bodies are more fragile than those of adults. However, because they are young and still growing they also have a greater ability to recover. Early medical intervention or therapy can often help to restore the use of damaged limbs or a disordered brain by 're-training' the developing system. It is therefore important that a child's disability is recognized as soon as possible. Early signs differ according to the type of disability involved – inherited conditions may be detected by genetic tests and developmental abnormalities may be spotted during routine postnatal tests to monitor a child's progress.

Children reach developmental milestones at different rates, so a child who seems to be lagging behind in things like crawling, walking or talking, may just be a late developer. Nonetheless, if parents notice that their child is different from others of the same age, they should take the child to a doctor for an assessment.

Obtaining assistance

Generally, all but the most severely disabled children are raised in the home environment. If a child is physically disabled, it may be necessary to provide aids such as a wheelchair or prosthetic appliances. Parents can usually get financial assistance with these, along with a disability caring allowance, from their local social services department. A number of high-tech devices have been developed for children who have severe movement and speech problems. They include electric wheelchairs, which allow the child to move around more independently and take part in most activities, including sports, and computers that can be operated by a

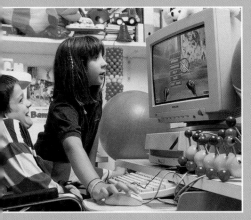

▼ **Self-expression**
Brain-activated computer technology can aid communication for people who are unable to use speech or the written word.

movement as slight as the blink of an eyelid. Such products are not widely available and parents may have difficulty finding them – charities devoted to the type of disability concerned are often the most fruitful sources of advice.

Equipment can also be obtained through Motability. This is a charity partnership between the Government and charitable and private sectors that helps disabled people to become more mobile. Most schools can accept disabled children, but special schools are available for those who are unable to attend mainstream classes.

Children with severe mental disabilities may need such intensive supervision and special care that it is not feasible for them to live at home. This is particularly true of those with severe autism, for whom there are special institutions where they can live safely.

DISABILITY AND AGEING
Advances in medicine have made it possible for people to live longer than they did in previous generations, and there is a greater proportion of elderly people in the community than ever before. The likelihood of developing a degenerative illness such as osteoarthritis, **Parkinson's disease**, **Alzheimer's disease** and **osteoporosis** increases sharply with age, and a disproportionate number of elderly people are therefore disabled.

Assistance in later life
Older people with minor disabilities can often live independently provided that they have immediate access to help if the need arises. Most local authorities, and some charities and private organizations, can provide a panic button, which is installed in the home or worn around the neck. A person can use it to summon help in an emergency. The local authority may provide a nurse or carer to call in on a daily basis to help with washing and dressing, or at less frequent intervals to help with household chores and shopping. Meal delivery services ensure that an elderly person's minimum nutritional requirements are met, and many charities provide volunteers to help elderly people with various aspects of living.

TREATMENT AND PREVENTION
Treatment of a disability will depend on its cause, and in many cases there is no cure. However, several experimental medical techniques provide some hope for people with disabilities that are currently untreatable. They include:
■ electrical implants, which have been used with some success to take over the functions of lost nerve cells (for example, in Parkinson's disease);
■ specialized techniques to repair nerves damaged by spinal injuries;
■ antitoxic drugs, which may help to prevent brain damage caused by the release of neurotoxins after **stroke**;
■ gene therapy, which is being developed to treat disorders caused by single-gene mutations, such as Huntington's disease;
■ stem cell therapy, which may be used to rebuild damaged or lost tissue resulting from degenerative diseases.

Prevention of age-related disabilities
Many of the most common causes of age-related disability can be prevented by good self-care and appropriate medical intervention when the disability is at an early stage of development.
■ Heart disease and **stroke**, for example, may be prevented by adherence to a regular exercise regime and a diet rich in antioxidants. A wide range of drugs is available to relieve symptoms of these diseases.
■ Osteoporosis can be prevented to some degree by **hormone replacement therapy** in women and a high intake (starting as early as possible) of calcium-rich foods and regular weight-bearing exercise.
■ Joint immobility can be minimized by undertaking exercise that gently stretches the limbs, such as swimming.
■ **Depression** may be prevented by mental activity, social interaction and antidepressant drugs.
■ Falls are a major cause of illness and subsequent disability in elderly people. The likelihood of falls can be reduced by using walking aids such as a walking stick or frame, and installing safety aids in the home.

SEE ALSO *Brain and nervous system; Cerebral palsy; Mental health and problems*

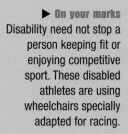

▶ **On your marks**
Disability need not stop a person keeping fit or enjoying competitive sport. These disabled athletes are using wheelchairs specially adapted for racing.

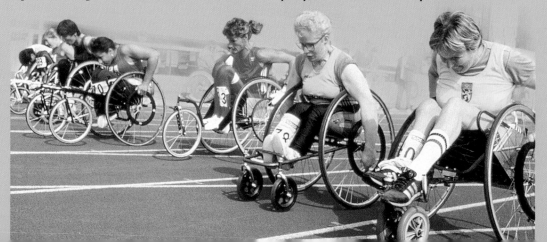

Diverticular disease

In the UK, 50 per cent of the population over 70 years old have diverticula, but in many cases the condition causes no trouble at all.

The term 'diverticular disease' describes conditions caused by sacs (diverticula) that protrude through the wall of the intestines. Diverticula occasionally form in the small intestine, but more usually in the colon. The cause is thought to be a lack of dietary fibre.

There are two forms of diverticular disease: diverticulosis and diverticulitis. Diverticulosis simply means that diverticula are present. Often there are no symptoms, but there may be **irritable bowel syndrome** with abdominal cramps and, occasionally, rectal bleeding. Treatment is with a high-fibre diet and antispasmodic **drugs**. Diverticulitis means that diverticula have become infected. Symptoms include pain, vomiting, fever and bowel problems, and **peritonitis** if the intestine perforates. Treatment is with antibiotics and, sometimes, surgery.

SEE ALSO *Bowel and disorders*

Dizziness

Dizziness is a common symptom, often defined as being a sensation of lightheadedness without the illusion of movement characteristic of **vertigo**. It often precedes fainting.

CAUSES
The causes of dizziness include:
- viral infection;
- low blood sugar;
- a drop in **blood pressure** on getting up (postural hypotension, which is common in elderly people and during pregnancy);
- reduced blood flow to the brain – seen in elderly people with osteoarthritis of the neck;
- anxiety and **hyperventilation**;
- intoxication with drugs or alcohol, and the effects of chronic alcohol misuse;
- occasionally, **carbon monoxide poisoning** (caused, for example, by a blocked flue in a domestic gas appliance).

DURATION
Dizziness usually starts suddenly, except in viral infection and anxiety, and lasts until the underlying cause settles down or is treated.

TREATMENT
The treatment varies depending on the cause. See your doctor if dizziness is continuous or recurs often. If other family members are affected, and domestic gas appliances are used, turn them off immediately and have them checked professionally for carbon monoxide emissions.

COMPLICATIONS
Usually none, unless the dizziness causes collapse resulting in injury.

Down's syndrome

Down's syndrome is a genetic disorder caused by the presence of an extra chromosome, giving a total of 47 instead of the usual 46. The extra chromosome is usually a duplicate of number 21, thus the most common form of Down's syndrome is also known as trisomy 21. This duplication mostly originates in the mother's egg, although in some cases it may be present in the fertilizing sperm.

Physical markers may include:
- a flattish face with downward sloping eyes, heavy eyelids, a broad flat nose, thick lips and small ears flattened back to the skull;
- a tongue which appears too large for the mouth cavity;
- thick, short hands and feet;
- undeveloped genitalia;
- short stature, weak muscles and slow growth.

Children born with Down's syndrome can have health problems, such as heart or inner ear defects, and may be more susceptible to anaemia and infectious illnesses.

There is always some degree of learning disability, but this varies considerably – IQ can be between 30 and 80, and is sometimes higher. The vast majority of Down's syndrome children learn to talk and an increasing number learn to read. Today, some even attend mainstream schools and go on to live semi-independent adult lives.

Overall, about one in every 1000 babies is born with Down's syndrome. The chance of having an affected child varies greatly according to the age of the parents, especially the mother. For women under 30 the likelihood is less than one in 1000, while for a woman over 45 the chance is more than one in 60.

OUTLOOK
In the past many people with Down's syndrome died in infancy, often as a result of untreatable internal abnormalities or infections. Today, most reach adulthood, thanks to medical advances and the greater willingness of health professionals to offer life-saving treatment, where necessary. Most children with Down's syndrome can now look forward to a lifespan of 60 years or more.

Down's syndrome is not a disease, so there is no treatment. However, greater understanding of the condition and changes in attitude towards it now mean that affected individuals are more likely to get the support they need to develop their potential and enjoy a full life.

SEE ALSO *Disability; Learning difficulties*

Drugs, misuse of

Drug misuse is the taking of drugs that can harm health, make it hard to function socially, or are simply illegal. It can lead to physical or psychological dependency on the drug, and may be a sign of other behavioural problems.

The misuse of drugs in the UK occurs in all sectors of society, particularly the taking of illegal drugs amongst younger people. Drug traffickers are known to target this age group providing easy access to cannabis, stimulants such as ecstacy, as well as a range of the more addictive drugs.

ADDICTIVE DRUGS

Not all drugs are addictive. Those that are will lead to a psychological – and sometimes physical – state which is characterized by a compulsion to take the drug. This is known as drug dependence. Addiction is a severe form of drug dependence. It is an actual physical need for the drug and results from changes in the body that have been caused by regularly taking that drug. Addiction is preceded by tolerance. Tolerance can develop to any drug if it is taken regularly. What it means in physical terms is that more of the drug is needed in order to achieve the same effects.

Some drugs, when used repeatedly, can cause withdrawal symptoms if suddenly stopped. In the case of opiates, withdrawal involves nausea, diarrhoea, pain and 'goose-flesh', though symptoms vary with the type of drug.

Psychological dependence is regarded as the compulsion to take a drug purely for the mind-altering effects, even in the absence of physical withdrawal symptoms.

Drugs producing major psychological and physical dependence include the opiates, nicotine, alcohol, benzodiazepines and barbiturates.

THE LEGAL POSITION

In the UK, drugs are regulated by the *Misuse of Drugs Act, 1971*, which makes illegal certain activities in relation to 'Controlled Drugs'. The penalties for offences involving the different drugs are graded broadly according to the perceived harmfulness of the drug when it is misused. For this purpose the drugs are defined as three classes, A, B and C.

Class A drugs are the most harmful. They include many opiates (opium, heroin, morphine, methadone, pethidine), cocaine, LSD, ecstasy, phencyclidine. They also include Class B drugs which have been prepared for use by injection.

Class B drugs include oral amphetamines, barbiturates, codeine and pholcodine.

Class C covers a broad of drugs related to the amphetamines, most benzodiazepines, and a number of drugs used in sport and body building, including androgenic steroids and anabolic steroids, and growth hormones (somatotropin, somatrem and somatropin).

In October 2001, the Government announced its intention of lowering the classification of cannabis to Class C. The main legal consequence of this is that the maximum legal penalties are reduced, for possession down to 2 years plus a fine, for supply down to 5 years plus a fine. This reclassification also reduces the powers of the police to stop and search anyone in the street for possession. It is expected that, in practice, the normal penalty for possession will simply be an informal police caution.

COMMONLY MISUSED DRUGS

Most drugs that can be described as being misued are taken to alter the user's state of mind. Some cause a depression or a calming of brain function, while others act as stimulants, elevating mood and reducing appetite and the need for sleep. Others have powerful hallucinogenic properties.

Relaxants and stimulants

The opiates, such as heroin, are some of the most powerful and popular relaxants. Initially they produce a state of euphoria, a general numbing of feeling and alleviation of pain. At higher doses, they bring drowsiness and sleep. A brown or white powder, heroin is often diluted with other substances and injected, sniffed or smoked.

Cannabis is also a relaxant, probably the most widely used. Although it causes some stimulation, giddiness and euphoria at first, this is quickly

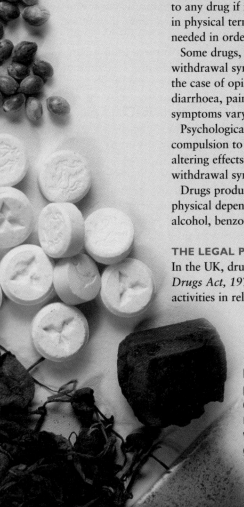

◀ Popular drugs
In the UK, over 50 per cent of the population under 24 have used illegal drugs more than once. Cannabis is the most popular drug with those over 16, while 11 to 12 year-olds prefer to sniff glue and other solvents.

followed by a feeling of calm and and an increased perception of the senses. Sedative-hypnotics such as benzodiazepines and the barbiturates, are also used to depress alertness, producing symptoms similar to those caused by large amounts of alcohol.

Nitrates, nicknamed 'poppers', are commonly used for an almost immediate, though short-lived, feeling of light-headedness, followed by a sense of relaxation and well-being. Some users also claim they have an aphrodisiac effect. But continued sniffing of such drugs can damage the circulatory system and the blood's capacity to carry oxygen, as well as causing skin problems around the mouth and nose. They are particularly harmful for people with anaemia, glaucoma, or breathing or heart problems, and may be fatal if swallowed. Mixing nitrates with Viagra is very dangerous.

There is also a range of powerful stimulants that act on the central and peripheral nervous systems to heighten alertness, creating a feeling of euphoria and of having boundless energy. These include cocaine, ecstasy and amphetamines ('speed') and their derivatives. Nicotine from smoking is also a stimulant, reducing the appetite and raising blood pressure.

Hallucinogenic drugs

Some drugs are used to produce changes in perception. A good example is LSD – a psychoactive drug with extremely powerful hallucinogenic properties. Mescaline, from the Mexican peyote cactus, and magic mushrooms have similar effects but are less potent. Some other drugs, such as cannabis, opiates and ecstasy, can promote vivid dreams and experiences, but are not regarded primarily as hallucinogens.

IF YOU THINK SOMEONE IS ABUSING DRUGS

There are often no definite signs that a person is misusing drugs. If you suspect that someone in your care has a drug problem, try not to be too alarmed; if you can, attempt to air your worries with them. Listen to what they have to say. Discuss the legal and health implications of drug taking – including alcohol and tobacco – and try to suggest ways of avoiding harm or preventing an escalation of the abuse.

If the person has a serious problem, it may help to discuss it with a health professional, perhaps your GP, in the first instance, or to phone one of the dedicated organizations that can offer advice and support.

SEE ALSO *Alcohol and abuse; Smoking*

DTP vaccine

DTP vaccine is a triple vaccine, used routinely to immunize children, that protects against the infectious diseases **diphtheria**, **tetanus** and pertussis (**whooping cough**). The first dose is given at two months followed by a second at three months and a third at four months. The vaccine is administered by an injection into a muscle or deep into the skin. It consists of a diphtheria vaccine and a tetanus vaccine, which neutralize the toxins produced by the bacteria causing these diseases, and a pertussis vaccine that works by reacting with the actual bacteria.

SEE ALSO *Immunization*

Duchenne muscular dystrophy

Duchenne muscular dystrophy is the most common and severe form of **muscular dystrophy**. Often referred to as DMD, this hereditary muscle disease almost exclusively affects boys. Its incidence is estimated to be between one in 3000 and one in 4000 boys born in the UK. The disease usually manifests between the ages of four and seven, and is characterized by a waddling movement and curvature of the lumbar spine. The calf muscles, shoulders and upper limbs often become firm and bulky. Most DMD patients die before the age of 30.

Dumping syndrome

Also called rapid gastric emptying, dumping syndrome is the excessively rapid movement of undigested food from the stomach to the lower end of the small intestine. It is usually the result of the disruption of the stomach's normal mechanisms by surgery (see **Gastrectomy**). It can sometimes be caused by stress.

If the stomach empties straight after a meal – early dumping – the symptoms include vomiting, bloating, diarrhoea and shortness of breath. Late dumping occurs one to three hours after eating; it causes weakness, sweating and dizziness as a result of a rise and then a fall in blood sugar levels. Some people experience both early and late dumping.

Treatment is primarily dietary: frequent small meals that are low in carbohydrates and sugars, and plenty of liquids consumed between meals rather than with them have been found to be helpful.

SEE ALSO *Digestive system*

Duodenal ulcer

An erosion in the wall of the duodenum, the first part of the small intestine, is referred to as a duodenal ulcer. In the UK, 10–15 per cent of people have a duodenal ulcer at some time in their life. It is more common in men than in women. Duodenal ulcers are two to three times more common than **gastric ulcers**.

The cause is an attack on the duodenal wall by acidic digestive juices, often when the bacterium *Helicobacter pylori* is present in the stomach. Cigarette smoking and the use of aspirin and other non-steroidal anti-inflammatory drugs (NSAIDs) contribute. Symptoms include abdominal pain – often at night – nausea and vomiting, tarry stools and weight loss.

Complications include an obstruction, perforation of the duodenum, **peritonitis** and bleeding. Treatment is with antibiotics and drugs such as cimetidine.

SEE ALSO *Ulcer*

Dupuytren's contracture

Dupuytren's contracture is a gradual puckering of the skin and bending of the fingers, which is caused by the painless thickening of the fibrous tissues of the hand. The ring and little fingers are usually affected, and may be drawn down onto the palm. It often occurs in both hands, and usually develops from the age of 40 onwards. It is more common in men than women.

SYMPTOMS

- A small lump develops on the palm, spreading to form a band of hard tissue under the skin, which may pucker.
- Over a period of months or years, the affected fingers gradually close over the palm in a fixed position.

CAUSES

The exact cause is unknown but abnormal activity of cell growth factors may be involved. The condition sometimes runs in families and it is more common in those suffering from **epilepsy** and alcoholic liver disease (see **Liver and disorders**).

TREATMENT

Surgery, in which the bands of thickened tissue under the skin are cut and separated, is the only effective treatment. The condition may return in time. Some sufferers benefit from exercise and warm water baths.

Complementary therapies

A combination of **acupuncture** and **homeopathy** may help. Some researchers in the USA have claimed that high doses of vitamin E can improve symptoms.

Dysentery

Dysentery is a bowel infection that causes severe **diarrhoea**. There are two forms: bacillary dysentery and amoebic dysentery. In the UK, between 2000 and 5000 cases are notified annually, mostly the mild form of bacillary dysentry caused by poor hygiene. Amoebic dysentery is very rare in the UK but common in tropical countries. Symptoms can include diarrhoea, stools streaked with blood, pus or mucus, vomiting, griping pains in the abdomen and an urgent desire to defecate. Rest and fluids may settle mild bacillary dysentery in a few days; severe cases can last for weeks. Amoebic dysentery needs at least ten days' treatment. Left untreated, it may persist for years.

CAUSES

- A group of bacteria called *Shigella* are the cause of the bacillary form.
- A parasite called *Entamoeba histolytica* is the cause of the amoebic form.
- Both types are spread by contaminated food and poor hygiene.
- Amoebic dysentery is also spread by water.

WHAT YOU CAN DO

- Take plenty of fluids.
- If the symptoms are not too severe, try an antidiarrhoeal medicine.

WHEN TO CONSULT A DOCTOR

- If symptoms are severe or persistent, or start to get worse.
- If blood, pus or mucus occur in the stools.
- If symptoms occur in a country where amoebic dysentery is present.

WHAT A DOCTOR MAY DO

- Send the patient's stools for testing.
- Prescribe antibiotics for bacillary dysentry and anti-microbial drugs for amoebic dysentery.
- Arrange for specialist treatment.

COMPLEMENTARY THERAPIES

Homeopathy and **acupuncture** may help when used alongside conventional treatments.

COMPLICATIONS

- The main risk is **dehydration**.
- Amoebiasis is more serious, because the parasite is hard to kill and may cause **abscesses** in the liver and lungs.

PREVENTION

- Strict hygiene measures if contact with dysentery sufferers is likely.
- Boil water in countries where amoebic dysentery occurs and do not eat raw food, salad or fruit that cannot be peeled.

OUTLOOK

The outlook for bacillary dysentery is good, but it is more difficult to cure amoebic dysentery completely.

Dyslexia

A person with dyslexia has problems acquiring reading and writing skills despite having average or high intelligence and normal opportunities to learn. The disorder can vary from a slight difficulty (which may not be recognized) to complete incomprehension of the written word. There may also be problems with basic mathematics, processing information and short-term memory. Dyslexia is nine times more common in boys than girls. It is thought to be caused by a developmental abnormality, with a strong genetic component.

Three kinds of dyslexia have been identified. It is unclear whether they are separate disorders or different manifestations of the same one:

■ Visual: the person can read individual letters but cannot put them together to make words.

■ Phonological: the person is unable to match written words to their sounds – an essential skill as normal reading involves internally 'speaking' words that are read and then understanding them by 'listening in' to this inner speech.

■ Semantic: the person is unable to match written symbols to their meaning; a rough meaning may be grasped, but a precise match is elusive – hence 'dog' may be read as 'cat'.

What's going on in the brain?
Different areas of the brain may be involved in different types of dyslexia. Visual dyslexia is linked with a functional abnormality in the magnocellular system – a nervous pathway that carries sensory information to the part of the brain concerned with directing attention.

Phonological dyslexia may also be due in part to such an abnormality, but another possibility is that people with this type of dyslexia process the visual component of writing satisfactorily but cannot transfer it from the part of the brain that 'comprehends' it to the part that turns it into articulated speech. Semantic dyslexia may similarly involve a blockage between the area of the brain that attaches meaning to a word and that which expresses the meaning.

TREATMENT
There is no medical treatment for dyslexia, but some studies have found that symptoms improved in children who took supplements, including fish oils, evening primrose oil, thyme oil and vitamin E.

People with dyslexia can be taught strategies to help them to overcome their problems. Some education authorities offer tuition for dyslexic children and may give them extra time in examinations.

The creativity connection

Dyslexia is often associated with left-handedness, which in turn is linked with visual creativity.

The human brain is divided into two hemispheres – the left is dominant for language, while the right mainly processes visual and emotional information. For right-handed people, this division holds true, but left-handers tend to process all kinds of information more equally across both hemispheres. The ability to bring both brain hemispheres to bear in this way is thought to be the key to their creativity, especially in the visual arts. Brain scans have shown that the same may be true of dyslexics, which is useful if the left hemisphere does not function properly and a word cannot be read – a signal can then be sent to the right hemisphere to process the word instead.

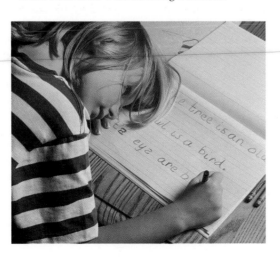

▶ Forming words
Writing skills are affected in varying degrees by dyslexia. One of the most common manifestations is misspelling – the right letters may appear, but in the wrong order.

Dyspepsia

Dyspepsia is the medical name for indigestion: a discomfort or pain in middle of the chest, often felt after eating but sometimes present at other times. Other symptoms include nausea, **heartburn**, bloating, flatulence and belching.

Generally the cause is eating too quickly or eating highly spiced or fatty foods, although stress may also be a factor. Sometimes dyspepsia is a symptom of another condition, especially when it persists or recurs. Often this is gastric ulcer or oesophagitis, but other possibilities include gallstones or a hiatus hernia.

SEE ALSO *Diaphragm and disorders, Gallbladder and disorders; Hernia; Oesophagus and disorders; Stomach and disorders*

Dyspraxia

Dyspraxia is due to an immaturity in the brain, resulting in difficulty in planning and carrying out complex movements. This disorder of the cerebral cortex affects at least 2 per cent of the population, and almost three-quarters of those affected are male.

Symptoms include clumsiness and poor posture, coordination and short-term memory. Children are often slow to develop, and their speech may be hard to understand. They may be of average or above-average intelligence, but their behaviour is immature.

Occupational and other therapies can help sufferers to overcome or minimize symptoms.

SEE ALSO *Occupational therapy*

Ear and problems

The ear is a dual-purpose organ. It is responsible for the sensation of sound as well as helping us to maintain our sense of balance. The external part of the ear is the gateway to an intricate piece of biological engineering made up of bones, membranes and channels. The ear normally does a superb job of keeping us in tune with the world around us. But its direct connection to the outside also makes it vulnerable to infection, while even minute disruptions in its workings may give rise to hearing loss or balance problems.

HOW THE EAR WORKS

To understand the workings of the ear, it is easiest to think of the way sound is conducted through its three major components – the outer ear, the middle ear, and the inner ear.

The outer ear consists of the auricle (or pinna), which is the part you can see, and the 2.5cm (1in) long auditory canal, which ends at the eardrum. While the curves of the auricle and the shape of the earlobe vary in subtle ways from person to person, they all have the function of collecting and channelling sound vibrations into the auditory canal. The auricle (except for the earlobe) is composed of a tough material called **cartilage**. Researchers are now

learning how to create cartilage in the laboratory and it may not be too long before they can fashion a replacement to repair ears that have been damaged through injury. The whole of the outer ear is lined with fine hairs (in some people, you can see these hairs sprouting) and glands that produce earwax – both of which have a protective function.

The outer ear is separated from the middle ear by a membrane called the eardrum, which vibrates when sound impinges on it. It is well supplied with blood vessels and nerves, which is why a punctured eardrum – caused by sudden exposure to very loud noise or a sharp blow to the ear – causes excruciating pain and bleeding from the ear. Sound is conducted through air in the outer ear, but through bone in the middle ear – chiefly through the auditory ossicles, three tiny linked earbones called the hammer (malleus), the anvil (incus) and the stirrup (stapes), which is the smallest bone in the human body. While the eardrum cuts off the middle ear from the outside, the middle ear space is filled with air from the Eustachian tube, which runs forwards and downwards from the middle ear to the back of the nose. Normally, the Eustachian tube is closed, but it opens up if you yawn or swallow. The Eustachian tube allows equalization of air pressure on either side of the eardrum, enabling it to function properly.

The base of the stapes lies up against a structure called the oval window, which separates the middle ear from the inner ear. From here on in, sound is transmitted through fluids contained within the complex structures

Anatomy of the ear
The ear is a complex organ divided into three sections – the outer, middle and inner ear.

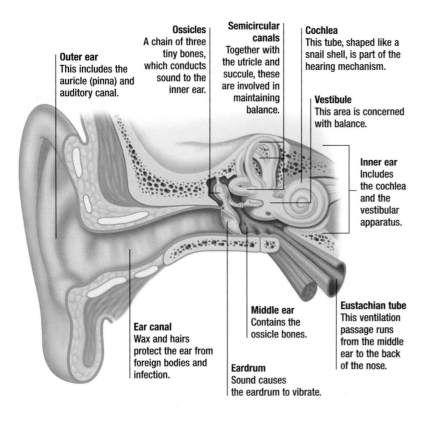

Outer ear
This includes the auricle (pinna) and auditory canal.

Ossicles
A chain of three tiny bones, which conducts sound to the inner ear.

Semicircular canals
Together with the utricle and succule, these are involved in maintaining balance.

Cochlea
This tube, shaped like a snail shell, is part of the hearing mechanism.

Vestibule
This area is concerned with balance.

Inner ear
Includes the cochlea and the vestibular apparatus.

Ear canal
Wax and hairs protect the ear from foreign bodies and infection.

Middle ear
Contains the ossicle bones.

Eardrum
Sound causes the eardrum to vibrate.

Eustachian tube
This ventilation passage runs from the middle ear to the back of the nose.

of the inner ear, which is also known as the labyrinth because of its intricacy. At the front is the cochlea, named after the Greek word for shell because of its shape. Inside the cochlea is a fluid-filled tube containing microscopic hairs. It is these hairs that form the interface between the ear and the brain. Stimulated by sound vibrations coming from the oval window, they send electrical impulses to the acoustic nerve, which are received and interpreted by the brain.

The auditory region of the brain can respond to the frequency, intensity (decibel level) and direction of a sound – thereby making sense of all the vibrations arriving at the eardrum; the brain can also readily distinguish between meaningful sound, carried by regular vibrations, and meaningless noise, where the vibrations are irregular.

Noise may have damaging health effects. Loud noise can impair hearing, but noise is also recognized as a stress factor, which can lead to learning difficulties in children.

According to research done in Sweden, noise can lead to an increase in blood pressure in adults, which raises the risk of heart disease and **strokes**.

Keeping a balance

The rear part of the inner ear is concerned with maintaining balance, re-orienting you relative to your surroundings whenever you change position. The three structures involved with balance are the saccule, the utricle and three semi-circular canals, which lie at right angles to one another and are connected to a cavity called the vestibule. The whole ensemble is known as the vestibular apparatus. The utricle and saccule help static (standing) equilibrium. The canals contain hairs that are bathed in fluid. Each responds to a different element of balance – such as gravity, acceleration, position or head movement. Nerve fibres interfaced with the hairs convey this information to the brain. The brain merges this information with that from the eyes and muscles. All this together keeps you balanced.

WHAT CAN GO WRONG

The ear is susceptible to a range of disorders which, in some cases, can cause deafness.

Ear infections

Both the outer and middle ear are vulnerable to infection by fungi, bacteria or viruses. An outer ear infection is often linked to swimming in infected water, or poking down the auditory canal. Middle ear infection (otitis media) occurs when bacteria infect the mucous membranes that line the spaces within the temporal bone, which surrounds this area. Acute otitis media is generally triggered by a cold or flu, which leaves the Eustachian tube swollen or blocked. The infection may become chronic and may then lead to rupture of the eardrum (see also **Glue ear**). Before the widespread use of antibiotics and **grommets**, complications from otitis media, such as mastoiditis (infection of the bone behind the ear) or even brain abscesses, were not uncommon.

The inner ear can be affected by **labyrinthitis**. This inflammation of the inner ear, believed to be caused by a viral infection, results in vertigo (see below), vomiting, loss of balance and deafness. Labyrinthitis may follow cold or flu-type infections and can last for six to eight weeks.

Hearing loss

A complete inability to hear is rare, and usually present from birth. Degrees of hearing loss occur from ear disease, injury or degeneration of the hearing process with age. Hearing loss is divided into two categories – conductive and sensorineural. In conductive deafness, there is a fault in the transmission of sound vibration from the outer to the inner ear. The most common cause is earwax blocking the auditory canal. Conductive deafness can also occur from **otosclerosis**, in which the stapes loses its mobility, this may be the result of otitis media, or from barotrauma – damage to the eardrum or middle ear occurring because of unusually rapid pressure changes in an aircraft or when diving.

Sensorineural deafness is linked to damage to the cochlea or inner ear, which degenerate in function as people age. It can also be caused by **Ménière's disease**, by acoustic neuroma (a benign tumour affecting the acoustic nerve) or by certain drugs, such as streptomycin.

Vertigo

Vertigo is a disabling sensation of spinning, falling or the feeling that the ground is moving beneath your feet. It occurs when someone is stationary, or the sensation will be quite out of proportion to the movement they are actually making. It is different from feelings of lightheadedness, dizziness or faintness, which have various causes. Vertigo is not a fear of heights (known as acrophobia). In the true sense it is linked to a problem in the vestibular system, such as labyrinthitis, a viral infection of the inner ear, or Ménière's disease. Vertigo is often accompanied by nausea and vomiting, and sometimes by **tinnitus**, a continuous ringing or buzzing sound in the ears.

SEE ALSO *Deafness*

Referred pain in the ear

Earache is not always the result of a problem in the ear. Problems occurring in other parts of the face may at first appear to be ear-related.

The cause of earache can be an obvious infection of the outer or middle ear, or a ruptured eardrum. But the nerves that serve the ear also connect into the face, jaw and neck. The brain may interpret an impulse coming from these regions as coming from the ear instead. Such referred pain is quite frequent. For instance, temporomandibular joint (TMJ) syndrome is a common cause of ear pain: caused by misalignment of the jaw, it is made worse by stress and teeth grinding. Other dental problems, such as tooth decay, could also cause referred earache. (*See Teeth and problems.*)

Ebola virus

Ebola, also known as haemorrhagic fever, is a severe and largely fatal infectious disease. It is caused by a virus of African origin, which was first recognized in 1976 when there were major outbreaks in the Sudan and the Democratic Republic of Congo (formerly Zaire). In 1995, there was another major outbreak in Congo.

The temperate climate and environmental conditions in the UK do not support the virus, although cases are occasionally imported.

Initial symptoms include muscle and joint pain, fever and headache, and there may be nausea, vomiting and diarrhoea. The disease progresses rapidly until there is massive bleeding either from the major organs or from tiny blood vessels within the digestive tract and in the gums.

Seven out of every ten people affected by the ebola virus die, usually within a week of contracting the disease. There is no readily available treatment but scientists are working on developing therapies against the virus.

SEE ALSO *Travel and tropical diseases*

E. coli

E. coli (*Escherichia coli*) is the name for a number of bacterial organisms found in the intestines of healthy human beings and animals. Most are harmless but one strain, *E. coli* 0157, which is found in the intestines of healthy cattle, can cause serious and sometimes fatal **food poisoning**. The bacteria are passed into the environment in the animals' faeces. If this fouls their hides or enters the water system, the bacteria can infect those who handle the cattle and even contaminate meat and other farm products entering the food chain.

People most commonly develop *E. coli* food poisoning from eating contaminated foods, particularly inadequately cooked minced beef. This is often in the form of beefburgers which, typically, have not been grilled, fried or barbecued until they are cooked through. Contaminated milk can also be a source of infection. Outbreaks have been linked to yoghurt, cooked meats, meat pies, cheese, dry-cured salami, raw vegetables, unpasteurized apple juice and water. Direct contact with farm animals, particularly with cattle, can also be a cause. Once caught, the infection can be passed from person to person.

SYMPTOMS
- Severe abdominal cramps (haemorrhagic colitis).
- Mild to bloody diarrhoea.

DURATION
- The incubation period, before the onset of diarrhoea, can range from one to 14 days.
- The *E. coli* bacteria are usually excreted from the body within a week, but the process can take much longer, especially in children and elderly people, who are more at risk from the infection.
- Those with mild symptoms usually recover within two weeks.

TREATMENT
See a doctor as soon as there are food-poisoning symptoms, especially if you notice blood in the stools or watery diarrhoea in children. The doctor may prescribe antibiotics. Serious cases may be referred to hospital.

COMPLICATIONS
Up to 10 per cent of people with *E. coli* develop haemolytic uraemic syndrome, which kills red blood cells and leads to kidney failure (see **Kidneys and disorders**). It usually affects young children and is a major cause of acute kidney failure in children in the UK. Some adults with *E. coli* develop haemolytic uraemic syndrome together with neurological complications.

PREVENTION
Government bodies have issued guidelines for the food and farming industries on minimizing the contamination of meat. Guidance on farm visits have also been issued to farmers and teachers. Preventive measures include the following:
- Cook all beef and meat products thoroughly. Minced beef, especially beefburgers, should be cooked until the juices run clear and there are no pink areas.
- Ensure good kitchen hygiene, and store raw and cooked foods separately. Wash your hands after handling raw meat.
- Do not drink unpasteurized milk.
- Do not touch manure and avoid handling animals on visits to farms or animal centres.
- Ensure children wash their hands thoroughly after stroking farm animals.

OUTLOOK
If the infection is severe, it can cause permanent kidney damage and may even be fatal. Those most vulnerable include babies, young children and elderly people.

SEE ALSO *Urinary system*

Eclampsia

Eclampsia is a condition affecting pregnant women. It is characterized by sudden convulsive fits that starve both the pregnant woman and her unborn baby of oxygen. These fits are followed by a period of coma and sometimes further convulsions. Eclampsia occurs in one in

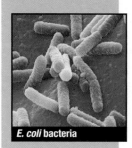

UNDER THE MICROSCOPE

Around 15 per cent of healthy cattle are thought to carry dangerous *E. coli* 0157 bacteria in their gut.

E. coli **bacteria**

2000 pregnancies; it is fatal for one in 50 affected women and one in 14 affected babies.

Eclampsia is more common among very young mothers, first-time mothers and women who are carrying more than one baby. The causes are not fully understood, but the condition can run in families.

SYMPTOMS

Eclampsia is usually preceded by pre-eclampsia, in which there is raised blood pressure, protein in the urine, and often swelling, headaches and visual disturbance. Eclampsia may develop so quickly that pre-eclampsia goes unnoticed.

TREATMENT

A woman with pre-eclampsia is advised to rest. She is closely monitored and may be admitted to hospital. Treatments include anti-convulsant drugs, low doses of aspirin and mild sedatives. If pre-eclampsia is severe and the pregnancy is sufficiently well advanced, the baby may be induced.

PREVENTION

High doses of vitamins C and E reduce the risk of eclampsia in high-risk women; low doses of aspirin may also help – but neither should be taken without medical supervision.

SEE ALSO *Pregnancy and problems*

Ectopic pregnancy

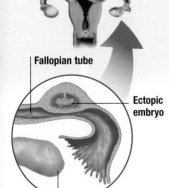

▼ **Doomed pregnancy**
A fertilized egg normally travels from the ovary to the uterus, where it can develop. An ectopic pregnancy occurs when the fertilized egg implants in the wall of the ovary, Fallopian tube or cervix.

Fallopian tube

Ectopic embryo

Ovary

If a fertilized egg implants outside the womb, the pregnancy is described as ectopic. In most cases, the egg implants in a Fallopian tube, but it may become attached to an ovary or the cervix, or in the abdominal cavity instead.

About one in 200 pregnancies are ectopic. Such a pregnancy has virtually no chance of lasting more than two months, and if not recognized and treated, it can be fatal.

CAUSES

Ectopic pregnancies have increased in the past 15 years, possibly owing to the rise in pelvic inflammatory diseases, such as those caused by **chlamydia** bacteria, which can damage the Fallopian tubes. Damage can also be the result of previous surgery. Other risk factors include the use of an intra-uterine contraceptive device, some types of fertility treatment and a previous ectopic pregnancy.

SYMPTOMS

Symptoms usually occur around the sixth week of pregnancy. An ectopic pregnancy may be signalled by vaginal bleeding and pain in the lower abdomen. Symptoms may subside briefly but worsen as the embryo grows. If it grows large enough, it may rupture the Fallopian tube, causing heavy bleeding, severe pain and shock.

TREATMENT

Diagnosis is confirmed by a positive pregnancy test, where necessary, followed by an **ultrasound** scan or laparoscopy, when a tiny telescope is inserted into the abdomen through an incision under the navel.

The embryo is removed, although the method depends on its size and location. This may involve **keyhole surgery** to remove the embryo on its own, or with a small section of Fallopian tube. It may also be possible to inject drugs during a laparoscopy to stop the embryo growing; the embryo dies and is reabsorbed into the body.

OUTLOOK

About 10 per cent of women who have had an ectopic pregnancy are left infertile, but 60 per cent become pregnant again within 18 months. A woman who has had an ectopic pregnancy is carefully monitored in future pregnancies.

SEE ALSO *Pelvis and disorders*

Ectropion

Ectropion is an outward turning of the eyelid or lids, away from the eyeball. It generally affects the lower lid. Ectropion is commonest in elderly people, whose muscles around the eye have lost their elasticity. It may also result from scarring of the surrounding facial skin or a loss of nerve function, for example, **palsy**.

Ectropion causes tears to flow onto the cheek, and the eyeball becomes dry, leading to grittiness and discomfort, occasional blurred vision, increased risk of **conjunctivitis** and, in severe cases, inflammation of the cornea. Rubbing the eye aggravates the condition.

Ocular lubricants or artificial teardrops may give temporary relief but a more permanent solution generally involves surgery.

SEE ALSO *Eye and problems*

ECT

ECT, or electroconvulsive therapy, is used to treat severe mental illness. Electric shocks are used to induce short seizures or fits, which have a beneficial effect on conditions such as serious **depression**. Although there is clear evidence of its effectiveness, ECT has side effects, including short-term memory loss, and is therefore used sparingly, with medication usually the first choice of treatment. Its use is confined to severe **depression**, mania and occasionally **schizophrenia**.

ECT may be offered as part of a package of care to people with severe mental illness. The patient will be under the care of a consultant psychiatrist, who will explain why ECT is being considered as treatment in this case, and answer any questions, before asking the patient to sign a consent form, as is usual for other medical and surgical procedures.

WHAT'S INVOLVED

ECT follows a clear pattern.
- The patient is given a general **anaesthetic**, with muscle relaxant.
- Electric pads are placed on the temples.
- A short controlled electric pulse is delivered to the electrodes.
- A mild fit occurs.
- Oxygen is usually given as the anaesthetic wears off.
- Consciousness is gradually regained.
- Immediate effects include headache, some confusion and memory loss.
- Between four and eight treatments is usual.

SEE ALSO *Mental health and problems*

Eczema

Eczema is an inflammatory condition of the skin. It causes scaly, red patches, itching and small fluid-filled blisters which burst, making the skin moist and crusty. The disease, also known as **dermatitis**, affects about one in ten people in the UK.

There are several types of eczema. The most common types are atopic and contact. Atopic eczema runs in families and often appears in the first year of life. Like other atopic diseases, it is caused by an overreaction of the immune system to an allergen – a substance that triggers an allergic response. This type of eczema is linked to other atopic diseases such as **asthma** and allergic rhinitis – more commonly known as **hay fever**.

Contact eczema is caused by contact with any of a wide variety of substances, ranging from washing powders to nickel watch-straps.

The discomfort caused by the condition can lead to extreme distress, which is made worse if the itching leads to sleep deprivation.

SYMPTOMS

Eczema commonly affects skin on the hands, inside the elbows and behind the knees, but it may be found anywhere on the body. Atopic eczema is commonly found in skin folds, whereas contact eczema is more usually seen on the hands. Seborrhoeic eczema affects areas such as the scalp and ears, and in men may also affect the back and chest. In severe cases it can spread to affect skin covering most of the body. Symptoms vary from mild to severe and can include:

- dry, scaly, thickened skin;

- redness;
- itching (skin may be rubbed raw by scratching);
- blisters;
- weeping sores that may become infected;
- crusting;
- a flaky scalp.

CAUSES

Although external factors can trigger a flare-up of atopic eczema, it is usually hereditary. One in every eight children and 1–2 per cent of adults suffer from it. If both parents have eczema, there is about a 40 per cent chance that their offspring will also have it.

Many factors can trigger eczema. A common cause of hand eczema in healthcare workers is an allergy to the latex rubber gloves that they sometimes wear.

Some people also find that eczema symptoms are brought on or made worse by eating certain foods, such as eggs or milk. There is, however, no firm evidence to show that diet plays a major part in causing flare-up of eczema.

Stress or anxiety can cause sudden flare-ups, however, although the cause of worry may not always be obvious, especially in children.

The skin bacterium *Staphylococcus aureusis* is associated with flare-ups of the condition, but eczema itself is not infectious.

TREATMENT

Dry and itchy skin should be treated with emollients, special moisturizers in the form of oils, lotions or creams that soothe, smooth and cleanse the skin. Eczema sufferers should wash with aqueous cream rather than soap, which can be very drying.

A doctor may prescribe a corticosteroid cream to reduce inflammation and to improve symptoms, but this will not cure the condition. Such creams should be applied as prescribed and should not used on the face or genitals.

Antibacterial bath additives help to reduce *staphylococcus* infection. Oral antihistamines may reduce itching and swelling in allergic eczema. In severe cases, immunosuppressive drugs may be prescribed in hospital.

Complementary therapies

Evening primrose oil contains gammalinolenic acid, an essential fatty acid that may help to

---

Different types of eczema

Eczema can appear anywhere on the body, but different types have different manifestations and tend to affect specific areas.

- **Atopic** – mainly affects the face, neck and inner creases of the elbows and knees. It is linked with an increased risk of asthma and hay fever.

- **Contact** – most commonly seen on the hands; it is caused by contact with nickel, for example.

- **Seborrhoeic** – affects the face or scalp; the greasy crusts of cradle cap are one example.

- **Asteatotic** – often on the legs of older people; it causes dry, crazy-paving skin patterns.

- **Stasis** – affects the lower legs; it is associated with poor circulation in the area.

- **Pompholyx** – mostly on the fingers, palms or soles of the feet; it causes small, itchy blisters.

- **Discoid** – usually on the legs and trunk; it appears as round – disc-shaped – areas of irritation.

- **Neurodermatitis** – a thickening of the skin known as **lichenification**.

- **Photo-allergic** – caused by the action of sunlight on skin sensitized by absorbed drugs or chemicals.

reduce itchiness and dryness in some people with essential fatty acid deficiency. It needs to be taken in large doses of around 240mg twice a day for at least three months before its effectiveness can be properly evaluated.

SEE ALSO *Skin and disorders*

EEG

An EEG (electroencephalogram) is a test that records the electrical activity of the brain. It can help in the diagnosis of many diseases affecting the nervous system, but is particularly useful in confirming the existence of **epilepsy** in someone with a history of **fits**, and in monitoring the progress of this condition.

The test is a painless procedure in which leads are applied to the scalp. These relay electrical transmissions from the brain, which are then converted into a brainwave tracing on paper. Normal brain activity is demonstrated by wave forms of predominantly two types – alpha and beta waves.

Abnormal waves are either much slower and of higher amplitude (that is, bigger) than normal, or consist of very fast spikes.

Interpretation of an EEG can pinpoint the area in the brain where discharges of abnormal electrical activity originate. This area is called the epileptic focus. The results of an EEG are highly relevant when deciding on treatment, whether with medication or with surgery.

Usually an EEG is carried out when a patient is resting but not sedated. However, brain activity may also be recorded during sleep, or when epileptic fits are deliberately provoked to aid diagnosis, or during anaesthesia to monitor brain function. In special circumstances, the absence of electrical activity on an EEG may aid in the confirmation of brain death.

SEE ALSO *Brain and nervous system*

Elbow and problems

The elbow is the junction of the upper arm and the forearm. It is made up of two joints. The main elbow joint is a simple hinge joint between the bone of the upper arm and the two bones of the forearm. The second joint, called the superior radio-ulnar joint, is a pivot; its function is to rotate. An arrangement of ligaments, tendons and muscles stabilize and move the joint.

WHAT THE ELBOW DOES
The movements that take place at the elbow's hinge joint are called flexion and extension – bending and straightening the elbow. Both

movements are limited – in the case of flexion by the upper arm and forearm muscles; and in the case of extension by the configuration of the joint's bones, which allow movement to only 180° – you cannot bend your elbow backwards.

A complex arrangement of bone and muscle
There are two joints at the elbow. A hinge joint that lies between the bones of the upper arm and the forearm and the superior radio-ulna joint which allows the bones of the forearm to rotate. Both are encased in a single fibrous capsule filled with lubricating synovial fluid.

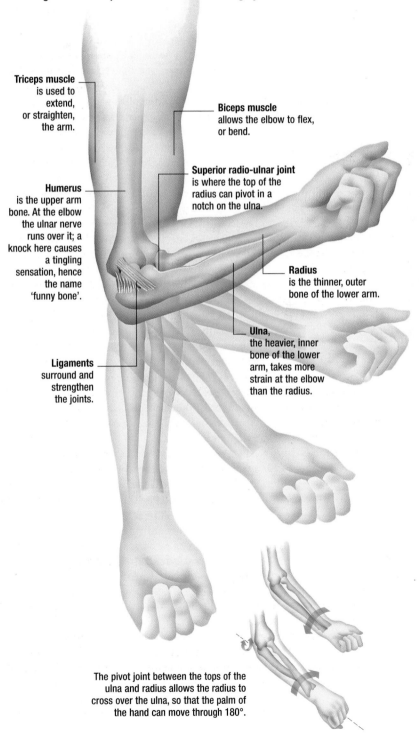

Triceps muscle is used to extend, or straighten, the arm.

Biceps muscle allows the elbow to flex, or bend.

Superior radio-ulnar joint is where the top of the radius can pivot in a notch on the ulna.

Humerus is the upper arm bone. At the elbow the ulnar nerve runs over it; a knock here causes a tingling sensation, hence the name 'funny bone'.

Radius is the thinner, outer bone of the lower arm.

Ulna, the heavier, inner bone of the lower arm, takes more strain at the elbow than the radius.

Ligaments surround and strengthen the joints.

The pivot joint between the tops of the ulna and radius allows the radius to cross over the ulna, so that the palm of the hand can move through 180°.

The only movement that takes place at the elbow's second joint – the superior radio-ulnar joint – is rotation. It is this joint, combined with the wrist joints, that allows you to turn your hand palm-down or palm-up.

WHAT CAN GO WRONG INSIDE THE JOINT

A number of conditions can arise within the elbow. They involve damage to the bones, tendons or nerves.

Osteochondritis dessicans

After the knee, the elbow is the commonest site of osteochondritis dessicans. In this condition, the cartilage that lines the bones where they meet at the elbow joint breaks down and eventually breaks away from the bone to form a 'loose body' (see below). The cause is unknown, but injury and a poor blood supply are thought to play a part.

Loose body formation

A loose body is any small, loose piece of bone, cartilage or fibrous membrane. The main causes are osteochondritis dessicans, osteoarthritis or a minor **fracture** in which a fragment of bone separates.

A loose body can also be caused by synovial chondromatosis, a rare condition in which the cells of a joint's fibrous inner lining turn into cartilage and detach themselves from the membrane, forming numerous minute loose bodies. The main symptom is a sudden 'locking' of the elbow during movement, accompanied by a sharp pain; this may be relieved by movement or it may clear up itself. If the locking happens frequently, treatment is by surgical removal of the loose body.

Rheumatoid arthritis

Rheumatoid arthritis frequently affects the elbows. The main symptoms are pain and swelling of the thickened synovial membrane surrounding the joint.

Pyogenic arthritis

Pyogenic arthritis is a rare condition that can occur if the humerus becomes infected. The sufferer has a raised temperature, and the elbow joint becomes inflamed, swollen with fluid and hot. A doctor will treat the condition by sucking out the fluid with a needle and syringe and prescribing a course of antibiotics.

WHAT CAN GO WRONG OUTSIDE THE JOINT

Several conditions can affect the outside of the elbow, which is especially vulnerable to damage caused by repetitive movements.

Tennis elbow

Tennis elbow is so-called because it can result from playing backhand strokes during tennis, but in reality its most common cause is ironing or polishing, because of the strenuous, repetitive movements of the forearm with the wrist held up that these activities entail.

Tennis elbow involves a tearing of the wrist extensor tendons at the elbow, where they are attached to the outside of the upper arm bone (humerus). Since this area is particularly rich in nerve endings, someone with tennis elbow feels acute pain, but there is also a dull ache felt as a broad band down the forearm. The condition makes it impossible to carry anything heavier than a sheet of paper, turn a doorknob or shake hands, for example.

Most cases of tennis elbow clear up of their own accord, but the process can take up to two years. Initial treatment involves the administration of anti-inflammatory drugs, with a hydrocortisone injection into the tendon. In severe cases, a surgeon may separate the tendon from the bone and re-site it.

Golfer's elbow

Golfer's elbow is similar to tennis elbow, but affects the wrist flexors (rather than the wrist extensors), where they attach to the humerus at the elbow. The condition is caused by overuse of the flexors when playing golf, but can also result from activities such as using a screwdriver. Golfer's elbow is treated in the same way as tennis elbow.

Student's elbow

Student's elbow is also known as olecranon bursitis. The bursa, a fluid-filled sac behind the funny bone (see **Bursitis**), can become inflamed as a result of minor injury – such as by leaning on a desk for extended periods of time. The bursa may also be affected by **gout** or blood poisoning. The condition is treated by sucking out any fluid, a hydrocortisone injection and, in persistent cases, surgical removal of the bursa.

Neuritis of the ulnar nerve

The ulnar nerve passes behind the bone of the upper arm (humerus) before passing down to the forearm and hand. It lies very close to the surface as it crosses the elbow and is easily injured by fracture or dislocation in this area. Osteoarthritis can also cause damage by putting prolonged pressure on the nerve, as can friction from a muscle tendon.

Once damaged, fibrous tissue is laid down over time and gradually the nerve ceases to function correctly. The result is neuritis, a condition characterized by numbness, pins and needles and muscle wasting.

Treatment is by surgery to free the nerve from the groove and move it so that it passes over the front of the elbow.

SEE ALSO *Arm and problems; Muscular system; Skeletal system*

> The most common cause of tennis elbow is not playing tennis but ironing.

Electrical injuries

An electric shock can cause effects varying from a minor tingling to instant death. Often an electric shock leaves **burns** – which can be deep and serious – where the current enters and leaves the body. The shock may also disrupt heart rhythm or breathing; children are particularly vulnerable to these symptoms. Such disruption may involve quivering of the heart muscles (fibrillation) or interference with a proper heartbeat, or the heart may stop altogether. If the injured person is still in contact with the electric current, rescuers are in danger, too.

The most common cause of electric shock is a faulty electrical appliance in the home. A lightning strike can cause similar injuries.

Anyone who has been unconscious or has suffered a burn due to electricity should go to hospital. Electrical burns can be more serious than they appear, and heart rhythm may need to be monitored for a while.

DEALING WITH AN EMERGENCY

If you are rescuing someone who has been electrocuted from a domestic supply, observe the following guidelines.

- Don't touch the person until contact with the electricity supply has been broken.
- Switch off the power at the socket or at the mains and pull out the plug.
- If it is not possible to disconnect the power, stand on some insulating surface (a rubber mat, thick towel or folded newspaper) and use a non-conducting implement – such as a wooden broom handle, walking stick or chair leg – to push the person away from the source of electricity, for example, by knocking the person's hand clear of the electrical appliance. Avoid anything wet or metallic.
- Check the affected person's breathing and pulse and start resuscitation if necessary and if trained to do so.
- Put the person into the recovery position.
- Look for and treat burns and **shock**.
- Call an ambulance.

PREVENTION

There are several precautions you can take to reduce the danger of electrical injuries.

- Have damaged cables and flexes mended before using an appliance.
- Never take electrical equipment into a bathroom.
- Don't touch electrical items with wet hands.
- Don't overload sockets or adaptors.
- Always have wiring jobs carried out by a competent professional.

SEE ALSO *FIRST AID; Heart and circulatory system*

Electromagnetic radiation

Electromagnetic radiation is the form of radiation given off by electrical devices. It is increasingly regarded as a form of pollution and has been linked with possible health hazards, but the evidence for such links continues to be a matter of scientific controversy.

Environmental sources of electromagnetic radiation include power lines and pylons, as well as domestic items such as microwave ovens, televisions, computers, satellite dishes, mobile phones and electric blankets. Children are thought to be particularly vulnerable to the effects of electromagnetic radiation, and there are reports of increased incidence of **leukaemia** among children living near power pylons and high-voltage lines. Other disorders suspected of possible association with electromagnetic radiation include **Alzheimer's disease**, birth defects, **cancers**, headaches, lethargy, memory loss, muscle pains and sleep disturbances, as well as such events as miscarriage, **sudden infant death syndrome** (cot death) and suicide.

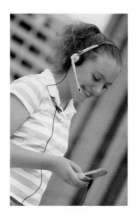

▲ **Keeping it short**
To limit the risk of radiation, mobile phones should be used for only a few minutes at a time. It is always advisable to use a hands-free device.

Minimizing exposure to radiation

If you are worried about your level of exposure to radiation, use a hand-held radiation monitor to measure the electric and magnetic fields in your home. To minimize risk, you can:

- avoid electric blankets;

- turn off appliances such as TVs and computers when not in use;

- restrict use of mobile phones to a few minutes at a time, or use a phone shield or a hands-free device;

- place children's beds away from walls that have a high concentration of electrical devices on the other side.

Elephantiasis

Elephantiasis is a rare disease of the **lymphatic system**, which causes massive swellings of a limb, the scrotum or the torso. The skin thickens and darkens, so that it resembles the skin of an elephant. It occurs most commonly in tropical regions, particularly in parts of Africa.

The most common cause of elephantiasis is small parasitic roundworms, which can be transmitted to human beings by mosquitoes; they then lodge in the lymphatic system and obstruct the lymph flow. Treatment usually involves surgery to remove the excess skin.

Emaciation

Emaciation is a wasting of the body, with loss of muscle as well as fat. The cause can be related to malabsorption syndromes, as in cases of intestinal surgery, **coeliac disease, Crohn's disease, irritable bowel syndrome** and other diseases that impair absorption of nutrients across the gut wall.

Other causes of emaciation range from a drastic reduction in food intake, as occurs in starvation or **anorexia**, to conditions such as **diabetes** and some cancers, where metabolic disturbances drastically affect the rate at which nutrients are absorbed by the tissues.

Embolism

An embolism occurs when part of a blood clot detaches and travels to lodge in an artery, cutting off an organ's blood supply. The lung and brain arteries are commonly affected. A blockage may occasionally be caused by fat (after a crush injury to bone) or air (after a diving accident or error in injecting into a vein).

Unless the circulation is quickly restored, the tissue may die (infarction).
SEE ALSO *Heart and circulatory system*

EMG

An EMG (or electromyogram) is a test in which the electrical impulses generated by muscle contraction are amplified and recorded. It is used in the diagnosis of nerve and muscle disorders, such as **muscular dystrophy** and myasthenia gravis.

The EMG involves inserting a needle electrode, attached to a recorder, into the muscle, or placing disc electrodes on the skin over the muscles being investigated. The electrical output is then displayed as a trace image on a computer screen or the trace is marked on paper. The trace indicates whether contraction is weaker than usual, and whether a weakness is due to degeneration of the muscle or damage to the nerves involved in its contraction.

Emphysema

Emphysema is a chronic obstructive pulmonary disease (COPD), a progressively disabling and life-threatening disease of the lungs. The disease is almost always associated with smoking cigarettes.

Smoking damages the tiny air sacs (alveoli) in the lungs, making breathing difficult. It is thought that only one in four cases of emphysema are diagnosed. It mainly afflicts men over the age of 45, although diagnosis in women is rising because increasing numbers of women smoke. Smokers in their late 20s may already have emphysema but attribute their symptoms to 'smoker's cough'.
SYMPTOMS
- Wheezing and breathlessness, mild at first;
- Increasing disability;
- Anxiety and depression.
CAUSES
In nearly all cases – about 98 per cent – smoking is the sole cause, though sometimes alpha-1 antitrypsin deficiency, an inherited condition, contributes. This is a disorder in which the liver produces too little or none of the protein alpha-1 antitrypsin, which protects the lungs. Without this protection, the lungs are damaged very easily by smoking.
TREATMENT
There is no cure, but treatment to relieve symptoms includes drugs to widen the airways and reduce inflammation, oxygen therapy, surgery to remove areas of damaged lung and fitness programmes.
What you can do
- Stop smoking.
- Avoid polluted air.
When to consult a doctor
See a doctor if you suffer from shortness of breath, wheezing, or if your symptoms become worse.
Complementary therapies
The following may help to ease symptoms:
- blowing up balloons;
- relaxation techniques;
- **massage**.
PREVENTION
Do not smoke.
OUTLOOK
Emphysema is a progressively debilitating disease that over many years results in increasing breathlessness, disability and eventually respiratory failure and death.
SEE ALSO *Lungs and disorders; Smoking*

Encephalitis

Encephalitis is a serious and sometimes fatal inflammation of the brain, usually caused by a viral or bacterial infection.
SYMPTOMS
A person with encephalitis usually has a feverish illness followed, perhaps days or weeks later, by varying degrees of disability as the

infection spreads to the brain tissue. Symptoms may include drowsiness, confusion, convulsions, involuntary movements, **paralysis** and **coma.**

The symptoms of encephalitis may be similar to those of **meningitis, encephalomyelitis** and encephalopathy, which is brain inflammation occurring as a result of drug overdose, liver failure and diseases such as brain cancer.

CAUSES

Encephalitis usually occurs as the result of a viral infection, but it can also be due to infection by bacteria and parasites. It may occur as a rare complication of the common viral infections **measles, mumps** and **rubella,** although an effective vaccination programme has caused this incidence to fall. Vaccination can also help prevent encephalitis caused by the rabies virus, Japanese encephalitis (a mosquito-borne viral disease that is widespread in Asia and to which travellers are vulnerable) and tick-borne encephalitis, which is common in forested parts of Europe and Scandinavia.

TREATMENT

Treatment usually focuses on alleviating symptoms. But encephalitis caused by the virus herpes simplex may be helped by the antiviral agent aciclovir.

OUTLOOK

Encephalitis may resolve itself completely, but some people suffer from permanent memory loss or muscle weakness. In severe cases, particularly those caused by the herpes simplex virus, the condition can be fatal.

SEE ALSO **Brain and nervous system**

Encephalomyelitis

Encephalomyelitis is an inflammation of the brain and spinal cord. Its symptoms are similar to those of **encephalitis** and myelitis (an inflammatory disease of the spinal cord).

SYMPTOMS

Encephalomyelitis usually begins with a feverish illness, headache and neck stiffness. Inflammation of the brain causes confusion, convulsions and **coma,** and inflammation of the spinal cord leads to paralysis in the limbs. Eyesight may also be affected.

CAUSES

Viral infections such as measles, smallpox, chickenpox, rubella and rabies can cause encephalomyelitis. Vaccination against these diseases can prevent the disease, but, in extremely rare cases, vaccination can also actually lead to encephalomyelitis. Smallpox vaccination is no longer recommended because the disease has been successfully eradicated from the world.

OUTLOOK

Most cases improve completely, but others may experience long-term weakness and some memory loss.

TREATMENT

Treatment is mainly directed at relieving the symptoms of encephalomyelitis.

SEE ALSO **Brain and nervous system; Viral infections**

Endocarditis

Endocarditis is a rare but serious, and sometimes fatal, infection of the lining of the heart cavity (endocardium), especially that of the heart valves. It is more common in developing countries.

SYMPTOMS

- Persistent fatigue, weakness and night sweats.
- Later there may be high fever, rashes, breathlessness and a rapid or irregular heartbeat.

DURATION

The infection can last several weeks.

CAUSES

- Bacteria or other micro-organisms enter the bloodstream (often during dental or medical procedures) and infect the heart.
- The infection usually affects people with pre-existing heart damage.
- People with lowered immune systems and intravenous drug users are also at risk.

TREATMENT

A cure may be possible with early treatment so seek medical advice at the earliest opportunity.

When to consult a doctor

Seek medical advice if you have any of the symptoms listed here, or if you have a high temperature without other symptoms or any apparent cause.

What a doctor may do

- Arrange tests, including blood analysis for bacteria.
- Refer you to hospital for intravenous antibiotics.
- Recommend heart valve surgery.

PREVENTION

People with pre-existing heart damage should take antibiotics before undergoing dental or surgical procedures.

COMPLICATIONS

- Heart failure.
- Kidney or other organ damage.

OUTLOOK

If the infection is treated early enough, a cure is often possible. However, about 25 per cent of sufferers die as a result of endocarditis.

SEE ALSO **Heart and circulatory system**

Endocrine system and disorders

The endocrine system is a complex communication network that governs the chemical processes behind our emotions and physical reactions. The hormones produced by the endocrine system control the way we grow and develop, as well as basic appetites such as hunger, thirst, sex drive and sleep.

The endocrine system is a sophisticated and sensitive system made up of a number of different organs or glands that secrete hormones. Hormones are chemical messengers, usually carried in the bloodstream, which speed up or slow down the activity of cells in other organs and tissues.

Hormones are responsible for a range of bodily reactions including response to stress, feelings of hunger or thirst, energy levels, mood, temperature and sexual desire. In childhood and adolescence hormones are essential for both growth and development. In adulthood, they control reproductive functions, including ovulation, menstruation, pregnancy and milk production in women and sperm production in men.

Most hormones are produced by the endocrine glands, but some are also produced by other body tissues. The major endocrine glands are the pituitary, thyroid, parathyroid, adrenal glands,

and the reproductive organs. The pancreas, the hypothalamus and pineal gland also contain endocrine tissue that produces hormones. Pockets of hormone-producing cells are also located in the small intestine, stomach, kidneys and the heart.

Hormonal levels rise and fall throughout the day. The stress hormone, cortisol, for example, peaks in the early hours of the morning, whereas growth hormone peaks while we sleep. Because hormones cannot be stored in large quantities, the brain programmes glands to produce them as needed in a biochemical cycle designed to keep our bodies in a state of balance. Hormonal production is controlled by a series of 'feedback loops', which operate in a similar way to the thermostat on a central heating system to raise or lower levels of hormones. The system is sensitive to many different factors. These can range from the food we eat, the amount of exercise we take, our feelings, illness, changes in body chemistry, pregnancy, ageing, temperature and even the time of day or season.

Although hormones are carried to almost all the body's tissues they can act only on specific 'target cells'. They do this by locking on to structures called receptors on the surface of or inside cells – like a door key fitting into a particular lock – and switching on or turning off the cell's activity. For example, when the stress hormone adrenaline binds to receptors on muscle cells in blood vessel walls it causes them to contract, preparing our bodies to fight or flee danger. All this takes place very quickly: a maximum of 11 seconds is needed for the blood to travel around the body and deliver a particular hormone.

THE MIND-BODY CONNECTION

The tiny pituitary gland at the base of the brain is often referred to as the 'master gland' because it plays a key role in co-ordinating the activities of the endocrine system. The pituitary looks rather like a pea on a stalk. The stalk is connected to the hypothalamus, an area of the brain about the size of a grape, which sends and receives hormonal messages between the brain and the rest of the body. The hypothalamus picks up information from the brain about a person's external or internal state and relays this by means of

► **Thyroid hormones**
The large molecule (in orange) is a hormone producer called a thyroglobin, which produces two thyroid hormones. These hormones are then carried into the bloodstream via the capillary network (in blue).

The glands and organs that produce hormones

More than 50 different hormones are produced within the body. The majority are produced by the endocrine glands, but several other organs, such as those in the reproductive system, also contain hormone-producing tissue.

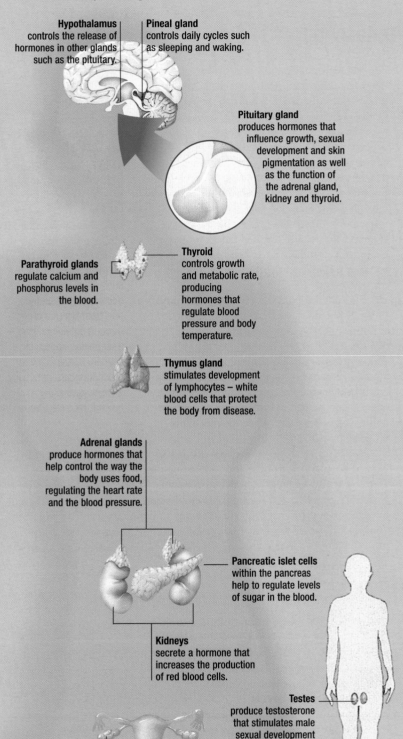

Hypothalamus
controls the release of hormones in other glands such as the pituitary.

Pineal gland
controls daily cycles such as sleeping and waking.

Pituitary gland
produces hormones that influence growth, sexual development and skin pigmentation as well as the function of the adrenal gland, kidney and thyroid.

Parathyroid glands
regulate calcium and phosphorus levels in the blood.

Thyroid
controls growth and metabolic rate, producing hormones that regulate blood pressure and body temperature.

Thymus gland
stimulates development of lymphocytes – white blood cells that protect the body from disease.

Adrenal glands
produce hormones that help control the way the body uses food, regulating the heart rate and the blood pressure.

Pancreatic islet cells
within the pancreas help to regulate levels of sugar in the blood.

Kidneys
secrete a hormone that increases the production of red blood cells.

Testes
produce testosterone that stimulates male sexual development and behaviour.

Ovaries
reproductive glands that secrete oestrogen and progesterone, which stimulate female sexual behaviour, development and menstruation.

hormones to the pituitary down the 'stalk'. This triggers the pituitary into stimulating or inhibiting the action of other glands (including the reproductive organs).

Not all glands are controlled by the pituitary. Some react to concentrations of chemicals such as glucose, fatty acids and minerals in the bloodstream, while others respond to neurohormones, chemical messengers produced by the nervous system.

DISEASES AND DISORDERS

Endocrine autoimmune disorders are conditions caused by the body's defence mechanisms turning against themselves. This involves antibodies attacking certain tissues within the body, believing them to be foreign material. Examples include Hashimoto's disease (a form of thyroid failure), Graves' disease (when the thyroid is overactive) and diabetes.

Tumours of the pituitary gland may occur. These are generally benign but may interfere with the normal functioning of the gland.

Multiple endocrine neoplasia (MEN) is an inherited disorder affecting 3 to 20 people in 100,000 in the UK. Tumours, usually benign (non-cancerous), develop, often all at the same time in a number of different endocrine glands. One common type involves the parathyroid, pituitary glands and the pancreatic islets.

CUTTING EDGE

Growing recognition of the links between hormones and the brain has led to the emergence of a field of study called psychoneuroendocrinology, dedicated to researching the links between hormones and our feelings and behaviour.

This field of research is throwing new light on medical conditions such as premenstrual syndrome (PMS), chronic fatigue syndrome, thyroid problems and irritable bowel syndrome (IBS). These have been recognized but insufficiently understood by the medical profession. Psychoneuroendocrinology is also offering fascinating insights into such phenomena as falling in love, sexual behaviour, parenting and addiction.

SEE ALSO *Adrenal glands and disorders; Diabetes; Digestive system; Kidneys and disorders; Ovaries and disorders; Pancreas and disorders; Pituitary gland and disorders; Reproductive system; Thyroid gland and disorders*

Endometriosis

With endometriosis, fragments of the uterine lining (endometrium) are deposited elsewhere in the body – typically in or on the Fallopian tubes, on the ovaries, behind the uterus, or on the bowel, bladder or pelvic wall, but sometimes in abdominal scars or even the lungs.

These fragments respond to monthly hormonal changes, growing and bleeding during each cycle. But, unlike the lining of the uterus, they have no means of escape, and this leads to inflammation and a build up of scar tissue.

Endometriosis can begin at any time from the onset of menstruation to the menopause. You are more at risk if you have a family history, a menstrual cycle shorter than 28 days and if your periods last more than a week. It is the second most common gynaecological condition, affecting between 10 and 15 per cent of women in their reproductive years – about 2 million women in the UK.

SYMPTOMS

The main symptom is pelvic pain. Other symptoms include bloating, fatigue, painful periods, painful sex, painful bowel movements, constipation, painful and frequent urination or blood in the urine during periods, and infertility. Diagnosis is confirmed by **laparoscopy**.

TREATMENT

There is no cure for endometriosis, but it usually disappears at the menopause. Treatment is aimed at relieving pain, shrinking or slowing the development of endometrial deposits, preserving or restoring fertility, and preventing or delaying recurrence. It may include hormonal drugs designed to stop ovulation and allow endometrial deposits to shrink; the combined oral contraceptive pill; and the Mirena, a T-shaped device made of light plastic that releases small doses of a progestogen.

Sometimes endometrial deposits are surgically removed or vaporized with a laser. In severe cases hysterectomy may be necessary.

What you can do

Relaxation and stress management techniques may help to reduce stress and fatigue. Acupuncture, aromatherapy, herbal treatments, homeopathy, reflexology, naturopathy and osteopathy may also help.

COMPLICATIONS

- Endometriosis may stick organs together with strands of tissue, called 'adhesions'.
- 'Chocolate cysts' filled with dark blood may form.
- Fragments of the endometrium may block the Fallopian tubes, making it difficult to become pregnant.

OUTLOOK

Research is being carried out into genes that may play a part in endometriosis and this could lead to new treatments.

SEE ALSO *Reproductive system*

Endoscopy

Endoscopy is a technique used by doctors to investigate and treat health problems by looking directly into the patient's body through a flexible fibre-optic viewing instrument known as an endoscope. Many major surgical procedures have now been replaced by endoscopy, allowing faster recovery time.

WHY IS ENDOSCOPY USED?

Endoscopy may be recommended for:
- diagnosis of medical problems through inspection of internal organs – **ulcers**, for example, are readily revealed from an examination of the stomach lining;
- taking specimens for pathological analysis – for instance, in colon disease;
- performing **keyhole surgery**, such as removal of the gallbladder, by attaching miniature surgical instruments to the endoscope.

WHAT'S INVOLVED

The endoscope is passed through the mouth, anus or penis, or through a miniature incision made in the abdomen. Since endoscopy often causes some degree of discomfort, the patient will usually be sedated while the procedure takes place.

New electronic endoscopes allow doctors to view almost any part of the body, including the digestive tract, the lungs, bladder, abdominal cavity, nasal cavity, and joints. Some endoscopes have a camera attached to them, allowing images of the interior of the body to be projected onto a large screen.

Enema

An enema is the introduction of fluid into the rectum. It may be given to relieve **constipation**, to clear the lower bowel before surgery, as part of an investigation (see **Barium investigations**) or as a means of introducing drugs.

HOW AN ENEMA IS GIVEN

A lubricated tube is introduced gently into the rectum while the recipient lies on his or her side with hips raised up by a pillow. Then the fluid, which has been warmed, is slowly pushed through the tube. Soap and water were used in the past, but nowadays special enema fluid is available. The procedure is not painful, although there may be some discomfort.

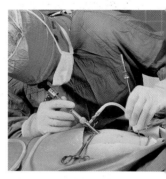

▲ **Endoscopy**
Surgical procedures such as endoscopy allow doctors to investigate and treat internal organs through small incisions – a technique known as keyhole surgery. These procedures are minimally invasive and allow a quicker recovery time.

POSSIBLE RISKS

Enema equipment is widely available, and some people give themselves enemas regularly, in the belief that doing so is conducive to good health. Frequent home enemas are inadvisable because both the lining and the muscles of the lower bowel may become damaged or infected.

Enteric fever

Enteric fever is an alternative name for both **typhoid fever** and **paratyphoid** fever. Typhoid is caused by infection with the bacterium *Salmonella typhi*, which can be transmitted to human beings via food or drinking water contaminated with faeces or urine from a carrier. A vaccine is available, which is needed when travelling to at-risk countries. Paratyphoid, caused by the bacterium *Salmonella paratyphi*, is similar to typhoid, but is usually much less severe.

SEE ALSO *Infectious diseases*

Enteritis

Inflammation of the small intestine, known as enteritis, can result in acute **diarrhoea**, loss of appetite, abdominal pain and, sometimes, vomiting. Possible causes include **food poisoning, salmonella**, exposure to contaminated water and **Crohn's disease**. Enteritis usually clears up without treatment in two to three days, although fluids should be taken to prevent **dehydration**.

Entropion

Entropion is an inward turning of the eyelid or lids, towards the eyeball. The condition may be present from birth, but it is most common in elderly people whose muscles around the eye have lost their elasticity. It may also result from scarring, usually of the surrounding facial skin, a common complication of **trachoma**.

With entropion, the eyelashes tend to rub against the cornea (see **Inturned eyelashes**), causing irritation, discomfort or more severe pain, blurred vision and watering of the eye. There is also an increased risk of conjunctivitis.

Special lubricants for the eye or artificial tears provide temporary relief. Taping the lid in the required position may reposition the lid margin and prevent further irritation but a more permanent solution usually requires surgery to realign the eyelid.

SEE ALSO *Ectropion; Eye and problems*

Epiglottitis

Epiglottitis is a relatively rare but serious illness that strikes suddenly. It mostly affects children aged between two and six years, but sometimes occurs in older children and adults. The infection causes inflammation of the voice box (**larynx**) and swelling of the epiglottis, the flap of cartilage at the back of the tongue. This obstructs breathing and, if not treated promptly, can cause death by suffocation.

Epiglottitis is usually caused by the bacterium *Haemophilus influenzae*. A vaccine against this micro-organism (which can also cause meningitis) is now included in children's routine vaccinations (see **Immunization**).

SYMPTOMS

Symptoms, similar to those of croup, include:
- fever;
- severe throat pain;
- hoarseness;
- difficult or noisy breathing, which is not relieved by steam inhalation;
- excess mucus in the mouth, with drooling.

TREATMENT

Always seek prompt medical treatment if a child has fever or breathing difficulties. If epiglottitis is suspected, the child will be admitted to hospital, where **X-rays** of the neck will be taken to confirm diagnosis. A tube may be passed into the windpipe to aid breathing, and oxygen may be necessary. Antibiotics will probably be given. The patient should begin to recover within 24 hours, once the breathing obstruction has been cleared.

Epilepsy

Epilepsy affects one in 130 people in the UK today and is characterized by recurrent **seizures** that occur suddenly for no apparent reason. The seizures are the result of excessive and disordered electrical activity in the brain, which produces a brief change in consciousness, behaviour, emotion, movement or sensation. Seizures are triggered by alcohol, stress, illness, skipping meals or occasionally by flashing lights, although they can occur without an identifiable trigger.

Each year, up to 10 per cent of people with epilepsy experience prolonged or repetitive seizures, with no recovery between attacks. This is called status epilepticus and can be fatal when the seizures are generalized.

There are also a number of epilepsy syndromes (for example, Lennox-Gastaut syndrome) in which people have a mixture of seizure types or have large numbers of seizures

Epilepsy affects one in 130, or 420,000 people in the UK. It is the most common of the serious neurological conditions.

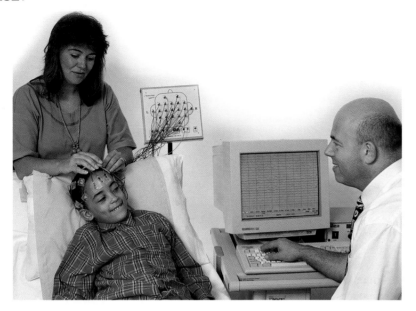

▲ **Brainwave activity**
An EEG machine can be used to detect tiny characteristic electrical impulses of brain activity that can help diagnose epilepsy.

each day. In children, these can be associated with learning difficulties.

SYMPTOMS

Symptoms range from small areas of numbness and tingling to widespread muscle spasms and convulsions, depending on the type of epilepsy. However, such symptoms can be due to other conditions – for example, certain heart conditions, **panic attacks** and breathing problems – and so anyone who is experiencing epilepsy-like seizures should be referred as soon as possible to a neurologist or other epilepsy specialist.

Some people with epilepsy know when they are about to have a seizure because they experience an aura – restlessness or an unpleasant feeling – before an attack. There are two types of epileptic seizures: generalized and partial.

Generalized seizures

The whole body is affected by generalized seizures, which are the result of abnormal electrical activity over a wide area of the brain. There are several types of generalized seizure.

■ Tonic-clonic (grand mal) seizures cause a person to lose consciousness and fall to the ground. At first the muscles contract and the body stiffens (the tonic phase), then the limbs twitch rhythmically for a time (the clonic phase) as the person goes into a deep sleep. Gradually the person regains consciousness, remembering nothing about what has happened. About 60 per cent of people with epilepsy have this type of seizure.

■ Absence seizures (also known as petit mal) occur mainly in children. There is a sudden, brief loss of conscious activity. The condition can easily go unnoticed as it may appear as though the sufferer is merely daydreaming. Other subtle symptoms include small chewing

movements, fluttering eyelids or trembling of the hands.

■ Myoclonic seizures produce a sudden brief single or repetitive muscle contraction, involving the whole body or just one part.

■ Atonic seizures are known as drop attacks because the brief loss of consciousness that they bring on causes children to drop to the ground for short periods. The sudden falls may result in head or other injuries.

Partial seizures

Partial seizures, also called focal seizures, are caused by abnormal activity in a small part of the brain. The location of the seizure in the body depends on which part of the brain is affected. However, a seizure can start in one part of the body and then spread.

Partial seizures are subdivided into simple and complex types. During a simple partial seizure, there is no loss of consciousness – a person may have muscle spasms, numbness or tingling for several minutes, but remains aware throughout. During a complex partial seizure, a person loses conscious contact with his or her surroundings for one or two minutes. The person may stare into space, move purposelessly and repetitively, make unintelligible sounds or appear confused. Usually the person will not be able to recall the episode.

Living with epilepsy

Between attacks, most people with epilepsy lead perfectly normal lives, and can work or go to school or college, and take part in everyday sports and activities.

■ Drug therapy stops seizures in about one-third of people with epilepsy and reduces their frequency in another third. The drugs are reduced gradually over time and about two-thirds of people with well-controlled seizures can eventually stop their drugs without having a relapse. It is not known why some people stop having seizures while others continue.

■ Women taking anti-epileptic drugs should take medical advice before becoming pregnant as their treatment may need to be changed to avoid harming the unborn child.

■ Very few jobs are unsuitable for people with epilepsy, although many of those affected find it hard to overcome employer fears and prejudices. Driving restrictions may make some jobs difficult. Anyone who has just been diagnosed with epilepsy must not drive by law. Anyone affected must inform the DVLA (Driver and Vehicle Licensing Authority) in Swansea, and can only reapply for a licence after he or she has been free of seizures for a year.

CAUSES

A tendency to develop epilepsy can be inherited, but there are numerous other causes, including strokes, brain tumours, head injury and meningitis. Epilepsy can also be brought on by alcohol and certain drugs. It is most common among children and the elderly. Some children stop having seizures as they get older.

DIAGNOSIS

Epilepsy is diagnosed mainly by the doctor listening carefully to a description of the way the seizure occurred, preferably by someone who saw it. An **EEG** (electroencephalogram) of electrical activity in the brain and a brain scan, usually by magnetic resonance imaging (MRI), provide additional information.

TREATMENT

People with epilepsy get to know which situations bring on a seizure and so to some extent can reduce the frequency of attacks by avoiding their own particular triggers. All but the mildest of cases will need treatment.

Medication

The aim of drug treatment is to control seizures with minimal side effects, preferably with a single drug. The exact choice and dose depends on the type of seizure, but most patients are likely to start with either sodium valproate or carbamazepine. Other drugs that may be used include the newer anti-epileptic drugs, lamotrigine and gabapentin. The older drug phenytoin tends to be reserved for hard-to-treat cases because of its unpleasant side effects.

Other drugs used in the treatment of epilepsy include tranquillizers and antidepressants, either to help to control primary symptoms or to relieve the side effects of treatment. Some types of complementary therapy, such as relaxation techniques, **massage**, yoga and aromatherapy may be helpful in this respect.

Surgery

A growing number of people are having surgery for epilepsy. This is especially true of younger people with simple partial seizures, originating in the temporal lobes of the brain cortex, which do not respond to drug treatment. MRI scans and other tests help to locate the precise area of the brain affected so that it can be removed.

SEE ALSO *Brain and nervous system; Fits; Seizure*

Episcleritis

Episcleritis is an inflammatory condition of the episclera, the outer layer of the white fibrous wall of the eyeball. It causes redness and discomfort. Common among young adults, it usually settles without treatment within a week or two. Episcleritis may recur. If concerned, you should see a doctor or optometrist to exclude other more serious causes of redness.

SEE ALSO *Eye and problems*

Erosion

Erosion is the wearing away of a tissue surface. Dental erosion reduces the protective enamel surface of teeth, caused by physical damage from excess brushing, or acid attack. Acid is present in carbonated drinks and citrus fruits, which also contain sugar. When sugar is present it is converted to acid by the bacteria that live in the mouth. In **bulimia nervosa**, when self-induced vomiting is frequent, the enamel on the back of the front teeth is attacked by stomach acid.

Cervical erosion is where the velvety lining of the cervical canal has become turned out and is visible at the opening to the vagina. The term 'erosion' isn't strictly correct; a more accurate name is 'ectropion', meaning 'turning out'.

Erysipelas

Erysipelas is a bacterial infection of the skin that spreads rapidly; it is a form of **cellulitis**. The infection starts as a small red patch, which is painful and swollen. It spreads within hours and blisters may form in the centre of the inflamed area. Other symptoms include a sudden fever, headache, shivering and vomiting. Erysipelas is caused by the bacterium *Streptococcus*, which may enter the skin via a wound, skin abrasion or ulcer, or fungal infection. Before the advent of penicillin, erysipelas caused many deaths; today, with prompt treatment, recovery can be rapid. If untreated, the infection may spread, causing blood poisoning, an **abscess** or **gangrene**, so it is important to see a doctor as early as possible.

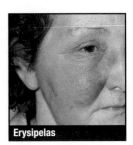

Erysipelas

▲ **Spreading rash**
Erysipelas affects the skin and underlying fat tissues. Headache, chills and fever often accompany the rash.

Erythrocyte sedimentation rate

The erythrocyte sedimentation rate (ESR) is the speed at which red blood cells fall through blood plasma. The faster the ESR, the greater the likelihood of significant inflammation within the body, indicating infections, cancers or autoimmune disorders. GPs routinely perform ESR tests on people with non-specific symptoms such as tiredness, joint pains and weight loss to see if more specific investigations are advisable.

Ewing's sarcoma

Ewing's sarcoma is a type of malignant tumour of bone. It is a **cancer** most commonly found in the long bones, especially the thigh bone (femur) and shin bone (tibia), and is more likely to occur in children, although adults may be affected. Typical symptoms include pain and swelling. Ewing's sarcoma is very resistant to treatment and so the cure rates are low.

Exhaustion

Exhaustion is a state of extreme tiredness. It is often experienced in both a physical and psychological sense, although the original cause may be either physical or psychological, and sometimes both. Physical causes include excessive exercise, dehydration, starvation, prolonged labour in childbirth, uncontrolled diabetes, and thyroid disease. Psychological causes include intense stress for longer than the individual can manage, uncontrolled psychotic illness and severe depressive illness.

Sleep deprivation has direct physical and psychological effects on the body because it deprives the muscles and joints of rest, as well as bringing on mental exhaustion.

Exposure

Exposure is the term used to describe the physical effects of being subjected to extreme weather – usually to intense cold, or cold combined with damp and wind. Exposure also covers the ill effects of extreme heat, radiation and environmental pollutants such as pesticides.

The human body is capable of surviving intense cold as long as it is warmly wrapped, fed and adequately sheltered. Clothing provides insulation, trapping air warmed by body heat. Since cold increases the rate at which the body uses energy, the body requires food to generate heat to keep warm.

Well-fed adults can maintain their core temperature of 37°C (98.6°F) for a long period in still air temperatures of -29°C (-84°F) or lower. If there is wind, however, it replaces the warm air around the body with cold, so the skin freezes and the core temperature drops. Water conducts heat away from the body faster than air, so if the clothing is wet from rain, snow or immersion in water of a temperature lower than 20°C (68°F), the core body temperature falls and death from **hypothermia** follows.

Medical treatment focuses on restoring the normal body temperature as a gradual process in order to maintain an even blood temperature.

PREVENTION

If you are at risk of exposure from cold, there are some simple measures you can take to protect yourself.

- Find or construct a shelter.
- Cover your body, head and extremities to insulate them from cold.
- If immersed in cold water, keep still. Moving prevents the body from warming a surrounding layer of water that could protect you.
- Drink water or other non-alcoholic drinks.

SEE ALSO *Frostbite*

Extradural haematoma

Extradural haematoma is a life-threatening brain haemorrhage resulting from a severe blow to the head. It often occurs at the same time as a skull fracture.

The trauma causes a tear in a major artery, which leaks blood into the outer covering of the brain (the extradural space), producing pressure on the brain. Brain swelling may cause the pupil of the eye on the affected side to dilate. The concussed patient recovers initially until deepening **coma** occurs minutes or hours later, necessitating prompt surgical treatment. This involves making a hole in the skull (burr hole) over the injury, removing the clot and tying the leaking artery.

SEE ALSO *Brain and nervous system*

Extrasystoles

Extrasystoles are extra heartbeats arising as a result of spontaneous electrical activity in the heart. They may interrupt the normal rhythm, producing the sensation of a 'missed beat'. This gives the heart longer to fill up, so the next scheduled beat becomes stronger and a 'thump' is felt. Extrasystoles can be identified by an ECG (electrocardiogram).

Some types of extrasystole are common in healthy people, and may be triggered by stimulants such as caffeine or stress. Ventricular extrasystoles may also be normal, but can be a sign of heart disease. Frequent extrasystoles may be the forerunner of other abnormal rhythms.

SEE ALSO *Heart and circulatory system*

Eye and problems

Problems affecting the eye range from infections and injuries to impaired vision and blindness. Any of the structures of the eye may be poorly developed or become diseased during a person's lifetime.

The eye has two main parts: an image-forming system consisting of the cornea, iris and lens, and the retina, which converts images falling onto it into electrical signals that are passed to the brain by the optic nerve.

Each eyelid acts as a protective shutter for the eyeball and, like the visible part of the eye itself, is lined by the conjunctiva, a thick membrane filled with blood vessels. Behind the lids lies the cornea – the 'window' through which light enters – and the sclera, or white of the eye. The conjunctiva and cornea are constantly bathed in tears secreted by the lacrimal and other glands to keep the front surface lubricated and protected.

The pupil, a hole of variable diameter in the centre of the iris (the coloured part), controls how much light enters the eye. The light is then focused by the lens, a firm, transparent, convex body behind the iris. The lens is made thinner or thicker by the action of a ring of muscle around it called the ciliary muscle. This focusing ability reduces throughout life (see also **Presbyopia**) due to a loss of elasticity of the lens – hence the need for reading glasses as we grow older.

The space between the cornea and the lens is filled by a watery fluid called the aqueous humour, which is constantly secreted and drained to maintain the eye's shape and internal pressure. If the drainage is blocked, it causes a rise in pressure in the eye, which can lead to **glaucoma**.

Light passes from the lens through the vitreous humour – a transparent, jelly-like substance that fills the interior of the eyeball.

Organ of vision
The eye is a complex and delicate structure that measures only 25mm (1in) in diameter. It supplies the brain with more information about the outside world than any of the other senses.

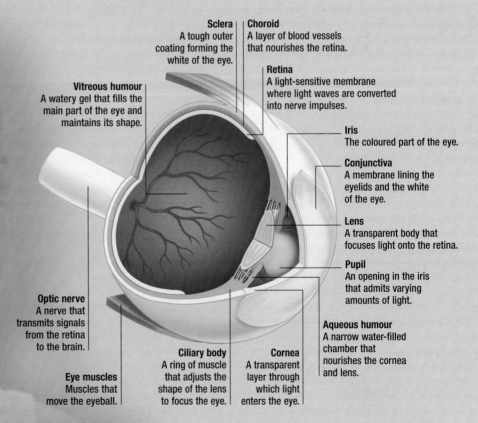

Sclera
A tough outer coating forming the white of the eye.

Choroid
A layer of blood vessels that nourishes the retina.

Retina
A light-sensitive membrane where light waves are converted into nerve impulses.

Vitreous humour
A watery gel that fills the main part of the eye and maintains its shape.

Iris
The coloured part of the eye.

Conjunctiva
A membrane lining the eyelids and the white of the eye.

Lens
A transparent body that focuses light onto the retina.

Pupil
An opening in the iris that admits varying amounts of light.

Aqueous humour
A narrow water-filled chamber that nourishes the cornea and lens.

Optic nerve
A nerve that transmits signals from the retina to the brain.

Eye muscles
Muscles that move the eyeball.

Ciliary body
A ring of muscle that adjusts the shape of the lens to focus the eye.

Cornea
A transparent layer through which light enters the eye.

From there, the light is focused onto the retina, a light-sensitive sheet of nerve cells and fibres lining the interior of the eyeball. Behind the retina is the choroid, a layer of blood vessels supplying the retina with nutrients.

The retina contains light-sensitive cells called photoreceptors that convert light into electrical signals. There are two types of photoreceptor cell: cones and rods. The cones are primarily responsive to colour and detail (and are faulty in **colour blindness**) and the rods respond to lower light levels and movement. The signals pass through retinal nerve fibres to a small area called the optic disc. Here the nerve fibres leave the eye and pass down the optic nerve. They carry the electric signals to the visual cortex on each side of the brain, where they are processed to allow perception of the image.

COMMON EYE PROBLEMS

External eye infections are usually related to **conjunctivitis**, an inflammation of the mucous membranes that line the eyelids. Other causes of redness and irritation are a persistent scaliness on the eyelid edges (**blepharitis**) and inflamed, painful bumps at the base of the eyelashes (**styes**). Inflammation may also result from injuries to the eye, allergies or irritants such as smoke.

Common problems affecting the lids and lashes include a turning out of the eyelid (**ectropion**), a turning in of the eyelid (**entropion**), **inturned eyelashes**, and swelling of a gland in the eyelid (chalazion). Tear problems are also common, and drainage of the tears may be disrupted, as happens with a blocked tear duct.

Diet and smoking

One of the keys to healthy eyes is general well-being – so, to keep your eyes in good condition, you need to maintain a balanced diet, take plenty of exercise and avoid smoking.

■ There is increasing evidence that a diet rich in antioxidants – contained in fresh fruit and vegetables, for example – may reduce the risk of degenerative diseases such as age-related macular degeneration.

■ A deficiency of vitamin A may lead to night blindness, so eat plenty of green vegetables and carrots.

■ A high-sugar diet has been linked with diabetes, the most common cause of blindness in people of working age.

■ Smoking increases the risk of age-related macular degeneration, which can cause blindness as well as cardiovascular disease.

Practical eye care

Some work and leisure activities expose the eyes to various dangers, but there are a number of practical steps you can take to minimize any risk.

■ Wear sunglasses with an adequate filter or tint, especially when skiing or taking part in other prolonged outdoor activities. Exposure to ultraviolet radiation can increase the risk of disorders such as corneal problems, cataracts and conjunctival degeneration.

■ Always wear eye protection when carrying out a task such as welding or garden strimming, which could result in injury.

■ When doing close work, ensure that you have good lighting and take regular breaks to reduce eye strain, which may cause discomfort and headaches.

■ If your work involves long hours in front of a computer screen, give your eyes plenty of opportunities to refocus by gazing into the distance at 20-minute intervals.

■ Have an eye test at least every two years to monitor the health of your eyes.

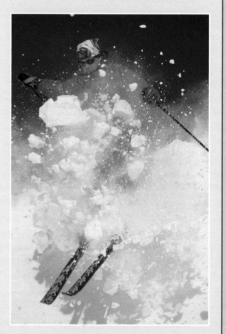

The cornea is vulnerable to damage by foreign bodies or abrasion and may become ulcerated (see **Cornea and disorders**). The sclera may become inflamed (scleritis or **episcleritis**), and the iris and ciliary body are also subject to inflammation (**iritis**).

VISION PROBLEMS

If the eye is not the right shape to allow normal focusing on the retina, a refractive error exists. For example, if the length of the eye from front to back – from the cornea to the retina – is too short, or the cornea is too flat, the eye will find it hard to focus on close targets; this is known as long-sightedness or **hypermetropia**.

If the focal length is too long or the cornea is excessively curved, the eye will have difficulty perceiving distant objects; this is called short-sightedness or **myopia**. If the eye is not spherical, **astigmatism** will result.

All these refractive errors can be corrected with focusing lenses, the powers of which are determined by the results of an **eye test**. **Laser surgery** can also be effective in correcting many refractive errors.

Double vision – seeing two images in place of one – when looking in certain directions indicates a squint, which can sometimes be corrected by a treatment programme that may include special eye exercises. An uncorrected squint in childhood can lead to amblyopia, in which the eye never achieves normal levels of vision.

The retina is vulnerable to many disorders, with symptoms ranging from night blindness to total blindness in conditions such as a **detached retina**. The central area of the retina with the highest concentration of photoreceptor cells is called the macular, and this often degenerates with age. Age-related macular degeneration is estimated to be responsible for about half of all registered sight loss in the UK.

Damage to the nerves carrying the signal out of the eye may occur, for example, in glaucoma or **optic neuritis**. Such damage is sometimes seen as a paleness of the fibres (optic atrophy).

Problems of the blood supply to the eye, its muscles or the structures within the visual pathway – as can occur in people with diabetes or high blood pressure, for example – may result in loss of normal eye function. In later life, the lens may lose its transparency (see **Cataract**).

SEEKING HELP
Optometrists, who are qualified to undertake **eye tests**, are listed in the Opticians Register, available from the General Optical Council. Most registered optical practices display a sign indicating the presence of a qualified optometrist on the premises.

Although the content of an eye test may vary depending upon the nature of the possible problem bring investigated, all tests should include an assessment of your vision and an eye health check.

Consult a doctor or optometrist if you experience any of the following:
- pain in the eyes;
- blurred vision;
- discharge;
- redness;
- visual phenomena, such as flashing lights or **floaters**.

See a doctor or report to your nearest eye casualty unit urgently if you experience:
- sudden loss of total vision or a portion of peripheral vision, with or without pain;
- severe pain;
- severe headaches, with or without loss of vision;
- sudden flashing lights or many floaters;
- haloes around lights;
- visual loss accompanied by feelings of general ill health;
- sudden onset of double vision.

SEE ALSO *Blindness; Contact lenses and problems; Eye test; Subconjunctival haemorrhage*

Eye test

An eye test is designed to assess an individual's level of vision and, if necessary, to prescribe spectacles or contact lenses. The health of the person's eyes is checked at the same time.

Such a test will generally be carried out by an optometrist (a specialist in vision defects) or an ophthalmologist (a specialist in eye diseases).

Regular tests are advisable because everyone's level of vision changes over time. This applies especially to elderly people, in whom conditions such as **cataract** and **glaucoma** are more common. Generally, a test every two years is adequate, but more frequent assessment may be advised, especially if you have **diabetes**.

Eye examinations are free on the NHS for children, full-time students up to the age of 19 and people over 60 – as well as those receiving certain health and social security benefits, those with glaucoma or diabetes, those over 40 who have a parent or sibling with glaucoma, and those who need a very strong correction.

WHAT'S INVOLVED
An eye test takes between 20 minutes and one hour, depending on the number of tests required. You will be questioned about your vision and any history of visual problems or symptoms. You will also be asked about your general health, and about any family members with eye or general health problems.

A series of tests will be carried out to check all aspects of your vision and to assess the health of your eyes. The optometrist will explain the results and advise you on general care of your eyesight, such as avoiding eye strain. He or she will also tell you when you should have your next eye test.

If you need help with your vision, you will be given a prescription specifying the strength of any spectacles or contact lenses required. You can take it to any optician where prescription spectacles are made up. Most opticians have a very wide selection of frames suitable for prescription lenses. If a health problem has been detected, the prescription will also indicate whether you should see your GP for further investigation.

SEE ALSO *Eye and problems*

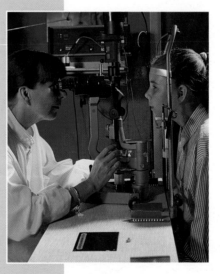

▲ **Health check**
As well as assessing your level of vision, an eye test can identify a variety of health problems.

Face and problems

The face is made up of 14 bones, including the two parts of the jaw. These are overlaid with specialized muscles that allow an enormous complexity of expression and communication. Women's faces are smaller than men's, with smaller teeth and jaws, more rounded contours, smoother facial bones, less prominent eyebrow ridges, sharper upper margins to the eye sockets and a more vertical forehead. The overall effect is that women are more 'baby-faced'; as with infants, such features tend to evoke protective instincts in adults – both men and women. Facial attractiveness is closely linked with facial symmetry: the more closely the two halves of the face match each other, the more a face is likely to be rated as attractive by observers.

The face is the front we present to the world and has vital importance to our sense of 'self', to emotional expression and to interactions with others. Any cosmetic deficiencies – whether real or imagined – can cause self-consciousness, low self-esteem, withdrawal from normal relationships and teasing or bullying from others.

SKIN COLOURING

Facial colouring is determined by the skin pigment melanin, which individuals have in varying amounts. This accounts for variations in skin tone among people of the same race, as well as for the differences in colour between people of different races. Alterations in skin pigmentation – either lightening or darkening – are sometimes much sought-after, but can cause considerable distress, particularly if the effects are patchy.

Factors that alter skin pigmentation include:
■ patchy darkening (melanoderma) caused by hormonal changes in pregnancy or the contraceptive pill (chloasma), sunburn, menopause, old age or various diseases including diabetes and malaria;
■ loss of pigment – known as vitiligo;
■ discoloration caused by carotenaemia – in which sufferers develop an orange skin colour as a result of consuming excessive quantities of carotene – or haemochromatosis ('bronzed diabetes'), a hereditary disorder in which iron is deposited in skin.

FACIAL DISFIGUREMENTS

Facial malformations evident at birth include **cleft palate and hare lip** and **birthmarks** such as strawberry marks (haemangioma) and port-wine stains. Malformations may be caused by more extensive disorders such as foetal alcohol syndrome, congenital syphilis, cretinism (lack of thyroid hormone), Down's syndrome, and some forms of muscular dystrophy. Causes of facial disfigurement developing after birth include:
■ bulbous red nose (rhinophyma) in **rosacea**;
■ deformity caused by fractures, especially of the nose;

Facial bones and muscles

The facial skeleton consists of 14 stationary bones (6 paired and 2 single), which provide attachments for the muscles that control facial movements.

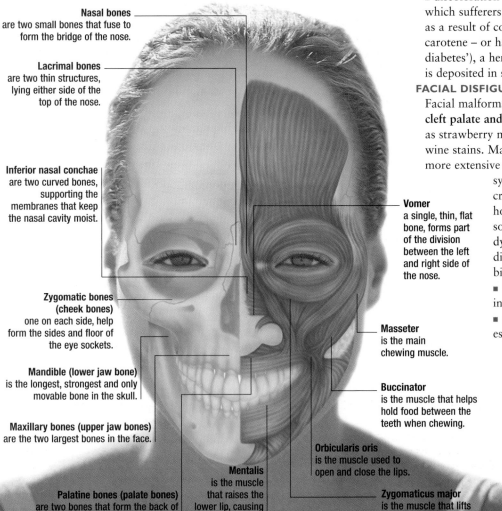

Nasal bones
are two small bones that fuse to form the bridge of the nose.

Lacrimal bones
are two thin structures, lying either side of the top of the nose.

Inferior nasal conchae
are two curved bones, supporting the membranes that keep the nasal cavity moist.

Zygomatic bones (cheek bones)
one on each side, help form the sides and floor of the eye sockets.

Mandible (lower jaw bone)
is the longest, strongest and only movable bone in the skull.

Maxillary bones (upper jaw bones)
are the two largest bones in the face.

Palatine bones (palate bones)
are two bones that form the back of the palate and floor of the nose.

Mentalis
is the muscle that raises the lower lip, causing it to protrude.

Vomer
a single, thin, flat bone, forms part of the division between the left and right side of the nose.

Masseter
is the main chewing muscle.

Buccinator
is the muscle that helps hold food between the teeth when chewing.

Orbicularis oris
is the muscle used to open and close the lips.

Zygomaticus major
is the muscle that lifts the corner of the mouth.

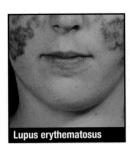

Lupus erythematosus

▲ **Diagnostic clue**
Red scaly patches on the face may be a sign of lupus erythematosus, a condition in which the connective tissue in the skin breaks down. The drug chloroquine (often used against malaria) can help, though most cases will improve with time.

■ drooping eyelids – many causes, including myasthenia gravis;
■ drooping of one side of the face due to muscle paralysis – **Bell's palsy**;
■ melanoma;
■ protruding or misaligned teeth;
■ rodent ulcer – a slow-growing skin tumour;
■ scarring due to **burns** or trauma;
■ squint.

'Invisible' facial problems include facial pain or frontal headache from sinusitis, trigeminal neuralgia, temporal arteritis and temperomandibular joint problems.

ENLARGED ADENOIDS

If left untreated, enlarged adenoids stop a child breathing through the nose. This tends to produce a characteristic facial expression – a gaping mouth with a vacant expression – associated with a nasal voice. Prolonged mouth breathing has been shown to reduce the levels of oxygen reaching the brain and can impair intelligence. (See also **Adenoids and problems.**)

PLASTIC SURGERY

Reconstructive surgery is used to repair or restore damage to the facial structure or skin. For example, people with severe burns to the face may need a number of skin-grafting operations or a badly broken jaw may need to be surgically rebuilt.

FACIAL CLUES TO BODILY AILMENTS

Many diseases are linked with abnormal facial features and can give doctors vital clues in making a diagnosis:
■ acromegaly – enlarged, coarse features;
■ Addison's disease and some cases of poisoning – dark pigmentation;
■ alcoholism – broken blood vessels apparent on the nose;
■ anaemia – pale skin;
■ chronic bronchitis – blueish complexion;
■ Cushing's syndrome or steroid treatment – enlarged 'moonshaped' face;
■ cyanosis – blue lips, dusky cheeks;
■ emphysema – reddish complexion;
■ hypothyroidism, also known as myxoedema – coarse puffy skin and eyelids;
■ jaundice – yellowed skin and the 'whites' of the eyes;
■ lupus erythematosus and rosacea – butterfly rash on the face;
■ mitral stenosis – prominent blood vessels on the cheeks;
■ thyrotoxicosis – staring, protruding eyes.

SEE ALSO *Cosmetic and plastic surgery; Endocrine system and disorders; Eye and problems; Mouth and disorders; Nose and problems; Skin and disorders; Teeth and problems; Thyroid gland and disorders*

Fainting

Fainting is when a person collapses due to loss of consciousness following a temporary reduction in blood supply to the brain. The effect of falling in a faint is to reduce the vertical distance between the heart and the brain, thereby helping to restore normal blood flow. Known medically as syncope, fainting is extremely common and can happen to anyone. Causes include emotional trauma and prolonged standing, particularly in hot, stuffy conditions – or a faint may follow injury or haemorrhage.

SYMPTOMS

There are common warning signs of an impending faint. The person feels lightheaded, giddy and sweaty, and vision may be blurred. Onlookers may notice that he or she looks pale, grey, clammy or sweaty. Eventually the person will become unsteady, lose consciousness and fall to the ground.

TREATMENT

Within a few minutes of being horizontal, most people recover consciousness and there are usually no after effects, unless the person is injured by falling. If fainting follows an injury, if other symptoms are present, or if repeated attacks occur with no obvious cause, medical advice should be sought.

PREVENTION

Someone who is about to faint should lie down or sit with the head between the knees, and breathe in some fresh air.

SEE ALSO *FIRST AID*

Fallen arches

Fallen arches (also known as flat feet) can cause poor posture as well as easily tired muscles in the feet and legs, low back pain and a burning sensation in the soles. In the long term, fallen arches can also lead to **arthritis** in the feet, knees and hips.

The feet have a natural arch shape at the insole, which acts as a shock absorber to protect the knees, hips and back. This arch can 'fall' as a result of the person being overweight, or if he or she stands relatively still for long periods of time.

Painless flat feet rarely need treatment. If the condition causes aching when standing or walking, individually moulded arch supports can be fitted inside the shoes. Exercises to strengthen the ligaments and muscles can help.

SEE ALSO *Foot and problems*

Fallopian tubes

The two Fallopian tubes are part of a woman's reproductive system. They carry eggs (ova) from the ovaries to the uterus. Each of these muscular structures is about 10cm (4in) long. The ovarian end opens into the abdominal cavity through a funnel-shaped structure edged with fringe-like projections called fimbriae. These direct the egg into the tube. Muscular contractions of the walls of the tube and the 'waving' of specialized lining cells then move the egg to the uterus.

The Fallopian tubes can be damaged by pelvic infection; abnormalities in the tubes account for up to 50 per cent of female infertility.

A fertilized egg sometimes implants itself in one of the Fallopian tubes rather than in the uterus. This is called an **ectopic pregnancy** and requires emergency medical intervention.
SEE ALSO *Infertility; Pelvis and disorders; Reproductive system*

Fallot's tetralogy

Fallot's tetralogy is a form of congenital heart disease in which an affected child is born with four heart defects that occur together. This results in the child appearing blue (cyanosis).

The condition develops progressively, usually from birth, and is usually diagnosed in the first month or two of life. The defects are a hole in the heart (ventriculoseptal defect), narrowing of the pulmonary valve, displacement of the aorta and a thickened right ventricle. Symptoms include **clubbing of the fingers or toes,** underdevelopment, and shortness of breath.

Fallot's tetralogy can often be treated with surgery, which is carried out before the child is five years old.
SEE ALSO *Congenital disorders; Heart and circulatory system; Heart surgery*

Farmer's lung

Farmer's lung is a lung disease caused by an allergy to the spores of fungus growing in mouldy hay or straw. It is a form of alveolitis, an inflammation of the tiny air sacs in the lungs. Farmer's lung occurs when someone who has developed a hypersensitivity to the fungi spores inhales them. The inflammation makes the lungs less efficient, causing breathlessness, fever, headache and muscle ache. Repeated exposure can make the condition chronic (long term). If it is not diagnosed early on, the lungs may be permanently scarred.

The risk of farmer's lung is reduced by ensuring that stored hay or straw is kept dry, and that farm workers wear protective masks and work in dry, well-ventilated areas.
SEE ALSO *Lungs and disorders*

Fatigue

Fatigue is a state of tiredness, which often becomes a normal part of everyday life. Its extreme stage is **exhaustion**. Causes include sleep deprivation, jet lag, prolonged stress or depression, work, exercise and illness.

Febrile convulsion

Also called **seizures** or fever fits, febrile convulsions are fits associated with a fever, and usually caused by a viral infection. They look like epileptic fits, but are not in fact a sign of **epilepsy**. Febrile convulsions may occur in a child aged between six months and five years if the child's temperature rises either too high or too quickly. The child may turn blue, the eyes may roll, and the limbs or whole body may start jerking or twitching.

In rare cases, a child may suffer febrile convulsions after receiving the **MMR vaccine**. In such a case, convulsion occurs eight to ten days after the vaccination. It is caused by the measles component of the vaccine, but this is responsible for fewer cases of febrile convulsion than measles itself.

Although they last for only 2–3 minutes, fits can be very alarming for parents. A child who has a fit should lie on his or her side on the floor. Do not insert anything into the child's mouth, and when the fit is over call a doctor.

To reduce a high temperature, give your child plenty of cool clear fluids, remove all clothing except a nappy or pants and vest, and keep the room cool.

Fetal alcohol syndrome

A woman who drinks too much alcohol during pregnancy may give birth to a child with a collection of characteristics and abnormalities known as fetal alcohol syndrome.

One in 500 babies born in Europe has fetal alcohol syndrome, and there is concern that this figure will rise as a result of increasing alcohol consumption among women.
SYMPTOMS
A baby affected by fetal alcohol syndrome may exhibit a number of problems, including:

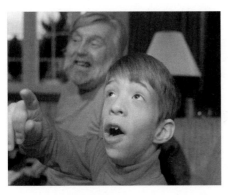

▲ **Uncertain future**
A child born with fetal alcohol syndrome has distinctive facial features and is likely to suffer from poor physical coordination.

■ a small size for its estimated delivery date;

■ small wide-set eyes, flattened cheekbones and bridge of the nose, and a shallow or non-existent groove between the nose and upper lip;

■ heart defects;

■ skeletal abnormalities such as fused joints, deformed fingers and toes, or curvature of the spine;

■ alcohol withdrawal after the birth, which may make the baby fretful.

PREVENTION

Fetal alcohol syndrome is most commonly associated with heavy drinking, but the 'safe' level of alcohol consumption during pregnancy is not known. Only a small number of babies born to women with alcohol problems suffer from fetal alcohol syndrome; the pattern of consumption and the mother's nutrition and genetic susceptibility also influence the risk.

Total abstention from alcohol throughout pregnancy prevents fetal alcohol syndrome, but some women drink alcohol before they realize that they are pregnant. This is unlikely to cause serious harm and should not lead to undue anxiety.

OUTLOOK

Fetal alcohol syndrome is the leading cause of mental retardation in the world, and children affected by the condition have irreversible damage to the central nervous system. They are likely to have developmental delays and learning and behavioural difficulties, as well as poor physical coordination.

Fever

Known medically as pyrexia, a fever is defined as a body temperature above 37°C (99°F), measured in the mouth.

Most fevers are triggered by the body's defence mechanism against either viral or bacterial infections, including typhoid fever, tonsillitis, influenza and measles. In these cases, proteins called pyrogens are released when the body's white blood cells fight the micro-organisms responsible for the illness. These pyrogens act on the temperature-controlling centre in the brain, causing it to raise the body's temperature in an attempt to destroy the invading micro-organisms.

Sometimes conditions that are non-infectious may be accompanied by a fever. These include dehydration, heart attack and lymphoma (a tumour of the lymphatic system). Why fever should be a feature of such conditions is not yet properly understood.

TREATMENT

Most fevers will not require any treatment, but it is advisable to drink plenty of fluids while the temperature lasts. Aspirin and paracetamol may help to relieve fevers caused by infections.

When to consult a doctor

■ If your temperature remains raised for longer than 48 hours or rises above 40°C (104°F).

■ If there are accompanying symptoms such as severe headache with a stiff neck or abdominal pain, which may be a sign of **meningitis**.

Complementary therapies

Feverfew is an old herbal treatment for the relief of fever, but it should not be taken by pregnant women.

SEE ALSO *Temperature*

Fibrillation

Fibrillation is characterized by cardiac muscle fibres contracting at different rates, producing a quivering effect instead of coordinated heartbeats. Atrial and ventricular fibrillation may be due to heart damage or other diseases; ventricular fibrillation after a heart attack or electrocution is often rapidly fatal. Drugs or electric shock treatment may restore normal rhythm.

SEE ALSO *Atrial fibrillation and flutter; Heart and circulatory system*

Fibroids, uterine

Also known as fibromyomas, uterine fibroids are benign (non-cancerous) tumours of the wall of the uterus. They consist of smooth muscle fibres and fibrous connective tissue. Their growth is stimulated by the hormone oestrogen and they vary considerably in size.

About 30 per cent of women over the age of 35 have fibroids. Childless women are at greater risk than women with children, and Afro-Caribbean women are at higher risk than white women. Fibroids do not develop before puberty and shrink after the menopause.

SYMPTOMS

■ Fibroids usually cause no symptoms and are often found during a routine pelvic examination.

■ The most common symptom of fibroids is heavy periods. There are other less common symptoms, which can include abdominal swelling, pain, frequent urination caused by pressure on the bladder, and **infertility**.

TREATMENT

Treatment is rarely needed for small fibroids that do not cause any symptoms.

- Women suffering from problematic fibroids are usually offered a **hysterectomy**. For those hoping to bear children, however, an operation to remove the fibroid while leaving the uterus intact (known as a myomectomy) is sometimes a possible option.
- Uterine artery embolization, a procedure that blocks the blood supply to the fibroid, may be offered as an alternative to surgery. This causes the fibroid to degenerate and form scar tissue.

OUTLOOK

Therapies currently being tested include using laser or an electric current to shrink the fibroid, and a treatment that combines a procedure to reduce oestrogen production with removal of the womb lining (endometrium) to control heavy periods.

SEE ALSO *Pelvis and disorders*

Fibrosis

Fibrosis is the irreversible thickening and scarring of connective tissue, usually caused by inflammation or injury. Fibrosis is normal in scar tissue, but becomes a problem in some types of scarring. In connective tissue disorders such as scleroderma, for example, the skin and other tissues progressively tighten and harden. In some cases disfigurement may occur, and when the underlying joints and muscles are severely affected there may be disability.

Fibrositis

Fibrositis is a common, sometimes severe, condition, also termed fibromyalgia, in which fibrous tissues and muscles are affected by pain and tenderness. Sufferers also experience sleep disturbance. Fibrositis may persist for months or years, but does no permanent damage.

SYMPTOMS

- Aching in muscles, tendons and ligaments.
- Stiffness in muscles.
- May affect one or more parts of the body.
- Fatigue or lack of energy.

If symptoms closely resemble those of ME (myalgic encephalomyelitis), consult a doctor as soon as possible.

TREATMENT

Treatment usually focuses on relieving symptoms.

What a doctor may do

- Advise or prescribe painkillers and non-steroidal anti-inflammatory drugs (NSAIDS).
- Administer steroid injection.

What you can do

- Avoid alcohol, tea and coffee late at night.
- Eat healthily and watch your weight.

- Identify and eliminate stresses.
- Exercise progressively.

Complementary therapies

Physiotherapy, **massage**, **acupuncture**, **homeopathy** and **chiropractic** may all help.

Fistula

A fistula is any abnormal channel between the interior and exterior of the body or two body organs. The most common form is an anal fistula, in which a channel between the rectum and anus allows mucus, pus and sometimes faeces to leak. The cause may be an injury, an abscess or **Crohn's disease**, ulcerative colitis or colorectal cancer.

Fits

Fits or seizures result from excessive nerve activity in the cortex of the brain. They can last for anything from just a few seconds to several minutes.

Fits may be recurrent or isolated and non-recurrent. Recurrent fits occur in **epilepsy**, for example. Non-recurrent fits can be caused by, for example, a head injury, **eclampsia** during pregnancy, or a childhood infection resulting in a high temperature (febrile seizure).

SYMPTOMS

Symptoms include altered consciousness and usually convulsions in which the body goes rigid and the limbs move rhythmically.

TREATMENT

Anyone experiencing a fit for the first time should seek urgent medical help.

Treatment of febrile seizures focuses on reducing fever. Seizures caused by infections, such as **meningitis** and **rabies**, are treated with anti-microbial therapy. In cases of eclampsia, it may be necessary to deliver the fetus early.

A variety of **drugs** are available to treat epileptic seizures.

PREVENTION

Vaccines are available against rabies and some forms of meningitis. Epileptic seizures may be prevented by regular medication. Alcohol- and cocaine-induced seizures may be prevented by reduction or withdrawal of intake.

COMPLICATIONS

Severe, prolonged or recurrent fits can cause brain damage.

SEE ALSO *Brain and nervous system; Epilepsy; Seizure*

Flat feet

Flat feet, also known as fallen arches, is a condition characterized by an absence of the normal arches of the feet, so that the soles lie flat on the ground. It is normal in toddlers, but should not persist into later childhood.

The condition can also develop in adulthood as a result of prolonged standing or obesity, and can lead, in the long term, to **arthritis** in the feet, knees and hips.

SEE ALSO *Foot and problems*

Flatulence

Flatulence – which affects everyone at times – is excess gas or wind in the digestive tract. Wind is brought up from the stomach through the mouth in a belch or passed through the anus.

CAUSES

The most common cause of gas in the stomach is swallowed air, which may be taken in while eating and drinking. Air swallowing is also often associated with nervous tension.

Gas in the bowel stems from bacterial fermentation of food, especially beans, peas, eggs and some vegetables, in the digestive tract.

Flatulence can be a sign of a gastro-intestinal disorder such as **gastroenteritis**, gastric ulcer, hiatus **hernia** or **irritable bowel syndrome**, or a condition affecting the **gallbladder**.

TREATMENT

Charcoal, available from pharmacies in tablet form, can be taken to absorb excess gas. Over-the-counter antacids or indigestion remedies may help.

When to consult a doctor
- If flatulence becomes socially troublesome.
- If it is accompanied by persistent pain, **constipation** or **diarrhoea**.

What a doctor may do
- Advise on diet.
- Prescribe an antacid liquid for belching.
- Check for any underlying causes.

PREVENTION

Avoid wind-producing foods, fizzy drinks, hurried meals and nervous tension.

SEE ALSO *Digestive system*

Floaters

Floaters are dark spots or specks in the field of vision. Most people see them occasionally, especially when looking at a light, even background, such as an overcast sky. Floaters are commonly remnants of the many blood vessels that filled the now transparent jelly in the chamber behind the eye lens (the vitreous humour) when the eye was developing in the womb. They may also be caused by damage to the retina or an inflammation of the eye.

ONSET AND DURATION

Once floaters are present, they remain, although they may not be noticed after a while. They are more noticeable when they drift into the centre of the eye, which is why people sometimes complain of intermittent floaters. Floaters are often reported after eye surgery, such as a **cataract** operation.

DIAGNOSIS

Any floaters seen for the first time (even if not in large numbers) should be investigated by a thorough eye examination in case there is an underlying disease that needs treatment, but most floaters are harmless.
- The sudden appearance of a large cobweb-like floater may be a result of the jelly inside the eye shrinking (a vitreous detachment). Consult a doctor or optometrist as soon as possible to rule out any damage to the retina.
- A sudden shower of floaters, accompanied by flashing or sparkling lights, may indicate retinal detachment. Report to your nearest eye casualty unit for urgent treatment.
- A gradual increase in large floaters together with a reduction of vision and a general feeling of malaise could indicate an inflammation in the eye. See a doctor if you have this combination of symptoms.

SEE ALSO *Eye and problems*

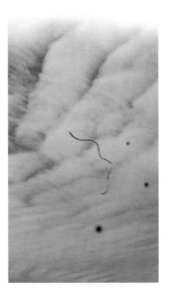

▲ **Spotted vision**
Floaters cast a shadow on the retina and are therefore seen as dark shapes. A large floater passing across the line of gaze may intermittently affect vision.

Fluid retention

Fluid retention is the accumulation of fluid in body tissue. It most commonly affects the feet and ankles, but can also affect the hands and face, in severe cases the legs, and sometimes the entire body. It occurs in many diseases in which sluggish circulation is a factor. Gravity tends to pull the fluid to the lowest point of the body. Fluid retention is common in premenstrual syndrome, occurring the week before the start of a period (see also **Oedema**).

SYMPTOMS
- Swelling of soft tissues.
- Weight gain.
- In severe cases, breathlessness and swelling of the entire leg.

DURATION

In premenstrual syndrome, fluid retention is resolved when the period begins. Otherwise the duration of the problem depends on what has caused it and what treatment is given.

CAUSES

Apart from premenstrual syndrome, there are several other causes of fluid retention:

- prolonged standing or sitting;
- varicose veins;
- pregnancy;
- heart, kidney or liver disease;
- malnutrition;
- allergy;
- side effects of some drugs, especially steroids and non-steroidal anti-inflammatory drugs (NSAIDs), such as aspirin or ibuprofen.

TREATMENT

If you suffer from fluid retention, keep your legs elevated while sitting. Take a mild diuretic, available from pharmacies. Avoid prolonged standing or sitting – if this is impossible, walk around for a few minutes every half-hour, and exercise the calf muscles by stretching the feet out and down, then back and up. This is especially important when undertaking any long-distance travel.

When to consult a doctor

- If the symptom is troublesome.
- If leg swelling is new, especially if it affects only one leg.
- If you are unwell.

What a doctor may do

- Examine and treat you as appropriate, refer you to a specialist, or admit you to hospital, urgently if necessary.
- Prescribe medication to alleviate premenstrual syndrome. Diuretics, evening primrose oil, hormones and vitamin B_6 (pyridoxine) can help. The antidepressant fluoxetine, which is useful in relieving the psychological effects of premenstrual syndrome, may also be prescribed.

Complementary therapies

- Herbal remedies include evening primrose oil and natural diuretics such as dandelion leaves and asparagus.
- A naturopath would recommend a wholefood, low-salt diet and greater consumption of foods containing gammalinoleic acid (the active ingredient in evening primrose oil). These include blackcurrants, redcurrants, gooseberries, oats, barley and borage oil.
- A homeopath would recommend Lacheis muta (lachesis) and Natrum chloratum (Nat. mur.) to relieve bloating in premenstrual syndrome.

PREVENTION

Regular evening primrose oil or vitamin B_6 can ease premenstrual syndrome generally and reduce the incidence of fluid retention.

SEE ALSO *Menstruation; Oedema*

Fontanelle

A fontanelle is one of two soft spots on a newborn baby's head, covering gaps between the plates of bone. These gaps later fuse together as the skull grows. During childbirth they allow a degree of overlap and movement of the bones so that the baby's head can pass through the birth canal.

The rear fontanelle is small and closes within six weeks of a baby being born. The front fontanelle is a larger, diamond-shaped area, measuring about 4cm (1½ in) by 2cm (¾ in), which closes at around 18 months of age. A fontanelle that appears sunken or depressed is a sign of dehydration – the baby should be offered more breast milk or small quantities of boiled and cooled water from a sterilized bottle.

SEE ALSO *Babies and baby care*

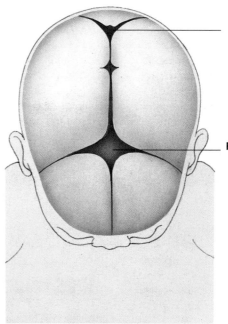

Rear fontanelle

Front fontanelle

◄ **Good protection**
A baby's pulse may be visible at the fontanelle, arousing worries that it is vulnerable to injury, but the baby's brain is protected by a layer of very tough cartilage.

Food poisoning

Food poisoning is usually an acute illness. It is generally caused by the recent consumption of food or drink contaminated by bacteria, viruses or parasites. Less common causes include the consumption of insecticide residues on fruit and vegetables; poisonous chemicals, such as lead or mercury; and poisonous berries or fungi.

Despite steadily improving methods of food preservation and storage, food poisoning is still common. It occurs particularly in the summer, when foods are less likely to be properly chilled, and at Christmas, when frozen poultry is sometimes inadequately thawed before cooking.

Symptoms can include vomiting, **nausea,
diarrhoea,** stomach **cramps** and **fever.** Consult
a doctor or call NHS Direct (0845 4647) if
symptoms persist for more than 24 hours.

HOW FOOD POISONING IS CAUSED

Food poisoning is often caused by the direct
invasion and infection of the intestinal wall by
any range of organisms including *E. coli,*
salmonella, campylobacter, enterotoxins
(poisons released by certain bacteria), and many
protozoa (single-celled parasites). The organism
produces a toxin that affects the gut lining, or
may be absorbed into the blood, causing fever
and affecting other parts of the body.

HOW TOXINS ARE PRODUCED

Some bacteria, such as *Bacillus cereus,* produce
a toxin in the gut after ingestion that causes
diarrhoea. Others, including *Staphylococcus
aureus* and *Clostridium botulinum,* produce
poisons as they multiply in food. Although the
bacteria are killed by heat when the food is
cooked, the toxins are heat-resistant and still
cause poisoning when eaten. *Staphylococcus
aureus* poisoning causes severe sickness and
diarrhoea, usually within six hours. But
Clostridium botulinum symptoms can take
up to a week to develop and can be fatal. This
toxin does not affect the gut, but attacks the
nervous system making it hard to swallow and
causing fatigue and double vision.

Foot and problems

In supporting the weight of the body, the feet
have to take a considerable strain. To cope with
this, they have a complex structure of bones,
muscles, tendons and nerves. Each foot contains
26 small, very delicate bones – the highest
concentration of bone structure in the human
body. To keep the bones in their correct
position and provide elasticity, there are four
times as many ligaments and muscles as there
are bones.

The largest bone in the foot is the heel bone,
the calcaneus. This is attached to the talus,
which forms part of the ankle joint, and to
various bones in front, which help to support
the arch of the foot.

The mid-section of the foot is made up of five
long bones known as the metatarsals. The big
toe (the hallux) has two small digit bones
known as phalanges, while the other four toes
each contain three bones, making 26 in total.

SHOES AND FOOT DAMAGE

Most foot problems are caused by wearing
the wrong type of shoes. If shoes are too tight
or too narrow, they cause bunions, corns and
calluses. If such shoes are worn for a long

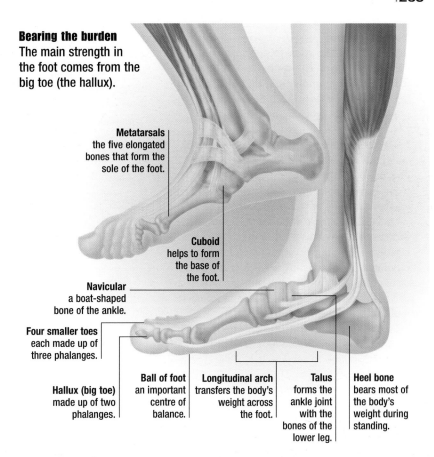

Bearing the burden
The main strength in
the foot comes from the
big toe (the hallux).

Metatarsals
the five elongated
bones that form the
sole of the foot.

Cuboid
helps to form
the base of
the foot.

Navicular
a boat-shaped
bone of the ankle.

Four smaller toes
each made up of
three phalanges.

Hallux (big toe)
made up of two
phalanges.

Ball of foot
an important
centre of
balance.

Longitudinal arch
transfers the body's
weight across
the foot.

Talus
forms the
ankle joint
with the
bones of the
lower leg.

Heel bone
bears most of
the body's
weight during
standing.

time, they will also cause malformation of the
feet. Shoes that are too big and do not support
the feet properly cause **blisters** and possible
flattening of the arches.

SKIN CONDITIONS

The most common problems to affect the feet
are skin and nail conditions including:
- fungal infections – for example, **athlete's foot;**
- bacterial infections – for example, those
associated with an **ingrowing toenail;**
- viral infections – for example, the infection
that causes verrucas;
- skin problems such as **calluses** and **corns.**

PROBLEMS AFFECTING BONES AND JOINTS

A number of structural problems can also occur,
such as **bunions** – harmless swellings of the
big-toe joints – and problems with the natural
arch shape of the foot at the insole. Fallen
arches can produce flat feet, and the shape of
the arch can become exaggerated in claw foot.

The foot may fail to develop normally in
a condition known as **club foot,** in which the
heel is drawn up and the sole of the foot is
turned inwards so the foot points downwards
and inwards. Club foot can be corrected with
splinting or, if necessary, surgery.

Pigeon toes are a minor abnormality that is
commonly seen in toddlers. The foot is rotated
so the toes point inwards when standing or
walking. The abnormality usually corrects itself
during childhood and rarely needs treatment.

NERVE DAMAGE

In a condition known as foot drop, damage to the nerves controlling foot movements causes the foot to hang limply from the ankle, so that the leg has to be raised high during walking to prevent the foot dragging on the ground.

FRACTURES

Fractures of the foot can occur during simple walking if the bones are weak or walking is prolonged, but, more often, fractures result from injuries: fracture of the heel bone is often caused by falling off a high ladder.

The heel bone may also develop a bony protrusion, known as a calcaneal spur. This usually follows injury, or occurs as a result of inflammation of the muscle sheaths in the sole of the foot (plantar fasciitis). But sometimes it can develop for no obvious reason in someone with otherwise healthy feet.

Treatment of foot fractures may involve immobilizing the affected foot in a hard plaster or fibreglass cast to encourage healing.

FOOT PAIN

A large number of conditions can cause painful feet, including:
- flat feet;
- **arthritis;**
- **gout;**
- tarsal tunnel syndrome (this condition is similar to **carpal tunnel syndrome**);
- plantar fasciitis (pain felt mainly under the heel and in the mid-line);
- erythromelalgia (the pain of this condition gives rise to the name 'burning feet syndrome');
- **metatarsalgia** (pain is felt mainly in the ball of the foot);
- conditions affecting nerve transmission, such as poorly controlled **diabetes.**

TREATMENT

Infections and skin problems affecting the feet can usually be remedied by a visit to a doctor or chiropodist/podiatrist (see **Chiropody**). Treatment of foot pain depends on the cause. Orthodox treatment of foot conditions often involves wearing heel pads, shoes and insoles moulded to fit your feet, **physiotherapy** and sometimes corticosteroid injections. Occasionally, a lack of B group vitamins causes burning feet syndrome, which may be relieved by dietary supplements.

Fractures

Any break in a bone is called a fracture. There are several different types of fracture, classified according to the shape and extent of the break.

CAUSES

Most fractures occur as the result of a fall, an injury or an accident, although prolonged stress

Types of bone fracture

There are several ways in which a bone may break. These have different classifications and require different forms of treatment.

Transverse

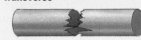

A straight fracture across the width of the bone, often in the long bone of the arm or leg. This type of fracture is usually caused by a severe direct blow.

Spiral

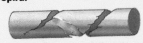

A break caused by a violent, rotating movement, for example, when the foot is caught and the leg twists excessively causing the shinbone to fracture.

Oblique

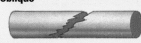

An angled, diagonal break across and through a bone, usually caused by a fall or a sharp, angled blow to the bone.

Greenstick

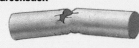

One side of the bone splinters and breaks, while the other side bends and stays intact; greenstick fractures tend to occur more commonly in children.

Depressed

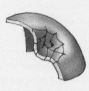

An area of bone is driven inwards, as in the case of a skull fracture. Usually caused by a heavy blow or severe impact. Common in road traffic accidents.

Comminuted or crush

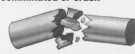

The fractured part of the bone shatters into several separate pieces. The cause is often a severe crushing blow, as may occur in a car accident.

A fracture may also be classified according to its effect on nearby tissues, including skin, other bones, blood vessels or body organs.

Closed, or simple

The broken bone does not pierce the skin and there is little or no damage to surrounding tissues.

Open, or compound

The skin is broken either by the original impact or by one or both ends of the fracture. A compound fracture is an open wound and therefore susceptible to infection.

Complicated

The fracture damages nearby tissues, such as blood vessels or body organs.

Impacted

One end of a broken bone becomes wedged or compressed into another bone.

to a bone, as occurs in long-distance running, can cause it to break. Some diseases of the bone, such as **osteoporosis** and certain **cancers**, can weaken bones so they fracture easily.

SYMPTOMS

One of the immediate symptoms of fracture is shock, characterized by dizziness, fainting, a fast, weak pulse, clammy skin and fast, shallow breathing. There will also be swelling, pain, muscle spasm around the fracture, deformity of the fractured area and an inability or extreme reluctance to move the affected area.

TREATMENT

The main aim of treatment for all fractures is to stabilize the bone in a position that will allow normal function of the limb when the bone has healed. In some cases, such as a rib fracture, holding the bone in position is impossible and it has to mend without support.

In the case of straightforward fractures, the ends of the bone are usually prevented from moving by a plaster or fibreglass cast. Comminuted fractures – where the bone is shattered – and unstable fractures may require screws, metal plates, wires, thick pins or the use of external fixators to hold the ends of the bones in position.

A complicated fracture, where nearby organs or tissues have been damaged, is treated as other fractures, but any severe internal injuries are treated before attention is paid to it.

A doctor will prescribe antibiotics in most cases of an open fracture – where one or both bone ends project through the skin – to protect the patient against infection of the bone (see **Osteomyelitis**) and surrounding area.

The healing process can take between three weeks and three months, but may take longer, depending on the site of the fracture.

COMPLICATIONS

Most fractures heal well without complications, but the bones may take longer to knit together if the blood circulation is poor. This complicates fractures of the neck of the femur (the hip bone), in particular, and a hip replacement operation may be necessary (see **Hip and problems**).

Fragile X syndrome

Fragile X syndrome is a genetic disorder that is responsible for about one in ten cases of **mental retardation** in boys. **Learning difficulties** associated with the syndrome vary from minor educational problems to severe mental handicap. Other symptoms, some of which do not appear until after puberty, include large ears, testes, jaws and forehead, speech defects and, sometimes, self-mutilation.

Roughly one boy in every 2000 is affected by fragile X syndrome, and half this number in girls. It has its origin in a region of the X chromosome that is unusually fragile and breaks, so that a portion of it is missing. No effective treatment is yet available.

Frostbite

Frostbite is tissue injury caused by exposure to extreme cold. It occurs at temperatures below freezing (0°C or 32°F) when ice crystals form beneath the skin. The lower the temperature the faster the damage is caused, and wind or blizzard conditions make the process faster still.

When the body is cold, blood is diverted from the surface to maintain the core temperature at 37°C, and without blood keeping them warm, the extremities – toes, fingers, nose and ears – freeze first. However, exposed skin anywhere can be affected, including the surface of the eyes and the lining of the airways into the lungs. Feelings of pins and needles or intense pain usually precede frostbite, but as cold stops the sensory nerves from working the skin goes numb, and frostbite can happen very quickly and without warning.

SYMPTOMS

The main symptom of frostbite is a raised white weal (blister) that may redden, swell and itch on rewarming. Blisters form if the blood vessels beneath have frozen. Soft waxy or black patches indicate dead skin, which eventually falls off. The area heals if circulation is restored, but if the tissues die and the affected area results in gangrene, the affected parts have to be amputated.

TREATMENT

Frostbite needs urgent treatment. The affected person must reach shelter and warmth to prevent the onset of hypothermia. If a doctor is not available, frostbite can be treated in the following way:

■ remove shoes, clothing and constricting items, such as rings or a watch, from the area affected by frostbite;

■ warm the area slowly and gently – tuck frostbitten fingers into the armpits or groin; cover with warm hands or clothing; or immerse the affected part in warm water that is no more than hand-hot (43°C/110°F);

■ cover with a sterile dressing.

PREVENTION

To prevent frostbite, keep the ears, mouth and nose covered; wear thick, comfortably fitting socks, shoes and gloves; and keep toes and fingers moving.

SEE ALSO *Exposure; Gangrene; Hypothermia*

Frozen shoulder

Frozen shoulder is a painful stiffness that gradually develops in the shoulder over a period of several weeks. It is a common complaint that affects middle-aged and elderly people, and may take months to a couple of years to resolve.

SYMPTOMS

- Painful restriction of shoulder movement.
- Ache in the shoulder and upper arm, which tends to worsen at night.

CAUSES

Frozen shoulder may occur for no apparent reason. Identifiable causes include:

- injury, including surgery, or other shoulder problems. The shoulder joint is particularly vulnerable to damage because it has such a wide range of movement, is in continual use, and is often subjected to bearing heavy loads;
- inflammation of tendons around the shoulder joint or of the fibrous capsule of the joint (capsulitis), or swelling of the joint bursa (a fluid-filled sac that cushions the joint).

TREATMENT

If the condition is not too severe, you may be able to ease it with a combination of gentle exercise and painkilling drugs. Ibuprofen, which has both analgesic and anti-inflammatory effects, is frequently recommended. Some people find that using a heat lamp or applying icepacks or bags of frozen peas can help to relieve the pain.

When to see a doctor

Seek medical advice if pain and stiffness persist and interfere with normal daily activities or prevent you from sleeping.

What a doctor may do

- Arrange an X-ray and blood test.
- Advise on maintaining mobility.
- Arrange physiotherapy, with gentle stretching exercises or heat treatment.
- Offer painkillers and anti-inflammatory drugs.
- If the pain is severe, arrange for you to receive injections of corticosteroids into the joint.

What you can do

If you are suffering from frozen shoulder, aim to keep the joint mobile by maintaining gentle movement. It is tempting to avoid using the joint if it causes pain, but immobility and stiffness can cause symptoms to spread down the arm and up into the neck.

Do not force movement that causes pain, and avoid repetitive movements and activities that place undue strain on the joint.

Complementary therapies

- Gentle **chiropractic** manipulation of the shoulder may shorten recovery time.
- **Herbal** celery supplement may help to ease symptoms.
- Aromatherapy treatment includes hot baths with essential oil of rosemary or pine.
- **Acupuncture** and **acupressure** on specific points can offer relief.

OUTLOOK

Provided that the shoulder joint is not allowed to seize up as a result of immobility, full recovery usually occurs eventually.

Fungal infections

There are more than 100,000 different species of fungi – parasitic life-forms that include moulds, mildews, yeasts, mushrooms and toadstools. Most of them are harmless or even beneficial to health, including various yeasts used in baking, some moulds that are the source of certain antibiotic drugs and various edible mushrooms and truffles. But there are also a number of fungi that can cause illness in human beings and sometimes even result in fatal disease.

TYPES OF INFECTION

Fungi grow most successfully in warm, moist areas of the body. Because of this, fungal infections are particularly common on the skin, genital area, scalp and nails. Types of infection include:

- **Tinea (ringworm)** Tinea is the term used to describe a group of common fungal infections of the skin, hair or nails, usually caused by fungi called dermatophytes, which are parasitic on the skin.
- **Athlete's foot** Known medically as *tinea pedis*, athlete's foot is a common form of ringworm that affects the feet.
- **Candida** Infection by the fungus *Candida albicans* is commonly known as candida, one form of which is thrush. The fungus is found in skin folds such as beneath the breasts and around the genitals and anal orifice. (See also **Candida**.)
- **Cryptococcosis** This rare infection is caused by inhaling the fungus *Cryptococcus neoformans*, found throughout the world in soil that has been contaminated with pigeon droppings. Infection by the *Cryptococcus* fungus can cause **meningitis** or growths in the lungs and skin.
- **Aspergillosis** Aspergillosis is an infection caused by *Aspergillus*, a fungus that grows in decaying vegetation. It can affect people with reduced immunity, triggering **asthma** symptoms or worsening an inflammation of the lungs. (See also **Aspergillosis**.)
- **Sporotrichosis** Sporotrichosis is a chronic infection caused by the fungus *Sporothrix schenckii*, which grows on moss and other

plants. It is usually contracted through a skin wound where an ulcer develops. An oral preparation of potassium iodide solution usually clears up the infection.

■ **Histoplasmosis** Histoplasmosis is an infection caused by inhaling the spores of the fungus *Histoplasma capsulatum*, which is found in soil that has been contaminated with bird or bat droppings in parts of the Americas, the Far East and Africa.

SYMPTOMS

The symptoms of any fungal infection will depend on where in the body the infection is.

■ When a fungal infection affects the skin, including the skin in the area of the genitals, symptoms usually include an itchy rash accompanied by inflammation.

■ A scalp infection often features hair loss and an area of red skin with fine scales and irritated skin.

■ With a nail infection, nails usually look white or yellow and opaque, and become thickened and brittle. Nail tinea may remain localized or may spread to other nails.

DURATION

■ Fungal infections may last anything from a week to several months, depending on what fungus has caused the infection and where it is in the body.

■ Athlete's foot and other localized inflammatory infections usually clear up on their own eventually, as the body fights them off. But this can take months or even years, so it is advisable to seek treatment.

CAUSES

Fungal infections result from contact with people, animals or soil on which the fungi are present. Infections transmitted to human beings from animals or from the soil are not generally passed on to other people. Fungi transmitted to human beings from other people tend to be highly infectious and can be spread by skin-to-skin contact, wearing contaminated shoes, sharing towels, or walking barefoot on floors which may be contaminated.

There is no clear-cut reason why some people develop fungal infections while others do not, but doctors believe that susceptibility may be due to differences in the efficiency of individuals' immune systems. This would explain why fungal infections tend to occur much more frequently in people whose resistance to infection is low, such as those with diabetes, or those taking long-term steroids or other types of medication that interfere with the working of their immune systems.

Skin type can also have an influence: people with oily skin can usually resist or fight off

UNDER THE MICROSCOPE

Disease-causing fungi – illustrated here by means of a technique called scanning electron micrography – most often affect the skin or lungs.

Trichophyton mentagrophytes is the cause of athlete's foot and ringworm. Both these infections are spread by fungal spores, shown here in orange.

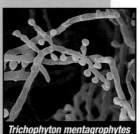

Trichophyton mentagrophytes

Repeated inhalation of the spores of *Aspergillus* (shown below) may cause aspergillosis, a hypersensitive lung reaction in asthmatics and those whose immune system is inefficient.

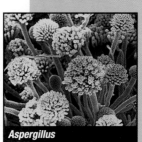

Aspergillus

Inhaled spores can lead to fungal growth on the lungs (shown below), which may then spread to other parts of the body.

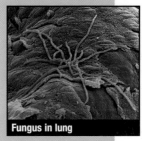

Fungus in lung

fungal infections, but those with sweaty and moist skin provide the perfect environment for the development of a fungal infection.

TREATMENT

Prompt treatment of any fungal disease is important to prevent the spread of infection.

When to consult a doctor

Always consult a doctor if you suspect that you have a fungal infection. Remember also that many skin diseases show the same symptoms as a fungal infection, but will require very different treatment.

What a doctor may do

■ To make or confirm a diagnosis, a doctor may take a scrape of the affected area for a microscopic examination and culture.

　■ You will probably be prescribed a cream or tablets. Creams usually contain imidazole, and tablets are likely to contain griseofulvin or terbinafine: all these are chemicals that will inhibit or kill fungal growth.

　■ A fungal infection of the nails is usually treated with tablets that will kill the fungus. Antifungal nail paints are sometimes applied.

Complementary therapies

　■ Take grapefruit-seed extract, which contains natural antifungal properties. Garlic has also demonstrated antifungal activity.

■ Taking a daily supplement of zinc for three to six months may be helpful for fighting fungal infections of the nails.

COMPLICATIONS

When a fungal infection affects the scalp, treatment should be started as quickly as possible. If it is left untreated for a period of time, it could result in more noticeable and long-lasting bald patches.

PREVENTION

The fungi that cause skin infections are everywhere and are virtually impossible to eliminate completely. However, there are certain precautions that can be taken to limit the chances of picking up a fungal infection:

■ Children should be prevented from playing with animals that have any round, scaly patches on their bodies.

■ Do not share towels.

■ Wash your feet every day and dry them thoroughly afterwards.

　■ Avoid walking around barefoot.

　■ Wear cotton or wool socks and change them every day or more often if they become damp.

　■ Avoid wearing shoes made of a synthetic material that can cause the feet to become sweaty and damp.

　■ Use antifungal dusting powder.

SEE ALSO *Athlete's foot; Candida; Hair, scalp and problems; Ringworm*

Gallbladder and disorders

The gallbladder is part of the **digestive system**. It stores bile, which is produced by the liver, and expels it into the intestine when bile is needed to break down fats.

The gallbladder is a small, pear-shaped muscular sac, about the size of a lime. It is attached to the base of the right lobe of the liver and lies immediately beneath it. The liver, which lies on the right side of the abdomen just below the diaphragm, makes about 1 litre (almost 2 pints) of bile a day.

WHAT THE GALLBLADDER DOES

The gallbladder stores any bile that is not needed immediately. Water is absorbed from bile through the gallbladder's lining, thereby concentrating the bile. When fatty foods and acidic gastric juices enter the duodenum in the small intestine, cells in the duodenum's lining produce a hormone called cholecystokinin. This hormone stimulates the gallbladder to contract and expel the concentrated bile into the bile duct. It then passes into the duodenum to help to break down and emulsify fats and neutralize gastric juices. This is a vital digestive function, because fat and the fat-soluble vitamins – A, D, E and K – cannot be absorbed by the intestines until bile has done its work.

Gallstones

Chemical changes can occur in the composition of bile, and this can lead to the formation of gallstones, a process known medically as cholelithiasis.

The most common change is for the level of **cholesterol**, which occurs naturally in bile, to rise and become out of balance with the level of bile salts. As a result, tiny crystals of cholesterol form and clump together as gallstones. Gallstones can vary in size from 1–24mm (½in) across; they can occur singly or there may be 20 or more.

In the UK, gallstones affect 22 per cent of women and 11 per cent of men. However, only about 30 per cent of those affected exhibit any symptoms, so most gallstones are discovered during imaging investigations such as **ultrasound** scans or **X-rays**, and in the course of postmortems.

If gallstones become stuck in the cystic duct – the exit duct from the gallbladder – they are likely to cause pain and inflammation. Sometimes the gallbladder itself becomes infected and inflamed; this is called acute cholecystitis. Repeated attacks of this infection can cause long-term damage to the gallbladder: its walls thicken and it shrinks and eventually ceases to function.

WHO IS AT RISK

Doctors look for the five 'Fs' as risk factors for gallstones: fair-skinned, fat, forty, female and fertile. This makes a typical sufferer an overweight, middle-aged woman. Obese women who have had numerous children and have been on the contraceptive pill are particularly at risk. And a family history of gallstones also makes the problem more likely, although anyone with a high cholesterol level has an above average risk of developing gallstones.

SYMPTOMS

Someone can have gallstones for years and be completely unaware of them. Other people can develop any of the following symptoms.

■ A pain in the upper right abdomen, just beneath the ribs, which develops a few hours after eating and lasts for some hours. This may be accompanied by nausea and vomiting. An attack may or may not recur, and may lead on to other symptoms.

■ Excessive flatulence and belching.

■ Severe pain, especially when breathing in, a fever and nausea and vomiting. These are signs of acute cholecystitis.

CAUSES

Around 80 per cent of gallstones are made of cholesterol crystals. Others, known as pigmented gallstones, are either black or brown and contain calcium and bilirubin, one of the breakdown products of red blood cells. This type of gallstone is associated with **cirrhosis of the liver** and some types of **anaemia**. It is possible to have both cholesterol and pigmented gallstones.

DIAGNOSIS

■ Gallstones that contain calcium deposits can be seen on an abdominal X-ray.

■ Gallstones that do not contain calcium can be detected by an ultrasound scan. They can also be seen using a technique called cholecystography. This is an X-ray taken after the patient has swallowed a solution containing iodine, which accumulates in the gallbladder and makes gallstones visible.

■ A blood test may be used to pinpoint a high white blood cell count, which can indicate acute cholecystitis.

TREATMENT

If gallstones are detected but the inflammation is not advanced, various treatments may be used to remove them and to prevent infection.

■ Lithotripsy – the use of ultrasound waves to dissolve the stones.

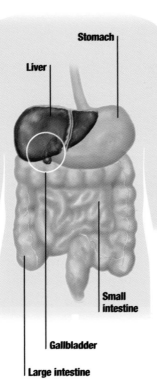

Stomach

Liver

Small intestine

Gallbladder

Large intestine

■ Medication – a derivative of bile salts is taken over a long period to dissolve gallstones; this method is effective only on small stones composed of cholesterol.

■ **Antibiotics** may be prescribed to prevent or fight infection.

■ **Analgesics** may be given for pain.

Following treatment you may be advised to follow a low-fat diet to prevent any recurrence of gallstones.

Treating cholecystitis

Prompt treatment is required in cases of acute cholecystitis. It may be necessary to remove the gallbladder by surgery (cholecystectomy). It is still possible to function without a gallbladder, however, because it is not essential to the digestive process: even without it, the liver's bile can reach the intestine.

COMPLICATIONS

In about 2–3 per cent of cases, an infected gallbladder becomes filled with pus. This may force its way out through an opening (a **fistula**). The pus may then leak into the small intestine, causing severe abdominal pain and fever. This condition is known medically as empyema.

Sometimes gallstones become lodged in the bile duct, causing inflammation and obstructing the flow of bile. The result can be **jaundice**, with pain, nausea and vomiting, a fever and a drop in blood pressure, and pancreatitis (see **Pancreas and disorders**).

Gallbladder tumour

A malignant tumour of the gallbladder is very rare. It is associated with a history of gallstones. Tumours tend to be confined to elderly people and generally show no symptoms, so by the time the disease is recognized the tumour has usually spread to the liver. The outlook is then bleak, with most of those affected dying within a year. The only treatment is to remove as much of the tumour as possible.

SEE ALSO *Digestive system*

Gamma globulin

Gamma globulin is the scientific term for antibody. It is also called immune globulin or immunoglobulin. Antibodies fight infection by recognizing the foreign cells and particles that enter the body and initiating their destruction.

Some infections can be prevented from taking hold by giving a specific antibody to a person. For example, in some types of viral hepatitis, antibodies derived from the blood plasma of people who have had the disease can be given to an individual. That person now has antibodies that will protect the body from hepatitis for as long as they last in the body. Gamma globulin given in this way provides what is known as 'passive immunity', since the person's body has done nothing active to produce the antibodies.

When a person produces his or her own gamma globulin against infection, induced by a vaccination, they are described as having 'active immunity'.

SEE ALSO *Blood and disorders; Immunization*

Ganglion

The term 'ganglion' describes a common condition in which a fluid-filled swelling or **cyst** grows on a tendon sheath, usually in the wrist, but more rarely a finger or foot. The cyst may be as small as a pea but it can grow as large as a golf ball. If a ganglion is painful or ugly, it can be surgically removed.

Ganglion is also the name for a group of nerve cells in the brain or spinal cord that control muscular movements or receive sensory messages.

Gangrene

Gangrene is the decay and death of part of the body following loss of its blood supply. It tends to affect the limbs, fingers and toes.

Several conditions and injuries can interfere with the blood supply, although these do not necessarily result in gangrene. They include **frostbite**, burns, thrombosis, atheroma, an embolism and certain skin infections. People with diabetes mellitus have a tendency to poor circulation and are also prone to gangrene of the legs or feet.

SYMPTOMS

■ The area suddenly becomes pale and cold, turning black within a few days.

■ In dry gangrene, the tissues die due to lack of oxygen and nutrients.

■ In wet gangrene, bacterial infection causes the flesh to rot and smell unpleasant; nearby tissue may become intensely painful.

TREATMENT

Simple ulceration of the feet or ankles can be nursed at home.

When to consult a doctor

If any digit or limb suddenly becomes cold and pale in appearance for more than two hours, or the ends become discoloured or ulcerated, you need to see a doctor as a matter of urgency. You may be at risk of developing gangrene which, if left untreated, can be fatal.

If a diabetic develops ulcers on the feet this needs urgent attention: diabetics are prone to infection and are more at risk of gangrene.

What a doctor may do
■ Antibiotics may be prescribed to prevent an infection from spreading.
■ Surgery may be needed to cut away the dead area before gangrene develops.
■ A finger, toe or limb affected by gangrene will almost certainly need to be amputated.

PREVENTION
■ Avoid extreme temperatures.
■ Stop smoking: smokers with arterial disease risk gangrene due to poor circulation.
■ Avoid wearing tight-fitting shoes, since these can interfere with the circulation of blood to the toes eventually causing the flesh to die.
■ If you have diabetes, it is important to treat infections of the feet promptly. Keep your toenails short and clean to minimize the risk of infection.

OUTLOOK
The affected part of the body cannot be salvaged once gangrene has set in. With prompt treatment, however, damage to the area can usually be limited and the person's life saved. This usually involves amputation of the affected fingers, toes or limb.

Gastrectomy

A gastrectomy is the removal of all or part of the stomach. It is a major operation performed under general **anaesthetic**. In a total gastrectomy the entire stomach is removed and the oesophagus is joined to the duodenum. In a partial gastrectomy, up to two-thirds of the stomach may be removed.

◄ **Surgical solution**
In a total gastrectomy, the stomach is removed and the oesophagus and duodenum connected to one another. In a partial removal, the duodenum is reconnected to the remaining stomach.

Oesophagus

Stomach

Total gastrectomy

Duodenum

Partial gastrectomy

WHY IT IS DONE
■ A total gastrectomy is usually performed in cases of stomach cancer, and sometimes in cases of Zollinger-Ellison syndrome (in which excess gastric acid is produced as a result of a pancreatic tumour).
■ A partial gastrectomy, in which the main acid-secreting area of the stomach is removed, may be performed to treat **peptic ulcers** that are severe or have not responded to drug treatment.

COMPLICATIONS
■ Weight loss, because you feel full quickly when eating, and your stomach cannot cope with much food.
■ **Dumping syndrome** in which palpitations and faintness occur after eating; this can happen as a result of the rapid passage of food into the intestine because of the absence of the stomach or its reduced size.
■ Pernicious anaemia, because a protein in the gastric juices – intrinsic factor – is needed for the body to absorb vitamin B_{12}, which has an essential role in manufacturing red blood cells.
■ **Malabsorption** – food passes through the digestive tract more quickly than normal impairing absorption of vitamins and minerals.
SEE ALSO *Stomach and disorders*

Gastritis

Gastritis is a broad term used to describe different conditions affecting the mucous membrane of the stomach.

TYPES OF GASTRITIS
There are three main types of gastritis: acute, chronic and atrophic.

Acute and chronic gastritis
Both acute and chronic gastritis cause the mucous membrane lining the stomach to become inflamed. This happens when the stomach is injured by infection or physical or chemical damage. Chronic gastritis rarely causes any symptoms apart from slight **heartburn**; acute gastritis, on the other hand, can cause nausea, stomach pain, loss of appetite and bleeding.

The most common cause of infection is the bacterium Helicobacter pylori, which is treated with antibiotics. Chemical irritation of the mucous membrane may be caused by long-term tobacco smoking or alcohol consumption, and medicines such as aspirin or anti-rheumatic NSAIDs. People on long-term therapy should always take these medicines with food and use paracetamol rather than aspirin as a painkiller.

Severe injury, or a heart attack or stroke can trigger the release of large quantities of gastric juices, which can 'burn' the mucous membrane. This can result in serious inflammation and the formation of numerous ulcers. These ulcers can bleed and may even perforate the stomach wall. Drugs may be prescribed to block the production of the acid in the gastric juices.

Atrophic gastritis

Atrophic gastritis is usually an age-related degeneration of the stomach lining. Half of those over 50 have some degree of atrophic gastritis. Patchy deterioration of the glands in the mucous membrane reduces the amount of gastric juices produced. Low levels of gastric juices make infections by bacteria, such as **salmonella**, more likely. Treatment is largely diet-related: avoiding indigestible foods, and taking extra care with food hygiene. Any infection needs to be treated with a course of antibiotics.

SEE ALSO *Digestive system; Stomach and disorders*

Gastroenteritis

Gastroenteritis is a violent short-term stomach upset that rarely lasts for more than two days. It is usually caused by eating or drinking contaminated food or water. It can also be triggered by an alcohol binge, food allergies and intolerances and, in some people, antibiotics.

SYMPTOMS

The nature of the illness and its severity depend on the cause. Symptoms can develop within one to twelve hours after infection, and include:

- vomiting;
- abdominal cramps;
- diarrhoea;
- dehydration.

TREATMENT

In healthy adults, gastroenteritis usually clears up within a few days. Antibiotics are rarely necessary and the only treatment is to take plenty of fluids to replace those lost and to re-introduce food slowly as the symptoms pass.

Factfile

Gastroenteritis in infants

Although gastroenteritis is usually mild in healthy adults, it can be fatal for young children.

In the UK, gastroenteritis is extremely common. It causes diarrhoea and vomiting which, in very young children, can quickly lead to dehydration. Replace lost fluids by offering cool boiled water. Oral rehydration sachets, such as Dioralyte, which replace vital sugars and salts, are available over the counter from pharmacies.

In frail, elderly or very young people, special care should be taken to prevent or treat **dehydration** by giving liquids containing dextrose and essential salts.

PREVENTION

Most episodes of gastroenteritis in the UK are caused by poor food hygiene, so being careful about food storage and preparation will prevent the majority of cases.

Anyone travelling to countries where diseases such as **cholera** are prevalent should obtain the appropriate vaccinations. Your GP surgery can advise you. Always drink bottled water if you are unsure about the local water supply.

SEE ALSO *Digestive system; Stomach and disorders; Travel and tropical diseases*

Genital herpes

Genital herpes is caused by the *Herpes simplex* virus (HSV Type I or Type II), which can also cause cold sores around the mouth. Genital herpes may be passed on through sex with an infected partner, or through oral sex from someone with an active **cold sore**.

SYMPTOMS

If symptoms develop, the incubation period is around five days. The primary attack is often accompanied by flu-like symptoms. Itching and tingling occur at the site of entry of the virus before a crop of painful blisters form. These burst to form shallow ulcers, which are intensely painful and heal after 10 to 14 days. Pain often makes urination difficult. During the first attack, the herpes virus travels up nerve endings to lie dormant in a nerve ganglion. There are recurrences in around 50 per cent of cases, but these are milder and usually heal within a week. Recurrent herpes may be triggered by stress, menstruation, other infections, or vigorous sex.

DIAGNOSIS

Genital herpes is diagnosed by swabbing a suspected viral blister and growing the virus in the laboratory. Blood tests that detect antibodies to the virus are now also available.

TREATMENT

A mild infection is treated by bathing the area with a salt-water solution. More severe symptoms may be treated with antiviral drugs such as aciclovir. If recurrences are troublesome, a three- to six-month course of antiviral drugs may be prescribed.

If active genital herpes sores are present when a pregnant woman goes into labour, a Caesarean section may be recommended to protect the baby from herpes meningitis.

SEE ALSO *Sexually transmitted diseases*

Genital warts

Genital warts are one of the most common sexually transmitted infections. They are benign skin tumours caused by the human papilloma virus (HPV), of which at least 60 different types exist.

The wart virus gains entry through minute cuts or splits in a person's skin during skin-to-skin contact – most usually this is during sex with an infected person. Once infected, the virus lies dormant in cells, and warts may appear from several weeks to 20 months afterwards, or they may remain dormant if a person has a natural immunity against them. Most carriers of the wart virus do not have active warts, so lack of visible warts on a sexual partner does not mean that they are free from infection.

Viruses stimulate overgrowth of skin cells to form warts that vary in shape and size from small, multiple, finger-like projections to single, large growths that are occasionally the size of a walnut – particularly during pregnancy. Warts may itch.

A doctor may surgically remove genital warts, or may treat them by painting on podophyllum or imiquimod (avoid during pregnancy), by freezing (cryotherapy) or by applying heat (**diathermy**). The immune system will usually bring the warts under control eventually.

As some wart viruses are associated with an increased risk of developing cervical cancer, women who have genital warts may be advised to have annual **cervical smear tests**. Using a condom reduces the chance of infection.
SEE ALSO *Cervix and disorders; Contraception; Sexually transmitted diseases*

Genu valgum

Genu valgum is an abnormal inward curvature of the legs at the knees so that, when standing, the knees are in contact, the lower legs splay out and the feet are apart. The condition, also known as knock-knee, generally affects both legs. It is very common in young children in their first two years of walking, but they usually outgrow it by the age of six or seven.

CAUSES

Knock-knee is nearly always caused by a slight inward rotation of the thigh bones at the hip joint. Other possible causes include:
■ bone softening – such as in **rickets** (due to a deficiency of vitamin D) and rare bone diseases;
■ bone injury involving damage to the growing end of the long bones (epiphyses) in childhood;
■ **arthritis**, if cartilage becomes thin.

TREATMENT

It is not usually necessary to treat genu valgum since the condition tends to right itself as the young child grows.

When to see a doctor
■ If a child still appears knock-kneed by the age of seven.
■ If one knee is normal and the other faces inwards.

What a doctor may do
A doctor may refer the child to an orthopaedic surgeon. If there is an abnormality of the knee joint or leg bones, splints or an operation may be suggested.

Sometimes, a child of ten or more still has severe knock-knee. As long as there is no underlying disease, it can be corrected surgically, using an operation called osteotomy, which involves cutting the tibia and realigning it to straighten the leg.
SEE ALSO *Knee and problems*

Genu varum

Genu varum is characterized by an abnormal outward curvature of the legs at the knees, resulting in a gap between the knees when standing. Also known as bow legs, it is very common in young children, who usually grow out of it. It becomes a problem only if it lasts into adulthood.

CAUSES

Most of the causes of genu varum are the same as those of genu valgum:
■ thigh bones that are a little outwardly rotated in the hip sockets;
■ bone softening – as in **rickets**, for example, or **Paget's disease**;
■ injury or abnormal growth of the growing end of the long bone (epiphysis) in childhood;
■ ligaments being stretched over prolonged periods, as in the bow legs developed by jockeys;
■ **arthritis**, if cartilage becomes thin.

TREATMENT

The condition is usually self-correcting, so treatment is rarely required. Consult a doctor only if you are anxious and need reassurance, or there are other symptoms that cause concern. Surgical correction by osteotomy (cutting the bone in two and realigning it to allow healing in the correct position) or other orthopaedic operations are possible for severe cases. If there is no underlying disease, especially where bow legs persist from childhood, treatment is advisable to prevent later development of osteoarthritis.
SEE ALSO *Knee and problems*

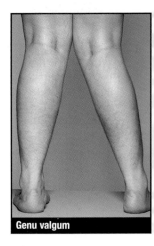
Genu valgum

▲ **Common curves**
A common condition in toddlers, knock-knee (genu valgum), usually corrects itself before a child reaches the age of seven.

▼ **Warning sign**
Bow legs (genu varum) that persist beyond early childhood may be an indication of abnormal growth or injury and need surgical correction.

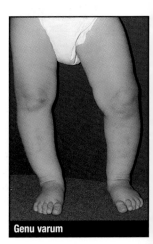
Genu varum

Giardiasis

Giardiasis is an infection of the small intestine caused by *Giardia lamblia*, a one-celled parasite that lives in the intestine of human beings and animals. The illness is most common in the tropics, but it is becoming more prevalent in developed countries.

In the developed world, giardiasis tends to occur in people who have been travelling in a tropical country, in homosexual men, in people living in institutions and in preschool children in nurseries. The parasite is spread through the stool of an infected person or animal, and is contracted by eating or drinking contaminated food or water, or by hand-to-hand or sexual contact with an infected person.

Symptoms of giardiasis include often foul-smelling diarrhoea or loose or watery stools, wind and stomach cramps. It usually clears up without treatment, but a doctor may prescribe metronidazole. This is an antibiotic that works quickly and stops the infection from spreading.

Gingivitis

Gingivitis is a redness and swelling of the gums caused by a buildup of bacteria in plaque. If left untreated, gingivitis can cause more serious problems (see **Gums and gum disease**).

The most obvious sign of gingivitis is that your gums bleed when you clean your teeth. To prevent it, you should brush carefully around the margins of the teeth and gums and floss to remove the plaque (see **Teeth and problems**).

Many dentists recommend using an electric toothbrush to guard against gingivitis; ask your dentist or dental hygienist for advice.

SEE ALSO *Dentists and dentistry*

Glandular fever

Glandular fever is a viral illness, known medically as infectious mononucleosis. The virus is spread from one person to another by fluid in the nose, and saliva in the mouth. Kissing is an obvious way by which glandular fever can be transmitted, which is why it is popularly known as the 'kissing disease'.

Young people aged between the ages of 10 and 25 years are most vulnerable to glandular fever. Its peak incidence is between the ages of 15 and 17. Infection is rare beyond the mid-20s. Once you have had glandular fever, you cannot catch it again.

SYMPTOMS

The symptoms are similar to those of flu. Typically, glandular fever starts with a headache and severe fatigue, followed by fever, sore throat and enlarged lymph glands. These can be felt as lumps in the neck, armpits and groin. There may also be a rash and often the tonsils swell and become inflamed, so that swallowing is difficult and painful.

DURATION

- The time between catching the virus and the appearance of the first symptoms is 30–50 days.
- The acute stage usually lasts for a week or two. Most people feel totally well after 4–6 weeks.

DIAGNOSIS AND TREATMENT

A doctor will diagnose glandular fever from the symptoms, but may often confirm the diagnosis with a blood test.

There is no specific treatment, but warm drinks can relieve a sore throat and plenty of fluids are needed during a **fever**. Someone with glandular fever needs plenty of rest. Physical activities should be resumed only gradually.

Over-exertion, such as strenuous exercise, should be avoided for about four weeks after symptoms have passed. This is because the spleen may be enlarged and therefore susceptible to damage.

COMPLICATIONS

Complications of glandular fever are rare, but they can include anaemia or jaundice. Sufferers may feel depressed and lack energy for two or three months after recovery. Some doctors believe that glandular fever can trigger **chronic fatigue syndrome**, but others disagree.

Glaucoma

Glaucoma is often associated with an abnormally high pressure of fluid inside the eye, producing a gradual loss of vision. The pressure damages the nerve fibres as they enter the back of the eye and spread out on the retina. Initially, this leads to a loss in peripheral vision which, if untreated, may lead to **blindness**. The most common form, primary open-angle glaucoma (POAG), affects one in 200 of the population aged over 40 and accounts for about 20 per cent of blindness in the UK and the USA. It tends to run in families, and to be associated with extreme short-sightedness (see **myopia**). It is rare in people under 40.

The other main type of glaucoma is an acute form known as primary closed-angle glaucoma (PCAG). This condition is characterized by a rapid rise in the pressure in the eye. It tends to occur in elderly people or those who are very long-sighted (see **hypermetropia**).

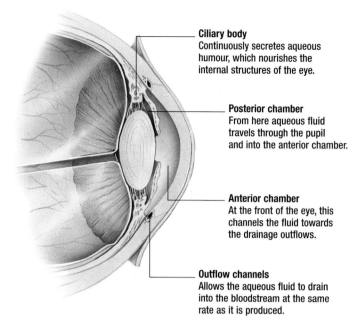

Ciliary body
Continuously secretes aqueous humour, which nourishes the internal structures of the eye.

Posterior chamber
From here aqueous fluid travels through the pupil and into the anterior chamber.

Anterior chamber
At the front of the eye, this channels the fluid towards the drainage outflows.

Outflow channels
Allows the aqueous fluid to drain into the bloodstream at the same rate as it is produced.

Drainage failure
In glaucoma, increased pressure in the eye is usually caused by a defect or a blockage in the drainage of the watery fluid, known as aqueous humour.

SYMPTOMS

POAG has no initial symptoms, but by the time your vision is reduced enough for you to be aware of it, it has reached an advanced stage. For this reason it is important to have regular eye tests, especially for people in the high-risk categories.

PCAG, on the other hand, will suddenly cause a very painful red eye, possibly with nausea. Vision is often cloudy. Before an attack, sufferers often report seeing haloes around lights.

DIAGNOSIS AND TREATMENT

There are three ways of detecting POAG during an eye test. An examination of the optic disc using an ophthalmoscope will show any existing damage or susceptibility to damage. The ophthalmologist can also use a device called a tonometer, which measures the pressure within the eyeball and indicates if glaucoma is present. In addition, a visual field test will reveal any areas of reduced peripheral vision.

POAG can be treated with eyedrops to reduce the pressure in the eye. To be effective, drops must be used regularly (perhaps twice a day), accurately and often for the rest of the person's life.

It is sometimes also necessary to open a drainage channel surgically. This removes excess fluid and reduces the pressure.

The acute form of glaucoma needs urgent treatment to relieve the pain – first with drugs, which may be prescribed as pills, eye drops or an intravenous drip, and then surgically. A laser can be used to make a hole in the iris painlessly to allow fluid to escape.

PREVENTION

Although prevention of glaucoma is not yet possible, early detection by regular **eye tests** can improve the success of treatments. Those at risk should have annual tests; these are usually free of charge.

COMPLICATIONS

Glaucoma is a progressive disease that can lead to blindness. Long-term use of eyedrops can cause side effects, such as irritation or an increase in pigmentation of the eye.

OUTLOOK

If the condition is diagnosed early and treated properly, the risk of deterioration is minimal and the outlook is good.

SEE ALSO *Eye and problems*

Glossitis

Glossitis is a swelling or inflammation of the tongue. It can have many causes. If the tongue is pale, the cause of the inflammation may be **anaemia**; if it is a fiery red, the sufferer may be deficient in B vitamins. Other causes of glossitis may be a bacterial or viral infection or a reaction to spicy food, mouthwash or other irritant. Sufferers should see a dentist or doctor for diagnosis and treatment.

SEE ALSO *Mouth and disorders*

Glue ear

Glue ear is a condition of the middle ear found mainly in children. Known medically as otitis media, it causes sticky fluid to collect in the middle ear cavity, and can affect a child's hearing. If parents and teachers are unaware that a child is not hearing properly, it can have a profound impact on the child's education.

An estimated 20–50 per cent of children have an episode of glue ear between the ages of three and ten. Boys and girls are equally susceptible, but boys seem to have more severe episodes.

CAUSES

■ Glue ear tends to follow exposure to other children through school, playgroup and nursery – suggesting a link with other respiratory infections such as colds and tonsillitis.

Factfile

Risk factors for glaucoma

Certain conditions make primary open-angle glaucoma more likely.

■ Age: it is more likely to occur in the over-40s.

■ Family history: about 10 per cent of those with a parent or sibling with the disease will develop it themselves.

■ Race: the condition is more prevalent among Afro-Caribbeans.

■ High myopia: severe short-sightedness is a risk factor for glaucoma.

■ Drugs: people on some medications, such as corticosteroids, may develop glaucoma.

■ Illness: diabetes and other illnesses can make glaucoma more likely.

■ If the child's adenoids become swollen, they can block the Eustachian tubes, which connect the middle ear to the throat. When this happens, mucus cannot drain away (see **Ear and problems**).

Allergic disease, such as asthma, is not thought to be linked to the risk of glue ear.

DIAGNOSIS AND TREATMENT

The first sign of glue ear is often a lack of responsiveness – a child who seems to be deliberately ignoring a request may simply not be hearing it. Glue ear is diagnosed by a hearing test, followed by examination of the middle ear through an otoscope – a viewing instrument used to look at the eardrums.

Decongestant nose drops may be enough to unblock the Eustachian tube so that the mucus can drain through it. In severe cases, the surgical insertion of small drainage tubes into the eardrum might be necessary (see **Grommet insertion**).

ADULTS AND GLUE EAR

Glue ear is rare in adults. When it occurs, it may be linked to a nearby tumour. Two-thirds of those with a tumour involving the nose or back of the throat develop glue ear, and it is also commonly found among people with AIDS.

Goitre

A goitre is a swelling in the front of the neck caused by an enlargement of the thyroid gland. Goitres vary in size from a small lump to a large swelling that interferes with breathing or swallowing. Many goitres will remain until treated.

CAUSES

■ A deficiency of dietary iodine, needed for the production of thyroxine, the hormone responsible for metabolism.
■ Puberty, pregnancy or menopause – all times of high demand for thyroxine.
■ Hyperthyroidism, a condition in which the thyroid gland produces excessive amounts of hormone.
■ Hypothyroidism, caused by under-production of thyroid hormones by the thyroid gland.
■ Thyroiditis, an inflammation of the thyroid gland.
■ Thyroid cancer, a very rare condition.

TREATMENT

You should consult a doctor if you have any lump or swelling in your neck.

What a doctor may do

■ Arrange tests to find the cause of the goitre.
■ Treat iodine deficiency with dietary changes.
■ Prescribe hormones for hypothyroidism.

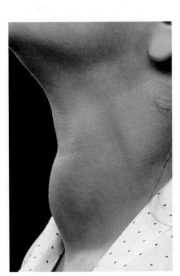

▲ **Lump in the neck**
Goitre is the enlargement of the thyroid gland. The condition has a variety of causes, including iodine deficiency and thyroid gland overactivity.

■ Prescribe drugs that inhibit the production of thyroid hormones to treat hyperthyroidism.
■ Recommend surgery to remove part of the thyroid gland to treat hyperthyroidism.
■ Recommend surgery and a course of radioactive iodine for thyroid cancer.

Complementary therapies

Herbalists might prescribe bugleweed or bladderwrack. Their effectiveness is unproven.

PREVENTION

Make sure your diet contains iodine – found in seafood, seaweed and iodized table salt.

COMPLICATIONS

A large goitre can make it hard to swallow or breathe freely.

Gonorrhoea

Gonorrhoea is a sexually transmitted infection caused by the bacterium *Neisseria gonorrhoeae*. It is popularly known as the clap. The infection is widely found in young adults who have had several sexual partners. More than 50,000 cases are reported in the UK each year.

SYMPTOMS

As many as 60 per cent of infected women and 10 per cent of infected males have no symptoms. But the first sign of infection is usually a heavily pus-stained discharge from the penis or vagina, or a burning pain on urination.

TREATMENT

To diagnose gonorrhea, swabs are taken from the urethra and cervix and examined for the presence of infectious bacteria. If the person has had oral or anal sex, swabs are also taken from the mouth or rectum.

Antibiotics are used to treat the infection. An infected person should not have sex for at least three weeks after treatment, and then not until they have been given the all-clear by the doctor after a repeat swab.

PREVENTION

Using a condom will protect against infection.

COMPLICATIONS

Gonorrhoea can spread to infect the prostate, the testicles or the female pelvic organs, where it can lead to infertility. In one per cent of infected males, gonococcal bacteria spread throughout the body to cause a skin rash, fever and joint pains. Untreated gonorrhoea can be passed from mother to baby during childbirth, causing **conjunctivitis**, which can cause scarring and blindness if left untreated.

Rarely, gonococcal bacteria multiply within the bloodstream to cause **septicaemia**.

SEE ALSO *Contraception; Pelvis and disorders; Prostate and problems; Sexually transmitted diseases*

Gout

Gout is a form of **arthritis** that particularly affects joints in the feet. It occurs when high levels of uric acid in the blood form a salt that crystallizes in joints. Men account for 95 per cent of cases. Gout is rare in under-35s, but its incidence increases with age. It used to be associated with drinking large quantities of port, but any heavy drinking can trigger an attack in someone with a tendency to gout.

SYMPTOMS
- Excruciating pain in the big toe.
- Pain in the knee, ankles, wrists and elbows.
- Swelling, redness and tenderness around a joint or joints.

Gout generally starts in one joint, but may affect others over time. Crystals can also build up in the soft tissues in the ears and around tendons, appearing as white spots called tophi.

TREATMENT
If you think you have gout, seek medical advice.

What a doctor may do
- Give a blood test to measure uric acid levels.
- Examine fluid from a joint for crystals.
- Prescribe a non-steroidal anti-inflammatory drug (NSAID) such as ibuprofen to reduce pain, and other long-term drugs if necessary.

What you can do
- Avoid foods that are high in substances called purines, which raise blood levels of uric acid. These foods include offal, poultry and pulses.
- Drink plenty of water.
- Avoid heavy alcohol drinking because this can precipitate an acute attack.
- Lose weight to reduce pressure on the joints.

Complementary therapies
Natural therapies to reduce uric acid levels include eating celery and drinking tea made from the herb devil's claw.

OUTLOOK
Treatment effectively controls acute attacks and prevents long-term complications.

Grommet insertion

Grommets are small tubes used in the treatment of severe cases of **glue ear**. An incision is created in each eardrum, and a grommet is inserted through the hole. This allows the equalization of pressure on both sides of the eardrum, so that the mucus buildup in the middle ear can drain away. Over 6–12 months, the hole closes and the grommet falls out.

Current medical opinion holds that it is safe for children with grommets to go swimming, but that they should avoid diving.

SEE ALSO *Ear and problems*

Growth and disorders

A child's growth is measured by height or length (stature), weight and the circumference of the head. Children should grow rapidly in infancy, so regular monitoring is important in order to identify any problems early on.

Growth is governed by a mixture of genetic, nutritional and hormonal factors. The heights and weights of children of the same age vary considerably and it is only when a child falls outside the normal range that there may be a cause for concern.

NORMAL GROWTH
There are three phases of growth: infancy, childhood and puberty. Children grow most rapidly during the first two years of life. There is then a much longer period of steady but slower growth, before a short, sharp period of rapid growth during puberty.

Girls are usually the first to begin their pubertal growth spurt, about two years earlier than boys. In boys, the slower childhood phase continues until the second half of puberty when they grow for a longer period and end up being on average 12.5cm (5in) taller than girls.

A child may be said to have slow growth if he or she is growing more slowly than would be expected for a child of his or her age with a similar lifestyle.

Growth charts
The weight, height and head circumference of a child under five years are normally monitored at a child health clinic. The measurements are entered into a child's personal health record book and compared against the national average for children of the same age using a centile or growth chart. The national average is represented on a centile chart by a line known as the 50th centile.

A child whose growth falls below the 3rd centile or above the 97th should be referred to a doctor, but as children vary a great deal, the chart is never considered in isolation from a child's general health.

Predictions can be made as to the height a child will attain in adulthood. Generally, give or take a few centimetres, a boy will eventually be twice

the height he is at two years, and a girl twice the
height she is at 18 months.

ABNORMAL GROWTH

The principal growth hormone is secreted by
the front part of the pituitary gland in the brain.
This controls the growth of bones, tissues and
organs. Production of growth hormone varies
considerably between individuals and its secretion
is influenced by many factors, including sleep
patterns, exercise, physical and emotional stress,
protein intake, blood sugar levels, malnutrition
and damage to the pituitary gland.

Growth assessment is part of the standard child
health surveillance programme; height and weight
are normally measured at developmental reviews
at 6–8 weeks, 18–24 months, 36–42 months and
school entry. Growth should also be checked if
a child has persistent or chronic health problems,
when parents or a professional express concern,
or when measurements on the centile chart
indicate cause for concern. Initial assessment of
abnormal growth is confirmed by two or more
accurate height measurements at an interval of
six months.

Investigations will include taking the child's
medical and family history and a blood test to
measure the level of growth hormone in the blood.

Short stature

When a child is shorter than average, factors
affecting growth could be:
- fetal – such as growth retardation in the uterus;
- genetic or chromosomal – for example, **Turner's
syndrome** or **Down's syndrome**;
- congenital conditions – for example,
achondroplasia (see below);
- inherited – the parents may have short stature;
- **malnutrition** – a poor diet or **malabsorption** can
lead to retarded growth;
- emotional – if a child is being emotionally or
psychologically abused or deprived, the stress can
inhibit growth hormone production and the
child's growth may be stunted;
- chronic disorders or illness – for example,
severe **asthma, coeliac disease** or renal failure
(see **Kidneys and disorders**);
- inactivity – long periods of inactivity without
exercise may restrict bone growth;
- hormonal – for example, growth hormone
deficiency or hypothyroidism (thyroid deficiency
that can retard growth; see **Thyroid and disorders**).

Tall stature

When a child is taller than is expected for his or
her age, the cause may be connected to:
- an excess of growth hormone;
- gigantism (see below);
- a genetic or chromosomal factor, such as
Marfan's syndrome or Klinefelter's syndrome
(see below);

- hormonal factors – for
example, excess growth
hormone or hyperthyroidism
(see **Thyroid and disorders**).

GROWTH DISORDERS

There are many disorders
that can affect growth. Most
of them are accompanied by
a range of other symptoms.

Achondroplasia

With achondroplasia, a short
stature is associated with a
shortening of the limbs, a
large head, a depressed
bridge of the nose and short
broad hands. It may occur
through an autosomal
dominant disorder, whereby
an affected parent carries an
abnormal gene on a pair of
chromosomes and may pass
the gene onto a child. In
50–80 per cent of cases there
is no family history, but a
chromosome defect occurs in
the sperm or ovum at the
time of conception.

Acromegaly

This rare condition, causing
tall stature, may occur at any
age and is a result of the
overproduction of growth hormone by the
pituitary gland. Certain bones, including those of
the hands and feet, may become enlarged.

Gigantism

Excessive tallness in childhood is called gigantism.
It may be caused by the overproduction of
growth hormone by the pituitary gland or by a
pituitary gland tumour. Treatment may include
a drug that blocks the release of growth hormone
or surgery to remove the tumour.

Growth hormone deficiency

This condition is rare, affecting just one in
3000–5000 children. Growth is usually normal
in the first two years, but then becomes stunted.
Early detection is very important as the condition
can be successfully treated with growth
hormone therapy.

Klinefelter's syndrome

In Klinefelter's syndrome, tall stature is caused
by a sex chromosome abnormality, which occurs
in one or two per 1000 boys. The child's height
is usually around the 75th centile (that is, 75 in
100 boys in the population as a whole are shorter
than someone with the syndrome tends to be).
The boy may also have small or undescended
testes and delayed puberty. Treatment may
include testosterone replacement.

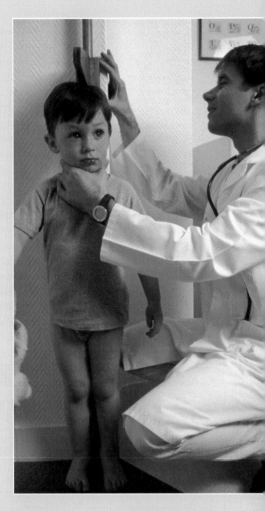

▲ **Measuring up**
A doctor records the
height of a young boy,
as part of a routine
check on his overall
development. Such
regular check ups mean
that abnormalities are
spotted early, which with
growth problems is
usually essential for
treatment to be effective.

Turner's syndrome

About one in 2500 girls suffers from Turner's syndrome, also a sex chromosome abnormality, which leads to short stature. Other signs and symptoms of the condition include neck webbing, widely spaced nipples, difficulties with feeding, and a number of problems such as heart, ear and eye disorders, and ovarian failure, which results in infertility. Treatment is with growth hormone from about the age of seven and oestrogen replacement at puberty.

GROWTH HORMONE THERAPY

Regular injections of human growth hormone have been proven to help children with growth hormone deficiency and disorders such as Turner's syndrome.

In the past children were given injections of growth hormone that had been derived from a human source. But after the discovery of **CJD** (Creutzfeldt-Jakob disease) in 1985 (and the associated risk of passing on the disease), a biosynthetic version has been used.

There is no risk of infection from biosynthetic growth hormone, which is given on prescription and administered by injection under the skin two to seven times a week. It is best given before bedtime as growth is stimulated by sleep. The injections are continued until the child reaches a mature adult height.

There is a slight risk of the injections provoking **diabetes** mellitus, and in a few cases the child's thyroid function may be impaired.

Some children who are shorter than average but otherwise healthy are prescribed growth hormone, even though they are not deficient in their own natural levels of the hormone. Studies have found, however, that this does not restore normal growth. Some experts also question whether it is ethical to subject these children unnecessarily to the trauma of daily injections.

Physical changes during puberty

The onset of puberty manifests itself in both boys and girls with the appearance of visible sexual characteristics such as the growth of body hair and changes in body shape.

Male

In boys, growth of the testicles is the first visible sign of puberty. Fine pubic hair begins to grow shortly after, followed by more general hair growth on the face, chest and limbs. Other physical changes include the growth of larger muscles and broader shoulders.

Female

The development of small lumps under one or both nipples signals the start of puberty. The breasts continue to grow and fat is deposited around them. Fine pubic hair appears, coarsening within a few years. The waist narrows and the hips widen.

Facial hair

Broad shoulders

Chest hair

Chest starts to widen

Enlarged penis and testicles

Coarse pubic hair

Breasts start to bud

Fat deposited around breasts

Wider hips

Coarse pubic hair

Testosterone level

8 10 12 14 16 18
Age in years

Oestrogen level

8 10 12 14 16 18
Age in years

Guillain-Barré syndrome

Guillain-Barré syndrome is a condition characterized by paralysis and impaired sensation. It usually starts with numbness or tingling and weakness in the toes and progresses over days to involve the legs and then the arms. Sometimes the muscles used in breathing and swallowing are affected. A viral or bacterial illness commonly precedes the condition by one to three weeks. Most people do not need specific treatment, but it may take weeks or even months to recover completely. Close monitoring in hospital may be necessary. **Physiotherapy** plays an important role in rehabilitation, and artificial ventilation may be required if respiratory failure occurs.

Gulf War syndrome

Gulf War syndrome is a much-debated term, covering a catalogue of conditions suffered by thousands of British soldiers since their return from the Gulf War in 1991. Sufferers claim that the syndrome is a single, all-encompassing illness arising directly from the war.

Symptoms include chronic fatigue, depression, memory loss, debilitating joint pains and gastric disorders. Illnesses range from post-traumatic stress disorder to **leukaemia** and other **cancers**.

Sufferers claim that Gulf War syndrome was caused by prolonged exposure during the war to low levels of chemical and biological agents. These substances are known to have delayed and chronic physiological effects. For many years Gulf War syndrome was not recognized as a specific illness, because it does not have a unique set of symptoms. However, in the UK in May 2002 a veteran was able to establish legally that it exists.

A British study published in August 2001, ten years after the conflict, reported that 17 per cent of Gulf War veterans believe they have the condition. This figure equates to 9000 British service personnel out of a complement of 53,000.

Gums and gum disease

Gum disease is far more prevalent in the UK than many people realize. An estimated 95 per cent of adults suffer from some form of gum disorder and of those 10 per cent have serious problems. In its early stages, gum disease (gingivitis) is easily treatable. The condition is a warning sign that plaque (a sticky film that contains bacteria) may be accumulating around the gum margins. Plaque produces toxins that irritate the gums, eventually destroying gum tissues. If plaque is not removed and it hardens, it forms tartar or calculus. Pockets of bacteria then build up underneath the gums, causing them to separate from the teeth and recede.

PERIODONTAL DISEASE

When the gums begin to recede, it marks the onset of periodontal disease, which is far more difficult to treat than gum disease. Periodontal disease exposes the roots of the teeth and breaks down the fibres that hold the teeth to the bone. Abscesses can form and pus may ooze from the pockets, resulting in bad breath (halitosis). Eventually, teeth become loose and in some cases may come out. In fact, more adults lose teeth because of periodontal disease than they do due to tooth decay.

Periodontal disease can also lead to an acute infection, called acute ulcerative gingivitis. This causes bleeding and ulceration around the gums and very bad breath. Smokers are particularly prone to ulcerative gingivitis, also known as trench mouth. If you are diagnosed with

Periodontal disease and diabetes

People with diabetes are at increased risk of developing periodontal disease.

This is thought to be because people with diabetes are generally more susceptible to contracting infections. Those people whose diabetes is not under control are most at risk. Also, diabetics who have periodontal disease often find it more difficult to control their levels of blood sugar.

periodontal disease, you may be referred to a hygienist, who will clean and scale the teeth to remove the calculus. The hygienist may also carry out root planing, a special cleaning of the root surface of the tooth. You might also be referred to a periodontist, a specialist who may prescribe antibiotics or mouthwashes to reduce infection. Surgery may also be recommended. This will involve a local anaesthetic so that the gums can be peeled back to expose the underlying bone. The inflamed tissue and the calculus are removed, then the gums are recontoured and stitched back into place.

GUM DISEASE IN PREGNANCY

Pregnant women are particularly susceptible to gingivitis and should take extra care with their oral hygiene and their diet. Expectant and new mothers should see their dentist regularly. Treatment for NHS patients is free during pregnancy and the following six months.

SEE ALSO *Dentist and dentistry; Teeth and problems*

Gynaecology and tests

Gynaecology is the study and treatment of diseases affecting the female reproductive system. The diagnosis of gynaecological disorders involves a variety of tests such as blood tests for **anaemia**, pregnancy tests, vaginal swabs, hormone profiles and **ultrasound** scans. Investigative procedures include **colposcopy, D&C, laparoscopy** and **laparotomy**, and hysteroscopy. If a serious problem is identified, it may lead to major surgery such as a **hysterectomy**.

COLPOSCOPY

A colposcopy is usually carried out if a routine **cervical smear test** has identified precancerous or early cancerous cells among those scraped from the cervix.

A magnifying instrument called a colposcope is inserted into the patient's vagina to examine the cervix in detail and identify the areas that have produced the abnormal cells. No anaesthetic is necessary for this procedure, which may be uncomfortable but not painful. Tissue samples (**biopsies**) for microscopic examination may be collected and any abnormal areas may be removed by **diathermy**, which uses heat produced by an electric current, or **laser surgery**.

D&C

D&C, which stands for dilation and curettage, has traditionally been used to investigate the cause of heavy menstrual bleeding. Under general anaesthetic, the cervix is dilated and a small tissue sample of the womb lining, the endometrium, is scraped away using a spoon-shaped instrument called a curette. The sample is then sent for microscopic examination.

D&Cs have now largely been replaced by out-patient procedures that can be performed without a general anaesthetic. An example is Vabra curettage, which uses a fine diameter tube and suction to remove a tiny sample of the uterine lining.

LAPAROSCOPY AND LAPAROTOMY

During a laparoscopy, the pelvic organs are examined through an illuminated tube called a laparoscope, which is passed through a small incision in the abdominal wall. A number of conditions, including **endometriosis, fibroids,** ovarian tumours, **salpingitis** and early **ectopic pregnancies,** may be diagnosed in this way. The procedure is carried out under general **anaesthetic**. It may not be possible for a laparoscopy to be performed if adhesions (scar tissue formed by previous infections) are present.

With an exploratory laparatomy, which is also performed under general anaesthetic, a larger incision is made in the abdominal wall. This enables doctors to examine the pelvic

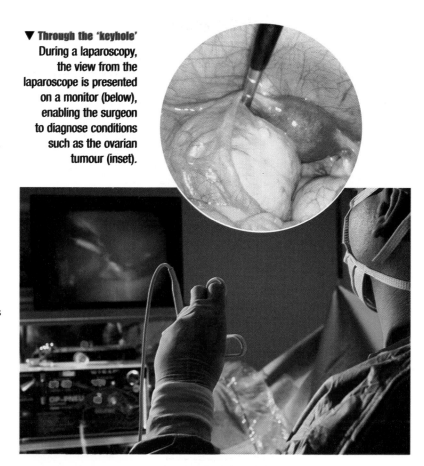

▼ **Through the 'keyhole'**
During a laparoscopy, the view from the laparoscope is presented on a monitor (below), enabling the surgeon to diagnose conditions such as the ovarian tumour (inset).

organs in more detail than is possible using a laparoscope.

HYSTEROSCOPY

An illuminated instrument is used to examine the interior uterus in cases of abnormal bleeding. It can be performed under general or local anaesthetic. Minor surgery, such as the removal or fibroids, can be done at the same time.

ULTRASOUND

Ultrasound scans produce detailed images of the pelvic organs on a television screen. Transvaginal ultrasound, using a transmitting probe in the vagina, gives very detailed pictures that are particularly useful for accurate diagnosis and treatment.

SEE ALSO *Internal pelvic examination; Reproductive system; Uterus and problems*

Gynaecomastia

Gynaecomastia is a condition in which one or both of a man's breasts increase in size. The usual cause is an excess of the female hormone oestrogen in the blood.

Gynaecomastia is seldom serious and affects 50–70 per cent of boys at some point during puberty; in older men it may be a symptom of another disease or a reaction to certain drugs.

Haematoma

A haematoma is a localized collection of blood that has leaked into the surrounding tissues and then clotted, forming a solid swelling. It may follow an injury or be due to a disorder of the blood vessels or clotting mechanisms. Most haematomas dissipate without any intervention, although a few require drainage. A haematoma within the skull may need urgent surgery to avoid pressure on the brain.

Haematuria

Blood in the urine is called haematuria. It may follow injury but is more usually the result of disease somewhere in the **urinary system**: the kidneys, ureters, bladder or urethra. Haematuria requires prompt medical attention. Causes include various kidney diseases, kidney stones, tumours or cysts in the bladder, prostate enlargement and tropical infections.
SEE ALSO *Kidneys and disorders*

Haemolytic disease of the newborn

If a mother's blood is Rhesus negative and the father and fetus have Rhesus positive blood, the mother develops antibodies that may pass into the fetal circulation, attacking the baby's red blood cells. This condition is referred to as haemolytic disease of the newborn or Rhesus haemolytic disease. It can result in the baby having severe **anaemia** and other problems such as **jaundice**. The condition does not usually occur in a first pregnancy, but to prevent it happening in subsequent pregnancies the mother should be given an injection of anti-D immunoglobulin soon after the birth. A Rhesus negative woman should also be given an injection of anti-D immunoglobin in the event of an abortion or miscarriage of a fetus that was Rhesus positive.
SEE ALSO *Blood and disorders*

Haemophilia

Haemophilia is an inherited disorder whereby the blood does not clot properly, leading to excessive bruising and bleeding even from a minor injury. Haemophiliacs are deficient in one of several clotting factors that are needed for the coagulation pathway, a sequence of reactions that cause blood to clot, to function.

Haemophilia generally affects only men. This is due to the way it is inherited. Women tend to be carriers, there being a 50 per cent chance that their sons will have the disorder and that their daughters will also become carriers. The most prevalent forms are haemophilia A and haemophilia B. Other forms are very rare.

HAEMOPHILIA A
Haemophilia A refers to a deficiency of clotting factor VIII and affects between one in 5000 and one in 10,000 boys and men in the West.

Individuals with at least 25 per cent of the normal level of factor VIII in their blood have few problems. Others with a lower percentage of factor VIII – down to about 1 per cent – experience abnormal bleeding and bruising from minor injuries; the condition may be suspected once they are toddling (and falling) or later. Sufferers with less than 1 per cent of factor VIII bleed spontaneously; the diagnosis is usually made rapidly at birth because of prolonged bleeding from the umbilical cord or unusually extensive bruising from the birth.

Severe haemophiliacs need intravenous infusion of factor VIII concentrate twice a day after even a minor injury. Otherwise, abnormal bleeding can destroy their joints, causing pain and distortion, and even lead to death. Sufferers from mild forms of haemophilia can lead mostly normal lives.

Families of haemophiliacs need genetic counselling about the risks of passing on the condition and advice on prenatal tests in future pregnancies.

HAEMOPHILIA B
Also known as Christmas disease, haemophilia B affects between one in 30,000 and one in 100,000 men and boys in the West. Sufferers lack clotting factor IX. The diagnosis, symptoms and treatment resemble haemophilia A, but treatment is with factor IX concentrate.
SEE ALSO *Blood and disorders*

Haemorrhage

Haemorrhage refers to the loss of blood from the body's circulation. It can be external and visible, or it can be internal, such as bleeding into a body organ, a muscle or a body cavity.

SYMPTOMS AND COMPLICATIONS
A sufferer may be pale and thirsty, and feel cold and clammy. There may be visible bleeding. Symptoms of shock may develop. In a severe haemorrhage, complications can include faintness, leading to collapse, unconsciousness and death. Types of haemorrhage include:
■ Aneurysm – a swelling of an artery, which can rupture and bleed.

- Bleeding from the stomach or bowel.
- Brain haemorrhage – caused by injury or a stroke.
- Injury causing bruising and/or bleeding.
- Injury to the abdomen, causing rupture to the liver, spleen, kidney or bowel.
- Pregnancy complication – miscarriage or ectopic pregnancy.
- Severe nosebleed.

TREATMENT

- Control external bleeding by pressing a clean dressing or pad on the wound for up to 15 minutes.
- If possible, raise and support the injured part.
- When bleeding stops, apply a sterile dressing.
- Watch for and treat signs of shock.
- If internal haemorrhage is suspected seek medical advice immediately.
- Call an ambulance if bleeding does not stop or shock develops.

Haemorrhagic disease of the newborn

Some newborn babies haemorrhage due to a lack of vitamin K, which is essential for blood clotting. The bleeding may occur up to the first eight weeks of life, and may result in bruises, other types of bleeding or sometimes a brain haemorrhage. A blood transfusion may be necessary to treat the condition, which is prevented by administering vitamin K routinely at birth to all babies, either by injection or by mouth. Breast milk is low in vitamin K, so breastfeeding babies who receive oral vitamin K at birth will need a further dose after four to seven days and then again a month later.

SEE ALSO *Birth and problems*

Haemorrhoids

Commonly known as piles, haemorrhoids are swollen or varicose veins outside or inside the anus. They are very common in both men and women. The risk of developing them increases with age, pregnancy and childbirth. Most cases clear up after a few weeks but may recur, sometimes becoming chronic until treated.

SYMPTOMS

People with haemorrhoids may experience bleeding from the anal passage with discomfort or pain during defecation. There may be a mucous discharge or itching. You may also feel or see small, bright red or blue-purple lumps just outside the anus. Pain may be extreme if the haemorrhoid becomes strangulated.

CAUSES

Haemorrhoids may result from constipation or straining to pass hard faeces, but there is no conclusive evidence. Most sufferers have normal bowel frequency, so constipation may follow, rather than precede haemorrhoids. There may be an inherited weakness of anal tissue.

They are more likely during pregnancy because the hormone progesterone, present in greater amounts during pregnancy, relaxes the veins and pressure on them increases as the womb enlarges.

TREATMENT

The treatment depends on the severity of the condition.

When to consult a doctor

- Any anal bleeding should be investigated.
- See a doctor if there is discomfort, pain or no improvement after a few weeks.

What a doctor may do

- Examine you to exclude more serious conditions.
- Recommend eating more fibre to loosen stools.
- Prescribe soothing ointments or suppositories.
- In more serious cases, use sclerotherapy (injection of an irritant liquid) or **cryosurgery** to shrivel swollen veins, or coagulate blood vessels by infrared treatment.
- Alternatively, the haemorrhoid may be surgically removed under general or epidural anaesthetic.

What you can do

- Eat plenty of fresh fruit and vegetables.
- Wash after every bowel movement.
- Take soothing hot baths.
- Use over-the-counter ointments or suppositories.
- With clean fingers, gently push any piles back into the anus.

PREVENTION

- Eat at least five portions of fresh fruit and vegetables a day.
- Eating a high-fibre breakfast may reduce the risk of haemorrhoids.

SEE ALSO *Anus and problems*

Hair, scalp and problems

Hair is made of a tough protein known as keratin. It provides warmth, reduces heat loss from the top of the head and helps to cushion the scalp from damage. Each hair grows out

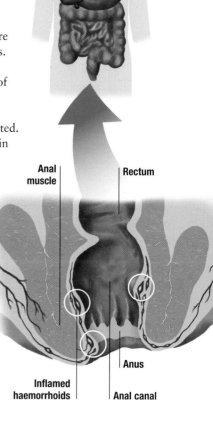

Anal muscle | Rectum

Anus

Inflamed haemorrhoids | Anal canal

▲ **Haemorroids**
Frequent constipation that causes repeated straining during bowel movements may cause the veins in the anal wall to become swollen.

of a hair follicle. Humans are born with around 100,000–150,000 hair follicles on their head.

When a hair is growing, its root is tightly surrounded by live tissue called the hair bulb, which contains a layer of dividing cells. As new cells are formed, older ones die and are pushed upwards to form the hair shaft. Active growth is followed by a resting phase in which the shaft remains attached to the scalp but does not grow. During this phase new cells are created in the hair follicle and active growth begins again.

Each hair shaft has a spongy core (the medulla), a middle layer (the cortex) and an outer cuticle made up of thousands of overlapping scales. A small muscle attached to the base of each hair follicle pulls the hair upright when it contracts. When this happens, the skin puckers to form a goose bump – for example, when you are cold. Near the top of each hair follicle are three to five small, oil-secreting (sebaceous) glands that secrete skin oils (sebum), which help to keep the hair in good condition.

Hair colour depends on the presence of the skin pigment melanin. Red melanin produces gold, auburn or red hair, while black melanin produces shades of brown or black depending on its concentration. In people with blond hair, melanin pigment is pale and only found in the hair cortex. In those with dark hair, pigments are found in both the cortex and medulla, which produces a greater depth of colour.

HAIR PROBLEMS

The condition of your hair is a good indicator of how healthy and well nourished you are. Your hair is often the first part of your body to show signs of lacking a particular vitamin, mineral or essential fatty acid. Nutritional deficiencies can rapidly lead to hair that:

- looks dull and lacklustre;
- is brittle, with split ends;
- feels dry and frizzy;
- looks limp and lifeless;
- is thinning;
- falls out, especially when combed.

Illness can also affect hair health, especially:

- serious illness such as cancer;
- an underactive thyroid gland (which can make hair dry, coarse, brittle and thinning);
- iron-deficiency **anaemia** (which can leave hair dry and thinning).

Cancer treatments such as **chemotherapy** can lead to hair loss.

Alopecia

Alopecia occurs when hair follicles fail to reactivate after the normal resting phase. The exact cause is unknown, but it is thought to be due to an overactive immune system attacking the hair follicles. Stress also plays a major role.

The condition is estimated to affect over 8.5 million people in the UK.

Hair loss in pregnancy

In some women hormonal changes during pregnancy prolong the growth phase of their hair, which becomes thicker than normal. After birth the growth phase reverts to normal, fewer hairs grow and much of the extra hair that grew during pregnancy falls out.

Some women become concerned if they appear to be losing more scalp hair than normal in the first three months or so after giving birth. At times of physical or emotional stress, hair life cycles can synchronize, so that hundreds or even thousands of hairs enter the resting phase of their life cycle together, rather than in a staggered pattern over time. As a result, many more hairs than normal fall out at the same time. This effect is noticed after major operations as well as after childbirth. If generalized, it can lead to widespread hair thinning. If localized, alopecia results.

If you are worried about hair loss, keeping your scalp clean and eating a well balanced diet should help to promote new hair growth.

Trichotillomania

People suffering from trichotillomania feel a recurring urge to pull out their own hair. In the UK the condition is thought to affect as much as 2 per cent of the population. The problem is commonly misdiagnosed as alopecia. Treatment involves cognitive behavioural therapy, counselling, antidepressants if appropriate, and weaving in of artificial hair fibres both to disguise hair loss and to make it more difficult to pull out hair roots.

Baldness

Male pattern hair loss produces a receding hairline, and/or a circular bald patch at the crown. A strong inherited link determines the age at which hair begins to thin and the pattern of **baldness** that follows. Several treatments are available to overcome male pattern baldness, including minoxidil lotion – a drug originally used in its oral form to treat high blood pressure. Operations to relocate hair follicles or transplant hair are also available.

SCALP PROBLEMS

Dry, scaly scalp conditions are common and affect at least one in four people at some time. They are usually due to **dandruff**, seborrhoeic dermatitis or **psoriasis**.

Dandruff is the name given to a buildup of unsightly white flakes in the hair. Around four in ten people suffer from dandruff at some point in their life, although the condition is often mild. More severe dandruff, associated with inflammation, redness, itching and dry or greasy scales, is known as seborrhoeic dermatitis. Dry or greasy scales form around the hairline and may extend to involve the ears, eyebrows, nose and chest as well as the scalp. Dead skin cells tend to clump together to form larger, visible flakes. In severe cases, a yellowish red crust may form.

Both dandruff and seborrhoeic dermatitis are thought to be triggered by a hypersensitivity to a yeast, *Pityrosporum ovale*, and usually respond to a shampoo containing antifungal agents. Other conditions that can trigger dandruff include stress-related skin scaling (neurodermatitis), contact **dermatitis** (due to an allergy to ingredients in a shampoo, for example), **eczema** and sunburn.

In scalp psoriasis, skin cells are produced up to ten times faster than normal, resulting in redness and scaliness on top of the head. Scales are normally tiny, but when large, overlapping flakes of skin form and remain attached to hair shafts; the condition is known as pityriasis amiantacea. Scalp psoriasis does not usually affect the hair itself, although more hair than usual may fall out during a flare-up so that thinning occurs. A variety of treatments are available on prescription, such as dithranol and calcipotriol creams or steroid ointments.

Halitosis

Halitosis is the medical term for bad breath. It is usually caused by bacteria in the mouth which produce volatile (and foul-smelling) sulphur compounds. Halitosis is usually a sign of ineffective oral hygiene: the solution is to improve brushing and flossing (see **Teeth and disorders**). Smoking and drinking large amounts of coffee can also cause halitosis. More rarely it can be a sign of gastro-intestinal problems.

If you are worried that you may suffer from bad breath, talk to your **dentist** who will be able to identify the cause of the complaint and may recommend treatments. When halitosis is the result of poor oral hygiene, you may be referred to a hygienist who will teach you how to brush and floss your teeth more effectively.

The bacteria that cause bad breath can become trapped around the margins of the teeth and **gums**, and are also found around the tongue, palate and cheeks. In people with healthy teeth and gums, the back of the tongue may be producing the odour. This should be gently and carefully cleaned with a brush or tongue scraper, which can be bought at some dental practices and specialist outlets. Also, mouthwashes can be a useful way of dealing with halitosis but should not be seen as a substitute for good brushing and flossing. Rinses containing chlorhexidine are particularly effective at killing bacteria but use over a long period may stain the teeth.

Bad breath can also be a side effect of a dry mouth (see **Salivary glands and disorders**). Smokers are more likely to be affected since smoking has a drying effect in the mouth, reducing saliva. Denture-wearers may also suffer from bad breath if they do not remove their dentures at night or clean them effectively.
SEE ALSO *Tongue and problems*

Hallucination

Hallucinations are what a person thinks they can see or hear when there is actually nothing there. They are a common feature of mental distress and can be confusing and frightening.
SYMPTOMS
- Screaming, hiding, confronting or running away from an unseen thing or person.
- Talking, shouting or swearing at voices others cannot hear.

CAUSES
Possible causes range from life events – hearing or seeing someone who has recently died is not unusual – to changes in brain chemistry. Hallucinations may be the result of drugs taken years before, or the withdrawal effects of certain drugs.

TREATMENT
Some people hear voices throughout their lives without any distress. Medical intervention is only normally necessary if the person becomes withdrawn, disturbed or frightened due to the hallucinations. A doctor may prescribe drug treatment, usually tranquillizers. Self-help and support groups for people with similar experiences may help to ease isolation.
SEE ALSO *Delusions; Mental health and problems; Psychosis*

Hand, foot and mouth disease

Hand, foot and mouth disease occurs mostly in children but can affect adults. Unrelated to foot and mouth disease in cattle, it is caused by a virus (usually the coxsackievirus) and is very contagious. Symptoms include blisters on the hands, fingers, feet and inside of the mouth, and a slight fever. Treatment is with mild painkillers.

Hand and problems

The hand performs two key functions: the whole hand is used to grasp, while the thumb and one or more fingers are used for pinching. But our hands suffer a lot of wear and tear and need looking after.

Each hand consists of 27 bones, giving it great flexibility and a wide range of movement. The four fingers and opposable thumb move independently, making possible two types of grip: grasping and pinching. As the human race evolved, the ability to perform these two actions gave us a huge advantage over other species when it came to making and using tools and weapons.

The four fingers on each hand each have three bones known as phalanges, which form hinge joints moved by tendons. The thumbs also consist of phalanges, but have only two each. Each finger and thumb is also connected to a bone in the palm of the hand called a metacarpal. The phalanx at the base of the thumb articulates with its metacarpal in a joint known as a saddle joint – in which two U-shaped bone surfaces fit together at right angles to rock back and forth and from side to side, although rotation is limited.

The wrist joint is made up of eight bones and allows movement in most directions. One of these bones, the scaphoid, is easily fractured if you fall

Intricate mechanism

The hand is a versatile tool. Its 27 bones form simple hinge joints – the knuckles – and more complex saddle joints – such as the base of the thumb – that act as hinges but also have some degree of rotation.

Wrist
The wrist has eight bones, or carpals. Four are linked to the bones of the arm; the other four are connected to the palm bones or metacarpals.

Saddle joint
The thumb's joint with its metacarpal is more flexible than a simple hinge.

Thumb
The thumb's opposability to the fingers allows for precision pinching movements.

Ligament
Strong ligaments bind the wrist bones together.

Tendon
The hinge joints are moved by tendons that attach the bones to muscles in the forearm.

Metacarpal
Each finger and thumb is connected to the palm by a bone called a metacarpal.

Phalanges
Each finger consists of three phalanges or sections joined to each other at the knuckles. The thumb has two phalanges.

Right and left-handedness

Babies are ambidextrous – they can manipulate objects using either hand – but by the age of 12 a preference is firmly established.

Ninety per cent of adults use their right hand for writing, while the other 10 per cent are either left-handed or ambidextrous. Right or left-handedness is largely determined by inheritance and depends on which hemisphere of the brain is dominant. Each hemisphere controls sense and movement on the opposite side of the body.

In the past, many children with an obvious tendency to left-handedness were trained to become right-handed so as to conform with the majority.

on an outstretched hand. This break is not easily spotted, even using an X-ray, and if it remains untreated it can lead to osteoarthritis and wrist pain. **Carpal tunnel syndrome** occurs when the median nerve becomes pinched as it passes through a bony tunnel in the wrist. (See also **Joints and problems; Wrist and problems.**)

CARING FOR YOUR HANDS
Many of us take insufficient care of our hands, exposing them to harsh chemicals, frequent wetting, cold, wear and tear, and to the risk of minor injury and subsequent infection.

For hygiene reasons, hands should be kept clean and germ-free. But repeated use of soap and water, and especially washing-up detergent, damages the top layer of the skin and can cause scaling or chapping. In extreme cases, chapping can lead to **eczema.**

Easing stiffness
If your fingers are stiff – caused by **arthritis,** for example – you may find hand exercises helpful both for regaining joint mobility and strengthening the muscles. Exercises can range from simple opening and closing of the fist, wriggling the fingers or squeezing a soft spongy object that fits into your palm.

People with rheumatoid arthritis find it helpful to exercise their hands in hot water first thing in the morning and throughout the day. Hot baths or showers are also soothing. Some people find hot or cold compresses helpful.

HAND DISORDERS
The hands and fingernails are always included in a medical examination because they can reveal signs of other health problems, including:
■ pale fingernail beds, a symptom of **anaemia;**
■ **clubbing,** a broadening of the fingertips that can be associated with certain **lung** diseases;
■ tremor and redness of the palms (erythema), sometimes a sign of **liver** disease.

Common problems that directly affect the hand include Dupuytren's contracture, ganglion, trigger finger and mallet finger.

Dupuytren's contracture
Dupuytren's contracture is a painless thickening of fibrous tissues in the palm of one or both hands. This causes puckering of the skin and a fixed bending forward of some fingers (usually the ring finger and the little finger). The affected fingers may be drawn right down onto the palm.

Ganglion
A ganglion is a small harmless swelling that forms within the sheath of tissues that contains tendons. Ganglions are most common in the wrist, fingers and feet, where they appear as a round lump beneath the skin. The lump contains a thick fluid and can disappear on its own. You can disperse the swelling yourself by applying firm finger pressure, but though the ganglion may disappear for a while, it will almost certainly recur; if it is painless it is best left alone. Consult a doctor if the ganglion is growing bigger and pressing on nerves, causing pain. The doctor may send you to a local out-patients' department, where the ganglion will be numbed with local anaesthetic and cut out. (See also **Tendons and disorders.**)

Mallet finger
Mallet finger is a deformity in which the fingertip cannot be straightened because the tendon controlling it has been snapped by injury. It can happen when a heavy blow to the fingertip – caused by, for example, stubbing the finger or trying to catch a hard, fast ball – forces the tip into a bent position. Mallet finger is treated by straightening the finger and putting it in splints to enable the tendon to heal properly.

Trigger finger
A trigger finger occurs when one or more fingers become locked in a bent position but can be released forcibly to produce a click. There is usually tenderness and swelling at the base of the affected finger. It results from inflammation of a tendon within its sheath. When the finger is bent, the swollen tendon slides out of the sheath and cannot re-enter it – with the result that the finger stays locked down until forcibly straightened.

Treatment involves injection of an anti-inflammatory corticosteroid drug, or surgery to widen the mouth of the tendon sheath.

Other finger disorders
One of the commonest infections on the hand is whitlow – a small **abscess** that forms on the fingertip, and can affect the finger pulp, the root of the nail, or the tendon sheaths running up and down the fingers. In acute cases, treatment is by cutting into the inflamed area and releasing the pus. A doctor may also prescribe antibiotics.

Other conditions affecting the fingers include:
■ a viral **wart;**
■ a **fracture;**
■ a dislocation;
■ chilblains (see **Foot and problems**);
■ osteoarthritis or rheumatoid arthritis.
■ **Raynaud's syndrome,** which when triggered by frequent use of pneumatic drills or chainsaws may be referred to as 'vibration white finger'.
SEE ALSO *Nails and disorders.*

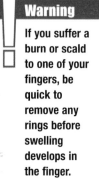

▲ Hand exercise
If you suffer from arthritis, this exercise will help to strengthen your hands and wrists and make them more flexible. Place a squash or tennis ball in one palm and firmly squeeze it with your fingers. Repeat until you feel the strain. Then rest and repeat with the other hand.

Warning
If you suffer a burn or scald to one of your fingers, be quick to remove any rings before swelling develops in the finger.

Hay fever

Hay fever, also known as **allergic rhinitis**, is an allergic reaction to pollens and moulds. It is a seasonal condition, usually starting in early June, that affects 15–20 per cent of people in the UK. Generally, hay fever is a manageable annoyance, but in more severe cases it can interfere with work, study and driving.

Anyone can develop hay fever at any time of life. But, if one of your parents suffers from hay fever, you have a one in three chance of developing it. If both parents have allergies, the risk increases to two in three.

The rise of hay fever

More people than ever suffer from hay fever and the reason could be to do with better hygiene.

The number of people suffering from hay fever has doubled in the UK since the early 1970s, but no one is sure why. According to the hygiene hypothesis, modern standards of living mean that we are no longer exposed to so many infectious diseases early in life, which would train our immune systems to tackle real dangers. Without this exposure our immune system lacks 'perspective' and produces an excessively strong response to harmless pollen.

SYMPTOMS
Hay fever has three groups of symptoms – associated with the eyes, nose and chest.
- The eyes may be watery and red, as well as feeling gritty and sore; there may also be itching and swelling of the whites of the eyes.
- Symptoms linked with the nose include sneezing – but, although people with hay fever sneeze a lot, it is not catching. The nose may also be runny, blocked or itchy, and there may be a headache caused by blocked sinuses.
- Symptoms in the chest include wheezing and a feeling of tightness (See **Asthma**).

CAUSES
Pollen and mould cause hay fever. The symptoms normally last for as long as the triggers are present.

In the UK, grass pollinates from May to August; trees pollinate in the spring; weeds pollinate in late summer; and mould spores are around in the late summer and autumn.

Headache

A headache can be an occasional, minor discomfort or a symptom of an underlying illness. But headaches are very rarely an indication of serious disease. The more sinister types of headache may occur along with other symptoms or signs.

DIAGNOSIS
A person's medical history and the frequency and severity of the headache is important in distinguishing an uncomfortable but safe headache from a more serious one. A doctor's consultation is likely to include these questions:
- When did the headaches start?
- Was the onset sudden?
- Is it one headache that is present all the time or does it come in bursts? If so, how long does each burst last?
- When do the headaches occur (for example, in the morning) and how often do they occur?
- Are they getting worse?
- What sort of pain is it – stabbing or aching?
- Where on the head does it occur – in one particular place or all over?
- Is there anything that seems to bring the headache on, make it worse or relieve it – certain foods, bending or coughing, for example?
- Does anything else occur with the headache?

CAUSES
Headaches occur for many reasons. Receptors responsible for the sensation of pain lie in blood vessels at the base of the brain as well as in the meninges, the protective coverings of the brain.

HARMLESS HEADACHES
The majority of headaches, however painful, are short-lived and are not a cause for concern.

Tension headache
A tension headache is the most common type and is experienced by most people at some time. The pain, often described as a band-like pressure around the head, tends to be fairly constant. The sufferer may be able to feel points of tenderness over the scalp. There is no associated vomiting or aversion to bright light (photophobia). The headache is generalized and can last for weeks or months, and for this reason is unlike **migraine**, which tends not to last for more than 72 hours.

Tension headaches can be brought on by stress, noise, fumes and concentrated viewing of TV or computer screens. Sometimes they arise because the body is dehydrated. The worry of having a headache may cause the pain to continue. It is important to remember that this type of headache is not dangerous.

To manage a tension headache:
- avoid precipitating factors if at all possible;
- relaxation and physical exercise may be helpful, as can **massage** and cooling packs;
- try drinking a glass of water if **dehydration** is suspected;
- painkillers available at the chemists may help, but they should only be used as prescribed and for the short term.

Migraine
Migraine headaches are characterized by a throbbing pain largely at the front of the head. This is often accompanied by vomiting, seeing flashes of light and sometimes a tingling sensation or numbness, moving across the body.

Most sufferers have a family history of the condition, but stress and certain foods, such as chocolate, can trigger attacks. Once trigger factors are identified, they should be avoided where possible. Aspirin or paracetamol are the best pain relievers, but avoid any containing caffeine, such as codeine, as these may cause further headaches once you stop taking them. While the headache lasts, sufferers usually prefer to be in a dark, quiet place.

Sinusitis

Sinusitis is often fairly easily diagnosed since the headache is associated with an upper respiratory tract infection or a cold with fever, runny nose and tenderness around the sinuses – at the top of the nose and around the eyes.

Simple steam inhalations or anticongestants can help, and in a few rare cases surgery is required. Antibiotics are sometimes needed to clear an infection.

Cluster headache

Despite being referred to as 'migrainous neuralgia', cluster headaches are not migraines. They are not common, men being about five times more likely than women to suffer from them. Usually beginning in the patient's 30s, they tend to disappear after the age of 35. The condition occurs more frequently among heavy smokers. Alcohol consumption may sometimes trigger an attack, although there appear to be no dietary triggers.

The symptoms are recurring attacks of extreme pain, located around one eye. Other symptoms include excess production of tears and blockage of the nostril on the side of the pain. There may also be vomiting. The patient tends to develop a pattern of pain at certain times in the day, for example, occurring every morning. It may even wake the patient up during the night.

Attacks can last for as little as 15 minutes, but can be up to 3 hours long. They usually last between 30 and 90 minutes. Sufferers often feel restless and need to walk about.

The attacks may occur several times over a number of weeks and then be followed by months of being free of symptoms before another cluster of attacks occurs. In severe cases, attacks occur several times a day. Painkillers and treatments for migraine tend to bring little relief. Frequent severe attacks of cluster headache may be prevented by taking prescribed doses of lithium carbonate, but this is quite a toxic drug with an array of unpleasant side effects –

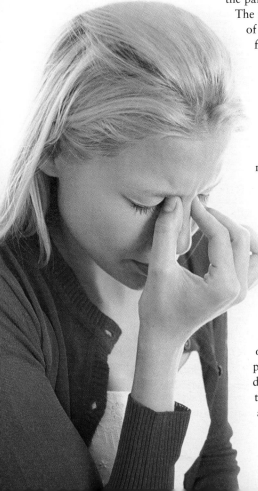

▼ Focused pain
A headache associated with sinusitis is often felt at the top of the nose and around the eyes.

including nausea, vomiting and tremor – that need to be set against its potential benefits. The patient will also require regular blood tests to monitor kidney and thyroid function.

Inhalation of concentrated oxygen can sometimes help to stop an attack.

Trigeminal neuralgia

Trigeminal neuralgia may be caused by damage to the trigeminal nerve, the main sensory nerve supplying the face. Sufferers tend to be middle-aged or elderly. Common causes of damage include infections such as shingles and diseases such as **multiple sclerosis** that affect the protective layer that encases the nerve fibres.

Factors that trigger trigeminal neuralgia include cold, touch or the actions of eating or drinking. The pain is often sudden and severe and may cause the patient to flinch.

Attacks may last only seconds or minutes but can occur several times a day. Bursts of pain may be followed by a dull, aching sensation.

People who suffer from trigeminal neuralgia should attempt to avoid trigger factors. Drug treatment with tricyclic antidepressants or anticonvulsants such as carbamazepine often proves highly effective. Destroying part of the nerve by either local injection of phenol or by surgery may also be effective but can lead to permanent numbness.

DANGEROUS HEADACHES

A headache may also indicate raised intracranial pressure, subarachnoid haemorrhage, meningitis or temporal arteritis – all of which require urgent medical attention.

Raised intracranial pressure

An increase in the pressure exerted on the brain can cause a severe headache. This can be due to an increase in the production of fluid within the brain, a decrease in its drainage (**hydrocephalus**) or a growth (for example, a tumour) within the skull. Other more obvious causes include headache following traumatic **head injury** or a heart attack, where there has been a reduction in oxygen supply to the body.

Apart from a headache, the symptoms include problems with speaking or writing, or difficulty with moving limbs. Typically, the headache is felt all over the skull, is most severe on waking and eases upon standing up. The pain tends to be made worse when coughing, straining, sneezing or bending forwards. Vomiting often occurs, usually in the morning.

The headache usually becomes progressively worse over a matter of days or weeks, but the speed at which the pain develops depends on the cause. Headaches caused by hydrocephalus tend to develop in hours or days, whereas pain due to a mass or tumour within the brain will progress over weeks or months.

Incidence of headache types

Only a small proportion of headaches investigated each year by doctors indicate dangerous diseases.

UNPLEASANT BUT SAFE	PER 100,000/YEAR
Tension headache	250
Migraine	250
Trigeminal neuralgia	5

DANGEROUS	PER 100,000/YEAR
Raised intracranial pressure	10
Subarachnoid haemorrhage	15
Meningitis	10
Temporal arteritis	5

Treatment of raised intracranial pressure depends on the cause – for example, a suspected tumour requires further investigation and, if necessary, surgery or radiation therapy to reduce the mass. Hydrocephalus requires the excess fluid around the brain to be drained off (often via a 'shunt' inserted from the brain into a major neck vein). Drugs that reduce swelling and excess fluid, such as dexamethasone, may be used to relieve the pressure within the skull.

Subarachnoid haemorrhage

A subarachnoid haemorrhage is signalled by a sudden, extremely severe headache that may be like being struck on the head with a hammer. The neck feels stiff and the patient may lose consciousness. It is caused by blood leaking from vessels and pooling under the protective coverings of the brain.

This is an emergency condition requiring immediate hospitalization and probable surgery to secure the bleeding vessel.

Meningitis

A severe headache may be a symptom of **meningitis**. Such headaches often develop over a matter of hours or days. Suspicion should be raised if the individual concerned also has fever, neck stiffness, irritability or varying levels of consciousness and possibly a rash.

Meningitis may be bacterial or viral in origin. Bacterial meningitis needs early treatment with antibiotics. Hospitalization is essential and a doctor should be consulted as soon as possible.

Temporal arteritis

Temporal arteritis is caused by inflammation of some of the blood vessels in the brain and can lead to blindness if vessels in the eye are affected. The headache develops over a matter of weeks, and pain may occur on one side of the head or all over. Women are twice as likely to be affected as men.

A typical symptom is that of pain in the jaw muscles when chewing. A quarter of those affected also have generalized joint and muscle aching. Diagnosis is made by blood tests and often requires a biopsy in which a small amount of tissue is taken from a scalp artery for study by a specialist.

Temporal arteritis needs prompt diagnosis and urgent treatment with high doses of steroids.

COMPLEMENTARY THERAPIES

It is important to ensure that your headache is not due to a serious illness before considering the use of any complementary therapy.

Therapies that induce a state of relaxation (such as aromatherapy, holistic **massage** and reflexology) may help to relieve tension headaches. Similarly, relaxing exercises, such as those of yoga and t'ai chi, may also be useful. Camomile tea and valerian, which have a calming effect, can also help.

Osteopathy and **chiropractic** often bring rapid relief when headaches are the result of poor posture or of muscle spasm.

If you suffer from migraines, a complementary therapist may recommend that you omit certain trigger foods (such as cheese, chocolate and red wine) from your diet. Eating fish rich in Omega-3 fatty acids (such as mackerel, salmon and tuna), may help to prevent migraines.

Certain supplements can also be beneficial to those affected by headaches. These include:
- feverfew, which may prevent or alleviate some types of headaches, including migraines, when taken over several weeks or months;
- riboflavin (a B vitamin) and a combined magnesium and calcium preparation, taken daily as a supplement, may be effective for persistent migraines.

SEE ALSO *Brain and nervous system; Head and injuries; Migraine; Subarachnoid haemorrhage*

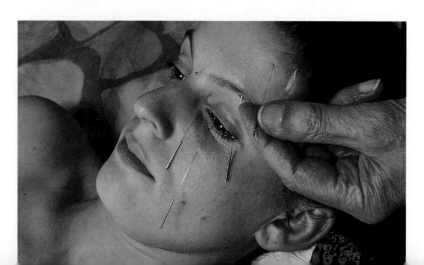

▼ **Acupuncture relief** Needles are inserted into points that correspond to a network of energy channels. According to traditional Chinese philosophy, the placing of the needles may assist the flow of energy and so cure the headache.

Head and injuries

Any injury to the head must be treated with great caution: it may be more serious than it at first appears. Even a minor blow can carry the risk of skull fracture or internal bleeding.

The head houses the brain, the control centre of the body, so any injury has the potential for serious and far-reaching complications. Head injuries may involve skull fracture or direct damage to the brain. There may be bleeding inside the skull, increased pressure in the brain, and fits or breathing difficulties.

Children are especially vulnerable to head injuries because they are more active and tend to be less coordinated than adults. They may also have poor judgement of speed and distance, requiring constant supervision in many activities.

The most serious cases of head injury result in **coma**, brain damage or death. Anyone who has been unconscious after a head injury, however briefly, should be assessed in a hospital.

UNCONSCIOUSNESS

People who become unconscious after head injuries may temporarily lose the normal reflexes that would prompt them to cough or turn over if something blocked their airways. There is a risk that they could inhale their own tongues or vomit and suffocate.

If someone is unconscious after a head injury, and you suspect a neck or back injury, do not move them. Otherwise place the person in the recovery position and call an ambulance. If the injured person regains consciousness, maintain close observation, but do not give the person anything to eat or drink (see also **First aid**).

CONCUSSION

Concussion is a temporary disruption of brain function due to a head injury. It occurs because the brain is a soft organ inside a hard case and has been 'wobbled' or shaken up by the blow

Mapping the brain

Brain injuries result in very different types of problems depending on the part of the brain affected, as indicated on this MRI image of a healthy brain.

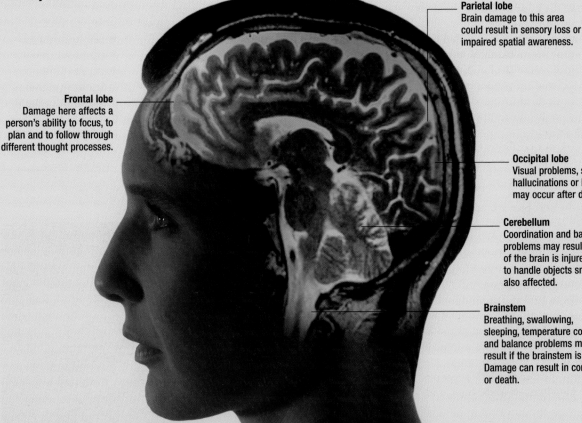

Parietal lobe
Brain damage to this area could result in sensory loss or impaired spatial awareness.

Frontal lobe
Damage here affects a person's ability to focus, to plan and to follow through different thought processes.

Occipital lobe
Visual problems, such as hallucinations or blindess, may occur after damage here.

Cerebellum
Coordination and balance problems may result if this part of the brain is injured. The ability to handle objects smoothly is also affected.

Brainstem
Breathing, swallowing, sleeping, temperature control and balance problems may all result if the brainstem is injured. Damage can result in coma or death.

itself and by the aftershocks of acceleration and deceleration forces within the skull. Concussion can also occur from a jolt or jar passing through the body – for example, after a fall from a height onto the feet, or a punch to the jaw.

Concussion almost always causes temporary unconsciousness, although it can be very brief. As well as headache, vomiting and confusion as the person comes round, it often also causes **amnesia** (loss of memory) relating to events leading up to, during or immediately after the accident.

Symptoms usually subside within a few days, with complete recovery, but mental symptoms, such as disorientation and forgetfulness, can persist for months after a head injury. Other long-term symptoms include headaches and giddiness.

SCANS AND TESTS IN HOSPITAL
Hospital doctors may use any of the following to establish the extent of the damage:
■ tests to assess consciousness and mental function and capability;
■ X-rays to look for fractures;
■ examination of the back of the eye (there may be haemorrhage in the retina after a head injury);
■ examination of any fluid leaking from the ears or nose to check whether it is cerebrospinal fluid, the liquid cushioning the brain and spinal cord;
■ a CT scan, which shows a cross-section of tissues of the brain, used to examine blood clots, bleeding, skull fractures and some brain tumours;
■ magnetic resonance imaging (MRI) to detect damage to the brain and soft tissues of the head;
■ an **EEG** (electroencephalogram) to measure the electrical activity of the brain. It is used if there is a suspicion of epilepsy after head injuries;
■ tests to measure blood flow and pressure within the brain.

TREATMENT
Even if there are no obvious complications, doctors may wish to observe someone overnight after a head injury. Severe head injuries may need intensive care, particularly if there is prolonged coma or raised pressure in the brain. Some patients need help with breathing. Drugs may be used to reduce pressure in the brain or to stop fits, and sometimes emergency surgery will be needed to deal with bleeding or haematoma.

Common head injuries
Severe head injuries may involve internal damage to the brain, fracture of the skull, or bleeding inside the skull. Bleeding from the scalp may also indicate a serious problem.

INTERNAL INJURIES TO THE BRAIN
Any blow to the head that results in a scalp wound or bruise can be severe enough to cause a skull fracture. Also, any head injury, with or without a fracture, can cause internal bruising, shearing of blood vessels or formation of a **haematoma** in the brain, as well as direct brain injury. Be particularly suspicious if there are signs of any loss of consciousness, such as a gap in the person's memory of the event – and bear in mind that loss of consciousness may have been so brief that the injured person may not be aware of it.

Skull fracture
The bones of the skull can be broken without there being any external signs of injury, and a fracture does not necessarily cause a person to become unconscious. Signs of a possible fracture include bleeding or leakage of clear fluid from the nose or ears, bleeding from the scalp, bloodshot eyes and bruising around the eyelids. If broken bones are visible through a wound, the injured person must get to hospital urgently. If you suspect a skull fracture, follow these guidelines:
■ Place an injured person who is unconscious in the recovery position.
■ Help an injured person who is conscious to sit in a reclining position, with the head and shoulders supported.
■ Call an ambulance.
■ If there is bleeding from the ear, cover with a sterile dressing held in place with a loop of bandage around the head. Don't put anything inside the ear.

Bleeding inside the skull
Blood vessels running between the membranes surrounding the brain can be torn by the movements involved in head injury. The thick, outer membrane (one of three) is called the dura, and vessels running beneath this are the most likely to be torn, leading to bleeding known as a subdural **haemorrhage**. In some cases, a minor head injury can produce a small subdural haemorrhage that continues to leak slowly over the following weeks or months, gradually producing a swelling called a subdural haematoma. Sometimes a haematoma may form outside the dura (extradural haematoma), and sometimes within the brain itself (intracerebral haematoma). Symptoms include gradually increasing headache, drowsiness and confusion, sometimes with limb weakness or speech difficulty. The swelling can press on the brain, damage important control centres within it, or raise the pressure within the skull as a whole. It requires urgent surgical treatment.

A chronic subdural haematoma can be very dangerous, because by the time symptoms appear the person may have completely forgotten about a minor blow to the head weeks earlier, and the symptoms may not be sufficiently specific to alert doctors to the true cause of the injury.

Signs of a head injury

Close observation of the injured person is very important, especially in young children. It can provide vital clues that may help a doctor or nurse with making a diagnosis and giving appropriate treatment, when the patient is taken to hospital.

Pressure inside the skull

If a head injury has caused internal bleeding, a depressed skull fracture (where a part of the bony plate is actually pressing down on the brain inside the skull) or swelling of the brain there is a risk that the pressure inside the skull will increase – a highly dangerous complication. If you notice any of following warning signs, seek urgent medical attention:

- falling level of consciousness, especially after a period of apparent improvement;
- shallow, noisy breathing;
- pupils appear unequal in size or both are very large and fail to constrict when light (such as a torch) is shone into them;
- slow pulse;
- weakness or paralysis on one side of the body.

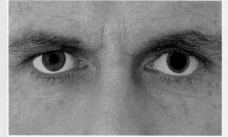

► **Eye warning**
Differing pupil size after a head injury may be caused by bleeding inside the skull or a brain tumour.

Delayed warning signs

Some head injuries show no serious signs for hours, days or even weeks after the injury. Always seek medical attention immediately if any of the following symptoms occur, especially any period of unconsciousness, after a blow or injury to the head:

- recovery from unconsciousness followed by a lapse into unconsciousness again;
- unconsciousness, however brief;
- loss of memory;
- headaches;
- confusion;
- nausea or vomiting;
- bleeding or leakage of clear fluid from the nose or ears – a sign of possible skull fracture.

Suspected neck injury

If a head injury includes damage to the bones of the neck, there is danger that any movement could damage the spinal cord, possibly leading to permanent paralysis. A neck injury may have occurred if the injured person reports neck or back pain, tingling or pins and needles in the hands or feet, or inability to feel or move any limb that has no obvious fracture. Take the following precautions:

- don't move the injured person unless there is an immediate threat to life, such as a fire risk;
- don't put the person in the recovery position;
- don't remove any safety headgear the person may have on unless you absolutely must – for example, to carry out mouth-to-mouth resuscitation;
- keep the person very still, steady the head with hands or padding, and await help;
- clear the mouth of any obstructions with your fingers and check the airway;
- if the injured person stops breathing, you will have to carry out resuscitation or the person will die. Do so as gently as possible and avoid moving the head sideways (see First aid).

Bleeding from the scalp

The scalp is well supplied with blood vessels and tends to bleed profusely, often seeming far worse than it really is. Nevertheless, bleeding is no guide to the severity of any underlying injury. As well as haemorrhage, blows to the scalp can lead to severe bruising or the formation of a haematoma on the scalp. If there is any loss of consciousness or signs of a more serious head injury seek immediate medical attention. Bleeding from the scalp should be treated as follows.

- Press the wound edges together with clean thumbs until the bleeding stops.
- Apply a large sterile dressing and secure it with a bandage or clean strip of material.
- Sit the person down and support his or her head and shoulders.

If bleeding persists seek medical advice.

PREVENTION

Many accidents are preventable. A few simple precautions could considerably reduce the risks.
- Supervise small children at play, especially on hard surfaces such as tarmac. If possible, choose a playground with a soft or protected surface such as rubber sheeting or wood chips.
- Ensure that children always wear a safety helmet when cycling or taking part in activities such as ice-skating or horse-riding.
- Ensure that stairs are well-lit and stair carpets well-fitting and secure.
- Have a handrail firmly fitted to staircases.
- Use a rubber mat in the bath or shower
- Secure rugs in place and watch for loose or broken floor coverings.

SEE ALSO *Brain and nervous system; Confusion; FIRST AID; Headache*

Healing

The body incorporates a remarkable system of self-repair, capable of dealing with most of the injuries and illnesses to which people are exposed during the course of their lifetimes.

The body is equipped to contain damage that occurs to it by stopping blood flow and preventing the spread of germs from one part of the body to another. It can also carry out longer-term repairs by such methods as replacing lost tissue. Many successful techniques of both orthodox and complementary medicine stimulate the body's capacity to heal itself. The treatment of a routine fracture, for example, aims to align the severed pieces of bone and keep them in a stable position while the body performs the task of reuniting the broken ends.

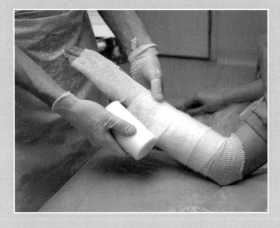

► Promoting healing
A doctor prepares a broken arm to take a plaster cast. This will keep the arm immobilized while the broken bone heals in the correct position.

THE FOUR STAGES OF HEALING
Traumas to the body, such as wounds, **burns** and **fractures**, cause damage in different ways. But the body's response often follows a similar pattern for both internal and external injuries, as in the example of a deep cut or wound.

Inflammation
The body's immediate response to injury is to open up the blood vessels in order to speed blood flow – and the body's defences – to the damaged area. Vessel walls become more permeable, allowing extra fluid and cells to pass through; a massive outflow of white blood cells pours from the blood into the tissues. This increased blood flow may also create a range of unpleasant but temporary symptoms, including:
- heat, from increased circulation;
- redness, caused by red blood cells passing into the tissues;
- swelling, caused by increased volume of fluid;
- pain, caused by the tension of extra volume within the tissues.

Clot or crust formation
After ten minutes or more, depending on the severity of the damage, blood starts to clot, sealing the edges of the wound together. The clotting also prevents excessive loss of blood.

Removal of dead tissue
The white blood cells then start the process of engulfing germs, dead cells and foreign material, clearing the site of all debris. Chemicals released by the injured cells further stimulate blood flow and draw more white blood cells to the site. Lymph vessels widen, ready to carry away fluid and cellular debris from the site of the injury. Dead white blood cells, full of ingested bacteria and debris, are removed by the **lymphatic system** or released as pus.

Repair and replacement
In the ensuing days, connective tissue grows to form a replacement skin surface. If the skin is badly damaged, permanent scar tissue may form at the site of the injury.

THE ROLE OF THE IMMUNE SYSTEM
The white blood cells not only engulf cellular debris and clear an injury site ready for self-repair with new tissue, but also produce antibodies, which help the body to fight infection.

The body is best at healing itself when the person is in an overall healthy state; a depressed immune system lowers a person's ability to deal with infection as well as impairing the body's healing ability.

Fever: a useful weapon
Most of the body's healing reactions affect only the immediate site of the injury. But if trauma is sufficiently severe, and especially if the injured area has become infected, a whole body response may also follow, including fever, a high pulse and distinct feelings of being unwell. Having a raised temperature makes us feel pretty miserable and is a key sign of illness, but a hot body is also a less hospitable place for invading micro-organisms. This temporary re-setting of the body's internal 'thermostat' is thought to be part of the body's protective mechanism, helping to fight infection and promote self-healing.

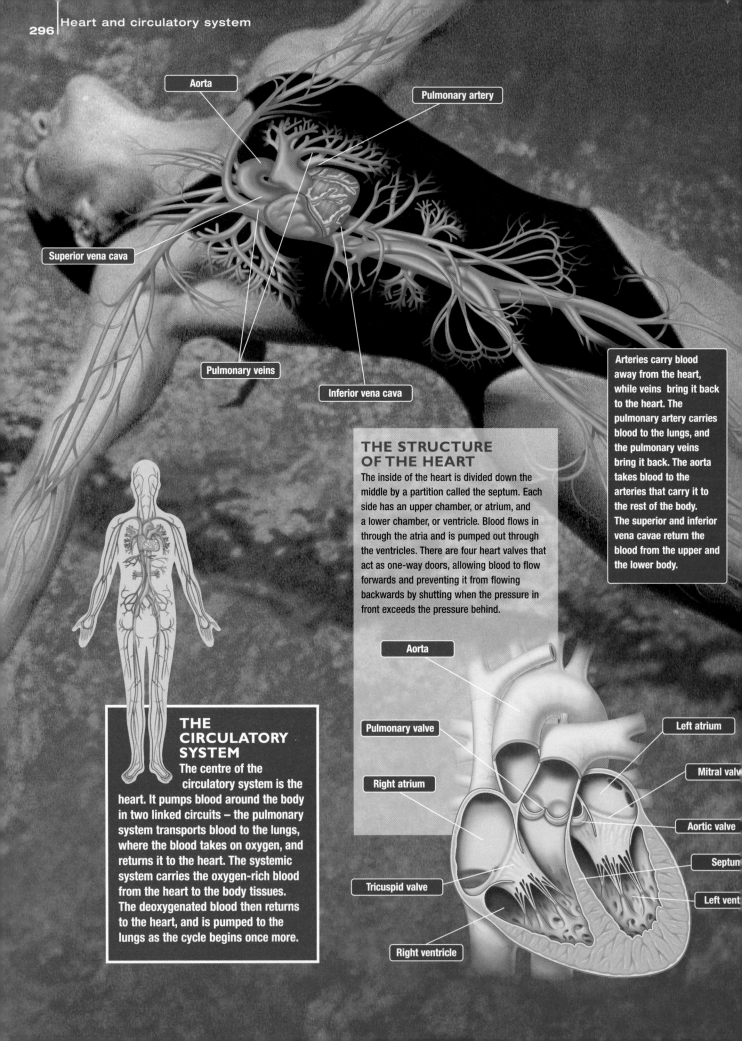

Aorta

Pulmonary artery

Superior vena cava

Pulmonary veins

Inferior vena cava

Arteries carry blood away from the heart, while veins bring it back to the heart. The pulmonary artery carries blood to the lungs, and the pulmonary veins bring it back. The aorta takes blood to the arteries that carry it to the rest of the body. The superior and inferior vena cavae return the blood from the upper and the lower body.

THE STRUCTURE OF THE HEART

The inside of the heart is divided down the middle by a partition called the septum. Each side has an upper chamber, or atrium, and a lower chamber, or ventricle. Blood flows in through the atria and is pumped out through the ventricles. There are four heart valves that act as one-way doors, allowing blood to flow forwards and preventing it from flowing backwards by shutting when the pressure in front exceeds the pressure behind.

Aorta

Pulmonary valve

Right atrium

Left atrium

Mitral valve

Aortic valve

Septum

Tricuspid valve

Left vent[ricle]

Right ventricle

THE CIRCULATORY SYSTEM

The centre of the circulatory system is the heart. It pumps blood around the body in two linked circuits – the pulmonary system transports blood to the lungs, where the blood takes on oxygen, and returns it to the heart. The systemic system carries the oxygen-rich blood from the heart to the body tissues. The deoxygenated blood then returns to the heart, and is pumped to the lungs as the cycle begins once more.

INSIDE A CAPILLARY

Oxygen and other nutrients pass from the blood through the permeable walls of capillaries to the body tissue. Waste products pass in the other direction, from the tissue to the blood, which returns through the system of small veins, or venules, to the circulation. Oxygen is carried by red blood cells attached to a protein called haemoglobin. Oxygenated blood is bright red, but turns a dusky blue when the oxygen is removed.

Red blood cell

White blood cell

Capillary wall

Heart and circulatory system

The muscular pump of the heart is the engine of the circulatory system, which delivers oxygen and nutrients, contained in blood, through the arteries to every cell in the body. The system also collects carbon dioxide and waste products, taking them through the veins to the lungs, liver and kidneys for excretion.

The large arteries that leave the heart branch first into smaller arteries, known as arterioles, and then into a set of very fine, thin-walled vessels called capillaries. Gases and chemicals are exchanged between the blood in the capillaries and the tissue fluid outside the capillaries. The blood then enters small veins, or venules, and begins its return flow to the heart via the network of veins. Most of the fluid and waste products of cell metabolism are picked up by the capillaries and venules, but about 10 per cent (2–4 litres/3.5–7 pints a day) is collected by a parallel system of tubes called the lymphatic system. The heart has its own blood supply delivered via the coronary arteries, which branch off the aorta, and is surrounded by a protective double-walled sac, called the pericardium. The heart's muscles gradually become less powerful with age.

How the heart works

Electrical impulses emitted by a specialized node in the heart regulate the pumping action that sends blood around the body.

The normal resting heart rate of a newborn baby is 120 beats per minute. By adulthood the rate has slowed to between 60 and 100 beats per minute.

A heartbeat is a set of contractions of cardiac muscle during which blood enters from veins, moves through the heart and is pumped out into arteries. One complete set of nerve signals and the muscle contractions they produce in the heart are known as a cardiac cycle (see box, below).

Electrical signals released by the sinoatrial node in the heart's upper right atrium regulate the heartbeat. These signals spread through the cardiac muscle in one big wave, forcing the heart to contract in a coordinated fashion. The cardiac muscle then recovers its normal electrical charge and relaxes, ready for another heartbeat. This happens very quickly, so that the heart can beat regularly, even at very fast speeds.

The sinoatrial node receives signals from the rest of the body, which tell it to speed up or slow down according to whether the body is resting or exercising. The sinoatrial node is also sensitive to hormones such as adrenaline (released by the body when you feel afraid) and to stimulants such as nicotine, alcohol, caffeine and amphetamines.

The atria and ventricles are made of muscle called myocardium, which is capable of working without ceasing. At an average of 72 beats per minute, the heart beats 4320 times an hour, 103,680 times a day and 37,843,200 times a year. By the age of 70, you will have had more than 2.5 billion heartbeats. The muscle on the heart's left side, which sends blood to the body, is three times thicker than it is on the right side, which sends blood to the lungs.

MEASURING THE HEARTBEAT

You can feel your heartbeat, usually about 2.5cm (1in) below the left nipple. Alternatively a doctor or nurse can listen to it using a stethoscope to amplify the sounds of the heart valves closing. The mitral and tricuspid valves produce the first heart sound – 'lub'; the aortic and pulmonary valves close more forcefully, producing the second sound –'dup'. A rapid heartbeat may be due to exercise, excitement, fear, fever, stimulants, heart disease or other illness.

Each heartbeat propels blood down the arteries, and this pressure wave can be felt at pulse points, where arteries lie just beneath the skin. You can feel the pulse at the wrist – with your palm facing you, put two fingers on the thumb side, between the wrist creases and where you might have a

Factfile

The cardiac cycle

The cardiac cycle has two main phases. In the first, known as diastole, the heart receives blood into the atria. In the second, known as systole, the heart pushes blood from the atria, through the ventricles and into the arteries.

1 Diastole. The heart is relaxed as blood flows in from the lungs and body. The incoming blood flows into the right and left atria.

2 Atrial systole. An electrical impulse from the sinoatrial node at the top of the right atrium makes both atria contract, pushing the blood through the mitral and tricuspid valves into the ventricles.

3 Ventricular systole. When the electrical impulse reaches the bottom of the right atrium, it activates the atrioventricular node, sending the electrical impulse through into the walls of the ventricles. This makes the ventricles contract and pump blood into the pulmonary artery and the aorta. The mitral valve and the tricuspid valves are closed, so blood cannot flow back into the atria.

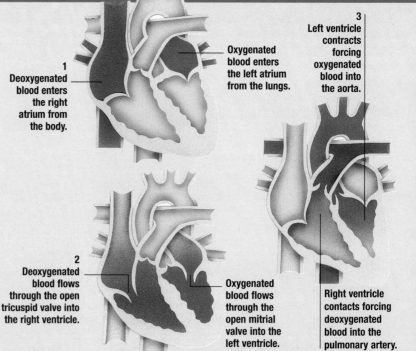

1 Deoxygenated blood enters the right atrium from the body.

2 Deoxygenated blood flows through the open tricuspid valve into the right ventricle.

Oxygenated blood enters the left atrium from the lungs.

Oxygenated blood flows through the open mitral valve into the left ventricle.

3 Left ventricle contracts forcing oxygenated blood into the aorta.

Right ventricle contacts forcing deoxygenated blood into the pulmonary artery.

watch strap. This is the radial artery. You can also feel the pulse at the elbow crease – with your arm straight and your palm facing upwards, the brachial artery pulse can be felt on the side nearest the body. Blood pressure is usually measured here.

A third place where the pulse can be felt is in the neck, beneath the angle of the jaw – never press both sides at once, as you risk tricking pressure receptors there into signalling to the brain that blood pressure is excessively high. This causes the heart to slow down, which can make you faint.

BLOOD PRESSURE
Blood in the arteries is under constant pressure. When the left ventricle of the heart pumps blood out into the aorta, pressure in the arteries reaches a maximum. This is called the systolic blood pressure. When the heart relaxes, the arterial pressure falls to a minimum. This is the diastolic pressure. Blood pressure can be measured using a device called a sphygmomanometer and is expressed as millimeters of mercury (mmHg). A reading of 120/80 – the average for a fit young person – means a systolic pressure of 120mmHg and diastolic pressure of 80mmHg. Disease, drugs and a person's emotional state can all affect blood pressure. There is no such thing as a 'normal' blood pressure, but people with higher than average blood pressure levels are described as suffering from hypertension (see **Blood pressure and problems**) and are more at risk of heart disease, stroke and other health problems.

Heart investigations

Treatment of heart and circulatory problems is greatly improved by a range of tests that can establish the cause of symptoms by producing clear images of the heart or recording its activity.

Electrocardiogram (ECG)
The electrocardiogram measures electrical conduction in the heart. Electrically sensitive patches are attached to the wrists and ankles and at six points across the chest. Twelve traces are produced, which provide clues to the rhythm, shape and health of the heart muscle and the conduction system.

Exercise tolerance (stress) test
Using a treadmill or exercise bike while an ECG is recorded shows how well the heart can cope with exertion. It may reveal an oxygen shortage (ischaemia) or irregular heartbeats (arrhythmias), which do not show up on an ordinary ECG. This helps in diagnosing angina or deciding if a patient needs coronary artery surgery.

The resistance and speed of the machine is gradually increased until the heart rate reaches a maximum, blood pressure falls, there is a marked change in the ECG reading or the person experiences chest pain or asks to stop. Blood pressure is also recorded. There is a slight risk of cardiac arrest – 1 in 10,000 – during this test.

Ambulatory ECG recording
When arrhythmias are thought to be the cause of a person's dizziness, faints or palpitations, he or she wears a small portable box that records the heart rate. The ECG is either recorded continuously for a 24-hour period or the person can trigger the ECG when he or she notices symptoms (event-recording).

Chest X-ray
An X-ray of the chest reveals the size and shape of the heart and may show signs of heart failure, or indicate non-cardiac causes of breathlessness and chest pain.

Echocardiogram (ECHO)
Ultrasound pictures of the heart can reveal the shape and thickness of heart structures such as the atria and ventricles, the heart valves and the aorta. Digitally produced false-colour pictures demonstrate muscle contraction, valve function and the direction and speed of blood flow. ECHO is used to investigate breathlessness, heart murmurs and heart failure. If you are related to someone who has **cardiomyopathy**, your doctor may suggest that an echocardiogram is carried out as a precaution.

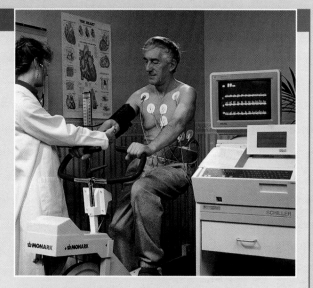

Coronary angiography
This detects coronary artery blockages that are suitable for surgical treatment. Dye is injected through a catheter inserted into an artery in the groin or arm. Coronary artery blood flow is monitored using an X-ray camera.

Radio-isotope scan
These are only used if ECHO and exercise-testing are inconclusive. Heart muscle function is monitored during an exercise test following an injection of radioactive thallium.

Magnetic resonance imaging
For magnetic resonance imaging, the entire body is placed in a special scanner. MRI gives a detailed scan that can reveal abnormalities in the functioning of the heart.

▲ **Heart tests**
A heart patient takes an exercise tolerance test. He is wearing electrodes that record the electrical impulses which precede the contractions of his heart and produce a reading on the screen (right). He pedals an exercise bicycle and the readings show how well his heart can cope with the exercise. His blood pressure is taken at the same time.

What can go wrong

Any disease or physical change that interferes with blood flow or the regularity of the heartbeat will have serious consequences.

An athlete's heart rate can be as low as 40 beats per minute. But in an unfit person a slow pulse may be a sign of heart disease, or an of an underactive thyroid, or of hypothermia or the effect of taking drugs.

The most common problems of the heart and circulatory system are caused by atheroma – degenerative changes in the walls of the arteries that restrict the flow of blood. If atheroma occurs in the heart or brain, causing a complete blockage of blood flow, it can lead to a heart attack or **stroke**. Even when the blockage is only partial, it can lead to **angina**, dizziness, disturbance of vision and collapse. Severe atheroma in the leg arteries may reduce the circulation to such an extent that **gangrene** develops in the feet.

Other problems are caused by degeneration or disease of the heart itself. The heart valves can become infected by bacteria and viruses in the bloodstream, leading to obstruction of blood flow. In some conditions, the mechanism controlling the heart's rhythm may be disturbed and the heart may beat very fast or irregularly. This may be due to a congenital abnormality or, in adults, to a deterioration in the nerves controlling the heartbeat. General diseases and infections can also affect the heart muscle.

HEART ATTACK
If part of the heart has its blood supply cut off, the affected cells die and the person has a myocardial infarction due to a coronary thrombosis, what is commonly referred to as a heart attack. More than 800 people have heart attacks in the UK every day, resulting in 300 deaths each day.

The commonest cause is coronary heart disease, leading to narrowing of sections of coronary artery. One of these sections can then suddenly become completely blocked by a blood clot or by a ruptured plaque (a fatty deposit that develops on the inner wall of an artery). Sometimes a heart attack occurs during another illness.

Heart attacks produce severe crushing pain in the centre of the chest, sometimes spreading to the arms or jaw, with breathlessness, faintness and profuse sweating. Sometimes heart attacks cause no symptoms, or produce pain elsewhere in the chest or abdomen. The heart pumps less effectively, and may beat too fast, too slowly or irregularly, as in the case of a heart block or an arrhythmia (see page 310).

If you or someone with you appears to be suffering a heart attack, dial 999 at once. Three out of ten sufferers die before they reach hospital,

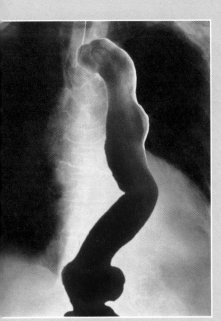

▲ **Aneurysm**
An angiogram shows two swellings in a person's aorta caused by weakness in the vessel wall. They can be symptomless, but are a risk – they can rupture, causing a haemorrhage.

and prompt treatment can save lives. Paramedics usually give 300mg aspirin to help prevent the formation of blood clots, oxygen and glyceryl trinitrate spray. Advanced life support (see page 302) will be needed if the heart stops. In hospital, an electrocardiogram (ECG) and blood tests usually confirm the diagnosis, and a 'clot-busting' drug such as streptokinase or alteplase is usually given as soon as possible. The heart is monitored for any signs of complications, such as irregular heartbeats or **heart failure**, and is treated with drugs. Very rarely, surgery is needed.

A hospital stay of around seven days is followed by cardiac rehabilitation, which consists of advice on lifestyle (see What can I do to reduce the risk?, below) and graded exercise. Lifelong treatment with drugs may be necessary in some cases.

Who is at risk of a heart attack?
You are more likely to have a heart attack if you have a family history of angina or heart attack, especially occurring before the age of 60 years, raised blood **cholesterol** or raised **blood pressure**. **Stress** appears to be bad for your heart and circulatory system in the long term. If you smoke, take very little exercise and are obese, you put yourself at risk of developing problems with your heart and circulatory system. People with **diabetes** are three times more likely than others to develop coronary heart disease.

Your gender is also significant – being a man aged under 50 years increases the statistical risk, although after the **menopause**, women quickly catch up and are twice as likely to die of heart or circulatory diseases than of cancer.

In the UK, death rates for coronary heart disease are highest in Scotland, Northern Ireland and Northern England, and 50 per cent higher in people of Indian, Pakistani, Bangladeshi or Sri Lankan origin than in other UK citizens. Rates are falling, but not as fast as in Canada, Finland, Sweden and Australia. Japan has the lowest death rates from coronary heart disease in the world.

What can I do to reduce the risk?
Coronary heart disease takes years to develop, and although family history cannot be changed, other risk factors can be reduced by changes to your lifestyle. Do not smoke. If you drink alcohol, keep within safe limits (see **Alcohol and abuse**). Follow a balanced diet and maintain a healthy weight, with a body mass index of 25 or under. Take regular exercise.

Reduce your stress levels – try to avoid stressful activities or consider using relaxation techniques, yoga or reflexology. Keep your blood pressure at a healthy level – have it checked every five years to the age of 65 years, thereafter it should be checked annually.

HEART BLOCK

A heart block is a complete or partial block at one of the places in the heart muscle where the electrical impulses occur that keep the pumping system of the heart working at a regular speed. The block causes the atria and ventricles to act independently of each other – the two main pumping chambers, the ventricles, pulse at a much slower rate than usual. Heart block is usually a sign of underlying heart disease and often develops after a heart attack. Partial blocks may not affect the heart's pumping rate and therefore cause few symptoms. The condition is then discovered only during an ECG.

If occasional beats (ventricular contractions) are missed (dropped), the patient may be aware of the irregularity. With more severe blocks, the circulation to the brain is reduced. This can cause dizziness, disturbance of behaviour and in some cases fainting and a small fit. All types of block reduce the usual performance of the heart and may result in chest pain, breathlessness and ankle swelling. The treatment for this condition consists of drugs to improve conduction, or a **pacemaker**, which takes over control of the ventricles from the sinoatrial node.

HEART DAMAGE

The heart can be damaged in a number of ways. Severe injury, electrocution or a heart attack can lead to cardiac arrest. A massive blow to the heart area – for example, in a road accident – may tear the coronary arteries or heart valves. Stab wounds to the chest may penetrate the pericardium or heart, so that blood pumps straight into the chest, or into the pericardium, compressing the heart.

HEART FAILURE

Heart failure affects one in ten people over the age of 65. The heart can be weakened by disease or overwork. The condition causes breathlessness on exertion, in bed or eventually at rest, coughing or wheezing, ankle swelling (**oedema**) and tiredness. Blood tests, ECG's and echocardiogram are used to the assess the severity of the failure. Additional tests may reveal the underlying cause.

Treatment is with drugs, but diet, exercise, stopping smoking and reducing alcohol intake are also important. Treating the cause may help significantly, but if heart failure is already very severe, prospects of improvement are limited. Heart transplantation is sometimes possible (see **Heart surgery; Transplants**).

ARRHYTHMIA

Arrhythmia means literally 'no heart rhythm', but the term is used to mean an abnormal heart rhythm. Occasional extra heartbeats, known as extrasystoles, commonly occur in normal hearts. The extra beat may not be felt, but there may be a slightly longer gap before the next heartbeat, allowing the heart to fill up more than usual, so the next heartbeat produces a detectable 'thump'. This type of arrhythmia has no effect on general health, but some types are more serious and can lead to shortness of breath, fainting or dizzy spells. They have major health implications.

If you have arrhythmia, your doctor will investigate it using an ECG or ambulatory ECG recording (see Heart investigations, page 299). If it is serious, the arrhythmia can be monitored and treated. In tachycardia, the heart feels as if it is racing; the condition is defined as a rate of

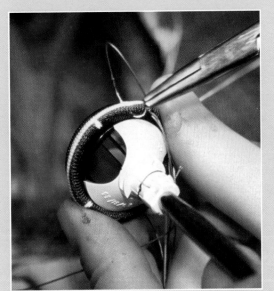

◀ **New valve**
If one of the heart's four valves becomes narrowed or begins to leak, surgery may be necessary to replace it. This valve has a soft fabric ring, which the surgeon is preparing to stitch into a patient's heart tissue.

more than 100 beats per minute, but rates of 160 beats per minute are not unusual. An ECG may show that the atria are contracting too rapidly. This can be caused by overstimulation by adrenaline, smoking, caffeine or an overactive **thyroid**. If an ECG shows rapid but weak contractions of the ventricles, at speeds of up to 200 beats per minute (ventricular tachycardia), the condition is far more serious. In such cases, treatment aimed at preventing heart failure is necessary.

PERICARDITIS

The double-layered protective sac that surrounds the heart – the pericardium – may become inflamed by infection with viruses, bacteria or **tuberculosis**, rheumatoid arthritis or after a heart attack. This produces a sharp pain that hurts more when you are breathing or lying flat. The

OTHER DISORDERS

Aneurysm

An aneurysm is a local swelling of an artery. It can develop if the artery is diseased or weakened, especially where the blood pressure is high. Aneurysms most commonly affect the aorta.

Angina pectoris

In angina, attacks of choking or throttling pain strike the upper part of the chest. They are due to a reduction in the blood flow through the coronary arteries that supply the heart muscle. Angina is usually brought on by exertion and relieved by rest.

Atrial fibrillation and flutter

Fibrillation is the term used for an irregular beating of the heart, and flutter is the term for a disturbance of the normal heart rhythm.

Stroke

A stroke is a sudden loss of function on one side of the body. Strokes are caused by an interruption in the blood supply to part of the brain. They are uncommon before the age of 50, but after that they become increasingly common with age.

condition, known as pericarditis, is controlled with anti-inflammatory drugs and treatment of the underlying cause.

The pericardium may fill up with fluid (pericardial effusion), or with blood leaking from a heart attack, **aneurysm** or heart trauma. The heart is compressed, producing breathlessness. Severe compression results in cardiac tamponade, a life-threatening emergency.

PROBLEMS WITH THE HEART VALVES

Disorders of the four valves of the heart – the tricuspid, mitrial, pulmonary and aortic valves – undermine their ability to control blood flow by acting as one-way valves. In mitral stenosis, the mitral valve narrows so the heart has to work harder to force blood from the left atrium into the left ventricle. In mitral incompetence, the mitrial valve leaks backwards, so blood has to be repumped. Both conditions strain the heart, and may lead to **atrial fibrillation**, blocked blood vessels, heart failure, or infections of the lining of the heart cavity (**endocarditis**). Symptoms include breathlessness and palpitations. A characteristic red flush may appear on the cheeks.

Rheumatic fever and **congenital disorders** of the heart are common causes of problems with the heart valves (see **Aorta and problems**).

Heart murmur

A heart murmur can be heard using a stethoscope when blood flow through the heart or a heart valve is slightly turbulent. It may be normal – the tricuspid valve is often slightly noisy in young people – or be a sign of a narrow or leaky heart valve, a narrowed artery or a hole in the heart.

CONGENITAL HEART DISEASE

Around one child in 100 worldwide is born with a structural abnormality of the heart. Some are slight and have no effect on day-to-day living, while others may be too serious for the child to live a normal life. In-between, there are many different abnormalities, which vary widely in their degree of severity.

Small abnormalities may sometimes become infected. Large abnormalities may interfere with the efficient pumping of the heart and cause progressive shortness of breath and heart failure. Contact your doctor if your child's skin turns blue when resting, crying or taking exercise, or if your child feels extremely tired or is failing to thrive. Your doctor may send the child for an ECG or X-rays, or for tests in a special heart unit. In some cases a heart operation will be necessary.

Holes in the heart

Holes may form during the folding and dividing that occurs as the heart develops. They are the most common congenital heart abnormality, and usually occur in the walls between the two atria

or ventricles. They may close naturally as the child grows, but corrective surgery is often necessary. (See **Congenital disorders**).

ENLARGED HEART

An enlarged heart is a sign of heart disease, except in athletes who have well-developed heart muscles. It is found in heart failure, valvular disease, aortic problems, raised blood pressure and heart muscle disorders (**cardiomyopathy**).

LIFE-SUPPORT TECHNIQUES

In the event of a cardiac arrest, basic life support in the form of cardiopulmonary resuscitation can maintain breathing and circulation with the kiss-of-life and external **cardiac massage** until skilled help arrives. (See also First aid.)

In advanced life support, an oxygen tube is passed down into the windpipe, and an ECG is taken to determine whether the heart is beating rapidly or chaotically (ventricular fibrillation) or has stopped beating altogether (asystole).

Ventricular fibrillation can be successfully treated by using electric shock treatment (cardioversion). An electric shock of between 200 and 400 joules, applied via special pads on the chest wall, may be able to jerk the heart back into a normal rhythm. Several shocks may be tried, alternating with cardiopulmonary resuscitation. Automatic defibrillators are now installed in many public venues, enabling trained members of staff to carry out ventricular fibrillation right there and then. If the heart has stopped beating, drugs may be fed directly into the circulation as a measure to restart the heartbeat, but this procedure is not always found to be successful.

Brain death will occur after three minutes without oxygen, so if you are a bystander when someone appears to be suffering a heart attack, act as speedily as possible. Send someone to dial 999 – go yourself if you are alone. Be aware of your own safety. If you are at the scene of a road traffic accident, for example, try to put out a warning light or order to alert any passing vehicles. If you have been trained, check the person's airway, breathing and circulation and carry out basic life support. Stay with the person and keep performing basic life support until the emergency services arrive.

THE FUTURE

Stem cells are the body's raw ingredients and can develop into many different types of organs. Transplanted adult stem cells, taken from bone marrow, can mimic the cells of the heart and improve heart function. Gene therapy may one day enable abnormal heart genes to be fixed or replaced with normal genes.

Heartburn

Heartburn is a painful burning sensation felt in the centre of the chest, which sometimes moves up to the throat. It is extremely common, especially in pregnancy – 25 per cent of pregnant women experience it daily, and half have heartburn occasionally. But although it is annoying and unpleasant, it is rarely serious.

CAUSES

Heartburn is caused by gastro-oesophageal reflux, also called acid regurgitation, in which the acidic stomach juices pass backwards into the oesophagus. This happens either because the sphincter of muscle between the oesophagus and stomach is weak or because it relaxes at the wrong time. A number of factors can contribute to this:

- eating large amounts of fried or fatty foods;
- drinking alcohol or coffee;
- eating chocolate or peppermint;
- smoking;
- obesity, because of the extra pressure on the stomach;
- pregnancy, for the same reason;
- constipation;
- lying down or bending over, because of gravity;
- a hiatus **hernia**, because the sphincter cannot work effectively when the upper part of the stomach is displaced.

TREATMENT

Occasional bouts of heartburn can usually be treated successfully by taking over-the-counter antacids and by using preventive measures to reduce the risk of recurrence. But if heartburn lasts for more than three weeks, you should consult a doctor, partly because there are risks associated with the long-term use of antacids. If a hiatus hernia is ruled out, drugs that reduce acid stomach secretions may be prescribed. In the very few cases that these are ineffective, surgery to strengthen the sphincter may be required.

COMPLICATIONS

Complications are rare, but sometimes chronic heartburn can cause oesophagitis, an inflammation of the oesophageal lining, which can lead to the formation of **ulcers** or bleeding. If scar tissue forms following repeated attacks, there is a risk that the gullet will become narrowed (a stricture), impeding swallowing.

PREVENTION

- Stop smoking.
- Lose weight, if necessary.
- Cut down on fatty foods, alcohol and coffee.
- Raise the head end of your bed.

SEE ALSO *Digestive system; Oesophagus and disorders*

Heart failure

In heart failure, the heart continues to beat, but does not function effectively and so is unable to keep the vital organs adequately supplied with fresh blood. Heart failure affects one in ten people over 65 years, and is the most common single cause of death in the UK. Each year, around 100,000 people are admitted to hospital due to heart disease.

SYMPTOMS

Heart failure can develop slowly or suddenly, and can affect the right or left side of the heart, or both. If the right ventricle is failing, blood tends to back up in the veins, raising **blood pressure**. If the left ventricle is failing, excess blood remaining in the heart can back up into the lungs, congesting them with fluid (congestive cardiac failure).

Symptoms can include:
- breathlessness on exertion, on lying flat, during the night, and eventually even at rest;
- coughing or wheezing;
- ankle swelling (**oedema**) due to salt and fluid retention;
- severe tiredness;

CAUSES

- Ischaemic heart disease (a reduction in the supply of blood to the heart as a result of coronary artery disease).
- Hypertension (raised blood pressure in the arteries).
- Valvular heart disease (ineffective or weak heart valves).
- **Myocarditis** (inflammation of the heart muscles) and cardiomyopathy (weakness of the heart muscles), especially in the young.

Drug treatments for heart failure

Depending on the cause of the heart failure, a doctor might prescribe one or more of the following types of drug.

- **Diuretics** ('water tablets' – furosemide, bendrofluazide, bumetanide, spironolactone) enable the kidneys to excrete retained salt and fluid.

- **ACE inhibitors** (angiotensin-converting enzyme inhibitors – enalapril, lisinopril, ramipril, losartan, irbesartan) affect salt and fluid regulation in the kidneys, and greatly improve chances of survival.

- **Beta-blockers** (atenolol, metoprolol) enable the heart to work more efficiently.

- **Nitrates** (glyceryl trinitrate, isosorbide mono/dinitrate) improve exercise capacity and survival.

- **Cardiac glycosides** (digoxin) slow the heart and enable it to fill and contract more effectively.

Oxygen and diuretic, nitrate and morphine injections may be used in severe acute left ventricular failure.

- Cor pulmonale (enlargement of the right ventricle of the heart caused by lung disease).
- Extra demand on the heart caused by anaemia, shock, thyrotoxicosis (excessive thyroid hormone in the bloodstream), blood loss or fluid overload.
- Arrythmias (irregularities in the heartbeat).
- Alcohol and drugs.

TREATMENT

Once the underlying cause of heart failure has been established, treatment may consist of medication, surgery or changes to lifestyle.

When to consult a doctor

Anyone who experiences any of the symptoms listed should seek advice from a doctor.

What a doctor may do

- Carry out blood tests, an ECG (electrocardiogram) and an echocardiogram (using ultrasound) to assess the severity of the heart failure.
- Perform additional tests to identify the underlying cause.
- Advise on lifestyle changes.
- Recommend immunization against **influenza** and **pneumonia**.
- Prescribe medication (see box, page 303).
- Suggest hospital admission for acute left ventricular failure or difficult-to-treat heart failure.
- Arrange exercise training and rehabilitation.
- Advise surgery – valve replacement, insertion of a pacemaker to regulate the heartbeat, a coronary artery bypass or, rarely, heart transplantation (see **Transplants**).

What you can do

- Stop smoking.
- Cut down on alcohol.
- Eat a nutritious diet.
- Exercise within your own limits.

COMPLICATIONS

- Arrythmias.
- **Stroke**, thrombosis and **embolism**.
- Liver abnormalities (see **Liver and disorders**).
- Muscle wasting (see **Muscular system**).
- Susceptibility to influenza, chest infection and pneumonia.

OUTLOOK

Roughly 50 per cent of people with severe heart failure and about 25 per cent of those with mild to moderate heart failure die.

SEE ALSO *Heart and circulatory system*

Heart-lung machine

Also known as a cardiopulmonary bypass, a heart-lung machine enables blood to bypass the heart and lungs during complex heart and lung surgery. The diverted blood is cooled to slow the body's metabolism and oxygen

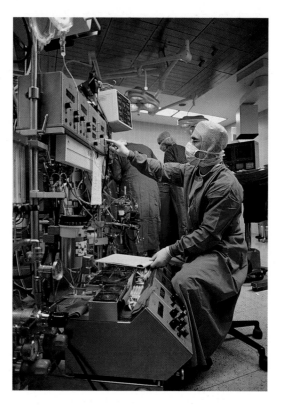

◀ **Critical condition**
A surgeon monitors a heart-lung machine while his colleagues operate in the background; the machine allows the patient's heart and lung functions to be temporarily suspended.

consumption; carbon dioxide is removed and oxygen is replaced. Chemicals to paralyze the heart, reduce energy requirements and prevent blood-clotting are also added. At the end of the operation, the blood is reheated and the heart is restarted.

Use of a heart-lung machine slightly increases the risks associated with open heart surgery, and may cause bleeding, blood clotting and occasionally death. There is also some evidence to suggest that the ventricles work better after surgery if use of a heart-lung machine is avoided.

New surgical techniques have made heart-lung machines unnecessary in some heart operations. However, there are still a large number that would be impossible to perform without them.

SEE ALSO *Heart surgery*

Heart massage

This is a life-saving technique used when the heart has stopped beating effectively – during cardiac arrest, for example. Blood is forced around the circulatory system by producing artificial heart contractions. In external heart massage, the heart is rhythmically compressed between the breastbone and backbone. In internal cardiac massage, the heart is directly massaged by hand.

SEE ALSO *FIRST AID; Heart and circulatory system*

Heart surgery

Some patients with serious heart disorders need surgery or, more rarely, a heart transplant. Modern techniques of heart surgery are quick and efficient and not only prolong life but improve its quality.

The main cause of death in the UK and the USA is heart disease. People whose diet is high in saturated fats and who smoke and lead a sedentary lifestyle are especially at risk.

The arteries that nourish the heart are very tiny, so they are particularly susceptible to blockages, which can lead to a heart attack. These blockages are the result of atherosclerosis – the buildup of fatty deposits within the artery walls.

In some cases, drug treatment, combined with taking regular exercise and a change of diet, might be sufficient to control or halt the progress of the disease. But sometimes you may need surgery to prolong or even save your life. A number of surgical procedures might be performed, including coronary artery bypass, valve replacement and heart **transplant**.

CORONARY ARTERY BYPASS SURGERY

In coronary artery bypass surgery, veins taken from the leg or chest are grafted onto a blocked artery to act as a bypass around the blockage. More than 25,000 such operations take place in the UK each year.

The procedure, sometimes known as coronary artery bypass graft or CABG, is used to treat several conditions. It can save the life of a patient with severe coronary artery disease; it can be used to relieve the suffocating chest pain brought on by exercise in someone who has severe angina, and whose illness cannot be helped with drugs; and it may also be recommended for those at high risk of fatal coronary thrombosis – in which the formation of blood clots in the coronary artery obstructs the flow of blood to the heart.

Cutting edge – new developments in heart surgery

Huge advances have been made in the field of heart surgery, and doctors continue to work towards less invasive forms of treatment.

■ An artificial heart has been successfully used in the USA for people who are unsuitable for heart transplantation. The plastic and titanium heart, called the Abiocar, weighs about 900g (32oz). It is powered by an external battery that has to be recharged every few hours and has no external wires or tubes.

■ Transplanted cells from the patient's own thigh muscles have been shown to improve weakened cardiac muscle function. This technique may become used with other forms of heart surgery.

■ Bone marrow stem cells have been transplanted from a man's pelvis and injected into arteries near his heart. The stem cells then travelled to areas damaged by a heart attack and turned into healthy, functioning heart muscle cells.

■ Further development in gene therapy may eventually replace or prevent the need for some forms of heart surgery.

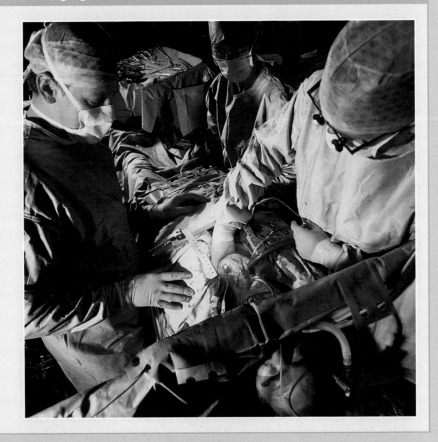

Questions to ask your doctor

Heart surgery is a major operation and you are bound to approach it with some trepidation. Knowing what to expect can be very reassuring.

- What are the general risks of my operation?

- Does my health history put me at risk of failure?

- What are the surgeon's personal results?

- Where does the hospital stand in the national league tables, and what factors may have affected its performance?

- How long is it likely to take to recover and resume normal daily activities?

- Will I need further treatment or medication?

An **X-ray** called a cardioangiogram can show the extent of damage to the coronary arteries and whether surgery will help. If, for instance, only one or two arteries are narrowed, an **angioplasty** may be simpler and safer than bypass surgery. In an angioplasty, a balloon catheter is fed into the artery and expanded to relieve the narrowing.

In conventional bypass surgery, the operation is performed through a 30cm (12in) incision. The heart is stopped with a paralysing solution so that it does not beat during surgery, and blood is piped to a **heart-lung machine**, which supplies oxygen, removes carbon dioxide and cools the blood, lowering the body's oxygen consumption and metabolic rate. The machine then returns the re-oxygenated blood to the body.

The veins to be used for bypassing the blockage or narrowing are surgically removed. These are then sewn on to the artery to bypass the obstruction. The heart-lung machine is then switched off and the heart is restarted.

The patient may spend a day or two in intensive care and, if all goes well, will leave hospital eight days later. Most return to normal activities within eight weeks, although they often need to take aspirin or other blood-thinning drugs for the rest of their lives. Sometimes people need repeat bypass surgery.

It may be possible to perform a less invasive operation, known as minimally invasive bypass surgery. The surgeon makes only a 12.5cm (5in) incision, or several smaller ones, there is no need for a heart-lung machine, and complications are rarer. Recovery time is also reduced: a hospital stay of two or three days and a return to normal after just two weeks. **Keyhole surgery** may eventually become routine for this procedure.

Assessing the risks of bypass surgery

Coronary artery bypass surgery improves **angina** symptoms and the working of the left ventricle, and reduces the risk of death in those with severe heart disease. Survival rates after bypass surgery are very good: 95 per cent of people are alive and well a year after the operation, 88 per cent after 5 years and 75 per cent after 10 years.

Any operation carries a level of risk, and bypass surgery is no different. There is a statistical one in 50 chance that you may die or suffer a post-operative heart attack or **stroke** – although the risk is five times greater in people over 75 than in those under 55. It is difficult to predict an exact risk for any individual; some patients are more vulnerable than others. At greatest risk are people who are having a repeat operation, those with **diabetes**, people with poor functioning of the heart's left ventricle (see **Heart and circulatory system**), people with kidney disease (see **Kidneys and disorders**) and those with peripheral vascular disease (see **Arteries and disorders**).

HEART VALVE REPLACEMENT

A narrowed or leaky heart valve places enormous strain on the heart, which has to work harder to keep the blood flowing forward through the atria and ventricles and into the aorta or pulmonary artery. Heart valves may be damaged from the stresses of long use, may be congenitally abnormal (that is, the condition is present from birth) or damaged as a result of **rheumatic fever**, heart failure or injury. The aortic and mitral valves are most commonly affected. In mitral valve prolapse, the valve flops back towards the left atrium but does not actually leak.

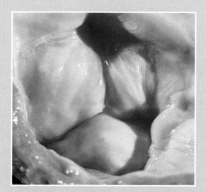

The symptoms of valve disease include palpitations, breathlessness, angina and dizziness. Heart failure may develop later (see **Heart and circulatory system**), and abnormal valves are also vulnerable to germs circulating in the bloodstream that can land on the valve and cause serious damage (see **Endocarditis**).

Only some types of valve may be repaired or replaced. The mitral valve, which controls blood flow from the left atrium to the left ventricle, is the most common. In valve repair, reconstruction of various components of the valve and its supporting structures is carried out through an incision in the chest. Narrowed valves can also be widened using a technique similar to angioplasty. A balloon-tipped catheter is inserted into the valve and inflated to widen the opening.

A valve that cannot be repaired is removed and replaced with an artificial mechanical valve. This is made of synthetic, hard-wearing materials such

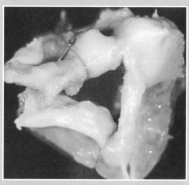

▲ **Valve damage**
The top picture shows a healthy heart valve. The heart valve below has been damaged by rheumatic fever, causing the valve opening to become narrowed.

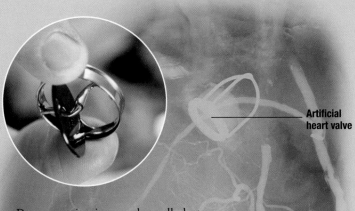

_____ Artificial
heart valve

as Dacron or titanium, and usually lasts a lifetime. It may produce audible clicking noises. Blood-thinning medication (anticoagulants) are used after surgery to prevent blood clots forming.

It is also possible to replace heart valves with transplants from pigs, cows or human donors. Such biological valves can be frozen for later use, allowing donors to be screened for infectious diseases. Occasionally, tissue from the person's own body can be transplanted – for example, the aortic valve can be replaced with the pulmonary valve. Biological valves can deteriorate with time, and may be rejected by the patient. For this reason, such transplants tend to be restricted to people who are older, have bleeding disorders, or cannot take anticoagulants.

▲ **New valve in place**
A mechanical valve made of metal and plastic has been used to replace a heart valve that is malfunctioning.

HEART TRANSPLANT

A heart transplant is a life-saving technique for people whose hearts can no longer pump effectively. It is used in severe heart failure, which is usually due to **coronary artery disease** or in cases of heart muscle weakness (**cardiomyopathy**), and occasionally in cases of congenital heart disease. About 300 heart transplants are performed each year in the UK. More than 50 per cent of heart transplant patients survive for five years or more. Some are still alive over 20 years after their transplant operation.

The biggest risk involved in heart transplant is rejection, which occurs because the body's immune system is programmed to recognize and destroy foreign tissue. Blood and tissue-typing tests are used to find the closest possible match between a donor heart and someone waiting for a transplant. People with transplanted hearts have to take immunosuppressant drugs for the rest of their lives in order to suppress the immune system and so prevent rejection. These drugs can increase the risk of infection.

Heart-lung transplants

Heart-lung transplants are performed in cases of severe disease of the heart and lungs. The recipient is given the donor's heart and lungs together, preserving the heart-lung connections. In some cases the recipient already has a healthy heart, in which case the heart section in the transplant can be given to someone else.

Hepatitis

There are two forms of hepatitis – acute or chronic. Both affect the liver, damaging and destroying liver cells (see **Liver and disorders**).

Acute hepatitis is the more common form. It appears suddenly and usually lasts for one or two months, although it can develop into the chronic form.

Despite the fact that chronic hepatitis is generally more serious, there may be few symptoms. It can be either persistent or active. Chronic persistent hepatitis progresses slowly and may cause little damage, but it sometimes turns into the active form, which can destroy the liver.

SYMPTOMS

The range and severity of symptoms depend on the type of hepatitis involved. In acute hepatitis there may be:
- tiredness;
- fever, with aching muscles and joints;
- nausea, vomiting and a loss of appetite;
- **jaundice**;
- pain in the lower right abdomen;
- **referred pain** in the right shoulder;
- in very serious cases, liver failure and **coma**;

Some forms of hepatitis complicate pregnancy and can be passed on to unborn children.

Chronic persistent hepatitis may cause no symptoms other than fatigue and general malaise. But if it progresses to chronic active hepatitis, **cirrhosis of the liver** may develop and eventually lead to liver failure and death.

CAUSES

The most common cause of hepatitis is a viral infection (see below). However, acute hepatitis can also be caused by:
- long-term alcohol abuse;
- overdose or abuse of certain drugs, such as paracetamol;
- interactions with certain prescribed medicines;
- exposure to certain toxic chemicals, such as dry-cleaning agents.

Chronic hepatitis may be triggered by an acute attack. Other causes include:
- an **autoimmune disease**, in around 20 per cent of cases;
- certain prescribed medications;
- some disorders of the **metabolism**.

Hepatitis viruses

Six hepatitis viruses – A, B, C, D, E and G – have so far been identified, but more are likely to be discovered. Hepatitis A and B are common in Africa, Asia and the Mediterranean. You can carry hepatitis, yet be free of symptoms.
- **Hepatitis A** is known as infectious hepatitis. It is excreted in faeces and contracted by eating or drinking contaminated food and water. Hepatitis A is always acute, never chronic.

■ Hepatitis B and D co-exist because the D virus cannot live independently and attaches to the B virus. The viruses are spread mainly by sexual contact and by contaminated needles. Hepatitis B used to be passed on through blood and blood products, when it was known as serum hepatitis. Hepatitis B is more serious than A, with about one case in 20 becoming chronic – sometimes bypassing the acute stage.

■ Hepatitis C is sexually transmitted; it is also carried in blood products and was passed on in transfusions of infected blood before donor blood started to be screened for the virus in the early 1990s. The virus can lie dormant for many years. There is a high risk of hepatitis C becoming chronic.

■ Hepatitis E is found mainly in developing countries. Like hepatitis A, it is contracted through contaminated food and water.

■ Hepatitis G is a mild chronic form of the virus, accounting for around 9 per cent of cases.

DIAGNOSIS

Hepatitis is diagnosed on the basis of symptoms reported by the patient. The diagnosis is confirmed with blood tests to look at levels of bilirubin and to identify enzymes released by damaged liver cells. Blood tests to detect antibodies can be used to pinpoint the virus.

TREATMENT

An attack of acute hepatitis will have to run its course – there is no treatment. Some high-risk cases are best treated in hospital: if the victim is pregnant, for example, or is very old, or has an especially severe bout of the infection.

Chronic hepatitis is treated with steroids, to reduce inflammation, and interferon, which attacks the virus directly.

OUTLOOK

The acute forms of hepatitis usually clear up within two to eight weeks, although the disease can develop into the chronic form. The condition is fatal in around one in 100 cases.

With treatment, the outlook for chronic hepatitis is generally good. However, there is a small risk of developing **cirrhosis** or liver cancer. Without treatment, the condition can be fatal.

PREVENTION

■ Practise safe sex; wash your hands regularly; when travelling in places where the virus is widespread, drink bottled water and beware of water-washed salads and ice in drinks.

■ Ensure that any needles, including tattooists' or acupuncture needles, are sterile.

■ Before travelling, ask your doctor about vaccinations. Although vaccinations against hepatitis A and B are available, they are usually recommended only for those especially at risk.

SEE ALSO *Sexually transmitted diseases*

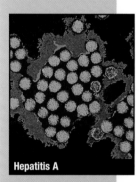
Hepatitis A

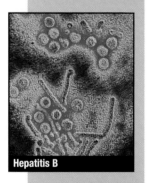
Hepatitis B

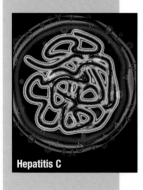
Hepatitis C

Herbal medicine

Herbal medicine is the use of plant extracts to treat disease and promote well-being. The earliest form of medicine known to mankind, herbal medicine is still used by over 80 per cent of the world's population, and until 50 years ago, some two-thirds of all medicinal drugs were based on herbs. Nowadays, the active therapeutic ingredients of many plants have been identified, and pharmaceutical companies have synthesized copies and patented new drugs to be used in orthodox medicine.

HOW IT CAN HELP

Herbalists will prescribe herbal medicines and herbal dietary supplements to help boost the efficiency of a body system rather than to combat a particular symptom or illness. There are herbal preparations to promote the health of the immune, nervous, circulatory, digestive, skeletal, muscular and hormonal systems, as well as the skin and hair and other body parts.

HOW IT WORKS

Herbal medicine, unlike orthodox medicine, uses the whole plant, or whole parts of a plant, rather than isolating one active ingredient. Herbalist believe that the collective power of the many different ingredients in plant leaves, roots, flowers, bark or stems is greater than that of each individual one. They call this the theory of synergy, claiming that remedies work better – more gently and with fewer side effects – when taken this way. One ingredient may act as a buffer for another that is effective but more abrasive, or it may help ensure that the active ingredient is absorbed or digested properly.

FINDING A PRACTITIONER

A wide range of over-the-counter herbal remedies are now available in high-street pharmacists and specialist shops, but you can also consult a professional medical herbalist. In the UK, herbalists undergo a rigorous three to five year training. Those who become Members of the National Institute of Medical Herbalists place the letters NIMH after their names.

A medical herbalist practises in a similar way to a mainstream medical practitioner, and some work with physicians to offer a complementary service. They treat disorders with a extensive range of herbal remedies, sometimes using powerful herbs that are restricted by law, in just the same way as an orthodox medical practitioner uses prescription-only drugs.

WHAT'S INVOLVED

The first consultation takes about one hour. The approach taken by herbalists is holistic and they take an extensive medical history as well as details of diet and lifestyle. The recommended remedies may be made up at the herbalist's surgery for you to take home, or may be obtainable from a reputable herbal supplier. Herbal preparations are available as tinctures (made by soaking the herb in alcohol), infusions (as 'teas', for example), whole plant extracts or as tablets and capsules.

Many people find that certain herbs have an unpleasant taste and prefer to take herbal medicines in the form of tablets and capsules. You can swallow these quickly without tasting the medicine itself. But in the case of the more pleasant-tasting herbs, tinctures, whole plant extracts and teas are becoming more common. Because these are liquids, they are absorbed more quickly and are often more potent.

WHAT YOU CAN DO

A variety of herbal dietary supplements and fresh, non-toxic herbs can be bought without consulting a professional herbalist. They can be used for first aid and to treat many everyday ailments, or to help boost the effectiveness of the immune system.

SEE ALSO *Chinese herbal medicine*

Hernia

A hernia develops when an area of the muscle that contains the abdominal organs becomes weakened or defective and allows a loop of the gut to protrude into a space. Most hernias form an external soft bulge. A hiatus hernia occurs internally when the top of the stomach protrudes into the diaphragm.

TYPES OF HERNIA

Common types of hernia include:
- inguinal hernia: most common in men and causes a bulge in the groin or scrotum;
- femoral hernia: mostly in women and causes a bulge at the top front of the thigh;
- umbilical hernia: most usual in babies and leads to a round swelling near the navel;
- incisional hernia: occurs when muscles are not properly rejoined after surgery;
- hiatus hernia: common in overweight adults and temporarily in pregnancy.

SYMPTOMS

Abdominal hernias often occur without any discomfort. Aching or severe pain may indicate that the hernia is obstructed or strangulated.

A hiatus hernia is not visible, and heartburn is common. This is caused by stomach acid flowing back into the gullet. It is usually worse on stooping, after heavy meals, and at night.

DURATION

Abdominal hernias tend to recur and persist until treated. Umbilical hernias in babies may disappear by the age of five. A hiatus hernia can heal on its own, after self-help measures (especially weight loss) or treatment.

CAUSES

In abdominal hernias, the muscle weakness may be present from birth, result from surgery or from strain through heavy lifting or substantial weight gain.

The causes of a hiatus hernia are not certain, but the risks is increased by obesity and smoking.

TREATMENT

Some abdominal hernias can be gently pushed back into the abdomen with the fingertips, but will still require treatment.

When to consult a doctor

Anyone who has a bulge in the abdomen, groin or scrotum, or who suffers from persistent heartburn or any other troublesome chest pain should consult a doctor.

What a doctor may do

An examinination will confirm an abdominal hernia. Surgery is usually recommended to repair the muscle weakness using tough internal stitches. These may be reinforced with the insertion of a fine nylon mesh to prevent recurrance. If surgery is not advisable, a truss may help to restrain some hernias.

A hiatus hernia can be diagnosed from an oesophagoscopy (a flexible telescope passed down the throat) or a barium swallow X-ray. Drug treatments reduce stomach acidity and protect the oesophagus. If treatment is unsuccessful, surgery is required.

What you can do

If you have a hiatus hernia, take sensible steps: stop smoking, lose weight if needed, avoid alcohol, hot drinks, spicy foods, and any food or drink that aggravates the heartburn. Avoid eating food four hours or less before bedtime.

Complementary therapies

Herbalists recommend slippery elm for hiatus hernia, to reduce stomach acidity.

PREVENTION

Abdominal hernias cannot easily be prevented. Exercises help to keep the muscles toned, and avoiding heavy lifting is a sensible precaution, as is stopping smoking.

Types of hernia

Hernias most commonly protrude through the abdominal wall and form a soft, round bulge.

When there is a weakness in the muscle that normally contains or supports internal organs, the soft tissue can push through the gap. Hernias are usually visible when standing upright but often diasappear when lying down.

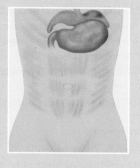

▶ **Hiatus hernia**
A weakness in the hiatus, the opening where the gullet passes through the diaphragm. This allows part of the stomach through the opening. Rising stomach acid causes heartburn.

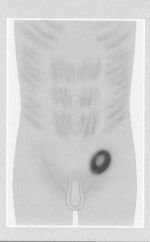

◀ **Inguinal hernia**
Usually occurs in men. There are two types of inguinal hernia. A direct inguinal hernia pushes through the muscle wall in the groin. An indirect inguinal hernia protrudes into the inguinal canal, which leads into the scrotum.

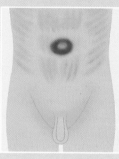

◀ **Umbilical hernia**
This type of hernia is more often caused by a congenital weakness, but strain from lifting a heavy weight may also cause the intestine to bulge at a point above the navel.

COMPLICATIONS

An obstructed or strangulated abdominal hernia is very painful, and urgent surgery is needed to resolve the protrusion and prevent gangrene. An obstruction is when part of the intestine becomes trapped, causing a blockage of intestinal matter. A strangulated hernia occurs when swelling cuts off the blood supply to the tissue within the hernia.

OUTLOOK

It is common for abdominal hernias to recur. Hiatus hernias can improve significantly if the doctor's advice is followed consistently, and prescribed medication is taken as advised.

Herpes simplex

There are two types of herpes simplex virus. Type 1 usually causes cold sores on the lips, mouth, nose and skin; *H. simplex* virus type 2 usually affects the genital area and is referred to as genital herpes. Attacks may be triggered by illness or by being tired or under stress. Herpes simplex viruses remain around a nerve for years and can cause recurrent attacks.

Cold sores

Cold sores are very common, particularly around the mouth and can last about 14 days.

SYMPTOMS

■ Tingling, burning or itching sensations around the lips or edges of the nostrils.
■ Fluid-filled blisters develop within hours.
■ The blisters burst within three to five days, and crust over within a week of the first symptoms, to form scabs.
■ Mild fever.
■ Enlarged lymph nodes ('glands') in the neck.

TREATMENT

There are various ways that you can treat the problem yourself.
■ Apply an antiviral medication such as aciclovir, available from a pharmacy.
■ Bathe the area in a warm salt solution, using 1 tablespoon of salt per pint of warm water.
■ Keep the area clean and moist and use a mild antiseptic cream to cover it.
■ Avoid kissing or touching the sore.
■ Apply essential oil of melissa, geranium, tea tree or lavender, diluted in a carrier oil.

If the symptoms are severe or are not resolved through the use of over-the-counter medications, consult a doctor. Antiviral medication, such as acyclovir, in cream or drug form, may be prescribed.

PREVENTION

■ Avoid physical contact with anyone who has a cold sore.
■ Strengthen your immune system and reduce stress.
■ Cover areas that are often affected with sunscreen in strong sunshine.

COMPLICATIONS

The viruses may infect the eyes and nose; first attacks may trigger mouth **ulcers**.

Genital herpes

Genital herpes is a **sexually transmitted disease** that results in a painful rash on the genitals.

SYMPTOMS

■ An itching, tingling, burning sensation where the sore is about to break out, usually on the penis for men and the labia for women.

■ Backache or a nerve ache in the affected area (for some), down the thighs or in the groin.

■ Sore blisters, which burst after 24–48 hours, leaving painful red ulcers. These crust over if they have formed on dry skin.

■ Feeling tired and generally unwell.

■ Swollen lymph glands in the groin.

DURATION

The symptoms may last for one to three weeks.

CAUSES

■ The *H. simplex* virus type 2, which is transmitted by sexual intercourse with an infected person.

■ You can also develop sores around your mouth by performing oral sex on someone with genital herpes.

■ Recurrent attacks can be triggered by illnesses, prolonged stress, or by being run down or tired.

TREATMENT

As soon as the warning signs appear, consult a doctor, who may prescribe an oral, antiviral medication, such as acyclovir or idoxuridine, or antibiotics. The symptoms can also be relieved by taking strong painkillers, or high daily doses of vitamin C . Elagen (a plant extract related to ginseng) or 200mg of vitamin E mau also help. Relief can also be gained from warm, salt-water baths, applying ice packs or dabbing vitamin E oil on the sores. Alternatively, apply Xylocaine gel, which is available from the pharmacist.

PREVENTION

■ Use condoms and dental dams during sex.

■ Reduce friction during intercourse by using a lubricant gel.

■ Wear loose cotton underwear and avoid tight trousers.

■ Try to reduce stress and boost the immune system by getting more sleep, including plenty of fruit and vegetables in your diet and supplementing with vitamins, minerals and herbal preparations such as echinacea (see **Herbal medicine**). Nutritional therapy, **homeopathy** and naturopathy may help.

COMPLICATIONS

Men may have difficulty urinating, and so retain urine in the bladder. Genital herpes can also cause **meningitis** or damage to nerve cells at the base of the spine (sacral radiculomyelopathy).

OUTLOOK

More than half of those who have one attack of genital herpes never get another.

Herpes zoster

Herpes zoster is an illness that causes a painful, blistered rash to erupt on the skin supplied by a particular spinal nerve – the condition is commonly known as shingles. Typical places for the rash to appear are on one side of the chest, face or forming a band around one side of the abdomen. It is rarely contagious.

SYMPTOMS

■ Early warning signs include itching, burning, tingling sensations just under the skin, which can be extremely painful.

■ The person feels tired and generally unwell, and develops a slight temperature.

■ Blisters appear two to five days after the first symptoms. They burst, weep, and turn into sores, which crust over, then slowly heal.

DURATION

Shingles can last for two to five weeks.

CAUSES

Herpes zoster is caused by *Herpes zoster* viruses, which initially cause **chickenpox**. Only those who have already had chickenpox may develop shingles. This is because when the body fights chickenpox (usually in childhood), the viruses retreat to lie dormant around the nerve that supplies the area. If reactivated, they return in the form of shingles. The trigger may be something that weakens the immune system such as overwork and tiredness, an illness or a shock.

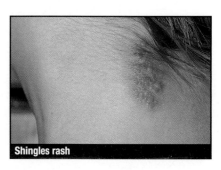
Shingles rash

TREATMENT

Although some self-help measures can relieve symptoms, shingles requires medical attention. As soon as you notice the warning signs, see a doctor because it is often more effective to treat shingles before the rash develops. It is essential to see a doctor if the rash appears near your eyes. Your doctor may prescribe antiviral drugs, such as aciclovir, and if necessary strong painkillers.

What you can do

In addition to taking your doctor's advice, apply ice packs. If clothing touches the site and causes discomfort, wrap cling film over the area, or ask your GP about a plastic spray called Opsite. This transparent dressing gives a bacteria-proof covering that minimizes irritation. Try a **TENS** machine to relieve pain. Taking vitamin B complex with L-lysine and vitamin C may also help.

COMPLICATIONS

Damage to the eyes and affected nerves can follow, resulting in numbness and pain.

▲ **Recognizing shingles**
A shingles rash most commonly appears as a long thin area over the ribcage, but can also appear on the face, neck and shoulder. Shingles affects about 250,000 people in the UK every year.

Hip and problems

The hip is a ball-and-socket joint at the top of each leg: the ball at the end of the thigh bone (femur) fits into a socket in the pelvis called the acetabulum. It is a synovial joint, meaning that it has a cavity filled with synovial fluid, an oily viscous fluid that acts as a lubricant to reduce friction between the two elements of the joint.

Unlike the shoulder joint – the body's other ball-and-socket joint – the hip is very stable. It is surrounded by a thick, strong joint capsule made of cartilaginous material, and is further strengthened by three ligaments. The largest and most important of these is the ileofemoral ligament, which prevents the hip from extending too far backwards. In addition, a small ligament called the ligamentum teres helps to keep the head of the femur in its socket.

WHAT CAN GO WRONG IN EARLY LIFE

The hip is subject to a wide range of ailments, some of which – such as congenital dislocation and developmental dysplasia of the hip – can begin before birth. Perthes' disease occurs in childhood. Arthritic tuberculosis of the hip usually affects children or young people who have been in contact with somebody who has pulmonary tuberculosis. Slipped femoral epiphysis is a condition of late childhood.

The construction of the hip.
The skeleton of the hip is formed from the ilium (hip bone), ischium and pubic bones, together with the sacrum at the base of the spine. The hip is the largest weight-bearing joint in the body.

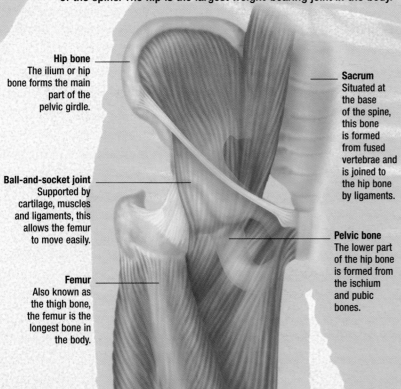

Hip bone
The ilium or hip bone forms the main part of the pelvic girdle.

Ball-and-socket joint
Supported by cartilage, muscles and ligaments, this allows the femur to move easily.

Femur
Also known as the thigh bone, the femur is the longest bone in the body.

Sacrum
Situated at the base of the spine, this bone is formed from fused vertebrae and is joined to the hip bone by ligaments.

Pelvic bone
The lower part of the hip bone is formed from the ischium and pubic bones.

Congenital dislocation

A spontaneous dislocation of the hip can occur either before or during birth or soon after it. In the West, it is one of the commonest congenital skeletal deformities (see **Congenital disorders**), occurring in around one in 1000 births.

Developmental dysplasia

Developmental dysplasia results from abnormal hip development in the womb. Rather than being cup-shaped, the acetabulum socket resembles a shallow saucer, so that the head of the femur can easily slip out of position. The condition is thought to be caused by a genetic tendency to joint and ligament laxity and is most common in girls, first-borns and babies who were born in a breech position.

The problem is usually picked up at birth, although hips that appear normal at birth can be found to be abnormal later, and in rare cases there may be no symptoms until early adulthood or even middle age.

The main symptoms of developmental dysplasia are hip joint instability and difficulty in walking. The early onset of osteoarthritis is likely if the condition is not treated.

Treatment depends on the age at which the disorder is diagnosed. Babies under six months may be given a simple harness to maintain the correct position of the ball and socket until the muscles and ligaments tighten around the joint. Infants and young children with dysplasia will be given manipulation under anaesthetic and then wear a body cast to maintain the position. Older children and adults require surgical treatment to increase the size and depth of the acetabulum. In severe cases, a hip replacement may be necessary if pain is a major problem.

Perthes' disease

In Perthes' disease, the head of the femur temporarily softens and may become deformed. It generally occurs between the ages of five and ten, and may lead to osteoarthritis later in life.

The cause of Perthes' disease is a temporary disturbance in the blood supply to the femoral head – but what causes the disturbance is unknown. Usually, only one hip is involved. Affected children complain of hip pain and, sometimes, groin or knee pain, but are otherwise in good health.

In mild cases the treatment is bed rest until the pain has subsided. In severe cases, when there is a risk of deformity, surgery is needed.

Arthritic tuberculosis

Arthritic tuberculosis of the hip used to be rare in the West, but has increased as more cases of **tuberculosis** are diagnosed as a result of war, homelessness and a lack of medical care.

The symptoms are pain in the hip, a limp and a general feeling of illness. Treatment is by a long course of antibiotics (often lasting six to nine months) and immobilization of the hip joint, usually in a plaster, for an initial period of three months.

If the cartilage and bones of the joint are intact and have not eroded by this time, gradual improvements are likely. But, if the bone or cartilage has been eroded, there is no possibility of maintaining the joint intact, and a full hip replacement will be needed once the patient has stopped growing.

Slipped femoral epiphysis

Slipped femoral epiphysis is a disorder of late childhood and adolescence in which the growth area (epiphysis) at the upper end of the femur is displaced from its normal position. The cause of this is unknown, but in around 50 per cent of cases it is associated with being overweight and with a problem in the **endocrine system.**

Either hip may be affected, but not usually both at the same time. Symptoms include a gradual onset of pain in the hip, and a limp, but the onset may be more rapid after a fall. Pain is sometimes felt in the knee. Some movements become restricted, but others remain normal.

As the condition develops, the head of the femur is displaced backwards and downwards. This is caused by the muscles pulling on the shaft of the femur and the pressure of bearing weight. Without treatment the head of the femur will eventually become fixed in the abnormal position. This causes a deformity of the joint and makes osteoarthritis more likely later on.

Diagnosis is confirmed by **X-ray**. Treatment is either by inserting wires or screws through the head of the femur to prevent any further slippage; or, if the slippage is severe, by cutting out a wedge of bone and returning the head of the femur to its correct position in the socket.

WHAT CAN GO WRONG LATER IN LIFE

Disorders occurring later in life most commonly stem from accidental dislocation, **arthritis** or fractures associated with **osteoporosis.**

Dislocation

The hip is not easily dislocated because it is a very stable joint. The most common causes of dislocation are road accidents, industrial accidents and falls from a height.

A hip dislocation is an extremely painful medical emergency. A surgeon will manipulate the hip back into position under a general anaesthetic and repair any damage done to the surrounding muscles. Even so, the dislocation can take up to three months to heal completely.

Osteoarthritis

Osteoarthritis of the hip is a common cause of severe disability in elderly people and is not uncommon even in younger patients, in whom it usually follows a previous disease or injury.

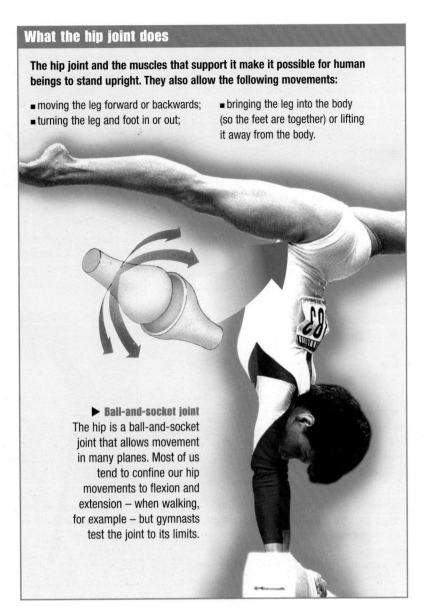

What the hip joint does

The hip joint and the muscles that support it make it possible for human beings to stand upright. They also allow the following movements:

- moving the leg forward or backwards;
- turning the leg and foot in or out;
- bringing the leg into the body (so the feet are together) or lifting it away from the body.

▶ **Ball-and-socket joint**
The hip is a ball-and-socket joint that allows movement in many planes. Most of us tend to confine our hip movements to flexion and extension – when walking, for example – but gymnasts test the joint to its limits.

There are three main reasons why the hip is especially vulnerable to osteoarthritis.
- It is a major weight-bearing joint.
- It has a poor blood supply.
- It is rarely put through its full range of movements; we tend only to flex and extend the joint – as when walking.

Lack of activity causes a reduction in the production of synovial fluid, increasing the hip's vulnerability. Without lubrication, the cartilage covering the bones becomes inflamed and damaged, and eventually hardens and is worn away, so that the head of the femur grinds on the socket with each movement. Bony, hook-like growths also form at the edges of the joint, limiting movement.

As the condition progresses, the head of the femur may be worn down to such an extent that eventually one leg can become shorter than the other.

The first signs of osteoarthritis are stiffness and pain, especially first thing in the morning and in cold weather. The pain is sometimes in the hip joint itself, but more frequently it is felt in the groin, down the front of the thigh and sometimes in the knee. The stiffness and pain increase until it can become difficult for the affected person to perform day-to-day activities and to sleep at night.

Osteoarthritis is to some extent a part of ageing, but there are ways to slow its onset.
- Reduce pressure on the joint by maintaining good posture and watching your weight.
- Take regular exercise that includes putting the hip joint through its full range of movements – examples include yoga, dancing and swimming (especially breaststroke).
- Take only moderate amounts of exercise that involves impact, twisting and turning – for example, football and squash – because these all increase wear and tear on the hip joint.

The only treatment for severe osteoarthritis is surgery to replace the hip joint. In most cases this relieves the pain entirely and restores freedom of movement. The treatment for moderate osteoarthritis is by anti-inflammatories, painkillers and **physiotherapy**, but this will only relieve the symptoms and cannot reverse the damage that has already been caused.

Rheumatoid arthritis
Rheumatoid arthritis does not often affect the hips, but when it does the consequent disability is serious. The main symptom is pain, aggravated by activity and limitation of movement. Eventually the disease causes no further damage, but any problems already caused are irreversible and may lead to deformity and secondary osteoarthritis.

Fractures
Hip fracture is most common in elderly people, usually occurring as the consequence of a fall. **Osteoporosis**, general frailty and lack of exercise increase the likelihood of a fracture. Treatment involves mending and securing the fracture with pins or plates, or in some cases replacing the head of the femur, followed by physiotherapy to restore mobility.

Trochanteric bursitis
Trochanteric **bursitis** of the hip is characterized by inflammation of a bursa, a small sac of fibrous fluid-filled tissue around the joint. Pain may be confined to the outer hip or move down the outer thigh to the knee. Any movement or held position may increase it, and rolling over onto the hip can be excruciating. The condition can affect anyone at any age, but is more common in middle-aged and elderly women. There are several causes:
- repeated minor injuries due to overuse;

A new hip

The hip is a major weight-bearing joint that is subject to huge wear and tear. Replacement of worn hip joints is therefore a common surgical procedure.

A hip replacement is designed to relieve pain when all other methods have failed, and to increase mobility. It is carried out when intense chronic pain is not relieved by anti-inflammatory medication, and when pain is so severe that it causes difficulty in carrying out day-to-day functions such as walking, climbing stairs and rising from a sitting position, and when sleep is disturbed.

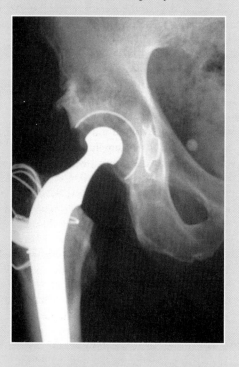

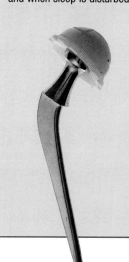

▲ **Replacement joint**
The diseased ball and socket are replaced with a metal ball and stem, inserted into the femur, and an artificial plastic-cup socket.

- disease of the lumbar spine or hip joint, such as osteoarthritis or rheumatoid arthritis;
- legs of unequal length, either present from birth or as a result of a **scoliosis** of the spine;
- a trauma, such as an accident or hip replacement operation;
- putting direct pressure on the bursa by lying on one side.

Treatment includes: using a cane to support the hip when walking; ice and non-steroidal anti-inflammatory drugs (NSAIDs) such as ibuprofen to reduce inflammation; weight loss to reduce pressure; cortisone injections; and physiotherapy to strengthen and stretch the muscles.

Transient osteoporosis
Transient osteoporosis of the hip is a painful but reversible condition. (It is distinct from osteoporosis, a progressive, generally painless disease of bone loss.) Two groups are most at risk: women in the third trimester of pregnancy, and men aged between 40 and 70. Symptoms include a sudden onset of pain for no clear reason, especially over the hip, front of the

thigh and the buttock. The pain increases with movement, weight-bearing and over time.

The cause is not known, but it usually resolves itself in 6–12 months. Diagnosis is confirmed by a bone scan or magnetic resonance imaging (MRI). Treatment aims to prevent damage occurring as the disease runs its course. It includes reducing weight-bearing activities – by rest and using crutches and walking sticks – and maintaining the joint's range of movements with controlled exercises, often involving hydrotherapy.

Osteonecrosis

Osteonecrosis of the hip is a condition in which the blood vessels that supply the head of the femur gradually close down, with the result that it is starved of nutrients and dies, then collapses. It is similar to transient osteoporosis of the hip in that the cause is unknown and there are few warning signs. Risk factors include being between 20 and 50 years old, a previous hip dislocation or fracture, alcohol abuse, glandular diseases such as rheumatoid arthritis, chronic pancreatis and **Crohn's disease**, and overuse of corticosteroid drugs. Treatment is a bone graft in the early stages or a total hip replacement.

Hip replacement and problems

The main treatment for hip joint problems is a hip replacement operation. The diseased bone and cartilage are removed and the head of the femur (ball) and the acetabulum (socket) are replaced with new, artificial parts (see box).

TYPES OF REPLACEMENT HIP

New hips are made of materials that allow a natural, gliding motion of the joint. Sometimes a special cement is used to bond the new parts of the joint to the existing, healthy bone. This is known as a 'cemented' procedure. In an uncemented procedure, the artificial parts are made of a porous material that allows the patient's own bone to grow into the pores and hold the new parts in place. Another option is a 'hybrid' replacement, with a cemented ball part and an uncemented socket.

An uncemented joint may last longer than cemented replacements because there is no cement to break away. The main drawback of an uncemented joint is the extended recovery period and thigh pain for several months after surgery. Cemented joints have repeatedly been shown to be effective in reducing pain and increasing joint mobility, usually with immediate results. Cemented replacements are more commonly used for older, less active people and people with weak bones, such as those who have osteoporosis.

Currently the demand for hip replacement far outstrips the NHS's ability to offer the operation.

SEE ALSO *Joints and problems*

Hirschsprung's disease

Hirschsprung's disease is a congenital disorder characterized by the absence of ganglia cells in the wall of the large intestine. It occurs in one in 5000 births. Ganglia cells control the passing of the bowel contents. Their absence results in faeces becoming trapped and building up in the colon, causing an obstruction.

Symptoms usually begin at birth, when the delayed passage of meconium (a baby's first faeces) becomes evident. Some form of surgery is usually needed to eliminate problems with constipation.

SEE ALSO *Babies and baby care*

Histoplasmosis

Histoplasmosis is a disease caused by the fungus Histoplasma capsulatum. The disease primarily affects the lungs and is not infectious. Its symptoms vary but can include a general feeling of illness, fever, chest pains and a dry cough. Antifungal medications are used to treat severe cases. Another form of the illness, called disseminated histoplasmosis, affects other organs, and can be fatal if it is left untreated.

SEE ALSO *Fungal infections*

HIV

SEE PAGE 316

Hodgkin's disease

Hodgkin's disease is a type of lymphoma, or **cancer** of the lymphatic system. There are about 30 types of lymphoma; all the others are known as non-Hodgkin's lymphoma.

Each year in the UK about 1500 people develop Hodgkin's disease, usually between the ages of 15 and 25. The disease can also develop later in life, in people over 60 – men are slightly more at risk than women.

The cause of Hodgkin's disease is unknown. People who have had glandular fever (an infection caused by the Epstein-Barr virus) may be slightly more likely to develop Hodgkin's disease, but more than half who develop the cancer have never had this infection. People whose immune system is suppressed – because of AIDS, for example, or after an organ transplant – are also at slightly increased risk.

SYMPTOMS

- Painless enlarged glands.
- Fever and sweats at night.

Continued on page 318

HIV

HIV is the human immunodeficiency virus that causes AIDS. Development of drug treatments has dramatically improved life expectancy for many people with HIV, but there is still no vaccine or cure.

HIV is a virus that affects cells in the immune system, gradually destroying them so that the person becomes susceptible to infections and cancers. People who have been infected with HIV usually remain in good health for several years – and may stay well for as long as 15 years. But after this time, the decline in the immune system accelerates and the person succumbs to various diseases, leading to a diagnosis of AIDS.

The virus is commonly spread by sexual contact, but may also be passed from an infected person via a blood transfusion, the sharing of needles, or through a mother's breast milk.

During the first three to five days after infection, the virus replicates in the lymph glands before spreading viral particles through the blood. The first stage of infection may go unnoticed, but 70 per cent of those affected experience brief flu-like symptoms such as fevers, night sweats, swollen glands, diarrhoea and rash. A blood test done at this time will show a high number of HIV viral particles – this is known as a high 'viral load'.

About three to six months after infection, the body begins to produce antibodies to the virus. An HIV antibody test checks for these antibodies in patients' blood. People whose blood contains the antibodies are said to be HIV-positive.

SYMPTOMS OF HIV

Apart from the initial symptoms at the time of infection, mild symptoms such as fatigue, weight loss, night sweats and oral thrush occur on average five to seven years after HIV infection. Within an average of ten years the immune system has suffered severe damage. Patients become vulnerable to a range of 'opportunistic infections'. These are caused by bacteria, fungi, protozoa and other infectious agents that an intact immune system can usually deal with, but which take advantage of the opportunity provided by weakened immunity to attack the body.

Infections commonly associated with HIV usually strike either the lungs or the central nervous system or the gastro-intestinal tract. They include **Kaposi's sarcoma** and types of lymphoma, as well as more than 20 infections such as oral candida (thrush), **tuberculosis** and *Pneumocystis carinii* **pneumonia**.

TRANSMISSION OF HIV

HIV is transmitted in many bodily fluids, including blood, vaginal fluid, semen and breast milk from an infected person. Although HIV has not been reported to be transmitted by tears or saliva, it has been reported after oral sex, especially where there are open sores in the mouth or gum disease. Using a condom for sex is the most effective way of protecting yourself against HIV infection. Be cautious about new sexual partners – an apparently healthy person may be HIV-positive and infectious. Sexual partners from sub-Saharan Africa are the highest risk.

Injecting drug users should never share needles or other equipment. People in the developed world are highly unlikely to be infected with HIV by blood transfusion. Since 1985 donated blood and blood products have been screened for HIV.

HIV is not passed on through everyday social contact with an infected person. Touching, shaking hands, hugging, coughing or sneezing cannot transmit the virus.

Who is at risk?

Anyone exposed to HIV infection through sex without a condom or contaminated blood can be infected with HIV. High-risk groups include homosexuals or bisexuals who engage in unprotected sex. This category represents 40 per cent of new cases in the UK. Injecting drug users constitute 3 per cent of new cases in the UK. Other high-risk groups are children born to infected mothers and adults in countries of high heterosexual HIV transmission – for example, countries in sub-Saharan Africa. Heterosexually acquired HIV is rare in the UK but accounts for nearly 90 per cent of cases worldwide.

HIV TESTS AND PREGNANT WOMEN

A pregnant woman who is HIV-positive may pass on the infection to her child. All babies born to HIV-positive mothers have antibodies to the virus in their blood, but most do not have the virus itself and will lose the antibodies by the age of 18 months. From about three months old, babies can take the PCR test, which looks for the virus rather than the antibodies identified in the HIV antibody test. Only one in six babies born to HIV-positive mothers has the virus.

An HIV-positive woman can protect her baby by taking drugs that reduce the chances of passing on the virus. She will be advised to have her baby by Caesarean section, which also reduces the chances of passing on the virus, and to bottle-feed rather than breastfeed her baby because the virus can be passed on in breast milk.

In some antenatal clinics all pregnant women are offered the HIV test. In others, women have to ask to take it.

Being HIV-positive does not affect your fertility. But if you decide to start a family and your partner is not HIV-positive, he risks contracting the infection during sex without a condom.

LIVING WITH HIV/AIDS
If you are HIV-positive, you can expect to live a normal life and feel healthy for many years and you will need only occasional monitoring of your HIV status. There is a real risk of passing on HIV, but it can only happen through unprotected sex or sharing injecting equipment. It is vital to understand HIV, the risks, and how to protect yourself and others. You need to decide whether and how to tell others about your condition.

As HIV progresses to AIDS you will need to plan your lifestyle and drug regime carefully to limit the effects of the likely infections, muscle wasting and loss of strength. Local and national charities and support groups can provide assistance at all stages to people suffering from HIV and AIDS.

TREATMENT
The outlook for HIV sufferers has improved in recent years with the introduction of Highly Active Anti-Retroviral Therapy (HAART). With HAART, patients take a combination of two or three anti-HIV drugs – research has shown this to be more effective than taking any single anti-HIV drug.

Currently available drugs slow the replication of the virus and subsequent immune damage. But there is still no cure or vaccine available for HIV/AIDS.

AZT, now called ZDV (for zidovudine), is the most widely used drug for HIV. Some people find ZDV ineffective or cannot tolerate its side effects, which include leg cramps, diarrhoea or anaemia. Alternatives include didanosine (ddI) or dideoxycytidine (ddC), but these, too, have potential risks.

The HIV virus can become resistant to particular anti-HIV drugs and sufferers may have to change the drugs or combinations of drugs they are using. The viral load test is used to check how well particular drugs are working. The test provides evidence of the number of viral particles

Monitoring the progress of HIV infection

If you think you may have been infected with HIV, visit a genito-urinary medicine (GUM) clinic for an HIV antibody test, freely available in the UK.

Before carrying out an HIV antibody test, staff at a GUM clinic will offer non-judgmental counselling and will discuss the consequences of a positive result. You will also be asked about the contact through which you believe you have been infected. If you test HIV-positive, you will be offered specialist monitoring of your HIV status.

When HIV enters the body, it seeks out certain white blood cells called T-cells, which usually defend the body against infection. The virus takes over a T-cell, causing it to die and releasing billions of copies of the virus back into the

blood. The new viruses then attach themselves to new T-cells – and the infection spreads.

HIV progress is measured in terms of the level of CD4 cells – one type of T-cell – in the blood of an infected person. A normal count is 500–1500 CD4 cells per microlitre of blood. People with a count above 500 need only regular monitoring. Once the level falls below 300, patients may be offered drugs to slow the progress of the HIV infection. A CD4 count below 200, plus several specific illnesses diagnosed by a doctor, defines AIDS.

in a patient's blood – the fewer particles, the more effective the drug.

In deciding whether to treat the initial stages of HIV infection, patients and doctors must weigh the benefit from HAART against the side effects and the risk of developing a drug-resistant virus early in the disease. Studies suggest that slowing the early rapid replication of the virus may delay the progression to AIDS. But HIV has not yet been eradicated by treating it in the early stage.

Treatment with trimethoprim-sulfamethoxazole (TMP-SMX) may protect people with AIDS against *Pneumocystis carinii* pneumonia (PCP), the most common respiratory tract infection to strike AIDS patients.

OUTLOOK
AIDS patients are vulnerable to infections, and it is these infections, rather than the virus itself, that can lead to death. A patient may recover from an infection only to succumb eventually to another one. Despite improving survival rates due to HAART, people with HIV still have a shortened lifespan.

SEE ALSO *AIDS; Blood and disorders; Infectious diseases; Lymphatic system; Sexually transmitted diseases; Travel and tropical diseases*

UNDER THE MICROSCOPE

When HIV invades the white T-cells, it kills the cells before releasing billions of copies of the virus into the blood. As time goes on, the body cannot produce enough T-cells to replace those that have been lost.

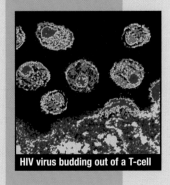

HIV virus budding out of a T-cell

Hodgkin's disease continued

- Weight loss.
- Tiredness.
- Cough or shortness of breath.
- Widespread itchiness.

The lymphoma cells grow mostly in the lymph nodes or glands, so the most common symptoms are enlarged lymph glands, which are often first noticed in the neck, armpit or groin but may be anywhere in the body. These are usually painless.

Occasionally enlarged lymph glands in the chest or abdomen cause other symptoms, due to pressure on internal organs.

The diagnosis is made by **biopsy**, when a gland is removed and studied in the laboratory to look for abnormal cells.

TREATMENT

The first step is to grade the tumour according to how malignant it is. This is done by examining the cells under the microscope to estimate how likely it is to spread and how fast. The lymphoma is also 'staged', which involves measuring how far it has spread in the body. For example, in Stage I only one group of lymph nodes is affected, while in Stage IV the disease has spread to distant sites such as liver, lungs or bone. The lymphoma is also coded A or B depending on whether there are symptoms such as sweats, fever or weight loss.

Grading and staging are vital to deciding the most appropriate treatment. The main treatments used are **radiotherapy** and **chemotherapy** (including steroids), sometimes in combination. In severe cases, high-dose chemotherapy may be used. But in high doses these powerful drugs can destroy the bone marrow. So they must be used along with stem cell support treatment. This involves collecting stem cells from the blood and returning these to the patient after chemotherapy.

Complementary therapies

Yoga, massage and aromatherapy may help sufferers to cope with the sleep disruption, anxiety and depression associated with undergoing treatment.

COMPLICATIONS

Treatment may be unpleasant and cause side effects such as nausea and hair loss, or complications such as infertility. Fortunately, there are drugs and other strategies that may help to prevent or minimize these problems.

PREVENTION

Hodgkin's disease cannot be prevented because the cause is not known. There is no screening test for the disease.

OUTLOOK

Even when Hodgkin's disease has spread, treatment is usually very successful. Most people (about 90 per cent) can be cured, or their disease can be controlled for many years.

Homeopathy

Homeopathy is a complementary therapy inspired by the natural tendency of the body to heal itself, and by the belief that 'like will cure like'. A homeopathic practitioner views the symptoms of an illness as signs of the body's attempt to heal itself, and treats the illness by prescribing minute doses of substances that could, in larger quantities, cause those very symptoms. The theory is that if the substance were given to a healthy person it would produce the symptoms of a particular disease, but in someone who is sick the remedy will boost the body's capacity for self-healing.

ORIGINS OF HOMEOPATHY

The theory of homeopathy was first expounded in the late 15th century, but was only developed some 300 years later by the German doctor Samuel Hahnemann. He observed that cinchona bark, which a fellow physician had claimed could be used to treat malaria, produced symptoms of the disease in healthy people. Conversely, the herb did indeed appear effective in treating those who were sick.

Hahnemann found in subsequent experiments that small doses of dilute herbs or their extracts were more effective than large ones in aiding the healing process. Such was the success of his treatments that the principles of homeopathy soon won widespread support.

By the middle of the 19th century a dedicated hospital, the London Homeopathic Hospital, had been founded in Britain. Homeopathy was embraced as a complementary medicine by the National Health Service when it was founded in 1948, and today there are five specialist homeopathic hospitals in England and Scotland – in Bristol, Liverpool, Tunbridge Wells, London and Glasgow.

HOW IT CAN HELP

A large number of conditions can be treated homeopathically. The main exceptions are those that require surgery or manipulation. Homeopathic remedies are commonly used to treat a wide range of disorders, for example, hay fever, asthma, migraine, headache, colds and flu, osteoarthritis, rheumatoid arthritis and chronic fatigue syndrome. You can use some remedies at home to treat first-aid problems such as cuts, stings, minor burns and bruises.

FINDING A PRACTITIONER

Practitioners may be medically qualified doctors trained in homeopathy or lay (non-medical) homeopaths. You may be referred by your GP, or choose to find a practitioner privately.

The initial consultation will usually last for about an hour, during which the patient will be asked to give a detailed personal and medical history. Follow-up consultations will assess how well the treatment is working and whether any adjustments are necessary.

WHAT'S INVOLVED

The aim of homeopathy is to treat the whole person rather than simply the illness. When prescribing medication, homeopaths take into account a patient's personality, feelings, habits, and likes and dislikes, as well as stress factors. As a result, two people suffering from the same illness may not be treated with the same remedy, and the same remedy can also be used to treat a range of symptoms, depending on the requirements of the individual.

If you take any prescribed or over-the-counter medicine regularly, you should tell your homeopath, since this may interfere with your homeopathic treatment.

Treatment usually involves taking remedies in pill, powder or granule form, although tinctures and creams are also available. The remedies contain minute traces of the original active ingredient (made from plant, animal or mineral extracts).

Remedies are available in three potencies – 6, 30 and 200. The higher a remedy's potency number, the more dilute – yet the more powerful – it is thought to be. For self-help, it is advisable to stick to lower potencies; a homeopathic practitioner may prescribe higher ones. In around 20 per cent of cases symptoms flare up briefly before receding.

How quickly results are seen depends on the nature of the problem and how your body responds to the treatment. Chronic complaints will not disappear immediately, although some improvement should be seen quite quickly. Acute complaints may improve more rapidly.

THE REMEDIES

There are more than 2000 homeopathic remedies, although fewer than 100 of them are generally used. The remedies include some plants and a number of substances that are highly poisonous in their undiluted form, such as belladonna (deadly nightshade) and arsenic. However, these are used in such a diluted form in homeopathic remedies that their effect is no longer toxic.

You may find that the same remedy might be used to treat any number of illnesses. This is because some illnesses produce quite similar symptoms. Someone with a cold, for example, might feel very hot, while someone with the skin condition psoriasis could experience a burning sensation in the skin. The remedy Arsenicum album (Arsen. alb) may be prescribed in both cases.

Conversely, two people might be prescribed different remedies for the same illness: one person might have a cough that is dry and tickly, and be given Aconitum napellus (aconite), while another person's cough might produce phlegm and be better treated with Kali bichromicum (Kali bich).

Listed below are five of the most commonly prescribed remedies, together with the symptoms they are used to treat.

■ **Aconite** This is helpful in situations where a patient has experienced some kind of shock. It might be prescribed to someone who has suffered an unexpected bereavement, for example, or to someone who is prone to anxiety-related panic attacks. It could be used as a first-aid treatment to help relieve shock or a feeling of panic following an accident. Other physical symptoms that it can be used to treat are sudden onsets of diarrhoea, and tickly coughs, earache or a chill following exposure to wind.

■ **Arnica** Arnica montana is particularly helpful for minimizing **bruising**. It might be taken following a tooth extraction, for example, or to reduce bruising with a sprain; some women take it to alleviate pain following childbirth.

■ **Arsen. alb** The symptoms that this remedy can treat are often associated with heat or cold in the body. It can be used to treat **cystitis**, the bladder infection that causes a burning sensation in the urethra; **hay fever**, where there is a burning nasal discharge; high temperature; mouth **ulcers** where the mouth feels hot and dry. It may also be used to treat any restlessness or chilliness, or to help someone who is suffering from feelings of anxiety or fearfulness.

■ **Belladonna** Like Arsen. alb, Atropa belladonna may be prescribed for conditions in which there is excessive heat – from sunburn, for example, or for the hot flushes experienced during the female **menopause**.

■ **Pulsatilla** Pulsatilla pratensis may be used to treat conditions as varied as **acne**, in which spots are aggravated by fatty food, bad breath (**halitosis**) in which the mouth feels overly dry, and feelings of tearfulness where a person is suffering from **depression**.

POSSIBLE SIDE EFFECTS

Homeopathic remedies do not cause side effects, and you cannot become addicted to them.

▼ **Homeopathic remedy**
Substances contained in a homeopathic kit are provided in minute doses to avoid any unwanted side effects.

Silica 30c
Contents: 1.4g sucrose pills

Hormone replacement therapy

By reversing the unpleasant symptoms of the menopause, hormone replacement therapy can improve the quality of a woman's life and protect against osteoporosis. But there is evidence that the therapy can slightly increase the risk of certain cancers, heart disease and strokes.

Strictly speaking, hormone replacement therapy (HRT) refers to replacing any of the body's hormones, including growth hormone in children, insulin in diabetes and thyroxine in thyroid disease. But it is usually used to describe the administration of oestrogen (and, perhaps, the synthetic hormone progestogen) to women at or after the **menopause**.

When women reach the menopause, their ovaries stop making the hormones oestrogen and progesterone. As a result, their periods stop. Many develop hot flushes, night sweats and vaginal dryness, accompanied by forgetfulness, depression and mood swings. Oestrogen helps to keep bones strong and so after the menopause the risk of **osteoporosis** increases. HRT replaces the lost oestrogen and can counteract some of the effects of the menopause.

PROS AND CONS OF HRT

In the past, HRT was mainly prescribed in the short term to alleviate menopausal symptoms. The recent trend has been to recommend it for longer, sometimes for the rest of a woman's life. Five or more years of oestrogen are needed to deter osteoporosis, but to maintain the benefit you need to go on taking the hormone.

In the short term, HRT is clearly effective in relieving hot flushes, night sweats and sleep disturbances, and alleviating vaginal dryness by increasing the thickness, elasticity and lubrication of the vagina. It may also help with problems such as stress **incontinence**, **cystitis** and **urethritis** by thickening the tissues of the urinary tract and perineum.

There is some evidence that hormone replacement therapy can also help to reduce mood swings and ease forgetfulness.

The long-term picture is less clear. Oestrogen certainly helps to prevent bone loss and reduce the risk of osteoporosis, although only while the woman continues to take it. But its effects on the heart and blood vessels are less categorical. Although some studies

suggest that HRT may protect against heart disease, others show that oestrogen increases the risk of heart attacks and **strokes**. It also encourages potentially dangerous blood clots (see **Deep vein thrombosis**).

People who take HRT for five years or more have an increased risk of breast cancer; the therapy also increases the risk of ovarian cancer. However, in both cases the risk is relatively small.

Deciding whether to take HRT involves assessing your individual risks on the basis of your lifestyle, medical history and other risk factors for breast or ovary cancer, heart attacks, strokes and blood clots.

You will be advised against taking HRT if you have unexplained vaginal bleeding, active liver disease or certain other liver problems, or have recently suffered a thrombosis.

New types of HRT are being developed to provide the benefits while minimizing the risks.

HOW HRT IS USED

Taking oestrogen on its own increases the risk of cancer of the lining of the womb. So, unless you have had a hysterectomy, you will also be prescribed the synthetic hormone progestogen to prevent an unhealthy buildup of the womb lining. Progestogen is similar to the progesterone that women produce in their ovaries. Progestogen causes monthly or three-monthly 'periods'. If your menopause was more than one year ago, you can choose a 'no bleed' formulation that reduces bleeding to spotting or eliminates it altogether.

HRT comes in the form of tablets, patches and creams or gels that are rubbed into the skin. Once you have started taking HRT, you need to have regular checkups by your GP or at a specialist clinic. You will be asked how HRT suits you, and you will be weighed and have your blood pressure tested. You will also be encouraged to be 'breast aware' so you can report anything unexpected to your doctor, and to have regular mammograms (see **Breasts and disorders**). The first formulation you try may disagree with you, but do not be discouraged: it can take trial and error to find your ideal brand.
SEE ALSO *Menopause*

HRT and weight gain

A variety of health fears are associated with the use of HRT, one of which is the risk of weight gain.

Many women believe they gain weight while on HRT, but research has failed to prove any connection – other than in those women who have a tendency to retain fluid while they are on oestrogen. Loss of muscle as we age encourages fat deposition, so it is important to eat a healthy diet and take daily exercise.

Huntington's disease

Huntington's disease is a progressive, incurable genetic disorder affecting the brain and nervous system. Also known as Huntington's chorea, it affects around one in 15,000 people.

SYMPTOMS

Symptoms usually begin to appear between the ages of 35 and 45, in the form of irritability, clumsiness, depression and forgetfulness, followed by slurred speech, grimaces, clenching and unclenching of hands and fists, and uncontrollable movements. Death, usually from **heart failure, pneumonia** or complications, generally occurs within 15 to 20 years.

OUTLOOK

The genetic mutation involved in Huntington's disease has been discovered and a test is now available. Due to the late onset of symptoms and the fact that there is no effective treatment, testing has raised some difficult and harrowing issues. People tested and found positive for Huntington's disease face not only a future of progressive and incurable degeneration, but may also lose health and life insurances, and career prospects. For these reasons many people with a known risk factor refuse to be tested.

Another issue is that parents who test positive for the disorder also have to deal with the complexities of the fact that all their children have a 50 per cent chance of having inherited Huntington's disease.

Hydatid cyst

A hydatid cyst is a slow-growing cyst caused by an infestation of the larvae of a small tapeworm, *Echinococcus granulosus*, which often settles in the liver, lungs or muscle. In rare cases, the brain or other organs are affected. The tapeworm, a parasite of dogs and sheep, is most common in sheep-raising countries; the eggs are excreted in their faeces and may be spread through contaminated food or water.

Hydrocephalus

Hydrocephalus is an abnormal increase in the volume of cerebrospinal fluid within any of the four fluid-filled ventricles (cavities) of the **brain.** In infants, this condition may cause enlargement of the head at a stage when the skull has not fully fused together. In adults, the skull forms a fixed protective shell, and an increase in volume inside the skull causes increased pressure on the brain. The condition is relieved by surgery to drain the excess fluid.

Hyperglycaemia

An abnormally high level of the blood sugar glucose is termed hyperglycaemia. It is most often caused by undiagnosed or uncontrolled **diabetes** mellitus. In people with diabetes, it can be a result of an insufficient amount of the hormone insulin being secreted by the pancreas, an excessive intake of food, insufficient exercise or physical activity, hot weather, illness, infection, injury or surgery. More rarely, it can be caused by other hormonal disorders. The symptoms of hyperglycaemia include increased thirst, frequent urination and weight loss.

TREATMENT

People with diabetes should monitor their blood sugar levels daily to ensure they remain healthy. High sugar levels can be brought under control by eating regular, healthy meals that are low in fat and high in fibre (fruit, vegetables and pulses); being more active; and, where necessary, adjusting insulin or other diabetic medication.

PREVENTION

If you have diabetes, you can largely prevent hyperglycaemia by eating a healthy diet, having regular meals, taking regular exercise and adjusting your medication as necessary.

COMPLICATIONS

Prolonged hyperglycaemia damages the large and small blood vessels leading to retinopathy (damaged blood vessels at the back of the eye), **cataracts**, heart disease, kidney problems, **impotence** and, in diabetics, foot problems.

OUTLOOK

Hyperglycaemia following meals may be a sign of glucose intolerance, which is thought to be the first phase in the development of Type 2 (late onset) diabetes. New drugs are being developed to combat this.

SEE ALSO *Adrenal glands and disorders; Blood and disorders; Diabetes; Endocrine system and disorders*

Hypermetropia

Hypermetropia (also known as hyperopia) is long-sightedness, or difficulty in focusing on objects that are near to you. It is caused by light rays focusing behind the retina and this happens when the eyeball is too short in relation to the focusing ability of the cornea and lense. The eye naturally becomes more long-sighted with age, which is why so many middle-aged people find it increasingly difficult to read small print.

SEE ALSO *Eye and problems*

Hyperpyrexia

Hyperpyrexia is very high body temperature and collapse. It is caused by failure of the body's heat regulation system due to heat stroke (excessive sun exposure) or stimulant drugs such as amphetamines, cocaine and ecstasy. There is a very rare reaction to general anaesthetic called malignant hyperpyrexia, in which body temperature rises by 1°C (1.8°F) every five minutes. A body temperature above 42°C (107.6°F) can lead to brain damage.

Hypertension

Hypertension is another term for high blood pressure – the elevation of the blood pressure in the arteries above the normal range expected in a particular age group. If left untreated, it may lead to heart disease, **stroke**, **dementia** or kidney failure. Treatment reduces the risk, but some types of damage also depend on whether other risk factors for arteriosclerosis (thickening of the artery walls) are present.

SEE ALSO *Arteries and disorders; Blood pressure and problems; Heart and circulatory system; Stress*

Hypertrophy

Hypertrophy is the excessive growth of an organ or tissue. This can be a result of excess physical stimulation (as in muscle hypertrophy in body-builders), or due to excessive hormonal stimulation or responsiveness to hormones. Hypertrophy of the fingers, toes and chin occurs in **acromegaly**. This is a condition in which these body parts increase in size as a result of a pituitary gland tumour secreting excess growth hormone.

Hyperventilation

Also known as overbreathing, hyperventilation is breathing that is too fast and too deep. Levels of carbon dioxide in the blood drop, leading to chemical changes that affect the way certain nerves work. People affected by hyperventilation start to feel unwell and may develop what can often be alarming symptoms, even though there is usually nothing physically wrong with them.

SYMPTOMS

In extreme cases, fainting may occur but more common symptoms include:
- shortness of breath;
- tingling around the lips and fingers;

Paper bag – does it help?

One widely known self-treatment for hyperventilation is breathing into a paper bag held loosely over the mouth and nose.

This helps to increase levels of carbon dioxide in the blood by breathing in exhaled breath, while also providing vital oxygen. However, in people for whom hyperventilation is a symptom of a respiratory or heart condition, it could cause a drop in blood oxygen levels from an already low level and, in very severe cases, a heart attack. Such people should therefore avoid this technique. Reassurance and calming can be just as effective – without any of these risks.

- dizziness;
- blurred vision.

CAUSES

The main causes of hyperventilation include anxiety, fear and strong emotion. Other rarer causes include an underlying respiratory condition, a heart attack and pulmonary embolism.

TREATMENT

Practise breathing exercises to develop steady, smooth, deep breathing. Meditation or yoga may also help.

If you are worried about your symptoms or they are getting worse, or if you suspect an underlying disease is the cause, consult a doctor, who may:
- examine your heart and lungs to make sure they are normal;
- treat any underlying physical condition;
- suggest counselling or mild tranquillizers for anxiety.

PREVENTION

If hyperventilation is recurring, you can practise relaxation techniques and breathing exercises on a regular basis. If you feel that you are likely to start hyperventilating, the techniques can be used as a preventive measure.

SEE ALSO *Respiratory system*

Hypnotherapy

Hypnotherapy is a treatment that uses hypnosis to relieve the symptoms of certain mental and physical problems. It can help to reduce agitation and anxiety associated with **depression**, to dispel **phobias**, to combat addictions such as **smoking**, and to provide symptom relief in medical conditions such as chronic pain, **migraine** and **irritable bowel syndrome**.

The essence of hypnotic technique is in persuading the subject to relax and to focus on an object or the hypnotist's instructions. A person who is hypnotized enters an artificially created state of altered consciousness that is neither wakefulness nor sleep.

Most hypnotized people are highly susceptible to suggestion. They comply with the instructions given by a therapist. This compliance continues after the session, whether or not the subject has a conscious awareness of what has been suggested.

WHAT'S INVOLVED

The number of hypnotherapy sessions required depends on the nature of the problem being treated. At the first session, your therapist will discuss the problem and explain how hypnosis may help. This is a good opportunity to ask questions. For example, you might want to know whether you will be asleep during the session or whether you are likely to behave strangely afterwards.

Once you agree to begin treatment, the therapist induces a hypnotic state in you by using a gently guiding voice. He or she gives clear instructions about controlling the problem, then gradually talks you back to a state of alertness.

Between hypnotherapy sessions you should keep a record of any changes in the mental or physical condition for which you are receiving treatment.

HOW IT CAN HELP

Hypnotherapy can be useful as part of a package of care from a doctor, dentist or clinical psychologist. It can be particularly useful when patients learn to induce the trance state themselves – self-hypnosis – and use this skill to manage their symptoms.

As only about 20 per cent of GPs offer access to complementary therapies on the NHS, you are likely to have to pay for hypnotherapy sessions. Check that a private therapist belongs to a professional body.

Hypoglycaemia

Hypoglycaemia refers to an abnormally low level of blood sugar. It most often affects people with insulin-treated diabetes as a result of too much insulin, not enough food or exercising without increasing food intake.

Symptoms include fatigue, nervousness, hunger, trembling, irritability, headache, cold sweats, rapid heart rate, blurred vision and confusion. Left untreated, it can lead to convulsions and coma.

SEE ALSO *Diabetes*

Hypospadias

Hypospadias is a congenital condition in which the penis fails to develop as it should. The opening of the urethra (from which a male urinates) develops in the wrong place – on the head, shaft or underside of the penis. It affects one in 300 male babies and is usually rectified by surgery before the age of two years.

SEE ALSO *Penis and problems*

Hypotension

Hypotension is the medical term for low blood pressure – lower arterial blood pressure than is normal at a particular age – which can reduce oxygen supply to the brain, causing faintness. It can affect pregnant women, elderly people and anyone who experiences shock, and may also be caused by medication, including anti-anxiety drugs, diuretics and painkillers.

Temporary hypotension may follow sudden or prolonged standing. Hypotension can be relieved by lying with raised feet, and treating the cause.

SEE ALSO *Blood pressure and problems; Pregnancy and problems*

Hypothermia

Hypothermia is an abnormally low body temperature: 35°C (95°F) or below. Normal body temperature is strictly controlled in the small range of 36.7–37.2°C (98–99°F).

The two groups of people who are most at risk from hypothermia are newborn babies (especially premature babies) and elderly people. In the UK, there were 38,000 cases of hypothermia in elderly people during the winter of 1996–7. Climbers and fell walkers, or those submerged in cold water, are also at risk.

SYMPTOMS

A person suffering from hypothermia will usually feel cold to the touch and there will be changes to their skin colour and pulse rate.

Babies

■ Lethargy; poor feeding; reddening of the skin; and feeling cold.

Elderly people

■ Slow pulse, skin looks grey and feels cold.

■ Shivering and confusion, with a temperature below 35°C (95°F).

■ Drowsiness but no shivering, with a temperature below 33°C (91.4°F).

CAUSES

Hypothermia occurs when there is insufficient warmth, but also has other causes.

Hypothermia is a potentially life-threatening condition and, if not caught and treated early on, can result in a rapid decline in the body's ability to function. Exposure to cold causes about 30,000 deaths a year in the UK.

Babies
- Sleeping in a cold room at night.
- Bathing in a cold room.

Elderly people
- Inadequate food, heating or clothing.
- Being unable to get up from a fall or get help.
- Alcohol or certain drugs, such as sedatives.
- Secondary conditions such as **diabetes**, hypothyroidism, immobility or **dementia**.

TREATMENT

Hypothermia is usually treated in hospital.

Babies

Babies are admitted to a special care baby unit for gradual warming in an incubator. Fluids and antibiotics (to prevent infections) may be given by infusion into a vein.

Elderly people

If the person's temperature is 32–35°C (89.6–95°F), he or she is nursed in a warm room, in a space blanket, to increase body temperature gradually. Too rapid a rise can cause too much blood to flow into the skin, producing a dangerous drop in blood pressure and damage to the body's organs. The heart rate is monitored as there is a risk of dangerous heart rhythms occurring during rewarming.

If an elderly person's temperature falls below 32°C (89.6°F) his or her breathing may need to be helped by the use of a ventilator. Fluids and antibiotics may be given by infusion into a vein.

PREVENTION

Premature or small babies should be born in a warm room and taken to a special care unit.

Keeping mobile, wearing sufficient clothing, eating well and using adequate heating are vital for elderly people. Regular visits from family, neighbours or home care agencies also help.

COMPLICATIONS

In babies with a temperature below 32°C (89.6°F), there is a 25 per cent risk of death.

In elderly people, hypothermia may result in coma and brain damage and there is a risk of pneumonia. There is a 5 per cent risk of death.

OUTLOOK

Emergency treatment is essential. There are usually no long-term effects, once the person is past the initial danger period.

Hysterectomy

A hysterectomy is the surgical removal of the womb (uterus). One in five women in the UK have had a hysterectomy before the age of 60. It can be a psychological as well as a physical trauma, as it means that a woman is no longer fertile and may feel unattractive and less feminine. For these reasons counselling is usually offered before and after the operation.

For women with cancer, it can be a life-saver. Menstrual periods will cease after the operation, and for some this brings great relief. A women may also find that her sex life is enhanced as her general health improves and she no longer fears an unwanted pregnancy.

WHY IT IS DONE

If a woman has cancer of the uterus or cervix, a hysterectomy may be necessary to save her life. But most hysterectomies are performed to correct persistent pain caused by, for example, severe menstrual problems or pelvic inflammatory disease (chronic salpingitis).

Very painful or exceptionally heavy periods can be caused by **fibroids** – benign growths on the wall of the uterus. These can sometimes be removed individually, but this is not always successful since fibroids have a tendency to recur. Your doctor may suggest that a hysterectomy is the only option that will alleviate the problem permanently.

Another cause of painful or heavy periods is severe **endometriosis**, when bits of the uterine lining – or endometrium – migrate out of the uterus and become embedded in other

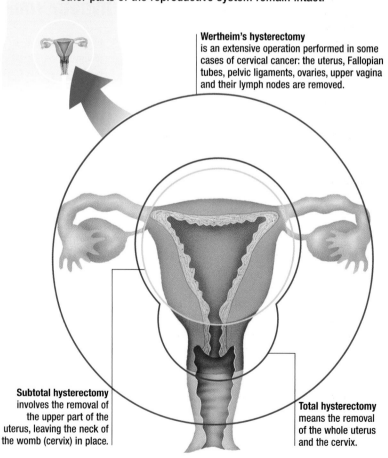

Types of hysterectomy
All types of hysterectomy involve the surgical removal of most or all of the uterus, but depending on the reason for the operation, other parts of the reproductive system remain intact.

Wertheim's hysterectomy
is an extensive operation performed in some cases of cervical cancer: the uterus, Fallopian tubes, pelvic ligaments, ovaries, upper vagina and their lymph nodes are removed.

Subtotal hysterectomy
involves the removal of the upper part of the uterus, leaving the neck of the womb (cervix) in place.

Total hysterectomy
means the removal of the whole uterus and the cervix.

Alternatives to hysterectomy

If a woman suffers from severe menstrual bleeding or pain caused by endometriosis or fibroids, she may prefer a less drastic solution to the problem than a hysterectomy.

The intrauterine system If a woman has endometriosis, she may benefit from a contraceptive device that releases tiny quantities of the hormone progestogen into the uterus. The insertion of the device can be performed as an out-patient operation. Mirena is the only version currently licensed in the UK (see **Contraception**). After a few months, the woman's periods will become light or cease altogether, thereby removing the source of pain and heavy bleeding.

Uterine artery embolization A technique that allows for possible pregnancy in the future is uterine artery embolization. This procedure blocks the blood supply to a fibroid causing the fibroid to degenerate and eventually to form scar tissue.

Myomectomy It may be possible to relieve menstrual problems caused by fibroids by undergoing a surgical procedure known as a myomectomy. This is an operation to remove any fibroids but leave the uterus intact. If there are a lot of fibroids, a myomectomy may not be effective. The advantage of the procedure is that it does not rule out later pregnancy.

Endometrial ablation In some cases, the only really effective treatment for endometriosis is to perform an endometrial ablation, a procedure to remove the lining of the uterus (endometrium). This can be carried out under a local **anaesthetic**. The operation causes periods to become light or to stop altogether and pregnancy is not possible afterwards.

---

abdominal tissues. If endometriosis does not respond to drug treatment or the surgical removal of any cysts caused by the condition, your doctor may recommend a hysterectomy. Fibroids and endometriosis cause no further problems after the menopause.

A hysterectomy may also be necessary to deal with a prolapse, when the uterus drops out of position because the ligaments that hold the uterus, bladder and rectum have become overstretched. In severe cases of prolapse the uterus descends into the vagina.

WHAT'S INVOLVED?

A hysterectomy is carried out under a general **anaesthetic**. The uterus is usually removed through an incision in the abdomen, but sometimes it is removed through the vagina. A vaginal hysterectomy is not possible if the uterus is very large or if it is affected by adhesions, and in some cases of cancer and endometriosis.

Keyhole hysterectomy, in which only a small incision is made, may be possible. This type of surgery means that recovery is faster and scarring is reduced, but a specially trained surgeon and specialist equipment are needed.

In premenopausal women, healthy ovaries are usually left in place, since removing them will bring on menopausal symptoms such as hot flushes and dryness of the vagina, and will increase the risk of developing cardiovascular disease and **osteoporosis**. Even if the ovaries are left in place, the menopause sometimes starts prematurely. **Hormone replacement therapy** (HRT) is therefore recommended for premenopausal women if their ovaries are removed or if they develop symptoms of the menopause at a younger age than expected with their ovaries in place.

AFTER THE OPERATION

Following a hysterectomy, a woman will usually need to spend up to a week in hospital; after keyhole surgery, she may be discharged after a day or so. Convalescence takes about six weeks. The lower abdomen will be sore while the muscle tissue heals, and there will be vaginal bleeding and discharge for a few days as the internal wounds heal. After the operation, it is inadvisable to lift anything heavy, to have sex, or to drive for a month or so, to avoid straining the abdominal muscles.

SEE ALSO *Cervix and disorders; Menstruation; Uterus and problems*

Hysteria

Hysteria is an outdated term, rarely used by health professionals today, for an emotional or anxious state in which the body develops problems without any physical cause. The word comes from the Ancient Greek word *hustera* meaning womb, as in the past a diagnosis of hysteria was given – usually by male doctors – to women whose emotions appeared to be out of control. Nowadays, the words **anxiety, panic** or **stress** are more likely to be used.

If someone has lost control of their emotions, and appears to be unaware of what is being said, speak to them in a calming voice, giving reassurance that the attack will pass. For people prone to anxiety and panic, it can be helpful to learn relaxation and breathing techniques.

SEE ALSO *Neurosis*

Idiopathic

The term 'idiopathic' is a medical label that is used when there is no known cause or origin for a condition. If, for example, a person went to the doctor with a set of symptoms that could not readily be diagnosed, that person might be sent for tests. Once all possible causes of the symptoms had been tested for and ruled out, the patient's condition would, as a last resort, be termed idiopathic, meaning that no certain diagnosis was established. It is really a shorthand way of saying that – in this instance – the doctors are uncertain about the cause.

Ileitis

Ileitis is an inflammation of the ileum, the lower portion of the small intestine. Its occurrence is relatively rare. The most common form is **Crohn's disease**, the cause of which is unknown. But some forms of ileitis may result from an abnormal reaction to an irritant, such as a bacterial infection.

Symptoms include abdominal pain, fever, loss of appetite, **anaemia**, constipation and diarrhoea. The problem may occur at any age, but young adults and elderly people are most likely to be affected. Some sufferers have only one or a few attacks, but others may have many. Treatment may include anti-inflammatory medication, special diets, and in cases where the intestine has become obstructed surgery may be necessary.

SEE ALSO *Bowel and disorders; Digestive system*

Ileostomy

An ileostomy is the removal of a part of the ileum, the lowest part of the small intestine. It is performed in the treatment of disorders such as **Crohn's disease**, polyposis of the colon and ulcerative colitis.

In a standard ileostomy operation, the ileum is connected to an artificial opening, known as a stoma, in the abdomen and a pouch is fitted to the stoma to collect liquid faeces. More often, a continent ileostomy is performed. In this procedure the remaining ileum is made into an internal pouch and drained through a valve.

In some patients who do not have Crohn's disease, another procedure – an ileorectal anastamosis operation – is carried out. This involves linking the ileum to the rectum, allowing a patient to pass loose stools normally through the anus.

SEE ALSO *Bowel and disorders; Colostomy*

Immunization

SEE OPPOSITE

Immunoglobulin

An immunoglobulin is an antibody that initiates the destruction of invading micro-organisms. There are five types of immunoglobulin, each with a distinct role. For example, IgG or Immunoglobulin G, destroys micro-organisms in the blood while IgA protects mucous membranes in the lungs and intestines. IgE is associated with allergic reactions in which histamine is released in previously sensitized people (see **Allergies**). Immunoglobulin injections are sometimes given to prevent or to treat infectious diseases. They are also given to people with immunodeficiency disorders.

SEE ALSO *Infectious diseases*

Impetigo

Impetigo is a highly contagious **skin** infection. It often appears around the nose and mouth, but can affect any area of the body. It is common in children, and more likely in warm weather.

SYMPTOMS

Infection causes the skin to redden, and small, fluid-filled blisters to appear. These break down, weep and then dry to form a characteristic golden-yellow crust.

CAUSES

Impetigo is caused by certain strains of a common skin bacteria, *Staphylococcus aureus*, which lives naturally in the noses of around one in three of the population. It enters broken skin through cuts, **cold sores** or **eczema**.

TREATMENT

The infection spreads very fast, so you should see a doctor as soon as symptoms appear. Antibiotics will be prescribed, to be taken orally or applied as an ointment. With treatment, impetigo should clear up in about five days.

Complementary therapies

Mild cases can be treated by applying tea tree essential oil regularly to the sores. When taking antibiotics, it is helpful to eat live bio yoghurt to promote healthy bacterial growth in the intestines. You could also take the **herbal medicine** echinacea to boost general immunity.

PREVENTION

Infection is passed on easily among family members and in schools; always keep infected children at home until symptoms disappear. Anyone infected should avoid sharing cups, face flannels and towels until symptoms have gone.

Immunization

Immunization is a technique for preventing certain infectious diseases. It involves deliberately exposing the body to a small dose of the disease, thereby equipping the immune system to destroy it at the next encounter.

People can develop a natural immunity after initial exposure to an infectious disease. The term 'immunization' describes the act of deliberately inducing immunity to prevent a specific disease from developing. There are two forms of immunization: active and passive.

In active immunization, more commonly known as vaccination, disease-causing micro-organisms are introduced into the body. The immune system identifies the micro-organisms as foreign and produces antibodies – specialized proteins that destroy them. The immune system retains a long-term memory of the micro-organisms and is able to produce antibodies again if they reappear.

Antibodies take time to develop after active immunization. For example, the **BCG vaccine** against **tuberculosis** only becomes effective ten weeks after it has entered the body, but it will then give long-lasting immunity.

In passive immunization, an immune serum is prepared from blood taken from someone who has been exposed to a disease and developed antibodies to it. The serum is used to inoculate other people who are at risk from developing the disease. Passive immunization gives immediate but short-term immunity, as the antibodies in the serum will only destroy the disease-producing viruses or bacteria that invade the body in the few weeks after vaccination. It is used to give protection when there is a danger of contracting a disease but no time for active immunization – for example, when someone is about to travel to a country where diseases such as rabies, tetanus and hepatitis B are prevalent.

Passive immunization also occurs naturally when antibodies in a mother's blood and breast milk give a baby temporary immunity.

Active immunization
Active immunization prompts the body to make its own antibodies against disease-causing bacteria and viruses.

1 Vaccination. The person is injected with disease-causing micro-organisms.

2 The immune system identifies the micro-organisms as foreign and produces antibodies against them.

3 The immune system remembers the micro-organism and can act fast if it encounters it again.

4 The antibodies take time to develop but they then give long-lasting immunity.

HOW IMMUNIZATION IS CARRIED OUT

Adult immunizations tend to be given by injection into a muscle or tissue beneath the skin of the upper arm. If there is a large volume of liquid, it may be injected into a buttock. Babies are usually injected in the thigh. Some types of vaccination can also be given orally; the polio vaccine, for example, is given on a lump of sugar.

How long do vaccines last?
Not all vaccines last forever. The **rubella** vaccine seems to give protection for life but the BCG vaccine protects for about 15 years and tetanus needs a booster every ten years.

The **cholera** vaccine given by injection is effective for only 12 weeks and the strains of **influenza** in circulation change so rapidly, that a new influenza vaccine has to be prepared every year to match the strains that are currently circulating.

The effectiveness of a vaccine depends on how well it stimulates the immune system to respond, and this may vary according to the way in which vaccines are prepared. It is possible to develop a disease after immunization but it is in a mild form.

POSSIBLE SIDE EFFECTS

Some vaccines, such as those for influenza, are commonly grown in cell cultures from hen's eggs; these cause reactions in people who are allergic to eggs. Some people are allergic to traces of antibiotics or chemicals in the vaccine. But side effects are usually mild and last for only a day or two. Symptoms may include tenderness and swelling at the site of the injection (in rare cases there may be abscesses and swollen glands), a fever, a rash, loss of appetite, nausea and vomiting, or lethargy and drowsiness.

You should contact a doctor if there is a marked rise in temperature, or if the person faints or has convulsions. If your baby seems ill or does not respond to you normally after having an immunization, call NHS Direct or go to your doctor's surgery.

IS IMMUNIZATION SAFE?

Some vaccines can produce serious complications. Immunization with the live polio vaccine can cause paralysis, for example. However, this is extremely rare – one in 2.5 million doses. Many parents fear DTP (**diphtheria**, tetanus, pertussis) and MMR (**measles, mumps**, rubella) because, in very rare cases, these combination vaccines for children can damage the nervous system. Some researchers have also linked the MMR vaccine to **autism** and inflammatory bowel disease, but all the evidence overwhelmingly refutes this.

Many parents become far more worried about the side effects of the vaccines than about the diseases they might protect their children from.

Childhood immunization schedule

The UK schedule for childhood immunization, shown here, changes from time to time, reflecting new developments in medical knowledge about immunization.

AGE	VACCINE
2 months	1st DTP (diphtheria, tetanus, pertussis/whooping cough), HIB (*Haemophilus influenzae* type B), polio, meningitis C
3 months	2nd DTP (diphtheria, tetanus, pertussis), HIB (*Haemophilus influenzae* type B), polio, meningitis C
4 months	3rd DTP (diphtheria, tetanus, pertussis), HIB (*Haemophilus influenzae* type B), polio, meningitis C
12–15 months	MMR (measles, mumps, rubella)
pre-school, 4–5 years	DTP booster, MMR booster, polio booster
10–14 years	BCG (tuberculosis) – skin test followed by one injection
16–18 years	Diphtheria and tetanus booster, polio booster

Immunization facts

Some immunizations are designed to protect whole populations and are aimed mainly at young children. Others protect people who may be at risk of exposure to unusual infections.

■ Pregnant women can safely have vaccines against tetanus and pneumococcal infection, and the HIB vaccination against meningitis, but TB, polio, measles, rubella, yellow fever, diphtheria and typhoid vaccinations can affect a fetus and should not be given.

■ Children should not be vaccinated if they have a fever.

■ Anyone with an immune-suppressing illness, for example, cancer or AIDS, should not be given a vaccine containing live micro-organisms such as that for yellow fever.

■ Plague, diphtheria, measles, cholera, typhoid and other deadly infectious diseases are endemic in many poorer countries. For advice on vaccination if you are travelling to such countries, see **Travel and tropical diseases**.

Doctors are anxious to point out the fact that the risk of serious complications in connection with the vaccines is very low compared to the risk if the child actually falls ill with one of the diseases. They warn parents that increasing numbers of unvaccinated children will inevitably lead to more of them catching that disease. Nevertheless, parents do need up-to-date information on which to base their decision.

THE FUTURE OF IMMUNIZATION

The resistance of diseases such as tuberculosis to antibiotics and the emergence of new infectious diseases such as AIDS has spurred research into immunization. Over 20 vaccines are currently being developed against infections such as **chlamydia**, tonsillitis, stomach **ulcers, gonorrhoea**, and the dengue fever virus, as well as cancers. Scientists are currently looking at ways to treat breast and prostate cancer by boosting an immunity to cancer cells.

In the future, vaccinations may be available to prevent diseases such as **malaria**, Alzheimer's disease, cancer-causing viruses and AIDS.

SEE ALSO *Infectious diseases; Travel and tropical diseases*

Impotence

Impotence – also called erectile dysfunction – is a condition in which a man is unable to attain or maintain an erection sufficient for satisfactory sexual activity.

The official estimate is that impotence affects about one in ten men in the UK at any one time. But some surveys have put it as high as one in four. The incidence of impotence increases with age: about one in 13 men aged under 30 years is affected compared with one in two men over 70.

CAUSES

It is important to see a doctor promptly in cases of erectile dysfunction as it is not, as many people believe, all in the mind. Three-quarters of cases have a physical component, some of which are very serious. Erectile dysfunction can be an early-warning sign of another disease or health problem including:

- heart disease;
- narrow arteries;
- high blood pressure;
- **diabetes**;
- Peyronie's disease, which causes the penis to bend at an angle during erection;
- **multiple sclerosis**;
- an injury to the pelvis or spinal cord;
- heavy drinking or smoking;
- drugs – either the side effects of prescribed drugs (for example, antihypertensive, antipsychotic and antidepressant drugs) or the abuse of non-prescribed drugs. In general, any drug that disrupts the blood flow to the penis may cause impotence.
- very rarely, low testosterone level.

TREATMENT

Research suggests that men do not seek help with erectile dysfunction because they think it cannot be treated. This is not true. In most cases treating the underlying cause will help. There are also specific erectile dysfunction treatments.

- Oral drugs – two drugs are licensed for the treatment of erectile dysfunction. One is a tablet taken one hour before sexual activity, the other is a tablet taken under the tongue 20 minutes before sexual activity. Both drugs are effective and do not cause an erection unless the man is sexually stimulated.
- Local applications – drugs may be injected into the base of the penis, or inserted as a small pellet, the size of a rice grain, into the urethra.
- Vacuum therapy – an erection is created using a vacuum pump.
- Penile implant – this is a mechanical device inserted into the erection chambers of the penis via surgery.
- Penile rings – these are helpful if an erection cannot be maintained.
- Testosterone patch – in cases where low testosterone levels are responsible for erectile dysfunction, a patch applied to the thigh and worn all the time will restore hormone levels.
- Sex therapy – there are sometimes major psychological or relationship issues that need to be addressed. Sex therapy aims to enhance the patient's sexual confidence and is particularly useful in cases of erectile dysfunction that are not found to have a physical cause.

Complementary therapies

- Some people advocate using aphrodisiacs for treating erectile dysfunction, but most doctors are sceptical about their effectiveness. The Brazilian bark catuaba, as well as ginger, ginkgo biloba, ginseng, and the South American herb *Muira Puama* ('potency wood') all have their advocates. Another oral treatment that is not licensed is yohimbine. It is derived from the bark of an African tree and several studies have suggested it helps to enhance erectile function.
- If stress or anxiety is part of the problem, aromatherapy, massage or other relaxing therapy will help.

Truths about impotence

Many men do not understand why they are impotent – and may feel too embarrassed to seek help. A doctor can usually identify the cause and recommend an effective treatment.

Impotence increases with age.
Impotence is associated with advancing age, as well as with a range of conditions including medication, obesity, coronary artery disease, high blood pressure and diabetes mellitus.

Smoking causes impotence.
Nicotine interferes with the blood's circulation including the flow of blood to the penis necessary to produce an erection. Smokers are 50–80 per cent more likely to become impotent than non-smokers.

Worrying about impotence contributes to it.
Impotence is purely psychological in only one in five cases but, in all cases, worrying about sexual performance can make it worse. Anxiety contracts the muscles and prevents blood entering the penis.

Relationship problems cause impotence.
If you can get an erection at night or when masturbating but not with your partner, you are not impotent. Your relationship problems are the most likely cause of erectile dysfunction.

COMPLICATIONS

Erectile dysfunction can have a major impact on the self-esteem of sufferers, especially on men who otherwise have a positive attitude to themselves. The condition often harms relationships. In one survey, one in five men felt that erectile dysfunction had led to the breakdown of his relationship. Prompt treatment is advisable even if the causes are believed to be purely psychological.

OUTLOOK

Very good. Virtually all cases of erectile dysfunction can be treated.

SEE ALSO *Penis and disorders*

Incontinence

Incontinence is an uncontrollable and involuntary passing of urine or faeces. About 3 million people in the UK suffer from urinary incontinence. As a person ages, the muscle surrounding the bladder opening becomes less efficient, making urinary incontinence more likely. The muscle also takes a battering during pregnancy and childbirth, so older women who have had children are particularly prone to leakage – especially when they cough or sneeze.

Any form of incontinence can be emotionally distressing, and lead to soreness and infection.

SYMPTOMS

There are four types of urinary incontinence and each type has different symptoms.

■ Stress incontinence is the release of small amounts of urine during coughing, laughter or physical exertion.

■ Urge incontinence is a desperate need to pass urine accompanied by the involuntary and uncontrollable emptying of the bladder.

■ Overflow incontinence causes intermittent dribbling. This happens when a person's bladder is always full as a result of an obstruction such as an enlarged prostate gland.

■ Total incontinence is rare, involving total loss of control due to a nervous system disorder.

■ Faecal incontinence often takes the form either of uncontrolled **diarrhoea**, or the passing of small lumps of faeces and faecal fluid.

CAUSES

The main cause of urinary stress incontinence is weak pelvic floor muscles. This can be the result of childbirth, or muscle thinning and loss of tone due to the **menopause**. Other causes of urinary incontinence include a prolapsed womb (uterus), an overactive bladder, a urinary infection such as **cystitis**, bladder stones, a bladder tumour and prostate enlargement. Sometimes incontinence is caused by spinal cord injuries or defects – such as **spina bifida**.

A **stroke** can also interfere with nervous control by the brain and result in **bedwetting**.

Faecal incontinence may be the result of an extremely severe stomach upset. It can also happen as a side effect of **constipation**: a newly toilet-trained child or an elderly person can become so constipated that the rectum becomes inflamed and faecal fluids and solid matter are passed involuntarily. Other causes include defects in the tone of the anal sphincter, **dementia** and **paraplegia**.

TREATMENT

The most helpful thing you can do for urinary stress incontinence is to exercise your pelvic floor. This involves squeezing and holding the pelvic floor muscles for several seconds at a time – as if you were stopping the flow of urine mid-stream. Other helpful measures might include going to the toilet only when the bladder feels full, and trying to keep your weight down as this puts a lot of pressure on the bladder muscles. Cutting out caffeinated drinks such as tea and coffee may also help.

The best remedy for faecal incontinence caused by impacted faeces is a high-fibre diet. Eating plenty of fresh fruit and vegetables and whole grain foods will help to prevent the constipation that causes the condition.

What a doctor may do

Your doctor can arrange tests to discover what is causing the incontinence. If you have urinary incontinence, a sample of your urine will be tested to make sure that there is no infection, that your bladder is not inflamed, and that you do not have undiagnosed **diabetes** mellitus. Other tests may include **ultrasound**, **X-ray** and cystoscopy, in which the bladder is viewed through an instrument inserted via the urethra.

Drugs can be prescribed for conditions such as cystitis that irritate the bladder, or your doctor may recommend an operation to tighten the muscles around the urethra. **Hormone replacement therapy** (HRT) can help women whose problem has been caused by the menopause. Bedwetting may be eased by using desmopressin, an inhaled drug that temporarily switches off urine production at night. An enlarged **prostate** gland can be corrected with drugs to relax the bladder or shrink the gland, or by surgery.

Where it is not possible to restore normal bladder function, the sufferer can wear incontinence pants with special disposable pads to absorb the urine. Some people prefer to learn self-catheterization, which involves inserting a sterile tube via the urethra into the bladder in order to empty it four or five times a day. A man can wear a penile sheath connected by a tube to a portable urine bag.

If you suffer from faecal incontinence, you may simply need treatment for constipation or diarrhoea. If the problem is caused by poor muscle tone, a psychological technique called biofeedback may help you to regain control. In a person with dementia or a nervous disease, the problem might be tackled with laxatives and **enemas**.

SEE ALSO *Bladder and disorders; Bowel and disorders; Pelvis and disorders; Urinary system*

Indigestion

Indigestion is also known as dyspepsia or an upset stomach. It is a common problem, involving chronic or recurrent pain or discomfort centred in the upper abdomen. Feelings of fullness, nausea, vomiting or bloating are often also present. Indigestion is rarely serious unless it is accompanied by other symptoms. Between 25 and 40 per cent of all people in the UK are regularly affected by it.

Indigestion is not the same thing as gastro-oesophageal reflux, although both can cause **heartburn** and acid regurgitation.

CAUSES

- Eating too much or too quickly, eating fatty foods or eating during stressful situations.
- Smoking.
- Drinking too much coffee or alcohol.
- Using medications that irritate the stomach lining, such as non-steroidal anti-inflammatory drugs (NSAIDs).
- Being tired and suffering from ongoing stress.
- A disease or a peptic **ulcer** affecting the digestive tract.

Some people have persistent indigestion that is not directly related to any of these factors. Called functional or non-ulcer indigestion, it may accompany **irritable bowel syndrome** (IBS). *Helicobacter pylori* **gastritis** is detected in about half of patients who are suffering from functional indigestion.

Indigestion with heartburn is very common in late **pregnancy** when the womb moves up and presses against the stomach. Pregnant women are advised to eat small meals at more frequent intervals, and to avoid typical triggers such as spicy food.

TREATMENT

Indigestion can be uncomfortable but, generally speaking, it is nothing to worry about.

When to consult a doctor

Occasionally indigestion can mimic or be a sign of a more serious disease. It is a good idea to see your doctor if you have:

Indigestion dos and don'ts

There are several things you can do to minimize the frequency of indigestion attacks.

Do

✔ Alter your diet by cutting out high-fat foods and avoiding those you know trigger your symptoms.

✔ Eat balanced meals at regular times.

Don't

✘ Smoke.

✘ Overuse anti-inflammatory drugs.

✘ Allow stressful situations to upset you.

✘ Drink large amounts of coffee or alcohol.

✘ Rush your meals or eat too much.

- vomiting, weight loss or appetite loss;
- black, tarry stools or blood in vomit;
- severe pain in the upper right abdomen;
- abdominal discomfort that is unrelated to eating;
- indigestion accompanied by shortness of breath, sweating or pain radiating to the jaw, neck or arm.

What a doctor may do

Persistent indigestion sometimes indicates a more serious underlying complaint, such as gallstones (see **Gallbladder and disorders**). Depending on your symptoms, a doctor may arrange for further investigation such as:

- an **endoscopy** – a slim, flexible fibre-optic device is passed down the throat and into the stomach, allowing the doctor to examine the lining of the gut;
- a **barium investigation** – the patient drinks a liquid that causes the outline of the stomach to show up on an X-ray;
- an **ultrasound** scan – a technique using reflected soundwaves to show the structure of the abdominal organs;
- a blood test – to detect **anaemia** or any other abnormality.

Drug treatment

Antacids can help to ease bouts of indigestion but they may inhibit the action of some drugs: if you are on medication, consult your doctor before taking over-the-counter antacids.

Research has shown that antacids are no more effective than taking a placebo in the treatment of functional indigestion. In such cases, your doctor may prescribe an alternative drug. However, drugs do not always help the condition.

SEE ALSO *Digestive system*

Infectious diseases

An infection occurs when harmful organisms such as bacteria, viruses, fungi or parasites invade the body. These cause infectious diseases, which may be passed from one person to another as the organisms spread.

Infectious diseases – which cause more than 50 per cent of deaths throughout the world – come in many forms, ranging from the common **cold** to HIV. Many can be passed from one person to another – as distinct from, say, cancer, which cannot be contracted from proximity to a cancer sufferer.

TYPES OF INFECTION
Bacteria and viruses are too small to be seen by the naked eye. Most bacteria are harmless, but some cause diseases – diphtheria, tetanus and botulism, for example. Whereas bacteria grow both inside and outside the human body, viruses can multiply only by invading a host cell within the human body. Viruses cause many infectious diseases, including the common cold, **influenza** (flu), chickenpox, **herpes** and **AIDS**.

Parasitic diseases are caused by parasites, which are organisms that live in human intestines and blood or on the skin. These diseases mostly occur in tropical climates, though infection with parasitic worms is common and is believed to affect more than 2 billion people worldwide.

Fungal infections are caused by fungi, micro-organisms that exist naturally on the skin and in the mouth but can cause problems in certain conditions. Warmth, moisture, irritation and chafing of the skin all help fungi to proliferate, and this can give rise to diseases. The skin, nails and genitals are most commonly affected, but, in rare cases, the lungs and other organs may be susceptible. Fungal infections are often mild, such as **athlete's foot**, which causes minor if persistent irritation in affected areas of skin. But infections can be severe in people whose immune system is seriously impaired – for example, those undergoing **chemotherapy**.

HOW INFECTIONS ARE SPREAD
Bacterial and virus infections may be transmitted by direct human contact, such as touching someone's hands when they have bacteria or a virus on them, or in airborne droplets that are released when an infected person coughs or sneezes. Consuming infected food or drink is another method of transmission. Some types of bacteria are transmitted primarily by sexual intercourse – for example, **chlamydia**, which causes a woman's Fallopian tubes or cervix to become inflamed.

Strictly speaking, diseases that can only be passed on by direct or indirect contact with another person are called contagious diseases, for example **gonorrhea** or flu. Diseases that can be spread without the need for any form of human contact – although they may be passed from person to person – are described as infectious, for example, **Legionnaire's disease** and pulmonary **anthrax**. However, in everyday speech 'contagious' and 'infectious' are often used interchangeably.

Fungal infections are spread by skin contact with an infected person, or by using an infected towel, or by walking on an infected floor and so on. They can also be transmitted by fungi present in drinking water or in any soil left on vegetables that have not been cleaned thoroughly.

Virus infections – colds and flu

Colds and flu are the most common viral infections in human beings. There are more than 200 viruses that can cause a cold, the most common of which is the rhinovirus. Most adults catch two to four cold-like illnesses each year.

The common cold and flu viruses attack the mucous membranes that line the respiratory tract. Infection is usually mild and temporary, but secondary infections can develop in the throat, ears or sinuses. These may be serious and require treatment, usually with antibiotics.

Many different viral infections produce flu-like symptoms but only three separate types of flu virus have been identified – types A, B and C. Type A flu is the most widespread. It infects both animals and human beings, and accounts for two-thirds of all flu cases. It is also the type that causes major pandemics (international epidemics). Type B is less severe and infects only human beings. Type C is milder. The flu virus also has the ability to change its structure and produce new strains to which few people have immunity.

Parasitic worms, such as hookworms and schistosomes, are spread through soil and can enter the intestine in infected food or water.

Some diseases are transmitted by animals or insects that are not themselves suffering from the disease. The animals or insects are then known as vectors. Insect vectors are responsible, for example, for the transmission of **malaria, yellow fever** and sleeping sickness.

TREATING INFECTION

Bacterial infections are treated by antibiotics, drugs that kill the disease-causing bacteria. To determine the type of bacteria involved, a doctor may perform a blood or urine test or take a swab or sample from the site of a bacterial infection.

Penicillin is used to treat certain types of bacterial infection. It is a member of a large group of antibiotics that includes ampicillin and amoxicillin. Another large group of antibiotics is the cephalosporins, which include cefaclor, cefalexin and cefuroxime. Some patients suffer from an allergic reaction to penicillin and cephalosporins. This is characterized by rashes, swelling and contraction of the airways. The heart rate may also increase and blood pressure may fall. In extreme cases, the allergic reaction can cause death. Doctors can use a skin test to detect the allergy, but this is not done routinely.

Antibiotics are used to treat many parasitic infections as well as bacterial infections. The full course of treatment must always be completed.

Antiviral drugs are effective against some viral infections, and many viruses are controlled by vaccines. There are vaccines against most virus diseases. These cause the virus to have less effect on the body when the person becomes infected. If you have a mild virus infection, the doctor will often treat the symptoms rather than the virus.

Fungal infections of the skin can be treated with tablets and creams. Tablets usually include the drug griseofulvin, and creams include imidazole.

LIFE-THREATENING INFECTIONS

Infectious diseases that are rife in some parts of the world can cause very serious illness and in some cases death, if they are not treated promptly. These include cholera, Q fever, cytomegalovirus (CMV) and tuberculosis.

Cholera

Cholera is an acute intestinal infection, which is caused by the *Vibrio cholerae* organism. It occurs mainly in developing countries and is contracted from contaminated food or water. Sufferers lose large amounts of fluid through diarrhoea and vomiting, which can cause severe dehydration and sometimes lead to death. It is important to make sure that you are vaccinated against cholera before you travel to any tropical country.

Q fever

Q fever is an infectious disease that affects animals. It is caused by a species of bacteria called *Coxiella burnetii*, which is excreted in the urine, milk, faeces and birth fluids of cattle, sheep and goats. Human beings can contract the disease either from ticks or by inhaling the bacteria from air that is contaminated with dust from these excretions. Farm workers, laboratory workers and veterinary surgeons are most at risk from Q fever. A person with Q fever usually becomes ill within two weeks of infection and develops a severe flu-like illness. Symptoms include a high fever (40°C/104°F), severe headache, nausea, vomiting, diarrhoea, chest pain and a cough. Some people also develop **hepatitis**.

Most patients recover without treatment in a few months. However, if the infection persists for up to six months, the condition becomes chronic and is much more serious. Chronic Q fever can develop up to 20 years after infection and may result in inflammation of the lining of the heart and of the heart valves (**endocarditis**). Most people who develop chronic Q fever already have vascular heart disease, and others are transplant recipients, cancer patients or people with chronic kidney disease. Around 65 per cent of patients with chronic Q fever may die.

The diagnosis of Q fever involves carrying out a blood test to detect the presence of antibodies to *Coxiella burnetii*. The antibiotic oxycycline is used to treat acute Q fever, and doxycycline and hydroxychloroquine can be used to treat chronic Q fever for up to three years. Surgery may also be required to repair any resulting damage to the heart valves.

A vaccine for Q fever in human beings has been developed in Australia and there is also a vaccine for animals. Pasteurization of milk, removing animals from human contact and routine animal testing can minimize the spread of the disease.

Cytomegalovirus

Cytomegalovirus, the most common virus transmitted to a baby before birth, belongs to the **herpes** virus group. It is found in all countries, but is most prevalent in developing countries and among lower socio-economic groups. When cytomegalovirus is contracted after birth, there are few symptoms or complications in healthy people, although the virus lies dormant in the body for life and may revive if a person's immune system is compromised by other health problems.

Cytomegalovirus can result in death in patients whose immune system is weakened, including people with HIV or cancer, or organ transplant recipients. Cytomegalovirus is also a danger to an unborn child. If a woman is infected with the virus when pregnant, her child is at risk of

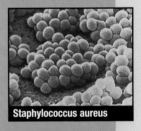
Staphylococcus aureus

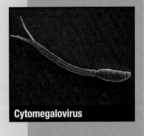
Cytomegalovirus

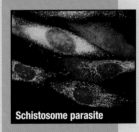
Schistosome parasite

Bacterial infections – Streptococci

Bacteria of the Streptococcus group cause many common diseases and disorders, from sore throats to meningitis. The bacteria are divided into groups A and B according to their characteristics.

Group A Streptococcus (GAS) is a bacterium that can be found on people's skin and in their throats, and often causes no signs of illness. Most GAS infections are mild and include 'strep throat' (a common throat infection) or the skin infection **impetigo**. The bacteria are spread through contact with the sores or mucus of infected people. People who carry the bacteria but who have no symptoms are not usually very contagious. Washing your hands can help prevent the disease spreading.

Severe or invasive GAS disease can occur if the bacterium gets into places where it is not usually found, such as the blood, muscles or lungs. People who use steroids or have chronic illnesses are particularly vulnerable to invasive GAS disease. One of the most serious forms of invasive GAS disease is **necrotizing fasciitis** (also known as cellulitis), an infection that destroys muscles, fat and skin. An infected wound combined with a fever can be a sign of the disease. GAS infections can be treated with a variety of antibiotics. In the case of necrotizing fasciitis, surgery may be required to remove the affected tissue.

Group B Streptococcal disease (GBS) is the most common cause of blood infections and pneumonia, as well as meningitis in newborn babies. Most cases in babies occur in the first week of life. One in 200 babies whose mothers carry GBS will develop symptoms and recover but one in 20 cases will be fatal. A woman can be tested for the disease during pregnancy by a swab of the vagina and rectum. If she tests positive, antibiotics can be given during labour. Some people carry GBS in the bowel, vagina, bladder or throat but do not become ill. Vaccines to prevent GBS are being developed.

being born with problems such as hearing loss, visual impairment and diminished mental and motor abilities.

Cytomegalovirus is transmitted in breast milk, saliva, urine and body fluids exchanged during sexual intercourse. It can also be passed on in organ transplants from an infected person. Infection is spread through intimate contact with an infected person and usually occurs when infected body fluids are absorbed through the nose or mouth, such as after handling nappies – so one way to guard against it is to wash your hands after changing a baby.

A doctor will suspect cytomegalovirus if a person shows signs of **hepatitis** but has negative test results for hepatitis A, B and C, or has symptoms of **glandular fever** (infectious mononucleosis) but has negative test results for both mononucleosis and the Epstein-Barr virus.

Legionnaire's disease
Legionnaire's disease is a bacterial infection, a form of **pneumonia** in which the lungs have become infected by the bacterium *Legionella pneumophila*. This bacterium thrives in places that are warm and moist, such as air-conditioning systems and water tanks, and outbreaks of the disease tend to occur in and around large public buildings.

Symptoms begin with headaches, fever and chills, and progress to pneumonia. As the disease develops, people find it increasingly difficult to breathe, because the air sacs in their lungs start to fill up with phlegm or fluid. If you develop any of these symptoms, you should visit the doctor, and do so urgently if you have been staying in a hotel where there has recently been an outbreak of Legionnaire's disease. The doctor will prescribe antibiotics for your infection, and in some cases hospital treatment may be required.

Erysipelas
Erysipelas is a serious infection of the skin and underlying fat tissues that occurs in the elderly, the very young and people whose immune systems have been damaged. It is caused by the *Streptococcus* bacterium (see box) entering the body through a scratch or leg ulcer or because a fungal infection has weakened the skin's normal defence mechanism. The infection appears as a red mark on the skin, localized at first but spreading within a few hours. Headache, chills and fever often accompany the rash. Antibiotics such as penicillin and erythromycin are usually given to treat the infection.

Tuberculosis
Tuberculosis (TB) is caused by the bacterium *Mycobacterium tuberculosis* and usually attacks the lungs. It is spread through the air from person to person. An infected person may not suffer any symptoms, but can develop the disease at a later date. If medication is taken when a person is first infected, the disease can be prevented from developing.

If the TB bacteria settle on the lungs and grow, the disease can move through the blood to other parts of the body and cause serious illness in anyone whose immune system is not fully functioning.

SEE ALSO *Bacterial infections; Fungal infections; Parasites and parasitic diseases; Travel and tropical diseases; Viral infections*

Infertility

Many people who have difficulty conceiving a child are often surprised to discover just how common fertility problems are. At least one in six couples in the UK will seek advice or treatment in order to start a family.

The desire to have a child is one of the most basic of all human instincts, and having a family is widely seen as a blessing. When something goes wrong, it is not surprising that many couples find it very difficult to accept. Sex can become a chore if it is being regulated by ovulation charts, and some men mistakenly believe that problems with their fertility indicate that they lack virility. In addition, although the treatment of infertility is improving all the time, it can be difficult and disappointing. Hormonal drugs may bring mood swings and a number of other unwanted side effects, and many couples find that, despite invasive tests and months of treatment, they still cannot conceive.

The World Health Organization defines infertility as the inability of a couple to achieve conception after a year or more of regular, unprotected sex. In those women who are still menstruating at the age of 50, the chance of becoming pregnant is just one in 20. Difficulties with conception are caused by problems with the woman's reproductive system in one-third of cases, infertility in the man in another third, and a combination of factors from both partners in the remaining third of cases.

> If 100 women under the age of 35 have regular, unprotected sex for a year, as many as 20 will fail to become pregnant.

FEMALE FERTILITY

When a baby girl is born, her ovaries already hold more than two million eggs, each of which has the potential to grow into a baby. At puberty, a surge of hormones stimulates rapid sexual development, the **ovaries** begin to function and the monthly menstrual cycle begins.

The **pituitary gland** produces two hormones, luteinizing hormone (LH) and follicle-stimulating hormone (FSH), which regulate ovulation and trigger a process by which follicles develop around some of the dormant eggs. One of these follicles grows more rapidly than the others and then ruptures, releasing an egg into the Fallopian tube. This is known as ovulation. Theoretically, if a woman is menstruating, conception is possible, but in reality there are only a few days in each menstrual cycle – just after ovulation – when conception is likely to occur. During a woman's reproductive life, only about 400–500 of her eggs are released and the longer eggs remain in the ovary, the more likely they are to deteriorate, with the result that fertility declines with age.

MALE FERTILITY

Men become sexually mature in their early teens, when a surge of the hormone testosterone stimulates rapid development and the testes begin to produce sperm. Unlike fertility in women, male fertility is not governed by a reproductive cycle. Men produce sperm constantly – around 125 million sperm a day – and in theory are capable of fathering a child at any time. But a number of factors, including alcohol consumption or poor nutrition, can affect the number of these sperm, their ability to move (motility) and their structure. Problems can include sperm with malformed tails or sperm that stick together.

Men have been known to father children in their 80s, but, like women, their fertility declines with age. On average, most men experience some drop in fertility from the age of 50.

FACTORS THAT AFFECT FEMALE FERTILITY

The complex nature of the female reproductive system means that many things can go wrong.
- If, for any reason, ovulation does not occur, there is no egg to fertilize.
- If the Fallopian tubes are blocked or damaged, sperm may not be able to reach an egg.
- Problems with the lining of the uterus can prevent a fertilized egg from attaching itself.
- Insufficient lubricating mucus around the cervix can prevent sperm from penetrating the uterus.

Disrupted ovulation

There are several reasons why a woman may not ovulate. The main ones are:
- polycystic ovary syndrome, caused by hormone imbalances. This condition is characterized by scanty or non-existent periods. Drugs such as clomifene can be given to increase egg production and stimulate ovulation. Low levels of follicle stimulating hormone are treated with injections of an ovarian stimulant called gonadatrophin;
- a previous ectopic pregnancy (see also **Ovaries and disorders**);
- being very underweight. Eating disorders tend to stop menstruation. To ensure ovulation, 25 per cent of a woman's bodyweight should consist of

fat – a body mass index of 23–24 is ideal for fertility. Extreme fitness training can also interfere with the menstrual cycle;

■ premature **menopause** may also be a cause of lack of ovulation.

When sperm cannot reach the egg

Sometimes a woman is ovulating successfully but her partner's sperm is unable to reach the egg. One of the most common reasons for this is blocked Fallopian tubes. The Fallopian tubes are very narrow and easily damaged by sexually transmitted infections such as **chlamydia**. This disease is symptom-free but, if left untreated, it can lead to pelvic inflammatory disease, or PID, which affects a woman's reproductive organs, scarring the Fallopian tubes. PID is responsible for one third of cases of female infertility. However, some tubal blockages can be repaired with microsurgery. (See also **Pelvis and disorders**.)

The Fallopian tubes and ovaries can also be damaged by **endometriosis**. This is a condition in which tissue similar to the womb lining is growing outside the womb. Endometriosis can be corrected with **laser** treatment or hormonal drugs such as gonadorelin.

The sperm may also be hindered by a woman's cervical mucus. Normally, mucus within the cervical canal acts as a holding reservoir for sperm and increases the likelihood of fertilization. Sometimes, the mucus is excessively alkaline or acidic, making it an inhospitable medium for sperm. In some women, the mucus contains antibodies that attack sperm. If tests show that female antibodies are destroying sperm, corticosteroids can be given to suppress this reaction. Sometimes there is not enough cervical mucus. This can occur when a woman has had part of her cervix removed for testing in a cone **biopsy** – in which a cone-shaped section of the cervix is surgically removed for testing – or if she has had repeated treatment for cervical abnormalities.

If fertility appears to be impaired by problems with cervical mucus, artificial insemination may be the best option.

Problems with the womb

In some cases, a woman ovulates normally and sperm reaches the egg, but the fertilized egg does not attach to the lining of the uterus. This can happen because of the presence of non-cancerous growths called **fibroids**, endometriosis, scarring as a result of infection, hormonal imbalances and congenital abnormalities.

About one in five women has what is known as a retroverted uterus. This means that the uterus tilts backwards instead of forwards. People used to believe that this condition might inhibit fertility, but there is no evidence to support this theory.

Female reproductive problems

Because the female reproductive system is neatly tucked away inside the body, damage by symptomless infections, such as chlamydia, can go unnoticed until a woman experiences difficulty getting pregnant.

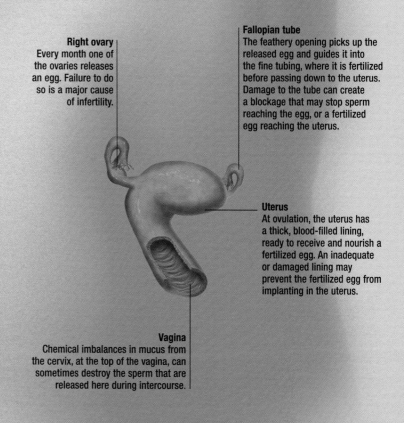

Right ovary
Every month one of the ovaries releases an egg. Failure to do so is a major cause of infertility.

Fallopian tube
The feathery opening picks up the released egg and guides it into the fine tubing, where it is fertilized before passing down to the uterus. Damage to the tube can create a blockage that may stop sperm reaching the egg, or a fertilized egg reaching the uterus.

Uterus
At ovulation, the uterus has a thick, blood-filled lining, ready to receive and nourish a fertilized egg. An inadequate or damaged lining may prevent the fertilized egg from implanting in the uterus.

Vagina
Chemical imbalances in mucus from the cervix, at the top of the vagina, can sometimes destroy the sperm that are released here during intercourse.

FACTORS THAT AFFECT MALE FERTILITY

Male infertility can be caused by a low sperm count, sperm abnormalities that affect the ability of the sperm to swim towards an egg, low levels of testosterone and problems with ejaculation.

Low sperm count

Factors that are known to reduce sperm count include alcohol, smoking, some medicines, narcotic drugs and poor nutrition, although doctors cannot always pinpoint the cause. If the problem is caused by low levels of testosterone, this can be corrected by hormone injections. Sometimes a man with a low sperm count produces just a few healthy sperm. In such a case, a technique known as intracytoplasmic sperm injection, or ICSI, can be used to fertilize an egg (see below).

Male fertility, like female fertility, is regulated by the hypothalamus and pituitary gland, and problems with either can cause hormonal imbalances. Some chromosomal conditions and kidney failure can also impair sperm production.

For maximum sperm production, the testes should be a couple of degrees cooler than the rest of the body – hence their air-cooled design. Any

Male reproductive problems

It is often assumed that failure to conceive is due to the woman, but the difficulty is just as likely to be caused by problems with the man's reproductive system.

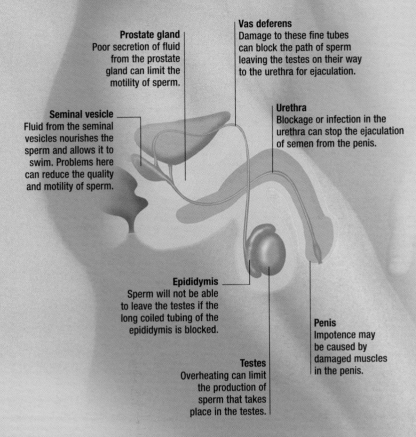

Prostate gland
Poor secretion of fluid from the prostate gland can limit the motility of sperm.

Vas deferens
Damage to these fine tubes can block the path of sperm leaving the testes on their way to the urethra for ejaculation.

Seminal vesicle
Fluid from the seminal vesicles nourishes the sperm and allows it to swim. Problems here can reduce the quality and motility of sperm.

Urethra
Blockage or infection in the urethra can stop the ejaculation of semen from the penis.

Epididymis
Sperm will not be able to leave the testes if the long coiled tubing of the epididymis is blocked.

Penis
Impotence may be caused by damaged muscles in the penis.

Testes
Overheating can limit the production of sperm that takes place in the testes.

rise in their temperature, such as that caused by wearing tight clothes, can reduce fertility.

Problems with sperm delivery

The most obvious problem that prevents sperm reaching the vagina is **impotence** – the inability to achieve or maintain an erection until ejaculation. This can have physical or psychological causes, and most men will experience it at some time in their lives. Another reason that sperm may fail to reach its target might be poor penetration as a result of faulty sexual technique.

One in four cases of male infertility is due to a genetic fault that causes sperm abnormalities. This affects the sperms' motility – in other words their ability to swim towards an egg. Sperm will also be unable to reach the egg if there is any blockage or abnormality affecting the vas deferens or epididymis, the tubes that transport sperm from the testes to be ejaculated from the penis. Problems with either the vas deferens or epididymis can often be corrected with microsurgery. The technique is also used to reverse a vasectomy.

In some cases men experience retrograde ejaculation in which the sperm travels backwards

into the bladder. This can be caused by certain prescription drugs, and changing medication may resolve the problem. It is also associated with urinary-tract surgery and **diabetes**; in such cases, retrograde ejaculation is rarely correctable.

Other factors

In the past, male infertility was less of an issue than it is today. This seems to be because people used to start their families when they were much younger. So if a man had a low sperm count or reduced motility, but his partner was a highly fertile 20-something, she would conceive anyway. These days, as more women delay having children until their 30s or later, when their own fertility is declining, any reduction in male fertility then becomes a significant issue.

Stress appears to affect fertility, but no one really understands why. It is known that many animals breed more successfully in the wild than in captivity, where they are under more stress. It is not unusual to hear stories of couples who adopt a child, and then conceive naturally as soon as they are free of the stress created by trying and failing to start their own family.

WHEN CONCEPTION DOESN'T OCCUR

As a general rule, you and your partner should speak to your GP if you have not conceived after a year of unprotected sex. However, some fertility specialists suggest that if you or your partner are in your 30s, if menstrual cycles are irregular or if there are any other worries, you should ask for advice sooner. A number of simple tests can be done to see if there is an underlying problem.

Most GPs can undertake sperm analysis to check count and motility and take blood samples to assess hormone levels and testosterone. Home-testing kits can also be used to check whether ovulation is taking place. Preliminary tests may pinpoint a simple problem that your GP can treat, but if nothing is revealed and infertility continues, both partners will be referred to a hospital or fertility clinic for further tests. There are around 80 units in the UK, operating in both the NHS and the private sector. They provide a complete range of assisted reproductive therapy (ART).

Further tests

If you are referred to a hospital or clinic, a very detailed medical history will be taken from both partners, and further blood tests will be done.

■ A detailed sperm analysis will be carried out to check the count and motility.

■ **Ultrasound** scans may be performed on the female partner to check for any abnormalities in the womb and to monitor the ovaries during the course of a cycle. Blood tests can be used to confirm ovulation is taking place.

■ A small sample of tissue from the lining of the womb may be taken for analysis. This is done via a probe inserted into the vagina. No anaesthetic is needed, although the woman may experience minor discomfort.

■ If a tubal blockage is suspected you may have a test called a hysterosalpingography, in which dye is injected into the cervix and **X-rays** are taken as it travels through the uterus and Fallopian tubes.

■ The pelvic area can also be examined via a **laparoscopy**, a test in which a flexible tube with a tiny camera is inserted into the pelvic cavity though a small incision in the abdomen.

■ A postcoital test may be carried out to see if the woman is producing antibodies that destroy her partner's sperm. In this case, the couple will be asked to have sex and around 12 hours later a sample of mucus will be taken from the woman and examined for signs of healthy sperm.

There are various treatment routes that your doctor may wish to explore before recommending assisted reproductive therapy. For example, hormonal drugs may be prescribed to increase egg production and stimulate ovulation, or hormone injections might be recommended for one or both partners. Microsurgery could be an option in cases of Fallopian tube blockage in the woman, or for problems with the vas deferens or epididymis in the man.

ASSISTED REPRODUCTIVE THERAPY

Assisted reproductive therapy, or ART, is an all-embracing term for infertility treatment. Before embarking on this route, it is important for couples to understand what is involved, and to have a realistic view of their chances of success. Counselling is therefore a large part of any infertility treatment. Counsellors encourage couples to be honest with each other about their fears and worries, and to face the fact that the treatment they are about to undergo may not succeed. The most widely known form of infertility treatment is in vitro fertilization (IVF), but there are several others.

Artificial insemination

When the woman ovulates, her partner provides a sample of sperm, either by masturbation or surgically. The sperm is then introduced directly into the cervical canal or, ideally, the uterus, via a fine tube. No anaesthetic is needed.

Artificial insemination can be used in cases of impotence, premature ejaculation, a vasectomy that cannot be reversed, retrograde ejaculation, low sperm count, blockages of the vas deferens or epididymis and problems associated with sperm getting through the cervix. Sperm from a donor may be used (see box).

To improve the chances of fertilization, seminal fluid can be treated before use to remove any dead or poor-quality sperm. A neutral fluid is added to the sperm sample; the sample is then

Donor sperm, eggs and embryos

In certain cases, sperm, eggs or embryos may need to be provided by donors if a couple is to have a chance of conceiving and bearing a child.

Donor embryos may come from couples who have produced more than three viable fertilized eggs during fertility treatment, or from the fertilization of donated eggs with donated sperm. Donor sperm is used in artificial insemination or in vitro fertilization in cases where the man has no sperm, or very poor sperm, or if there is a risk that he will pass on a hereditary illness. Some clinics also use donor sperm to impregnate single or lesbian women. The donor may be anonymous, or may be an acknowledged donor known by those seeking help. Donor eggs are used in IVF when the woman produces no eggs or eggs of poor quality, or if there is a risk of her passing on an inherited disease. Many donor eggs are provided by women who are themselves undergoing fertility treatment. This is because these women have been given follicle-stimulating drugs as part of their treatment so they often produce more eggs than they can use. These spare eggs can then be frozen for future implantation or donated to other women. Eggs may also be donated by women who have completed their own families and are being sterilized, or by women who simply want to help others.

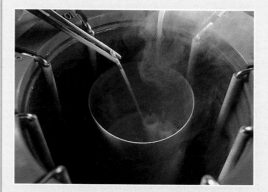

◄ **Sperm banks**
Donor sperm is stored in containers of liquid nitrogen, which keep it at a temperature of -200°C (-328°F). When needed, it is thawed and checked for quality before being used to help treat infertile couples.

put in a centrifuge (a device that rotates rapidly and separates fluids of different densities) to obtain a concentrated sample of healthy sperm.

In 15 per cent of cases artificial insemination works at the first attempt and in most suitable cases, the couple conceives within six months.

In vitro fertilization (IVF)

In vitro fertilization involves mixing eggs and sperm outside the body, in the laboratory. In most cases, the woman is first given fertility drugs to stimulate the production of several eggs. These are harvested using one of two methods. Under general **anaesthetic**, a laparoscope – a fine tube with a tiny camera – is inserted into the pelvic cavity through a small incision in the abdomen and the eggs are drawn off. Alternatively, ultrasound is used to guide a needle through the abdomen to draw off the egg-containing follicles. This can be done under local anaesthetic.

The eggs are mixed with semen in a laboratory dish and incubated for 48 hours. If fertilization occurs, the eggs will have formed into embryos containing four, or possibly eight, cells. These embryos are examined for abnormalities and put into the uterus with a syringe. No anaesthetic is needed. The woman may be advised to remain lying down for up to four hours.

No more than three embryos can be placed in the womb under UK law; any extra embryos may be frozen. If all three embryos implant, doctors may recommend removing one or two, as the risks of prematurity, birth defects, low birth weight and other long-term problems are increased with a multiple pregnancy. The success rate of IVF is only around 15 per cent.

This technique can be carried out using donor sperm, eggs or embryos (see box, left).

Gamete intra-Fallopian transfer (GIFT)
Gamete intra-Fallopian transfer is a form of IVF used when no cause can be found for female infertility, or if men have low fertility. Eggs and sperm are collected, mixed together and then transferred directly to the Fallopian tubes without waiting to ensure that fertilization has actually occurred. GIFT can also be carried out using donor sperm or eggs. The success rate using this technique is 25–30 per cent.

Zygote intra-Fallopian transfer (ZIFT)
Zygote intra-Fallopian transfer works in the same way as GIFT, the difference being that technicians check that eggs are fertilized before they are injected directly into the Fallopian tube. This method is used if it is thought that female antibodies are attacking sperm. The success rate for ZIFT is 25–30 per cent.

Intracytoplasmic sperm injection (ICSI)
Intracytoplasmic sperm injection is the technique most often used to address problems with sperm motility or low sperm count. Sperm and eggs are collected as for in vitro fertilization (see above), but a single sperm is then injected directly into the egg to ensure fertilization.

There have been reports that children conceived in this way may have birth defects or be infertile themselves. There is conflicting evidence about the risk of abnormalities, but it is known that many of the men who benefit from ICSI are infertile because of a chromosomal problem that affects their sperm, and this will be passed on to any male children, making them infertile, too. ICSI now accounts for more than one third of all fertility treatments in some centres in the UK. The success rate is 22 per cent and rising.

Surrogacy
Sometimes when a woman is unable to carry a pregnancy, she and her partner may enter into a surrogacy agreement with another woman who is prepared to carry the child. This is usually done using sperm from the partner.

SEE ALSO *Reproductive system; Menstruation; Miscarriage; Pelvis and disorders; Pregnancy and problems*

Infestation

Infestation occurs when a part of the body is invaded or inhabited by animal parasites. Mites, ticks or lice, for example, may be present on someone's skin or in hair or clothing, while particular types of worm, such as tapeworms and hookworms, live inside the body. These parasites, called ectoparasites, depend on another organism for nutrition, and can survive only inside or outside of that organism.

The term 'infestation' can also be used to describe the presence in the body of large intestinal parasites, such as intestinal worms, but this is more often referred to as infection.

SEE ALSO *Parasites and parasitic diseases*

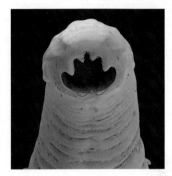

◀ **Toothed parasite**
A hookworm uses its hook-like teeth (shown magnified) to attach itself to the small intestine. Up to a quarter of the world's population is thought to be infested by hookworms, but it is rare in the UK.

Inflammation

Inflammation is a protective reaction of the body to injury. Its purpose is to destroy, dilute and isolate whatever is causing the injury and the injured tissues themselves.

The common signs of inflammation are redness, heat, swelling, pain and loss of function in the inflamed area. Complex tissue changes take place microscopically.

Cell damage leads to the release of the chemical histamine and other compounds from specialized immune cells called vasoactive amines. These cause the smallest blood vessels – the arterioles, capillaries and venules – to dilate and become leaky. Blood flow to the area is increased, causing redness and heat. Fluid leaks into the tissues, making them swell, and white blood cells are able to enter the tissue through the leaks to attack infecting organisms or foreign material and to clear up damaged tissue. The tissue damage and white cells release chemicals that in turn trigger nerve pain receptors, increasing the pain of the injury and making it difficult to use the inflamed part. Since the inflamed part hurts, it tends to be kept still or not used, which aids recovery.

ACUTE INFLAMMATION
Inflammation is acute when it develops suddenly, as in a fingernail bed infection.

The fingertip becomes red, hot, painful, and swollen, making it very difficult to use the finger. Acute inflammation is frequently accompanied by pus formation – a mixture of live and dead white cells as well as bacteria and fragments of dead tissue.

If the infection is not treated, or the pus cannot leak out naturally, the body rapidly forms a wall around it to contain the pus. This is known as an abscess. If an abscess neither bursts nor is lanced, it remains as a painful lump, which may gradually settle in time and leave scar tissue.

CHRONIC INFLAMMATION

Chronic inflammation is usually less intense than acute inflammation, but it continues for a longer time. It tends to form scar tissue, which makes it harder for the person with inflammation to use the affected part of the body. An example is a damaged tendon, where scar tissue causes the tendon to stick to its sheath, resulting in pain and loss of function for weeks or even months.

Influenza

Influenza, commonly called flu, is an acute respiratory illness. It is caused by a virus, which attacks the lining of the air passages, the nose, throat, windpipe and lungs, leading to inflammation. The virus is usually passed from one person to another through the air, and the illness often breaks out as an epidemic, quickly spreading from town to town and country to country. The epidemic conditions usually last for a period of four to six weeks before they ease off.

Every few years a new strain of flu appears that spreads so rapidly that precautions cannot be developed in time. This can lead to pandemics – international epidemics – which threaten millions of lives.

SYMPTOMS

Many people confuse flu with the common **cold**. Both colds and flu are caused by a virus but the symptoms of flu are usually much more severe than those of a cold and include a high temperature. Flu also tends to have a more sudden onset than a cold.

Flu symptoms include:
- fever (a temperature of 38–40°C);
- a cough;
- a sore throat;
- headache;
- lack of appetite;
- severe muscle aches and pains;
- extreme fatigue;
- later, a runny nose and sore throat.

DURATION

One to two days after being infected, the person suddenly becomes ill. The illness usually lasts about a week but can continue for a longer period.

CAUSES

Flu is caused by the flu viruses A, B and C. Type A is the most serious, and has the most acute symptoms. It is also the commonest form, usually breaking out every two or three years. Type B has similar symptoms but is not as serious; the outbreaks happen every four to five years. Type C is the mildest form, with symptoms similar to those of a cold.

When a person is infected with flu, the body forms antibodies against the particular type of the virus. If that same type infects the person again, he or she will be less severely affected because of protection from these antibodies. The problem with the flu virus is that it constantly mutates into slightly different versions of itself, allowing the virus to cause another severe infection in the same person. One reason why vaccinations against flu are sometimes ineffective is because they are made with the previous season's variant rather than the current one.

Flu usually occurs in winter. Damp or cold cannot cause flu, but sudden changes in temperature may cause the symptoms to appear more quickly.

How the virus is spread

A single infected person is able to transmit the virus to a large number of people via mucus from the nose and throat expelled during sneezing, coughing or talking.

The virus may also pass through hand-to-hand contact or through touching a contaminated object such as a door handle or piece of paper, although the virus cannot live for long on objects.

It is possible to pass the infection on to other people, from the day before the symptoms first develop until the day after the fever has disappeared.

TREATMENT

The majority of healthy people with flu can treat the illness themselves.
- Paracetamol can relieve the high fever and aches and pains.
- Plenty of bed rest and sleep are needed, in a well-ventilated, warm room.
- Drinks such as hot lemon with honey can ease a cough.
- Plenty of juices and water are needed – the fever causes sweating and dehydrates the body.
- Avoid smoking or drinking alcohol.

When to consult a doctor

Seek medical advice if the illness continues for more than a week or symptoms are very severe.

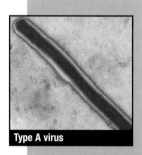
Type A virus

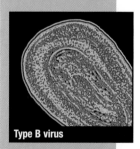
Type B virus

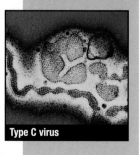
Type C virus

Elderly people and those suffering from diabetes or a lung, heart or kidney condition should consult a doctor as soon as the first symptoms appear.

What a doctor may do

A doctor may prescribe antibiotics if you develop any complications, such as bacterial infection in the lungs. Antibiotics are not effective against the flu virus itself, which will be dealt with by the body's own defences.

There are two antiviral drugs, zanamivir and oseltamivir, which can be used to treat flu. But they are not widely prescribed because they have been shown to reduce the duration of flu by only one day. To be effective, they have to be taken within 36 hours of the onset of flu.

Very serious cases of flu may be referred to hospital for treatment.

Complementary therapies

There is some scientific evidence to indicate that the herbal supplement echinacea boosts the effectiveness of the immune system by stimulating the activity of white blood cells. Taking 1–2g of vitamin C a day may also have a beneficial effect.

COMPLICATIONS

Complications include bacterial infection of the lungs, including life-threatening **pneumonia**, or sinus problems, causing difficulty in breathing. Individuals at higher risk of suffering from complications include elderly people, especially those who live in residential homes where there is an increased risk of contagion through close daily contact with others. People with long-standing lung, heart or kidney conditions, as well as those with diabetes, are also more likely to develop complications. Those most at risk are advised to get a flu vaccination every year.

PREVENTION

Vaccines for the most recent types of flu viruses have some protective effect. These are normally administered at the start of the flu season, in the autumn. Elderly people and those with chronic diseases qualify automatically for a flu vaccine on the NHS. Some high street pharmacists also offer flu vaccination.

Following a healthy diet and lifestyle may help to strengthen your immune system and make it more effective in fighting off the virus; some healthy people who are infected with the virus do not develop any flu symptoms at all.

If you are infected, good personal hygiene can help you to avoid infecting others, particularly those with whom you live. You should also stay away from work to avoid passing the infection on to colleagues.

OUTLOOK

Most people who develop flu recover fully provided that there are no complications.

Factfile

Reducing the spread of infection

Influenza is an air-borne infection that spreads rapidly. The virus is released into the air when those people already infected cough and sneeze.

Vaccination against flu is now widely available, not only from your doctor, but also in high street pharmacists. It does not guarantee that you will not catch flu, because new strains of flu virus are constantly appearing, but if you are infected, your symptoms will be much milder.

The best time to be vaccinated is between late September and early November each year. You should seriously consider vaccination if you are aged 65 or over, especially if you live in an old people's home or nursing home, or if you have one of the following conditions:

- a chronic heart or chest problem, including asthma;
- chronic kidney disease;
- diabetes;
- weakened immunity, perhaps due to cancer treatment or taking certain drugs – check with your doctor.

There are no permanent side effects. But, in some people weakened by age or disorders such as lung disease, flu can be fatal. Flu and the complications linked to it kill hundreds of people in the UK each year.

SEE ALSO *Lungs and disorders*

Ingrowing toenail

An ingrowing toenail occurs when the edge of a nail (usually on the big toe) presses into the soft flesh on one or both sides of the nail, causing painful inflammation. This usually results from wearing too-tight shoes, neglect of the nails, or from cutting the nail incorrectly.

If you have an ingrowing toenail, bathe the affected foot in a warm, diluted antiseptic solution for 15–20 minutes. After softening the flesh, carefully tuck a small wisp of cotton wool under the ingrowing corner of the nail using a blunt pair of scissors. Every day, replace the old piece of cotton wool with a fresh wisp, slightly larger if necessary. The cotton wool helps lift the nail edge away from the flesh it is digging into and encourages it to grow properly.

You should also see your doctor if the toe is severely infected or if you suffer from diabetes because, in severe cases, nail surgery may be necessary to correct the problem.

To help to prevent ingrowing toenails, trim the nails straight across, avoid picking your toenails, wear comfortable shoes with sufficient room to wiggle your toes and walk barefooted at home as much as possible.

SEE ALSO *Foot and problems*

Insomnia

Most people have short-term sleeping problems at some time in their lives, but five million people in the UK suffer from chronic insomnia, in which they are deprived of proper sleep most nights or every night.

The amount of sleep we need varies with age and between individuals. Some adults require only three to four hours a night, while others cannot function properly on fewer than nine hours each night. People with insomnia – who are unable to go to sleep or to remain asleep – fall short of the amount of rest they need and can become distressed and exhausted.

Insomnia may be long-standing with no obvious trigger, or recent and have a clear cause. In the UK, more than half of us develop short-lived insomnia at some time in our lives, and one in ten adults suffers long-term (chronic) insomnia. Insomnia affects men and women of all ages, but those most likely to be affected include shift workers, people with a history of **depression**, elderly people and post-menopausal women.

Some people fall asleep normally but wake abnormally early and then find that they cannot go back to sleep. Early morning waking is a common pattern in elderly people, but is also a symptom of depressive illness.

Many sleeping problems can be linked to a disruption in biorhythms – the natural periodic cycle exhibited by the body in response to environmental changes or to various internal control mechanisms.

If you often find it hard to sleep at night and think that you are getting less sleep than your body needs, there are many self-help techniques and relaxation therapies that may help. But, if you have tried several of these and the problem remains unresolved, seek medical advice. Your doctor may refer you to a specialist sleeping clinic or prescribe a short-term course of sleeping pills.

CAUSES OF INSOMNIA

Depression, stress or constant worry may prevent you from getting to sleep at night. Other common causes of insomnia include the following.
- Pain caused by a chronic physical illness such as osteoarthritis.
- Hyperstimulation caused by over-consumption of caffeine or nicotine – or by watching exciting television films.
- **Jet lag** and shift work, leading to a disruption in biorhythms (delayed sleep phase syndrome).
- Irregular sleeping routines.

- Stimulant drugs.
- Chronic excessive alcohol intake.
  Less common causes include:
- Breathing problems (most commonly congestive heart failure, but also **asthma** and chronic lung disease such as **emphysema**).
- An overactive thyroid (hyperthyroidism).
- Legs that tingle or feel uncomfortable unless moved (**restless leg syndrome**).
- Withdrawal from benzodiazepines or other hypnotic drugs (rebound insomnia).
- Nightmares, night terrors and sleep walking (parasomnias).
  Rare causes include:
- **Malnutrition** and low body weight.
- Post-traumatic stress disorder.
- Agitated psychiatric illness (mania).
- Temporary interruptions to breathing during sleep (sleep apnoea).

Delayed sleep phase syndrome
Delayed sleep phase syndrome occurs when the biorhythms are disturbed, usually where sleeping and waking times are delayed and cannot be changed back to an earlier schedule.

Restless leg syndrome
Restless leg syndrome is a condition in which prickling or mild pain in the legs makes them uncomfortable when still and prompts the individual to shift position repeatedly. It usually occurs in older people.

Rebound insomnia
Rebound insomnia is common when hypnotic drugs – for example, benzodiazepines – are withdrawn or reduced after long-term use. It can be avoided by reducing the dose slowly over the course of a few weeks.

Sleep apnoea
In obstructive sleep apnoea, a disturbance to the mechanisms governing breathing causes someone temporarily to stop breathing, provoking a reflex struggle to breathe that causes waking several times each night. People with sleep apnoea often feel extremely tired by day.

The problem of obstructive sleep apnoea has been linked with heart disease. A rare cause is brain damage from head injury or infection damaging the hypothalamus, the part of the brain that establishes the biorhythms.

PREVENTING AND TREATING INSOMNIA

The following measures may help you to get
a good night's rest.

■ Avoid caffeine, strong spices and monosodium
glutamate within six hours of bedtime.

■ Talk over anxieties or problems with friends
or family.

■ Exercise during the day and avoid daytime
naps; avoid evening exercise.

■ Have a warm milky drink and a light snack
at bedtime.

■ Stay calm and relaxed in the hour before
bedtime, and try not to talk on the telephone
at this time.

■ In the bedroom, arrange soft lighting, ensure
minimal noise, adequate ventilation and a
comfortable room temperature.

■ Do not read or watch television in bed.

■ If you cannot sleep after 30 minutes, get up and
do something relaxing until you feel sleepy.

When to see a doctor

If you suffer from chronic insomnia and there
is no obvious self-treatable cause, consult your
doctor. It is also advisable to seek medical advice
if you experience occasional but disruptive
insomnia (for example, as a result of working
shifts) or if you suffer from depression.

Sleeping pills

A doctor may prescribe a short course of sleeping
pills to provide temporary relief from chronic
insomnia, but sleeping pills do not offer a cure
and must be used with caution. The main group
of sleeping pills are the benzodiazepines such
as diazepam (valium). They can be addictive and
should be taken for short periods only. Moreover,
benzodiazepines have side effects and can cause
withdrawal symptoms that may cause more
discomfort than the original problem. Most
pharmacists carry a range of sleep-inducing
remedies that are non-addictive and available to
buy over the counter.

Complementary therapies

Relaxation techniques such as hypnosis, listening
to soothing audio tapes and doing appropriate
exercises can all help to relieve insomnia.

Acupressure can be used to encourage the
release of endorphins – natural painkilling
chemicals released by the body – and induce
a feeling of relaxation. You can buy from
pharmacists plasters or cones that are designed
to be applied to acupressure points on the wrist.

Other useful complementary remedies include
herbal preparations such as valerian tincture,
catnip tincture, camomile tea and hop pillows,
aromatherapy oils such as neroli, lavender and
myrtle – either inhaled or added to bath water –
and naturopathic combinations such as valerian,
camomile and passion flower.

SEE ALSO *Anxiety*

Internal pelvic examination

An internal pelvic examination enables a doctor
to assess the size and position of a woman's
uterus and to locate swellings or tender areas
in the pelvis. The technique is also used during
labour to assess the dilation of the cervix.

For the examination the woman lies on her
side with her thighs apart, enabling the doctor
gently to insert the index and middle fingers of
one hand into the vagina while pressing the
lower abdomen with the other hand. An
instrument known as a speculum is inserted into
the vagina so the vaginal walls and cervix can
be viewed.

Intertrigo

Intertrigo is an inflammation of skin areas
such as those found beneath the breasts, in
the armpits, between the fingers or toes, and
between the thighs. Inflammation may result
from rubbing, or from infection developing
in these warm, moist areas.

The infection may be fungal or bacterial.
The affected skin becomes red and moist and
may develop blisters or dry scales along with
an unpleasant odour. Intertrigo is most common
in those who are overweight, and in visitors
to tropical countries.

Treatment is with antifungal or steroid
creams. Carefully drying these areas, and
particularly the skin between fingers and toes,
after washing, paying good attention to
personal hygiene, wearing loose clothes made
from natural fibres, and losing excess weight
all help to prevent the problem.

SEE ALSO *Skin and disorders*

Inturned eyelashes

Inturned eyelashes, also known as trichiasis,
is a condition in which the eyelashes rub
against the cornea, causing discomfort and
sometimes infection.

True trichiasis is a result of faulty positioning
of the lash follicles and may be congenital; it
is more common in people from the Far East.
Pseudotrichiasis, in which the follicles are in the
correct position but the lid has turned in,
accompanies **entropion**. The offending lashes
may be removed by an optometrist or doctor.
A longer-term solution may be electrolysis to
remove the lashes permanently.

Intussusception

Intussusception is a condition in which part of the bowel collapses into an adjoining part, causing severe pain, vomiting of blood and mucus in the stools. It is most common in babies, and may follow a viral infection; in adults it may be due to an intestinal polyp. A **barium** enema is used for diagnosis and may correct the problem; if not, surgery is necessary.
SEE ALSO *Bowel and disorders*

Iritis

Iritis is the inflammation of the iris, the coloured part of the eye. In its acute form, it causes a sudden, very painful red eye, often with excessive watering. It requires prompt treatment with a drug to dilate the pupil and anti-inflammatory drugs such as corticosteroids. Chronic forms tend to be less painful, but still require examination. Iritis is associated with general inflammatory conditions such as **Crohn's disease** and some forms of acute **arthritis**.

Iron test

Iron testing checks the blood for iron-deficiency **anaemia**. It involves measuring levels of the iron-containing pigment haemoglobin – which transports oxygen to the tissues – and the examination of a blood sample, which may reveal red blood cells that are smaller and paler than is normal, due to lowered haemoglobin levels.

Irritable bowel syndrome

Irritable bowel syndrome (IBS) is a persistent intestinal disorder of unknown cause. Symptoms include wind, bloating and cramps. Bowel movements are often erratic, varying from diarrhoea to constipation. Sufferers are thought to have a colon that is highly sensitive, especially to stress. Avoiding certain foods, such as dairy products, high-fat foods, caffeine and spicy dishes, and managing stress can help.
SEE ALSO *Bowel and disorders; Digestive system*

Ischaemic bowel disease

Ischaemic bowel disease is a condition in which the supply of blood to the bowels is reduced. The cause may be a clot in an artery that is supplying the bowel, a weakening of the pumping action of the heart, or shock. The problem occurs most often in elderly people and those suffering from atherosclerosis (see **Atheroma**) or **diabetes**.

Symptoms may include abdominal pain, bloody diarrhoea and, in the worst cases, **gangrene**.
SEE ALSO *Bowel and disorders*

Ischaemic heart disease

Ischaemic heart disease is a condition in which the heart is damaged by a reduction in its blood supply due to **coronary artery disease**. There may be no symptoms, but insufficient oxygen in the heart's muscles may lead to angina, heart attack, irregular heartbeats, cardiac failure or death. Treatment is based on reducing the risk factor, medication or surgery.
SEE ALSO *Heart and circulatory system*

Itching

Itching is an intense irritation that can be widespread or restricted to just one area of the body. It produces a strong desire to scratch the affected area, which can sometimes lead to skin infections. The exact cause of itching is unknown, but it may be associated with an irritation of the sensory nerve endings in the skin or underlying areas.
SEE ALSO *Skin and disorders*

IVF

In vitro fertilization (IVF) is a method of overcoming infertility. A woman's eggs are harvested and fertilized with her partner's sperm outside the body. In some cases donor sperm may be used.

If fertilization is successful, two or three embryos are transferred to the woman's womb in the hope that one will implant and continue to grow, resulting in a successful pregnancy.

Couples may produce more fertilized eggs than can be transferred to the womb at the first attempt, they may then decide to keep their extra embryos in cold storage, and use them in future attempts at pregnancy.
SEE ALSO *Infertility*

Jaundice

Jaundice is a yellowing of the skin and the whites of the eyes. In adults, it is a symptom of one of several underlying diseases, notably **hepatitis**. In babies, it can often be of little significance and pass within a few days, or be a sign of **haemolytic disease of the newborn**.

Normally, the spleen breaks down dead red blood cells into the pigments bilirubin, which is yellowish, and biliverdin, which is greenish. They are then broken down further by the liver. An accumulation of bilirubin in the blood causes the yellowing and is an indication of a liver disorder.

Treatment of jaundice depends on the cause. Babies requiring treatment will undergo a course of phototherapy, in which exposure to special lights breaks down the excess bilirubin.

SEE ALSO *Liver and disorders*

Jet lag

The body follows a circadian rhythm in which it adjusts to the 24-hour cycle of the rising and setting of the sun. Without this constant change of stimulus from light to dark, it follows its own 25–27 hour cycle.

Jet lag is the disruption of the normal cycle of waking and sleeping caused by rapid crossing of time zones. A businessman, for example, might leave London on a 9am flight, cross five time zones in seven hours and arrive in New York around 11am – in good time for an afternoon meeting. Yet the businessman's body clock has already registered a full day's work, and will be preparing body and mind for rest. This changing of time zones causes the body to be out of synch with the usual cycle of day and night. The body may want to sleep, but the brain will be saying that it is not time yet. It is this that leads to symptoms such as:
- disruption of normal sleep patterns;
- a general feeling of overtiredness;
- an inability to concentrate, reduced alertness and impaired performance;
- disruption of regular body functions, such as the desire to eat and to defecate;
- headache and other signs of **stress**.

The body adjusts naturally to the new cycle of waking and sleeping in three days, but repeated disruption to the circadian rhythms causes chronic stress.

PREVENTION

There is no treatment for jet lag, but the following steps will minimize disruption.

Before the journey
- Build up a sleep reserve by getting as much sleep as you comfortably can during the week before the flight.
- Sleep as close as you can to the normal bedtime at your destination for a day or two before you fly.

During the flight
- Eat as close as possible to normal mealtimes at your destination.
- Vitamin B-complex and antioxidants may help the body to adjust.

On arrival
- After a westward journey, stay awake until bedtime at your destination. The body adjusts naturally to a longer daily cycle.
- Spend as much time as possible out of doors. Sunlight is thought to slow the body clock.
- If possible, nap when overtaken by sleepiness, or before an important event. Napping for up to 45 minutes raises the body's level of alertness and concentration.
- Relaxation techniques can diminish stress and help to induce sleep when required.
- Sleeping pills may help to overcome the temporary **insomnia** associated with jet lag. However, they are best avoided during the flight because the deep sleep that they induce prevents natural movement and may lead to circulation problems (see **Deep vein thrombosis**).

Melatonin is a natural chemical in the body that helps regulate sleep cycles. It can be taken in pill form to induce sleep and reduce jet lag, but it is a controversial and complex treatment not available in the UK. If it is taken too early in the day melatonin may cause sleepiness and delay adaptation to local time. It is not recommended for people with epilepsy or for anyone taking warfarin.

Self-help
Keeping your circulation moving

Perform the following exercises at regular intervals during a flight to help to reduce discomfort and keep your blood circulating.

1. While sitting in your seat, flex your feet so that the toes are pointing upwards. Hold for several seconds. Repeat several times.

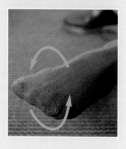

2. Raise one foot a little way off the ground and point your toes forward. Rotate your foot in one direction, then the other. Repeat several times, then with the other foot.

Joints and problems

When two or more bones meet they form a joint, or articulation. All body movement occurs at joints, from the small movements of the fingers to the large movements of the shoulder. The bones are held together by fibrous or cartilaginous connective tissue and are moved by the contraction and relaxation of muscles.

The shape of the articulating bones and the flexibility and strength of the surrounding ligaments determine the strength, stability and range of movement of the joints. Bones with curved surfaces that fit tightly to each other form strong, stable joints with less freedom of movement. Bones that have little curvature but articulate loosely with each other form joints that are less stable but allow greater movement.

TYPES OF JOINT

Joints are classified into three main groups.
■ Fibrous joints do not allow movement. The bones fit tightly together, held firmly by fibrous tissue. There is no cavity within the joint. The body's only fibrous joints are found in the skull.
■ Cartilaginous joints allow a small amount of movement. The bones are connected by a disc of fibrocartilage (see **Cartilage**), but again there is no joint cavity. There are only two types of cartilaginous joint in the body: the symphysis pubis, between the two pubic bones in the pelvis; and the joints between the vertabrae of the spine.
■ Synovial joints allow a wide range of movements, limited only by the shape of the articulating bones, their position and the strength of the surrounding connective tissues. All the other joints in the body are synovial.

Synovial joints

The shape and range of movement of synovial joints vary, but they share certain characteristics:
■ a joint cavity – a space within the joint;
■ hyaline cartilage – cartilage that covers the surface of the articulating bones, reducing friction and allowing smooth movement;
■ a joint capsule – a fibrous capsule that surrounds the joint like a sleeve. It holds the bones together and encloses the joint cavity;
■ ligaments – strong bands or sheets of fibrous tissue that strengthen the capsule on the outside of the joint. They are sometimes found inside a joint, for example, in the knee and hip, where they further stabilize and strengthen the joint;
■ a synovial membrane – a membrane that lines the inside of the capsule and secretes synovial fluid into the joint cavity;
■ synovial fluid – a fluid that lubricates and feeds the bones, cartilages and inner ligaments.

Some joints have additional features that improve the fit of bones, absorb impact or

Types of synovial joint

Synovial joints are freely moveable joints. There are six types, classified according to their structure and the range of movement they allow.

Slippery cartilage over the ends of the articulating bones and constant lubrication from the synovial fluid help to minimize friction and keep all movements smooth.

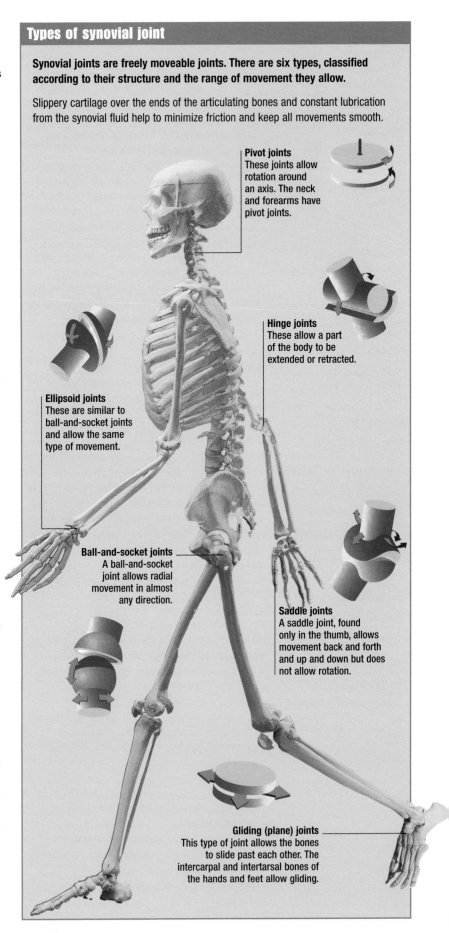

Pivot joints
These joints allow rotation around an axis. The neck and forearms have pivot joints.

Hinge joints
These allow a part of the body to be extended or retracted.

Ellipsoid joints
These are similar to ball-and-socket joints and allow the same type of movement.

Ball-and-socket joints
A ball-and-socket joint allows radial movement in almost any direction.

Saddle joints
A saddle joint, found only in the thumb, allows movement back and forth and up and down but does not allow rotation.

Gliding (plane) joints
This type of joint allows the bones to slide past each other. The intercarpal and intertarsal bones of the hands and feet allow gliding.

Flexion
Bending of a joint to bring the bones that form it towards each other.

Extension
Extending or stretching to straighten a limb.

Abduction
Movement of a limb away from the mid-line of the body.

Adduction
Movement of a limb towards the mid-line of the body.

Circumduction
The circular movement of a limb.

Medial rotation
Turning in towards the body.

Lateral rotation
Turning out, away from the body.

reduce friction. For example, some joints contain fibrocartilage pads called discs. They are attached to the articulating bones and give the joint a better fit as well as cushioning the impact of movement. Examples include the intervertebral discs of the spine.

Bursae, sacs filled with synovial fluid, are found in and around joints; they reduce friction, usually between bones and tendons.

WHAT CAN GO WRONG
Many conditions can affect the joints, either singly or in combination.

Types of arthritis
Osteoarthritis can affect any joint in the body but is more common in weight-bearing joints such as the hip, knee and lumbar spine. Rheumatoid arthritis commonly starts with the peripheral joints, such as the hands, wrist and elbows. **Ankylosing spondylitis** affects the spine, starting from the lumbar spine and gradually moving up to the neck (see also **Arthritis**).

Deformities
Deformities present from birth include **club foot**, bow legs, knock-knees, congenital dislocation of the hip and **spina bifida**. Acquired deformities can be caused by arthritis, poor posture, **fractures**, dislocations, shortening of **tendons** or **ligaments**, and muscular imbalance caused by **paralysis**.

Soft tissue disorders
Soft tissues, such as muscles, tendons and the synovial tissues around joints, connect, support or surround other structures of the body. Disorders affecting the synovial tissues around joints include **bursitis** and soft tissue tumours.

Fractures or dislocations
The joints may be affected by **fractures** of the bones, or by dislocation problems.

Neurological disorders
The joints can be affected by neurological disorders such as **poliomyelitis** and **cerebral palsy** (see also **Brain and nervous system**).

Bone disorders
Some bone disorders may also cause joint problems, for example, **osteomyelitis, tuberculosis** infection and osteochondritis.

Joint replacement
A joint replacement, or arthroplasty, is an operation to construct a new moveable joint or to adapt an existing one. Not every joint can be reconstructed successfully, and in practice arthroplasty is performed only on the hip, knee, elbow, shoulder, certain joints in the hands and the metatarso-halangeal joint of the big toe.

The decision about whether a joint replacement operation is practical or advisable depends on the joint concerned and the degree of pain and disability. However, an operation

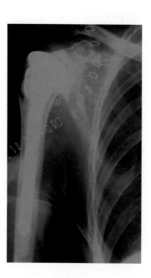

◀ **New shoulder joint**
A ball-shaped implant can be cemented onto the top of the upper arm bone to replace a damaged area that has been caused by injury or a disorder such as arthritis.

may be necessary to treat joints affected by severe osteoarthritis and rheumatoid arthritis. Surgery may be used to correct some types of deformity, such as hallux valgus, which affects the big toe. It may also be used when **fractures** of the head of the thigh bone in elderly people have not united.

WHAT'S INVOLVED
There are three main techniques of arthoplasty:
■ Hemi-arthroplasty involves cutting away and replacing one of the two articulating bones with a similarly shaped artificial version (prosthesis). This is usually made of metal and held in place by acrylic joint cement. This technique is often used on elderly people to treat a femur fracture.
■ Total replacement arthroplasty replaces both articulating surfaces with prostheses. In large joints, such as the hip and knee, one component is usually made of metal, the other of a tough polyethylene. In the hip joint, for example, the socket of the pelvis is deepened to receive a ball socket made of polyethylene which is fixed into position with acrylic cement.
■ Excision arthroplasty cuts away the surfaces of the two articulating bones to enlarge the joint space and remove any bony spurs. Then the space between the bones is filled with soft tissue. At the hip, for example, a part of the gluteus medius muscle may be sewn between the enlarged joint cavity to act as a cushion between the pelvis and the femur. This method is usually used only as a salvage operation on the weight-bearing joints, such as the hip, after a previous total replacement arthroplasty has failed.

COMPLICATIONS
A prosthesis can work loose or wear out over time and need replacing. The average life of a joint replacement is ten years. There are long waiting lists for hip replacement operations on the NHS in many areas.

SEE ALSO *Bone and problems; Skeletal system*

Kaposi's sarcoma

Kaposi's sarcoma is a condition in which small, purplish-black tumours develop on the skin, mucous membranes or the internal organs. These tumours are often malignant and may be life-threatening when they develop on organs.

The condition is caused by an infection with the human herpes virus 8 (HHV-8), which can be **sexually transmitted**. Kaposi's sarcoma is most commonly associated with **HIV** infection, when it may develop at any stage. But it can occur in people who are not HIV-positive.

Kaposi's sarcoma may not need treatment in the early stages, but the condition progresses. Treatment of underlying HIV and improving immune function may get rid of the tumours. Otherwise, people with the condition will be prescribed topical creams, **radiotherapy** and **chemotherapy**. Some tumours can be removed or destroyed by freezing.

SEE ALSO *Cancer*

Keratosis, actinic

Also known as solar keratoses, actinic keratoses are inflamed, silver scaly patches on the skin that have a conical surface and red base. They are usually surrounded by inelastic, wrinkled and mottled skin and are a symptom of sun-induced skin damage. They are premalignant conditions that may develop into skin **cancer** if left untreated. The patches can be removed by freezing or by being treated with an anticancer cream (5-fluorouracil).

SEE ALSO *Skin and disorders*

Keyhole surgery

Keyhole surgery means using tiny cameras and miniature surgical instruments to perform investigations and operations through very small incisions in the body. The development of keyhole techniques is one of the major medical advances of recent years. The process causes less scarring and usually allows for a much faster recovery than traditional surgical operations. A wide range of operations, including hernia repair, minor heart operations, knee operations and a large number of gynaecological operations can all be performed by keyhole surgery.

A typical example of keyhole surgery is the operation to remove the gallbladder for gallstones, a procedure known as a laparoscopic cholecystectomy. A small, thin tube with a video camera at its tip (a **laparoscope**) is inserted through a tiny cut made just below the navel. The surgeon can see the gallbladder on a television screen and perform the surgery with tools inserted in three other small cuts, each 5–10mm (⅕–⅜in) long, made in the upper-right part of the abdomen. The abdomen is inflated with carbon dioxide gas to allow the surgeon to see the internal organs more easily. The gallbladder is taken out through one of the cuts.

There have been many recent advances in the techniques of keyhole surgery, but it is not possible to perform every type of operation in this way. For many complicated types of surgery, it would mean a far longer operation, which often is not practical or in the patient's best interest. Keyhole techniques also take a long time to learn and not all surgeons have been trained in them.

There are also a number of individual reasons why keyhole surgery may not be performed in certain cases. For example, not everyone can have his or her gallbladder removed by keyhole surgery. If a person has previously had surgery in the area of the gallbladder or has a problem that would make it difficult for the surgeon to see the gallbladder, then open surgery might be the safer option. Surgeons will always discuss the reasons for and against any operation with each patient.

Kidneys and disorders

The two kidneys form the uppermost part of the **urinary system**. They are situated at the back of the abdomen, high up, on either side of the spine. The right kidney is a little shorter and wider than the left one, and sits slightly lower down. Each kidney has a tough, protective coating connected to the kidney within by blood vessels and fibrous tissue.

FILTERING THE BLOOD

The kidneys' main function is to filter the blood and excrete waste products and excess fluid from the body in the form of urine. They also regulate the volume and composition of body fluid, including the acidity of the blood. The kidneys produce hormones and prostaglandins, hormone-like substances that are involved in the metabolism of vitamin D and some small proteins.

The kidneys filter fluid from the blood at a fairly constant rate of 120–130ml per minute. The average adult produces 170–180 litres of filtered fluid per day. This vast amount is necessary to eliminate toxins and wastes such as urea, which are present in low concentrations in the blood. Important nutrients and up to 80 per cent of the filtered water is reabsorbed so that the body can conserve energy and fluid.

The amount of urine excreted each day is around 1–2 litres. The amount of urine you pass depends on how much you have drunk, and on the effects of certain hormones that help to regulate salt and water balance in the body.

HORMONE PRODUCTION

The kidneys produce the hormone renin, which is involved in blood pressure control. Production of the hormone is boosted when specialized muscle cells in the kidneys' filtering units (the nephrons) detect a fall in the pressure of blood entering the kidney.

The kidneys also produce the hormone erythropoietin, which stimulates the production of red blood cells in **bone marrow**. Lack of erythropoietin – caused by kidney failure, for example – leads to **anaemia**; while overproduction – perhaps as a result of kidney

cancer – can cause too many red blood cells to be produced. A synthetic version of the hormone is now used to help to prevent anaemia in people with renal failure.

WHAT CAN GO WRONG

Many diseases can affect the kidneys. The body can function well with only one kidney, which means that kidney disease is rarely life-threatening unless both kidneys are affected. When this is the case, **dialysis** treatment, in which the individual's blood is filtered artificially, is recommended.

Polycystic kidney disease

Polycystic kidney disease is an inherited disorder in which multiple fluid-filled cysts gradually replace most of the tissue within both kidneys. The kidneys become progressively larger and their ability to function gradually declines. There is a juvenile form of the condition, which is usually diagnosed at or before birth. In adults, the disease quite often appears before the age of 45, causing pain in the lower back or abdomen, blood in the urine, high blood pressure, **subarachnoid haemorrhage** or, more rarely, cysts in the liver or pancreas. This can lead to kidney failure in the person's late 50s. Careful control of high blood pressure, which can result from poor kidney function, may help to slow damage to the kidneys.

Single cysts

Single kidney cysts can also develop as fluid-filled sacs. They are usually benign and of little significance. The doctor may decide to send you for a procedure in which the fluid is withdrawn and tested to rule out the possibility of cancer.

Kidney stones

Kidney stones occur when salts in the urine crystallize. The stones are known medically as calculi. They may be caused by chronic infection, continually drinking insufficient fluid or eating a diet high in substances called oxalates, which are found in rhubarb, spinach, leafy vegetables and coffee. They can also be the result of hormone disorders caused by an excess of salt in the bloodstream.

Kidney stones range in size from tiny particles to large formations up to 50mm (2in) across. Large stones may take years to develop, but smaller ones may form within a week or two.

The stones often cause severe pain, which starts in the back and spreads to the front of the abdomen down in the scrotum, penis or vulva. The pain builds to a climax, lasts about a minute before it eases and then returns in a few minutes. Other symptoms are difficulty passing urine and, sometimes, blood in the urine.

In some cases there are no symptoms. Although kidney stones can grow very large,

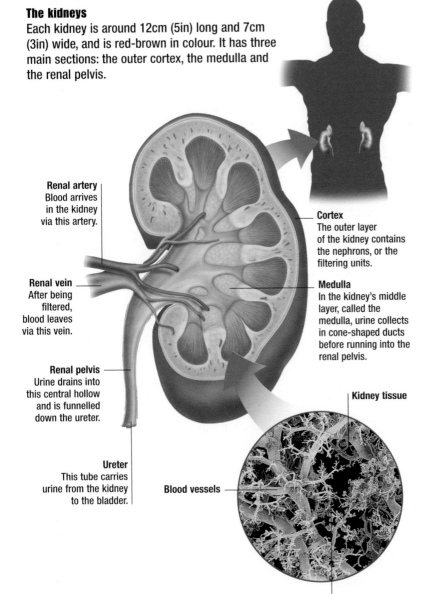

The kidneys
Each kidney is around 12cm (5in) long and 7cm (3in) wide, and is red-brown in colour. It has three main sections: the outer cortex, the medulla and the renal pelvis.

Renal artery
Blood arrives in the kidney via this artery.

Renal vein
After being filtered, blood leaves via this vein.

Renal pelvis
Urine drains into this central hollow and is funnelled down the ureter.

Ureter
This tube carries urine from the kidney to the bladder.

Cortex
The outer layer of the kidney contains the nephrons, or the filtering units.

Medulla
In the kidney's middle layer, called the medulla, urine collects in cone-shaped ducts before running into the renal pelvis.

Kidney tissue

Blood vessels

Capillaries

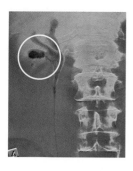

▲ **Kidney stones**
This kidney stone can be seen as an orange lump in the kidney (circled). In an intravenous urogram (IVU) test, the individual was injected with a radio-opaque liquid. This makes the stone visible on the X-ray as the kidneys process the liquid in order to excrete it in urine.

they may remain unnoticed as long as they stay in place. On the other hand, a tiny stone may cause excruciating pain if it leaves the kidney and tears the lining of the urinary tract on its way to the bladder.

See your doctor if you develop any of these symptoms. He or she will test your urine and may give you a pain-relieving injection and refer you to a hospital for **X-rays** and examination by a specialist. The doctor will also seek to treat any underlying cause of the problem such as **gout** or infection.

Small kidney stones are passed as fine gravel in the urine. The larger stones can be shattered by a shock-wave treatment known medically as **lithotripsy**. Alternatively, they can be removed surgically.

Pyelonephritis

Pyelonephritis is an infection of the kidney that can be either short-term (acute), or long-term (chronic). Acute pyelonephritis is usually a complication of **cystitis** and is caused by bacteria that live in the bowel such as **E. coli**.

This form of the disease is more common in women. This is because the urethra, the tube leading from the bladder to exterior of the body, is much shorter in women than in men – so bacteria can enter the bladder more easily and move up to the kidney. In addition, sexual activity can push bacteria up into the woman's urethra. During pregnancy, hormonal changes relax the muscle fibres lining the urinary tract, which also makes it easier for bacteria to move up towards the kidneys.

Chronic pyelonephritis usually occurs when the normal flow of urine is blocked and becomes stagnant. The commonest cause of chronic pyelonephritis is a leaky valve at the bottom of the tube that links the kidney to the bladder (the ureter). This condition is known medically as vesico-ureteric reflux, and is present from birth. The condition also occurs in children with spina bifida and adults with paraplegia. Other common causes of chronic pyelonephritis include a kidney stone, a tumour in the bladder or an enlarged prostate gland.

The symptoms of pyelonephritis can include the following in adults:
- fever and being unwell;
- chills and shakes;
- a sudden onset of pain in the back and sides, in the region of the waist, and sometimes in the lower abdomen;
- burning, stinging or discomfort when passing urine;
- passing of cloudy or bloodstained urine.

Babies and young children may simply have a pale appearance and a fever and fail to put on weight as expected. In pregnant women,

there are often no symptoms and the disease is discovered during routine antenatal visits.

Pyelonephritis is treated with antibiotics, which clear up most cases within 14 days. You should also drink plenty of fluids, take painkillers in recommended doses to relieve the pain, and get as much rest as possible. Rest in bed if you can. Raising the foot of the bed by 15cm (6in) may help to relieve severe pain.

Your doctor will recommend tests after treatment to check that your urine is completely clear of bacteria. Sometimes surgery is needed to correct anatomical abnormalities or to remove stones or blockages.

Acute pyelonephritis can lead to complications such as blood poisoning (see **Septicaemia**). Take care if an ageing relative develops acute pyelonephritis – it is especially liable to become chronic in elderly people. Chronic pyelonephritis can last for many years, causing high **blood pressure** and, if left untreated, occasionally leading to kidney failure and death.

Glomerulonephritis

'Glomerulonephritis' is the term used for a group of **autoimmune diseases** that result from a buildup of antibodies in the glomeruli (the coils of capillaries within the nephrons, the kidneys' filtering units). This buildup causes inflammation and may be due to the body's response to a concentration of foreign substances (antigens) in the glomeruli. Alternatively, it may be that the antibodies are actually attacking the glomeruli themselves as part of an autoimmune disease.

The inflammation means that the glomeruli cannot work properly as filters. They become leaky, so that blood cells and proteins enter the liquid that the glomeruli filter from the blood. The kidney's ability to remove wastes and excess water is also affected.

Glomerulonephritis can follow a viral or bacterial illness – it sometimes occurs about ten days after an acute throat infection. The condition tends to come on suddenly in children but more slowly in adults. Chronic cases may be due to **lupus** erythematosus. Chronic glomerulonephritis can follow acute attacks, or develop slowly and go unnoticed over a period of many years.

Symptoms of glomerulonephritis can include:
- reduced urine output in the early stage;
- frothy or cloudy urine (as a result of the presence of protein);
- blood in the urine;
- severe headache and backache;
- thirst;
- feeling lethargic;
- puffiness of the face, eyes and legs;

- shortness of breath (because of fluid building up in the lungs);
- high blood pressure.

Consult your doctor at once. He or she will order urine tests and check your blood pressure. You may be sent to hospital for further tests.

Treatment of glomerulonephritis depends on the cause. It can include using antibiotics, corticosteroids and immunosuppressant drugs. Your doctor may recommend that you reduce your intake of fluids and follow a low-salt diet. Acute glomerulonephritis usually improves within two months. Chronic glomerulonephritis may grow worse over months and years and, in some cases, can cause kidney failure.

Conditions such as glomerulonephritis, which allow protein to leak into the urine, can lead to a condition known medically as nephrotic syndrome, in which there is a severe loss of protein from the body. The reduction of protein in the blood causes excess fluid to accumulate in the body tissues, leading to uncomfortable and unsightly swelling of the legs and face, with puffiness around the eyes. Fluid can also accumulate in the chest cavity, a condition known as pleural effusion, or in the abdominal cavity, a condition known as ascites (see **Liver and disorders**). Nephrotic syndrome can also result from severe allergic reactions to bee stings, poison ivy, pollen and cow's milk as well as from kidney damage.

Cancer of the kidney

Cancers of the kidney are rare, and usually occur in people over the age of 40 years. The most common form is renal cell carcinoma, a malignant tumour in the kidney cells. Symptoms include blood in the urine, loin pain, abdominal swelling, fever and weight loss. Renal cell carcinoma is often diagnosed late, with the result that the cancer has spread into other parts of the body before treatment. Because of this, only 25 per cent of people diagnosed with the disease survive for more than five years.

Wilms' nephroblastoma is a tumour that mainly affects children under the age of four years. It accounts for about ten per cent of cancers in young children. Its symptoms include a lump in the abdomen and sometimes abdominal pain. If the condition is diagnosed and treated early, more than 80 per cent of those affected recover.

Transitional cell carcinoma is a cancer that arises in the cells lining the renal pelvis, where fluid collects before leaving the kidney via the ureter. It is most likely to occur in smokers and those who have used painkillers in high doses for many years. The most common symptom is blood in the urine, but it can also cause enlargement of a kidney – felt as a lump – due to blockage of urine. Survival rates vary, depending on when the disease is diagnosed. A kidney that is cancerous will be removed and anticancer drugs may also be given.

Other disorders

Kidney disease can result from any condition that blocks the normal flow of urine through the urinary system. An enlarged prostate gland, a bladder stone or a congenital obstruction in the ureter can result in urine building up in the bladder. This can cause a swollen, fluid-logged kidney, a condition known medically as hydronephrosis. Treatment depends on whether the kidney is still healthy. If so, the blockage is surgically removed and kidney function may return to normal. If not, the kidney is surgically removed. In reflux nephropathy, the kidney is damaged by irritation and scarring as a result of the backflow of urine from the bladder.

Kidney failure

Kidney failure is an inability of the kidneys to filter wastes and remove excess fluid properly. This leads to a buildup of waste products, fluid and salts in the body, raised blood pressure and a reduction in urine output. It can occur suddenly, following severe injury, or be the result of a long-term condition such as glomerulonephritis.

If untreated, kidney failure leads to nausea, loss of appetite, weakness, vomiting, itching of the skin, drowsiness and swelling of the face and body. These symptoms may develop rapidly or gradually. The condition needs to be treated with renal **dialysis**, to filter the blood and lower the levels of waste products in the body artificially, or a kidney **transplant** may be necessary. If left untreated, kidney failure eventually leads to coma and death.

KIDNEY TESTS

The efficiency of the kidneys is usually tested by measuring the blood levels of creatinine, a substance that the kidneys normally excrete. A high concentration means that the kidneys are not functioning properly. The kidneys are also involved in maintaining the body's salt balance, so blood levels of sodium, potassium and chloride ions are usually measured as well.

Kidney imaging assesses the size and structure of both kidneys. It helps to diagnose anatomical abnormalities and problems such as scarring, kidney stones and renal tumours.

There are various techniques for kidney imaging. Initial screening is usually done by **ultrasound** scanning. This has greatly improved in recent years and has the advantage of not exposing the patient to radiation. CT and MRI scanning provide detailed cross-sectional images of the kidneys. The workings of the kidneys can also be seen with an intravenous urogram (IVU), also known as an intravenous pyelogram (IVP). An iodine-based dye is injected into a vein and X-rays are taken as the dye reaches the kidneys and the ureters. X-rays are also taken to show the bladder before and after emptying.

SEE ALSO *Bladder and problems; Cancer; Dialysis; Transplants; Urinary system*

Knee and problems

The knee has two main functions. The first is to bend and therefore to make walking, running, sitting and kneeling possible. The second is to support the body in an upright position without buckling or the need for excessive muscular effort. Anatomically, the knee is a synovial hinge joint (see **Joints and problems**). It is straightened by the quadriceps group of muscles at the front and sides of the thigh, and is bent by the hamstrings at the back of the thigh and the calf muscles in the leg (see **Muscular system**).

Positional support is provided by small rotational movements of the knee joint brought about by one of the quadriceps muscles, the vastus medialis. When the knee is braced back – when walking, for example – the thigh bone is rotated slightly inwards and locked firmly onto the shin bone so that little muscular effort is required to maintain the position.

WHAT CAN GO WRONG

Conditions affecting the knee can lead to severe pain. They are caused by inflammation of the cartilage or other elements, or by wear-and-tear damage to the joint.

Arthritis

All the arthritic disorders can trouble the knee, but it is affected by osteoarthritis more often than any other joint (see **Arthritis**).

In osteoarthritis, the bones become eroded and the cartilage wears away. The condition is especially common in elderly, overweight women. Often both knees are affected at the same time, causing severe pain and great difficulty moving about.

Consult a doctor if pain in your knee is interfering with your normal activities. The doctor may arrange for a blood test, an **X-ray**

The body's largest joint

The knee is formed by the junction at the bottom of the thigh bone (femur) and the top of the two bones of the lower leg – the shinbone (tibia) and the outer leg bone (fibula). It enables the leg to bend and allows a small amount of rotation.

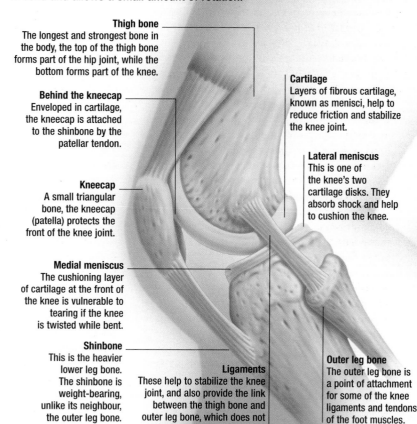

Thigh bone
The longest and strongest bone in the body, the top of the thigh bone forms part of the hip joint, while the bottom forms part of the knee.

Behind the kneecap
Enveloped in cartilage, the kneecap is attached to the shinbone by the patellar tendon.

Kneecap
A small triangular bone, the kneecap (patella) protects the front of the knee joint.

Medial meniscus
The cushioning layer of cartilage at the front of the knee is vulnerable to tearing if the knee is twisted while bent.

Shinbone
This is the heavier lower leg bone. The shinbone is weight-bearing, unlike its neighbour, the outer leg bone.

Cartilage
Layers of fibrous cartilage, known as menisci, help to reduce friction and stabilize the knee joint.

Lateral meniscus
This is one of the knee's two cartilage disks. They absorb shock and help to cushion the knee.

Ligaments
These help to stabilize the knee joint, and also provide the link between the thigh bone and outer leg bone, which does not form part of the knee joint.

Outer leg bone
The outer leg bone is a point of attachment for some of the knee ligaments and tendons of the foot muscles.

or a magnetic resonance imaging (MRI) scan to check that no other disorder is responsible for your symptoms. In the early stages, the doctor will recommend **physiotherapy** to strengthen the quadriceps muscles in the thigh, and prescribe anti-inflammatory drugs and painkillers. He or she may discuss strategies for losing weight and recommend a diet high in fruit and vegetables. In advanced cases, a total knee replacement operation may be necessary. Some people find that **acupuncture** helps with arthritic knees.

Baker's cyst

The knee joint is surrounded by a lubricating layer known as the synovial membrane. When this becomes inflamed, a severely painful condition known as a Baker's cyst occurs. This is a secondary condition to rheumatoid arthritis or osteoarthritis of the knee.

Bursitis

Bursae are sacs containing small amounts of lubricating fluid, which are found in parts of the body where there is a great deal of movement and friction. There are ten bursae around the knee joint and these can become

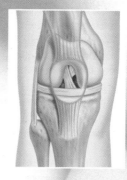

▲ **Front view of the knee**
Two knuckle-like protuberances on the bottom of the thigh bone fit into depressions on the head of the shinbone. They are separated by a layer of cartilage.

inflamed, causing severe pain. One of these, the prepatellar bursa, sits in front of the kneecap and the tendon that holds it in place. When it becomes inflamed, it causes the condition commonly known as housemaid's knee, in which the knee swells, becomes tender and is sometimes also hot to the touch.

Bursitis of the knee joint is called housemaid's knee because it is caused and aggravated by kneeling. If you have to kneel repeatedly, using a rubber mat will help to prevent the condition from developing. If you do develop it, try to rest and avoid pressing on your knee. The condition may last a few days or many months. Some people who suffer from housemaid's knee find pain relief through acupuncture, **massage** and wearing compresses of comfrey or slippery elm (see **Herbal medicine**). Consult a doctor if the swelling persists for more than two weeks or grows bigger. The doctor may use a local **anaesthetic** to numb the knee and then remove excess fluid from the bursa using a fine needle. He will prescribe antibiotics if there is infection. In more serious cases, the doctor may send you for a minor hospital operation in which the bursa is removed under local anaesthetic.

Cartilage problems

The menisci are cartilages that sit between the thigh bone and the shinbone in the knee joint. They can tear when the knee is twisted while it is bent or partly bent. Footballers frequently suffer these tears because their knees often become twisted while they are running or competing for the ball.

After a twisting movement, there is a sudden pain in the knee joint that reduces mobility, and the knee cannot be fully extended. A day later, the knee swells and becomes painful. The medial meniscus at the front of the knee tends to tear more frequently than the lateral meniscus at the rear of the joint.

If you tear your menisci, you will be advised to rest. The condition will subside over a couple of weeks. However, you may never fully recover your ability to extend and lock your knee fully – after the first injury, your knee is likely to give way more easily.

The doctor may recommend treatment by **keyhole surgery** either to repair or remove the menisci, followed by physiotherapy to strengthen the quadriceps muscles. If you tear one of your menisci or have one of them removed, you are more likely to develop osteoarthritis of the knee (see above).

Chondromalacia patella

Chondromalacia patella is a condition affecting the cartilage around the kneecap. It makes any movement of the knee joint extremely painful, especially going up or down stairs.

The condition, also referred to as anterior knee pain, mainly affects adolescent girls.

Doctors do not know for certain what causes the problem, but it is thought to be due to the quadriceps muscles in the thigh pulling on the kneecap at an incorrect angle. As a result, this results in the kneecap grinding against the thigh bone instead of gliding over it. This wears away the cartilage around the kneecap, which means that movement of the knee joint causes pain. If you develop this condition, the doctor will advise you to wear a knee support, take painkillers in recommended doses and rest until the symptoms pass. After that, you will be advised to follow an exercise programme to strengthen and stretch the quadriceps muscles.

Cruciate ligament tears

The two cruciate ligaments in the knee joint help to bind the thigh bone to the shin bone. One is at the front of the joint and is called the anterior cruciate ligament. It stops the shinbone sliding forwards on the thigh bone. The other, at the rear of the joint, is called the posterior cruciate ligament and stops the shinbone slipping backwards against the thigh bone. The cruciates can tear when the shinbone is jerked or twisted while the thigh bone is in a fixed position – for example, when you land on a leg while turning at the same time or when you are kicked on the back of the leg. Unsurprisingly, footballers often suffer from torn cruciate ligaments – as do those who engage in sports that require a pivotal action, such as discus throwing.

The cruciate ligaments have a poor blood supply and, as a result, even minor tears heal badly. Even when the initial injury has healed, the knee joint never fully recovers. The torn ligament is weakened and the joint is unstable. This instability often leads to other knee problems such as damage to the layer of cartilage between the thigh bone and shinbone. If you tear your anterior cruciate ligament completely, it may be replaced surgically by means of a graft from either a hamstring tendon or from the tendon that holds the kneecap in position at the front of the knee joint.

Dislocation of the patella

The kneecap may become dislocated from the outside of the knee when the knees are flexed – for example, when standing up, playing bowls or skiing. In some people, the dislocation happens only once, but in others it becomes recurrent and disabling.

A tendency to this problem seems to be congenital – and girls are more likely to suffer than boys. Both knees can be affected, and the first dislocation usually occurs during adolescence. The following people are more likely to be affected:

■ those who are double-jointed – they have an inherited tendency to loose ligaments;

■ those who have a small kneecap bone;

■ people who have shallower than normal protuberances (femoral condyles) on the base of their thigh bone;

■ people whose kneecap sits abnormally high above the knee joint;

■ people with knock-knees (see **Genu valgum**).

The doctor will recommend physiotherapy to strengthen the quadriceps muscles and especially the vastus medialis muscle, which lies on the inner side of the thigh. If dislocations keep recurring, the patellar tendon that helps to hold the kneecap in position may be moved surgically further down, in the middle of the shaft of the shinbone. This alters the angle at which the quadriceps muscle pulls on the kneecap.

Osgood Schlatter's disease

Osgood Schlatter's disease is a painful enlargement of the protuberance at the head of the shinbone. It is caused by excessive and repetitive pulling by the quadriceps muscles in the thigh at the point where the shinbone is attached to the patellar tendon. This condition occurs most often in boys aged 11–16, and especially among those who play sports frequently.

A painful swelling develops below the knee at the top of the shinbone. The pain is at its worst during and after exercise. Boys and others suffering from the disease develop a marked limp and find it increasingly difficult to move the knee joint at all. The condition usually resolves itself over time, although playing sports may not be possible until this has happened. A doctor may recommend immobilizing the knee joint in plaster for six to eight weeks to encourage recovery.

Osteochondritis dissecans

Osteochondritis dissecans is a condition in which an area of bone and cartilage in a joint loses its blood supply – possibly because of an injured blood vessel – and dies. Eventually, the dead area separates but remains inside the joint.

The condition can affect any joint, but it strikes the knee more than any other and occurs most often in the medial condyle, one of the two protuberances at the base of the thigh bone. It causes swelling and pain in the knee, which may lock unexpectedly. The problem generally affects young adults and tends to run in families, suggesting a genetic cause. The symptoms are worse after exercise.

The treatment you will receive varies, depending on how far the condition has developed. If the dead area has not separated, the treatment is to wear a knee support and refrain from strenuous exercise. If separation has already occurred, the fragment of dead tissue will be removed by **keyhole** surgery.

SEE ALSO *Joints and problems; Leg and problems*

Korsakoff's syndrome

Korsakoff's syndrome is a disorder of the brain that results in intellectual impairment, usually as a late complication of long-term alcoholism. The disorder evolves as a result of chronic deficiency of thiamine (vitamin B_1). Less commonly, it occurs as a result of head injury or poisoning with heavy metals, such as lead (found in paint), mercury (present in dental fillings) and cadmium (found in batteries). The sufferer shows signs of **dementia** and memory lapse, and is prone to fabricating events. A person with Korsakoff's syndrome has a complete lack of insight into the condition, although some aspects of intellect, such as problem-solving or understanding the spoken and written word, remain intact.

Varying degrees of recovery can occur, although the condition is not completely curable. In chronic alcoholism, the affected person often shows other signs of the disease, such as **jaundice**, tremor, red palms, wasting, unsteady gait and impaired sensation in the fingers and toes. In this situation, Korsakoff's syndrome can increase the likelihood of developing Wernicke's encephalopathy – a condition in which mental confusion or **delirium** occurs along with difficulty walking and paralysis of the eye muscles.

SEE ALSO *Alcohol and abuse*

Kyphosis

Kyphosis is an excessive outward curvature of the spine, producing a hump or rounded back. This uncommon condition may be caused by a number of underlying diseases. These include osteochondritis, where pressure on an area of softened bone can produce deformity, particularly in children. In later life, kyphosis may be the result of **osteoporosis**, a disorder common in post-menopausal women, in whom thinned and weakened bones cause the spine to curve. Treatment depends on the underlying cause and may include **physiotherapy**, bracing and, in some severe cases, even surgery.

SEE ALSO *Back and back pain; Spine and disorders*

Korsakoff's syndrome may take 20 years to develop in men and about half that time in women.

▼ **Spinal weakness**
The slight 'hunchback', or kyphosis, of this teenage boy was probably caused by inflammation in his spinal region, resulting in weak or softened bones.

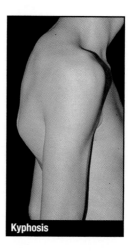
Kyphosis

Labyrinthitis

Labyrinthitis is a viral or bacterial infection of the labyrinth – the part of the inner ear concerned with balance. Symptoms include **vertigo**, **nausea** and vomiting. **Tinnitus** (ringing or buzzing in the ears) and hearing loss may also be experienced. Viral labyrinthitis usually occurs as a complication of flu, measles or mumps. Bacterial cases are linked to infections of the middle ear (otitis media) that have not been thoroughly treated and, occasionally, to head injury.

Viral labyrinthitis tends to clear up without treatment, although this may take several weeks. The bacterial form needs immediate medical attention and treatment with antibiotics because the infection may spread to cause **meningitis**, or it may lead to permanent hearing loss.

SEE ALSO *Ear and problems*

Laparoscopy

A laparoscopy allows the inside of the abdominal cavity to be examined without the need for major surgery. A viewing instrument called a laparoscope is inserted through a small incision in the abdominal wall. To create more space in the abdomen and make viewing easier, carbon dioxide gas is pumped in via a hollow needle that is inserted into a another small incision under the navel. The procedure is carried out under general **anaesthetic**.

Operations such as removal of the appendix or gallbladder, and female sterilization, are now often done using laparoscopy rather than conventional surgery to avoid making a large incision. A miniature video camera is attached to the tip of the laparoscope, allowing an image to be enlarged and viewed on a television monitor during the operation. Gynaecologists also use laparoscopy to examine the Fallopian tubes and ovaries, and to investigate **infertility**.

SEE ALSO *Endoscopy; Keyhole surgery*

Laparotomy

Laparotomy is an exploratory operation that is generally carried out to diagnose problems in the abdominal cavity. It involves making an incision through the abdominal wall.

Today, non-invasive methods, such as a CT scan, **ultrasound** and **laparoscopy**, are often used instead. But laparotomy has a place when complications develop after conventional or **keyhole** surgery, or when patients have had previous abdominal operations. For instance, adhesions between segments of bowel may arise, causing abdominal obstruction; a laparotomy allows the surgeon to cut through these to relieve the obstruction.

Laryngoscopy

Laryngoscopy is a technique used to examine the **larynx** (voice box) in order to detect abnormalities in the vocal cords. It involves putting a viewing tube into the patient's throat to see persistent infection, nodules or tumours.

In a direct laryngoscopy, the patient lies down, extending the neck, and the doctor presses down the tongue using a rigid or flexible tube (laryngoscope). Use of a rigid laryngoscope requires a general **anaesthetic**, but with the flexible tube the patient needs only mild sedation. In an indirect laryngoscopy, the patient sits or stands while a mirror is held behind the tongue. No sedation is needed.

Larynx and disorders

The larynx, also known as the voice box, is an organ located at the upper end of the windpipe and at the front of the oesophagus. It is responsible for producing your voice, and it prevents choking by stopping food entering the airway when you swallow. This function is performed by the epiglottis, which forms a protective lid over the top of the larynx.

It is easy to find the larynx, because it forms a protuberance known as the Adam's apple just beneath the skin in the front of the neck. The Adam's apple is far more prominent in men, and begins to enlarge from puberty.

THE VOICE BOX

The larynx makes speech possible. It is made up of strips of cartilage, between which are stretched two flaps of tissue called the vocal cords. As air passes through the larynx, the vocal cords vibrate, producing sounds. They are controlled by a set of muscles that can generate different degrees of contraction in the tissue, producing a range of sounds of different pitch. The loudness of the sound depends on the amount of air passing over the vocal cords, which, in turn, is regulated by the pressure applied to the lungs by the chest and the abdominal muscles.

Because men have longer, thicker and less taut vocal cords than women, their voices tend to be deeper. And a person's voiceprint – an electronic analysis of the sound he or she produces – is as individual as a fingerprint. The voice derives its unique quality from the shape

The larynx
The main job of the larynx is to channel air into the windpipe and produce the voice, but it also helps to filter the air and prevents choking.

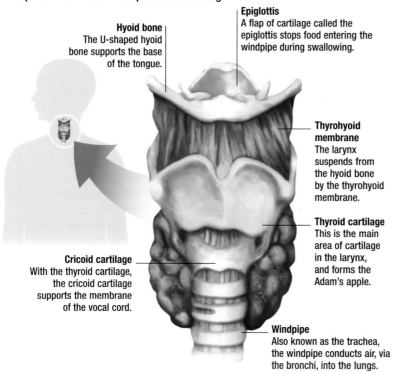

Hyoid bone
The U-shaped hyoid bone supports the base of the tongue.

Epiglottis
A flap of cartilage called the epiglottis stops food entering the windpipe during swallowing.

Thyrohyoid membrane
The larynx suspends from the hyoid bone by the thyrohyoid membrane.

Thyroid cartilage
This is the main area of cartilage in the larynx, and forms the Adam's apple.

Cricoid cartilage
With the thyroid cartilage, the cricoid cartilage supports the membrane of the vocal cord.

Windpipe
Also known as the trachea, the windpipe conducts air, via the bronchi, into the lungs.

of the nasal cavity and the sinuses, while the vast repertoire of speech comes from the lips, tongue and soft palate modifying the sounds produced by the larynx.

WHAT CAN GO WRONG
Most problems with the larynx cause hoarseness because they affect the vocal cords. Other symptoms of laryngeal disease include coughing and breathing difficulties.

Laryngitis and epiglottitis
When the vocal cords are swollen, infected or have growths on them, the flow of air past them is affected and the voice sounds hoarse, breathy or husky. There may also be a harsh noise on inhalation. Known medically as stridor, the noise is caused by turbulence as air passes through distorted vocal cords. Most commonly, hoarseness indicates laryngitis, an inflammation of the larynx. This often follows an upper respiratory infection, particularly when it is accompanied by a sore throat and fever.

Laryngitis is best treated with rest, plenty of fluids and painkillers. But see your doctor if symptoms are severe or if they persist. Laryngitis is usually caused by a virus, but persistent laryngitis may have a bacterial cause, in which case antibiotics might be prescribed.

Epiglottitis, an inflammation of the epiglottis, is a rare disease that can obstruct breathing. Symptoms include fever, hoarseness and noisy

breathing, which are similar to those in **croup** but are not relieved by steam inhalation. It can be fatal if untreated, especially in young children. Treatment is with antibiotics and sometimes with artificial ventilation.

Growths and tumours
If hoarseness persists for more than two weeks, seek medical attention. There may be a growth or tumour on the larynx. Although most of these growths are benign (non-cancerous), they should always be looked at to exclude the possibility of cancer. There are various types of laryngeal tumours.

- **Vocal cord nodules** – or 'singers' nodes' – are smooth, benign tumours on the vocal cords. They are usually found in professional singers and people who overuse their voice.
- **Polyps** – these are benign tumours that often occur in smokers. They may also affect people who have been exposed to a chemical irritant.
- **Warts** – these are benign tumours caused by a virus. They sometimes develop on children's vocal cords.
- **Ulcers** – these may occur in people with acid indigestion. A weakened stomach valve allows acid from the gut to travel up the oesophagus and corrode the mucous membranes of the oesophagus and larynx, causing ulcers.
- **Squamous cell carcinoma** – this is a malignant growth and the most common form of **cancer** of the larynx. It tends to occur in people who smoke tobacco and drink alcohol in large quantities. Besides hoarseness, symptoms include coughing up blood, pain on swallowing, weight loss, ear ache and swollen neck glands.

Any of the above conditions may require a **laryngoscopy**, which allows doctors to view the larynx. It may be necessary to remove nodules or to take a **biopsy** sample so that any growths can be investigated for signs of cancer.

Leukoplakia
A common cause of hoarseness among smokers is a disorder called laryngeal leukoplakia. A **biopsy** may reveal a precancerous cell change called dysplasia. Around 5 per cent of cases of mild dysplasia develop into cancer; in severe cases, up to 60 per cent will progress to cancer. Giving up **smoking** can reverse dysplasia.

Vocal cord paralysis
Occasionally, a tumour, an infection or surgery in the throat area damages one or more of the nerves serving the larynx, resulting in vocal cord paralysis. This causes loss of voice and can interfere with breathing. In some cases, surgery is performed to remodel the voice box by moving the affected vocal cord.

Removal of the larynx
If someone has a large cancerous tumour on the larynx, the larynx has to be removed along with

the tumour through an incision in the neck. This is known as a laryngectomy. The airway below the larynx (the trachea) is then sewn to the skin around the incision to make an artificial opening called a stoma, through which the patient then breathes.

The person can be taught, using speech therapy, to speak in a new way – swallowing air, and then expelling it. The so-called oesophagal speech produced this way is gruff, but recognizable. Alternatively, some form of artificial larynx can be used.

Laser surgery

Laser surgery is performed using a high-energy light beam. The energy from the light beam bombards the tissue cells until their structure is destroyed. A laser light source can cut like a scalpel, destroy diseased tissue and seal small blood vessels. Since it can be focused precisely on very small areas, a laser can be particularly useful in surgical procedures where the surrounding tissue needs to be preserved. It also reduces the scarring normally associated with such operations.

A recently developed technique involves scattering laser light over the operation site, which shows up the natural contour lines of the skin. The surgeon can make the incisions along these lines, which minimizes any scarring. Many people find that they need no pain relief after minor laser surgery, especially if a local **anaesthetic** is given during the procedure. Major surgery using lasers causes less discomfort than conventional surgery because bleeding and swelling are reduced.

WHY IT IS DONE

Laser surgery has many uses, including:
- removal of tumours (such as in the brain or liver);
- ear, nose and throat surgery, including procedures to relieve snoring and operations on the ear and removal of tonsils;
- treatment of eye conditions, such as **cataracts**, diabetic and age-related eye disease;
- vision correction for people who do not want to wear glasses or contact lenses;
- clearing out decay in teeth and gum surgery;
- sealing of small blood vessels to reduce bleeding;
- sealing of lymph vessels to reduce swelling and prevent the spread of malignant cells;
- sealing of nerve endings to reduce pain;
- cosmetic surgery, such as the removal of tattoos, warts, moles, wrinkles and other skin blemishes or flattening of scars;
- removal of unwanted hair.

COMPLICATIONS

Apart from the risks associated with any general anaesthetic, laser surgery may result in complications typical of skin wounds, such as bleeding and infection.

Laser exposure to skin can result in burning and redness, particularly in sensitive areas such as the face. Such burning and redness usually disappears after about a week. Long-term scarring and burns and lasting discoloration of the skin can occur, but are quite rare.

Exposure to strong sunlight before and after laser surgery should be avoided to reduce the likelihood of these complications.

SEE ALSO *Surgery and surgical techniques*

Lassa fever

Lassa fever is a dangerous, sometimes fatal, infectious disease caused by a virus. It was first identified in the 1960s after an outbreak in Lassa, Nigeria. Infection occurs mainly through contact with the faeces of infected rodents deposited on floors or beds or in food or water. The illness starts with a fever, headache, muscular aches and a sore throat. Later, severe diarrhoea and vomiting develop.

The condition is diagnosed by a blood test. Infected people must be isolated, and are treated by the relief of symptoms and by injections of the antiviral drug tribavirin and of a serum containing antibodies active against the virus. About a quarter of all people treated in hospital for Lassa fever die from the illness.

SEE ALSO *Travel and tropical diseases*

Lead poisoning

Lead poisoning is caused by the inhalation of lead fumes or dust, usually from industrial processes. It may be acute or chronic.

Symptoms of acute lead poisoning take hold rapidly after exposure. They include abdominal pain, diarrhoea and vomiting, sometimes accompanied by convulsions and paralysis.

Chronic lead poisoning is caused by cumulative exposure to low doses of lead – for example, from lead waterpipes or lead-based paints. The telltale sign of chronic poisoning is a blue line on the gums. Symptoms include **anaemia** and abdominal pain, and there may be kidney or nerve damage. In both acute and chronic cases, complications include mental disturbances. Treatment is with a chemical agent called edetate, or EDTA, which chemically binds to the lead and allows the body to excrete it.

Learning difficulties

People with learning difficulties find it hard to pick up skills or to process information. They are no less intelligent than other people, but they may appear so. Early assessment and help resolves most problems.

People with learning difficulties may well know more than they can express. However, they may be incapable of providing answers if questions are presented in ways that they cannot grasp.

Learning disorders are distinct from learning problems caused by poor vision or hearing, emotional disturbance or mental disabilities such as **autism** or **Down's syndrome**. They are also not the same thing as 'slow' learning, where a child simply lags behind its peers in development. Slow learners eventually catch up, but people with learning difficulties remain at a disadvantage all their lives, in that they have to work harder, or find alternative mental strategies, to do things that come naturally to others.

An abnormality may affect the way in which an individual understands information, such as the appearance of written words. Or it may affect the way in which a person's intention (for example, to move the hand in order to write a word) is translated into appropriate muscle commands.

In some cases there is a failure in the bodily mechanism governing attentiveness. This results in an inability to focus on particular information and therefore to take it in and act on it.

CAUSES OF LEARNING DIFFICULTIES

Learning difficulties start with a problem in one or more of the intellectual processes involved in the laying down, retrieving and handling of information. Many learning difficulties are thought to originate in prenatal development, when the embryonic brain is organizing the neural pathways that process information. One possible cause is oxygen deprivation while in the womb or during birth.

This failure to process information properly is caused by an abnormality in brain structure or function. Different types of information are processed along different pathways in the brain. Learning difficulties show up in various ways, depending on which pathway is affected. The development of the brain may be arrested temporarily if a fetus is deprived of oxygen. This sometimes occurs during pregnancy or birth if the umbilical cord becomes wrapped around the baby's neck, or if there is a very difficult or prolonged labour.

Genetic factors may also contribute, and learning disorders often run in families. A child with a language problem, for example, tends to have a parent with a similar history. However, the parent may have, for example, **dyslexia** – the inability to understand written words or to express oneself in writing – while the child may have dyscalculia – an inability to carry out mathematical calculations.

Some researchers believe that there is a pattern of genetic inheritance that tends to produce certain types of brain dysfunction which will manifest themselves in one of several forms. For example, geneticists have identified a gene that is essential for the normal development of language, but – in contrast to what might have been expected – its absence has not been linked specifically with dyslexia.

Toxins (poisons) may also be a cause of the brain abnormalities that lead to learning difficulties. Drugs such as alcohol, nicotine and cocaine taken by the mother during pregnancy may affect brain development in the child directly – or indirectly, by causing premature birth, which in turn makes the baby more vulnerable to brain dysfunction. Environmental toxins may affect

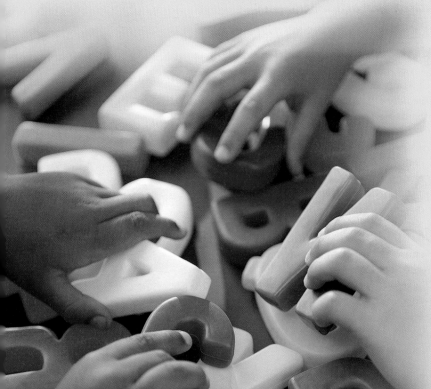

▼ Development through play
Long before children are ready for formal teaching, playing with large, brightly coloured plastic letters and numbers can help establish basic literacy and numeracy skills.

brain development after birth. For example, learning difficulties are more common in children born in areas with a high concentration of lead pollution from vehicle-exhaust fumes.

TYPES OF LEARNING DIFFICULTIES

Learning difficulties take the form of language disorders, academic skills disorders, attention disorders or dyspraxia, which affects coordination. A whole host of different language and academic skills disorders have been identified. These disorders have similar-sounding names. However, they all describe related but distinct problems.

Language disorders

Speech and language problems are often the earliest indicators of learning disabilities. Children may fail to produce normal speech sounds, use words inappropriately or fail to understand what other people are saying.

Such characteristics are normal in infants when they first start to use language. A learning difficulty should be suspected only when the mistakes persist in a child long after they have ceased to occur in others of similar age.

Developmental articulation disorder (DAD) is marked by a difficulty in speaking words correctly or controlling the rate of speech. Infantile pronunciation may persist – for example, a six-year-old may say 'wabbit' for 'rabbit' or 'thwim' for 'swim'. Developmental articulation disorder may disappear naturally, as children learn to correct themselves, or it may be helped by speech therapy.

Factfile

How common are learning difficulties?

About 5 per cent of school-age children in the UK are estimated to have learning difficulties, and many continue to have problems as adults.

It is impossible to say precisely how widespread learning difficulties are because there is no routine screening and a perceived learning problem is frequently mistaken for general slowness or, in children, naughtiness.

Learning difficulties are much more likely to be recognized in families where a high level of academic achievement is expected than in those where doing badly at school is unremarkable. Highly intelligent children (and adults) cope with learning disabilities by working exceptionally hard or by finding imaginative ways of achieving results that others arrive at easily. These people may therefore appear 'average' and their special talents may be overlooked.

In the case of developmental expressive language disorder (DELD), the problem is finding the correct words and stringing them together rather than simply saying them. A five-year-old who speaks only in two-word phrases or a six-year-old who cannot answer a simple question with anything more than yes or no may have developmental expressive language disorder.

Developmental receptive language disorder (DRLD) manifests itself as a failure to understand what other people say. The lack of understanding may apply to all speech, but sometimes it is only certain types of words that are misunderstood. For example, a child may mix up nouns – and pass a cup, say, when you have asked for a ball. Developmental receptive language disorder is often mistaken for hearing dysfunction, but the problem lies not in speech discrimination but in speech understanding – the word is heard correctly but is 'scrambled' in the brain. As using and understanding language are closely related, people with DRLD often have DELD, too.

Academic skills disorders

Students with academic skills disorders are often years behind their classmates in standards of reading, writing and arithmetic. Each of the 'three Rs' has a specific diagnosis associated with it.

Dyslexia, or developmental reading disorder (DRD), is probably the most common type of learning difficulty. It is marked by the inability to comprehend the written word or to express ideas in written form. Various types of information-processing problems cause developmental reading disorder. One is the inability to connect single letters to make words – for example, a child may be able to read out the letters b-a-t but be unable to string them together to form the word. Another is the inability to translate a written word into a concept – a child with this form of dyslexia may be able to read the word 'bat' but be unable to connect it with the object itself.

Developmental writing disorder (DWD) is characterized by an inability to express words in written form. Children with developmental writing disorder may be unable to write down words spoken to them – even though they may be able to read them. They may also be unable to compose grammatical sentences on the page. Developmental writing disorder is closely linked with developmental reading disorder and often occurs with it.

▲ **Developmental arithmetic disorder**
Some children have great difficulty relating numbers to the symbols that represent them, and cannot work out how to do the most basic sums.

Developmental arithmetic disorder (DArD), also known as dyscalculia, is marked by an inability to do even the simplest calculations. Mathematical skills may seem distinct from language skills, but both depend on recognizing and manipulating symbols, and both depend on certain common information-processing pathways. For this reason, developmental arithmetic disorder may occur in conjunction with other learning difficulties. But some aspects of maths – those concerned with geometric comprehension, for example – are dealt with in a separate part of the brain, so this disorder may appear in isolation, too. If one part of the brain is 'underperforming', another part may be overactive – so a person who is very bad at language may be very good at certain aspects of maths, and vice versa.

Attention disorders

The attention system in a child's brain takes time to develop. The symptoms of an attention disorder are the normal state for very young children, but behaviour normal in a two-year-old is abnormal in an older child, and five- or six-year-olds who cannot turn their attention to a single topic and focus on it may have an attention disorder. There are two types: attention deficit disorder (ADD) and attention deficit hyperactivity disorder (**ADHD**). ADD is characterized by a failure to concentrate, and children with the disorder are often passive and prone to day-dreaming. ADHD is marked by a failure to remain focused on an outside stimulus such as an academic task or a teacher's instruction. It manifests itself as constantly flickering attention, impulsive behaviour, and physical and mental agitation. Both disorders can make academic learning extremely difficult.

One in 200 children in the UK is believed to suffer from attention deficit hyperactivity disorder, while in the USA one in twelve has been diagnosed as having the condition.

Dyspraxia

Dyspraxia is a disorder of the system that coordinates hand, body and brain (see **Brain and nervous system**). The system allows people to carry out complicated and precise movements; when it fails to work properly the person becomes clumsy and physically uncontrolled. Dyspraxia may affect children's ability to do simple things such as getting dressed or throwing a ball. It may also prevent them from making the fine hand movements used in writing or drawing.

RECOGNIZING LEARNING DIFFICULTIES

Parents are usually the first people to notice delays in their child's development or more subtle signs of learning difficulties. Some problems are apparent before a child starts school, while others may not reveal themselves until a child starts at secondary school. The first few years of life are signposted by milestones such as the start of babbling (the precursor to speech), crawling, first steps, first words and so on. Although all children develop at a slightly different pace, these early markers occur at fairly precise ages – within months rather than years of each other. So, if a child is a full year behind others of the same age in skills such as talking or walking, there may be some reason to suspect a learning difficulty. By the time children start school, parents have a fairly good idea about their general intelligence – one sign of a learning difficulty is if children fail to do as well as might be expected given their intelligence levels. Regular contact with teachers is essential to identify particular problems.

TREATMENT

As a group, children with learning difficulties have the same range of intelligence levels as other children – and most can achieve average academic performance (or higher) with the help of special tuition. If a learning difficulty is suspected at school, parents may ask for a formal assessment from their local education authority. If the child is found to have such a problem, he or she may be defined as having special educational needs and assigned to a special school or given extra tuition – a process known as 'statementing'. The resources available for such children differ from area to area.

A child who suffers from language disorders or academic skills disorders should be given detailed hearing and sight tests, as defects in these areas often exacerbate learning difficulties. A doctor will refer your child for these tests.

Children with attention disorders may benefit from prescription amphetamine-derived drugs such as Ritalin, which enhance concentration. In some children they provoke side effects, including headaches, disturbed sleep and loss of appetite.

Changes in diet appear to improve behaviour in some children with attention disorders, although there is no scientific proof of this. Some children with an attention disorder may have a food **allergy** or be unable to metabolize substances such as preservatives and artificial colours in processed foods. It may be worth avoiding cow's milk, chocolate, sweetened fizzy drinks and foods rich in additives. Before making changes in a child's diet, discuss them with your doctor.

There is some evidence that children with language problems may be helped by a diet rich in fish oils.

Behaviour therapy and cognitive behaviour therapy may help children with attention disorders to control their behaviour by means of both positive encouragement and reward schemes.

SEE ALSO **Dyslexia**

Leg and problems

Our legs support most of our body weight, so they have to be strong as well as flexible and responsive. Some problems affecting the legs can seriously restrict mobility, and hence may have an impact on our whole way of life; others, such as **cramp**, can cause temporary – although intense – pain.

HOW THE LEG WORKS

The thigh bone, or femur, is the longest and one of the strongest bones in the body. It forms a ball-and-socket joint with the pelvis at the hip and a hinge joint with the shin bone, or tibia, at the knee. The tibia, another long bone, goes down from the knee and its lower end forms part of the ankle joint. A thinner bone, the fibula, lies on the outside of the leg, next to the tibia, and also forms part of the ankle joint – but it plays no part in the knee joint; its top end is attached to the tibia by ligaments.

The bones and joints of the leg are supported, stabilized and moved by groups of ligaments and large, powerful muscles. The largest of these muscles are the quadriceps group at the front of the thigh, the hamstrings at the back of the thigh and the calf muscles (the soleus and gastrocnemius). There are many other smaller muscles, especially around the foot.

BLOOD SUPPLY TO THE LEG

The main blood supply to the leg is from the femoral artery, which comes through the abdomen and then passes through the groin and down the inner thigh to the knee. As it passes behind the knee, it becomes the popliteal artery, which in turn divides into two arteries called the anterior and posterior tibial arteries. The anterior tibial artery supplies blood to the front of the leg and the top of the foot, while the posterior tibial artery supplies the calf and the sole of the foot.

Blood returns up the leg through a network of deep-lying veins and the large saphenous vein, which runs up the inner side of the leg, and joins the femoral vein at the groin.

Two factors prevent gravity from forcing blood to flow backwards when an individual is standing or sitting. Firstly, the veins of the leg contain one-way valves; secondly, the muscles of the lower leg force blood back up to the heart when they contract – this type of mechanism is described as 'muscle pump'.

Nerves in the leg

The main nerve in the leg is the sciatic nerve, which is the longest nerve in the body. It runs down the back of the thigh to the knee and can be affected by spinal problems in **sciatica**.

At the knee the sciatic nerve divides into the tibial and common peroneal nerve. The tibial nerve runs down the calf into the foot, and the smaller common peroneal nerve crosses over the fibula and runs down the outside of the leg, making it vulnerable to damage.

WHAT CAN GO WRONG

A large number of conditions can affect the leg. They include injuries, fluid retention, nerve damage, numbness, arthritis of the hip and knee, cramp, varicose veins, ischaemia, leg ulcers, bow legs and knock-knee. Symptoms of leg problems are also very varied, but mainly involve aches and pains, and general lack of mobility.

Leg muscles and bones
Because legs have to support the entire weight of the human body, they contain some of our strongest bones and most powerful muscles.

Quadriceps
These powerful muscles at the front of the thigh cause the thigh to bend at the hip and the leg to swing forward.

Knee joint
A hinge joint, reinforced by strong ligaments, the knee joint links the bones of the thigh and lower leg.

Fibula
The thinner lower leg bone, the fibula is not part of the knee joint, but is linked to the tibia at both ends.

Calf muscles
These strong muscles at the back of the lower leg allow the foot to bend downwards, providing the thrust for moving forward.

Hamstrings
These muscles at the back of the thigh help pull the thigh back and cause the knee to bend.

Femur
The longest bone in the body, the femur, or thigh bone, links the pelvis with the knee.

Patella
A flat, triangular bone, the patella, or kneecap, covers and protects the front of the knee joint.

Tibia
The thicker of the two lower leg bones, the tibia, or shinbone, forms a joint with the femur at the knee. At its lower end, it forms part of the ankle joint.

Ankle joint
A hinge joint is formed at the ankle between the tibia and the talus bone in the foot.

Arthritis of the hip and knee

Arthritis of the hip and knee is extremely common. Both the knee and the hip joints are frequently affected by osteoarthritis and rheumatoid arthritis, often leading to severe disability requiring joint replacement.

Injuries

Leg injuries, such as **fractures** and torn tissues, are often caused by accidents, falls or direct blows – motorcycle or riding accidents often result in serious leg injuries. Leg bone fractures, especially those of the femur, tend to take a long time to heal.

Cramp

Cramp is a painful spasmodic contraction of a muscle or group of muscles. It usually affects the calf muscles and the hamstrings at the back of the thigh. The causes are not fully understood, but excessive salt loss as a result of sweating, strenuous exercise and taking drugs, such as amphetamines, can lead to cramp.

Varicose veins

In the UK, more than 500,000 people consult their GP about varicose veins each year. Five times more women than men are affected. The presence of enlarged, and often twisted and distorted, veins near the surface of the leg is caused by weak valves in the veins that carry blood away from the leg back into the femoral vein. Some blood therefore flows backwards into the veins, putting extra pressure on them. Treatment is required in all but minor cases to prevent complications such as ulceration. (See **Veins and disorders.**)

Numbness

Numbness of any part of the leg can be caused by a disorder affecting the nervous system as a whole or by damage to nerves that serve the affected area. An example of a disorder that affects the whole nervous system is a **stroke**, which can cause paralysis as well as numbness. **Sciatica**, which can cause numbness down the back of the thigh, knee, calf and the sole of the foot, is an example of damage to a nerve.

Sometimes a circulatory problem can limit the blood supply to an area and make it impossible for the nerves there to function correctly.

Swelling

Some causes of a swollen leg are trivial, such as an insect bite, but others are life-threatening – a **deep vein thrombosis**, for example. There are four main causes.

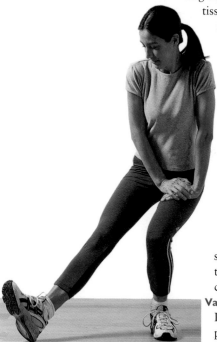

▲ **Take time to stretch**
Always stretch before and after exercise sessions. This 'warms up' the muscles, avoiding strain, and helps to avoid soreness afterwards.

■ Heart failure or kidney failure, both of which cause fluid retention.

■ Weakness in the veins that prevents them from carrying blood efficiently out of the leg and into the femoral vein with each heartbeat, causing some of the blood to leak backwards. The medical term for this is venous insufficiency. It is more likely to be the cause of swelling in the ankles and legs but not the feet; ulceration is also associated with problems in the veins. If the valves in the veins of the leg are damaged or become malformed, or if the muscle pump is inadequate, venous blood collects in the veins, which places pressure on the capillaries. This forces fluid from the capillaries into nearby tissues.

■ Damage or obstruction to the **lymphatic system**, which helps drain tissue fluid in the lower leg. It relies on the pumping action of the leg muscles to remove much of this fluid, so any weakness in these muscles can lead to fluid retention and swelling.

■ Allergy, injury or disease. A swelling in one area with no general symptoms may be the result of an allergic reaction to an insect bite. It can also be a sign of a serious condition such as a deep vein thrombosis, which is difficult to detect but requires immediate treatment. Some forms of rheumatism also cause swelling, but other symptoms, such as swollen and painful joints, are usually felt as well.

If you have a swollen leg, see a doctor for a diagnosis. If any infection is detected, antibiotics will be given to reduce further damage to the veins or lymph vessels. Lymphapress treatment – in which a machine massages the leg mechanically from ankle to thigh, mimicking the effect of muscular activity – may be offered.

Support stockings and special exercises may also be recommended to help reduce swelling. Try to keep the foot higher than the pelvis whenever possible to promote drainage of fluid.

Leg ulcers

Ulcers of the leg are common, especially in elderly and disabled people. In 95 per cent of cases the cause is a circulatory problem, generally relating to a vein.

Venous ulcers are common around the ankle joint, while ulcers linked to problems with arteries are usually found on the foot and are more likely to be painful. Other causes of ulcers are nerve damage caused by diabetes or **alcohol abuse**, infection, injury and pressure sores (see **Bedsores**).

The underlying cause needs to be treated, but you can promote healing of the ulcer by:
■ keeping it clean and dry;
■ washing it with salt water;

- wearing support stockings;
- using paraffin dressings as directed by your doctor.

People with leg ulcers should not use steroids or antibiotic creams. Severe, deep ulcers may require surgical cleansing before any form of healing treatment can start.

Ischaemia

Ischaemia is an inadequate supply of blood to an area of the body – in this case, the lower leg. As a result, the muscles become deprived of oxygen. It is usually due to a blockage of an artery as a result of arteriosclerosis, in which fatty deposits are laid down on the arterial walls, or damage. The lower leg and the heart are two areas of the body most often affected.

The symptoms of lower-leg ischaemia include:
- cramplike pain when walking;
- absent or weak pulse at the groin, knee, ankle or foot, either during exercise or just after;
- pain when at rest, especially at night;
- skin becoming colourless;
- cold legs and feet.

See your doctor if you are suffering from any of these symptoms. He or she may recommend one of the following procedures in order to confirm a diagnosis.
- An ankle pressure unit, similar to a normal blood pressure gauge, is used to take the pulse at the ankle, before and just after the patient finishes exercising. If it is weaker or absent after exercise, the person has ischaemia. The length of time it takes for the pulse to return to normal also indicates the likely number of blockages and their location. A recovery time of less than 15 minutes usually indicates a single blockage, while a longer recovery time suggests that there is more than one.
- Arteriography is a procedure in which a radio-opaque substance is injected into the arteries so that they are visible when an **X-ray** is carried out. Any narrowing of the space within the arteries can be seen. This procedure is used to pinpoint the site or sites of a blockage.

How ischaemia is treated depends on the patient's overall health, because people with lower-leg ischaemia often also suffer from heart ischaemia and this may need to be dealt with first. Treatment of ischaemia includes the following:
- drugs in the form of vasodilators, which widen the blood vessels by relaxing the muscle in their walls;
- surgical reconstruction, in which the affected area of the artery is replaced by either an artificial tube or a length of vein taken from another part of the body;
- rarely, amputation, which may be necessary in very serious cases as a preventive measure.

When there are areas of dead tissue, surgery is carried out to stop any infection from spreading to unaffected parts of the leg (see **Gangrene**).

Bow legs and knock-knee

Bow legs and knock-knee are both common in childhood. Bow legs, known medically as genu varum, usually correct themselves over time. Mild cases of bow leg are so common as to be considered normal in children between the ages of one and three.

Knock-knee, which is known medically as genu valgum, is common in children between the ages of three and five and usually corrects itself as the child develops.

Treatment may be required if either condition is severe or persists long after an age when it would be considered normal. There are a number of possible underlying causes. These include:
- a fracture of the lower part of the femur or of the upper part of the tibia that has not healed properly;
- the uneven development of part of the femur or tibia in children;
- rheumatoid arthritis or osteoarthritis;
- **rickets, Paget's disease** or osteomalacia (see **Bones and disorders**).

Children are not usually treated until after they have reached the age of ten, unless the cause of the problem is an underlying disease. If the bones are developing abnormally, the bones on one side of the knee (the epiphyseal plates) are then pinned to slow down growth, and a wedge is placed on the other side to increase the bone's length.

In adults, the only treatments are surgery, known as osteotomy, or to wear remedial shoes to equalize the length of the bones.

SEE ALSO *Ankle and problems; Foot and problems; Hip and problems; Knee and problems*

Legionnaire's disease

Legionnaire's disease is a form of **pneumonia**, and has symptoms that are similar to those of severe flu. The disease takes its name from the first known outbreak, which killed 29 members of the American Legion in a US hotel in 1976.

The bacterium responsible for the disease, *Legionella pneumophila*, thrives in warm, moist conditions, including those commonly found in water tanks, air-conditioning systems and shower heads. Outbreaks usually occur in or around large public buildings.

The infection is contracted when tiny droplets of contaminated water in the atmosphere are breathed in. The disease becomes increasingly

UNDER THE MICROSCOPE

Inhaling air infected with the bacterium *Legionella pneumophila* can not only cause Legionnaire's disease, but may also lead to disorders of the liver and kidneys.

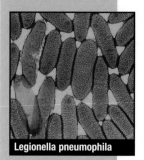

Legionella pneumophila

severe within a few days unless it is treated. Serious breathing problems can develop, which may lead to complete respiratory failure. After treatment, the person will take several weeks to make a complete recovery.

People over the age of 50 are most likely to be affected. In 1997, 226 cases occurred in England and Wales, resulting in 28 deaths.

SYMPTOMS

Early symptoms of Legionnaire's disease include headache, muscular aches and abdominal pain. Other symptoms include:
- fever, shaking and chills;
- nausea, vomiting and diarrhoea;
- dry cough, sometimes accompanied by chest pains;
- pneumonia, in which breathing is difficult as the air sacs in the lungs fill up with fluid or thick phlegm.

TREATMENT

If you suspect that you may have Legionnaire's disease, especially if you have been staying in a hotel or have spent time in a public place where cases have occurred, consult a doctor immediately.

What a doctor may do
- Refer you for sputum and blood tests to confirm the diagnosis.
- Send you for a chest **X-ray**, which will reveal any patches of pneumonia.
- Prescribe antibiotics, such as erythromycin and rifampicin.

PREVENTION

Hotels and other public buildings should keep their water tanks and air-conditioning systems at temperatures of either above or below 20–50°C. This is the ideal temperature for the bacteria, at which they multiply rapidly.

OUTLOOK

Younger people frequently make a full recovery from Legionnaire's disease. But the condition can be fatal, particularly in elderly people, if respiratory failure develops.

SEE ALSO *Infectious diseases*

Lentigo

Lentigo is a flat, brownish discoloration of the skin, similar to a freckle. The spots may occur singly or in groups. They are not sun-related and they do not fade in winter. Lentigines – the plural of lentigo – are considered harmless and no treatment is usually necessary. However, any changes should be reported to a doctor because, rarely, a lentigo may progress to form a malignant melanoma (see **Skin and disorders**).

Leprosy

Leprosy is a bacterial infection, also known as Hansen's disease. It attacks the nervous system, especially the nerves in the hands, feet and face, and may also lead to skin damage. It is caused by a bacterium, *Mycobacterium leprae*, spread in droplets of nasal mucus. Leprosy is a painful condition, but it is curable; when it is left untreated, it can leave sufferers deformed and crippled.

The World Health Organization estimates that there are 830,000 cases of the disease worldwide. It mostly occurs in poverty-stricken areas of Asia and Africa but is very rare in the UK and other developed countries.

SYMPTOMS
- Chronically stuffy nose.
- Many skin lesions and nodules on the front and back of the body.
- Loss of sensation that starts at the fingers and toes and may affect only a small patch of skin at first, before becoming more widespread in some forms of the disease. This can lead to unnoticed injuries, which may in turn become infected.
- In advanced cases, **gangrene** will set in and the skin will rot.

Types of leprosy

There are three types of leprosy, each with distinct symptoms.
- The generalized form, lepromatous, attacks peripheral nerves in the skin, the hands and feet, and the mucous membranes such as the lining of the nose and the eyes.
- Tuberculoid leprosy causes only a few skin lesions. The loss of sensation will affect only a small patch of skin.
- The third type is dimorphous leprosy. It causes skin lesions that affect only a small patch of skin as well as lesions that cause widespread numbness.

TREATMENT
- Early diagnosis of the disease is essential to prevent permanent disfigurement and disability.
- Diagnosis is made by a physical examination and can be confirmed by a skin **biopsy**, the removal of a sample of skin tissue for analysis.
- Treatment is with strong antibiotics, such as dapsone, rifampicin and clofazimine. A combination must be used because the leprosy bacteria can develop resistance to antibiotics very quickly.

OUTLOOK

With treatment, the disease is curable. But most cases occur in places where there may be little medical help available, and so many of those affected are not treated early enough.

Leukaemia

Leukaemia is a cancer that causes abnormal white blood cells to proliferate and damage the blood. The disease can be fatal, but with advances in treatment, many more people are now making a full recovery.

There are many types of leukaemia, most of which disrupt blood-cell production, causing faulty white blood cells to be produced in large numbers in the bone marrow. These cells inhibit the production of normal white blood cells, red blood cells and platelets.

Normal white blood cells are an important part of the body's defence mechanism, so a reduction in the number lowers the person's resistance to infection. A lower level of red blood cells affects the blood's ability to carry oxygen around the body (see **Anaemia**). And a reduction in the number of platelets affects the blood clotting process, with the result that the person may suffer from abnormal bleeding (thrombocytopenia). The cancerous white cells can spread to the lymph nodes, liver and spleen.

HOW LEUKAEMIA DEVELOPS

New blood cells are constantly being formed in the bone marrow, inside the bones, from a supply of mother cells known as precursor or stem cells. In leukaemia this process goes wrong, and large numbers of one particular type of cell are produced. What triggers this process is not yet known, but there are several factors that put people at risk.

Risk factors for leukaemia

- Gender: men are slightly more susceptible than women to developing leukaemia.
- **Smoking**: more than one in four cases of acute myeloid leukaemia can be attributed to the carcinogens in cigarette smoke.
- Previous cancer, especially lymphoma or childhood leukaemia.
- A previous blood disorder which has damaged bone marrow for example, aplastic **anaemia**.
- Exposure to radiation (from previous **radiotherapy**, or in certain occupations such as those associated with nuclear reactors).
- Exposure to carcinogens (such as benzene among fuel workers).
- Genetic factors: there are some genetic links, for example, leukaemia is relatively common in people with **Down's syndrome**.
- Exposure to strong electromagnetic fields, such as living close to electricity pylons, may be a risk factor, but the link is not proven.

THE MAIN TYPES OF LEUKAEMIA

Depending on how fast the cancer develops, leukaemia is defined as being either acute or chronic. In cases of acute leukaemia, immature blood cells are produced very rapidly and accumulate in the blood and tissues, disrupting normal function. Chronic leukaemia is slower to develop: the blood cells mature but do not function very well.

Around 6000 new cases of leukaemia are diagnosed in the UK each year. It is the most common cancer in childhood, but nine out of ten cases affect adults. There are four main types, which are classified according to the type of white blood cell that is spreading abnormally.

Acute myeloid leukaemia (AML)

This involves the granulocytes – the white blood cells that normally fight infection. It may develop very rapidly and people may be very sick by the time the diagnosis is made – with the result that only one in three of those affected survives. Acute myeloid leukaemia affects about one in 10,000 people, and is most likely to affect those over the age of 60.

Acute lymphoblastic leukaemia (ALL)

This form of leukaemia involves a type of white blood cell known as a lymphocyte. It is the most common cancer to affect children. The higher the initial levels of white blood cells – known as the white cell count – the more difficult the disease is to treat and cure. Acute lymphoblastic leukaemia can progress rapidly, but cure rates are generally better than for acute myeloid leukaemia. Children affected by either form of leukaemia respond better to treatment than adults, and the majority of children with acute lymphoblastic leukaemia make a full recovery.

Chronic myeloid leukaemia (CML)

Chronic myeloid leukaemia accounts for 15 per cent of leukaemias, and occurs most often in middle age. In about 95 per cent of cases, the person has a specific genetic abnormality called the Philadelphia chromosome.

The course of chronic myeloid leukaemia is variable but usually it has two phases: chronic and acute. The chronic phase may last months or years, during which time the person has few

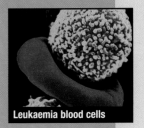

Leukaemia blood cells

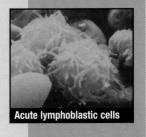

Acute lymphoblastic cells

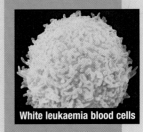

White leukaemia blood cells

Leukaemia in children

Around 400 children are diagnosed with leukaemia each year in the UK, most commonly with acute lymphoblastic leukaemia.

In children, certain types of leukaemia are more common than in adults, symptoms may be different and cure rates are generally higher than for adults.

■ Around 80 per cent of children with acute lymphoblastic leukaemia and many with acute myeloid leukaemia will be cured. Survival rates continue to rise.

■ Symptoms may be particularly hard to spot in children. They may complain of tiredness and pains in their limbs. They may have swollen glands, be generally grumpy, or even have problems at school. At first, the disease may seem to be a viral infection.

■ Children all react differently to their illness. Some seem to cope, but most experience fear and anxiety. It is vital to acknowledge these emotions and to give children plenty of encouragement to talk. Specific problems for children can include disruption of growth and interrupted schooling.

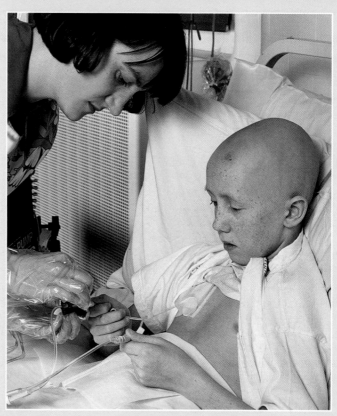

▶ **Life-saving chemotherapy**
A young boy undergoes chemotherapy for leukaemia. Many children are very distressed by the sickness and hair loss that usually accompany this treatment.

if any symptoms. After this, a change to the cells known as blast transformation takes place. Once that change has taken place, the disease moves into the acute phase. Treatment can only help in the chronic phase of the disease.

Chronic lymphocytic leukaemia (CLL)
This type of leukaemia affects the mature lymphocyte white blood cells. It accounts for about 25 per cent of cases of leukaemia – making it the most common form. It usually affects people over 50, and twice as many men as women. Chronic lymphocytic leukaemia cannot be cured, but it is not necessarily fatal.

One in four people with CLL has no symptoms and the disease is often discovered when a person has a blood test for some other reason. This form of leukaemia usually progresses slowly – some people do not get any worse for years and may even improve. Without treatment, the lymph nodes usually slowly enlarge, and the person may eventually die of the disease.

SYMPTOMS AND DIAGNOSIS

In cases of acute leukaemia, there are no obvious identifiable symptoms. But there are a number of more general indications that the cells of the blood are not functioning properly. These include tiredness due to **anaemia**; loss of weight; fever;

abnormal bleeding of the gums or blood in the urine; a high incidence of bruising; frequent infections such as colds and flu (because the white blood cells do not function well enough to fight infection); bone pain; shortness of breath; enlarged lymphatic glands and spleen. Many of these symptoms are common problems that are not usually due to cancer. But if they persist for over a week, see a doctor as soon as possible.

Several different tests are used in the diagnosis of leukaemia. Samples of blood and cells are taken from the bone marrow under local **anaesthetic** (see **Bone marrow and disorders**). Blood tests are performed to check numbers of the different cells present, to gauge the levels of certain chemicals in the blood which indicates whether other organs in the body have been affected, and for an analysis of the DNA or chromosomes. In a lumbar puncture or spinal tap, a sample of the spinal fluid is taken, under local anaesthetic, from around the spinal cord in the lower back. This is examined for signs of leukaemia cells.

X-rays are performed to look for problems in the chest or for hot spots of leukaemic cells in the bones. Bone scans may also be carried out to look for leukaemia hot spots. **Ultrasound** scans are performed to check organs such as the

In the early 1970s, only three in ten children and adults with leukaemia survived longer than five years. Advances in treatment meant this figure had risen to almost seven out of ten by the late 1980s.

lymphatic glands and spleen, which become enlarged in cases of acute leukaemia. CT or MRI scans are carried out to check for any enlarged lymph nodes.

Before deciding on the best treatment, doctors consider how far the leukaemia has spread. Acute leukaemia will also be classified or graded according to the appearance of the blood cells under the microscope as well as the results of chromosome and DNA tests. These enable doctors to predict the possible spread of the disease, possible complications and the patient's likely response to different treatments.

TREATMENT

Some of the following treatments will be used, depending on the type of leukaemia diagnosed, its stage and grade:

■ **Chemotherapy** – anticancer drugs are usually given in cycles. A combination of different drugs at high doses is taken as tablets or injections.

■ **Steroids** – given alongside chemotherapy.

■ **Immunotherapy** – the anticancer drug interferon may be given, especially for a rare type of leukaemia called hairy-cell leukaemia.

■ **Growth factors** – these are proteins that bind to the cell surface, and regulate tissue growth and the division of cells. They are given to increase the numbers of white blood cells and stem cells from which normal blood cells are produced.

■ **Radiotherapy** – this treatment is usually given in cases where the leukaemia has spread to the brain and spinal cord.

■ Bone marrow or stem cell transplants.

Treatment is given in several phases. The first phase, known as remission induction, aims to destroy as many of the leukaemia cells as possible and to get rid of all signs of leukaemia in the bone marrow. It uses a combination of different chemotherapy drugs given over a number of days. During this time, most of the normal bone marrow cells are also destroyed, and the cancer patient becomes especially vulnerable to infection and bleeding. Normal bone marrow cells will be produced within two to three weeks and will then start to produce new blood cells.

Because leukaemia sometimes spreads to the brain and spinal cord, preventive chemotherapy (known as intrathecal chemotherapy) may be given by injection into the spinal fluid. Radiotherapy may also be given to the head.

Without further treatment the leukaemia is likely to return, so follow-up treatment with high-dose chemotherapy, known as consolidation therapy, is vital.

When leukaemia cells are still present in bone marrow after treatment, the leukaemia is termed 'resistant'. If a remission occurs, but the leukaemia returns after successful treatment, this is called a relapse. Further courses of different combinations of treatment are then given.

LIFE AFTER DIAGNOSIS

'What are my chances?' is something that a person with cancer almost always wants to know. Statistics are based on averages from studies of large numbers of patients and so do not predict what will happen to any individual. There is no substitute for discussing your individual case with your own specialists.

Overall, the survival rate for leukaemia is still only about 30 per cent but it is steadily rising, by more than 10 per cent each decade. Some types of leukaemia are more responsive to treatment than others. Stage of tumour, general health and other factors are also important.

BONE MARROW AND STEM CELL TRANSPLANT

Blood cells are made mostly in the bone marrow from immature or precursor cells, known as stem cells. One way to treat leukaemia is to destroy all the diseased stem cells with very high doses of chemotherapy, then to restore the blood with a transplant of healthy stem cells or bone marrow. The aim of a bone marrow or stem cell transplant is to provide a new source of immature cells from which healthy blood cells can be made.

The transplant – known as an allogeneic transplant – may be done using a donation of bone marrow or stem cells from someone else. A brother or sister whose bone marrow is a close

---

Bone marrow tests

To diagnose leukaemia, a sample of cells from the bone marrow must be examined under the microscope in the laboratory, as leukaemia cells may not show up in the bloodstream.

Carrying out a bone marrow test involves a minor operation. The cells are removed, usually from the hipbone or from the breastbone. There are two ways of removing the cells. Sometimes both are performed.

■ Cells in the liquid marrow may be sucked out through a syringe and needle. This is called a bone marrow aspirate.

■ Cells may be taken out as a fine core of bone and cells using a larger needle. This is called a bone marrow biopsy.

Although bone marrow tests are generally done under local anaesthetic, they can still be very uncomfortable. There may be a feeling of pressure during the test. And after the procedure has been carried out, the bone may feel bruised and sore for several days.

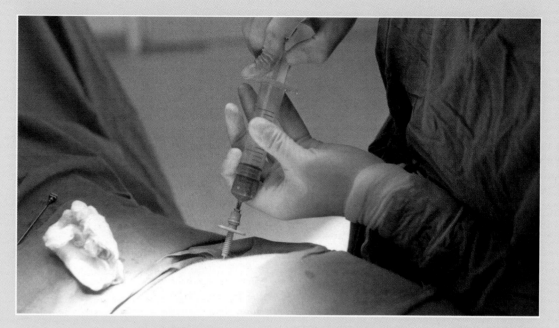

match is usually the best donor, but sometimes stem cells from a matching but unrelated donor may be used.

If stem cells are to be transplanted, the donor is given treatment with growth factors, which will stimulate the production of stem cells. The donor is then connected to a machine known as a cell separator. The donor's blood is passed through the machine, which extracts the healthy stem cells from the blood. It is then returned to his or her body. The extracted cells can be frozen and stored until they are needed.

Factfile

Donating marrow

Matching bone marrow is carried out by blood tests. The best match usually comes from a brother or sister.

Any one of us may be asked to donate our marrow to save the life of a relative. And many people are on a register of volunteers and are prepared to donate their marrow if they provide a good match for someone who needs it.

A donor should be in good health. You will be given a thorough medical check-up. One or two pints of blood may be taken from you a week or so before your bone marrow is collected. This can then be given back if you need a transfusion.

The operation usually involves a 48-hour stay in hospital during which time your bone marrow is collected under general anaesthetic. Afterwards, you can get back to normal activities, although you will probably need painkillers for a few days as the area from which the marrow was taken will feel sore.

A transplant can also be performed using the person's own stem cells (known as an autologous transplant). These cells are taken from the blood while the person is in remission.

How the transplant is performed

1 High doses of chemotherapy or radiotherapy are used to destroy every cell in the patient's bone marrow and so ensure that any abnormal cells which were still there cannot re-establish the cancer.

2 If bone marrow is to be transplanted, this is removed from the donor under general **anaesthetic**. Otherwise, previously collected stem cells are prepared for use.

3 The donated marrow or stem cells are given through an intravenous drip, or central line. They recolonize the bone marrow with healthy versions of every cell type. The transplant takes a few weeks to settle into the bone marrow and start producing healthy blood cells. In the period before the new marrow has established itself, the patient may become anaemic. He or she will have little immunity and be vulnerable to infections, so must stay in an isolation room in the hospital.

There is a risk that the transplanted cells will reject their new body. This condition, called graft-versus-host disease, can occur up to six months after the transplant. It may cause life-threatening complications, although the transplant can be treated with drugs.

SEE ALSO *Blood and disorders; Bone marrow and disorders; Transplants*

Lice

Lice are small, wingless creatures that feed by sucking human blood. There are three types, head lice, body lice and crab lice (also known as pubic lice). Head and crab lice lay eggs called nits that attach to hair, while body lice lay their eggs on clothing.

SYMPTOMS

The main symptom of lice is intense itching at the affected areas, causing the person to scratch. Infection is then common, resulting in blisters, redness and swelling. With head lice, whitish nits can often be seen at the hair shaft near the roots. The grey or brown lice are more difficult to spot, except in blonde hair. Crab lice are so-called because they look like tiny crabs. They are most often found in pubic hair, but are also found in other areas where hair grows, such as under the arms, or on beards and eyelashes. Body lice live on clothing and visit the body only to feed.

DURATION

The eggs take about seven days to hatch and each louse may live for several weeks.

CAUSES

■ Lice are spread from person to person by close physical contact, or by contact with shared items, such as clothing, bedding and hair brushes.
■ Head lice will often spread very rapidly among young children including those at nursery and infant school.
■ Crab lice are usually spread by sexual contact, but can also be passed on by almost any type of close physical contact, if other parts of the body have become affected.
■ Body lice only affect people who rarely change and wash their clothes.

TREATMENT

Treatment varies, depending on the type of lice involved.

What you can do

■ To clear head lice, wash the hair with ordinary shampoo, then apply plenty of hair conditioner. While the conditioner is still on the hair, comb through from the roots with a fine toothcomb. Clear the comb of lice between each stroke. Repeat every three to four days for two weeks. You can buy a kit which includes combs and details of this wet-combing technique, or you can buy an insecticide shampoo. Both are available from pharmacists (see also **Nits**).
■ To clear crab lice from the eyelashes, smear the lids with white petroleum jelly (such as Vaseline) twice a day for ten days.
■ To rid clothes and bedding of crab lice, put them into a hot tumble dryer for several minutes, then wash thoroughly.

Complementary therapies

A number of herbal products, including tea tree oil, are suggested for head lice.

When to consult a doctor

See your doctor if home treatment fails, if you develop a skin infection, such as crusting, swelling or redness, in the affected area, or if you think that you may have crab lice.

What a doctor may do

For crab lice, your doctor will prescribe insecticide lotions containing malathion. Any sexual partner should also be treated. For all lice, your doctor will prescribe a medication to cure any resulting skin infections.

PREVENTION

■ If you have young children at nursery or school, check their hair weekly while it is wet, using a detection comb from a pharmacy.
■ Body lice are prevented by washing clothes and bedding regularly in hot water. Bathing does not help to prevent head or pubic lice.

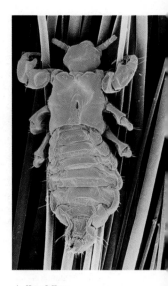

▲ **Head lice**
The head louse lives on the hair of the head, glueing its eggs (called nits) to individual hairs.

Lichen planus

Lichen planus is a recurring, itchy skin disease. Symptoms are small, raised, purplish spots on the wrists, forearms, legs and torso that combine to form larger, scaly patches. Patchy baldness of the scalp sometimes occurs. Blueish white sores may form on the inside of the mouth, with blotches on the tongue. The cause of lichen planus is unknown, but it may be the body's response to certain chemicals or drugs.

Mild cases of lichen planus require no treatment. Any skin lesions that develop are usually treated with steroid creams. Lichen planus in the mouth may be treated with steroid lozenges or mouthwashes. Most lichen planus clears within 18 months and does not usually come back, although some patients may have a recurrence many years later.

Ligaments and problems

Ligament are strong bands of slightly elastic, white, fibrous tissue. They run from one bone to another, and stabilize and reinforce a joint. Ligaments may also form part of a capsule that surrounds a joint like a sleeve (a synovial joint capsule), as in the **knee**.

Ligaments are tough but flexible and pliant. They offer no resistance to normal movements, but they become taut at the end of normal movement range in order to prevent excessive or abnormal motion. Problems with ligaments often stem from the fact that they are not designed for prolonged tension. Like a strong

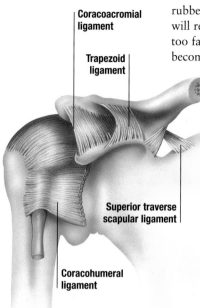

Coracoacromial ligament

Trapezoid ligament

Superior traverse scapular ligament

Coracohumeral ligament

▲ **Shoulder ligaments**
The hardworking shoulder joint is protected by ligaments that are particularly strong and flexible.

rubber band, a ligament can be stretched and will return to its original length, but if stretched too far or for too long, it loses its elasticity and becomes flabby. Overstretching by sudden movement can also tear or snap it. Ligaments have a poor blood supply, so they have a tendency to heal slowly or incompletely.

WHAT CAN GO WRONG
Ligaments are prone to various disorders, usually caused by over or underuse.

Tight ligaments
Most people suffer from tight rather than loose ligaments. This is normally the result of underuse of the joints. Tight ligaments bind a joint too firmly, restricting movements and, in particular, the small accessory movements that keep joints healthy. As a result, the joint becomes stiff and prone to osteoarthritis. Stretching exercises or activities such as yoga or swimming help to stretch tight ligaments.

Loose ligaments
Loose ligaments (hypermobility syndromes) are inherited conditions in which the protein that makes up the supporting tissues of a joint is more flexible than usual. **Marfan's syndrome**, for example, is a rare genetic disorder that affects connective tissue, leading to excess height and abnormally long fingers and toes. Another disorder, called benign joint hypermobility syndrome (BJHS), allows some or all joints to move through a greater range than is normal. This may be an asset for ballet dancers or gymnasts, who are very fit, but for most people, loose ligaments give inadequate protection to the joints, resulting in pain, inflammation and early osteoarthritis. The treatment is to strengthen the muscles

A new treatment

Ligament damage can now be treated by a series of injections that stimulate new tissue.

Proliferative therapy, or sclerotherapy, is a new treatment designed to strengthen weakened, damaged or lax ligaments. A non-toxic natural substance called 'proliferant solution' is injected into the ligament to create inflammation in the tissue. Repeated injections are given over a period of weeks. This sustained inflammation triggers the body to produce more ligament tissue, eventually increasing its bulk and, therefore, strength. This technique is still being evaluated and is not yet practised by many orthopaedic specialists in the UK.

to provide extra support for the joints through special exercises or activities such as swimming.

Sprains
If a joint makes a movement outside its normal range, the ligaments stabilizing it are likely to be overstretched or to tear. The result is a sprain. The ankle is most commonly affected – it usually twists inwards and so wrenches the ligaments on the outside of the joint. Wherever a sprain occurs, the effects are the same: pain, inflammation and swelling. The surrounding muscles go into spasm to protect the joint from further damage.

Treatment is with RICE (rest, ice, compression and elevation – see **First Aid**), and with **ultrasound**. The aim is to relax the muscles so that controlled movements can be made, which will prevent scar tissue from forming in the ligament. Scar tissue reduces ligament flexibility and makes future sprains more likely.

Ruptures or tears
Certain ligaments, especially those of the knee and ankle, can be badly torn or ruptured by a sudden twisting movement. A **whiplash injury** often involves a ligament rupture, but the tibial and medial ligaments of the knee are the most vulnerable of all. Treatment is by immobilizing the joint to allow healing, or surgical repair.

SEE ALSO *Joints and problems; Skeletal system*

Lips and problems

The lips are fleshy tissues around the opening to the mouth. They have a copious nerve supply, making them very sensitive. Their colour is due to a profuse supply of blood vessels, which is why one of the earliest signs of shortage of oxygen in the blood is blue lips (**cyanosis**). The lips can appear pale in **anaemia**.

Human lips are unique among primates in being everted (turned out). This is what makes them both very visible and 'kissable'. The lips may play a role in sexual signalling; they become fuller and redder during sexual arousal.

WHAT CAN GO WRONG
Minor problems are common, but sometimes signal a more serious underlying disease.
■ Chapped lips are usually caused by cold or excessive licking, especially in babies; they also occur in chronic illness.
■ Cracking and soreness at the angle of the mouth may be due to malnutrition, vitamin deficiency or ill-fitting dentures.
■ **Cold sores** are recurrent blisters due to infection with the herpes simplex virus.
■ Inflammation of the lips (cheilitis) is an infection, particularly with staphylococcal bacteria or candida fungus.

■ Swollen, cracked, red lips (cheilosis) are often a sign of nutritional disorder, particularly a deficiency of vitamin B_2.

■ Blood blisters can arise from biting or injury.

■ Sunburn: since they are covered with very delicate skin, the lips can easily get burned. They need protection with sunscreen.

■ Blue lips (cyanosis) may be due to cold exposure, or to heart, lung or blood disorders.

■ Cleft lip or hare lip – a split in the upper lip – is a birth deformity (see also **Cleft palate and hare lip**).

TREATMENT

Seek medical advice if:

■ soreness or cracking of the lips persists for more than a week despite using lip creams;

■ there are pronounced cracks at the corners of the mouth;

■ lips are persistently blue, even when not cold;

■ symptoms affect the mouth or tongue as well.

SEE ALSO *Mouth and disorders; Tongue and problems*

Listeria

Listeria is a bacterial infection common in animals, including poultry. It may also affect human beings; the infecting organism has been found in dust, mud, sewage and animal stools. The incidence of human infection caused by *Listeria monocytogenes* is low but increased in the 1980s, when cook-chill foods, one of the main sources of infection, became popular. Tighter controls on their storage were introduced in the 1990s, and the number of people affected by listeria began to decrease.

SYMPTOMS

Most healthy adults who are infected with the listeria organism do not suffer any ill effects and it rarely leads to serious problems.

People who are at high risk of suffering complications if they are exposed to the bacteria include pregnant women, infants and people with poor defences to infection, including cancer patients, kidney-transplant patients, diabetics and elderly people.

CAUSES

Infection occurs from eating food contaminated with the bacteria, including poultry, eggs, cow's milk, cook-chill food and soft cheese. Listeria is not killed by cold temperatures and can multiply at refrigerator temperature – that is, 4–6°C (39–43°F).

Doctors believe that the bacteria is spread from the gut to various parts of the body, probably through the bloodstream. In pregnant women, the organisms pass from the infected mother to the fetus.

TREATMENT

People diagnosed with listeria who are believed to be at risk of complications are usually admitted to hospital. Severe forms of the disease are treated with antibiotics.

PREVENTION

Pregnant women and people with disorders that lower resistance to infection must avoid eating meat-based pâté and soft cheeses, such as goat's cheese, Camembert, Brie and blue cheeses.

Heat all cook-chill foods and ready-prepared poultry thoroughly. Storage instructions and sell-by and eat-by dates of food products should be strictly observed.

COMPLICATIONS

In the high-risk groups, listeria can cause fever, chills, fatigue and muscle pain. In pregnant women, infection may lead to **miscarriage** or stillbirth. (See also **Pregnancy and problems**.) In a newborn baby, listeria may cause a chest infection, breathing difficulties and **meningitis**.

SEE ALSO *Food poisoning*

Lithotripsy

Lithotripsy is a method of breaking up stones in the kidney, bladder or ureter (the tube that connects the kidney and bladder) using highly concentrated ultrasonic waves. The waves are focused onto the precise location of the stone, and do no damage to surrounding areas of the body. Once the stone is shattered into minute pieces, these are passed naturally by the body or removed by surgery.

There are two methods of lithotripsy. In one, a machine called a lithotripter delivers focused **ultrasound** through the skin. The patient usually receives a general or epidural **anaesthetic** and might experience some bruising or blood in the urine. In the other method, a viewing instrument (nephroscope) is inserted into the kidney through a small incision and an ultrasound probe introduced through this to break up the stone. The surgeon then extracts the fragments through the nephroscope.

Liver and disorders

The liver is the body's chemical regulator, and performs more than 500 chemical functions daily. To keep the body working, the liver refines and detoxifies much that enters it. It converts food into forms the body can use as well as making, storing and regulating important substances used by the rest of the body. It detoxifies poisonous chemicals to help in their removal from the body, and breaks down drugs that have been absorbed in the digestive tract. It also helps to fight against infections in the body.

The liver and nutrition

Blood enters the liver laden with important nutrients. The liver processes this blood to remove the substances that are important for metabolism. Carbohydrates are broken down into glucose and stored both in the liver itself and in the muscles as glycogen. Between meals, or in an emergency when the body needs energy, the liver is triggered by hormones to convert the glycogen back into glucose, which the body can use more easily.

Proteins arrive at the liver already broken down into amino acids, their building blocks. They are either stored there, converted into energy for the muscles or changed into urea, which is excreted in the urine.

Minerals are removed from the blood entering the liver. They are stored or used. In particular, the liver stores iron, which is obtained from the breakdown of oxygen-carrying haemoglobin, in worn-out red blood cells.

Fats are broken down in the intestine by bile, which is a thick digestive fluid produced by the liver. Enzymes in the intestine then break the fats down further and they are absorbed into the blood through the walls of the intestine. Vitamins A, D, E and K, which dissolve in fats, are stored after being broken down by bile.

Detoxification

Substances that can affect or harm the body include medication, alcohol and poisons (known as toxins) released by bacteria. All these pass through the liver before reaching the blood that circulates to other organs. The liver breaks down these substances, rendering them harmless, or in the case of drugs such as barbiturates, modifies them so that they can work effectively. Most of the waste products are excreted in the bile, although some pass out of the body as urine or sweat. The liver cannot break down some toxins, such as the venom of certain snakes, which must be treated with antivenom drugs as a matter of emergency. (Snakebites are rarely venomous in the UK.)

What the liver makes

As well as secreting bile, the liver creates a whole range of proteins that are vital constituents of blood plasma, the straw-coloured fluid in which the blood cells float. These include the following:

■ complement, a group of proteins that are part of the immune system;

■ albumin, which controls the exchange of water between tissues and blood. Some people with liver disease have very low albumin levels in their blood, and so too much water escapes from the blood into the cells of body tissues – causing swollen legs (**oedema**), for example;

■ globin, part of the pigment haemoglobin that carries oxygen in the blood;

■ coagulation factors, which cause clotting when the wall of a blood vessel is damaged;

■ cholesterol and proteins that help to regulate how fat stores are transported around the body.

Fighting infections

The liver plays a key role in resisting infections, especially bowel infections. It activates the macrophage system, a part of the body's defence mechanism. Macrophages are mobile scavenger cells, which destroy any bacteria with which they come into contact. The liver contains more than half the body's supply of macrophages.

SYMPTOMS OF LIVER DISEASE

General feelings of ill health and weariness are commonly associated with liver disease. Other typical symptoms include abdominal pain, nausea and vomiting, loss of appetite and the development of visible blood vessels in the skin (spider naevi). But liver disease can have no symptoms at all in its earlier stages.

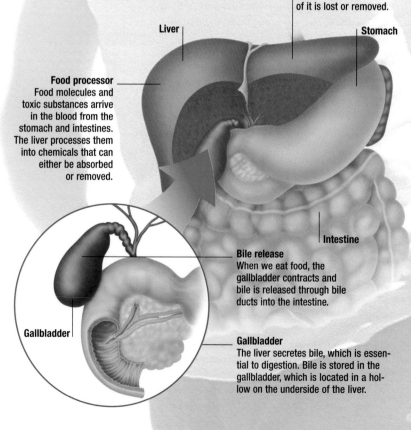

Detoxifying the body
The liver is the body's largest gland. It weighs about 1.25kg (2lb 12oz), and sits just below the heart and lungs, mainly on the right side of the abdominal cavity. Its underside is in contact with the stomach, intestines and right kidney.

Renewable organ
The liver can grow new cells to replace damaged ones. It can regain its normal size and function even if three-quarters of it is lost or removed.

Liver

Stomach

Food processor
Food molecules and toxic substances arrive in the blood from the stomach and intestines. The liver processes them into chemicals that can either be absorbed or removed.

Intestine

Bile release
When we eat food, the gallbladder contracts and bile is released through bile ducts into the intestine.

Gallbladder

Gallbladder
The liver secretes bile, which is essential to digestion. Bile is stored in the gallbladder, which is located in a hollow on the underside of the liver.

As the disease progresses, the following symptoms may occur.

■ **Jaundice** The skin and whites of the eyes turn yellow when there is an obstruction of a bile duct (by gallstones or a tumour, for example) or if the liver is unable to process bilirubin (a yellow pigment formed from haemoglobin). The urine may darken and stools become paler when there is obstruction. If the bilirubin is forced back into the bloodstream, it can be deposited in the skin and may cause itching.

■ **Portal hypertension** Cirrhosis of the liver (see below) may hinder the flow of blood from the stomach and intestines. This leads to a buildup of pressure in the portal vein, which carries blood into the liver from the stomach and intestines, and this may cause fluid to collect around the abdominal organs (ascites, see below) or result in the widening of the veins surrounding the lower end of the oesophagus (see **Oesophagus and disorders**). Treatment is required urgently if the veins around the oesophagus are affected, because they may burst, causing internal bleeding.

■ **Ascites** When cirrhosis of the liver is advanced or a blood vessel near the liver becomes blocked, fluid slowly builds up around the organs in the abdominal cavity. Those affected may include an increase in girth, abdominal discomfort and breathing difficulties. Sufferers are usually advised to rest in bed and to reduce their intake of fluids and salt. In advanced cases of ascites, doctors may advise draining the fluid.

■ **Impaired brain function** When the liver is severely damaged, certain toxic substances may not be removed from the bloodstream. When these substances are carried to the brain, they can cause slurred speech, memory lapses and even unconsciousness.

TYPES OF LIVER DISEASE

There are many types of liver disease, but among the most important are cirrhosis of the liver, hepatitis, liver cancer, gallstones and liver disorders in children.

Cirrhosis of the liver

In this chronic disease, knobbly fibrous scar tissue replaces normal tissue in the liver, impairing its function. Cirrhosis is often associated with excessive alcohol consumption, but can be caused by hepatitis. If the disease can be stopped in time, the undamaged part of the liver can regenerate itself back to a normal state. However, if a person develops cirrhosis of the liver but does not stop drinking alcohol, the destruction of his or her liver will continue and death will eventually follow. Cirrhosis of the liver causes 6000 deaths a year in the UK.

Excessive alcohol consumption does not lead to liver damage in all people, even though alcohol is directly toxic to the liver. This is probably due to genetic differences between individuals.

Always keep to safe levels of alcohol consumption. If you are worried about your drinking, discuss the matter with your GP. (See also **Alcohol and abuse.**)

Gallstones

Gallstones are solid masses, like pebbles, that are found in the gallbladder and in the bile duct leading to the gallbladder from the liver. They form as a result of long-term inflammation of the gallbladder. They are more likely to develop if a person has some abnormality in the make-up of their bile or if the gallbladder becomes blocked. One in ten people and one in five of those aged over 40 have gallstones. (See also **Gallbladder and disorders.**)

Hepatitis

Hepatitis is an inflammation of the liver. It can be caused by long-term abuse of alcohol or overuse of certain drugs such as paracetamol, but is most often a viral infection. Viral hepatitis can be caused by six different viruses. Hepatitis A is most common in children and young adults. The virus is found in the faeces of infected individuals and is transmitted by contaminated food or water. Hepatitis E is also spread in this way, usually in the developing world. Hepatitis B, C and D are spread by contact with blood or body fluids and can be passed on during sexual contact. Hepatitis G is a mild version that often occurs alongside other forms of the condition. There is no hepatitis F.

Liver cancer

There are two types of liver cancer: primary and secondary. Primary cancer develops in the liver itself (a hepatoma) or in the bile duct (a cholangio-carcinoma). A secondary cancer is one that has spread to the liver from elsewhere in the body. In the UK, hepatomas usually arise as a complication of cirrhosis. Only 700 people are affected in the UK each year. Secondary cancer is much more widespread, affecting about 14,000 people each year. It spreads to the liver from the surrounding organs, where it may have remained unnoticed.

Liver cancer may be accompanied by weight loss, lack of appetite, **jaundice** and weakness. Tumours can be detected with **ultrasound** scanning and their presence confirmed with a liver **biopsy**. The latter involves a very small sample of liver tissue being removed for microscopic analysis.

A liver transplant or removal of the tumour may cure primary liver cancer, as it may remain restricted to the liver for a long time. Anticancer drugs to prolong life have very limited effects.

UNDER THE MICROSCOPE

The most common disorder in heavy drinkers is excess fat in the liver. In regular heavy drinkers, a fatty liver will begin to cause discomfort in the upper-right abdomen as the liver swells. Jaundice may follow.

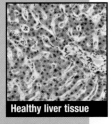
Healthy liver tissue

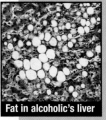
Fat in alcoholic's liver

Liver disorders in children

There are more than 100 types of liver disease that can affect children. These are the more common ones.

■ Chronic active hepatitis is a little-understood allergy-like process by which liver cells are destroyed and replaced with scar tissue.

■ Galactosaemia is a hereditary disorder that leads to **cataracts**, cirrhosis of the liver and brain damage. Milk sugar builds up in the liver and other organs because an enzyme needed to digest it is missing.

■ In biliary atresia, the bile ducts are either too small or absent. Without the ability to release bile, internal bleeding and cirrhosis usually lead to death by the age of two.

■ In Wilson's disease, cirrhosis and brain damage are caused by an inherited abnormality that leads to the buildup of a large amount of copper in the liver.

TESTS AND CHECKS

Liver function tests are blood tests carried out to check for liver damage, and sometimes to see how well a patient is responding to treatment. Different liver complaints can be diagnosed by gauging the levels of substances in the blood. Bilirubin, alkaline phosphatase and prothrombin are used as test substances to help to determine if there is a blockage in the bile ducts, while a low blood level of albumin (one of the proteins made in the liver) indicates that a disorder may be long term.

A biopsy is the only direct way in which doctors can determine the extent of any liver damage, when symptoms or liver function tests have shown that there is a problem. A thin, hollow needle is inserted through the skin and a small sample of liver tissue is taken. As the procedure can be quite uncomfortable, a local **anaesthetic** is used. You will normally be expected to stay overnight in hospital, although some people are able to leave the same day. The tissue sample is then examined under the microscope.

A variety of methods are used to precision-guide the needle. Ultrasound or computed tomography (CT) scanning may be used to find small tumours. Then a **laporoscopy** may be performed. This involves making a small incision in the abdomen that allows a fibre-optic tube to be inserted and directed to the exact point of sample. The needle is then passed down the tube. Alternatively, the needle may be guided down from the neck to the liver through the hepatic vein. Fewer than one per cent of people who undergo a liver biopsy experience any complications.

In some cases of severe liver damage, a liver transplant may be the only option.

Lordosis

Lordosis is an exaggerated inward curve of the spine in the lower back. A slight curve is normal but lordosis, sometimes called hollow back, is usually a sign of poor posture and weak abdominal muscles. It may lead to lower back pain or a slipped disc. Lordosis can be corrected by adopting better posture and strengthening the abdominal muscles.

SEE ALSO *Back and back pain; Spine and disorders*

Lumpectomy

Lumpectomy is a treatment for breast cancer in which only the obvious lump along with the surrounding tissue, rather than the whole breast, is removed. It is usually supplemented with **radiotherapy** and **chemotherapy**. Research suggests that lumpectomy gives survival rates at least as good as **mastectomy**. In the latest trial, nearly 900 women with breast cancer were treated either with a lumpectomy or with a modified radical mastectomy. Ten years later, there was no significant difference in overall survival rates between the two groups – 66 per cent for the mastectomy group and 65 per cent for the lumpectomy group.

WHO IT CAN HELP

In general, women who have a single breast tumour of less than 3cm (1¼in) diameter will benefit. If there are several tumours and the lymph glands are involved, more extensive surgery is necessary.

WHAT'S INVOLVED

An incision is made over the breast lump, which is cut out together with a 1cm (½in) margin of tissue. The tissue is sent to the pathology lab to check that the margin is free of cancer. Some or all of the lymph nodes under the armpit, where cancer often spreads, are often removed at the same time, as a precaution. Lumpectomy is usually followed with radiotherapy to mop up any remaining cancer cells.

SEE ALSO *Breasts and disorders*

Lung function tests

Lung function tests (also termed pulmonary function tests) are used to assess how well the lungs are working – in particular, to diagnose any respiratory disorder, measure how severe it is and to monitor the course of the disease. Simple tests use peak-flow meters, spirometers – many family doctors now have these – and more specialized equipment in chest clinics and

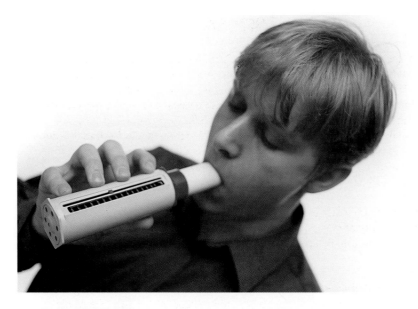

▲ Testing lung capacity
The patient is asked to breathe out as hard as possible through a peak-flow meter. This device measures the rate of air flow from the lungs, and is used to diagnose and to monitor disorders such as asthma, which constrict the lungs' airways.

teaching hospitals. These can measure the total volume of air in the lungs, how much of it can actually be used, how quickly the patient can breathe in and out, and levels of oxygen and carbon dioxide in the blood.

SEE ALSO *Lungs and disorders; Respiratory system*

Lungs and disorders

The lungs are large sacs sited either side of the heart in the chest cavity. They expand and contract with the movements of the diaphragm and ribcage, rather like old-fashioned bellows. During breathing the diaphragm, which is below the lungs, contracts downwards while the ribs expand outwards. This creates a vacuum in the chest, which causes air to rush down through the air passages into the lungs. Then, as the diaphragm and chest relax, the air in the lungs is forced out. This breathing action is controlled by part of the nervous system.

The lungs allow oxygen to be transferred from the air to the bloodstream, supplying the body with the oxygen it needs to convert nutrients into energy. The carbon dioxide that this produces is expelled by the lungs into the atmosphere. This exchange of gases takes place in the alveoli, small air sacs lined with tiny blood vessels, or capillaries, that are situated deep in the lungs. In order to supply enough oxygen to meet the body's needs, the lungs of an adult move approximately 10,000 litres (2200 gallons) of air each day.

The nose, mouth, upper throat, and larynx (voice box) are all involved in the routing of air to the lungs. They also filter out any germs and particles of dirt, which is why **colds**, runny noses and sore throats are so

common – the nose and throat trap any infection and localize it before it has a chance to reach the lungs and develop into a serious disease such as **pneumonia** (see **Respiratory system**).

Lower down, in the trachea and bronchi, particles can be trapped by lung secretions, or mucus. This is then coughed up, and most of it is automatically swallowed. As the air travels down into the lungs, it becomes moist and warm, as can be seen when breathing out through the mouth on a cold day.

WHAT CAN GO WRONG
The lungs can be affected by a wide range of diseases and problems, and it is estimated that around 8 million people in the UK suffer from some sort of lung ailment.

There are three main ways in which problems affect the lungs.
■ By obstructing the airflow to and from the lungs, particularly in asthma, chronic bronchitis and emphysema. These illnesses have most effect on the bronchi and bronchioles (airways).
■ By restricting the ability of the lungs to hold air. Scarring can occur in part of the lungs following infections such as pneumonia, or over the whole of the lung as in pulmonary fibrosis. Such damage particularly affects the alveoli, or breathing sacs.
■ By the alveoli filling up with infection, as in pneumonia, or with fluid, as in heart failure. This makes it difficult for oxygen to get into the bloodstream.

The people who are most at risk of developing a lung disease are smokers and the people who live or work with them, babies and young children, frail and elderly people, and those who are suffering from chronic ill-health due to other causes.

SYMPTOMS
Symptoms of lung disease in adults include:
■ breathlessness and wheezing;
■ cough (though a cough is often due to throat rather than lung problems);
■ the production of large amounts of phlegm;
■ coughing up blood (only occasionally serious);
■ chest pain (not always due to lung problems).

Symptoms in children
Breathing problems affect children faster than they do adults. As well as the adult symptoms, children may also display:
■ a blueish tinge to the skin, particularly around the mouth – this is a key symptom to look out for in babies;
■ in babies, being too breathless to feed;
■ a barking cough;
■ in children of one year or younger, sucking in of the neck and the spaces between the ribs when breathing.

The respiratory system

The respiratory system is the means by which oxygen in atmospheric air is carried into the body and carbon dioxide is expelled. As the air is drawn through the upper respiratory tract, it is warmed or cooled to body temperature and dust particles and microbes are trapped in the membranes that line the passageway. Disease can affect any part of the system.

Alveoli
Tiny air sacs lying deep in the lungs, the alveoli are lined with fine blood vessels, in which the exchange of oxygen and carbon dioxide occurs.

Bronchioles
The narrowest airways, leading off the bronchi, are known as the bronchioles. They run directly into the alveoli.

Upper respiratory tract
All the airways from the upper part of the trachea upwards, including the larynx and nasal cavity, are referred to collectively as the upper respiratory tract.

Trachea
Tough rings of cartilage protect and help to keep the trachea or windpipe open. It leads down into the chest, where it divides into smaller airways, called bronchi.

Bronchi
Beyond the trachea, the airways divide first into two bronchi, one to each lung, then into a series of increasingly narrow tubes, ending in the fine bronchioles, that reach into all areas of the lungs.

Pleura
The lungs are enclosed by a double-layered sac called the pleura. The space between the two layers – the pleural cavity – is filled with a lubricating liquid.

Lower respiratory tract
All the airways, from the lower part of the trachea downwards and including the bronchi, bronchioles and alveoli, are known collectively as the lower respiratory tract.

Children are most likely to be affected by asthma and bronchiolitis. Babies can be born with premature lung disease. This occurs when the lungs are not developed and lack sufficient surfactant – the substance that lines them and stops them collapsing. It can also occur when complications in pregnancy cause lung damage.

LUNG PROBLEMS

Lung disorders can be caused by infection, allergy, tumours or injury. Elderly people and babies are most at risk from lung infections.

Acute respiratory distress syndrome

Acute respiratory distress syndrome (ARDS) is a serious disorder of the lungs in which inflammation and increased fluid accumulation cause breathing difficulties, which then leads to a deficiency of oxygen in the blood. It can affect premature babies whose lungs have not developed sufficiently to cope with independent breathing. Almost 90 per cent of babies survive the condition.

In adults, acute respiratory distress syndrome is a rare and life-threatening condition that involves treatment in intensive care. It usually affects those who have suffered a major injury, such as may occur in a car accident. Of those adults who develop acute respiratory distress syndrome, half die from it while most survivors will develop scarring of the lungs.

Asthma

Asthma is a condition in which the airways are oversensitive and react in two ways. First, chemicals are released which cause the lungs to tighten up, making it difficult for air to get in and out. This results in symptoms of breathlessness and wheezing, that respond to drugs called bronchodilators. Secondly, the airways become inflamed, causing a cough; steroid inhalers are often recommended to ease the problem.

Asthma is often brought on by virus infections, exercise, and triggers such as cat hair, pollen, dust mites or cigarette smoke. There are more than 5 million people with asthma in the UK and it is one of the main causes of lung problems in children.

Bronchitis

Bronchitis is an inflammation of the bronchi. The main causes are infection by a virus, which may also cause a sore throat, cold and fever; and irritation from smoking or being in a smoky or polluted environment. The first sign of bronchitis is usually a cough, which starts off dry but becomes wet, with phlegm, later on.

Bronchiolitis

Bronchiolitis is a viral infection of the bronchioles, which become inflamed and filled with mucus. The symptoms are similar to a cold, followed by a wheezy cough. Most children can be treated at home with over-the-counter pain relief to bring down fever. The condition is serious only if breathing difficulties develop. It most often affects children under one year, and occurs in epidemics.

Chronic obstructive pulmonary disease

Chronic obstructive pulmonary disease (often abbreviated to COPD) is the collective term for chronic bronchitis and emphysema. It causes persistent obstruction to the flow of air to and from the lungs.

The condition is almost entirely caused by smoking; for this reason it is also known as 'smoker's lung'. It affects around 2–3 million people in the UK, but most are recognized late because symptoms only become apparent when the disease is advanced. About 30,000 people die from the disease every year.

The symptoms include a chronic cough, and later bringing up mucus every morning. Viral infections lead to attacks during the winter, along with recurrent chest infections. As the disease progresses, increasing wheeziness and increasing breathlessness may also develop. Respiratory or heart failure may result.

The main treatment is to give up smoking. Although the damage caused by COPD is irreversible, stopping smoking will prevent any further damage and slow down the progression of the disease. Drugs such as antibiotics are used to treat the chest infections, and bronchodilators (used in asthma) are also used to alleviate symptoms.

Lung cancer

Lung cancer is a very serious disease and is the biggest cause of cancer deaths in the UK. Half of those affected die within six months of diagnosis and only about ten per cent of people diagnosed with lung cancer survive for longer than five years. This is because the disease is often diagnosed at a late stage. It is therefore essential to seek medical advice immediately if you suspect that you might have the disease.

The main symptoms of lung cancer are:
- recent or worsening cough or breathlessness;
- coughing up blood;
- unexplained weight loss;
- pains in the chest.

To make a diagnosis, **X-rays** may be taken of the lungs. These will be followed by a bronchoscopy, in which the bronchi are examined using a fibre-optic viewing tube (see also **Endoscopy**). Alternatively, a needle **biopsy** will be performed. This procedure involves removing a small piece of tissue to be examined under a microscope to detect cancerous cells.

The treatment depends on the type of lung cancer and whether it has spread. Some cancers can be cured by surgery, and improvement in others can follow a course of **radiotherapy** or **chemotherapy**. (See also **Cancer**.)

Occupational lung disease

Occupational lung disease is the collective term for lung conditions that are caused by exposure to dust and chemicals at work. Conditions include pneumoconiosis, **asbestosis**, **farmer's lung**, beryliossis and **byssinosis**.

Pneumonia

Pneumonia is an infection of the tiny alveoli in the lungs. It is caused by bacteria, viruses or other organisms. It starts suddenly with fever and cough, often accompanied by chest pain or breathlessness. Mild cases of pneumonia can be managed at home; others need hospitalization. Most people recover but sometimes the disease is fatal.

Tuberculosis

Tuberculosis (TB) is a severe bacterial infection of the lungs. It used to be called consumption, and was the main cause of death in adults until effective treatment became available 50 years ago. However, in Europe it has began to resurface, particularly among the homeless, immigrant and refugee populations. Worldwide, tuberculosis is a huge problem – one-third of the world's population is thought to be infected. The disease kills about three million people each year.

Other lung conditions

There is a variety of other, less common, conditions that can affect the lungs.
- **Pleurisy** is an infection of the pleural sac that envelops the lungs.
- A pulmonary embolism is a blockage in the supply of blood of the lungs. It is normally caused by a blood clot from the legs.
- **Cystic fibrosis** is a genetic condition that causes the mucus produced in the lungs to be particularly thick and sticky, making it difficult to clear the airways. It causes breathing problems and leads to increased chances of infection. It is one of the most common reasons for a lung transplant.
- Bronchiectasis is a condition in which the lower airways remain widened, making

Factfile

Smoking and lung disease

Smoking causes around 120,000 premature deaths each year. About one quarter are from lung cancer and one fifth from chronic obstructive pulmonary disease (COPD). Some 13 million people smoke in the UK.

Respiratory illness and smoking are closely connected. Smoking causes:

- 90 per cent of lung cancers in men and 73 per cent of those in women (numbers of deaths every year: 21,000 and 9500 respectively);

- 86 per cent of cases of COPD in men and 79 per cent of those in women (numbers of deaths: 15,100 and 9300 respectively);

- 25 per cent of pneumonias in men and 11 per cent of those in women. Pneumonia is more likely to be fatal in people who smoke (numbers of deaths: 5800 and 4100 in men and women respectively).

If you can quit smoking, your risk of developing lung cancer will drop by up to 50 per cent after five years and will return to that of a non-smoker within ten years.

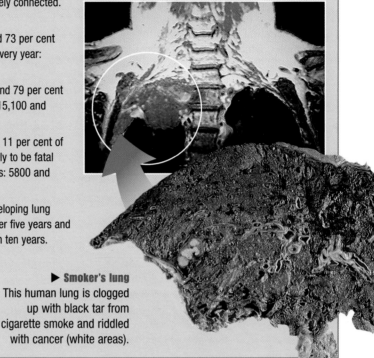

▶ **Smoker's lung**
This human lung is clogged up with black tar from cigarette smoke and riddled with cancer (white areas).

---

it difficult to clear mucus. The mucus may become infected, leading to multiple chest infections and breathlessness.

- Sarcoidosis is an inflammation in the lungs resulting in breathlessness and a dry cough; it sometimes affects other parts of the body, too. It is not known what causes the disease. Usually it clears up without treatment within a matter of weeks, although it may last for years and some patients need treatment with steroids.

- Fibrozing alveolitis is the progressive scarring of the lungs. The cause is unknown.

THE EFFECTS OF SMOKING

All lung disorders are aggravated by smoking and so it makes sense to stop smoking and avoid smoky atmospheres if you have any disease associated with the lungs.

Smoking is the single most preventable cause of death in modern society. Half of all smokers will die from their habit if they continue to smoke, and smoking reduces life expectancy by 10–12 years. For every six people smoking 20 cigarettes a day, one will die 10 years prematurely, during retirement, and one will die 25 years prematurely, before he or she retires. Tobacco smoke is bad for the lungs in two ways: it contains tiny particles of tar that

damage and clog up the airways; and it contains toxic gases such as carbon monoxide and oxides of nitrogen. When tobacco smoke is breathed in, the cells in the airways of the lungs react to the poisons it contains in two ways:

- The tar in smoke damages the cells, which may then grow in an uncontrolled way, leading to cancer – either of the larynx or of the lung.

- The cells are destroyed by the smoke. These dead cells release substances, which cause more harm to the structure of the lung, leading to chronic bronchitis and emphysema.

Tobacco smoke also endangers the defences of the lungs and the airways by:

- destroying the muco-ciliary action – the movement of thousands of tiny hair-like structures that help to clear the lungs of foreign bodies trapped in the mucus;

- damaging the cells in the nose and throat, making colds and other infections more likely;

- irritating the mucus-producing cells so they produce excess mucus, which can clog airways;

- stimulating the protective response, causing the airways to narrow.

SEE ALSO *Chest pain; Cough; Respiratory system; Smoking*

Lupus

Lupus, known more fully as systemic lupus erythematosus, is an **autoimmune disease**. That means that the condition results from the production of autoantibodies, which attack the body's own cells and tissues. Symptoms vary, depending on the cells affected, and the condition usually affects women aged 20–40 years.

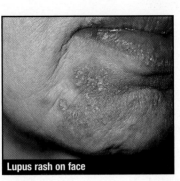

Lupus rash on face

SYMPTOMS

The symptoms of lupus can include:
- painful, swollen joints and fever;
- marked skin changes, such as an abnormal sensitivity to sunlight (photosensitivity) or an itchy red rash;
- shortness of breath and chest pain when breathing in;
- **anaemia**;
- blood clotting problems;
- **Raynaud's** phenomenon;
- hair loss.

CAUSES

The causes of lupus are unknown, but are likely to include one or more of the following:
- an inherited predisposition;
- immune system disorders;
- drugs, including hydralazine and procainamide;
- recent infection.

TREATMENT

See your doctor if you experience any of the symptoms listed.

What a doctor may do
- Test your blood for antibodies.
- Advise you to avoid the sun and use a sunscreen.
- Prescribe anti-inflammatories for pain or corticosteroid creams for irritated skin. More severe disease may require immunosuppressants.

OUTLOOK

The disease may come and go over several years. Drug-induced lupus usually subsides when the drug is stopped.

Lyme disease

Lyme disease is caused by a bacterium that is transmitted to human beings by bites from ticks. It is also known as borreliosis. Climate changes have been blamed for a rising number of cases of Lyme disease in the UK.

SYMPTOMS
- Drowsiness.
- Headache.
- Mild fever.
- Joint and muscle pain.
- Swollen lymph glands.

CAUSES

Lyme disease is caused by an infection from a micro-organism, *Borrelia burgdorferi*. It is transmitted by a bite from the wood tick, a blood-sucking parasite that normally lives on deer. The wood tick is found in many areas, particularly in forests where deer are common. When the tick has found a suitable place on the body (it prefers warm, moist and dark places, such as the crotch or armpits), it sticks in its probe to draw up blood, exposing the person to the risk of infection.

TREATMENT

See a doctor as soon as possible. If it is caught early, the disease is treatable with antibiotics, but in the later stages Lyme disease does not respond so well.

COMPLICATIONS

A range of complications can develop with late-stage Lyme disease, including joint inflammation. Complications include conditions that affect the heart, such as myocarditis and heart block (see **Heart and circulation system**), or the nervous system, such as **meningitis**.

Lymphanogranuloma venereum

This **sexually transmitted disease** occurs mainly in tropical regions. The infection is caused by *Chlamydia trachomatis* serotypes 1, 2 and 3, and is closely related to the chlamydia that causes NSU (**non-specific urethritis**).

Small, painless ulcers or lumps appear on the genitalia, the anus or mouth 7 to 21 days after infection. These may pass unnoticed because they quickly heal leaving no scar. Fever, headache, muscle and joint aches and a rash sometimes also occur. This stage is short-lived and is occasionally symptomless.

Three to twelve weeks after infection, the disease progresses to cause massive swelling and inflammation of the lymph nodes in the groin; these are known as buboes. **Abscesses** may form, with ulcers on the overlying skin. These take several months to heal unless antibiotic treatment with doxycycline is applied for at least two weeks. Left untreated, chronic infection with scarring and abscesses can occur.

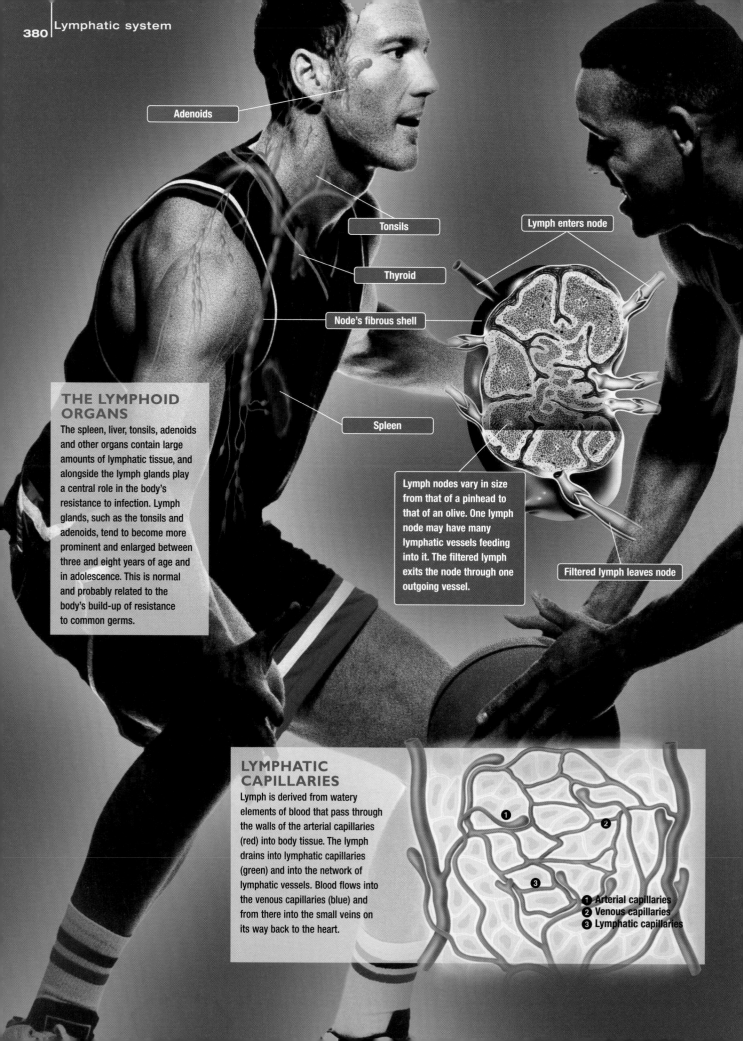

Adenoids

Tonsils

Thyroid

Node's fibrous shell

Spleen

Lymph enters node

Filtered lymph leaves node

THE LYMPHOID ORGANS

The spleen, liver, tonsils, adenoids and other organs contain large amounts of lymphatic tissue, and alongside the lymph glands play a central role in the body's resistance to infection. Lymph glands, such as the tonsils and adenoids, tend to become more prominent and enlarged between three and eight years of age and in adolescence. This is normal and probably related to the body's build-up of resistance to common germs.

Lymph nodes vary in size from that of a pinhead to that of an olive. One lymph node may have many lymphatic vessels feeding into it. The filtered lymph exits the node through one outgoing vessel.

LYMPHATIC CAPILLARIES

Lymph is derived from watery elements of blood that pass through the walls of the arterial capillaries (red) into body tissue. The lymph drains into lymphatic capillaries (green) and into the network of lymphatic vessels. Blood flows into the venous capillaries (blue) and from there into the small veins on its way back to the heart.

❶ Arterial capillaries
❷ Venous capillaries
❸ Lymphatic capillaries

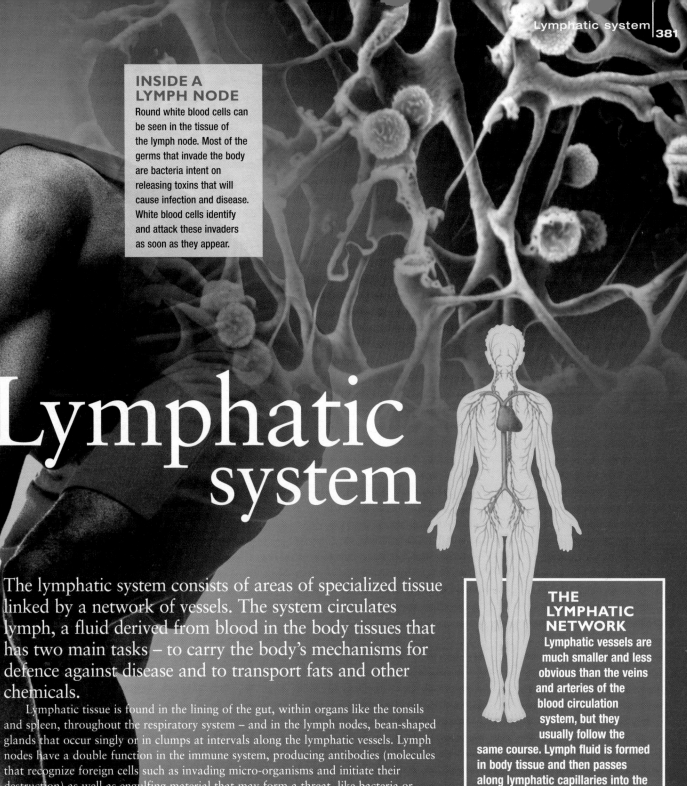

INSIDE A LYMPH NODE

Round white blood cells can be seen in the tissue of the lymph node. Most of the germs that invade the body are bacteria intent on releasing toxins that will cause infection and disease. White blood cells identify and attack these invaders as soon as they appear.

Lymphatic system

The lymphatic system consists of areas of specialized tissue linked by a network of vessels. The system circulates lymph, a fluid derived from blood in the body tissues that has two main tasks – to carry the body's mechanisms for defence against disease and to transport fats and other chemicals.

Lymphatic tissue is found in the lining of the gut, within organs like the tonsils and spleen, throughout the respiratory system – and in the lymph nodes, bean-shaped glands that occur singly or in clumps at intervals along the lymphatic vessels. Lymph nodes have a double function in the immune system, producing antibodies (molecules that recognize foreign cells such as invading micro-organisms and initiate their destruction) as well as engulfing material that may form a threat, like bacteria or foreign body particles such as smoke. Lymphatic vessels in the walls of the small intestine absorb fats and fat-soluble vitamins and deliver them to the blood circulation system. Disorders of the intestinal lymphatics affect fat absorption, causing weight loss, fatty diarrhoea and deficiency in vitamins A, D, E and K.

THE LYMPHATIC NETWORK

Lymphatic vessels are much smaller and less obvious than the veins and arteries of the blood circulation system, but they usually follow the same course. Lymph fluid is formed in body tissue and then passes along lymphatic capillaries into the lymphatic vessels, which carry it through lymph nodes and other collections of lymphatic tissue in body organs, before emptying into the jugular veins in the neck. Smooth muscles in the walls of the lymphatic vessels contract, propelling the fluid along the vessels. Contractions occur between two and ten times a minute. This is much slower than in blood vessels.

Disorders of the lymphatic system

Swelling caused by blockages to the system can be difficult
to treat, while lymphatic cancers may often be cured.

A major problem affecting the lymphatic system
is swelling of the body's soft tissues caused by
lymphoedema, the pooling of lymph fluid that
has not drained properly. This can affect the
oxygenation of the surrounding tissues, making
it more likely that these tissues will become
infected, (**cellulitis**), or that the lymph ducts will
become infected, a lymphangitis.

Causes of lymphoedema

Primary lymphoedema occurs when a person's
lymphatic drainage system has not developed
properly. It may cause a limb to swell up and
is difficult for doctors to treat effectively.
Secondary lymphoedema is caused by damage
to or blockage of the lymphatic system by
infection, injury, surgery or radiation. Doctors
will decide on treatment depending on the cause,
but the outlook is often poor, with recurrent
swelling and damage to the soft tissues. The risk
of damage is high if lymph nodes are removed
during surgical treatment of a cancer – the
surgery itself or subsequent scarring can disturb
the flow between ducts. Secondary lymphoedema
may also develop after blood vessel damage such
as development of a blood clot (thrombosis).
People considering surgery or radiotherapy
should discuss the risk of lymphoedema with
their doctor.

Lymphoedema can be caused by worm infection
of the lymphatic ducts, a major problem in
many undeveloped countries (see **Travel and
tropical diseases**).

Stages of lymphoedema

There are three stages of lymphoedema. In stage I
(spontaneously reversible lymphoedema), the limb
is normal in the morning, but swells when moved.
The swelling goes down when you rest the limb.
In stage II (spontaneously irreversible), swelling
no longer goes down when you rest the limb, and
the skin and soft tissue harden. Once stage III
(lymphostatic elephantiasis) has set in, the
swelling canot be reduced. The limb is noticeably
enlarged and its tissues may have grown hard.

Treatment

The earlier treatment begins, the more successful
it is, so see your doctor as soon as symptoms
start. Treatment begins with managing the
underlying cause, where possible. Doctors should
promptly investigate and treat any possible
infection and thrombosis. Wearing stockings and
long gloves can reduce swelling in the legs and
arms, while exercises and **physiotherapy** can
maintain suppleness. Skin care techniques and
dietary changes can help to maintain skin
condition and keep further skin damage to
a minimum. Complementary therapies include
manual lymphatic drainage and self-massage.

LYMPHOMA

Lymphoma is cancer of the lymphatic system.
Cells called lymphocytes grow in a rapid,
disordered way and because they move easily
within the system, the cancer can spread very
quickly to other parts of the body such as the
liver, spleen and bone marrow.

Lymphomas are divided into **Hodgkin's** and
non-Hodgkin's lymphomas, depending on the
cells involved. Both Hodgkin's lymphoma and
non-Hodgkin's lymphoma cause painless swelling
of the lymph glands, fever and tiredness. They
make sufferers more susceptible to infection.
About 30 per cent of AIDS patients contract
lymphoma (see **HIV**).

Key questions to ask your doctor

**If you think you may have a problem with your
lymphatic system, consult your doctor as soon
as possible. This checklist of questions may
serve as a useful prompt.**

- Why are my glands swelling?

- If the swelling is due to recurrent infection, why
do I keep getting infections?

- Should I have a blood count or diabetes test?

- Is there another cause that I should be tested for?
For example, should I be checked for either cancer
or for HIV?

- What can I do to help myself?

If there is swelling of your limbs or soft tissues:

- Is this lymphoedema, and if so is it primary
or secondary?

- What else might be the cause?

- What investigations do you plan to cnduct?
For example, do I need blood tests or should
I have a lymphogram?

If lymphoedema has been diagnosed:

- What has caused it?

- What are the current treatments?

- What exercises will help?

▶ **Lymphangiography**
To view the abdominal lymph glands, a dye is injected before a series of X-ray pictures are taken. The pale blue patches show enlarged lymph glands in an abnormal pattern.

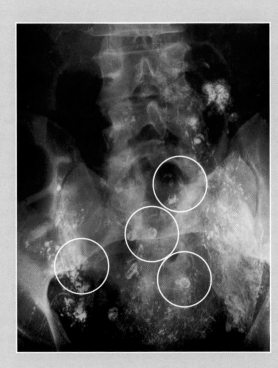

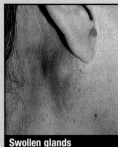

Swollen glands

▲ **Lymphoma**
Swelling behind the ear can indicate a swollen lymph node, possibly a symptom of lymph cancer. This swelling, in a 51-year-old woman, was caused by non-Hodgkin's lymphoma.

Other disorders

Lymphangitis
This is inflammation of the lymph vessels. The most common cause is a bacterial infection with *Streptococcus*. Lymphangitis is treated with antibiotics.

Glandular fever
This condition, which affects young adults and teenagers, is marked by enlargement and soreness of most lymph glands in the body, with sore throat, fever and general malaise. Recovery takes place without any special treatment, during two to four weeks.

Lymphadenitis
Inflammation of the lymph nodes or glands, which can swell up and become painful, hot and tender. In infants inflammation of the lymph nodes around the intestine is a cause of abdominal pain during infectious illness.

Hodgkin's lymphoma

Hodgkin's lymphoma is a cancer that is often associated with chronic viral infection – such as with the Epstein-Barr virus (EBV, which causes **glandular fever**), which appears in 40–50 per cent of cases. **HIV** and **hepatitis** also increase the risk of developing Hodgkin's. In general, the disease affects those between the ages of 15 and 30 and the over-50s. Approximately 1300 new cases of Hodgkin's lymphoma occur every year in the UK. The cancer may also attack the liver, spleen and bone marrow. Both **chemotherapy** and **radiotherapy** are very effective methods for the treatment of Hodgkin's lymphoma, and most people affected make a complete recovery.

Non-Hodgkin's lymphoma

The cancer affects a wide age range of people, from 30-year-olds to the over-70s. A small percentage of cases occur in people whose immune systems are not working properly – for example, after they have had a transplant or because they have HIV infection. Some cases of lymphoma may develop after treatment for cancer with chemotherapy or radiotherapy. In most cases, no clear cause can be identified but the cancer may start after exposure to a trigger – for example, an environmental factor such as industrial chemicals and toxins such as pesticides. Your doctor may recommend chemotherapy or radiotherapy to treat non-Hodgkin's lymphoma. But in most cases, a policy of 'watch and wait' often applies.

Stages of lymphoma:

There are four stages of lymphoma. In stage I, there is one cancer site and the bone marrow is not affected. In stage II, there are two affected sites, either above or below the diaphragm, and the bone marrow is not affected. In stage III, there are sites both above and below the diaphragm, and the bone marrow is not affected. In stage IV, either the bone marrow is affected or the cancer cells have spread outside the lymphatic system.

OTHER LYMPHATIC DISORDERS

Lymphadenopathy is a general term for disease of the lymph nodes. It is used to describe painful swelling of the nodes due to an infection, and painless swelling due to the spread of cancer cells to the node.

Lymphadenitis is the inflammation of a lymph node or nodes. It occurs when bacteria, which have been transported to the node through the lymphatic drainage system, then infect the tissue of the node itself. The node swells, becomes hot, red and painful and an **abscess** may develop. Doctors may recommend treatment with antibiotics or surgical drainage.

Acute lymphoblastic leukaemia is a type of cancer that affects the lymphocytes and lymphocyte-producing cells in the **bone marrow**. The number of working lymphocytes falls and patients are susceptible to infection. Treatment through chemotherapy can sometimes cure the condition.

Macular degeneration

'Macular degeneration' is a term covering a group of conditions that affect sight. It involves the gradual death of tissue in the centre of the retina – or macula – resulting in the reduction or loss of central vision in both eyes.

The risk increases markedly with age, and age-related macular degeneration (ARMD) is the most common cause of impaired vision and eventual **blindness** in elderly people. The more widespread, dry form, results in central blurring and makes reading difficult; it is untreatable. The wet form, caused by blood vessels leaking under the macula, results in a more dramatic loss of central vision. If detected early enough, it may respond to drug or **laser** treatment.

Malabsorption syndrome

Malabsorption syndrome is a condition that impairs the ability of the small intestine to absorb certain nutrients from food. Common symptoms include **diarrhoea**, weight loss and **anaemia**, as well as stomach cramps, bloating, flatulence and abdominal distension (swelling). Malabsorption may also lead to impaired growth and development in children, and even **malnutrition** in advanced cases of the condition.

CAUSES

Malabsorption is caused by a range of diseases that affect the digestive system, or by surgical removal of part of the gut. Depending on the cause, the body may be unable to absorb carbohydrates, proteins, fats, or vitamins and minerals. In certain cases, a range of dietary nutrients cannot be properly absorbed. Causes of malabsorption include:

- **Cystic fibrosis**, which damages the **pancreas** and disrupts its production of enzymes.
- Pancreatitis, which also damages the pancreas.
- Lactose intolerance, in which the enzyme lactase is missing.
- **Coeliac disease**, which damages the intestinal walls, hampering nutrient absorption.
- Tropical sprue, which also damages the intestinal walls, leading to deficiencies of folic acid and vitamin B$_{12}$.
- **Cirrhosis of the liver** or obstruction of the bile duct, both of which impede the flow of bile, so that fats are not broken down and absorbed.
- **Surgery**, to remove parts of the small intestine.
- **Parasites** such as *Giardia lamblia*, which causes **giardiasis**.

TREATMENT

If a patient does not appear to be absorbing dietary nutrients properly, a doctor may recommend various tests.

- Stool examination: a stool test is taken to look for globules of fat and meat fibres, which can indicate a pancreatic disorder; bulky, loose greasy stools may be a sign of coeliac disease; and examination under the microscope may reveal the presence of parasites.
- Absorption tests: these are used to test for carbohydrate malabsorption. After a period of fasting, the patient is fed a test food. Urine or blood is then checked to see if the intestine has absorbed it.
- Blood tests: these can detect iron deficiency anaemia and deficiencies in other nutrients.
- **Barium investigations**: the small intestine may be examined for abnormalities using an X-ray.
- Small-intestine **biopsy**: mucus obtained using **endoscopy** is examined to determine microscopic abnormalities.

Treatments vary depending on the underlying cause, but can include drugs such as antibiotics, changes to diet and, sometimes, surgery.

SEE ALSO *Digestive system; Nutritional disorders*

Malaria

Malaria is a serious and sometimes fatal tropical disease. It is caused by the malarial parasite, which is usually transmitted to human beings by bites from infected mosquitoes. There are 500 million new cases a year worldwide. In the UK, about 2500 people return from abroad every year with the disease, and an average of 12 people each year die from it. Malaria occurs in more than 90 countries: malarial areas include large parts of Central and South America, Africa, the Indian subcontinent, Southeast Asia, the Middle East and Oceania.

SYMPTOMS

At the beginning, malaria may be difficult to distinguish from **influenza**. Symptoms usually occur ten days to four weeks after the initial infection, although they can begin eight days after being infected or up to a year later. They include:

- fever;
- shivering;
- headache;
- repeated vomiting;
- diarrhoea;
- generalized convulsions;
- pain in the joints;
- backache.

Cycles of chills, fever and sweating usually occur every one to three days. The person's temperature may be constant or variable.

There are four types of malarial parasite: *Plasmodium falciparum*, *P. vivax*, *P. ovale* and

Malaria-risk areas and antimalarials

Travellers to risk areas should check the latest information on which antimalarials to use; in some areas, the parasite is immune to certain drugs.

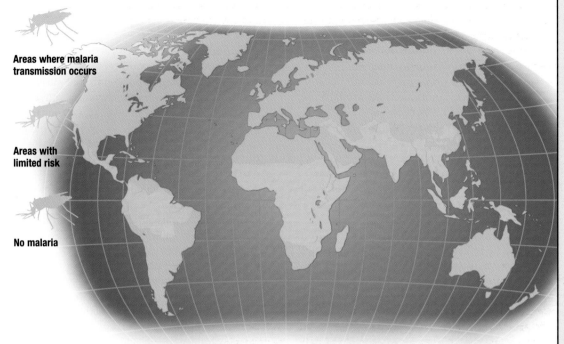

Areas where malaria transmission occurs

Areas with limited risk

No malaria

P. malariae. Vivax malaria is the mildest form, while falciparum is the most life-threatening, accounting for most malaria deaths.

DURATION

With treatment, malaria lasts for 10 to 20 days. Untreated ovale or vivax infections can recur every two to three months for 10 years.

CAUSES

Malaria is usually transmitted to a person by the bite of an infected female mosquito of the *Anopheles* type. When an infected mosquito bites someone, the malarial parasites are injected into his or her blood. The parasites find their way to the liver, where they multiply. Some parasites lie dormant in the liver and may only become active years later. However, they are usually released from the liver after ten days to two weeks, when they enter the bloodstream and invade the red blood cells. Here, they quickly reproduce and grow, causing the red blood cells to rupture and release more parasites into the bloodstream.

It is both the direct action of the parasite and the body's response to the parasitic infection that leads to the symptoms of malaria.

TREATMENT

See a doctor as soon as you develop symptoms, even if they appear months after visiting a country where malaria is present.

■ You may be admitted to hospital either for testing or for treatment.

■ Malaria is treated with antimalarial drugs. The choice of drug depends on the type of malaria, the resistance of the parasite to the drugs and the severity of the disease.

PREVENTION

Travellers to malarial countries should see a doctor or travel clinic to obtain the best antimalarial tablets for where they are going. There are currently six drugs used for preventing malaria and different ones work in different areas (see malaria-risk areas, above).

■ Antimalarial drugs may have unpleasant side effects, including headache, nausea and diarrhoea. Some people report psychological effects too, such as mood swings and paranoia.

■ Most antimalarial drugs need to be taken one week before travelling and often need to be continued for a month after you have returned.

■ Mosquitoes have developed resistance to certain drugs. For example, chloroquine-resistance in the malarial parasite *P. falciparum* exists throughout sub-Saharan Africa, Southeast Asia, the Indian subcontinent and large areas of South America. It is spreading to new areas.

What you can do

Try to avoid being bitten by mosquitoes, particularly at twilight and night when they are most likely to bite. Use mosquito-repellent cream containing diethyl toluamide (DEET), which is the most effective bite-preventive treatment. Sleep in rooms that are properly screened with gauze over the windows and

---

Antimalarial drugs

Chloroquine is taken weekly. It is effective in the Middle East, Central America and the Carribean, which do not have chloroquine-resistant malaria. In areas with a slight risk, it is taken in combination with a daily dose of Proguanil. Both of these drugs can be bought over the counter.

Proguanil can be used on its own in areas with chloroquine resistance. The parasite has also developed resistance to proguanil over the years.

Malarone is an effective alternative to mefloquine. You take it daily, for up to 28 days, to prevent falciparum malaria, which is often resistant to other antimalarial drugs.

Doxycycline is as effective as mefloquine but not advised in pregnancy. You take this drug daily, starting two days before you travel and continuing for four weeks after leaving the malarial area.

Mefloquine (Larium) gives good protection in areas with chloroquine-resistant malaria. These are Asia, Africa, India, the Pacific Islands and South America. Taken weekly, the course is started two or three weeks before departure. It can cause unpleasant side effects, which may include paranoia and mood changes.

Maloprim is taken weekly. It has been largely superseded by newer drugs, but it gives some protection in chloroquine-resistant areas for people with epilepsy, particularly children, who can react to other drugs.

doors. Air-conditioning also discourages mosquitoes. Spray rooms with an insecticide before you go in, to kill any mosquitoes that have entered during the day. Suspend a mosquito net impregnated with an insecticide around your bed. If you are worried about fumes, use pyrethrum, a harmless substance based on extract of chrysanthemum.

Complementary therapies
■ Homeopathic antimalarials are available but their effectiveness is not proven.
■ Apply refined lemon-eucalyptus oil to the skin to repel mosquitoes.

COMPLICATIONS
People with severe falciparum malaria may develop bleeding, kidney or liver failure, central nervous system problems and coma.

OUTLOOK
Most people infected with the vivax, ovale and malariae forms of malaria recover completely, but being infected once does not give you immunity. Falciparum malaria can be fatal.

In October 2002, scientists announced that they had mapped the genetic blueprint for the parasite that causes malaria and for the mosquito that transmits it to people. This will speed the development of new antimalarial drugs and vaccines and could also lead to the creation of environment-friendly insecticides.

SEE ALSO *Parasites and parasitic diseases; Travel and tropical diseases*

> Malaria kills more than 2 million people worldwide each year. The majority are children under the age of five.

Malnutrition

Malnutrition is the result of inadequate nutrition. In poor and undeveloped countries, disease linked to malnutrition is the major cause of death. Lack of nourishment may also stunt the physical and mental development of large numbers of the population. In richer, developed countries, malnutrition affects mainly those who suffer from eating disorders, are chronically sick or have absorption difficulties, caused by conditions such as **coeliac disease**. Elderly people, alcoholics or those following rigid diets are also vulnerable.

INDICATORS OF MALNUTRITION
The Body Mass Index (BMI) and the circumference of a person's upper arm can be used as indicators of malnutrition.

SEVERE MALNUTRITION
Severe malnutrition can be divided into three main types.
■ Nutritional dwarfism This form of malnutrition stunts a person's growth. Individuals may appear normal, so that it is only when the age of the person is known that the lack of growth is apparent.

■ Kwashiorkor In this condition, the energy content of the diet is sufficient but there is severe lack of protein. It most commonly occurs in children. The characteristics are fine, brittle, discoloured hair, a skin rash, which is more obvious in dark-skinned people, oedema and an enlarged liver.
■ Marasmus or starvation Affected individuals lose a large amount of body mass and muscle tissue, particularly from the shoulders and buttocks. There is almost no subcutaneous fat, and the skin becomes thin, atrophied and hangs in folds. The person's face has the pinched look of an older person.

CAUSES
Anyone is theoretically at risk of malnutrition if the diet is not sufficient in the basic requirements of carbohydrates, protein, fats (known as macronutrients), and minerals and vitamins (micronutrients).
■ The main cause of malnutrition is insufficient food. It is most likely to affect people living in countries where there are inadequate food supplies or those dependent on others for their nourishment, including infants, children, the elderly, disabled people and mentally ill people.
■ People in affluent countries are more likely to become malnourished because of diseases that negatively affect appetite, digestion, absorption or assimilation of nutrients. These include **Crohn's disease**, **irritable bowel syndrome** (IBS), **coeliac disease** and pancreatic insufficiency (see **Pancreas and disorders**). Self-inflicted malnutrition from eating disorders, such as **anorexia nervosa**, is increasing.

Mammoplasty

Mammoplasty is a surgical procedure to reinstate the breast, increase or decrease its size or to enhance its appearance. It is often of great psychological benefit to women who have had surgery for breast cancer and for those who are uncomfortable about having very large, small or asymmetrical breasts.

BREAST REDUCTION
Surgery can considerably alter the appearance of very large breasts and relieve problems such as back and neck pain, and the **fungal infections** that can flourish in the moisture that collects under the breasts. Very large breasts commonly cause embarrassment and make it difficult for a woman to carry out everyday activities or participate in sport.

What's involved
■ Breast reduction is a major operation performed under a general **anaesthetic** when the breasts are fully developed.

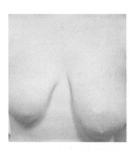

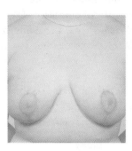

▲ **Mammoplasty**
Through mammoplasty breasts of unequal size and shape (top) can be reconstructed to appear more symmetrical.

■ An incision is made around the nipple. The nipple and surrounding pigmented area (the areola) are then moved upwards and excess glandular tissue, fat and skin is removed.

After the operation

■ Post-operative swelling and bruising subside after a few weeks, but the breasts may take a year to settle into their new shape.

■ Some scars are inevitable but are usually not visible under a normal bra or bikini top. They fade considerably with time.

■ Breastfeeding is unlikely to be possible since most of the ducts linking the nipple to the milk-producing glands are severed. However, some ducts may join up again to allow a milk flow.

■ The nipple and surrounding skin may be less sensitive than normal.

■ Breasts will still undergo the normal changes in size that are associated with pregnancy, weight gain and age.

BREAST ENLARGEMENT

Breast enlargement is the most common cosmetic operation performed on women in the UK. For many, the operation improves self-esteem and, therefore, their quality of life.

What's involved

■ The operation usually involves the insertion of synthetic implants surrounded by a firm, silicone elastic shell. Fillings available in the UK include silicone gel, saline, hydrogel and PVP (polyvinyl pyrolidine) solution. Implants are designed to last ten years, but have been left in without any problems for much longer.

■ Under a general anaesthetic, an incision is made below the breast, around the nipple or in the armpit. A pocket is then created in the tissues of the breast to hold the implant.

After the operation

■ As with breast reduction, there is swelling, bruising, and some scarring.

■ Since the implant lies deep in the breast, it does not interfere with breastfeeding.

COMPLICATIONS

Concerns about the safety of silicone have been raised in recent years, in particular its link with breast cancer, **autoimmune diseases** (in which the body's immune system attacks its own cells) and rheumatoid **arthritis**. However, extensive studies have found no evidence to support this.

■ After the operation, scar tissue forms around the implant, which may shrink. This can cause noticeable hardening of the breast and sometimes pain. It affects about one in 10 women with an implant and may lead to the implant being replaced or completely removed. The recent introduction of textured silicone shells has reduced the risk of this complication.

SEE ALSO *Breasts and disorders; Cosmetic and plastic surgery*

Manic depression

Manic depression is a severe mental illness in which periods of deep depression alternate with periods of overactive, excited behaviour, or mania. The medical name for manic depression is bipolar disorder, meaning that the illness is characterized by directly opposite states of mind.

A person suffering from manic depression may have gaps in-between the highs and lows, or these extreme states may come directly after one another. Some people have frequent episodes of manic depression, whereas others may have only one or two in their life, and feel fine the rest of the time. When a person has four or more episodes a year it is sometimes called rapid cycling.

Hypomania is a less severe form of mania. People with hypomania may not have a depressive episode afterwards.

About one per cent of the general population of the UK is diagnosed with manic depression. The illness usually appears during a person's 20s or 30s, although some people develop it during their teens.

SYMPTOMS

If you have manic depression, you will have times when you are manic, times when you are depressed, and times when you are neither. Although the highs can be enjoyable (and people often say they are very creative during mania), they can also be very disruptive. You may spend large amounts of money and build up debts, or make big changes or decisions that you later regret.

The symptoms of mania can include:

■ feeling very happy or sometimes very angry;

■ having lots of energy – being very active and talkative;

■ feeling restless and irritable;

■ having racing thoughts;

■ having strange or unfounded thoughts or beliefs, called **delusions**;

■ hearing voices or seeing things that are not there (**hallucinations**);

■ being unable to sleep much.

The symptoms of depression can include:

■ feeling very low and negative;

■ being unwilling to do things that you have previously enjoyed;

■ having difficulty in concentrating and remembering things;

■ having little energy;

■ feeling suicidal.

CAUSES

The cause of manic depression is unknown, although scientists have found that people with the illness have different chemicals in their brain from people who have never had the condition.

There are several possible causes.
- Genetics – a person has a higher risk of developing manic depression if a close relative has it.
- Stressful life events or physical illness can be triggers for the illness.
- Family background – problems in early life increase a person's risk.

TREATMENT

Medication is usually given to control the symptoms and to help people to live with the illness. Lithium is the most common treatment; it prevents mood swings for about 60 per cent of people. Carbamazapine is given when lithium does not work. Antipsychotics are given for severe symptoms of mania, or antidepressants for underlying depression. The medication may take several months to work.

Talking therapies such as counselling or cognitive behaviour therapy can give support and help in living with the illness.

A person who has particularly severe symptoms or is suicidal may need a short stay in hospital.

PREVENTION

- Try to recognize and avoid stressful events or other triggers for the illness.
- Notice early signs that you are becoming unwell, and seek help or support.
- Talk to someone about your feelings.
- Look after yourself physically – eat well and exercise regularly.
- Join a support group or self-help group.

OUTLOOK

Manic depression cannot be cured, but medication and talking therapies can help to control the symptoms, and may help an affected person to carry on with life as normal.

SEE ALSO *Depression; Mental health and problems*

Marfan's syndrome

Marfan's syndrome is a genetic disorder that mainly affects the skeleton, eyes, heart and blood system. People with the syndrome have distinctive physical characteristics. Someone with Marfan's is likely to be unusually tall and have a protruding breastbone; the face may be long and narrow. Sight problems such as a detached retina and near-sightedness are common. The wall of the aorta is often weakened and may rupture, causing death.

Marfan's syndrome is inherited, with 50 per cent of children born to a person who has the disorder inheriting it. It affects about one in 10,000 people. There is no reliable method of prenatal diagnosis.

Massage

Therapeutic massage has evolved from one of the most important and instinctive human needs – to touch and be touched. Paintings in Egyptian tombs show people being massaged. The emperor Julius Caesar was accustomed to have a daily massage for his neuralgia, and the physicians of ancient Greece and Rome valued the power of touch as a method of relieving pain.

Massage also plays a part in sophisticated Eastern healing systems, including those of China, Tibet, Japan, Indonesia and India (see **Ayurvedic medicine**).

In the West, massage is increasingly used therapeutically and in clinical settings by professionally trained masseurs and healthcare workers such as nurses. It is also routinely used within the NHS in intensive care units for people with cancer, heart disease and AIDS, for children and premature babies, for elderly people, and in ordinary healthcare centres, pain clinics and drug dependency clinics. Nine out of ten hospices in Britain also offer some form of physical therapy, including shiatsu, reflexology and massage.

Doctors usually regard massage as a complementary therapy in addition to medical treatment, rather than as a separate therapy in its own right.

HOW IT CAN HELP

Massage can bring about improvements in the health of people with a wide range of problems, including:
- stress-related conditions such as **headaches,** premenstrual syndrome and **insomnia;**
- joint and muscle disorders, such as **back pain, arthritis** and many types of sports injury;
- pain in general;
- high **blood pressure** and certain heart problems;
- **anxiety, depression** and poor body image;
- problems with the **digestive system,** such as irritable bowel syndrome and constipation.

Research findings

Results of trials at London's Royal Marsden Hospital in 1995 suggested that massage can reduce anxiety and improve quality of life for people with cancer. At Miami University's Touch Research Institute, regular massage has been demonstrated to have the following beneficial effects.
- It encourages weight gain in premature babies, making possible earlier hospital discharge.
- It increases the number of immune system fighter cells in **HIV**-positive men.

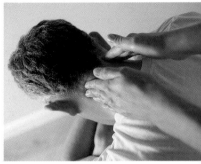

▲ **Tension relief**
A circling massage on either side of your partner's neck will ease tension. Place your fingers on the muscles either side of the spine and make small circling motions moving downwards from the base of the skull. Repeat this three or four times.

- It helps children with **asthma** to breathe more easily and reduces the number of their attacks.
- It reduces glucose levels in children with **diabetes**.

Additional research in the USA in 2000 further supported the theory that massage may also relieve premenstrual syndrome.

HOW MASSAGE WORKS

Basic massage techniques can stimulate both physical and emotional healing.

Physical effects

The pressing, squeezing, moving and stroking that take place during massage enhance blood circulation so that more oxygen and nutrients flow to the body's organs and tissues. There is also stimulation of the lymphatic system, which is believed to encourage the efficient excretion of waste products.

Massage can be relaxing or stimulating, depending on which techniques are used. The basic ones are effleurage (meaning to touch lightly, or stroke), petrissage (kneading, and wringing with a controlled twisting action), and percussion (a pounding stoke, used to stimulate muscular or fleshy areas).

Massage also stimulates reflex action. This is an automatic reaction by one part of the body in response to the stimulation of another part. For instance, a relaxing back massage can calm tense lower back muscles that are irritating the sciatic nerve – and may as a result relieve leg pain.

Emotional effects

Massage is a physical therapy, but it can also have powerful emotional effects. Stroking can stimulate the release of endorphins – the body's natural painkilling chemicals – which promote feelings of relaxation and well-being. It is also thought that massage can set free emotions previously held in, by releasing any muscle tension and stiffness associated with them.

The Austrian psychoanalyst Wilhelm Reich came up with the theory of body armouring to explain the emotional effects of massage. He believed that feelings such as distress or anger are held in the body as muscular tension, causing the person to become stuck in a defensive or aggressive posture.

WHAT'S INVOLVED?

The sort of massage treatment that you receive depends very much on the nature of your problem, your personal preferences and the therapist's particular skills.

During an initial consultation, a masseur will ask you about your general heath, diet and medical history. Some masseurs make home visits; others work in complementary health clinics, spas, health farms, and in medical settings such as hospitals.

A Western (Swedish) massage usually takes place with the subject lying on a special high couch. It is usual to undress, although for comfort and modesty you will be covered by warm towels and you can wear underpants. A full body massage takes 60–90 minutes; a shoulder or back massage takes around 20–30 minutes. You may feel deeply relaxed, sleepy, light-headed or even emotional for a while afterwards.

For an aromatherapy massage, the therapist selects appropriate essential oils based on information provided by clients about their current physical state, and any illnesses or injuries that may affect the massage. Geranium oil, for example, may be chosen to treat menopausal and menstrual problems. The selected oils are then blended into a base massage oil and usually used as part of a traditional Swedish massage. The blend will vary with each visit to meet changing needs.

Biodynamic massage combines Swedish massage techniques with other movements such

Types of massage

Some massage techniques may have different beneficial effects, such as relieving muscular spasm or injury or improving blood circulation.

MASSAGE	BENEFITS
Swedish massage	The Swedish Treatment Movement was founded in the early 19th century by Per Henrik Ling. Solidly grounded in anatomy, the massage devised by Ling forms the basis of Western massage techniques. Ling put great emphasis on therapeutic massage, which he called medical gymnastics, to keep the body functioning well.
Manual lymphatic drainage (MLD)	MLD is a gentle form of massage that speeds up the removal from the body of waste products and toxins by encouraging efficient lymph drainage.
Biodynamic massage	Biodynamic massage was developed by Norwegian-born psychologist and physiotherapist Gerda Boyesen. She agreed with Wilhelm Reich that the body could harbour suppressed emotions in the form of physical tension. Both massage and discussion are used to release this bio-energy from the muscles and gut.
Aromatherapy massage	Aromatherapy massage uses the healing power of aromatic essential oils to relax or stimulate, detoxify and regenerate the body. The essential oils are inhaled by the subject during the massage and also absorbed through the skin. They are blended to meet a client's individual needs, and can help to relieve a wide range of chronic conditions, including stress, fatigue, menstrual or menopausal problems, digestive disorders and joint stiffness.

as manipulating the legs or arms to release trapped energy. You can receive the massage clothed or unclothed, depending on how you feel most comfortable. The therapist applies a stethoscope to the abdomen to listen to any sounds from the intestines – these are thought to mirror psychological change. There is also an opportunity to discuss any issues or feelings that arise during the massage.

SAFETY PRECAUTIONS

Seek medical advice before having a massage if you have **phlebitis** (inflamed veins), varicose veins, or severe or acute back pain or if there is any chance that you have a **deep vein thrombosis**. People with cancer need to be treated by specially trained practitioners.

Avoid massage on areas of the body where there are swellings, bruises, fractures or skin infections because pressure on these areas might cause further harm or spread infection to other areas. Massage of the legs, abdomen and feet should be avoided during the first three months of pregnancy, when the risk of miscarriage is at its highest.

HOW TO FIND A PRACTITIONER

Anyone can call himself or herself a massage therapist and set up in commercial premises, at their own home or visit clients in their homes. It is important to check that your masseur has professional qualifications and is registered with a reputable organization.

SEE ALSO *Osteopathy*

Mastectomy

This is the surgical removal of the breast, usually because of breast cancer. The extent of the operation varies according to the size and site of the tumour and whether it has spread. In a partial mastectomy, the tumour and a wide margin of surrounding tissue are removed. In a simple mastectomy, the breast is removed, although the skin and nipple are sometimes preserved. A radical mastectomy is an extensive operation involving the removal of the breast, skin, underlying chest (pectoral) muscles and lymphatic tissue from the armpit. A modified radical mastectomy, which preserves the pectoral muscles, is more often performed.

SEE ALSO *Breasts and disorders*

Mastitis, nodular

Nodular mastitis is a benign (non-cancerous) breast condition in which the whole or part of the breast feels lumpy and sometimes uncomfortable. Both symptoms usually worsen before a period and improve afterwards. Also called benign breast change or breast nodularity, is so common that it can be regarded as a normal result of changes in oestrogen and progestogen levels during each menstrual cycle. The term 'mastitis' is misleading as it implies there is infection or inflammation, neither of which is present. Breast nodularity and pain often improve spontaneously with time, but some women have persistently nodular breasts.

SEE ALSO *Breasts and disorders*

Mastoiditis

Mastoiditis is the inflammation of the prominent bone behind the ear lobe (the mastoid process). It is usually caused by a bacterial infection that spreads out from the middle ear. The inflammation reaches the mastoid bone via the mastoid antrum, the air space that connects it to the middle ear.

SYMPTOMS

Before mastoiditis sets in, there is usually a two- or three-week period of infection in the middle ear, with discoloured discharge from the ear and varying degrees of hearing loss. A fever develops, together with a general feeling of ill health and a dull pain behind the ear as the infection spreads into the mastoid antrum and attacks the inner part of the mastoid bone. The skin covering the mastoid bone becomes red, swollen and tender as an **abscess** forms in the bone. There is a progressive loss of hearing and increasingly severe pain. Eventually the abscess breaks out of the mastoid process, producing a creamy discharge from behind the ear.

A CT scan can be used to see if the air spaces in the mastoid process are filled with fluid.

MASKED MASTOIDITIS

One form of the condition, masked mastoiditis, sometimes follows an ear infection that has been partially treated with antibiotics. The pain and inflammation of the middle ear heal, but hearing fails to return to normal and the eardrum remains slightly bulging and opaque. Gradually, over the next two weeks, there is increasing fever, a feeling of ill health, and progressive deafness. In this case, an abscess behind the ear does not form and the condition may progress so 'silently' that the first marked symptoms of a problem are when serious complications such as **meningitis** or a brain abscess develop.

TREATMENT

High doses of antibiotics are administered immediately. A sample of the discharge from the ear or the abscess is analysed to identify the organism causing the infection. The antibiotic treatment is adjusted accordingly and continued for two weeks. Often the swift application of antibiotic drugs is enough to stem the infection. If an abscess has formed, an operation may be necessary. This involves a small incision behind the ear so that the cortex and damaged tip of the mastoid process can be removed. Hearing generally returns to normal after treatment.

COMPLICATIONS
Untreated mastoiditis can lead to **deafness**, **meningitis**, brain abscess, sepsis and death.
SEE ALSO *Ear and problems*

Measles

Measles is a highly contagious viral disease. It affects mainly preschool children, causing a rash, and is one of the most unpleasant and dangerous childhood illnesses because of the potential complications.

Anybody who has not already had measles can be infected. However, infants up to four months old will not be infected if the mother has had measles herself because they will be protected by her antibodies. One attack of measles gives you lifelong immunity: once you have had measles, you can never catch it again.

The disease is usually more severe in adults than children and is particularly dangerous for pregnant women: measles during pregnancy results in death of the fetus in about one-fifth of cases. Measles may be particularly severe in people with poor defences against infection, including those with AIDS or cancer.

SYMPTOMS
Symptoms develop 10–14 days after infection. There may be:
- a high temperature of about 39°C/102°F;
- a runny nose;
- a sore throat;
- swelling of the lymph nodes ('glands') in the throat;
  - sensitivity to light
  - sore, red eyes;
  - a cough.

Blotchy, red spots appear within a week. They usually begin on the face, then spread down the body to the trunk and limbs. At first the spots are very small, about 2mm ($^1/_{16}$in) in diameter, but they rapidly double in size and begin to join together. The rash usually lasts for two to five days.

The temperature may reach 40°C/104°F and stay that high for a couple of days. The cough is often the last symptom to disappear.

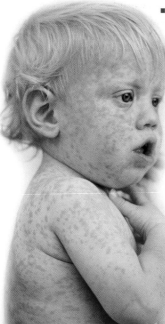

▼ Tell-tale rash
The spots easily identify measles, but the child will have been unwell, and infectious, for four days before they emerge.

DURATION
- The incubation period, the time between the infection and the outbreak of the condition, is usually one to two weeks. You are infectious from four days before the onset of the rash until five days after it first appears.
- Most people get better within seven to ten days unless complications occur.

CAUSES
Measles is caused by a virus that passes very readily from person to person. It spreads via airborne droplets of infected mucus from the mouth and nose, expelled during sneezing and coughing. It enters the body through the nose and mouth, multiplying in the lining of the airways. It then spreads through the blood to various parts of the body, including the skin, where it produces the rash. Even if the sick person is isolated, the disease may still spread from room to room.

TREATMENT
The treatment is usually the same for both adults and children.

What you can do
It is important to keep the sick person's temperature down. When infants experience high temperatures, there is a risk of a fit. Plenty of fluids should be drunk and paracetamol may be given (see also **Fever**).

Keep the person in bed in a cool room without any bright lights. Children with measles should stay away from school or childcare until they are fully recovered and their temperature is back to normal.

When to consult a doctor
- Once measles is suspected.
- If the temperature of a child with measles remains high.

What a doctor may do
- Check for complications.
- Give children under the age of one an immunity injection within five days of exposure.

PREVENTION
In the UK, all children aged 12–18 months are offered the MMR vaccination, which aims to protect them against measles, mumps and rubella; a second, booster dose is given to the child between the ages of three and five.

COMPLICATIONS
Complications from measles are rare but can be serious. The most common are chest and ear infections, such as inflammation of the middle ear. If a persistent cough remains, then an **X-ray** of the chest may be carried out to rule out pneumonia. If the doctor thinks that the person has pneumonia, a course of antibiotics will probably be given. Very rarely, an infection in the brain (**encephalitis**) may occur.
SEE ALSO *Immunization*

Memory loss and distortion

Memory loss or distortion, also called **amnesia**, is an inability to retain and recall short- or long-term memory.

Memory is controlled by an area of the brain known as the cerebral cortex. Any disease or condition that adversely affects the normal functioning of the cerebral cortex can distort the memory processes and cause memory loss and dysfunction.

Memory loss can occur rapidly, as in some types of **head injury** or in toxic states such as **meningitis** or **drug misuse**. In conditions that progress slowly such as **senile dementia** or where the person has a slow-growing tumour of the brain, the symptoms may be less obvious. Confusion or emotional disturbance will often occur when there is memory dysfunction.

SEE ALSO *Brain and nervous system*

Ménière's disease

Ménière's disease is a condition characterized by a periodic buildup of fluid in the inner ear, which disrupts a person's hearing and sense of balance. Ménière's disease affects about one person in 1000 in the UK. Its cause is unknown.

SYMPTOMS
Symptoms may come on suddenly and be very severe for a few hours. They include:
■ vertigo (giddiness) with a sensation of spinning or falling;
■ a sense of fullness in the head;
■ nausea and sometimes vomiting;
■ hearing loss and **tinnitus**, at first intermittent and later persisting between attacks;
■ in some cases, nystagmus;
■ in some cases, sweating, **palpitations**, anxiety or diarrhoea.

DURATION
Attacks last from a few minutes to 24 hours. Periods between attacks vary from a few days to many years.

TREATMENT
If you think that you may have Ménière's disease, seek medical advice.

What a doctor may do
■ Examine your ears and eyes and test your hearing and nervous system.
■ Prescribe medication to reduce the number and severity of attacks.
■ Suggest a tinnitus masker or hearing aid.
■ In severe cases, where medication is not effective, suggest an injection of a drug through the eardrum (intra-tympanic gentamicin) or surgery, to relieve vertigo.

What you can do
You can reduce the likelihood of an attack by avoiding stress and cutting down on salt, caffeine and alcohol, all of which influence body fluid levels. If you have an attack, try to rest and keep still while it lasts.

Complementary therapies
There is clinical evidence that a homeopathic remedy, Vertigoheel, helps to relieve vertigo symptoms in Ménière's disease, and some people find ginger root tea helpful for nausea. Ginkgo biloba and niacin (vitamin B_3) have been found helpful for tinnitus in some trials. They should be taken under medical supervision as they may interact with other medicines or have side effects.

OUTLOOK
Treatment can help to control symptoms and reduce but not prevent attacks. These may become more or less frequent over time. Hearing impairment often increases and may become permanent. Balance problems of varying severity may develop.

Meningitis

Meningitis is the inflammation of the three protective membranes that surround the brain (the meninges). It is most commonly caused by viral or bacterial infection. The symptoms are similar whatever the cause of meningitis, but the severity of the disease and the seriousness of complications depend on the infecting organism. Anyone concerned about meningitis should seek urgent medical advice.

Viral infection occurs in small epidemics but does not usually have serious consequences. On the other hand, bacterial meningitis, although rare, is extremely serious. It is fatal in one in ten cases, and one in seven survivors is left with a severe disability such as brain damage or deafness. A complication is multiple organ failure arising from the blood-borne infection **septicaemia**.

Since infectious bacteria can be spread by droplets travelling over short distances, clusters of meningitis cases can occur where social conditions lead to close contact within crowded environments, for example, in university halls of residence, army barracks, prisons and daycare centres.

Some conditions that weaken the immune system predispose a person to meningitis. These include HIV/AIDS, immunosuppressant therapy (after major organ transplants, for example), tuberculosis and malfunctioning defence systems – affecting, for example, people without a spleen and those suffering from sickle cell disease. Other predisposing conditions are alcoholism and diabetes mellitus.

VIRAL MENINGITIS

About 500 cases of viral meningitis are reported every year in the UK, but the true figure is probably higher because its mild, flu-like symptoms mean that the disease is not always accurately identified and may be mistaken for a cold or other mild viral infection. No treatment is necessary and painkillers and bed rest are usually recommended. Antiviral drugs such as aciclovir may be used in some cases.

Viral meningitis may be a consequence of **mumps** or **measles**, but childhood vaccination programmes against these diseases have considerably reduced the incidence of meningitis contracted in this way.

Infections tend to occur during summer.

BACTERIAL MENINGITIS

Three organisms are responsible for 80 per cent of bacterial meningitis infections. They are found naturally in the back of the nose and throat, or in the upper respiratory tract. People of any age can carry the bacteria for days, weeks or months without becoming ill.

The most frequent culprit is *Neisseria meningitidis*, the cause of meningococcal meningitis and septicaemia, which can affect people of any age. The other two types of infection tend to occur in certain age groups. *Haemophilus influenzae B (HIB)* affects children under 5 years old. *Streptococcus pneumoniae*, the cause of pneumococcal meningitis, most commonly affects very young and very old people.

The meningitis bacteria can be passed from person to person by prolonged close contact or by sneezing, coughing or intimate kissing. They cannot live for long outside the body. The incubation period is between two and ten days. Bacterial meningitis is more prevalent during the autumn and winter months.

Around 3000 cases of bacterial meningitis and septicaemia occur annually in the UK. It has become less common following meningitis vaccination programmes, and increased public awareness has alerted people to seek help in the early stages of the infection.

SYMPTOMS

In bacterial meningitis and septicaemia, symptoms can develop quickly, sometimes in the space of a few hours. In the later stages of the disease, drowsiness may be followed by **fits**, confusion and unconsciousness. In more than 50 per cent of cases of meningococcal disease, septicaemia is present and a rash of red or brown pinprick marks occurs. If the rash does not disappear when pressed with a glass, contact a doctor immediately.

The main symptoms of meningitis and septicaemia are:

- fever;
- severe headache;
- nausea and vomiting;
- aversion to light (unusual in small children);
- a stiff neck (unusual in small children);
- irritability;
- rapid breathing;
- joint or muscle pain;
- cold hands and feet.

In babies and young children, meningitis can cause high temperature, vomiting, refusal to feed and a high-pitched moaning cry.

TREATMENT

If bacterial meningitis is suspected in a patient, a doctor will administer an antibiotic by injection and arrange immediate hospitalization. The hospital doctors will carry out tests, including blood tests and sometimes a lumbar puncture, whereby a thin needle is inserted into the spinal cord to remove some cerebrospinal fluid. Analysis of the fluid usually gives a definitive diagnosis and identifies the bacterium responsible for the illness.

If the cause of the meningitis is confirmed as bacterial, high-dose antibiotics are continued. The antibiotics used include forms of penicillin and cephalosporins, but the precise choice depends on the type of bacterium involved and the age of the affected individual.

Other treatments may involve steroids to reduce inflammation, and intravenous fluids if necessary.

PREVENTION

Meningitis and septicaemia remain uncommon, but they often seem to strike at random. Since 1992, babies in the UK have been immunized against HIB in their first year, greatly reducing the incidence of the illness. A vaccine against one form of meningococcal meningitis has recently been introduced.

If someone contracts meningitis or septicaemia, the spread of the disease can be controlled by giving antibiotic treatment to people with whom the infected individual has been in close contact.

SEE ALSO *Brain and nervous system; Immunization; Infectious diseases*

Factfile

A sign of septicaemia

In about half of meningococcal meningitis cases, a rash of small red or brown marks appears on the limbs, indicating septicaemia. If left untreated, the marks join up to resemble bruises.

A 'glass test' can help to identify a septicaemia rash. If you press the side of a drinking glass firmly onto the spots or bruises, they will not fade. If you suspect meningitis, do not wait for the rash to appear but get medical help urgently.

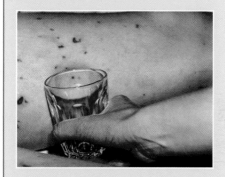

Menopause

The experience of menopause is a highly individual one. It affects women at different ages, and while some sail through it with few or no problems, others may be incapacitated by unpleasant symptoms.

Menopause is the term doctors use to describe the time in a woman's life when ovulation (release of eggs from the ovaries) and **menstruation** (periods) cease and she is no longer able to bear children.

Menopause most often occurs between the ages of 45 and 55 (in the UK the average age is 51). But it can happen as early as the 20s or 30s or as late as the 60s. A woman commonly goes through menopause around the same age as her mother or grandmother. On average, smokers tend to experience menopause earlier. Medically, menopause is considered to have occurred only when a woman has been without menstrual periods for one year.

Women vary tremendously in how they view the menopause. For some it is a welcome change and a time to discover a new-found sense of freedom: there is no longer the need to worry about contraception, or engage in decision-making about whether or not to have any more children. Furthermore, there are no more periods, which for some women have made a few days each month of their fertile lives hard to endure. Other women feel sad and mourn the loss of their fertility. But a life expectancy of around 80 years means that, however a woman feels, she can expect to live more than one-third of her life after the menopause.

WHY MENOPAUSE HAPPENS

Menopause happens because the 2 million or so eggs that a woman is born with run out. The process begins around three to five years before menopause, when about 1000 eggs remain. At this point, a woman's periods may become erratic and irregular (a time known as the perimenopause). As the eggs become fewer, the ovaries produce less oestrogen and progesterone and ovulation becomes irregular. It is not known exactly why the symptoms of menopause occur, but it is thought to be linked to this fall in hormone levels, particularly oestrogen.

SYMPTOMS

The precise symptoms and their severity vary from one woman to another, but many women experience a number of common problems.

Hot flushes

Hot flushes are the most common symptom of menopause. Typically they begin with a feeling of extreme heat that starts in the centre of the chest and spreads, particularly to the shoulders, neck and face. They may be accompanied by sweating. Most last for a few minutes, but can last for anything from half a minute to half an hour.

Doctors do not know exactly what causes hot flushes. In fact, one of the mysteries about menopause is that some women are severely affected by hot flushes while others never have them at all. They are thought to be linked to the effect that fluctuating levels of oestrogen have on the body's temperature-control mechanism.

Irregular periods

Some women experience a sudden cessation of periods, but in general the periods become more erratic. The menstrual cycle may lengthen or shorten, and periods may get lighter or heavier before they stop altogether.

Decreased fertility

As ovulation becomes more unreliable, fertility declines and a woman is less likely to conceive. However, it is still possible to become pregnant if you have ovulated. Ovulation may be erratic during the perimenopause, but it still happens, so it is important to continue using contraception until you are quite certain you have passed through the menopause. Once you have definitely passed through the menopause, and it is a year since your last period, it is impossible to conceive.

Insomnia and sleep disturbances

Around one in four women experiences sleep disturbances, such as night-waking for no apparent reason or **insomnia**, around menopause. These may be worsened by night sweats, which are often, but not always, linked to hot flushes.

Vaginal dryness

Another very common consequence of the decrease in oestrogen is vaginal dryness. This can make sexual intercourse uncomfortable or even painful. Vaginal dryness may be accompanied by an increased risk of vaginal infections, **cystitis** and other urinary problems such as stress **incontinence** – which causes the leakage of a small amount of urine when you cough, sneeze, laugh or lift anything heavy.

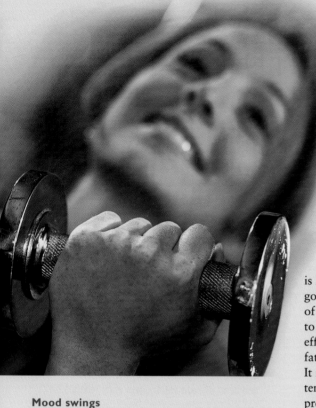

◀ **Weights help**
Improve the strength of your bones and lessen the risk of developing osteoporosis by taking regular weight-bearing exercise.

Mood swings

Many women complain of mood swings, forgetfulness, irritability and other emotional upsets during menopause. It is not known whether these are directly attributable to hormonal changes, or whether they are, at least in part, coincidental. These symptoms could, for example, be a response to crucial life changes that tend to take place in a woman's late 40s and early 50s – her parents may become ill or die, or her children might be leaving home.

Changes in appearance

Women can be upset by changes in the way they look that seem to happen at menopause. Some of these changes are caused by shifting hormone levels, but others are simply part of the natural process of ageing. Women often put on some weight at this time, especially round the waist – but taking exercise and watching what you eat can help to stop this from happening. The breasts may be less full and the skin is generally drier – this is a good time to buy a well-designed bra and effective moisturizing cream. A few women may find that their facial hair seems a little coarser and more noticeable – a problem that can be dealt with by a beautician. Thinning hair is also common, but it does not lead to baldness. The hair loss will stop, and having regular haircuts will keep the hair looking thick and healthy.

EFFECTS ON WOMEN'S HEALTH

After the menopause, women are more at risk of certain medical conditions, in particular heart disease, **stroke** and **osteoporosis**.

Until they reach menopause, women's risk of developing heart disease or having a stroke is lower than men's. After menopause, the risk goes up, eventually becoming the same as that of a man of the same age. This may be partly to do with the fact that oestrogen has positive effects on the blood vessels and levels of blood fats – benefits that disappear after the menopause. It is also linked to other risk factors such as the tendency to put on weight and the fact that blood pressure increases with age in both sexes.

You can lessen the risks of heart disease and strokes by eating carefully: try to keep to a low-fat diet, and eat lots of fibre in the form of fresh fruit and vegetables. You should keep your intake of salt to a minimum in order to keep your blood pressure down. If you smoke, stop. You should also take regular exercise. **Hormone replacement therapy** (HRT) was once routinely prescribed to help to protect against heart disease and stroke. But recent studies suggest that there is not enough evidence to recommend its use in this way.

Osteoporosis

Throughout our lives, calcium is lost from the bones and regained in a constant cycle. However, during the year following menopause, calcium is lost from a woman's bones at a faster rate than it is rebuilt, increasing her risk of developing the bone disease **osteoporosis** to one in four. It is vital to obtain sufficient calcium at this time (1500mg daily), and to take regular weight-bearing exercise to help to strengthen the bones. HRT and bone-building drugs can also help.

MANAGING THE MENOPAUSE NATURALLY

Going through the menopause does not consign you automatically to a life on a cocktail of hormones and drugs. Several foods and supplements are rich in phyto-oestrogens – plant oestrogens that may help to alleviate menopausal symptoms. They include soya, chickpeas, lentils and other pulses, linseeds, wholegrains, some fruits and vegetables and the supplement red clover. Vitamin E may help to maintain a healthy heart, and calcium supplements can help to protect you against osteoporosis.

Medical terms

Climacteric
Another word for menopause. It is sometimes used to describe the period leading to menopause.

Perimenopause
The period approaching menopause during which a woman is still ovulating, but may be experiencing menopausal symptoms.

Postmenopause
The years following menopause when a woman's ovaries no longer produce oestrogen and progesterone, and release no eggs.

Wild yam cream, which is rich in progesterone-like chemicals, is sometimes recommended as a form of natural HRT. However, more research is needed before it can definitely be established that it helps. Black cohosh, a herb used by Native American women, is sometimes recommended for hot flushes. It can be poisonous, however, so it should only be taken under the supervision of a qualified herbal practitioner (see **Herbal medicine**).

THE HRT DEBATE

HRT is the administration of oestrogen and, perhaps, progestogen (a progesterone-like preparation) to women at or after the menopause. HRT replaces the lost oestrogen and can counteract some of the effects of the menopause. But the decision to take HRT is an individual one: the benefits of alleviating flushes and vaginal dryness in the short term, and protecting against osteoporosis in the long term, must be balanced against the slightly increased risk of breast cancer and ovarian cancer. And while some studies suggest that HRT may protect against heart disease, others show that oestrogen increases the risk of heart attacks and strokes, and encourages potentially dangerous blood clots.

For those women who decide against taking HRT, there are drugs available that prevent and treat osteoporosis. There are also drugs, known as selective oestrogen receptor modulators, which have some of the beneficial effects of oestrogen but do not increase the risk of breast cancer.

Some types of HRT cause a monthly bleed, rather like a scanty period. But any postmenopausal bleeding not associated with

▼ **HRT options**
HRT can be taken in several different forms: as tablets taken daily, gels or cream used in combination with oestrogen tablets and as patches worn on the upper thigh and replaced twice weekly.

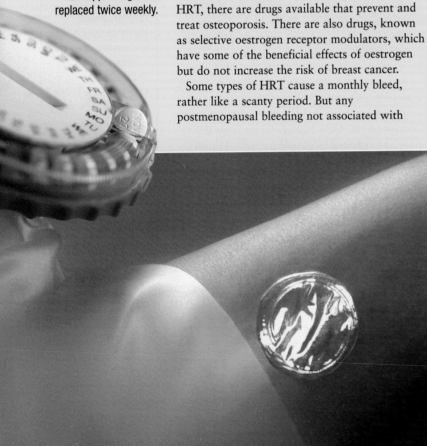

Managing the menopause

There are certain things you should and should not do to make the menopause a healthy and forward-looking time in your life.

Do

✓ Eat a healthy diet that is low in saturated fat and rich in fruit, vegetables and grains.

✓ Take regular exercise for strong bones, a healthy heart and flexible joints.

✓ For hot flushes, wear cotton and use a light-weight duvet. Avoid hot drinks and spicy foods.

✓ Use a lubricant such as Senselle or KY jelly for vaginal dryness. Staying sexually active helps.

✓ Relax – try yoga and meditation.

✓ Ask your doctor about HRT.

Don't

✗ Smoke – it increases the risks of osteoporosis and heart disease and triggers early menopause.

✗ Neglect your health. Have regular medical checks such as mammograms and cervical smears.

✗ Neglect your pelvic floor exercises. They can stop stress incontinence.

HRT, or bleeding between periods in the perimenopausal period, may be a sign of more serious problems and you should discuss this with your doctor.

EARLY MENOPAUSE

Early or premature menopause is when the menopause occurs at a much earlier age than usual – in a woman's 20s or 30s, for example. It is a very distressing event for a young woman, especially if she wants children. It can be a result of hormonal abnormalities or it may be triggered by a radical **hysterectomy**, in which the ovaries are removed with the uterus, or by **chemotherapy** or **radiotherapy** treatments for cancer.

Women who have had an early menopause are usually advised to take HRT to prevent osteoporosis. Researchers are investigating the possibility of preventing early menopause by injecting ovarian cells into the forearms of women who have received treatment for ovarian cancer.

Menstruation

Menstruation refers to the monthly shedding of an unfertilized ovum or egg together with the endometrium (lining of the uterus or womb). The menstrual cycle is defined as the time from the first day of a menstrual period to the first day of the next one. This cycle is governed by a series of different hormones that, unless suppressed, for example, by pregnancy, breastfeeding or a contraceptive pill, prepare the body for conception each month.

THE PHASES OF THE MENSTRUAL CYCLE
The menstrual cycle has three phases.

■ In the follicular phase, a hormone causes a dormant egg cell or follicle to begin to ripen in the ovaries. Oestrogen is released, causing the endometrium to thicken in preparation for fertilization. The pituitary then secretes another hormone, luteinizing hormone (LH). This triggers ovulation, in which the ripened follicle bursts releasing an egg (ovum) that travels down the Fallopian tubes to the uterus.

■ During the luteal (or secretory) phase, the supporting cells remaining after ovulation start to secrete progesterone. This hormone increases blood supply to the uterus, creating an environment that is rich in blood and nutrients in preparation for a potential embryo. If fertilization does not occur, progesterone levels will fall. This deprives the endometrium of oxygen and nutrients, causing the cells to die.

■ Finally, during the menstrual phase (or menstruation), the endometrium is shed as a period and the whole cycle begins again.

WHAT CAN GO WRONG
Menstruation depends on the complex interaction of hormones that govern the menstrual cycle. Anything that disrupts this, such as disease, diet or weight changes, emotion or faulty development of the reproductive organs, can cause menstrual problems.

Premenstrual syndrome (PMS)
Most women experience some physical and mental changes in the week or so before menstruation. However, some women find that these symptoms are severe enough to disrupt their everyday lives. Symptoms include mood swings, irritability, depression, anxiety, insomnia and physical symptoms such as bloating, tender, swollen breasts and weight gain. They usually all disappear as soon as menstruation begins. A low-salt, wholefood diet, exercise and supplements such as B$_6$ and evening primrose oil can often help to control PMS (see also **Herbal medicine**). A variety of drugs, ranging from diuretics to hormonal drugs, are sometimes used to treat more severe cases.

Some women experience a severe form of PMS called premenstrual dysphoric disorder (PMDD), in which mood symptoms are a particular problem. SSRI antidepressants may be helpful in this case.

Dysmenorrhoea (painful menstruation)
An estimated 50 per cent of women experience pain before or during their period and some 10 per cent suffer severe pain. The pain is typically experienced as fluctuating cramps, similar to early labour pains, in the lower abdomen. These may spread to the thighs and lower back. In severe cases, there may be nausea, vomiting, diarrhoea, dizziness and headaches. There are two kinds of dysmenorrhoea – primary dysmenorrhoea and secondary dysmenorrhoea.

Primary dysmenorrhoea affects women of any age, but is often relieved after childbirth. There is no identifiable underlying cause, although some experts believe it may be linked to high levels of hormone-like substances called prostaglandins, which cause the uterus to contract. The pain generally begins with menstruation and tends to be worse on the first day or so of the cycle. Drugs that quell prostaglandins, including aspirin, can help. Other medications may include the oral contraceptive pill.

Secondary dysmenorrhoea tends to affect older women and may be caused by a number of underlying physical disorders such as **fibroids**, polyps, **endometriosis**, adenomyosis and pelvic inflammatory disease (PID) (see **Pelvis and disorders**). Occasionally, the problem is due to narrowing of the opening from the cervix into the vagina. Treatment depends on the underlying cause, but may include hormonal drugs and surgery such as **hysterectomy**.

Cycle disturbances
Few women menstruate exactly every 28 days, and anything from 21–42 days can be normal for a particular woman. Cycles often become erratic as a woman nears the **menopause**, but this can also be a sign of overgrowth of the endometrium (endometrial hyperplasia) caused by lack of ovulation. In mild cases, progestogen may be prescribed, but in more severe cases, surgery may be needed. Low levels of reproductive hormones may cause extremely short cycles with frequent bleeding (polymenorrhoea), which may also result from other hormonal disorders such as **thyroid** problems. Long regular cycles may be normal for some women. However, in other cases, particularly where the cycles are irregular, there may be a problem such as ovarian **cysts** or an underlying hormonal disorder.

Menstrual cycle

Approximately every 28 days, throughout a woman's reproductive life, an egg matures in one of her ovaries and her womb prepares for pregnancy. If the egg is not fertilized, the womb sheds its blood-rich lining, another egg starts to mature, and a new cycle begins.

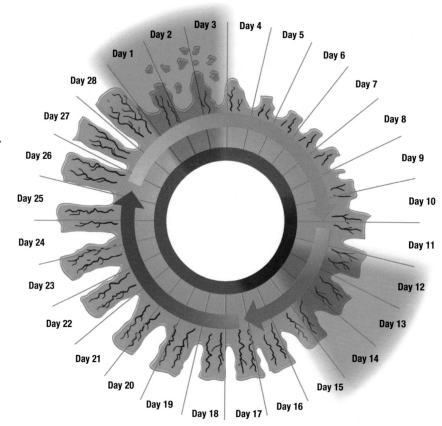

■ Oestrogen
■ Luteinizing hormone (LH)
■ Progesterone
■ Follicle stimulating hormone (FSH)

Menorrhagia (heavy periods)

Heavy periods are defined as the loss of 80ml (2¾ fl oz) or more of menstrual blood each period (the average is 30–40ml/1–1½ fl oz or 6 to 8 teaspoons). In practice, this means having to change pads or tampons extremely frequently, together with the passage of large clots. There may also be cramplike pains. Persistent menorrhagia can lead to **anaemia**.

In many cases menorrhagia has no identifiable cause. In others, the cause may be **fibroids** or fibromyomas, or an IUD (intrauterine device). Heavy periods tend to be more common following sterilization. **Obesity** and hormonal abnormalities may also be a cause.

Treatment depends on the underlying cause, but may include the oral contraceptive pill or a specialized IUD that releases progestogen (called Mirena). A number of hormonal medications and, in severe cases, removal of the endometrium or uterus (hysterectomy) may also be recommended.

Amenorrhoea (lack of periods)

There are two type of amenorrhoea – primary amenorrhoea, defined as failure to begin menstruating by the age of 16, and secondary amenorrhoea, a temporary or permanent failure of menstruation in a woman who has previously had regular periods.

Primary amenorrhoea affects about 3 girls in 1000. It is normally simply a case of beginning puberty late and may be hereditary.

In some cases, it may be a result of a disease such as **tuberculosis**, **meningitis** or **encephalitis**. Alternatively, it may be a result of abnormalities in the **reproductive system**, or may indicate a disorder of the **endocrine system**. Other possible causes include excessive exercise, **anorexia nervosa** and excessive weight loss, which causes insufficient ovary-producing hormones to be produced, leading to low levels of oestrogen.

Secondary amenorrhoea can have a number of different causes. In a sexually active woman who has previously menstruated regularly, pregnancy is the most common cause. In a woman over the age of 40, **menopause** may be the cause. Other possible causes include tumours, ovarian cysts, significant weight gain or loss or a number of hormonal disturbances, which affect ovulation. Polycystic ovary syndrome, for example, is a hormonal disorder in which multiple cysts form in the ovaries, leading to menstrual disturbances or absence of menstruation (see **Ovaries and disorders**).

OUTLOOK

Research into premenstrual problems has shown that both magnesium supplements and electrical nerve stimulation may reduce prostaglandin-induced menstrual pain.

For heavy periods, an IUD called Mirena, which releases small doses of a progesterone-like substance, can help to treat heavy bleeding.

SEE ALSO *Contraception; Infertility; Pituitary gland and disorders*

Mental health and problems

Mental health problems are as common as heart disease and three times as common as cancer. They affect about 6 million people in the UK, and can be as painful and debilitating as physical illness. The various treatment options range from talking to someone about your problem to taking medication.

Mental health problems are disorders that affect one or more functions of the mind, causing suffering to the patient or others. Mental health problems cover a range of experiences, and come in many forms. They all affect the way that people feel, think or behave and they limit their ability to cope with life. Feelings of depression, anxiety or confusion are a normal response to difficulties or problems. These feelings become a problem, however, when they are so extreme, or last so long, that it becomes difficult to cope with everyday life. A person may then be described as having a mental health problem, or even a mental illness, and may be given a diagnosis.

Your mental health is influenced by several factors. These include your physical health, your feelings or emotions and the environment in which you live. You may suffer from a chronic health problem or physical disability, or you may feel isolated from close family if you do not live near them. Most mental health problems seem to happen as a result of life events and how we cope with them. When you are feeling vulnerable, perhaps because of a death or the loss of a job, you may experience mental distress. Some people go on to develop conditions such as **depression** or **schizophrenia**. Around one in five children also suffer from mental health problems.

Most of us will experience some mental distress in our lives or know someone else who has. Many people struggle on alone, but one in ten will seek professional help, most often for depression, anxiety and other stress-related problems. One in 50 people will have severe psychotic illness such as **schizophrenia**.

The word 'psychotic' is used to describe someone who cannot tell the difference between what is real and what is imaginary, especially if this involves hearing voices or seeing things that are not there. The effect of hearing or seeing things that other people don't can be distressing: we are used to believing what we see and hear, and it is difficult not to react.

A mental health problem is not something to be ashamed of nor is it a sign of weakness. But many people do not understand mental health problems and sufferers can find it difficult to be open about what is happening to them.

Anyone who is worried about their own or a relative's mental health should contact their GP. Most people make a full recovery – half of those who visit their GP with mental health problems get well in less than a year. Sometimes people come out of the experience feeling stronger and wiser. Others get over the worst, but remain vulnerable and relapse from time to time. Even those who do not recover may not have severe symptoms all the time.

SIGNS OF MENTAL HEALTH PROBLEMS
The following are common indicators of mental health problems.
■ Hearing or seeing things that others don't (see also **Hallucination**).
■ Mistaken beliefs, for example, that someone is about to hurt you, is laughing at you or is trying to take over your body (see **Delusions**).
■ Changes of behaviour – changed sleep patterns or appetite, feeling more energetic or more

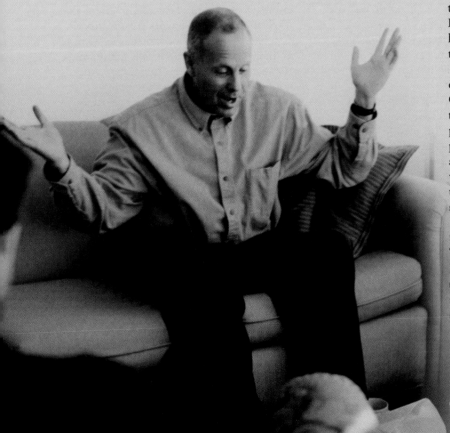

▼ **Talking therapies**
Many people with depression find talking therapies a helpful form of treatment. These may be given on a one-to-one basis by a therapist or in a group of people with similar problems.

Hearing voices

Research has show that many people hear voices – some people cope with them well whereas others need help to deal with them.

Hearing voices can be confusing and frustrating when you realize that other people don't hear them. But many people hear voices all their lives without it causing them any difficulty or distress. In some cultures, voices are viewed in a positive way. Voices or visual hallucinations usually come to the attention of others only when it becomes a problem.

People who see things react in different ways depending on what they see. In response to something frightening, for example, they may freeze or scream. Others may try to hide or escape.

Such reactions can be unnerving for the people around them, but it helps if you try to understand what the person is feeling or experiencing. For example, a person who is ranting or hurling abuse may be responding to internal threatening voices.

lethargic than normal, finding it difficult to get on with people.

■ Extreme or quickly changing moods – for example, feeling energetic, creative or 'high'; or feeling lethargic, depressed or 'low'. Moods may alternate or one mood may dominate.

■ Self-harm: some people find that they can release pent-up emotions by physically hurting themselves; others may attack themselves because of a mistaken belief, for example, that a snake is wrapped around their arm.

■ Eating disorders: a person's life becomes centred on food – avoiding it, overeating, or eating then purging – as an expression of emotional distress.

TYPES OF MENTAL HEALTH PROBLEMS

Mental health problems come in many forms. If you seek help, a diagnosis may be possible, but having a diagnosis can be a problem if it is incorrect or if you feel labelled as a set of symptoms rather than as an individual. And some problems are difficult to diagnose. The more common mental health problems are listed below.

Anxiety

Most people feel anxious from time to time, but **anxiety** becomes an illness when it feeds on itself and dominates your life. Doctors describe chronic fear, tension and **panic attacks** as 'anxiety states'. Some people have panic attacks – a rapid buildup of anxiety where your heart pounds, and you overbreathe or find breathing difficult.

Dementia

This is caused by brain cells wasting away. People with **dementia** become anxious, forgetful and confused as the disease progresses. **Alzheimer's disease** is a particular type of dementia.

Depression

Most of us get depressed at some time in our lives and it is often a natural reaction. Life events such a bereavement, divorce or redundancy may cause symptoms of depression but these reduce in time. A depressive disorder or clinical depression is where symptoms of depression, such as loss of energy, suicidal thoughts or sleep problems, continue for a long time or are extreme, going beyond normal mood changes.

Eating disorders

Anorexia nervosa, where people starve themselves, and **bulimia nervosa**, a combination of overeating and vomiting, are types of eating disorder. Both are often ways of coping with psychological or emotional problems. Eating disorders mostly affect young females but also affect young men.

Manic depression

Manic depression involves extreme mood swings, from severe depression and exhaustion to extreme happiness, energy and overactivity. These mood swings can happen several times in a week, or only once or twice in a year.

Phobias and obsessions

These are both linked to anxiety. A **phobia** is an uncontrollable fear of an object or situation, such as a fear of certain insects or of enclosed spaces. **Obsessions** are recurring thoughts or ideas that are often accompanied by rituals, or compulsions, which the person carries out to ward off the imagined danger.

Schizophrenia

This term is used to describe a dramatic disturbance in a person's thoughts and feelings, accompanied by behaviour that seems bizarre to others, hearing voices, seeing things that are not there, or believing they are being persecuted by other people.

CAUSES OF MENTAL HEALTH PROBLEMS

Just as there are many types of mental health problems, there are many possible causes or combinations of causes. No one knows why some people have a greater reaction to life events than others. Opinions vary about whether our personalities and ability to cope are shaped by our life experiences or determined by our genes, passed on from our parents. However, it does seem clear that some of us are more prone to mental health problems that are triggered by stressful events.

Some possible causes of mental health problems are listed below.

■ Difficult family background. Growing up feeling uncared for, excessively criticized, frightened of a parent, or being sexually abused can lead to insecurity and make you more vulnerable to mental distress.

■ Suppressed feeling. Feelings that are held back and not expressed may cause tensions that affect our physical and mental health.

■ Stressful life events. These may affect people immediately, or years later. Sexual or physical abuse, accidents, war or other disasters can cause distress. Childbirth, the breakup of a relationship, or a death of someone close, can cause depression, grieving, or low self-esteem. For some people, this understandable distress goes well beyond bearable limits.

■ Chemical changes. There is some evidence that mood disorders, such as depression or manic depression, are connected to changes in the chemicals in the brain, but it is unknown what comes first, the mood change or the chemical change. The chemical adrenaline is produced when we are frightened or under pressure. If it is not used up in physical activity, our minds and bodies remain tense and overactive (see **Stress**).

■ Genes or inherited factors. Parents pass on physical characteristics to their children through their genes. Genes may also affect personality, and there may be genes that make you more vulnerable to mental health problems.

■ Spiritual or religious explanations. Some cultures or religions interpret and accept some mental health problems in the context of their beliefs. This gives them a meaning that may be missed by people outside that culture or religious group.

GETTING HELP OR TREATMENT

For some people, all that is needed is a talk with someone who understands and is supportive. But when things are more serious or don't get any better, professional support may be needed. If you feel there is something wrong, seek help as soon as possible. Don't wait until things are really bad.

The first step is to contact your GP. Remember you are not alone; one in eight people visits his or her family doctor to talk about emotional problems each year. If you feel you would prefer not to see your GP, you can contact your local social services office and ask to speak to a mental health worker.

Your GP may be able to help you personally, or may refer you to a counsellor or nurse in the practice. Sometimes, your doctor will refer you to a specialist mental health professional, such as a psychiatrist, psychologist, or a community psychiatric nurse.

There are many things that can be done to help to ease mental health problems, including talking therapies, medication, **complementary therapies** and self-help strategies. They can be used on their own or in combination. Medication can help

Community care

Community care offers people with long-term mental health problems support to live independently.

Following the introduction of the Community Care Act in 1990, long-stay hospitals for people with mental health problems have closed down. Many of the services once provided within the hospitals are now provided by other agencies within the community. Community mental health teams are responsible for supporting the vast majority of people with mental health problems in the UK. These teams include community psychiatric nurses, social workers, psychologists, doctors, occupational therapists and support workers. With their help, it is sometimes possible to support someone through a mental health crisis either at home or in a residential crisis centre instead of in hospital. Other community care services include day centres, housing with care and support, help with employment, and welfare rights advice.

Media reports tend to focus on seriously ill people living in the community and harming others. These incidents are rare, as very few people with mental health problems are violent or a risk to others.

some people to recover, but other treatments, such as counselling or therapy, may be needed as well, to discover the underlying problem. You may need to try several treatments to find out which one suits you best.

The main types of available treatment for mental health problems are listed below.

Drug treatment

The most common type of treatment for mental health problems is prescribed medication, given by a GP. A number of drugs may be used – to help you sleep, calm you down, lift depression or control disturbing thoughts. They work by affecting the chemical balance in the brain. Medication helps some people, but not in all cases. It can ease the symptoms of mental health problems and help people to keep going – working and looking after their children, for example.

Some drugs can be addictive and have side effects that make some people feel worse. The dosage of drugs given is important – too little may mean the drug doesn't work and too much may cause side effects. Some drugs have withdrawal effects – if you cut down or stop taking them, you experience a range of unpleasant symptoms and these withdrawal effects can be mistaken for a relapse of the mental health problem.

The main drugs given for mental health problems are:

- minor tranquillizers (such as Librium, Valium, Mogadon), given for anxiety, agitation or to help with sleep problems;
- antidepressants (such as Anafranil, Gamanil, Parnate, Prozac), given for depression;
- lithium (Priadel) or carbamazepine (Tegretol), given for both high and low mood swings (manic depression);
- antipsychotic drugs (such as Largactil, Stelazine, Haldol). These are given for delusions, hallucinations and manic or disturbed behaviour.

Talking therapies

There are many different types of talking therapy, which will help you make sense of your problems.

Counsellors and psychotherapists are specially trained to help people to understand themselves better and overcome difficulties in their lives. They can help you to work out a plan of action for tackling your problems. Many GPs now employ counsellors, or can refer you to one.

Counselling looks at what you are feeling now and helps you to adjust to life events such as bereavement or a relationship breakdown.

Cognitive behaviour therapy aims to help you to change negative thoughts and replace them with positive ones.

Psychological therapies may help you to find the reason for your problems, usually by looking at your past and childhood experiences.

Electroconvulsive therapy (ECT)

ECT is sometimes given to people with severe depression or other serious mental health problems and who have not responded to drug treatment. It is a controversial treatment, which some people find helpful and others find extremely distressing. It involves an electrical current being passed through the person's brain while he or she is under an **anaesthetic**. Side effects include memory loss, drowsiness, confusion, headaches and nausea. ECT should only be given as a last resort.

Complementary therapies

These therapies can be helpful for emotional problems because the emphasis is on you as a whole person – mind, body and spirit. Treatments such as aromatherapy, **massage** or **acupuncture** can be pleasant and relaxing. Some people find meditation, yoga or spiritual healing helpful. A complementary practitioner will spend time talking to you about how you are feeling, and many people find this therapeutic in itself.

These treatments can be used alongside orthodox medical treatments, but you should tell your doctor about them.

Self-help and support groups

Self-help groups are especially helpful for people who have a particular problem shared by members of a group. Finding somebody you can talk to – a friend or family member or someone from a support group – can help you to overcome your problems. Contact your local branch of Mind, or another voluntary organization or group that focuses on your specific problem, such as Cruse for bereavement.

IMPROVING YOUR MENTAL HEALTH

Many factors that affect mental health are beyond our control, but there are strategies you can adopt to improve your mental health.

- Recognize your triggers. Certain events or situations can be difficult. If you identify them, you can either avoid them or learn strategies to deal with them and their effect on you.
- Get support. There are many local support groups for different types of mental distress at which sufferers, relatives and friends can share experiences and strategies for coping with and understanding situations that may arise.
- Learn to relax. There are many books and tapes available. Yoga, meditation, massage and aromatherapy can all help.
- Look after yourself physically. Follow a healthy diet, get plenty of sleep and take regular exercise: physical well-being affects mental health.
- Learn to express your feelings openly. Allow yourself to get angry, to cry or shout if you are upset. Letting feelings out in this way can reduce the buildup of stress and tension inside.
- Face up to problems and make changes if they are needed. Don't ignore problems and hope they will go away.

HOW OTHERS CAN HELP

Mental health problems are difficult for carers, family and friends to cope with as well as for the individual concerned. There may be marked changes in the person's behaviour, such as social withdrawal or aggression, which can be difficult to deal with. The way that others help and respond to the situation can be very important in the person's recovery.

- Be sensitive and reassuring. The person may be frightened and need someone he or she can trust and open up to.
- Don't judge. The person needs support and acceptance, and not to be told 'pull yourself together'.
- Encourage the person to discuss his or her feelings, and to work out an effective strategy for managing them.
- Encourage the person to get help. Investigate support groups where feelings and experiences can be shared with others.
- Get some support for yourself – from family members, support groups or carers' groups. And make sure you have some time for yourself.

Mental retardation

Mental retardation is a very general term that can be applied to a wide range of intellectual disabilities. In the UK, the term '**learning difficulties**' is now in more general use, and mental retardation is no longer recognized as a specific medical condition. But the term is still used to identify people who have learning difficulties that result from a general disability rather than a specific problem.

In the USA, the term is more commonly used, and is defined by three criteria:

■ an IQ below 75;
■ significant limitations in two or more of the following areas – communication, self-care, home living, social skills, leisure, self-direction, and basic skills such as reading and writing;
■ a condition that is present from childhood.

About 3 per cent of the population in the USA is estimated to be mentally retarded. Equivalent statistics are not available in the UK, because mental retardation is included in the statistics for learning difficulties, but the percentage is likely to be similar.

CAUSES

Mental retardation has a number of possible causes, ranging from genetic diseases and problems during pregnancy or birth to childhood diseases, accidents and poisoning.

■ Genetic – more than 500 genetic diseases are associated with mental retardation. The most common are **Down's syndrome**, (a chromosome disorder) and **Fragile X syndrome**.
■ Problems during pregnancy – malnutrition and use of alcohol (leading to fetal alcohol syndrome) or drugs by the pregnant mother. Other risks include maternal illnesses during pregnancy, such as toxoplasmosis, **rubella**, **HIV** (human immunodeficiency virus), **cytomegalovirus** and syphilis (see also **Pregnancy and problems**).
■ Problems at birth – lack of oxygen to the infant's brain during delivery is now rare, thanks to improved obstetric care. But low birth weight and prematurity are still associated with mental retardation (see **Birth and problems**).
■ Problems after birth – childhood diseases such as **whooping cough**, **chickenpox**, **measles** and **meningitis** can damage the brain, as can accidents such as a blow to the head or near-drowning. Lead, mercury and other environmental toxins may cause irreparable damage to the brain and nervous system.

DIAGNOSIS

Children are diagnosed using a standardized IQ test. Their ability to reason, to respond emotionally and to carry out general skills are also assessed.

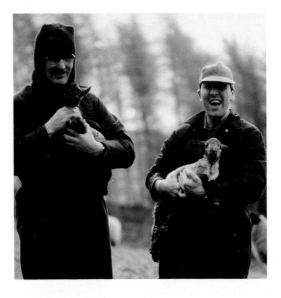

◄ Working life
Community care schemes can provide the training and support necessary for people with learning difficulties to develop to their maximum potential and lead fulfilling lives.

PREVENTION

■ Taking folic acid supplements before and in the early months of pregnancy reduces the risk of neural tube defects.
■ Screening in early pregnancy gives parents the option of terminating a pregnancy that will result in a mentally retarded child (see **Pregnancy, termination of**).
■ Screening of newborn babies can pick up treatable diseases such as **phenylketonuria** (PKU) and congenital hypothyroidism, which are known to cause mental retardation. This allows prompt intervention. In the case of PKU, this involves ensuring an appropriate diet, while congenital hypothyroidism is treated with the thyroid hormone thyroxine (see also **Congenital disorders**).
■ Childhood vaccination (against measles, mumps and rubella, for example) prevents diseases that may cause brain damage (see **Immunization**).

OUTLOOK

Children with mental retardation who are at the higher end of the IQ range are slower than average in learning new information and skills, but their mental retardation may not be identified until they enter school. As adults, many are able to lead independent lives in the community, to work, marry and bring up families.

People in the middle IQ range (that is, with a score of 50–65) may need special schooling. Some may later work in intellectually undemanding jobs and be able to look after themselves within a supportive community.

In the lower IQ range, people are likely to need help with day-to-day living, and those with an IQ beneath about 20 require constant supervision.

SEE ALSO *Disability; Learning difficulties*

Mercury poisoning

Mercury is a silvery metal that becomes liquid at room temperature. Breathing in its vapour, swallowing or simply touching it can cause harm. In high doses, it causes acute mercury poisoning, also known as mercurialism, and kidney damage. Symptoms include vomiting, abdominal pain and diarrhoea with bleeding. Prolonged low-dose exposure to mercury results in chronic poisoning, characterized by mouth ulcers, gum inflammation, anaemia and loose teeth. There may also be abdominal disturbances, kidney disorders, tremors, mental disturbances and balance problems. For example, pregnant women are advised not to have amalgam fillings because of concerns about the toxic nature of mercury.

Mercury is rarely used nowadays because it is so poisonous. Treatment of accidental exposure is with a drug called dimercaprol.

Mesenteric adenitis

Mesenteric adenitis is an inflammation of lymph nodes in the mesentery, the inner membraneous lining of the abdominal wall. The cause is often an infection by the bacterium *Yersinia enterocolitica*, carried to the mesentery from the intestines by the **lymphatic system**. It is more common in children than adults.

The symptoms are very similar to those of **appendicitis**. They may appear suddenly or develop slowly, and include pain in the lower right abdomen, sometimes with fever, diarrhoea, tiredness, loss of appetite, nausea and vomiting. Treatment by antibiotics is usually successful, but sometimes a surgical investigation – a **laparotomy** – is needed to rule out appendicitis.

Metabolism and disorders

The term 'metabolism' covers all the chemical reactions within our bodies that are necessary for life. It includes the digestion, absorption and elimination of food, respiration, circulation, temperature regulation and all the processes by which our bodies generate and use energy.

Metabolism involves two phases, known as anabolism and catabolism. In anabolic processes, the body builds up complex substances from simpler ones. For example, the simple blood sugar glucose is converted into glycogen and fat under the direction of insulin. In catabolic processes, complex substances are broken down into simpler ones, releasing energy. For example, glucose is broken down to produce energy together with carbon dioxide and water. Our bodies are constantly breaking down and building up molecules at an incredible rate.

THE METABOLIC RATE

The rate at which the body uses energy, and produces heat, is known as the metabolic rate. The energy you expend at rest when you have not eaten for 12 hours and are mentally and physically relaxed is known as the basal metabolic rate (BMR). This indicates the rate at which the body needs to produce energy simply to keep you alive.

Metabolic rate is controlled by a number of different hormones, which regulate the speed at which chemical processes take place within the cells of the body. The most important of these hormones, in regulating and determining the basal metabolic, rate is the thyroid hormone thyroxine.

Body temperature and metabolic rate tend to rise and fall together. A fever caused by an infection, for example, raises the metabolic rate. Stress is another factor that can trigger a rise in someone's metabolic rate, by stimulating the breakdown of fat for energy. However, the biggest rises in metabolic rate are triggered by exercise. Even a slight increase in the work that muscles do can speed up the metabolic rate, which is why regular exercise will help to maintain a healthy weight. Conversely, fasting or severe limitation on the intake of food slows down the metabolic rate, leading to a slower breakdown of body reserves such as fat. The body wants to keep its precious stores of energy, so it preserves any stored fat by lowering its metabolic rate whenever its food intake is greatly reduced. This is the reason why very low-calorie diets are often counterproductive.

Metabolic rate gradually declines with age, as a result of muscle and bone wasting, together with reduced hormonal action.

Diet and the metabolism

Throughout life the food we eat is vital to provide our bodies with the raw materials needed for efficient metabolism. A nutritionally poor diet that is lacking in proteins, carbohydrates and fats, over- or undereating, heavy drinking and certain drugs can all upset the metabolism.

WHAT CAN GO WRONG

Metabolic disorders include a large number of conditions in which different aspects of the body's internal chemistry have been disturbed in some way. They include several relatively rare, inherited disorders known as inborn errors of metabolism. These are caused by an error in a gene that affects a particular enzyme

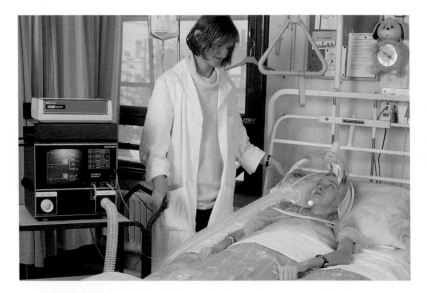

Your metabolic rate can be measured by monitoring how much oxygen and carbon dioxide you breathe out – the amount of oxygen your body consumes at rest can then be calculated.

needed for the metabolism of a certain substance. Examples of these disorders include **cystic fibrosis, phenylketonuria** and **porphyrias**.

The accumulation of a substance that the body is unable to metabolize can cause a variety of symptoms, depending on the nature of the fault. Some of these substances can lead to severe developmental delay if they are not controlled. These disorders include carbohydrate metabolic disorders such as galactosaemia, which is caused by a missing liver enzyme that is needed to convert lactose, or milk sugar, into glucose; lipid metabolic disorders, including hyperlipidaemia, which lead to the accumulation of high levels of fats in the blood; or mineral metabolic disorders such as hypercalcaemia, in which abnormally high levels of calcium build up in the blood.

Treatment often involves changes to a person's diet, which again are determined by the particular metabolic fault. Children suffering from these disorders are usually closely monitored by a dietitian.

Metabolic and endocrine disorders are closely intertwined, because of the crucial effect hormones have on the metabolism (see **Endocrine system and disorders**). Among the metabolic disorders that result from the deficient or excessive production of a hormone are Cushing's syndrome, **diabetes** mellitus, hypothyroidism and hyperthyroidism (see **Thyroid and problems**) and insulinoma, caused by a rare benign (non-cancerous) pancreatic tumour (see **Pancreas and problems**).

Treating metabolic disorders

Currently, many metabolic disorders are treated by changes to the person's diet. A clinical nutritionist will devise a diet plan that is specific to a particular disorder. In addition, a patient may be prescribed daily medication.

Research is also investigating gene therapy, which involves inserting copies of a normal gene into the body. This offers the potential of permanently correcting any faulty genetic mechanism, which would allow sufferers to enjoy a normal diet and lifestyle.
SEE ALSO *Nutritional disorders*

Metastasis

Metastasis is the process by which cells from a malignant tumour spread to other parts of the body. This occurs by three main routes: the cells grow out and invade nearby tissues in other body cavities; the cells break off and travel through the bloodstream; or the cells break off and make their way through the body via the lymphatic system.

A metastasis also describes the new tumour that has formed away from the original, or primary, site. It may be abbreviated to a 'met', and is often described as a secondary tumour.
SEE ALSO *Cancer*

Metatarsalgia

Metatarsalgia is a pain in the foot originating in one or more of the five metatarsal bones that make up the middle section of the foot, between the heel and the base of the toes. It may be caused by fracture of a metatarsal bone, from increased pressure as a result of **fallen arches** and flat feet, or from pressing on a neuroma – a benign tumour on a nerve within the foot.
SEE ALSO *Foot and problems*

Microencephaly

Microencephaly is a condition in which a person has a very small brain, typically less than half the normal size. It is usually associated with severe **mental retardation**. Some cases of microencephaly are due to a genetic fault that prevents the growth of the upper part of a baby's head during pregnancy. Babies born with this condition have a characteristic appearance: the lower part of the face is normal but the forehead and skull are shrunken and pointed. Other cases are usually due to developmental problems in pregnancy caused by a disease in the mother such as German measles. Sometimes a baby is born with a normal brain that then fails to mature as a result of brain injury or disease in infancy.

Migraine

Migraine is characterized by severe disabling headaches. Some migraines are heralded by an aura of flashing lights or zigzags; other symptoms are nausea, vomiting and increased sensitivity to light and sound.

Migraine has three components – severe headache, nausea and sickness, and an increasing discomfort with light and sound. An attack typically begins with a feeling of general illness and irritability. Patients then often describe seeing flashes of light or silvery zigzag lines that move across their field of view. This is known as an aura, and it can last for between 10 minutes and a half hour before a severe headache starts. About one-third of migraine sufferers experience auras which are thought to be caused by a wave of increased activity of brain cells. The visual disturbances move across the field of vision and there may also be a sensation of tingling or numbness that is usually one-sided.

A migraine sufferer will want to be in a quiet, dark room and sleep during the headache phase of the attack. The throbbing pain usually occurs over the front part of the head, but may also affect the back. It often improves after vomiting.

▼ Migraine alert
You may be warned of an impending attack by a visual blind spot, flashing lights, zigzag patterns in front of your eyes and a dislike of bright light.

There is often a family history of migraine, suggesting a genetic element to the condition. It is more common among women than men, with about 20 per cent of women compared with 6 per cent of men experiencing migraine in their lifetime. Migraine attacks in women may be affected by their periods. Other trigger factors include some foods – particularly the four 'Cs': chocolate, cheese, caffeine and citrus – and **stress**. Attacks caused by stress tend to occur after, rather than during, the stressful event. Another factor may be changes in sleep pattern such as shift work or sleeping longer at the weekend.

DEALING WITH MIGRAINE

Many migraines are triggered by specific factors and if you can identify these triggers, it makes sense to avoid them. Try monitoring your diet and keep a diary of your attacks. Some women find that changing their **contraceptive** pill helps, as hormones can influence the attacks.

A drop in the body's level of blood sugar may bring on an attack, so it is a good idea to eat regular and fairly frequent light meals and avoid going without food for more than twelve hours. It will also help to drink plenty of water. People who experience a warning aura can sometimes prevent the headache by sucking a barley sugar or eating a spoonful of honey.

Avoid painkillers that contain codeine and caffeine as these can cause rebound headaches and may increase the number of headaches suffered. Aspirin, ibuprofen or paracetamol are better for pain relief. Antisickness medicine may help to relieve nausea and absorb painkillers.

People who have frequent attacks can take ongoing preventive medication, such as low-dose antidepressants and specific migraine therapies such as pizotifen. Sumatriptan drugs such as Imigran can be prescribed for acute attacks.
SEE ALSO *Headache*

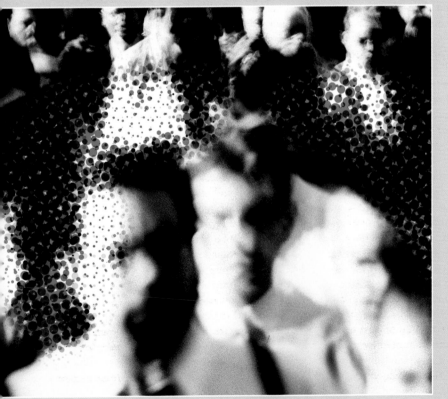

Miscarriage

A miscarriage is the premature end of a pregnancy before 24 weeks' gestation. If a pregnancy fails after 24 weeks it is known as a stillbirth. Miscarriages are quite common – more than one in four pregnancies ends in this way. But most women who have a miscarriage will have no trouble in carrying their next baby to term – only one woman in 36 has two miscarriages in a row. Nevertheless, the impact of a miscarriage can be devastating, and women may feel a sense of bereavement and of guilt. The first step towards recovery can be to discuss your feelings with someone who is close to you.

SYMPTOMS

Seek medical help at once if you are pregnant and have vaginal bleeding or cramps, or if your waters break (see **Pregnancy and problems**).

CAUSES

In most cases the cause of miscarriage is not known. Triggers include infections such as **listeria**, **salmonella**, toxoplasmosis and **rubella** and low levels of certain pregnancy hormones. Other possible triggers include immune system problems that make the mother's body reject the fetus and prolonged exposure to gases used in general **anaesthetic**.

RISK FACTORS

In most early miscarriages (occurring in pregnancies of up to about 14 weeks' gestation), the embryo or fetus is expelled because it has a serious abnormality. One in four late miscarriages (between 14 and 24 weeks' gestation) is associated with cervical incompetence, when the **cervix** begins to open (dilate) before time. This usually occurs because the muscle in the cervix is weak and the pressure of the growing baby makes it give way. The condition can be caused by previous surgery, such as a cone **biopsy** to treat precancerous cells, or by having several terminations.

Other risk factors include having had multiple pregnancies and drug abuse. Vitamin C deficiency appears to be a factor in some cases. But there is no evidence that using computer monitors increases the risk of miscarriage as is sometimes thought.

TREATMENT

If the embryo or fetus is not completely expelled, you may need a surgical operation called a D&C – dilatation (expansion) of the cervix and curettage (scraping) of the uterus. If an infection then occurs, antibiotics will be prescribed.

SEE ALSO *Ectopic pregnancy; Pregnancy and problems*

If you have recently had a miscarriage, it is sensible to avoid strenuous physical exercise in the first 12 weeks of your next pregnancy

MMR vaccine

The MMR vaccine is a combination vaccine against the viral diseases of **measles, mumps** and **rubella** (German measles). MMR is given to children at 13 months and again before they reach five years. MMR contains live organisms and may cause mild side effects, such as slight fever, a rash and a mild form of mumps.

Children who catch measles, mumps or rubella can suffer complications, such as **convulsions, meningitis** and **encephalitis,** which can be fatal. These complications can also occur after an MMR vaccination, but the risk is greatly reduced. Reports of a link between the MMR vaccine and autism and bowel disease have been discounted by the World Health Organization after studies carried out in several countries.

SEE ALSO *Immunization*

Motion sickness

Motion sickness is the nausea and vomiting experienced by many people, particularly children, when travelling. It occurs when the vehicle's movement temporarily upsets the relationship between what the eyes see and the balance mechanism of the inner ear. The eyes adjust to the movement, while the inner ear does not, and the brain receives conflicting messages.

SYMPTOMS

Motion sickness may produce a range of symptoms including:
- rapid breathing, sweating and feeling faint;
- nausea and vomiting;
- loss of appetite;
- pale or greenish complexion and diarrhoea;
- slight abdominal pain.

TREATMENT

There are many simple self-help remedies.
- Try over-the-counter antisickness medicines. These may cause drowsiness, so experiment to find a remedy that works.
- Eat a light snack an hour before travelling.
- Drink small amounts of cool water regularly to prevent dehydration.
- Fresh air and exercise help. Make regular stops on a car journey. If at sea, go out on deck.
- If symptoms are severe, lie down with eyes closed, keeping the head still.

Complementary therapies
- There is evidence that ginger tea, a herbal remedy, dissipates nausea.
- **Acupressure** devices that apply pressure to a point above the wrist help some people.

When to consult a doctor

See a doctor if there is severe abdominal pain and vomiting.

Motor neurone disease

The term 'motor neurone disease' covers a group of progressive conditions that cause degeneration of the motor nerves. These nerves carry messages from the brain to the muscles, and their degeneration causes muscle weakness, twitching and other problems. Motor neurone disease affects about 5000 people in the UK, most over the age of 40. The condition is most common in people aged 50–70, and slightly more men are affected than women. About 1000 new cases are diagnosed each year, and as there are a similar number of deaths from the condition, the overall rate of motor neurone disease remains the same. The cause is not known. The condition is not infectious – it does not spread from person to person.

In most cases, the disease has no apparent cause and there is no link to a family history of motor neurone disease. But in 5–10 per cent of cases, there is a family history of the disease, which suggests an inherited genetic factor. Scientists are still researching this genetic link. One very rare form of motor neurone disease can develop in children.

The most common form of motor neurone disease is called amyotrophic lateral sclerosis. This form affects both the upper motor neurones, which carry messages from the brain to the spinal cord, and the lower motor neurones, which carry messages from the spinal cord to the muscles. Amyotrophic lateral sclerosis accounts for 8 out of 10 cases of motor neurone disease.

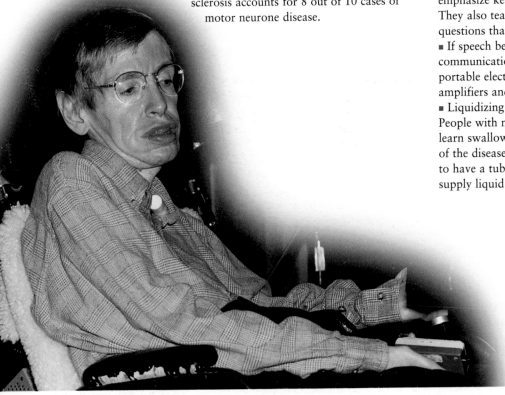

SYMPTOMS

The symptoms of motor neurone disease depend on which motor neurones are affected and how the condition progresses, so there is a great deal of variation between individuals. Common symptoms include:

- muscle weakness;
- cramps, stiffness and twitching;
- gradual wasting of the muscles;
- problems with speech, chewing and swallowing;
- feeling profoundly tired.

It is often difficult for doctors to distinguish the early stages of the disease from the very many other conditions that also produce fatigue and muscle weakness. There is no specific test for motor neurone disease. Diagnosis is usually made by a neurologist and is based on the symptoms, a physical examination and neurological tests. The neurologist will usually order blood tests, X-rays and a magnetic resonance imaging (MRI) scan.

TREATMENT

Doctors focus treatment on relieving symptoms, and so making people with the disease as comfortable as possible.

- Muscle relaxants and **physiotherapy** help to relieve cramps and boost muscle function.
- Painkilling drugs relieve discomfort.
- If speech is affected, speech therapy can relieve the distress caused by the inability to communicate. For example, speech therapists coach people with motor neurone disease to emphasize key words and speak more slowly. They also teach carers and relatives to ask questions that demand short responses.
- If speech becomes impossible, many communication aids are available, including portable electronic devices such as voice amplifiers and speech synthesizers.
- Liquidizing food can make swallowing easier. People with motor neurone disease can also learn swallowing techniques. In the later stages of the disease, people with the disease may need to have a tube inserted into the stomach to supply liquid nutrition. This greatly reduces the

◀ **A great mind**
Motor neurone disease does not affect the intellect. Astrophysicist Stephen Hawking was diagnosed with the disease at the age of 21, but became one of the leading scientists of his generation.

Case study

Maintaining communication

Susan developed a rare form of motor neurone disease in her mid-50s when she was working as a teacher. She has now had the disease for three years and uses a speech synthesizer.

The first problem Susan had was with clearing her throat, but soon afterwards she found that she had trouble making herself understood in the classroom. Then she began to laugh or cry for no reason and without feeling emotional. She was diagnosed with progressive bulbar palsy. This is a rare form of motor neurone disease that affects the muscles of the face, throat and tongue as well as the part of the brainstem that governs physical expressions of emotion such as crying and laughing.

Susan retired from her job. She found physiotherapy and speech therapy a great help with breathing and swallowing as well as with speaking. But eventually she needed a speech synthesizer. With this, she was able to chat to her former pupils when she visited for their leaving play at the end of the summer term.

risk of lung infections, which can occur if food gets into the lungs as a result of choking when food is swallowed.

■ Physiotherapy can be helpful for those with motor neurone disease who find it difficult to breathe and cough as well as to improve muscle function (see above). People are taught to improve their seated posture and to use breathing exercises. Other options include ventilation through a mask or through a tube attached to a ventilator machine.

■ Riluzole (Rilutek) is the only drug currently licensed in the UK aimed at treating or preventing the nerve damage that occurs in the disease. Your doctor will refer you to a specialist in the management of the disease before prescribing it. Riluzole works by inhibiting the release of glutamate, a nerve transmitter that excites motor neurone cells. Excessive stimulation of glutamate receptors is thought to play a role in the destruction of motor neurones in motor neurone disease. Rilutek does not cure motor neurone disease, but may help people with the disease to live longer. Rilutek usually has no side effects, but some people have skin rashes and feel tired.

Complementary therapies

Some people find relaxation and visualization techniques helpful in relieving the symptoms of motor neurone disease and improving their overall well-being. Aromatherapy and massage may also prove soothing and relaxing.

Living with motor neurone disease

A range of specialist medical, nursing, therapy and social support services may be available. If you or a friend or relative are diagnosed with motor neurone disease, ask your doctor for help in developing a plan of action to combine and make the most of these services.

Contact the Motor Neurone Disease Association for advice. The Association loans equipment to those who have been diagnosed with the disease – including electric riser/recliner armchairs, rotating car seats and portable pumps to remove excess mouth saliva. If your health worker or social worker agrees you need this or similar equipment, the Association may also be able to award a grant to help you to buy it.

Motor neurone disease is a serious progressive illness and people with the condition may experience considerable psychological and emotional distress. They may understandably become frightened, anxious and depressed by the onset of worrying symptoms and fears about becoming a burden. They often want to talk about their fears and, if family and carers find this difficult, a counsellor or psychological therapist can help. Antidepressant drugs may also be helpful.

As people reach the end of their life, they may want to put their affairs in order and talk about what will happen to their family after they are gone. This is upsetting for everyone, but many hospitals have palliative care teams of doctors, nurses and others who can help and support families through this difficult time.

OUTLOOK

There is no cure for motor neurone disease. Most of those affected survive for two to five years, but some sufferers live for ten years or even longer after diagnosis. The English physicist and bestselling author Stephen Hawking has lived with amyotrophic lateral sclerosis for more than 35 years.

Research is underway into potential new treatments for the disease. Researchers are investigating the importance of glutamate and other neurotransmitters to the progress of motor nerve damage and they are developing nerve growth factors that may help motor neurones become more resistant to degeneration. They are also testing the effects of antioxidants, such as vitamin E, in preventing nerve damage.

SEE ALSO *Brain and nervous system; Disability*

Mouth and disorders

The primary purpose of the mouth is to provide a route of entry for food into the body and to carry out the first stage of digestion. It also plays an important role in vocal communication and speech and contributes to facial appearance and recognition. The mouth is surrounded by muscles, and it is the enormously varied movements of these that enable us to express such a range of emotional expressions.

The mouth is roofed by the hard palate, which separates the mouth from the cavity of the nose. The tongue, which provides taste sensation and aids chewing, swallowing and speech, is attached to the soft floor of the mouth. At the front, the teeth are set in the gums and anchored into the upper and lower jawbones, which provide chewing and grinding motions. At the back of the mouth, the throat is the entranceway to the oesophagus, leading to the stomach. On either side are the masses of lymphoid tissue that form the **tonsils**. The inside of the mouth is lined with mucous membrane, which is kept moist by constant secretion of saliva from the salivary glands, to aid chewing, swallowing and digestion of food.

The salivary glands

The mouth contains three pairs of salivary glands, which secrete saliva. This is an alkaline fluid that softens food, moistens the mouth and helps swallowing. Saliva also contains an enzyme called salivary amylase, which begins the process of digesting the starch we eat.

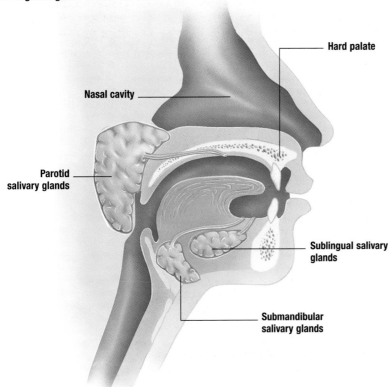

Hard palate

Nasal cavity

Parotid salivary glands

Sublingual salivary glands

Submandibular salivary glands

A HEALTHY MOUTH

A healthy mouth has a glistening, moist surface with a clean, pink tongue, and gums and teeth that are free from disease and decay. The best way to maintain the health of the mouth is to eat a balanced diet and to ensure good dental hygiene, which involves thoroughly cleaning the teeth twice a day and making regular visits to a dentist. (See also **Dentists and dentistry.**)

SYMPTOMS

Symptoms may indicate a local problem (in the mouth) or a disorder elsewhere in the body.

Thirst

Abnormal thirst may be due to:
- reduced fluid intake;
- excess salt consumption;
- increased fluid loss, due to fever, sweating or diarrhoea;
- lack of normal saliva flow;
- **diabetes;**
- **kidney** failure.

Increased salivation

An increase in saliva production may be due to:
- irritations in the mouth, such as stomatitis, teething in babies or ill-fitting dentures;
- nausea;
- infection;
- rarely, poisoning.

Taste disturbances

Loss of taste is most often caused by an obstruction in the nose – including having a cold. An obstruction may cause a loss of the ability to detect more subtle flavours, which depend on the sense of smell. But they leave intact the capacity to detect strong tastes of sweetness, bitterness, sourness and saltiness, which are sensed on the **tongue.**

Heavy smoking or nervous system problems may also cause loss of taste.

Difficulty in speaking, chewing or swallowing

This may be due to a dry mouth, dental problems or any source of pain or discomfort in the mouth. Very rarely, it is due to neurological conditions.

Soreness or pain

Pain tends to occur especially on eating, or when taking very hot or cold food and drinks. It is most often due to dental disease; other causes include ulcers, inflammation and infection.

Swelling or lumps

A swelling in the mouth may be due to a salivary gland problem, infection, a dental abscess or ill-fitting dentures. Lumps may be caused by an abscess or by tumours.

COMMON PROBLEMS IN THE MOUTH

The most common condition affecting the mouth is dental disease (see Gums and gum disease; Teeth and problems). Another common problem is halitosis, which is also known as bad breath. This is usually due to recently eaten food that is strongly flavoured, poor dental hygiene or stomach problems. Other causes include breathing through the mouth rather through the nose, throat infections, sinusitis or lung infection. The mouth is also affected by a wide range of other problems.

Mouth ulcers

Ulcers are tiny white or red spots, appearing singly or in groups. They are painful and may cause discomfort when eating. Ulcers are extremely common, especially on the tongue, but can occur anywhere in the mouth. The cause is unknown but they often appear during times of stress and are made worse by emotional tension. There may be some hereditary component – a tendency to ulcers runs in families. Hormones also play a part – ulcers often appear first at puberty, may tend to occur with menstrual periods and usually disappear in pregnancy.

Ulcers usually clear up without treatment and within a few days. An ulcer that does not go away may signal an infection, Crohn's disease or cancer.

Candida infection

The mouth is susceptible to infection by the fungus Candida albicans, which causes soft white patches and soreness on the palate, tongue or inside of the cheeks. It often follows antibiotic treatment, or may occur in people with immune system deficiencies or **diabetes**. Treatment is with an antifungal drug. (See also **Candida**.)

Dry mouth

A dry mouth is usually due to reduced saliva flow (see **Salivary glands and disorders**). It also occurs with mouth-breathing due to nasal obstruction and as an acute reaction to fear. It can lead to secondary symptoms, such as speech problems, difficulty swallowing and sore throat. When persistent, it can contribute to gum disease and dental caries (decay).

TREATMENT

Treatment varies depending on the cause. Seek medical advice if you have any of the following:
■ any lump or swelling in the mouth or on the face or jaw;
■ difficulty in eating or swallowing, or a mouth ulcer that persists for more than 14 days or is accompanied by ulcers or blisters on the skin or other bodily symptoms;
■ any unusual bleeding, especially from an ulcer or lump;
■ signs of candida infection.

SEE ALSO *Face and problems; Nutritional disorders; Speech disorders; Throat and problems; Tonsils and disorders; Tongue and problems*

Mucus and mucous membranes

The mucous membranes are the moist pink membranes that line most of the body's cavities and hollow organs, including the mouth, nose, digestive tract, eyelids and vagina. The moistness comes from a slimy jellylike substance called mucus, which is secreted by goblet cells embedded within the membrane.

Mucus is made up of water, various salts and a protein called mucin, which gives it stickiness. It has protective and lubricating functions.
■ It stops acids and enzymes from dissolving the walls of the stomach and intestines.
■ In the respiratory system, it traps matter such as smoke, which would irritate the lungs.
■ It lubricates the oesophagus, making swallowing easier.
■ It helps with the passage of bowel contents.
■ During the reproductive years, a woman's vagina is moistened by mucus, which facilitates sexual intercourse.

DISORDERS

Ulcers form when the mucous membrane is broken, as a result of infection, injury or irritants such as smoke. Mouth ulcers are a common type: they usually clear up quickly with simple treatment. More serious are ulcers occurring lower down the digestive tract. If the stomach and duodenum are infected with the bacterium Helicobacter pylori stomach acid can break through the mucous membrane. This may cause an ulcer to form in the wall of the stomach or duodenum. Aspirin blocks mucus secretion in the stomach, and long-term use of this or related drugs can lead to stomach bleeding in those susceptible. New drugs – known as the superaspirins or COX-2 inhibitors – do not affect mucus secretion and so are kinder on the stomach.

In ulcerative colitis, the large intestine becomes extensively ulcerated and inflamed. The affected section of intestine has to be surgically removed in severe cases, and sufferers can run an increased risk of bowel **cancer**.

After the **menopause**, a decrease in mucus secretion and thinning of the vaginal walls can lead to painful intercourse in around 20 per cent of women.

Mucus can become infected – as in many upper-respiratory infections. This is a particular danger among people with **cystic fibrosis**, who have a genetic defect that results in production of abnormally sticky mucus. This becomes infected very easily, and daily physiotherapy is needed to remove mucus secretions from the lungs to prevent infection.

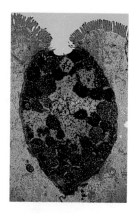

▲ **Goblet cells**
Goblet cells line the small intestine and secrete mucus (in dark blue here), which protects the lining of the intestine. Projections called microvilli (in green here) increase the surface area of the intestine, thus allowing more nutrients to be absorbed.

Multiple sclerosis

People with multiple sclerosis can develop severe problems with movement, sight and other functions. Their condition is caused by damage to the sheath of tissue that protects nerve fibres in the central nervous system.

Multiple sclerosis affects approximately 85,000 people in the UK and is usually diagnosed when people are in their late 20s or early 30s. It affects more women than men and is more common in temperate, northern European countries than in hotter places. Despite its disabling effects, MS does not usually have any significant impact on life expectancy.

The symptoms vary greatly from one patient to another. They may start with numbness, tingling or muscle weakness, and later affect many bodily functions, causing one or more of the following: blurred or double vision; loss of balance and coordination; movement problems; speech difficulties; overwhelming fatigue; loss of bladder and/or bowel control; loss of sexual function; increased sensitivity to heat; and psychological problems such as confusion and forgetfulness. Dealing with such a disabling condition makes some people anxious and depressed.

The early symptoms of multiple sclerosis may be vague and perhaps last only a few days, so that it can often take some time to make a firm diagnosis. A specialist will take a detailed medical history to help identify previous symptoms and will carry out a number of neurological tests, including a magnetic resonance imaging (MRI) scan to look for inflammation and damaged nerves. Multiple sclerosis will only usually be diagnosed after a person has experienced two or more episodes of the symptoms associated with the condition and if evidence of nerve damage shows up on an MRI scan.

TYPES OF MULTIPLE SCLEROSIS

There are four types of multiple sclerosis and each develops in different ways.

People with benign multiple sclerosis have a small number of mild attacks, but are not permanently disabled. This type accounts for about 20 per cent of cases.

People with relapsing – remitting multiple sclerosis suffer attacks that last at least 24–48 hours and are then followed by complete or partial recovery over a few weeks. The attacks recur but do not grow worse each time. Relapsing – remitting multiple sclerosis accounts for about 25 per cent of cases.

In people with primary progressive multiple sclerosis, the symptoms and disability grow progressively worse. The sufferers occasionally reach a plateau on which symptoms and disability no longer worsen but they have no chance of permanent recovery. Primary progressive multiple sclerosis accounts for about 15 per cent of cases.

The fourth type, secondary progressive multiple sclerosis, at first produces intermittent attacks that do not grow worse (similar to relapsing – remitting multiple sclerosis). But after the initial period, the attacks become more serious. People with secondary progressive disease occasionally enjoy periods of remission in which symptoms ease, but these are few. This type accounts for about 40 per cent of cases.

LIVING WITH MULTIPLE SCLEROSIS

The key to living as full a life as possible with multiple sclerosis is learning to manage your symptoms. Your GP can offer advice on drugs and help you choose the right combination of medical, nursing and other services.

Factfile

Drugs for symptom relief

Your doctor may prescribe the following types of drug to relieve particular symptoms:

- analgesics to relieve pain;

- muscle-relaxing drugs (for example, baclofen, botulinum toxin and tizanidine) to relieve muscle spasms;

- anticholinergic drugs to reduce your production of urine if MS makes you incontinent;

- antidepressants for depression;

- corticosteroids to reduce inflammation in the brain and spinal cord in severe episodes of MS and to shorten the period of relapse. This treatment does not affect the progression of the disease;

- Viagra, injections and vacuum-pump devices for men whose multiple sclerosis leads to erectile dysfunction.

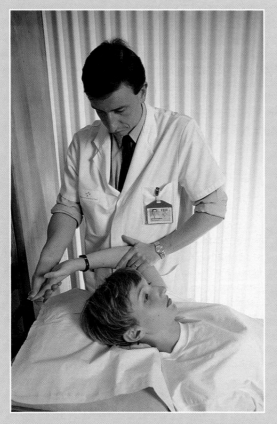

▶ Manipulating muscles
A physiotherapist manipulates an arm that has become temporarily paralysed during an episode of multiple sclerosis. It is important to keep the muscles active during this time to avoid loss of muscle tone.

Being diagnosed with multiple sclerosis can have a heavy emotional impact. Many people feel frustrated or angry as they come to terms with any necessary changes. Psychological therapy and counselling may help. You should try to keep as active as possible – it is important to maintain the function of your nerves and muscles. If you can, take exercise and carry on your normal work routine. Discuss this matter with your GP.

If you are suffering from fatigue, **physiotherapy** and **occupational therapies** can help to improve your movement and make everyday activities easier. A physiotherapist will devise appropriate exercises to help you to strengthen and relax your muscles. An occupational therapist will advise you on planning your daily routine: you may need to set aside periods of rest or arrange for help with some activities. These therapies will also help you to deal with stiffness and spasms.

Some people with multiple sclerosis find water exercises (aquatic therapy) helpful. **Speech** therapy will help if you have trouble speaking. If you are finding it difficult to eat well, seek advice from a dietitian specializing in multiple sclerosis. Small studies have shown that a diet high in polyunsaturated fats (such as those found in sunflower margarine, vegetable oils and fish oils) may help to prevent the progression of multiple sclerosis. The benefits of other supplements are unproven. The Multiple Sclerosis Society runs short courses on managing your symptoms that cover advice on diet and appropriate exercise, techniques to combat frustration and depression and advice on managing fatigue and pain.

Some people find complementary therapies such as aromatherapy, relaxation techniques and massage helpful. Others advocate cannabis to relieve pain and muscle spasms that do not respond to other therapies, but the drug is not legally available in the UK. Studies are currently being undertaken to investigate further the medical benefits of cannabis use, and it is possible that a licensed cannabis drug may soon be available to people with multiple sclerosis.

TREATMENT

A series of studies published between 1993 and 1998 showed that the drug beta interferon could slow down the progression of some forms of MS, notably relapsing-remitting and secondary progressive disease. The studies suggested that beta interferon reduced the incidence of relapses by about one-third and delayed the progression of the disease and any associated disability.

Exactly how beta interferon works remains unclear. It appears to inhibit the activity of T-lymphocytes – white blood cells whose normal function is to fight infection but which in multiple sclerosis sufferers seem to trigger inflammatory reactions around the myelin sheaths of the nerve fibres in the central nervous system.

Further studies of multiple sclerosis sufferers have revealed that a second drug, glatiramer acetate, can also reduce the incidence of relapses as well as delaying the progression of disability by working to limit the activity of T-lymphocytes. In 2000, glatiramer acetate was approved for use in the treatment of multiple sclerosis in the UK.

Both beta intereferon and glatiramer acetate are expensive to prescribe. Also, although treatment with these drugs is effective in some cases, others fail to respond to them. In October 2001, the NHS's advisory body, the National Institute for Clinical Excellence, decided that the drugs should not be prescribed on the NHS because of uncertainty over long-term cost-effectiveness.

However, the four UK health departments subsequently agreed with the drug manufacturers a national 'prescribe and monitor' scheme to provide the drugs at prices that will vary according to their long-term results. The Association of British Neurologists has produced guidelines for prescription. Patients with relapsing-remitting MS are considered for treatment if they can walk independently and have had two attacks in the past three years. Some people with secondary progressive MS are also considered if they are still experiencing relapses.

SEE ALSO *Brain and nervous system; Disability*

Mumps

Mumps is a viral infection that mainly affects children, but can also affect adults. It is much more uncomfortable if contracted by men in their teens or as adults. The virus thrives in the parotid salivary glands, which lie in the cheeks just in front of the ears, hence the swelling in the face that characterizes the disease.

Although all small children can catch mumps, the disease is most common in those over the age of two. Most children are protected against mumps by the **MMR vaccine** (for measles, mumps and rubella).

SYMPTOMS
- Initially, an increasing temperature rising to 40°C/104°F.
- An uncomfortable feeling in the region of the parotid glands before they swell.
- Swelling occurs unevenly, on one side of the face before the other.
- Pain on swallowing.

DURATION
- Mumps has a long incubation period, about three weeks from infection to outbreak.
- In mild cases, the swelling may last only three to four days but it can continue for a week and sometimes longer.

CAUSES
- Mumps is caused by the paramyxo virus, which is spread by airborne droplets from the nose or throat. It is passed from one person to another only by close contact.
- The virus enters the body through the airways, then passes around the body in the bloodstream. It can end up almost everywhere – the kidneys, thyroid gland, sexual glands and salivary gland. But it thrives in the parotid salivary glands.

TREATMENT
- Consult a doctor to confirm diagnosis and if complications develop.
- Apart from staying in bed when the swelling and temperature are at their peak, mumps demands no special attention. The illness can be regarded as a normal part of childhood.

COMPLICATIONS
- The most serious complication is the possible infection of other organs. In up to 30 per cent of adult men with mumps, the disease infects the testicles (a condition known as **orchitis**), causing swelling, pain, soreness and a higher temperature. This often occurs about a week after the disease has broken out and is a serious infection that may cause sterility. However, among the few sexually mature men who contract mumps, only half of them develop orchitis, and of these only 10 per cent are affected in both testicles. Even then, the condition does not necessarily cause sterility, and there is still a chance that fertility may be restored.
- Less common complications include inflammation of the pancreas (pancreatitis, see **Pancreas and disorders**), or of women's ovaries (see **Ovaries and disorders**). The latter does not affect fertility.
- Mumps can also cause **meningitis**, an inflammation of the membranes of the brain or spinal cord that may appear three to ten days after the onset of mumps. Although meningitis is usually a serious disease, when it occurs in connection with mumps, it is generally mild.

PREVENTION
In the UK, MMR vaccination is offered to all children between 12 and 18 months. A second, booster dose is given between the ages of three and five, before the child starts school.

OUTLOOK
After one attack of mumps, people have lifelong immunity to the disease.

SEE ALSO *Salivary glands and disorders*

Munchhausen's syndrome

Munchhausen's syndrome is a psychiatric condition in which people pretend to be ill. They might fake a seizure or abdominal pain, for example, or exaggerate or worsen an existing problem – perhaps by interfering with a wound so it does not heal. Alternatively, they may bring on an illness – for example, by injecting themselves with bacteria to cause an infection. The result is that the person may be given treatment, in the form of tests, hospital care and even surgery, that is not needed. Munchhausen's is also known as hospital-addiction syndrome.

People with Munchhausen's syndrome appear to crave the attention, care and status they receive as patients. It is a serious and disabling mental health problem that has become better understood in recent years.

More men than women suffer from Munchhausen's syndrome. Sufferers may be offered psychiatric help, but are often unwilling to pursue treatment. Occasionally people with Munchhausen's syndrome also suffer from **depression**, which can be treated.

In Munchhausen's syndrome by proxy, an individual makes another person sick. The person suffering from Munchhausen's secures attention and status by being the sick person's carer (usually parent). This is a form of abuse in which children are the usual victims.

SEE ALSO *Mental health and problems*

Muscular system

SEE PAGE 416

Muscular dystrophy

The muscular dystrophies are a group of hereditary diseases in which muscles grow weaker and waste away as their tissue is replaced by fat and connective tissue. The most common and serious form is Duchenne muscular dystrophy, named after Guillaume Duchenne, the French neurologist who first described the condition in 1861.

CAUSES

Duchenne muscular dystrophy affects between one in 3000 and one in 4000 babies, and is almost always restricted to boys. A problem in a particular gene leads to the absence of the protein dystrophin in the muscle cells, which causes the muscles to waste away.

The discovery of the dystrophin gene in 1986 led to the development of a prenatal test for the condition, which can also be used to identify carriers in families who are affected by the disorder.

SYMPTOMS

The symptoms of Duchenne muscular dystrophy become apparent when a child is between the ages of two and four, and are likely to include awkward walking, stumbling and problems with getting up from the floor, running and climbing stairs.

TREATMENT

The condition is incurable, but medication can relieve stiffness of muscles, **physiotherapy** can delay muscular weakening and orthopaedic equipment can assist mobility.

The identification of the dystrophin gene has stimulated research into gene therapy for the condition. This involves using viruses, which are adept at invading cells, and the version of the gene found in people without muscular dystrophy. Technicians remove the disease-causing part of the virus and replace it with the dystrophin gene. The viruses are then used to 'infect' the patient and carry the dystrophin gene into muscle tissue affected by its absence. Clinical trials of this treatment are taking place in the USA and in France.

Another possible treatment being explored for muscular dystrophy is the use of the protein utrophin as a substitute for dystrophin. Researchers are working on methods to stimulate the production of this protein in people with Duchenne muscular dystrophy to compensate for the absence or defective production of dystrophin.

OUTLOOK

Duchenne muscular dystrophy progresses rapidly and most of those affected need to use a wheelchair by the time they reach their teenage years. About one-third show some mental retardation. People with the condition tend to die of respiratory failure before the age of 30.

OTHER FORMS OF MUSCULAR DYSTROPHY

There are several other forms of muscular dystrophy.

- Becker's muscular dystrophy is caused by a different mutation in the dystrophin gene and results in there being too little dystrophin rather than none at all. The disease appears later in life. Symptoms are much less severe.
- People with limb girdle muscular dystrophy develop weak shoulders or hip joints. The problem may appear at any time from childhood to early adulthood. The condition usually progresses slowly, but by early middle age most of those affected are unable to walk. Life expectancy is slightly shortened. Several mutations may be responsible for the condition.
- Facio-scapulo-humeral dystrophy weakens the muscles in the face, shoulders and upper arms. The condition generally becomes apparent in the teenage years. It usually progresses slowly. Although the condition is very rare, it is inherited and is liable to appear in almost every generation of an affected family.

Myelomatosis

Myelomatosis, also known as multiple myeloma, is a cancer that develops from plasma cells in the bone marrow. Plasma cells usually produce immunoglobulins, or antibodies, which fight infection. In myelomatosis, myeloma cells overproduce faulty immunoglobins, which develop in different sites of the marrow and make the patient vulnerable to infection. The abnormal cells take over the marrow and destroy bone tissue, causing pain and fractures. Other symptoms include **anaemia** and lesions on the kidneys.

Myocarditis

Myocarditis is an inflammation of the heart muscle. The cause is often unknown, but it can be the result of an **autoimmune** reaction to viral infection. There may be no symptoms, or there may be breathlessness, chest pain, irregular heartbeat, **palpitations** or **heart failure**. Abnormalities may show up on an ECG.

SEE ALSO *Heart and circulatory system*

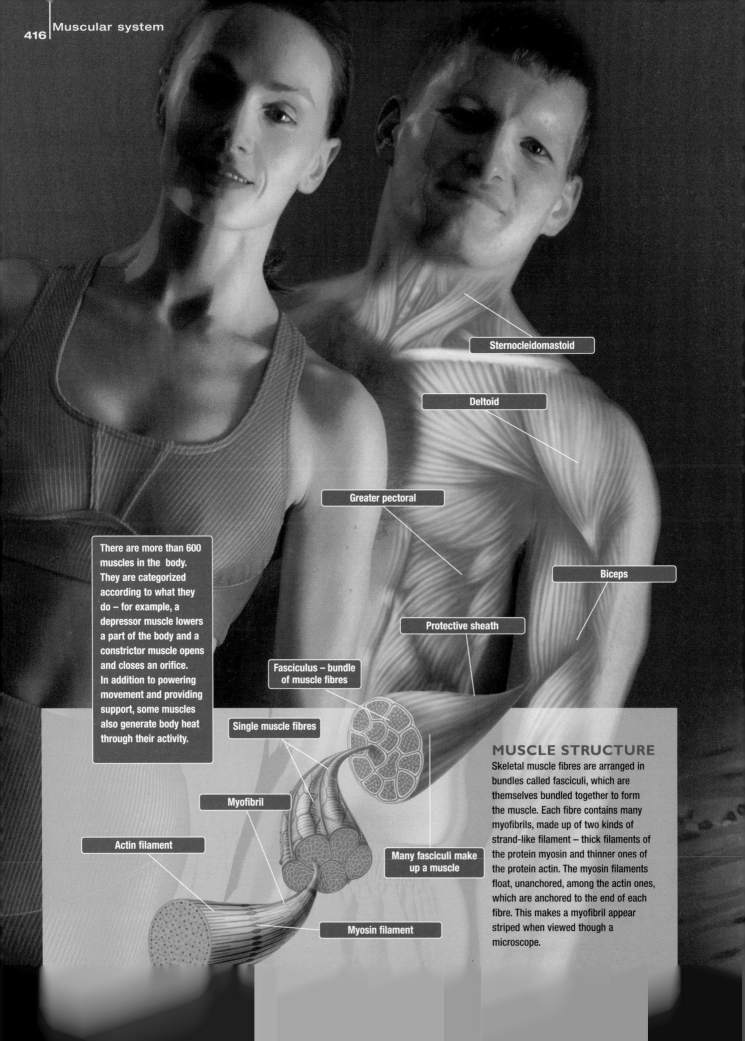

Sternocleidomastoid

Deltoid

Greater pectoral

Biceps

Protective sheath

There are more than 600 muscles in the body. They are categorized according to what they do – for example, a depressor muscle lowers a part of the body and a constrictor muscle opens and closes an orifice. In addition to powering movement and providing support, some muscles also generate body heat through their activity.

Fasciculus – bundle of muscle fibres

Single muscle fibres

Myofibril

Actin filament

Many fasciculi make up a muscle

Myosin filament

MUSCLE STRUCTURE

Skeletal muscle fibres are arranged in bundles called fasciculi, which are themselves bundled together to form the muscle. Each fibre contains many myofibrils, made up of two kinds of strand-like filament – thick filaments of the protein myosin and thinner ones of the protein actin. The myosin filaments float, unanchored, among the actin ones, which are anchored to the end of each fibre. This makes a myofibril appear striped when viewed though a microscope.

Muscular system

Muscles enable the body to move, and they also support the body by maintaining a level of tension that allows us to hold a chosen position – for example, to sit up straight. There are three types of muscle in the body – the skeletal muscles, the smooth muscles and the cardiac muscle. The skeletal muscles are attached to the bones. The cardiac muscle powers the heart. Smooth muscles are found in the walls of blood vessels and many other places, where they contract or relax according to need.

The skeletal muscles are under the conscious or subconscious control of the nervous system. When we use these muscles to move our body, we have made a conscious decision to do so. The work that the skeletal muscles perform in maintaining our posture does not require conscious control, but it does need alertness – this is why you cannot sleep standing up. Neither the cardiac muscle nor the smooth muscles are under this level of control because their work is, by necessity, automatic and continuous. For example, smooth muscles in the wall of the stomach and intestine move food forward though the digestive system without our needing to think about it. Similarly, the cardiac muscle contracts rhythmically, without deliberate effort on our part, for a lifetime – by the time you are 70 it will have relaxed and contracted more than 2.5 billion times.

Smooth muscle, which consists of irregularly grouped fibres, can work for long periods without getting fatigued.

Cell nucleus

Grouped fibres

MUSCLE POWER

The great majority of muscles are skeletal muscles – each has its own nerves that connect it to the spinal cord and brain. Skeletal muscles form the flesh of the body. The fibres in skeletal muscles vary in length depending on the type of muscle from a few millimetres to about 300mm (12in). Smooth muscles that perform involuntary actions are found in the blood and lymph vessels, stomach, intestines, ureters, urinary bladder, gallbladder, womb and Fallopian tubes, trachea, bronchial tubes, the eye's ciliary muscle and iris and the dartos muscle in the scrotum. Cardiac muscle is found in the myocardium, the muscular layer of the heart.

How muscles work

Muscles are controlled by the nervous system. They spring into action when stimulated by nerve impulses.

Most skeletal muscles are connected at both ends to a bone or organ by a tendon. One of the two tendons is normally more rigid than the other. The end of a muscle at which the rigid tendon links it to a bone is known as the origin, while the end where the less rigid, more mobile tendon lies, is known as the point of insertion. When a muscle contracts, the bone at the point of insertion is usually moved towards the origin. For example, the point of insertion of the main calf muscle runs via the Achilles tendon to the heel bone, while the muscle's origin is connected to the two protuberances at the lower end of the thigh-bone. So when this muscle contracts, the heel rises – as when you are walking.

CONTROL AND COORDINATION

Each muscle fibre obeys a law that can best be described as 'all or none'. When a nerve sends an impulse to a muscle fibre to trigger it to contract, the fibre contracts to its full extent – it cannot half-contract. Whether a muscle as a whole contracts strongly or weakly depends on how many fibres are stimulated, not on the strength of the nerve signal.

Although each muscle is supplied by its own nerve or nerves, the brain recognizes groups of muscles rather then individual muscles – the brain does not have a control centre for each individual muscle. This is because all types of movement involve more than one muscle, and most types involve many muscles, which either contract or relax to move a joint or simply maintain tension to stabilize it.

A muscle is said to be the prime mover or agonist when it contracts. When you bend your elbow, the biceps muscle of the upper arm acts as the prime mover. But as the biceps contracts, the triceps, at the back of the arm, relaxes and elongates – muscles relaxing as the triceps does in this instance are known as antagonists. Other muscles, usually small ones, are known as fixators. These surround a moving joint and stabilize it to prevent any unnecessary movements, which allows the desired movement to be controlled and exact – as, for example, when you put your finger on your nose.

Another group of muscles, called synergists, comes into play if a contracting muscle passes over two joints. For example, the biceps passes over both the shoulder and the elbow joint. If movement at the elbow alone is required, the synergists contract to prevent movement at the

shoulder. Any muscle can act as a prime mover, antagonist, fixator or synergist depending on the nature of the movement that is desired.

SLOW-TWITCH AND FAST-TWITCH FIBRES

There are two types of muscle fibre. Red, slow-twitch fibres contract slowly but repeatedly over a long period. White, fast-twitch fibres, contract strongly, tire rapidly and are used for short bursts

Factfile

How muscles contract

Inside each muscle fibre, or cell, is a chemical soup known as the sarcoplasm. Into this are packed, lying parallel to each other, the strands of tissue known as myofibrils, which in turn are made up of two types of protein filament – the thick myosin and thinner actin myofilaments (see page 416).

While a muscle is relaxed, there is some distance between individual myofilaments. When a nerve signal stimulates the muscle, hooks on the myosin filaments catch on to the actin filaments and pull them along. This causes the actin and myosin filaments to slide over each other, so that the muscle shortens and contracts.

In general, muscles are hardly ever fully relaxed. There is usually some degree of contraction. This tension, known as muscle tone, is essential, in order for the body to maintain its posture. A muscle that has little or no tone is described as flaccid, while one that has too much tone is said to be spastic. If a muscle is underused, it will rapidly lose its tone and become flaccid, but if a muscle is used frequently, it may increase in bulk and tension but it will never become spastic.

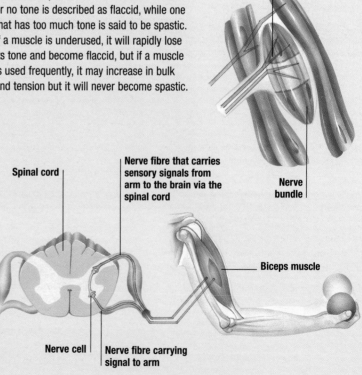

Nerve fibres

Nerve bundle

Spinal cord

Nerve fibre that carries sensory signals from arm to the brain via the spinal cord

Biceps muscle

Nerve cell

Nerve fibre carrying signal to arm

of activity, such as fast running or other forms concentrated exercise.

Most muscles contain both red and white fibres, but red fibres predominate in the muscles used in endurance activities, such as jogging and swimming, while white fibres predominate in muscles that are used in short bursts – sprinting, for example. The difference between the fibres can be seen if you look at a roast chicken: the dark meat of the legs is full of red fibres, which allow the chicken to perch for long periods, while the breast meat contains white fibres that allow the chicken to flap its wings intermittently and fly for short distances.

HOW MUSCLES DEVELOP

All the muscles of the body develop from cells in the central layer of the embryo called the mesoderm. Each muscle fibre develops from a single, specialist cell called a sarcoplast, although not all sarcoplasts turn into muscle fibres as the body grows. Many remain undeveloped, lying between the muscle fibres. Muscles continue to grow and develop through childhood and adolescence, and in boys until early adulthood. Once the body is physically mature, further muscle growth is still possible, because each skeletal muscle can increase in size, and therefore strength, the more it is used. Smooth muscle can also develop to meet bodily needs – the womb grows from 30–40g (1–1½oz) to 1kg (2lb) during pregnancy.

A muscle can also repair itself when damaged – any muscle fibres that remain unaffected by the damage will either increase in size or split to form new fibres. The undeveloped sarcoplast cells can mature when needed to provide another source of new fibres.

MUSCLE FATIGUE

When we make muscles work for long periods, they start to ache. This is because chemical side products of the work – notably lactic acid – accumulate in the muscle. The chemicals have an effect on the nerves that control the muscle, and this causes the ache. Blood flow moves the chemicals out of the muscles, and the ache goes away. This is why you feel better after a rest. Gentle massage of the affected area and a hot bath both increase blood flow through the muscles, and flush the chemicals more quickly. If your muscles are strong they generate fewer chemicals, so when you are fit your muscles ache less after a run.

What can go wrong
Warming up before exercise can prevent muscle strains, cramps and tears.

We can be acutely aware of our muscles after a run, a day's crosscountry walk or a bout of lifting work to which we are not accustomed. Taking care to avoid sudden movements and to stretch before and after exercise may prevent muscle strains, cramps and tears.

Cramp
Cramp is a painful, sudden contraction of a muscle or muscles that affects most people at some time. It can occur during exercise, when a muscle is tired or when it is held in a particular position – for example, when you are asleep. Doctors do not know what causes the sudden contraction. If you have cramp, try to stretch the affected muscle. and massage it gently.

Muscle strain
Muscle strain is more commonly known as a pulled muscle. It occurs when an excessive demand is suddenly placed on a muscle's tissues – for example, when a footballer tries a full-out sprint without having warmed up properly and pulls a hamstring muscle. A muscle strain is more likely when a burst of activity follows a period of inactivity – when you decide to dig the garden after ignoring it for several weeks – or when using a sudden, jerking movement.

The damage can range from overstretching a few muscle fibres to partially tearing them. The surrounding muscle fibres go into spasm to protect the damaged ones, but this can cause painful nodules in the muscle. The treatment is to reduce the inflammation by RICE (Rest, Ice, Compression, Elevation), where you can, and by massage and **physiotherapy** treatment.

Ruptured muscle
A muscle may be either completely or partially torn. A complete rupture is very rare, but a rupture of some of the muscle fibres is common. The cause is usually a sudden movement of a muscle that is already fully contracted, or a direct blow. The torn fibres bleed into the surrounding tissues causing swelling and pain and the formation of a **bruise** inside the muscle. The treatment is the same as for a pulled muscle. A bruise may also need deep friction, applied by a physiotherapist, to break down the blood clots and aid reabsorption. You may need to follow a programme of exercises to rebuild the muscle's strength and resilience – ask a physiotherapist.

Inflamed muscle
Inflammation of muscle tissue is called myositis. It causes pain, tenderness and weakness. The simplest type is localized (in one area only) and

Muscle-relaxant drugs are prescribed to reduce spasm and excess muscle tension in both smooth and skeletal muscles.

Muscle spasms caused by an injury can be treated with diazepam (the benzodiazepine drug once known as Valium, which is an anti-anxiety drug, as well as a muscle relaxant) and a painkiller. Excess muscle tension that results from a stroke or spinal injury, or from conditions such as multiple sclerosis, cerebral palsy or Parkinson's disease can be helped by a muscle-relaxant called Dantrolene.

Spasms in smooth muscle can be reduced by drugs that disturb the transmission of a nerve impulse to muscle fibres (anticholinergics) and so reduce the muscle's ability to contract.

Anticholinergic drugs may cause drowsiness, a dry mouth, blurred vision and, on rare occasions, liver damage.

Benzodiazepines should be taken only with medical supervision. They may cause drowsiness, dizziness and confusion and can be addictive. However, you should consult your doctor before stopping a course, in case of withdrawal symptoms.

results from a strain or rupture. Other types include inflammation of the muscles of the ribcage (pleurodynia) caused by a virus, and **autoimmune diseases** that cause myositis throughout the body (polymyositis).

Compression syndrome

Compression syndrome occurs when a muscle retains too much fluid. It is caused when you take unusually vigorous exercise without warming up or cooling down afterwards. Wearing compression bandages, lifting the affected muscle up and massage help to disperse the excess fluid.

The phrase 'compression syndrome' is sometimes used to refer to the compression of a nerve, which causes it to lose its ability to send messages to and from the muscles it serves. This leads to wasting of the affected muscles – as, for example, in **carpal tunnel syndrome**.

Myasthenia gravis

Myasthenia gravis is an **autoimmune disease** in which the body develops antibodies to the chemical that allows transmission of nerve impulses at the nerve endings to the muscles (acetylcholine). This stops the nerves from receiving the instruction to contract. It affects both skeletal and smooth muscles.

The main symptoms of this serious condition are muscle fatigue and rapidly becoming tired

when you have to perform muscular work. One in 30,000 people in the UK develop myasthenia gravis, and two-thirds of those affected are women. In women the symptoms first appear in early adult life, while men tend to develop the disease in middle age.

In some cases of myasthenia gravis the thymus gland is enlarged and surgical removal of the thymus can help. Removal of the thymus can bring about a marked improvement that increases each year after the operation, sometimes to the point at which symptoms disappear. Otherwise, treatment is designed to increase the levels of acetylcholine and suppress the production of the antibodies.

Tumours

Tumours are rarely found in muscles, whether benign or malignant. The most common benign tumour of muscle occurs in the uterine muscle and is called a fibroid (see **Fibroids, uterine**). Malignant tumours of muscle are called myosarcomas (see **Cancer**).

Infections

Infections rarely affect muscles directly. However, viral infections, such as flu, can cause muscles to become stiff and painful (myalgia), and the toxins produced by some bacteria – those responsible for **tetanus**, for example – can make the muscles go into spasm.

Genetic disorders

Genetic disorders can cause progressive muscular weakness and physical disabilities. The majority of disorders are diagnosed at birth or when a child is in infancy, although a few rare cases develop in later life (see **Muscular dystrophy**).

Nervous system disorders and muscles

Muscles can be affected by many disorders that primarily affect the nervous system. For example, diseases such as **poliomyelitis** affect the motor fibres of nerves and lead to muscle weakness and a loss of muscle tone (the capacity of the skeletal muscles to maintain tension and so support our posture). Other nervous system disorders lead to either too much or too little muscle tone and sometimes to paralysis. They include **Parkinson's disease, multiple sclerosis, cerebral palsy**, a **stroke** and **motor neurone disease**.

Other disorders

Carpal tunnel syndrome

In carpal tunnel syndrome severe aching and muscular weakness in the hand is caused by compression of the median nerve that passes through the wrist.

Poliomyelitis

Poliomyelitis is a viral infection that causes fever, muscle cramps and weakness and in some cases permanent paralysis. Immunization to prevent the spread of polio was introduced in the UK in the 1950s.

Tic

A tic is an involuntary, habitual muscular spasm or twitch thought to have a psychological origin. Tics are common in children but can be hard to treat in adults. Psychotherapy can help in some cases.

Trichinosis

This condition is caused by infection with the larvae of the roundworm Trichinella spiralis, which is found in undercooked infested meat. It can cause severe muscle pain, fever, nausea and diarrhoea.

Myopia

Myopia is the medical term used for short-sightedness. It allows objects nearby to be seen in clear focus, while distant objects are blurred because the eye cannot focus on them. It is a result of either the eyeball being longer from front to back than normal or of the eye's focusing structures overworking, so that the focusing point falls short of the retina. Myopia tends to be inherited. It usually occurs between the ages of 8 and 20 and is corrected by wearing glasses or contact lenses. High myopia increases the risk of **glaucoma** and a detachment of the retina.

SEE ALSO *Eye and disorders*

Myxoedema

Also referred to as hypothyroidism, myxoedema is a disease in which the thyroid gland does not produce sufficient thyroid hormones. This leads to a lack of energy and a thickening of the skin.

Myxoedema affects about one per cent of the adult population and is more common in women. It usually develops between the ages of 30 and 60.

SYMPTOMS

Symptoms appear gradually and may not be noticed for months or even years. They include:
- intolerance of cold;
- coarsening of the skin and other tissues, especially on the face;
- dry skin;
- thinning and loss of hair;
- hoarse voice and slow speech;
- slowed thinking;
- apathy and fatigue;
- aching muscles and pins and needles in the hands;
- **constipation;**
- weight gain;
- periods may become heavier;
- **goitre**, a swelling of the neck due to an enlargement of the thyroid gland.

DURATION

Myxoedema usually lasts for life, so the treatment has to be lifelong too. Once treatment has been started, the symptoms will usually disappear fairly quickly.

CAUSES

The condition is most commonly caused by an **autoimmune disease**, which leads to the body destroying its own tissues – in this case, those in the thyroid gland. Sometimes, the treatment for hyperthyroidism – in which the thyroid produces excessive amounts of hormones – will involve much of the gland being removed by surgery or destroyed by radioactive iodine treatment. This can lead to myxoedema developing. Other causes include a lack of iodine and a disorder of the pituitary gland (see **Pituitary gland and disorders**).

TREATMENT

Treatment is aimed primarily at correcting the levels of thyroid hormone in the body.

When to consult a doctor

A doctor should be consulted when the symptoms are first noticed. Early symptoms may be vague, but should always be reported. Often friends and relatives may be the first to realize that someone is ill.

What a doctor may do

- Blood tests to check thyroid function.
- Prescribe tablets containing thyroxine, a synthetic form of one of the main thyroid hormones.
- Take occasional blood samples to ensure that the correct dose of thyroxine is being taken.

PREVENTION

A doctor may prescribe thyroxine tablets after treatment for thyroid overactivity to prevent the development of myxoedema. There is no other means of prevention.

COMPLICATIONS

Myxoedema can cause several complications. These include **hypothermia**, excessively low body temperature, in the elderly; heart disease; and if untreated, mental disturbances. Personal neglect, coma and eventually death may occur.

OUTLOOK

With treatment and regular medical checks, the outlook is excellent.

SEE ALSO *Thyroid and disorders*

Myxoviruses

A myxovirus is a type of virus that affects mucous tissue, such as that in the throat, mouth, or lungs. Myxoviruses are responsible for infections in the respiratory tract and include the **influenza** viruses A, B and C.

A large number of diseases are caused by viruses, often the smallest known types of infectious agent. These are spread mainly by the fine spray of respiratory droplets that is coughed and sneezed by those affected. They invade and take over cells of other organisms, in order to make copies of themselves.

Other groups of disease-causing viruses include paramyxoviruses, which cause mumps and measles; herpes viruses, which cause cold sores, genital herpes, chickenpox, shingles and glandular fever; and the retroviruses, which cause AIDS.

SEE ALSO *Viral infections*

Nails and disorders

The nails are specialized skin structures made of keratin, a tough protein that is secreted by active cells at the base and sides of each nail. These growing areas are protected by folds of skin, called cuticles. At the base of the nail is a pale, half-moon area, known as the lunula, which contains some nail-making cells, while the rest of the nail bed looks pink because of the underlying blood vessels.

Nails help to strengthen the tips of the fingers and toes, protecting them from damage and splinting the end of the fingers so that the fingertips are more sensitive to touch. A fat pad behind the nails helps to cushion the sensitive fingertip.

WHAT CAN GO WRONG

If you develop a nail problem, it is important to consult a doctor for a proper diagnosis. Nail disorders have a number of causes, from localized nail or nail-bed infection to more widespread illness.

A serious illness can produce multiple horizontal ridges in the nails due to changes in nail growth rates. Psoriasis can cause roughness and pits in the nails. Iron deficiency can cause splitting, brittleness, pallor and, if the deficiency is severe, a spoonlike curvature known as koilonychia. White markings on the nail are common, and most are due to knocks and bruises on the nail bed. Sometimes white marks are linked with nutrient deficiencies and can also occur with paronychia, a nail-bed infection. A blueish tinge to the nails can be a sign of heart or lung disease.

Ingrowing toenails

Ingrowing toenails are common. They are most likely to occur on the big toe when tight shoes are worn or the nail is cut too short. This problem can lead to infection of the skin around the nail, which needs prompt treatment.

Paronychia

Paronychia is an infection of the skin fold at the side or base of the nail. It affects the fingernails and most often occurs in women with poor circulation, and whose work involves repeated wetting or washing of their hands. It leads to redness and swelling of the skin and often a brownish discoloration of the nail. If there is just one infected nail, the likely cause is an acute bacterial infection. If several nails are affected, this is probably the chronic form of the disease, and the cause is more likely to be a combined bacterial and fungal nail infection involving the yeast *Candida albicans*. The condition causes soreness around the edge of the nail, which can spread to cause worsening nail problems.

Treatment of paronychia can include antifungal cream or tablets and, if a bacterial infection is also present, oral antibiotics. If paronychia remains untreated, it can cause:
- loss of cuticles;
- a brownish discoloration of the nail due to infection of the matrix cells that produce the plate of the nail;
- thickening of nail folds;
- unsightly ridges on the nail;
- brittle, flaking, split nails;
- white patches on the nails – although most white markings are due to knocks and bruises;
- lifting of the nail from its bed;
- thickened, distorted nails.

Whitlow

A whitlow is a small abscess that forms on the fingertip, or rarely, on a toe. It can affect the root of the nail or the tendon sheaths of the fingers. Whitlows most commonly occur around the edge of the nail and are usually due to a bacterial infection, often caused by *Staphylococcus aureus*. The infected area becomes swollen, red and painful, and throbs. A collection of pus then forms.

In the early stages, a whitlow can be treated with antibiotics alone. Once pus is visible, the abscess can be incised and drained as a minor operation under a local **anaesthetic**. Care should be taken when handling food – an infected finger can be the root cause of an outbreak of **gastroenteritis**.

In rare instances, an untreated whitlow may infect the bone and cause **osteomyelitis**.

Occasionally, a whitlow is due to the **Herpes simplex** cold sore virus. This produces fluid-filled blisters, which are extremely painful. A herpetic whitlow should not be incised and drained because of the high risk of spreading the infection. The pain can be relieved by

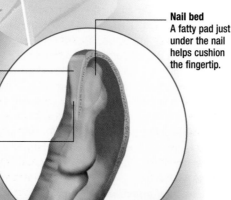

Nail structure
Nails form a protective layer at the tips of the fingers and toes. They grow throughout life and even continue after death.

Nail bed
A fatty pad just under the nail helps cushion the fingertip.

Nail body
It takes about six months for a nail to grow from cells produced at its base.

Lunula
Nail cells are produced in the pale area at the base of the nail.

applying an antiviral ointment such as aciclovir, which should not be applied to broken skin.

Fungal nail infections

Fungal nail infections are thought to affect up to 3 per cent of the population at any one time. There are various forms of fungal infection, many of which are mild and painless. This means that they are often ignored or go unnoticed, particularly if hidden by shoes or nail varnish. As a result, the fungal infection spreads, sometimes to the skin on the hands and feet when it becomes more difficult to eradicate.

You can also pass on the infection to other members of your family.

If the problem is severe and causes breakdown and distortion of the nail plate, then the nail can start to lift off from its underlying bed.

If your doctor suspects that you have a fungal infection, he or she may arrange for your nail clippings to be sent for analysis. Simple infections can be treated by applying antifungal creams, or with the use of an antifungal nail lacquer that hardens to protect the nail while it treats the infection. Alternatively, tablets may be taken by mouth, but long courses are often needed.

Damage to the old nail cannot be repaired, and it is difficult to kill the fungal infection within the nail plate. The aim of treatment is therefore to protect new nail growing through. As the new nail plate develops, it looks pink and healthy compared to the scarred, discoloured nail slowly moving further away from the nail bed. Treatment then must be continued until the old nail has grown through completely and been cut. If treatment is stopped too early, the fungus or yeasts usually grow down into the nail bed from the old infected nail and treatment has to be started all over again.

SEE ALSO *Hand and problems*

Fungal infection of the toenails

▲ **Treatment needed**
These discoloured and poorly growing toenails are affected by tinea, a fungal infection that is also responsible for athlete's foot. An antifungal cream or tablets will be needed to clear up the condition.

Narcolepsy

Narcolepsy is a sleep disorder that causes abnormal daytime sleepiness and episodes of involuntary sleep. The disorder can sometimes be inherited.

SYMPTOMS

The main symptom of narcolepsy is excessive daytime sleepiness, which can be severe and lead to 'sleep attacks' at abnormal sleeping times, such as in the middle of the day, an affected person may suddenly collapse into a state of deep sleep for a few seconds or for more than an hour.

About three-quarters of people with narcolepsy also suffer from cataplexy. This is a sudden loss of muscle tone that lasts for a few seconds and causes the person to collapse while fully conscious. It is triggered by laughter, strong emotion, surprise or sexual arousal.

Sleep paralysis is another symptom of narcolepsy. It is a brief muscular paralysis that occurs during the period between sleeping and waking and it can render the sufferer unable to speak or move for a matter of minutes, even though he or she is fully conscious.

Some narcoleptics have hypnagogic hallucinations, realistic and often frightening dreams that occur while falling asleep or waking up. These hallucinations may seem to continue on from events that actually occurred before the onset of sleep.

It is possible to suffer from sleep paralysis and hypnagogic hallucinations even if you are not narcoleptic. But if you have sleep attacks, episodes of cataplexy, sleep paralysis and hallucinations, you almost certainly have narcolepsy. The diagnosis can be confirmed by examining the electrical activity of the brain using an **EEG** (electroencephalography).

Diagnosis is less easy when a person has only isolated symptoms. Patients who are reported by a witness to have had an attack where they were unable to move or speak, but whose eyelids and muscles were noticeably twitching may be misdiagnosed with **epilepsy**.

TREATMENT

At present, there is no cure for narcolepsy, so treatment is aimed at relieving the symptoms. Antidepressant drugs may help to reduce the incidence of cataplexy. Daytime sleepiness may be controlled by taking frequent naps and through the use of prescribed stimulants.

Nausea

Nausea is the unpleasant sensation that is experienced just before vomiting: it causes a 'sick' feeling, an aversion to food, a sensation of fullness in the abdomen, and an overwhelming feeling that vomiting is about to start.

Other accompanying symptoms include:
- an urge to swallow frequently;
- excessive salivation;
- clammy, sweaty feeling;
- lightheadedness.

Certain other physical changes prepare the body for vomiting. The muscles of the stomach wall slacken; there is a decrease in the usual waves of contraction (peristalsis) in the wall of the stomach; the muscular ring (pyloric sphincter) that controls stomach output tightens; and the oesophageal sphincter, the equivalent muscular ring at the inlet to the stomach, slackens.

CAUSES

Nausea can have several causes ranging from overindulgence in alcohol to infection. The main triggers are:

■ aversion to certain foods and very bad smells, such as rotting flesh;

■ **motion sickness**;

■ unpleasant emotional experiences;

■ extreme physical pain;

■ **morning sickness** during pregnancy.

The causes of nausea that are associated with ill health include:

■ **gastroenteritis** and gastritis;

■ inner ear disorders, such as **labyrinthitis**;

■ **anxiety** states;

■ alcoholism (see **Alcohol and abuse**);

■ **migraine**;

■ viral **hepatitis**, in which it is an early sign;

■ **heart failure** with liver congestion;

■ **chemotherapy** and **radiotherapy** treatments for cancer;

■ some drugs (both normal and excessive doses). Antibiotics, such as digoxin; erythromycin; opiates, such as morphine; and NSAIDs (non-steroidal anti-inflammatories) can all bring on nausea.

TREATMENT

See your doctor if the cause is not obvious, if it is connected with a prescribed treatment or any underlying illnesses, or if the nausea is particularly prolonged. Treatment will depend on the underlying cause.

Complementary therapies

Ginger preparations, available in health food shops, can help to relieve motion sickness and morning sickness.

Acupressure wrist bands have a button that presses on a specific point on the inside of the wrist. Royal Navy researchers have found them to be more effective than a dummy treatment. These wrist bands are available in pharmacies.

PREVENTION

■ Avoid known triggers, such as food smells.

■ Use over-the-counter travel-sickness tablets.

■ When travelling by car as a passenger, focus your vision on the horizon. Looking anywhere inside the car – reading, for example – 'tells' the brain that there is no overall movement. This clashes, however, with the true signals from the balance organs that are telling you that there is movement. This confuses the brain and causes the feeling of nausea.

■ Wear a protective mask if exposure to repulsive smells is unavoidable.

Neck and problems

The neck is the part of the spine that runs from the base of the skull to the top of the back. Consisting of seven vertebrae placed one on top of the other, the neck supports the head and allows it considerable freedom of movement. It protects the spinal cord as it leaves the skull, supplies the brain and skull with blood and nutrients, and provides points of attachment for ligaments and muscles.

The neck vertebrae differ from the vertebrae lower down the spine in that they have a wider, triangular-shaped vertebral canal to accommodate the spinal cord – which is larger at the top of the spine than it is at the bottom. Each of the seven vertebral bodies in the neck is separated from its neighbour by an intervertebral disc; these are relatively thick and contribute to the curved position of the neck.

THE ATLAS AND THE AXIS

The two vertebrae at the very top of the spine – the atlas and the axis – are different from the other vertebrae in the neck. The atlas bears the weight of the head. It is essentially a bony ring with several projections, which enable the neck to articulate with the skull. The axis has an elongated body (the dens), which projects up into the hollow atlas, rather like a peg. This allows the head and atlas to turn from side to side. The dens is held in position within the atlas by a strong transverse ligament.

MUSCLES AND NERVES

Various muscles allow the neck and head to extend back or forwards; while the sternomastoids, at the side, make it possible to bring the ear down to the shoulder and vice versa. All these muscles also help with the rotation of the head and neck.

The neck is a vulnerable area because it contains numerous blood vessels and nerves. Among them is a network of nerves called the brachial plexus, which extends behind the collarbone and into the armpit. These nerves stimulate and control the muscles and skin of the chest, shoulders and arms.

WHAT CAN GO WRONG

The neck can be affected by many problems, the most common of which are caused by awkward movements or poor posture. **Physiotherapy**, wearing a collar or taking anti-inflammatory drugs can help to resolve many conditions, but in some cases surgery is the only option. Although neck surgery remains potentially dangerous, new techniques and instruments have improved the outlook considerably.

Acute neck

Acute neck is a problem that occurs suddenly as the result of a **whiplash injury**, an awkward movement – when swinging at a golf ball, for example – or something as trivial as sleeping on an uncomfortable pillow.

Since the neck muscles are relaxed when the unexpected movement or action occurs, they fail to restrict it adequately, causing the dislocation of a facet joint in a vertebra – one facet slips off the other (see **Spine and disorders**). This results in minute tears in the joint capsule and ligaments, as well as inflammation and swelling. Muscle spasm – in which the neck is held rigidly by the muscles to avoid any sudden movements – increases the pressure on the damaged joint.

A person with acute neck may be advised to wear a foam collar to support the neck and allow the muscles to relax. This relieves the pressure on the facet joint, which usually corrects its position.

Repeated attacks of acute neck increase the likelihood of cervical spondylosis (see below).

Muscle and ligament problems

Muscle and ligament problems are a frequent cause of chronic neck pain. Poor posture – rounding the shoulders, for example, while pushing the head forward – puts tremendous strain on the muscles and ligaments. They become overstretched, but at the same time have to contract to hold the head in position. After a while, parts of the muscles go into spasm, causing neck and shoulder pain and a tension headache. The ligaments lose elasticity and offer little support to the cervical spine, making it vulnerable to an attack of acute neck.

Habitual poor posture may also lead to the early onset of osteoarthritis (see **Arthritis**).

Cervical spondylosis

Cervical spondylosis is the medical name for osteoarthritis of the neck, which commonly affects the bottom three neck vertebrae. Most people over the age of 50 who have a neck X-ray show some signs of the condition.

The first symptoms are stiffness and pain. The intervertebral discs are the first part of the neck to be affected, followed by the facet joints.

As the condition progresses, the growth of bony spurs at the margins of the joints can cause pressure on the spinal nerves, resulting in **referred pain** in the shoulder and down the arm, with numbness and pins and needles. Sometimes pressure may be placed on the spinal cord itself, leading to a condition called central stenosis (see **Spine and disorders**).

In elderly people, the two arteries that run through the vertebrae on each side of the neck are sometimes thickened by arteriosclerosis, which impedes blood flow (see **Arteries and disorders**). In someone who also has cervical spondylosis, blood flow may be further impeded by the formation of bony spurs at the edges of the facet joints. The flow of blood may stop completely for short periods, causing **blackouts**, **vertigo** and visual disturbances. The problem generally occurs when the head is being tilted back, since this movement reduces the size of the channels through which the arteries pass.

Treatment for cervical spondylosis is usually limited to pain relief, anti-inflammatory drugs,

The neck

The neck not only supports the head, it forms a highway of blood vessels and nerves that relay nourishment and information to the brain.

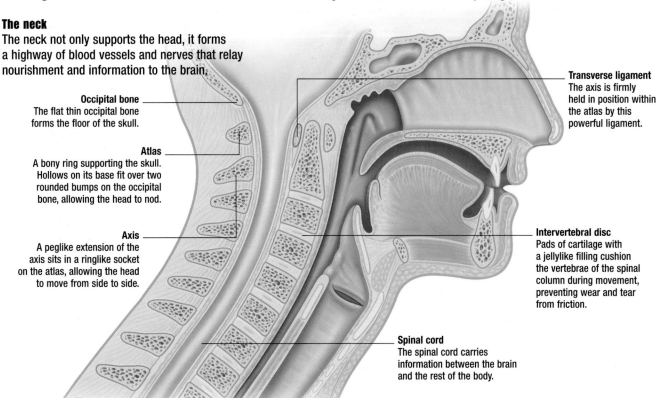

Occipital bone
The flat thin occipital bone forms the floor of the skull.

Atlas
A bony ring supporting the skull. Hollows on its base fit over two rounded bumps on the occipital bone, allowing the head to nod.

Axis
A peglike extension of the axis sits in a ringlike socket on the atlas, allowing the head to move from side to side.

Transverse ligament
The axis is firmly held in position within the atlas by this powerful ligament.

Intervertebral disc
Pads of cartilage with a jellylike filling cushion the vertebrae of the spinal column during movement, preventing wear and tear from friction.

Spinal cord
The spinal cord carries information between the brain and the rest of the body.

a neck collar and physiotherapy. In the few cases in which the spinal cord is affected, surgery may be needed to cut away parts of the vertebrae (a laminectomy), to free the spinal cord, and to fuse the vertebrae.

If the person with osteoarthritis also suffers from arteriosclerosis, it may be necessary to immobilize the neck with a firm collar to prevent the head from tilting back.

Rheumatoid arthritis

Rheumatoid arthritis can lead to the destruction of the intervertebral joints in the neck, allowing one vertebra to slip off the vertebra below it – with the risk that pressure may be placed on the spinal cord. This condition is particularly dangerous when the joint between the axis and atlas is affected. This is because the peglike dens of the axis may slip forward within the ring of bone that forms the atlas, spiking the spinal cord, and causing paralysis.

In the early stages of the condition, the neck can be supported by a collar to prevent further deterioration; later, an operation to fuse the vertebrae may be needed.

Ankylosing spondylitis

Ankylosing spondylitis, also known as bamboo spine, affects the whole spine, causing stiffness. It starts in the lumbar region, but eventually creeps up the spine to affect the neck as well.

Brachial neuralgia

Brachial neuralgia is the irritation of a nerve in the neck. It is characterized by a lancing pain, similar to that of **sciatica** but felt down the arm.

As the nerves of the neck leave the spinal cord, they pass close to the facet joints in the vertebrae before interweaving to form the network of nerves that extends from behind the collarbone into the armpit (the brachial plexus). If one of the nerves is pinched or stretched by an inflamed facet joint, or, more rarely, by a disc prolapse, it becomes irritated and fires off signals that are felt as acute shooting pains along its course.

Depending on which of the cervical nerves is affected, there may be no pain in the neck but continuous pain down one side of the arm, which is relieved only if the arm is held above the head. When the arm is held above the head, the stretch on the nerves of the brachial plexus is reduced – and so, too, is the pain.

Brachial neuralgia is relieved by treating the underlying cause.

Disc prolapse

Commonly called a slipped disc, a disc prolapse occurs much less frequently in the neck than it does in the lower back.

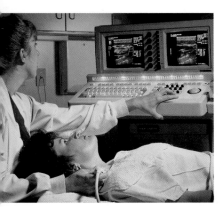

▲ Ultrasound scan
Doppler ultrasound scanning can be used to detect problems in the neck area, such as arteriosclerosis that can affect blood flow to the brain, causing vision problems and blackouts. The procedure causes no pain and is harmless.

The neck discs most often affected by a prolapse are those between the fifth and sixth and the sixth and seventh vertebrae. The cause is usually a jarring injury, such as whiplash, and the result is chronic neck pain, sometimes accompanied by brachial neuralgia (see above).

The discs usually bulge out to the back and side. A small bulge may press on one of the ligaments of the spine, causing neck pain; a larger one may impinge on a nerve, causing brachial neuralgia. Rarely, a prolapsed disc bulges into the spinal canal and presses on the spinal cord causing more extensive neurological symptoms, which may include paralysis.

Treatment focuses on relieving pain using analgesic drugs. Someone with a prolapsed disc will be advised to wear a collar and to have physiotherapy, including ultrasound, gentle mobilizations and graduated exercises to restore muscle strength and mobility. Surgery is considered only if there are indications of central stenosis.

Cervical spondylolisthesis

Cervical spondylolisthesis is a rare condition in which one neck vertebra slips forwards, over one below it. There are three causes.

■ A congenital defect that allows the atlas to slip off the axis, or stops it healing properly after injury.

■ An inflammation – caused by, for example, rheumatoid arthritis or a bad infection of the ear or throat – which leads to stretching of the ligament that holds the peglike body called the dens in position inside the atlas. This allows the atlas to slip forward within the joint.

■ Joint instability from a previous injury, or arthritis that allows a vertebra gradually to slide forward over the one below it.

Symptoms include a stiff neck, muscle spasm and, if the slipped vertebra is pressing on the spinal cord, neurological signs that may range from brachial neuralgia to bowel and bladder disorders, muscle weakness and paralysis.

The diagnosis is confirmed by an X-ray. Treatment depends on the symptoms. If the spinal cord has been compressed, treatment includes immobilization with a plaster cast and surgery (laminectomy and vertebral fusion).

Cervical rib

A cervical rib is a congenital overdevelopment of the seventh vertebra. This extra rib may be fibrous or bony, small or complete, and may cause no symptoms. But it can affect the brachial plexus and the subclavian artery, both of which pass over it. This may result in pain and damage to the nerves of the forearm and hand, especially on the little-finger side. Small clots may form in the artery, reducing blood supply and making the wrist pulse weak.

Physiotherapy in the early stages can help to strengthen the muscles, but the extra rib may need to be removed surgically if symptoms affect the nerves or the circulation of blood.

Infantile torticollis

Infantile torticollis becomes apparent soon after birth because the baby's head is tilted abnormally due to a shortening of the sternomastoid muscle on one side of the neck. It is thought to be caused by interference in the blood supply to the muscle during birth. The condition has become less common with improvements in obstetric practice.

Gradual but repeated stretching of the muscle by a physiotherapist can be helpful in the early stages. If the condition persists, fibrous tissue starts to replace parts of the muscle, in which case surgery may be needed.

Tumour

A tumour may affect the bones in the neck, the spinal cord, its membranous linings or a spinal nerve. Tumours in the actual vertebrae are usually cancerous and secondary to a primary tumour elsewhere in the body. Tumours of the nervous system are often primary and can cause spinal compression or affect the brachial plexus. In both cases there are neurological symptoms and considerable pain. Treatment includes surgery, chemotherapy and radiotherapy.

SEE ALSO *Back and back pain*

Necrotizing fasciitis

Necrotizing fasciitis is a rare and often fatal form of bacterial infection, which spreads rapidly, killing body tissue. It can be caused by a variety of micro-organisms, in particular *Streptococcus pyogenes*, the bug more usually responsible for **scarlet fever** and the skin infection **impetigo**.

Every year, up to 60 people develop the condition in England and Wales. Although apparently healthy people can develop it, it is more likely to affect people with circulatory problems or whose immune systems have been weakened by disease, drugs or alcohol.

SYMPTOMS
- Those affected rapidly become very ill, developing fever and shock.
- Other symptoms include cold, clammy skin, fast, shallow breathing and confusion.
- When the infection follows a skin injury, the site becomes exceptionally painful, turns dusky purple and may blister.

CAUSES
The infecting bacteria usually enter the body via a minor skin injury or surgery, but in some cases the route of entry remains unknown.

TREATMENT
- Although the diagnosis of necrotizing fasciitis can be confirmed with blood and tissue tests, doctors treat it as soon as it is suspected because it spreads so rapidly.
- Treatment is with surgery to remove areas of dead and dying tissue, which may mean amputation and high-dose antibiotics.

OUTLOOK
About two-thirds of people affected by necrotizing fasciitis will die as a result.

Nephropathy

Any disease or condition affecting the kidneys comes under the term 'nephropathy'. Examples include analgesic nephropathy, which is due to the abuse of painkillers, **AIDS**-related nephropathy, diabetic nephropathy, **gout** nephropathy and hypertensive nephropathy. Other examples include obstructive nephropathy, which is kidney damage caused by pressure from urine unable to exit the bladder, and reflux nephropathy that results from urine flowing backwards up the ureters and can then cause damage and scarring to the kidney.

SEE ALSO *Bladder and disorders; Kidneys and disorders*

Nephrosis

Also known as nephrotic syndrome, nephrosis is a disorder of the kidneys in which large amounts of proteins (especially albumin) are lost from the blood and excreted in the urine. Nephrosis may be caused by conditions such as **diabetes** mellitus, severe high **blood pressure** and inflammation of the filter units in the kidneys, but in many cases the cause is unknown.

SEE ALSO *Kidneys and disorders; Urinary system*

Nephrostomy

Nephrostomy is the drainage of urine from the kidney using a sterile, narrow tube called a catheter. This is passed into the kidney through an opening in the surface of the skin, and allows urine made in the kidney to escape without passing through the ureters or bladder. Nephrostomy is often used to allow the ureter to rest and to heal more quickly after an operation – for example, when a kidney stone has been removed.

SEE ALSO *Kidneys and disorders, Urinary system*

Nephrotic syndrome

Nephrotic syndrome is a condition in which damage to the filtering units of the kidneys (the glomeruli) results in severe loss of protein from the body through the urine. Reduced protein concentration in the circulation leads to the accumulation of excess fluid in the tissues of the body (**oedema**), with severe swelling of the legs and face, and puffiness around the eyes. Fluid can also accumulate in the abdominal cavity (ascites), and in the chest cavity (pleural effusion).

Nephrotic syndrome can result from kidney damage associated with persistent high **blood pressure**, inflammation of the glomeruli (glomerulonephritis), poorly controlled **diabetes**, abnormal protein deposits in the kidney (amyloidosis) and toxic kidney damage caused by some poisons and drugs. Severe allergic reactions to bee stings, poison ivy, pollen and even cows' milk can also lead to nephrotic syndrome in some cases.

SEE ALSO *Allergies; Kidneys and disorders*

Nervous system and disorders

The nervous system is the body's control centre. It is in charge of automatic processes such as breathing, and also governs conscious and complex activities such as playing sport.

There are two parts to the nervous system. The peripheral nervous system consists of countless nerves throughout the body.

▼ **Communicators**
There are numerous nerve cells in the brain and spinal cord. Each nerve cell has many branches. These receive nerve impulses from other cells, interpret the message and pass it on, forming a continuous chain of communication.

These collect raw data, which is routed along the spinal cord to the brain. The brain and the spinal cord constitute the central nervous system, which processes and interprets the data, and formulates a response.

Disorders of the central nervous system such as a **coma** resulting from a **head injury,** may shut-down the system, whereas diseases such as **Alzheimer's** and **Parkinson's** can delete or block the path of neural data.

Damage to the peripheral nervous system impairs communication between the central nervous system and the body and can affect automatic activities, leading to symptoms such as blurred vision or **incontinence**. General symptoms may include pain and problems with movement. Damage may also be caused by infections such as botulism, metabolic disorders such as diabetes and diseases such as cancer.

SEE ALSO *Brain and nervous system*

Nettle rash

Nettle rash is a skin condition which is also known as hives and urticaria. It results in raised, itchy reddened areas of skin that look like nettle stings. It is caused by the release of histamine into the skin, and usually goes away within four hours.

CAUSES
Common causes include:
■ an infection;
■ recently started medication;
■ something eaten or drunk in the previous 24 hours;
■ insect stings or bites;
■ contact with cosmetics, creams, plant saps or chemicals;
■ exposure to the sun or a sun lamp;
■ extreme heat or cold;
■ emotional upset.

TREATMENT
In most cases nettle rash can be treated by simple first aid.
What you can do
■ Take an over-the-counter antihistamine tablet.
■ Hold ice cubes or ice wrapped in cotton material against the affected skin, for 5–10 minutes. Do not apply for longer or you risk causing frostbite. Then apply calamine lotion.
■ Take a cool bath. Add a little baking powder or cornstarch to the water, or put some oatmeal into a sock and suspend it under the tap as you fill the bath. Do not use soap. Wrap yourself in a towel (avoid rubbing) and then apply calamine lotion or an unscented moisturizer.
■ Establish the trigger and avoid it in future, if possible.

When to consult a doctor
- Immediately, if you experience any swelling around the face, lips, tongue or throat, or if you develop other symptoms, such as wheezing, joint pains or a fever.
- If the rash persists for longer than a few days.

Neuralgia

Neuralgia is pain caused by irritation of, or damage to, a nerve. The pain can be very severe but is usually brief, and can often be felt coursing along the path of the nerve. There are several specific types of neuralgia.
- Post-herpetic neuralgia can occur following an attack of shingles. The pain is severe and disabling, and will occur at the site of the original infection.
- Trigeminal neuralgia (or tic douloureux) is the most common type of neuralgia. It affects the trigeminal nerve that supplies sensation to the face, and causes intense lancing pain on one side of the face. The attacks last from between 30 minutes to an hour. The causes of trigeminal neuralgia are not known with certainty (see also **Headache**).
- People who suffer from **migraine** often have a neuralgia that affects the area around the eye.

CAUSES
Inflammation, systemic diseases, compression and physical disruption can all cause the irritation or damage to the nerve that causes the pain. The location of the pain is dependent on the underlying problem and the nerve involved.

TREATMENT
There are several ways of treating neuralgia. Some forms respond well to anticonvulsant drugs such as carbamazepine. Analgesic drugs (painkillers), such as paracetamol, can also be used. Various drugs may be used in the treatment of post-herpetic neuralgia, and surgery is sometimes considered.

Complementary therapies
A good diet with foods rich in B vitamins may be useful. **Acupuncture** has also been reported to be very effective. **Homeopathy** and certain **herbal medicines** may be beneficial.

Neural tube defect

In a human embryo, the neural tube is the structure that eventually forms the nervous system, with the brain at one end of the tube and the spinal cord extending from it. When the neural tube fails to close completely, congenital defects occur, the most common being **spina bifida**. Folic acid, taken prior to pregnancy and during the first 12 weeks, has been found to reduce the incidence of neural tube defects.

DIAGNOSIS
A blood test at 11–14 weeks of pregnancy allows early detection of high-risk pregnancies. Termination of pregnancy may be offered if further tests confirm fetal abnormalities.

IMPACT ON FUNCTION
The impact of spina bifida depends on the site and severity. There may simply be a minor depression in the backbone, with a patch of hair or other skin defect over the site. This will have no impact on everyday function.

In more severe cases, a sac of tissue containing meninges (the protective membrane surrounding the brain and spinal cord) and cerebrospinal fluid may protrude through the vertebral column (meningocele). In the most severe form of the defect, this sac additionally contains neural tissue (meningomyelocele). A severe meningomyelocele is likely to result in paralysis; the individual will be unable to walk and there will be no bladder and bowel control. He or she may also have **hydrocephalus**, which occurs when the circulation system for the cerebrospinal fluid is impaired. This can have implications for intellectual functioning.

Between these two extremes, there is a range of possible disability. The condition does not get worse as the child gets older – for example, weakness in the legs diagnosed early in infancy may make learning to walk more difficult, but is not likely to deteriorate further.

TREATMENT
Surgical treatment aims to prevent further problems by repairing the defect, and controlling hydrocephalus by the insertion of a 'shunt' to allow the cerebrospinal fluid to drain effectively. Medical treatment is focused on management rather than cure.

OUTLOOK
Children born with severe damage to the brain or spinal cord have a reduced life expectancy, but those with only a minor defect can expect to live as long as anyone else. Legislation enacted in the *Disability Discrimination Act*, better access to buildings and public transport, together with changing attitudes, can all contribute to ensuring excellent quality of life for people facing physical challenges.

Neurasthenia

Neurasthenia describes varying degrees of nervous exhaustion. Symptoms may include dizziness, headache, sleep disturbance and an inability to relax. Severe anxiety may induce disabling physical symptoms such as

palpitations, shortness of breath, wheezing and chest tightness. Chronic neurasthenia can lead to muscle weakness, exhaustion, and a lack of motivation and concentration. Predisposition to neurasthenia depends on personality type and is associated with anxiety disorders.

SEE ALSO *Anxiety; Panic attack*

Neuritis

Neuritis is the inflammation of a nerve, resulting in pain, numbness or tingling over the site of the nerve. Certain abnormalities occur if specific nerves are affected – for example, there may be muscle wasting of the arm in brachial neuritis and visual problems in **optic neuritis.** Both commonly occur in **multiple sclerosis.**

Neurofibroma

A non-cancerous swelling, or tumour, attached to a nerve is called a neurofibroma. It may occur in isolation or as one of a collection in the congenital disease **neurofibromatosis.**

Painless non-symptomatic neurofibromas are often left alone. But those causing severe symptoms, such as deafness if the acoustic nerve is involved, may be removed surgically.

▼ **Patchy skin**
Coffee-coloured patches on the skin are a symptom of the genetic condition neurofibromatosis.

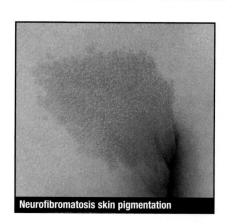

Neurofibromatosis skin pigmentation

Neurofibromatosis

Neurofibromatosis is a hereditary disease in which clusters of non-cancerous swellings, known as neurofibromata, occur along a nerve. It is also known as von Recklinghausen's disease. The condition results in patches of pigmented skin, and can occur throughout the body. Those affected may also suffer from **epilepsy.** In severe cases, the skin may appear gnarled. Most cases are mild and treatment is rarely required. But surgery may be done for cosmetic reasons or if individual tumours cause other symptoms.

Night blindness

Night blindness is the reduced ability to see in low light levels, such as in dim evening light or at night. It may be due to a dietary deficiency of vitamin A, which is a significant problem in developing countries. In the UK,

night blindness is generally the result of rare inherited conditions, the best known of which is retinitis pigmentosa. This is characterized by loss of the light-sensitive rod cells of the retina, which are responsible for vision in low light levels. The first sign of retina pigmentosa is a difficulty getting around at night time. If you have this problem, see your doctor. He or she will arrange investigative tests.

Nits

An infestation of head lice is commonly called nits, although technically nits are the empty eggshells that remain attached to hair after the lice have hatched. Anyone can catch head lice, but they are most common in children aged 4–11 years. Girls are more likely to be affected than boys. Head lice spread by head-to-head contact. They are found on both dirty and clean hair, and on long and short hair. In most cases, there are fewer than ten lice on the head.

The female louse lays about six to eight eggs a day, and these are glued onto the hair shafts close to the scalp. The eggs take seven to ten days to hatch.

SYMPTOMS
The only reliable method of identifying a current infestation is to find live lice, although these can be difficult to see in the hair with the naked eye. However, you should also look out for any of the following signs and symptoms:
■ The presence of tear-shaped eggs or empty egg shells – these tend to be found lower down the hair shaft and can sometimes be mistaken for dandruff.
■ Itching, which is often the only symptom, though it may not begin until weeks or months after the infestation.
■ A rash on the back of the neck, which is caused by an allergic reaction to louse faeces.
■ Louse droppings, which are sometimes seen as black specks on pillows or collars.

TREATMENT
Head lice can be removed by wet combing or by the use of insecticide shampoo treatment.

Wet combing
Wet combing involves washing the hair in the normal way before applying a large quantity of hair conditioner. The hair should then be combed through with an ordinary comb. After this, use a very close-pronged, plastic comb to work your way around the head, slowly combing from the roots of the hair to the tips. Wipe the comb with a tissue after each stroke. If you find lice, repeat the procedure every three to four days for two weeks, in order to remove any newly hatched

lice. Alternatively, if you do find lice, you may wish to kill them by applying an insecticide (see below).

Insecticides

Insecticides used to treat head lice contain malathion, phenothrin, permethrin or carbaryl. Carbaryl treatment can be obtained only on prescription. Check with a doctor if an affected child is under six months old, or if he or she suffers from **asthma** or **eczema**. Follow the product instructions very carefully. If live lice can still be seen or are seen within a day or two of treatment, the lice may be resistant to the insecticide. In this case, use the wet combing method or switch to a product with a different ingredient. A second application of the same treatment is recommended seven days after the first one, so that any eggs that were missed and have now hatched are killed.

Complementary therapies

Several complementary and other treatments are available, including battery-operated combs, herbal remedies and tea tree and other essential oils. There is no reliable evidence to show that any of these are effective. Some essential oils may irritate the skin or may not be suitable for children. Always read the manufacturer's notes on usage, and do not use essential oils as a preventive measure.

Nocturia

A frequent urge to pass urine at night is described as nocturia. Anyone who wakes more than twice during the night to pass urine may be said to have the condition. Drinking large quantities before sleep, especially alcohol, coffee or tea, can cause nocturia. But if the urge to empty the bladder several times a night persists, see your doctor. The condition is usually the result of some underlying disorder, such as **cystitis** or an enlarged prostate gland. It can also be a sign of **heart failure, diabetes** or **kidney** disease. Nocturia is more common in elderly people and many people have it without realizing that there is a problem.

SEE ALSO *Heart and circulatory system; Kidneys and disorders; Prostate and problems*

Nocturnal myoclonus

'Nocturnal myoclonus' is a term used to describe jerking movements of the legs that a person can sometimes experience while falling asleep. The affected person is usually totally unaware of these spasms. Anticonvulsant drug treatment can help to relieve the symptoms.

Non-specific urethritis

Doctors say a man has non-specific urethritis (NSU) when he is suffering irritation of the urethra and discomfort when urinating. There is usually a discharge from the urethra that may contain pus cells, indicating infection. NSU is a collection of symptoms rather than a disease – doctors are usually uncertain of the cause of the man's genital irritation and use NSU as an interim diagnosis.

CAUSES

The most common infection identified in men with these problems is **chlamydia**. The doctor will take a swab from your penis and a urine sample and send them for antigen testing in the laboratory. The test results are usually given within seven to ten days.

In the meantime, you will probably be treated on the presumption that you have a chlamydia infection.

The most common form of chlamydia infection is *Chlamydia trachomati*, which is a **sexually transmitted** infection. It often produces no symptoms, but an infected man may notice a discharge from his penis, or discomfort on passing urine, which usually starts within one to six weeks of exposure to the infection. This discharge is typically present early in the morning and clears during the day. Staining of the underclothes with mucus or a slightly pus-stained discharge is another sign of *Chlamydia trachomati* infection.

If the test is negative, you will probably be told you have NSU with cause unknown. Either way, your doctor is likely to continue with the same treatment. The unknown cause may be infection with the *Ureaplasma* micro-organism, which is not checked for in the tests but which responds to the same antibiotics as chlamydia.

TREATMENT

Chlamydia infection is treated with antibiotics including oxytetracycline, doxycycline, erythromycin and azithromycin. It is important that sexual partners are also treated to prevent the infection from being passed back and forth between partners.

PREVENTION

Using barrier contraceptives – such as condoms – will protect you from sexually transmitted infections.

SEE ALSO *Urinary system*

Nose and problems

The nose has two important roles. It is the organ of smell and it also acts as the body's air-conditioning unit for the lungs. It forms a passageway that leads from the nostrils at the front, and extends back for about 7.5cm (3in) into the upper region of the throat (the nasopharynx).

The nose is made up largely of bone and cartilage – the tough, gristly material that is also found in the ear, the windpipe and various other parts of the body. It is divided into two separate compartments at the nostrils by the septum, which consists of cartilage at the front and bone at the back.

The bones of the skull create the inner part of the nose. The bridge of the nose – where spectacles balance – is formed by the nasal

bones, while the skull bones make up the roof of the nose. The walls of the nose are formed from part of the upper jaw bone and its floor is made from the hard palate, or roof of the mouth.

The bones that make up the nose contain a number of air-filled spaces called the sinuses, or sometimes the paranasal sinuses. There are four pairs of sinuses. They are lined with mucous membranes, and their mucus fluid drains into the nasal cavity.

The function of the sinuses is not entirely clear. They may, perhaps, reduce the weight of the skull, or insulate the brain from damage, acting rather like the airbags of a car. Along with the nasal passages, they form a space where sound from the larynx resonates, giving the human voice its individual quality – which is temporarily lost when someone has a heavy cold that produces nasal congestion.

The nasal cavity acts as a drain in other ways. The Eustachian tube, which allows the equalization of pressure on both sides of the eardrum, opens up into the nasopharynx. The nasolacrimal duct, which drains the tears that continually bathe the eyeball, also drains into the nasal passages. That is why your nose tends to feel congested when you cry.

FILTERING AND CONDITIONING

The nose filters, warms and moistens air entering the body through the nostrils, and by doing so, it plays an important protective role for the respiratory system. Just inside the nostrils there are small hairs – which are very noticeable in some people – that trap dust and dirt. Also, all incoming air passes over the nasal mucous membranes, and any potentially harmful micro-organisms become trapped within the mucus. This then flows backwards into the throat and is eventually swallowed, so that the micro-organisms are destroyed by strong stomach acid.

THE SENSATION OF SMELL

Olfaction – the sense of smell – is the most primitive of all our senses, being linked inextricably to the emotions. At the same time, smell is highly specific and remarkably sensitive. Human beings are able to distinguish between some 10,000 different odours, and we can detect certain unpleasant odours, such as those of sulphur compounds, down to a concentration of one part in 30 billion. That makes the sense of smell about 20,000 times more sensitive than the sense of taste. But the two senses are intimately connected, because chewing food releases odour molecules so the mouth and nose are working together – literally sampling the chemical composition of the dish. When you have a cold, or some other form of nasal

Inside the nose

As well as containing odour-sensitive receptors, the interior of the nose is designed to function as a cleansing device, and a warming and lubricating channel for the air we breathe in.

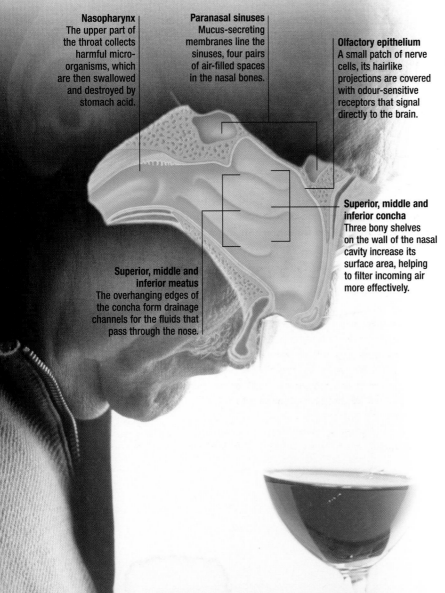

Nasopharynx
The upper part of the throat collects harmful micro-organisms, which are then swallowed and destroyed by stomach acid.

Paranasal sinuses
Mucus-secreting membranes line the sinuses, four pairs of air-filled spaces in the nasal bones.

Olfactory epithelium
A small patch of nerve cells, its hairlike projections are covered with odour-sensitive receptors that signal directly to the brain.

Superior, middle and inferior concha
Three bony shelves on the wall of the nasal cavity increase its surface area, helping to filter incoming air more effectively.

Superior, middle and inferior meatus
The overhanging edges of the concha form drainage channels for the fluids that pass through the nose.

congestion, food tends to lose its flavour. But, in reality, it is the sense of smell that is impaired, rather than the sense of taste.

Odours are the result of small, volatile molecules of a substance entering the nose on convection currents in the surrounding air. The detection system is a 5cm² (2sq in) patch known as the olfactory epithelium. It contains about 50 million specialized cells and is located high up in the nasal cavities.

When you sniff, currents are created within the air passing through the nose, which force more odour molecules upwards to hit the olfactory epithelium. Sniffing is a reflex action that occurs whenever our attention is attracted by an odour, making the nose more sensitive to what might be a danger signal, such as the smell of burning.

Once an odour molecule has become bound to the olfactory epithelium, it generates an electrical stimulus that travels to the olfactory bulb, which lies just above and behind the nose and is the part of the brain that processes smell signals. Smell is unique among the senses because the electrical signals that are generated by the olfactory epithelium go directly to their target in the brain, the olfactory bulb. Signals from the body's other senses travel through the thalamus, the brain's relay station. In fact, you could say that the nervous system has a far more immediate contact with the outside world

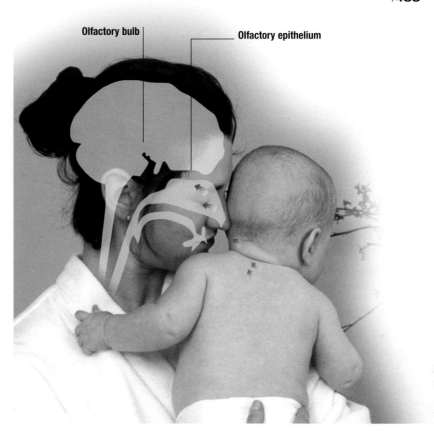

Olfactory bulb | Olfactory epithelium

▲ **Smell mechanism**
Smells detected by the olfactory epithelium are sent directly to the olfactory bulb in the brain for processing. Because the olfactory bulb also has links to memory and emotion, babies quickly learn to recognize their mother by smell alone.

through smell than it does through any of the other senses.

What is more, the olfactory bulb is part of the inner limbic system of the brain, an area which also contains structures that are very closely involved with both the emotions and memory. There are a large number of neural connections between these structures and the olfactory bulb – which may explain why smells can be so evocative.

WHAT CAN GO WRONG?

The nose, being quite a complex structure and one that is connected to several other important areas of the body, such as the lungs and the ears, is subject to a wide range of disorders. These range from infection and injury to congenital malformations and **cancer**.

Rhinitis

Rhinitis is the inflammation of the mucous membranes that line the nasal cavity. It leads to nasal congestion (a blocked nose), nasal discharge, sneezing and a reddened skin.

The common **cold**, which is a viral infection, is the most usual cause of rhinitis. **Allergic rhinitis** is triggered by allergens, such as pollen – which gives rise to the seasonal form of the disease, commonly known as **hay fever** – animal fur, house-dust mites and various foods, including wheat, eggs and nuts.

Injury

Because of its prominent position on the face, the nose is particularly prone to injury. A blow

---

Factfile

Examination of the nose

Most nasal examinations can be done quickly and easily by your GP. A hospital appointment will be made for an endoscopy if necessary.

■ A doctor uses a speculum to open up the nostrils to examine the inside of the nose. A more detailed examination is done, under local anaesthetic, using an endoscope – a miniature telescope on a flexible probe, which is inserted through the nostrils.

■ The nasopharynx area can be investigated with a mirror. This is held behind the soft palate to one side of the uvula while the tongue is depressed. This allows a doctor to see the back end of the nasal septum, the Eustachian tube openings, and the roof of the nasopharynx.

■ The extent of any nasal congestion can be assessed by holding a cool polished surface, such as a metal tongue depressor, below the nostrils. The area of condensation – caused by breathing out – from each nostril can be compared and any differences investigated.

Nosebleeds: what you can do

A nosebleed can be alarming, and it helps to know what to do if one occurs.

1 The correct position for someone whose nose is bleeding is sitting and leaning slightly forward so that blood or clots cannot obstruct the airway.

2 Pinch the lower part of the nostrils for about 15 minutes, while the person breathes through his or her mouth.

3 When the bleeding stops, the person should avoid touching or blowing the nose.

4 If bleeding does not stop within 20 minutes, seek medical advice.

5 Always get urgent medical attention if a nosebleed starts after a heavy blow to the head – this could indicate a fractured skull.

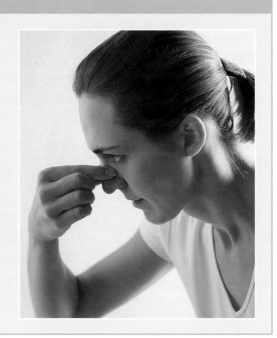

to the nose – often a sports injury – might produce a fracture in one of the nasal bones. This is one of the most common reasons for people attending casualty departments, and the doctor's priority is to investigate whether there is an accompanying skull or spinal fracture, which would be potentially far more serious.

Nosebleeds are common, too (see box above). They frequently occur for no apparent reason, although very high **blood pressure** can be a cause among older people.

Young children often insert foreign bodies into their nasal cavity, and if these get stuck they may elicit a strong inflammatory response, which results in a foul-smelling nasal discharge. Many cases of mysterious nasal symptoms in children can be explained by the discovery of a foreign body. The object is usually inserted without the parents' knowledge and there may be a delay before symptoms start to emerge.

Septal deviation and perforation

It is rare for the septum to divide the nasal cavity with perfect symmetry. Minor degrees of deviation rarely cause problems; however, injury to the nose during birth – or later in life – can produce a more pronounced degree of deviation that may result in nasal obstruction, recurrent sinus infection, or even chronic middle ear infection. For instance, the septum may take on an S-shape, which causes considerable distortion of the nasal cavity.

Another cause of damage to the septum is repeated sniffing of cocaine: this results in perforation, which in turn may cause nosebleeds

and produce a whistling sound when the person breathes in. Septal deviation can be repaired by surgery if it is causing problems, but septal perforations are almost impossible to repair.

Growths in the nasal cavity

Nasal polyps are swellings that occur within the nasal passages on both sides. They are usually caused by the overproduction of fluid by the mucous membranes lining the sinuses in response to an allergen. They are nearly always benign (non-cancerous). If polyps have a tendency to appear only on one side of the nose, your doctor may recommend further investigation, especially if they start to bleed or become ulcerated.

Skin **cancer** can develop in the area around the nostrils. The most common types are called basal cell carcinoma and squamous cell carcinoma, although other tumours may arise inside the nose, such as nasopharyngeal carcinoma. This type of cancer has been linked to infection with the Epstein-Barr virus, which causes **glandular fever**. It rarely gives rise to any symptoms until it is quite far advanced, and is treatable by radiation

Another malignancy of the nasal area is T-cell lymphoma, which rapidly invades the face, sinuses and nose. If you notice symptoms such as a lump in the nose or neck or a bloodstained nasal discharge, visit your doctor without delay.

SEE ALSO *Respiratory system*

Nutritional disorders

If the body does not receive the nutrients it needs, it cannot thrive. Nutritional deficiencies and disorders occur if the diet is unbalanced and unhealthy or there are special nutritional needs that are not met.

Few people in the developed world are short of food or suffer from a severe lack of essential nutrients. The majority of nutritional disorders and deficiencies in developed countries such as the UK are caused by poor dietary habits or conditions that prevent digestion and absorption, limiting the body's ability to draw the required nutrients from food.

SYMPTOMS

General symptoms of nutrient deficiency include tiredness, pale skin, listlessness, gastric upset, changed bowel habits and lack of stamina. Nutritional disorders can affect your mood and mental performance, leading to depression, anxiety, emotional problems, an inability to concentrate and poor memory.

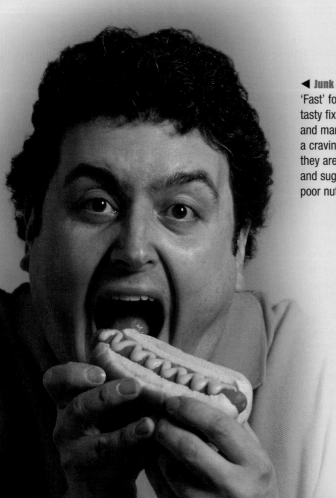

◀ Junk food
'Fast' foods offer a quick, tasty fix for hunger pangs and many people develop a craving for them. But they are often high in fats and sugars and are of poor nutritional value.

These symptoms could be caused by any of a number of conditions that limit the absorption of nutrients by the body's **digestive system**. For example, in cases of pancreatic insufficiency, the pancreas produces too few digestive enzymes, while in **Crohn's disease** areas of the gastrointestinal tract become inflamed and cannot absorb nutrients.

When the digestive tract does not absorb fats properly, the body excretes excessive amounts of fat in the stools (steatorrhoea). **Coeliac disease** is caused by an intolerance of gluten, which damages the villi, the finger-like extensions on the surface of the intestine; this reduces the body's ability to absorb nutrients. If the digestive tract becomes infected by bacteria such as Salmonella and Campylobacter and parasites such as Giardia lamblia, it will try to reject these bacteria and in doing so will not absorb nutrients from food (see Food poisoning).

Nutrient deficiency can also result from structural problems in the digestive system. In some people the opening from the stomach to the small intestine (the pylorus) is narrow, and this interferes with the passage of food. In young babies, this condition (**pyloric stenosis**) can produce sudden and violent vomiting. (There are many other less serious reasons why a baby may be vomiting – see **Babies and baby care**.) If one of the ducts that carry bile from the liver to the gallbladder or from the gallbladder to the intestine becomes blocked, the bile – which contains salts needed to emulsify fats – is unable to reach the intestine and this interferes with digestion.

Disorders such as **diabetes**, **thyroid disease** and lymphoma can also limit the absorption of nutrients. Some drugs – for example, antibiotics and laxatives – also interfere with nutrient absorption during digestion.

TREATING NUTRITIONAL DISORDERS

You should always consult a doctor for diagnosis and treatment if you suspect you have a nutritional disorder. Conventional treatment varies widely, but can include the use of drugs such as antibiotics or steroids and surgery. Changes to your diet may also help, depending on the disorder.

Nutritional therapy may effect a cure in mild cases of certain conditions and may alleviate symptoms in more serious cases. Generally, the earlier a condition is treated, the more successful the therapy.

RISK OF NUTRIENT DEFICIENCY

Certain groups of people may be more at risk of developing nutritional deficiency, including elderly people, pregnant and nursing women, children and adolescents. Some disorders in pregnancy make it difficult for women to meet the nutritional needs of the fetus.

Children and adolescents

Children's nutritional requirements are much greater during phases of rapid growth. Children have small stomachs and can fill up quickly, making it important that they have regular meals which are high-energy and nutrient-dense. Children can become faddy with food, and may benefit from taking spcially formulated multivitamin and multimineral supplements that include Vitamins A, C and D.

Among adolescents, image is often more of a concern than health, and high-sugar, high-fat foods and drinks can replace nutritionally balanced meals. They may also have a significant intake of alcohol and smoke cigarettes. To counter the effects of this they will need antioxidants in their diet and should be encouraged to increase their intake of antioxidant-rich fresh fruit and vegetables. It may also be advisable to take a multivitamin and multimineral supplement.

Elderly people

Research indicates that a significant number of elderly people do not reach the recommended daily allowance for many essential nutrients, particularly, vitamin D. They may be on medication, which can interfere with the body's ability to absorb nutrients, or their digestive system may be inefficient. If you look after elderly people, encourage them to take care with their diet and suggest they take a multimineral and multivitamin supplement.

Alcoholics

People who drink alcohol every day in amounts well beyond recommended levels may develop pancreatic and liver problems, which lead to poor digestion. The body's detoxification processes stop working properly. The effects of alcohol include increased urine production, which leads to the loss of water-soluble nutrients such as minerals and some vitamins. Alcohol also affects the body's metabolism of carbohydrate, fat, protein and sex hormones. Some alcoholics stop eating properly and may suffer from malnutrition for this reason. Taking a multimineral and multivitamin supplement may prevent these problems, but alcoholics should always be encouraged to seek help to overcome their addiction.

Poor nutrition in pregnancy has been shown to cause premature birth and low birthweight, both of which have been linked to a higher risk of serious illness in adult life.

Anorexics and bulimics

People suffering from **anorexia** and **bulimia** have an extremely low intake or retention of all nutrients. In addition, prolonged self-inflicted starvation can cause psychological disturbances. Anorexics and bulimics are extremely anxious about choosing food, and this anxiety leads to impaired digestion. In some cases, it may be appropriate for an anorexic to take multivitamin and multimineral supplements, but it is perhaps most important to address the psychological causes of the illness.

Pregnant and breastfeeding women

Both pregnancy and breastfeeding create an increased need for nutrients, especially protein, essential fatty acids, vitamins and minerals. Some nutritionists estimate that your need for vitamin B complex, vitamin C, calcium, zinc and magnesium rises by more than 30 per cent during pregnancy and breastfeeding and that your general food intake needs to increase by around 15–20 per cent. Your doctor or midwife can give you advice on your diet and whether you would benefit from additional supplements. Nutritious food is essential for the well-being both of the mother and of the fetus.

Nausea caused by changes in hormone levels is usually restricted to the first three months after conception, but in some women it continues throughout pregnancy. Because they feel sick, women eat less – which could mean that they and their baby are not getting enough nutrients.

Another threat to fetal nutrition arises if a mother has iron-deficient anaemia. This condition is caused by low intake or poor absorption of iron and can usually be prevented by consumption of high-iron foods such as dark green vegetables and cocoa. But pregnant women should not eat liver, despite its high iron content, because it also has a high concentration of Vitamin A. Sometimes an iron supplement will be prescribed.

Mothers with a food intolerance may have to limit their diet. Even where no intolerance or allergy exists in the mother, it is possible for an infant to develop an allergy because of diets followed by the mother in pregnancy, or because of allergens contained in the mother's milk.

Deficiency of folate before conception and during the first 12 weeks of pregnancy has been associated with spina bifida in the fetus. Foods rich in folate include wheatgerm, rice germ, black-eye peas, soya flour, kidney beans, asparagus, lentils, spinach, walnuts, oranges and dark green vegetables, such as broccoli, Brussels sprouts and spinach. Many women are advised to take folic acid supplements for three months before conception and during the first months of pregnancy.

Obesity

Food is plentiful in the western world, and a lot of it is much higher in calories than the human body was designed to cope with. So eating more than your body needs is easy – and obesity is becoming more common.

Obesity is life-threatening. Obese people are more likely than others to develop dangerous conditions such as cardiovascular disease, gallbladder diseases and certain cancers. They are also at greater risk if they undergo surgery. The body mass index (BMI), which relates your weight to your height, is used to define obesity – a body mass index of 20–25 is generally defined as healthy, but more than 30 is defined as obese.

Statistics gathered by the Worldwatch Institute in Washington, DC, show that in the United States 23 per cent of adults are obese, 55 per cent are overweight and 20 per cent of children are obese or overweight. The USA is the most obese nation in the world, but the UK is fast catching up: one in five British women and one in six men are obese, with 45 per cent of men and 33 per cent of women being overweight. Obesity is also

increasing among children and teenagers. The scale of the problem was brought into sharp focus by research published in February 2002, which showed that four obese British teenagers had been diagnosed with Type 2 **diabetes**, a form of the disease that occurs when fat and muscle cells lose their sensitivity to insulin. The teenagers were the first white British children to develop the disease. Previously, it had been known only in obese adults and in obese children from ethnic minorities, who are known to be at increased risk for genetic reasons.

BODY WEIGHT AND OBESITY

Most people step on the bathroom scales to check that they are not putting on weight. But the weight of the body only gives part of the story; it is body composition that is important in terms of health. Take, for example, two men of the same height who each weigh around 76kg (12 stones), since muscle tissue is heavier than fat, one could be plump and have a high percentage of body fat, while the other could be lean.

There are several ways of measuring how much of a person's total weight is fat and how much is muscle. Two of these methods – underwater weighing and Duel Energy X-ray Absorptiometry (DEXA) – require equipment usually found only in research laboratories or hospitals. Other methods – such as bioelectrical impedance analysis and skinfold measurements – are less accurate, but more accessible. Bioelectrical impedance analysis, for example, is routinely used by health clubs and fitness centres. It works on the principle that lean tissue is a good conductor while fat causes electrical resistance. A very mild electric current is passed through the body to measure conductivity and the proportion of fat is calculated electronically.

THE LINK TO HEALTH

Research carried out at Loughborough University in 1992 showed that the risk of ill health is closely linked to the percentage of body fat. For women, the percentage that carries least risk was 18–25 per cent body fat, and for men, the figure was 13–18 per cent. But it is also known that the distribution of your body fat is as important

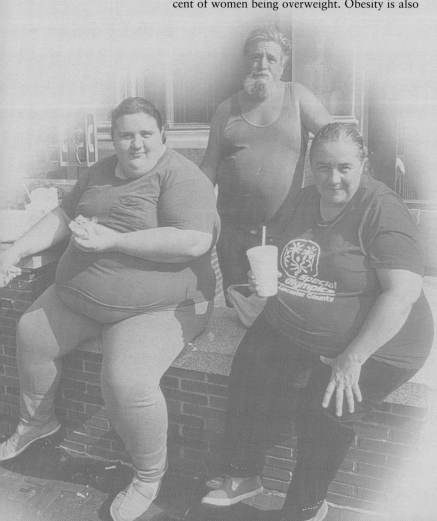

Check your Body Mass Index (BMI)

Locate your height and weight and follow the boxes across and up until they meet. The number shown is the BMI indicator.
For example, a person measuring 1.75m (5ft 9in) and weighing 81.6kg (180lb) has a BMI of 27 – slightly overweight.

HEIGHT m & (ft, in)	45.4 (100)	47.6 (105)	49.9 (110)	52.2 (115)	54.4 (120)	56.7 (125)	59.0 (130)	61.2 (135)	63.5 (140)	65.8 (145)	68.0 (150)	70.3 (155)	72.6 (160)	74.8 (165)	77.1 (170)	79.4 (175)	81.6 (180)	83.9 (185)	86.2 (190)	88.5 (195)	90.7 (200)	93.0 (205)	95.3 (210)	97.5 (215)	99.8 (220)	102.1 (225)	104.3 (230)	106.6 (235)	108.9 (240)	111.1 (245)	113.4 (250)	115.7 (255)	117.9 (260)	120.2 (265)	122.5 (270)	124.7 (275)	127.0 (280)	129.3 (285)	131.5 (290)	133.8 (295)	136.1 (300)
1.93 (6'4")	12	13	13	14	15	15	16	16	17	18	18	19	20	20	21	21	22	23	23	24	24	25	26	26	27	27	28	29	29	30	30	31	32	32	33	34	34	35	35	36	37
1.92 (6'3")	13	13	14	14	15	16	16	17	18	18	19	19	20	21	21	22	23	23	24	24	25	26	26	27	28	28	29	29	30	31	31	32	33	33	34	34	35	36	36	37	38
1.88 (6'2")	13	14	14	15	15	16	17	17	18	19	19	20	21	21	22	23	23	24	24	25	26	26	27	28	28	29	30	30	31	32	32	33	33	34	35	35	36	37	37	38	39
1.85 (6'1")	13	14	15	15	16	17	17	18	19	19	20	20	21	22	22	23	24	24	25	26	26	27	28	28	29	30	30	31	32	32	33	34	34	35	36	36	37	38	38	39	40
1.83 (6'0")	14	14	15	16	16	17	18	18	19	20	20	21	22	22	23	24	24	25	26	27	27	28	29	29	30	31	31	32	33	33	34	35	35	36	37	37	38	39	39	40	41
1.80 (5'11")	14	15	15	16	17	17	18	19	20	20	21	22	22	23	24	24	25	26	27	27	28	29	29	30	31	31	32	33	34	34	35	36	37	37	38	38	39	40	41	41	42
1.78 (5'10")	14	15	16	17	17	18	19	19	20	21	22	22	23	24	24	25	26	27	27	28	29	29	30	31	32	32	33	34	35	35	36	37	37	38	39	40	40	41	42	42	43
1.75 (5'9")	15	16	16	17	18	18	19	20	21	21	22	23	24	24	25	26	27	27	28	29	30	30	31	32	33	33	34	35	36	36	37	38	38	39	40	41	41	42	43	44	44
1.73 (5'8")	15	16	17	18	18	19	20	21	21	22	23	24	24	25	26	27	27	28	29	30	30	31	32	33	34	34	35	36	37	37	38	39	40	40	41	42	43	43	44	45	46
1.70 (5'7")	16	16	17	18	19	20	20	21	22	23	24	24	25	26	27	27	28	29	30	31	31	32	33	34	35	35	36	37	38	38	39	40	41	42	42	43	44	45	46	46	47
1.68 (5'6")	16	17	18	19	19	20	21	22	23	23	24	25	26	27	27	28	29	30	31	32	32	33	34	35	36	37	38	39	40	40	41	42	43	44	44	45	46	47	48	48	49
1.65 (5'5")	17	18	18	19	20	21	22	23	24	25	26	27	28	29	30	31	32	33	34	35	36	37	38	38	39	40	41	42	43	43	44	45	46	47	48	48	49	50			
1.63 (5'4")	17	18	19	20	21	22	22	23	24	25	26	27	28	29	30	31	32	33	34	35	36	37	38	39	40	40	41	42	43	44	45	46	46	47	48	49	50	51	52		
1.60 (5'3")	18	19	20	20	21	22	23	24	25	26	27	28	29	30	31	32	33	34	35	36	36	37	38	39	40	41	42	43	43	44	45	46	47	48	49	50	51	51	52	53	
1.57 (5'2")	18	19	20	21	22	23	24	25	26	27	27	28	29	30	31	32	33	34	35	36	37	38	38	39	40	41	42	43	44	45	46	47	48	49	49	50	51	52	53	54	55
1.55 (5'1")	19	20	21	22	23	24	25	26	27	27	28	29	30	31	32	33	34	35	36	37	38	39	40	41	42	43	44	44	45	46	47	48	49	50	51	52	53	54	55	56	57
1.52 (5'0")	20	21	22	23	23	24	25	26	27	28	29	30	31	32	33	34	35	36	37	38	39	40	41	42	43	44	45	46	47	48	49	50	51	52	53	54	55	56	57	58	59
1.50 (4'11")	20	21	22	23	24	25	26	27	28	29	30	31	32	33	34	35	36	37	38	39	40	41	42	43	44	45	46	47	48	49	50	51	52	53	54	55	56	57	58	59	60
1.47 (4'10")	21	22	23	24	25	26	27	28	29	30	31	32	34	35	36	37	38	39	40	41	42	43	44	45	46	47	48	49	50	51	52	53	54	56	57	58	59	60	61	62	63

WEIGHT kg & (lb)

UNDERWEIGHT	HEALTHY WEIGHT	OVERWEIGHT	OBESE	VERY OBESE

▲ BMI
The Body Mass Index (BMI) is a useful and simple method of classifying body fat content based on the ratio of weight to height squared. Using this calculation, the resulting figure is the BMI indicator (see above).

as the total amount of fat. This distribution is determined partly by genetics and partly by the influence of hormones. Men tend to deposit fat around the abdomen and internal organs (heart and kidneys) and between the shoulder blades. Excess fat in these areas leads to the 'apple' body shape traditionally associated with overweight men. This pattern of fat distribution carries a much bigger risk of heart disease.

Women have higher levels of oestrogen, which promotes the accumulation of fat around the hips, thighs, breasts and upper arms. This gives a 'pear' shape. The fat deposits are less mobile and less easy to shift, but carry a lower health risk. But after the menopause oestrogen levels decline and fat is more likely to be deposited around the abdomen, increasing women's risk of developing heart disease and Type 2 diabetes.

WHY PEOPLE ARE OBESE
Your basic body shape, like all your physical characteristics, is inherited from your parents. But the extent to which obesity is genetically determined is not clear. It has long been known

that there is a gene that triggers obesity in mice and in 1994 a similar gene was identified in human beings. Exactly how this gene operates is the subject of intense research – it does not follow that if you have the gene you will become obese, and that if you don't have it you won't. What is known is that only 25 per cent of very obese people can blame their genes for the condition. In fact, the UK as a nation is getting much fatter much more quickly than can be accounted for by genetics alone.

The metabolic rate
Your metabolic rate is the speed at which your body can burn energy. It has long been assumed that thin people have a high metabolic rate, while fat people have a sluggish rate, which makes it easier for excess calories to be deposited as fat. Studies carried out at the Dunn Nutrition Centre in Cambridge were designed to test this. Groups of fat and thin people were given an extra 1250 calories above their normal daily requirements. After 42 days, the fat group had put on weight – but so had the lean group. In addition, the individuals who were originally overweight were

found to have a higher metabolic rate than the thin people. This means that they burned calories at a faster rate than the thin people. The irony is that overweight individuals need more calories. They have more muscle tissue and the body uses more energy to move a heavier weight compared with a light one.

Your metabolic rate naturally declines as you get older. The rate is at its fastest at around the age of 25 and then gradually slows down. After the age of 30, we need to consume 50 calories less a day in order to maintain our weight. Part of the reason for this decline in metabolic rate is the loss of muscle mass that comes with ageing. This can be prevented by regular exercise including toning or strengthening routines to retain muscle mass.

Some women going through the menopause gain weight while on **hormone replacement therapy** (HRT). However, HRT does not affect a woman's metabolic rate. At menopause, the metabolic rate often decreases naturally; in addition, many women take less exercise as they get older, so weight gain is inevitable. Similarly, some women on the Pill find that they gain weight. Again, research has shown that the Pill itself has no effect on the metabolic rate.

Lack of exercise and diet

Lack of exercise is a major cause of obesity in the Western world. The UK National Food Survey, carried out in 2000, showed that total energy intake had decreased in the decade 1990–2000 and yet the number of obese children and adults had risen. The main reason for this was reduced general activity and exercise.

Eating patterns have also changed. Food manufacturers have responded to the needs of people with busy lives by producing highly processed fast foods and snacks. It is easier to grab these and eat them quickly than to spend time preparing a healthy meal. Such highly refined foods are usually concentrated sources of calories and low in nutrients. Unrefined foods such as fresh fruits and vegetables and whole grains, which are as close as possible to their natural state, are filling, nutritious and more difficult to overeat.

It takes time to become obese, and successful treatment is also a long-term process. Part of the treatment must involve understanding the reasons for the weight gain: genetic factors, lack of activity, snacking habits or comfort eating.

If you are overweight, a doctor can refer you to a qualified dietitian who will examine the causes of your weight gain and develop an all-embracing approach to lifestyle and dietary changes with you. Only in very serious cases will a doctor consider other approaches, such as jaw wiring, stomach stapling and drugs.

Losing weight the healthy way

Small, short-term goals are much easier to achieve than grand designs. Set yourself reachable targets, and reward yourself as you meet each one.

Do

✔ Keep a food diary. For at least three consecutive days, write down what and how much you eat, when and with whom. The information will make you more aware of your eating habits.

✔ Set a target. A steady loss of not more than 1kg (1–2lb) per week is healthy. High rates of weight loss often mean that muscle tissue rather than fat is being lost.

✔ Find out what works for you. Some people find low-fat diets to be very effective, while for others low-carbohydrate diets work better.

✔ Limit your consumption of alcoholic drinks to recommended levels (see **Alcohol and abuse**).

✔ Combine your diet with an increase in physical activity – such as taking a 30-minute brisk walk each day. But check with your doctor before starting a new form of exercise.

Don't

✗ Be tempted to follow a quick-fix diet programme, based on milkshakes instead of meals, herbal tablets or strange and limited combinations of foods (such as the cabbage-soup or boiled-eggs-and-beetroot diet). You may lose weight, but you will put it on again.

✗ Eat processed or synthetic foods. Include in your diet wholefoods such as brown rice, wholemeal bread, brown pasta, fresh vegetables and fruit.

✗ Rely on diet or light versions of foods such as low-fat margarine, yoghurt or cheese, low-sugar fizzy drinks, 'lite' breads, or low-calorie chocolate, biscuits, cakes or soups.

✗ Give up. A slow and steady weight loss is better for you than a dramatic fall, and you are more likely to keep off those unwanted pounds.

DRUGS THAT COMBAT OBESITY

A number of slimming drugs have been developed that aim either to suppress appetite or to interfere with the body's absorption of nutrients. Fenfluramine-based appetite-suppressants were withdrawn after they were linked with heart-valve abnormalities.

Sibutramine acts on the central nervous system to suppress the appetite, but unwanted side effects include insomnia, mood changes and raised blood pressure. Another drug, orlistat, interferes with fat-digesting enzymes. Orlistat has to be taken as part of a low-fat diet; otherwise, it has unpleasant side effects including a bloated and painful stomach and oily diarrhoea.

Other drugs designed to act directly on the metabolism of fat are currently being developed. The so-called Advanced Obesity Drug (AOD) acts on the body's fat cells to enhance the breakdown of stored fats and inhibit the synthesis of new fat – similar to the slimming effects of physical exercise. The drug is undergoing clinical trials and could be on the market in 2005.

SEE ALSO *Blood pressure and problems; Diabetes; Heart and circulatory system*

Obsessions and compulsions

Obsessions are repetitive thoughts or ideas that are distressing or frightening. They seem to force themselves into the mind, making the affected person anxious and fearful. Examples of obsessions are worrying excessively about death, germs or illness, fearing there is going to be a disaster, or fretting that you may cause harm to others. Sufferers cannot control these thoughts, even though they may know them to be absurd or unrealistic.

Sometimes, the anxiety caused by obsessions can only be relieved by performing a particular action or ritual to ward off imagined danger. These rituals are called compulsions because sufferers cannot stop themselves performing them. Examples of compulsion are excessive cleaning, counting, checking, measuring, and repetition of tasks or actions. But the relief from anxiety provided by such actions is temporary – the obsessive thoughts always return.

WHAT IS AN OBSESSION?

Minor obsessions and compulsions, such as the urge to count or check, are common and are experienced by around 80 per cent of the population. We all worry sometimes about whether the gas is turned off, or the door locked. Many of us have everyday rituals we perform without thinking, such as throwing spilt salt over our left shoulder, touching wood or avoiding the path of a black cat. And many people have some small compulsive behaviour such as insisting that books are arranged in a particular way on a shelf.

The distinction between obsessions and compulsions and ordinary, everyday behaviour is one of degree. If our thoughts or actions are not causing anxiety or disrupting our life, they are not a problem. Help is only needed when obsessions and rituals severely impede normal life – for example, if checking rituals mean it takes an hour to leave the house. Compulsions can also lead to physical problems, such as chapped skin through excessive handwashing.

Obsessions differ from addictions – to gambling or alcohol, for example. Addicted people are physically or psychologically dependent on a substance or activity; they 'need' it to feel normal. Obsessions, by contrast, are not something the sufferer seeks, but a thing to be feared – they are unwanted thoughts that force their way into the mind.

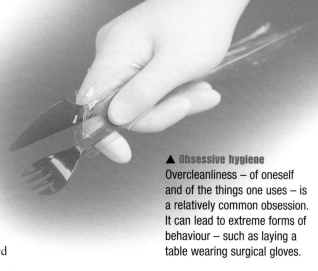

▲ **Obsessive hygiene**
Overcleanliness – of oneself and of the things one uses – is a relatively common obsession. It can lead to extreme forms of behaviour – such as laying a table wearing surgical gloves.

OBSESSIVE-COMPULSIVE DISORDER

Obsessions and compulsions often go together, but not always. A doctor may diagnose you as having obsessive-compulsive disorder if you experience obsessions or compulsions, or both, to such a degree that it affects your everyday life or causes you distress.

A classic example of obsessive-compulsive disorder is a man with an obsession about cleanliness who believes that his hands are contaminated. This recurring thought will compel him to wash his hands needlessly hundreds of times a day. Other sufferers may spend hours each day dressing or undressing or going up and down stairs. They are compelled to repeat these actions by the fear that it was not done properly the last time.

Obsessive-compulsive disorder is an anxiety disorder and has similar symptoms to **phobia,** including rapid heartbeat, churning stomach, dizziness, shortness of breath, sweating and trembling. Most people can relate to the fears that cause phobias, but many are unable to understand the anxieties that underlie obsessive-compulsive disorder. A fear of being confined in enclosed spaces (claustrophobia), for example, is more widely understood than an obsessive concern with cleanliness. But sufferers cannot avoid their recurring obsessional thoughts in the way that people with claustrophobia can avoid enclosed spaces. Children can also experience obsessive-compulsive disorder, with a problem often starting at the age of four or five.

CAUSES

There are many theories as to what causes obsessions and compulsions. Some experts believe they stem from childhood experiences – sexual abuse or obsessional behaviour by parents can often lead to fears or anxiety as an adult. Memories of traumatic events may also trigger obsessive-compulsive behaviour.

Personality may well also play a role – people who are by nature perfectionists are perhaps more prone to obsessions. Chemical changes in the brain have also been blamed but there is disagreement among experts about this.

TREATMENT

There is no immediate cure for obsessions and compulsions. But there are things you can do to help yourself to overcome them. The vital first step is to seek help. Your doctor may refer you to a psychologist or a psychiatrist. You may be given talking treatments, drugs or a combination of both. Alternatively you may prefer to seek help outside the NHS from a private therapist, or from a self-help or support group.

Talking treatments

Behaviour therapy and cognitive behaviour therapy help sufferers to develop practical skills to manage their thoughts and behaviour. Psychologists use this approach to help people to face their fears and reduce their rituals. Some people find relief through a combination of behaviour therapy and low doses of medication.

Psychotherapy and counselling aim to help you to look for the causes of your problems, as well as to develop coping strategies. It is not always useful for people with obsessions or compulsions to look for reasons, but different things work for different people. This type of treatment is available on the NHS, privately or through voluntary organizations.

> Between one and three per cent of the UK population may have symptoms of obsessive-compulsive disorder, but only the worst affected seek help.

Medication

Medication can help on its own, or when used alongside other treatments. Tranquillizers may be prescribed in the short term to reduce anxiety, but they can be addictive in the long term. Antidepressants called selective serotonin reuptake inhibitors (SSRIs) can help to relieve any depression that is making behaviour therapy more difficult. They can, however, take several weeks to work. The disadvantage is that most of these drugs have unwanted side effects.

Psychosurgery

Psychosurgery involves surgery to remove minute areas of brain tissue that are thought to affect emotional control. It seems to have little benefit and is now rarely used. But it has been used in severe cases of obsessive-compulsive disorder if all other treatments have been unsuccessful.

SEE ALSO *Mental health and problems; Phobia*

Occupational therapy

Occupational therapy is a programme of mental or physical activity to assist people who are disabled or recovering from disease or injury. It can help people to get the most out of their lives when, for whatever reason, they are unable to carry out everyday tasks.

Occupational therapists work with people who have physical, mental or social problems, regardless of whether the problem has been from birth or is the result of an accident, illness or ageing. The purpose of occupational therapy is to work out what people want need and want to do for themselves in their daily lives, and to maximize their ability to achieve this; however, it may not always be possible to achieve or restore all the function they may desire.

WHAT'S INVOLVED

To establish exactly what the individual person wants to achieve, the occupational therapist begins with a thorough assessment of his or her needs and lifestyle. The therapist also seeks to establish the reason why a person is unable to perform certain tasks. He or she may then adapt the living or working environment of the person, teach different ways of coping with particular difficulties, or recommend therapeutic activities to improve coordination, concentration or strength. For example, a person who has suffered a **stroke** may learn woodwork in order to re-establish good muscle control.

Treatment is always tailored to the individual and a large proportion of the occupational therapist's work will take place in a person's

---

Self-help

Dealing with obsessive behaviour

There are several things you can do to help yourself to cope with your fears:

■ Talk to someone you trust about your fears; this will make those fears feel less powerful and overwhelming.

■ Share your experiences and ways of coping with other people who have similar problems. Find out about self-help or support groups from the organizations listed at the end of this book.

■ Use relaxation techniques to help rid your body and mind of tension and improve your breathing. Books and tapes will enable you to follow your own programme at home.

If you know someone who suffers from obsessive-compulsive disorder, you can help:

■ Try to give sympathetic support: sufferers may find it hard to talk about fears and may feel that their thoughts are unacceptable. Accept that their fears are real for affected people, and don't try to reason with them or talk them out of it.

■ Contact a voluntary organization for information, or help a person work through a self-help programme.

■ Accept that caring for someone with obsessive-compulsive disorder can be distressing, and ask for help if you need it.

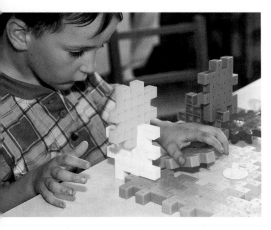

▲ Play therapy
Occupational therapists may use play to help a child to overcome neurological or physical problems.

own home or work environment. Making simple adjustments such as repositioning furniture and equipment, or changing its height, can make a significant difference to someone's independence.

As a person's level of functioning improves, the occupational therapist will focus on other aspects of life – for example, meal preparation, leisure and social interests, or employment opportunities.

Since recovery rates vary, the occupational therapist will design a personalized treatment plan, based on the individual person's lifestyle and ability.

Where occupational therapists work

Occupational therapists combine medical and social care, working in a variety of different settings. These may include:
- the patient's home;
- GP practices, health and day centres;
- social services departments;
- hospitals;
- residential and nursing homes;
- industrial and commercial organizations;
- charities and voluntary organizations;
- the prison service.

HOW IT CAN HELP

When people first come into contact with occupational therapy, they may be surprised at the ordinariness of the activities they are working on; everyday tasks that are normally taken for granted, such as making tea and getting dressed, may be a starting point. But as the occupational therapy sessions develop, clients begin to realize the real significance that achieving these ordinary everyday activities can have on their health and well-being.

Occupational therapy can be a stressful and emotional experience for people who are trying to perform activities that they find difficult, and perhaps embarrassing. They are not just relearning basic skills, but are having to confront their own limitations and may be struggling with extremes of hope and despair. They need to be prepared to become fully involved both mentally and physically.

People that benefit from occupational therapy include those suffering from:
- long-term physical disability;
- disability as a result of accident;
- stroke;
- learning disabilities;
- mental disorders.

SEE ALSO *Physiotherapy*

Oedema

Oedema is an abnormal collection of fluid (mainly water) that has leaked from the circulatory system and accumulated in an area of the body's tissues. It is most commonly seen around the ankles – due to the force of gravity – but can also appear in other parts of the body, especially in the spaces in the lungs and around the abdominal cavity. It may be the result of an injury, but it also occurs as a symptom of diseases of the circulatory, respiratory and urinary systems.

SYMPTOMS

The symptoms of oedema are puffiness and swelling of the tissues, either localized or generalized. When you press an affected area with your finger, the indentation will only slowly return to normal as the fluid seeps back.

DURATION

Depending on the cause, oedema may last for a few days only or much longer.

CAUSES
- **Heart failure.**
- Kidney failure (see **Kidneys and disorders**).
- **Nephrotic syndrome.**
- **Cirrhosis of the liver** (the most common cause is alcoholism).
- Reactions to certain drugs, such as corticosteroids and oral contraceptives.
- Injury.
- Pre-eclampsia in pregnancy.

TREATMENT

Oedema is treated by the use of diuretic drugs, which will increase the amount of urination, and by correcting the cause, if possible. When a large amount of fluid accumulates in the abdomen, for example, the fluid may sometimes be drained out through a tube. This procedure can be carried out painlessly with the use of a local **anaesthetic**.

When to consult a doctor

If you notice any unexplained swelling of limbs or respiratory pain or problems.

What a doctor may do
- Determine the cause of the oedema and then treat the underlying condition.
- Prescribe diuretic drugs and reduce salt intake to make the kidneys produce more urine and so excrete the excess fluid.

What you can do

This will depend on what is causing the oedema; for swollen ankles, for example, you should try to rest with your feet raised above heart level.

COMPLICATIONS

Oedema of the lungs can become so serious that the person literally drowns in his or her own body fluid. It needs urgent treatment.

Oesophagus and disorders

The oesophagus is also known as the gullet. It is the muscular tube that connects the back of the throat with the stomach. It lies at the back of the chest beside the windpipe and just in front of the spine. Muscular valves at both ends, called sphincters, open to allow food and drink to pass. As food is chewed it is directed towards the back of the throat. The process of swallowing closes the epiglottis over the windpipe to prevent food and drink entering the lungs. Meanwhile, cells on the inner lining of the oesophagus produce mucus that helps to ease the food into the digestive system. Muscles in the oesophageal wall contract in waves to move the food along – this process is called peristalsis.

WHAT CAN GO WRONG

Swallowing difficulties, chest pain, **heartburn** and regurgitation of acidic stomach juices into the oesophagus are the most common symptoms of oesophageal disorders in general.

Oesophagitis

Oesophagitis is inflammation of the oesophagus due to gastro-oesophageal reflux. It is one of the most common complaints reported to GPs. Abdominal pressure, as a result of overeating, for example, or a weakness of the lower sphincter, as a result of a hiatus **hernia**, can lead to oesophagitis. Other, less common causes include bacterial, viral or fungal infections, surgery and exposure to caustic substances.

Symptoms include heartburn, difficulty swallowing, mild fever and even joint pain. A diagnosis is made using **endoscopy** (in which a flexible tube containing optical fibres is inserted into the oesophagus and transmits images onto a screen). **X-rays** and **biopsy** may also be used to diagnose oesophagitis. Treatment is aimed at the underlying cause, and a drug may be prescribed to reduce acid production in the stomach. If left untreated, oesophagitis may lead to acute inflammation, stricture (see below), ulceration, scarring or Barrett's oesophagus.

Oesophageal varices

Oesophageal varices are dilated veins surrounding the lower end of the oesophagus. Varices are the result of increased pressure within the hepatic portal vein in the liver, which is often due to excessive alcohol consumption (see **Liver and disorders**). Increased pressure in the hepatic portal vein, which carries blood to the liver from the digestive tract, has a knock-on effect, increasing blood flow through other veins in the digestive system. The lower oesophageal veins are most likely to be affected. Increased pressure may cause the thin walls of the veins to rupture, leading to vomiting blood (which is potentially fatal), and black stools. Symptoms of severe liver disease may also be present. X-rays and endoscopy are used to confirm the diagnosis.

As an emergency measure, a balloon catheter can be inserted into the oesophagus. In the longer term, drug therapy includes the use of vasopressin, a synthetic hormone that narrows blood vessels, and sclerosants, which seal off the affected veins. Liver surgery may be needed.

Oesophageal stricture

Narrowing of the oesophagus can occur due to oesophagitis and other oesophageal disorders, such as gastro-oesophageal reflux, infections and swallowing caustic substances. Symptoms include difficulty in swallowing and loss of weight. Treatment may involve widening the oesophagus using a balloon catheter. This is inserted into the oesophagus and inflated for a short time. Once the oesophagus is widened the

Epiglottis
When food and drink are swallowed, the epiglottis closes the windpipe.

Oesophagus
Food and drink are moved down the oesophagus by a process called peristalsis.

High speed
Once it is swallowed, food takes 6–8 seconds to reach the stomach.

The food pipe
The oesophagus is a muscular tube – 23–30cm (8–12in) long in adults – that leads from the throat to the stomach. It is lined with mucous membranes, which lubricate food as it travels to the stomach.

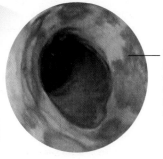

Oesophagitis
Inflammation of the oesophagus is most commonly due to acid regurgitation from the stomach.

balloon is deflated and then withdrawn; the procedure is repeated later using a larger balloon. When a stricture is severe and extensive, it is removed surgically and either replaced with a segment of the colon or by part of the stomach, which is drawn up into a tube.

Oesophageal atresia

Oesophageal atresia is a rare, but serious developmental abnormality in which the oesophagus is either narrowed or blind-ended in both directions. Babies diagnosed with this condition usually have immediate surgery. It affects one in 2500 births in the UK, and is linked with other digestive or heart disorders.

Oesophageal diverticulum

Oesophageal diverticulum is a relatively rare condition in which a pouch forms in the oesophageal wall. There are two types. Traction pouches occur in the mid-gullet; symptoms are rare and treatment not usually necessary. Pulsion pouches occur below the upper sphincter. If this does not relax properly during swallowing, the throat muscles continue working, which causes the gullet's lining to be pushed through its wall. The pouch grows as food becomes trapped in it, causing swallowing difficulties, **halitosis** and regurgitation. A **barium investigation** is carried out to confirm diagnosis, and the pouches removed surgically.

Oesophageal spasm

Oesophageal spasm is an uncommon condition that causes erratic contractions of the oesophageal muscles, with the result that food cannot be swallowed properly. There may also be pain in the chest and abdomen. The cause is often unknown, although other oesophageal disorders may be associated with the problem. The spasms are more common in women and occur in one in 1000 people in the UK.

An endoscopy is performed to check whether any specific disorder is causing the spasms, and barium investigations can be used to view them. Treatment is aimed at any underlying cause, and may involve taking muscle-relaxant drugs.

Oesophageal cancer

A malignant tumour may grow from the lining of the oesophagus, making it progressively harder to swallow. Oesophageal cancer is the third most common type of cancer in the digestive tract, and is more frequent in men over 50. The risk is increased by alcohol consumption, and gastro-oesophageal reflux. Oesophageal cancer often has no symptoms until it has reached an advanced stage so the prognosis is usually poor. But the cancer can be surgically removed if caught early enough.

There are two types of oesophageal cancer. Squamous carcinoma starts in the squamous (skin-like) cells that make up the lining of the

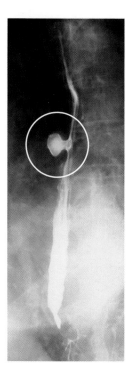

▲ **Diverticulum**
A diverticulum forms when the lining of the oesophagus bulges out through a weak point in the wall.

oesophagus and mainly occurs in the upper two-thirds section. In this condition, the cells lining the oesophagus change to look more like the cells lining the stomach. Adenocarcinoma occurs lower down. Adenocarcinomas are associated with Barrett's oesophagus, in which stomach cells replace squamous cells.

As the tumour grows, swallowing difficulties increase so that even fluids are hard to get down. Loss of weight, choking and chest complaints are common symptoms. A barium investigation, endoscopy and biopsy are used to investigate the extent of blockage and damage.

It is most important that treatment is given as early in the tumour's development as possible. In the UK, this usually involves surgery in which the affected section of the oesophagus is removed together with the surrounding lymph glands. A tube is then made out of the stomach and drawn up into the chest or neck, where it is joined to the remainder of the oesophagus.

Radiotherapy and **chemotherapy** are used in conjunction with, or as an alternative to, surgery, and endoscopic laser treatment may also be used. A new therapy, photodynamic therapy, may also prove effective. In this treatment the patient is given chemicals that react to certain types of light; this can then be activated to destroy the cancer cells.

Surveillance programmes for oesophageal cancer have been established in the UK in an attempt to identify precancerous changes and enable treatment before the disease develops. **SEE ALSO** *Digestive system*

Oliguria

Oliguria is abnormally low urine output – less than 300ml (10fl oz) of urine per day. It is most often a sign of kidney disease or of an obstruction affecting normal **urinary** flow. But the condition may also be due to poor fluid intake, excess sweating (in a hot climate, for example), low blood pressure, or having lost a large volume of fluid (through haemorrhage, for example). These factors trigger a fall in urinary output in order to conserve body water.

Onchocerciasis

Onchocerciasis is a tropical disease of the skin caused by larvae of the parasitic worm Onchocerca volvulus, which are transmitted to human beings by the black simulium fly. If the dead remnants of this worm pass to the eye they can cause partial or total blindness, a disease known as river **blindness** in Africa.

Ophthalmia neonatorum

Ophthalmia neonatorum, also known as neonatal conjunctivitis, causes swelling of the eyelids in a newborn baby and a discharge of yellow pus. It is caused by a bacterial infection and can be transmitted to the baby's eyes from the mother's vagina during birth if she has a sexually transmitted infection, such as **chlamydia** or **gonorrhoea**.

Optic neuritis

Optic neuritis is an inflammation of the optic nerve. If the inflammation affects the part of the nerve that reaches the eyeball, it is called optic papillitis. When the part of the nerve behind the eye is affected, it is known as retrobulbar neuritis. The condition affects young adults and may be triggered by a temperature change – a hot bath, for example.

Symptoms of both types include a reduction in the colour of objects, which look washed out, followed by a rapid reduction in vision. Eye movement may cause discomfort and pupil reactions are slow. In retrobulbar neuritis, there is more likely to be pain when the eye moves.

The condition usually resolves within weeks, although there may be some optic atrophy, with reduced vision and field of vision.

In some cases, retrobulbar neuritis may be an early symptom of **multiple sclerosis**.

SEE ALSO **Eye and problems**

Orchitis

Orchitis is inflammation of one or, more rarely, both testes, usually as a result of a bacterial or viral infection. Common causes include **mumps** – approximately one in four men who catch mumps develop orchitis – and **sexually transmitted** infections such as chlamydia and gonorrhea. In epididymo-orchitis, the epididymis – the sperm-carrying tube attached to the testes – is also affected.

SYMPTOMS
- Swelling in the scrotum, testicle or groin area.
- Pain and a sense of heaviness in the testicle.
- Pain when urinating or ejaculating.
- Discharge from the penis.
- High temperature and fever.

TREATMENT
Men concerned they may have orchitis should consult their GP promptly so that more serious conditions can be ruled out. The doctor will perform a physical examination and may order urine and blood tests to help with diagnosis.

Doctors may prescribe antibiotics in the case of a bacterial infection and recommend painkillers in the case of a viral one. They will also advise the use of a support bandage and ice packs on the affected areas and, ideally, bed rest. If the infection was sexually transmitted, sexual partners should also be treated.

PREVENTION
Two measures reduce the risk of orchitis:
- immunization against mumps;
- using barrier contraceptives such as condoms to prevent sexually transmitted diseases.

COMPLICATIONS
Orchitis may cause shrinkage of the testes or, more rarely, **infertility** (which may not be permanent).

OUTLOOK
The symptoms of orchitis generally improve within a week to ten days.

SEE ALSO **Testicles and disorders**

Osteochondritis

Osteochondritis is an inflammation of bone and cartilage at a joint, which results in pain, swelling and constricted movement. It mainly affects young adults and is thought to be caused by an impairment to the blood supply to the area affected. The most commonly affected joints are the knees and elbows, and the only treatment is rest until the inflammation has gone. The problem tends to run in families.

SEE ALSO **Bone and problems; Joints and problems; Skeletal system**

Osteomyelitis

Osteomyelitis is an infection of the bone marrow. The disease is most common in children, especially boys. It affects the long bones of the leg or arm, causing inflammation and pain in the area, and a sudden high temperature. Sometimes a joint next to the affected bone swells and stiffens.

Osteomyelitis is usually caused by the bacteria *Staphylococcus aureus* or salmonella, which get into the bloodstream via a **boil**, cut or skin infection, or enter the bone through a **fracture**.

If the disease is not treated promptly, there is a risk of blood poisoning (septicaemia). Also, the inflammation may block blood vessels inside the bone, depriving an area of bone of blood and oxygen. This can impair bone growth which, in a child, may mean that one limb ends up shorter than the other. Weakness in the affected bone can make further fractures much more likely.

TREATMENT

Intensive antibiotic treatment is needed to stop the condition becoming long-term (chronic) when abscesses may form and cause severe bone damage. Treatment of osteomyelitis is aimed at killing the infecting bacteria and saving the affected bone. As well as antibiotics, which are given via an intravenous drip, it involves:

- bed rest in hospital;
- sometimes, splints on the affected bone;
- in serious cases, surgery to drain any pus and so relieve pain.

COMPLICATIONS

The chronic form of osteomyelitis can develop. The infected bone becomes thicker because it contains pus and dead bone tissue. There may be an open wound on the skin surface, discharging pus, but this may heal up intermittently though not permanently.

Osteopathy

Osteopathy is one of the most respected and widely used **complementary therapies**, particularly for musculo-skeletal problems and back pain. Osteopaths seek to improve the mobility of the joints and soft tissues by using physical manipulation and massage.

The therapy was originally developed in the late 1880s by Andrew Taylor Still, a medical doctor. Still believed that medicine should offer more than drugs, and advocated the use of a physical manipulative treatment for which he coined the name 'osteopathy'.

Still identified the musculo-skeletal system as a key element of health. He also emphasized the body's ability to heal itself and the importance of preventive medicine, eating properly and keeping fit.

Osteopaths believe that if a person's joints and muscles are correctly aligned and working properly, all the body's systems will function well, and the body will be healthy. But **stress**, both physical and emotional, injury or poor posture can adversely affect the muscles and skeleton, causing pain and affecting nerves – either locally, where the original difficulty is, or elsewhere in the body.

WHO IT CAN HELP

Osteopathy is often used for back pain, neck pain, sports injuries, headaches, sciatica, painful periods, repetitive strain injury, digestive problems and asthma. In Britain, one in three doctors refer their patients to osteopaths, usually for musculo-skeletal problems.

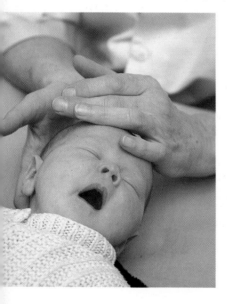

▼ Soothing therapy
Cranial osteopathy can be used on very young babies to help with problems such as extreme restlessness and infantile colic.

WHAT'S INVOLVED

When you visit an osteopath for the first time a full medical history will be taken and you will be examined. You will probably be asked to take off some of your clothing and to carry out a simple set of movements. The osteopath will then use a touch technique, called palpation, to identify any points of weakness or excessive strain in your body. He or she may also require additional investigations such as an **X-ray** or a blood test. This will allow a full diagnosis so that a treatment plan can be developed for you.

To help to realign the body, an osteopath can use a range of techniques. These include massage; gentle manipulation; vigorous joint manipulation, using short sharp pushes; and visceral manipulation, in which the osteopath uses touch to locate and relieve a problem in an internal organ such as the liver. Other important techniques involve lifts and stretches to open up or decompress the spine; and muscle release techniques, which involve the patient pushing against specific resistance provided by the osteopath.

The first consultation usually takes between half-an-hour and an hour. Thereafter, sessions will last about 20 or 30 minutes.

SAFETY

You should not have any vigorous manipulation if you have a badly prolapsed disc. Also, avoid any osteopathic treatment if you have a bone or joint infection, or suffer from bone cancer.

Osteopathy is totally safe for women who are pregnant: it can help the body to adjust to its changing posture and is useful for treating any back problems that may occur during the pregnancy and postnatally.

CRANIAL OSTEOPATHY

Cranial osteopathy is sometimes called paediatric osteopathy, because it is especially suitable for young babies and children. The technique developed from the discovery in the 1930s that small tolerances of movement exist within the human skull.

The technical approach used involves extremely gentle, but specifically applied adjustments of the skull and spinal bones. The adjustments can barely be felt but they affect the pressure and the natural pulse of the cerebrospinal fluid that bathes both the spinal cord and brain.

Osteopaths using this approach can help with a wide range of conditions, including certain cases of **glue ear**, **migraine**, dizziness and the after-effects of difficult or prolonged deliveries, as well as orthopaedic and spinal conditions for which other, more vigorous osteopathic techniques would be inappropriate.

SEE ALSO **Chiropractic**

Osteoporosis

The bone disorder osteoporosis is becoming increasingly common as people live longer and lead more sedentary lifestyles. Women are most at risk of the disease – but one in 12 men in the UK suffers from it, too.

Bones are not solid. They are composed of a thick, compact outer shell and a strong inner bony mesh – rather like the struts and girders that support the weight of a tall building beneath its façade.

Throughout life, our bone mass is continually being eaten away – releasing calcium into the bloodstream – and replaced. When we are young, the bone is replaced as quickly as it is used, but as we grow older, we lose more calcium from our bones than we put back and the strong honeycomb mesh inside becomes less dense and therefore weaker. In osteoporosis – which means porous bones – the bones become weak and brittle so that sufferers are vulnerable to fractures even after minor falls. The areas most at risk are the hips, wrists and spine.

PREVENTING OSTEOPOROSIS

To help to prevent osteoporosis it is essential to build strong, healthy bones during childhood and adolescence. Although your genes determine the potential height and strength of your skeleton, lifestyle factors can influence the amount of bone you invest in your bone 'bank' during your youth and how much you save in later life.

Bones need a calcium-rich diet that is well balanced and incorporates minerals and vitamins from different food groups. Dietary levels of calcium during adolescence are especially important for maximum bone density and strength in adulthood. The best sources of calcium are milk and dairy products, such as cheese and yoghurt. Non-dairy sources include green leafy vegetables, baked beans, bony fish and dried fruit.

The body also needs vitamin D in order to absorb calcium. The main source of this vitamin is sunlight on the skin, but it is also found in eggs and oily fish, and in some fortified breakfast cereals and margarines.

Exercise is vital. In common with muscles and other parts of the body, bones suffer if they are not used. They need regular weight-bearing exercise that exerts a loading impact and works the muscles, stimulating bone to strengthen. Good bone-building exercises include running, skipping,

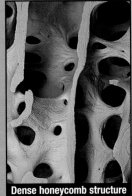

UNDER THE MICROSCOPE

The difference in these pictures shows why bones weakened by osteoporosis break so easily. Healthy bone mass has degenerated into a fragile latticework that will crumble on impact.

Dense honeycomb structure

Weak honeycomb structure

Risk factors for osteoporosis

Low oestrogen levels in women increase the risk of osteoporosis, as the hormone slows down the rate of bone loss. Other factors also increase risk.

- Close family history of osteoporosis.
- Early menopause or hysterectomy including the removal of ovaries before the age of 45.
- Long-term use of corticosteroid drugs for health problems such as asthma and arthritis.
- Low body weight, which puts less stress on bones – stress on bones increases their density.
- Missing periods for six months or more as a result of too much exercise or excessive dieting – such as in female athletes or women with **anorexia nervosa.**
- Smoking, which hampers oestrogen production.
- Excessive alcohol and salt consumption, because these hasten calcium loss.
- Low testosterone levels in men.

aerobics, tennis and brisk walking. Try to exercise for a minimum of 20 minutes at least three times a week. People who have osteoporosis should also take exercise because this will help to prevent further mineral loss from the bones. It will also improve strength, muscle tone and balance, making the chances of falling less likely.

Smoking has a toxic effect on bone in men and women. Because it also interferes with oestrogen production, it can cause women to have an early menopause and may increase the risk of hip fracture in later life. Stopping smoking will help your bones and your general health and fitness.

Drinking too much alcohol damages bone turnover. It is best to limit your alcohol intake to a weekly maximum of 28 units for men and 21 units for women. Diets high in protein and salt also contribute to calcium loss, so reducing your intake of both can also help.

SYMPTOMS

Often there are no symptoms and osteoporosis is discovered only when a bone is fractured.

Warning signs can include back pain, pain in the hip joints, loss of height and sometimes a stooped posture as weakened bones in the spine become compressed. Osteoporosis is permanent and progressive unless treated.

Around 3 million people in the UK suffer from osteoporosis and the number is growing. Of people aged 50 or over, one in three women and one in 12 men are affected by the disease. Women have a much higher risk of osteoporosis because they have less bone mass to begin with and, at menopause, they lose the protective effect of the hormone oestrogen, which slows bone loss. Younger women with low oestrogen levels can also suffer from osteoporosis.

TREATMENT

The medical treatment of osteoporosis aims to slow down or stop the bones from getting weaker.

When to consult a doctor

If you have broken a bone easily, you may need surgery. Your doctor will then want to talk to you about the possibility of osteoporosis. You should also see the doctor if you have back pain and fall into one of the risk categories (see Risk factors box). Early detection and treatment of osteoporosis can slow down its progress.

What a doctor may do

Your doctor will probably arrange for you to have a bone density scan. Known as a dual X-ray absorptiometry (DXA) scan, this is a reliable means of assessing the strength of bones. DXA machines are usually used to scan several bones in the lower spine and one hip, two of the main areas at risk from osteoporotic fractures. Other bones, however, can also be assessed, using this procedure, including the forearm and the heel. The technique is painless and uses a low radiation dose, similar to natural background radiation. It takes between 10 and 20 minutes.

You may also be referred to a specialist – an endocrinologist for hormone problems such as low oestrogen levels, or a rheumatologist for back pain, for example. A number of sessions with a physiotherapist may be recommended to help improve your mobility following a fracture.

Your doctor might prescribe painkillers and possibly calcium and vitamin D supplements, or biphosphonates to halt bone loss. He or she may also wish to discuss **hormone replacement therapy**, or an alternative therapy known as selective oestrogen receptor modulators or SERMs. A synthetic hormone, calcitonin, is also sometimes prescribed.

Osteoporosis is not, in itself, painful. However, broken bones cause a lot of pain in the short term and discomfort and disability in the long term. A break usually takes between six and eight weeks to heal, and if you have fractured your wrist, hip or spine, you may be in a lot of pain. You will be prescribed painkilling drugs and may also find heat pads (for muscle relaxation), ice packs (to reduce inflammation) and **TENS** (transcutaneous electrical nerve stimulation) helpful.

The effects of drugs and supplements

Biphosphonates are non-hormonal substances that improve bone density by slowing down the rate at which bone is lost, helping the bone-building cells to work more efficiently.

Calcium and vitamin D supplements have been shown to benefit older people as they can reduce the risk of breaking a hip.

Calcitonin is a hormone made by the thyroid gland. It prevents the cells that break down bone from working properly, improving the action of the bone-building cells. It also has a painkilling effect and can be prescribed to help with acute pain after a fracture in the spine.

Hormone replacement therapy (HRT) replaces oestrogen lost after the menopause, and reduces bone loss at any age after the menopause. For men who have low testosterone levels, testosterone replacement may help to maintain bone density.

Selective oestrogen receptor modulators (SERMs) are drugs which act in a similar way to oestrogen on the bone, helping to maintain bone density and reduce fracture rates specifically in the spine.

Complementary therapies

Complementary therapies do not improve bone density but may help in the management of pain. As osteoporosis makes the bones very frail, manipulative treatments, such as osteopathy and chiropractic, should be used only with extreme caution. If pain is severe following a new fracture, **acupuncture** can stimulate the nerves to stop pain signals reaching the brain, or can cause endorphins (the body's natural pain relievers) to be released.

Massage, with or without essential oils, can help to ease tension.

Hydrotherapy, a form of exercise performed in lukewarm water, is effective for relaxing tight muscles and easing joints. A physiotherapist can devise a series of exercises to help individuals to improve muscle strength, balance and coordination as well as reduce fear of falling (see **Physiotherapy**).

OUTLOOK

Osteoporosis is not in itself a life-threatening disease, but the damage it does cannot be reversed. Treatment can halt bone loss and reduce the risk of broken bones, while positive management of chronic pain can greatly improve a sufferer's quality of life.

SEE ALSO **Bone and problems**

Otitis externa and media

Otitis is an ear infection. Such infections are defined according to the part of the ear affected. In otitis externa, the outer ear is infected and it becomes hot, inflamed and painful. Otitis media is a middle ear infection; one form of this condition, **glue ear**, commonly affects children.

Otitis may be acute or chronic. Chronic otitis externa often occurs in people who swim regularly and is nicknamed swimmer's ear. It is usually treated with antibiotics and eardrops. Applying warmth to the ear with a hot water bottle may be helpful. The infection can be avoided by keeping the ear clean and dry, avoiding sticking anything into the ear canal and taking care not to swim in polluted water.

SEE ALSO *Ear and problems*

Otosclerosis

Otosclerosis is a disorder of the middle ear that gradually leads to deafness. It tends to run in families, mostly affecting women between 15 and 30. It can be triggered by pregnancy.

The disorder causes an abnormal growth of bone in the middle ear area. Normal bone is replaced by spongy bone that prevents the stirrup-shaped stapes from vibrating properly in response to soundwaves. Someone with otosclerosis may also suffer from **tinnitus** and **vertigo**. Their hearing is often better in a noisy environment.

Severe hearing loss can be treated by an operation called stapedectomy, in which the stapes is replaced by an artificial one.

SEE ALSO *Ear and problems*

Ovaries and disorders

From puberty until the menopause, a woman's ovaries develop and release eggs and produce the female sex hormones, oestrogen and progesterone. The ovaries lie in the pelvis on either side of the uterus, below the outer ends of the Fallopian tubes. The outer layer of each ovary contains many fluid-filled sacs called follicles, each with an egg inside.

WHAT CAN GO WRONG

In some babies the ovaries are small or absent as a result of genetic abnormalities. In **Turner's syndrome**, for example, girls have only one X chromosome instead of two, and poorly developed ovaries.

A condition that affects young women of childbearing age is polycystic ovary syndrome, in which multiple cysts grow in the ovaries.

Female reproductive system
The ovaries are glands lying on either side of the uterus immediately beneath the openings of the Fallopian tubes. The ovaries produce egg cells and the hormones oestrogen and progesterone.

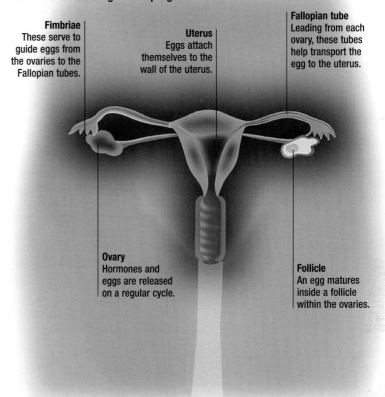

Fimbriae
These serve to guide eggs from the ovaries to the Fallopian tubes.

Uterus
Eggs attach themselves to the wall of the uterus.

Fallopian tube
Leading from each ovary, these tubes help transport the egg to the uterus.

Ovary
Hormones and eggs are released on a regular cycle.

Follicle
An egg matures inside a follicle within the ovaries.

The biggest problem associated with the ovaries is the growth of tumours. These can be solid or fluid filled, in which case they are known as **cysts**. Most ovarian tumours are harmless, but about 25 per cent are cancerous. Ovarian cancer is the fourth most common cancer in women in the UK. It is most likely to occur after the **menopause**.

Polycystic ovary syndrome

Polycystic ovary syndrome, or PCOS, is a complex condition that causes both ovaries to become enlarged by fluid-filled cysts. It is associated with a hormonal imbalance that can be detected in a blood test. A woman with this condition rarely ovulates and may be much less fertile than normal. The condition also causes hormonal disturbances. It affects around 5 per cent of women of childbearing age in the UK.

SYMPTOMS

Women with PCOS have irregular periods, which may affect fertility. They also experience other hormonal changes that may lead to weight gain, the appearance of facial hair and acne. The main symptoms are:

■ absent or infrequent periods. Periods can be as frequent as every five to six weeks, but might only occur once or twice a year, if at all;

■ infertility – infrequent or absent periods are linked with rare ovulation;
■ increased facial and body hair, usually found under the chin, on the upper lip, on the forearms, lower legs and abdomen;
■ greasy skin and acne, usually only on the face;
■ overweight or obesity;
■ miscarriage, sometimes recurrent.

CAUSES

The underlying cause of polycystic ovary syndrome is unknown, though it seems to run in families. Researchers are trying find out whether there is a gene for PCOS. They have discovered that when the condition is passed down the male side of the family, the men are not infertile but they have a tendency to go bald before the age of 30.

TREATMENT

Your family doctor will be able to suggest various drug treatments available. These aim to improve several aspects of the syndrome:
■ fertility can be improved by stimulating ovulation;
■ hormone imbalances can be corrected;
■ excess hairiness can be reduced.

Your doctor will probably suggest that you lose weight, which will help both the symptoms and hormonal abnormalities; and you may be referred to a specialist for **laser** or **diathermy** (heat) treatment to the surface of the ovary.

COMPLICATIONS

Excess oestrogen inhibits ovulation and sometimes overstimulates the lining of the womb so that it becomes abnormally thick. This is associated with a small increased risk of developing cancerous changes (see **Uterus and problems**).

Women with polycystic ovary syndrome may develop an abnormal resistance to the effect of insulin in controlling their blood sugar levels. This puts them at risk of later developing non-insulin dependent **diabetes** and cardiovascular disease.

OUTLOOK

Even without treatment, polycystic ovary syndrome usually settles down at menopause.

Non-cancerous growths

Small ovarian growths usually cause no symptoms and are often discovered when a woman is being examined for another purpose.

CAUSES

Growths can occur for several reasons. In women of childbearing age, a developing ovarian follicle sometimes does not release its egg and forms a harmless temporary cyst. Some cysts are caused by **endometriosis**, in which the same type of tissue as that lining the uterus

grows in the pelvis or abdomen. If there are numerous cysts, they may be due to polycystic ovary syndrome (see above).

TREATMENT

Small tumours or cysts may persist for years without symptoms, and most cysts vanish without treatment. A doctor may request an **ultrasound** scan to check growths are harmless.

COMPLICATIONS

A growth may twist or rupture, causing acute abdominal pain.

Ovarian cancer

An ovarian tumour may be cancerous, growing and sometimes spreading to other organs.

SYMPTOMS

There may be no symptoms at first, although a woman might feel unusually tired and feel discomfort in her lower abdomen. The growth may be discovered because the tumour has grown so large that she can feel it, or because it is pressing on her bladder causing a need to urinate frequently. Fluid caused by spread of cancer can cause an expanding waistline.

CAUSES

Doctors do not know what triggers the majority of ovarian cancers. Most ovarian growths are benign and remain so, but some may later become malignant. Some are malignant from the beginning while some have spread (metastasized) from cancers originating in other organs of the body. Rarely, ovarian cancer runs in families, in which case there may be a genetic cause for the disease.

Women who have used oral contraceptives and those who have had children have a reduced risk of ovarian cancer. The disease is rare in women under 40.

Risk factors for ovarian cancer

Those most at risk of ovarian cancer are:
■ menopausal women over 50 years of age;
■ women with a family history of ovarian, breast or bowel cancer;
■ women who have had breast cancer;
■ those who have never been pregnant;
■ women who started menstruation early;
■ those whose first pregnancy was after 30;
■ women taking fertility drugs;
■ those who had a late menopause.

TREATMENT

Ovarian tumours need to be surgically removed. If the cancer is advanced and cannot be completely removed, a surgeon may still cut out part of the tumour to improve the woman's response to chemotherapy.

PREVENTION

Screening women for early ovarian cancer, with blood tests to pick up abnormal antibodies or ultrasound scans, has so far proved

Polycystic ovary syndrome affects around one in 20 women of childbearing age in the UK.

▼ **Ovarian cancer**
A coloured MRI scan through the abdomen shows ovarian cancer (brown). The cause of a malignant ovarian tumour is unknown. Treatment includes surgical removal of affected tissues, with radiotherapy and chemotherapy.

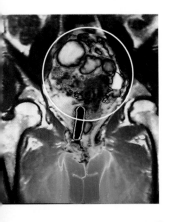

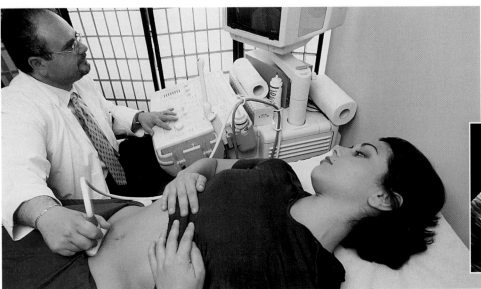

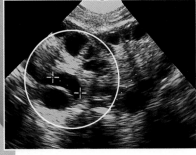

◄ **Ultrasound view**
A coloured ultrasound scan of the young woman's abdomen shows an ovarian cyst (marked with two crosses). This is a fluid-filled swelling inside an ovary.

unreliable, but methods are being improved. If your GP thinks you are at risk of developing the cancer because of family medical history, he or she can refer you to a specialist or NHS family cancer clinic to assess whether screening is appropriate.

OUTLOOK

Many simple cysts stay the same for years while others develop complications. Survival rates for ovarian cancer vary according to the stage of the tumour at diagnosis. With cancer confined to the ovary, up to 90 per cent of women are still alive five years later and many women live for many years after that. With advanced cancer, only about 10 per cent of those affected live for five years or more.

Other problems

The health and normal functioning of the ovaries can be affected by other factors.

Reduced oestrogen production

Women who lose an excessive amount of weight may produce less oestrogen in their ovaries. This causes ovulation to cease and periods to stop. The condition may affect female athletes as well as women with **anorexia nervosa** and other eating disorders. Gaining weight reverses the process. If weight gain is impossible, you may be advised to take oestrogen in the form of the Pill in order to protect against **osteoporosis**.

Early ovarian failure

The ovaries normally stop producing oestrogen at about the age of 50, resulting in the menopause. A premature menopause may occur in much younger women spontaneously, or after chemotherapy or radiotherapy or the surgical removal of the ovaries. Oestrogen replacement therapy will relieve menopausal symptoms and reduce risks of osteoporosis and heart disease.

Ovarian hyperstimulation syndrome

This rare condition is a potentially dangerous side effect of an **infertility** treatment that involves high doses of the hormone human chorionic gonadotrophin. Large cysts temporarily appear in the ovaries, and abdominal pain, swelling and gastro-intestinal symptoms may occur. Occasionally, women with ovarian hyperstimulation syndrome develop blood clots. This may necessitate treatment in intensive care while the condition resolves itself.

SEE ALSO *Menstruation; Reproductive system; Uterus and problems*

Ovulation syndrome

Ovulation syndrome is lower abdominal pain during ovulation, which is experienced by some women. When an ovarian follicle ruptures and releases an egg from the ovary, fluid from the follicle irritates the membrane lining the abdominal cavity (peritoneum). The pain – sometimes referred to as Mittelschmerz, meaning 'middle pain' – typically occurs about 14 days before the next period is due and is aching or sharp. It is occasionally severe enough for the woman to be seen as an emergency – when the symptoms may be confused with **appendicitis** – but usually vanishes within 24 hours. A woman suffering from ovulation syndrome will find sexual intercourse uncomfortable during ovulation.

Treatment of the acute pain involves analgesics. If the pain recurs each month, it can be avoided by taking the combined contraceptive Pill, which prevents ovulation.

SEE ALSO *Menstruation; Reproductive system*

Pacemaker

A pacemaker is a temporary or permanent device that makes the heart contract regularly.

Normal heartbeats are triggered by electrical signals that spread through the heart's central conducting system and heart muscle, producing a coordinated contraction (see **Heart and circulatory system**). But in some circumstances, this normal pattern becomes disrupted.

■ In heart block, the signals get blocked and the lower chambers (ventricles) then contract at their own very slow rate.

■ If the conducting system is damaged by a heart attack, the electrical signals spread haphazardly through the heart muscle; different areas then contract at different times.

■ In some cases, an electrical signal develops outside the central conducting system causing the heart to contract out of its normal timed sequence. This disruption can lead to faintness, breathlessness, arrhythmia (abnormal heart rhythms), **heart failure** or cardiac arrest.

TEMPORARY PACEMAKER

A temporary pacemaker is sometimes used to regulate the heartbeat in cases of:
■ myocardial infarction (heart attack);
■ drug overdose;
■ arrhythmia;
■ heart failure;
■ cardiac arrest.

An electrical wire is inserted into a large vein in the groin or upper chest, and guided through the veins to the heart. **X-rays** are then used to check that it becomes lodged in the correct part of the heart, usually the right atrium (upper chamber). The wire is then attached to an external pacemaker, worn on a belt, and remains in place until it is no longer needed or is replaced by a permanent pacemaker.

PERMANENT PACEMAKER

A permanent pacemaker is needed when tests show that the heart's conducting system is irreparably damaged.

The electrical pacing wire is usually inserted into a vein near the shoulder or neck and is connected to an internal pacemaker. This weighs about 50g (2oz), and is worn in a pocket constructed between the skin and the chest muscle. An X-ray checks that the device is correctly positioned. Occasionally, the wire is directly attached to the surface of the heart.

There are two different types of pacemaker. A 'fixed rate' pacemaker sends out regular impulses at a steady rate that stimulate regular contractions, irrespective of the heart's activity. A 'demand' pacemaker checks first to see if the heart is beating normally, and sends out a signal as required, such as when the heart rate slows or a beat is missed.

A pacemaker has its own battery, which lasts for five to ten years and is checked annually at a hospital. Replacing the battery involves a minor operation. Contact sports and certain electrical equipment, such as airport security systems, can damage pacemakers. Driving is usually permitted once symptoms have settled.

▼ **Keeping pace**
Pacemakers are usually implanted under the skin below the collarbone and connected to the heart via a wire guided down into the heart.

Paget's disease

Paget's disease is chronic bone disease, affecting up to a million, mainly elderly, people in the UK. Accelerated bone growth, particularly in the skull, pelvis, spine, thigh and shinbone, causes pain, bone deformity and fractures. The cause is unknown but it may be viral or genetic in origin. Drugs called biphosphonates can help to calm the condition and promote normal bone growth. But when the skull is affected, blindness or deafness may result.

Palpitations

Palpitations are characterized by a heartbeat that is felt to be rapid or irregular. This may be caused by stimulants such as caffeine or cigarettes, by anxiety, or by illness such as anaemia, **fever** and thyroid disease, or by heart disease. Palpitations may cause faintness, breathlessness or **chest pain**. Treatment is directed at the underlying causes. Drugs can be used to regulate the heartbeat.

SEE ALSO *Heart and circulatory system*

Pancreas and disorders

The pancreas is a gland – which means that it is able to make and secrete chemical substances such as enzymes and hormones. Endocrine glands release hormones directly into the bloodstream, while exocrine glands discharge their secretions via ducts into other organs or the body's surface.

The pancreas has both exocrine and endocrine functions. It produces digestive enzymes that are released via the pancreatic duct into the duodenum – the first part of the small intestine. Here, they play an important role in breaking down food molecules. The other main function of the pancreas is the production of insulin and glucogen. These hormones regulate the amount of glucose in the blood.

WHAT CAN GO WRONG

The pancreas contains exocrine tissue, which secretes enzymes via the pancreatic duct into the duodenum, and endocrine tissue, which secretes insulin and glucogen into blood vessels. When the pancreas fails to produce a sufficient quantity of insulin, the result is **diabetes**. Other diseases affect the pancreas's exocrine function. For example, most people with **cystic fibrosis** are unable to produce sufficient enzymes to break down proteins and fats. This leads to malabsorption syndrome and steatorrhoea. The main disorders to affect the pancreas itself are pancreatitis and pancreatic cancer.

Pancreatitis

Pancreatitis is inflammation of the pancreas. The inflammation can be either acute or chronic, and both forms cause severe pain in the abdomen and back, with vomiting and fever. Pancreatitis affects 10,000 people a year in the UK, and is fatal in about 10 per cent of cases.

Acute pancreatitis is usually caused either by alcohol abuse or gallstones. Attacks are sudden and may last up to two days. The inflammation and a buildup of fluid around the gland (a pseudocyst) prevent enzymes from leaving it, which leads to further inflammation and damage to the gland's exocrine tissue. If you develop pancreatitis, you will need immediate hospital treatment. You will probably be given intravenous feeding to allow the gland to rest. Most people recover within a few days. If your case is severe, you may need to have damaged parts of the gland removed surgically.

Chronic pancreatitis may develop after the primary cause of acute pancreatitis has been treated, but is most commonly caused by excessive consumption of alcohol. It leads to the formation of permanent scar tissue in the gland, which reduces or halts enzyme production. Symptoms include **jaundice**, loss of weight and back pain that lasts days or weeks. Diabetes may develop in the later stages. If you develop chronic pancreatitis, you will be prescribed painkillers and enzyme supplements and advised to follow a low-fat diet.

Role of the pancreas in digestion

The pancreas produces enzymes that help in the breakdown of food, sodium bicarbonate, which neutralizes stomach acid, and the hormones glucogen and insulin, which regulate the amount of glucose in the blood.

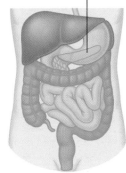

Digestive system
The pancreas sits beneath the stomach and liver and above the small intestine.

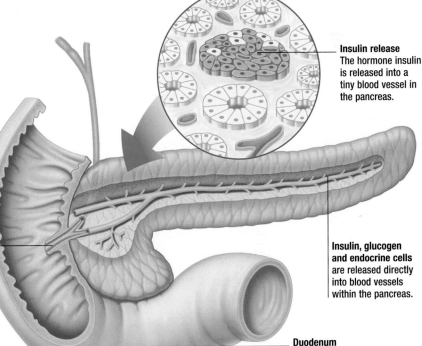

Insulin release
The hormone insulin is released into a tiny blood vessel in the pancreas.

Pancreatic duct
Digestive enzymes are released into the duodenum down a narrow tube.

Insulin, glucogen and endocrine cells are released directly into blood vessels within the pancreas.

Duodenum
In the first part of the small intestine, enzymes made in the pancreas and bile made in the liver work to break down food molecules.

Cancer of the pancreas

Pancreatic **cancer** is the fifth leading cause of death from cancer worldwide. It affects about 7000 people in the UK each year but is becoming more common. More men than women are affected and it is more likely to develop in those aged over 50. The cause is unknown, although it is associated with chronic pancreatitis, smoking, alcohol abuse and a high-fat diet. Symptoms may include abdominal pain, weight loss, nausea and constipation.

In many cases, the disease is not detected until it has reached an advanced stage – with the result that nine out of ten people die within a year of diagnosis. But the cancer can be surgically removed if it is diagnosed early enough. Ongoing studies with a new chemotherapeutic agent – gemcitabine – also look promising.

SEE ALSO *Digestive system*

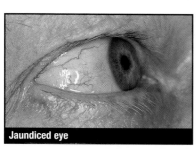

Jaundiced eye

▲ **Pancreatic cancer**
A jaundiced eye is a key symptom of pancreatic cancer. The cancer usually develops in the head of the pancreas and often blocks the bile duct, causing jaundice and itchy skin.

Panic attack

A panic attack is an exaggeration of the body's normal response to fear, stress or excitement. People experiencing an attack may develop very rapid breathing and heartbeat, chest pains, dizziness, sweating, tingling or numbness in the hands and feet, or hot or cold flushes. They may feel terrified and out of control. Some people think that they are going mad or are about to have a heart attack.

Panic attacks can happen to people with **anxiety, phobias** or **obsessions** or they can come out of the blue. A person may feel fine one minute and the next be deeply distressed and in the grip of a panic attack.

People who have panic attacks often develop a fear of fear and may begin to avoid places and situations in which attacks have occurred. This can develop into **agoraphobia** or a fear of social situations.

DURATION

Most panic attacks last between 5 and 20 minutes. Some people may have one or two attacks and never have another, whereas others may have several attacks each week or month.

CAUSES

Anxious people are more likely to have panic attacks, as are people who are critical or disapproving of themselves.

Childhood incidents or life changes and crises can cause attacks, sometimes much later on. Physical factors such as unstable blood sugar levels, dieting and fasting, **hyperventilation** (overbreathing), taking antidepressants or withdrawing from drugs can all lead to panic attacks.

TREATMENT

Treatment is normally with cognitive behaviour therapy or behaviour therapy. You can help yourself to feel in control of your bodily reactions by learning relaxation techniques or breathing exercises. **Complementary therapies** can help to boost feelings of well-being.

SEE ALSO *Anxiety; Phobia*

Papilleodema

Papilleodema is a swelling at the start of the optic nerve (the optic disc or optic papilla). It is due to raised pressure within the skull and is always a sign of an underlying condition. This could be a buildup of cerebrospinal fluid or the presence of a tumour or large aneurysm (swelling or defect in an artery wall) in the head. These conditions are potentially fatal.

Symptoms include headache, vomiting, mood changes and double vision. But 10 per cent of cases are symptomless and papilloedema is detected only during a routine eye test.

People with papilloedema need immediate medical attention. If you develop the condition, you will given a head scan to determine its cause. If you have a buildup of cerebrospinal fluid you may need to have the pressure reduced by removing some fluid from the spine. If you have an aneurysm or tumour, surgery may be recommended to correct the problem.

PREVENTION

There is a link between the buildup of cerebrospinal fluid and **obesity**, and aneurysms are more likely in those with cardiovascular disease, so a healthy diet and lifestyle may reduce the risk. Further research is needed into the possible link between excessive use of mobile phones and tumours within the skull.

Papilloma

A papilloma is a tumour that develops on the surface of the skin or the mucous membranes of the gut, breathing passages or urinary tract.

Papillomas tend to look like fleshy warts and may be flat or protruding on a stalk. Although usually benign, they may be unsightly if they form on the skin, and they can cause physical problems – especially in the bowel, where they can cause bleeding, or on the larynx or voice box, where they cause hoarseness. Papillomas are usually easily removed by surgery. Occasionally a papilloma becomes cancerous.

Paralysis

A muscle is said to be paralysed if it is unable to contract in the normal way. The condition occurs when control of a muscle is lost somewhere along the route from the brain, via the nerves, to the muscle itself (see **Brain and nervous system**).

If there is no stimulation of the muscle whatsoever, the muscle is floppy and soft and the condition is known as flaccid paralysis. If there is some stimulation from reflex nerve activity, as sometimes occurs following a **stroke** or in **cerebral palsy**, the muscle is tight, making the limbs rigid. This is called spastic paralysis. If muscular control is only partially lost, the condition is known as paresis.

Paralysis may be permanent or temporary. Sometimes it is accompanied by loss of feeling.

CAUSES

Paralysis may be caused by damage to the brain, to the nerves in the spinal cord, or to the nerves of the peripheral nervous system, which connects the brain and spinal cord to the rest of the body.

Damage to the brain

Voluntary movement is controlled in an area on the brain's surface called the motor cortex. There are two motor cortexes, one on each side of the brain – the left cortex controls the right side of the body, while the right cortex controls the body's left side. If one motor cortex is damaged, the use of muscles in the associated area of the body is damaged. For example, a stroke or brain injury affecting the left motor cortex, or nerve fibres linking it to the spinal cord, may leave the right side of the body partially or wholly paralysed.

Cerebral palsy, viral or bacterial infection of the brain and **multiple sclerosis** can all cause damage to the motor cortexes, resulting in paralysis.

Damage to the spinal cord

The spinal cord may be damaged if the vertebral column that protects it is fractured, if the spinal cord itself is damaged by **cancer** spreading from elsewhere, or by some forms of stroke. Damage in different regions is likely to cause paralysis in particular parts of the body (see box, right). This generally affects the sensory nerves and the motor nerves and there is usually loss of sensation as well as paralysis. Viral infections such as **poliomyelitis**, bacterial infection and **motor neurone disease** can all damage the spinal cord and cause paralysis.

Damage to peripheral nerves

A peripheral nerve leading to a single muscle or a small group of muscles can be damaged as a result of a cut or crush injury, or by conditions

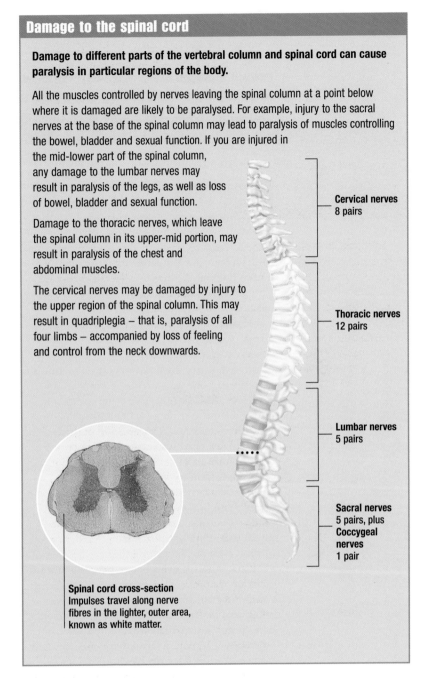

Damage to the spinal cord

Damage to different parts of the vertebral column and spinal cord can cause paralysis in particular regions of the body.

All the muscles controlled by nerves leaving the spinal column at a point below where it is damaged are likely to be paralysed. For example, injury to the sacral nerves at the base of the spinal column may lead to paralysis of muscles controlling the bowel, bladder and sexual function. If you are injured in the mid-lower part of the spinal column, any damage to the lumbar nerves may result in paralysis of the legs, as well as loss of bowel, bladder and sexual function.

Damage to the thoracic nerves, which leave the spinal column in its upper-mid portion, may result in paralysis of the chest and abdominal muscles.

The cervical nerves may be damaged by injury to the upper region of the spinal column. This may result in quadriplegia – that is, paralysis of all four limbs – accompanied by loss of feeling and control from the neck downwards.

Cervical nerves
8 pairs

Thoracic nerves
12 pairs

Lumbar nerves
5 pairs

Sacral nerves
5 pairs, plus
Coccygeal nerves
1 pair

Spinal cord cross-section
Impulses travel along nerve fibres in the lighter, outer area, known as white matter.

that affect only the peripheral nerves, such as neuritis. This will cause a flaccid paralysis of the muscle, but because opposing muscle groups in the limb remain intact and are then unbalanced, the limb may be held in a distorted way. An example is ulnar nerve damage in the arm. This causes claw hand, a deformity in which the fingers are permanently contracted and the joints between them are extended.

TREATMENT

The treatment of paralysis depends on its cause. **Physiotherapy** and **occupational therapy** are often useful to help recover some lost function, and make the most of any remaining function. Psychological therapies may also be used.

Paranoia

People with paranoia are suspicious without reason, often believing that others are trying to ridicule or persecute them. They may fear some future event such as a personal betrayal or a violent attack.

Paranoid people can interpret any event irrationally so that it fits in with their delusions. Some think their life is in danger, because their food is being poisoned, for example. Some feel constantly under threat and unable to trust anyone – for this reason, paranoia tends to lead to isolation. Others fear that their thoughts or actions are being controlled – they may hear voices in their head telling them what to say or commenting on what they have done.

Some people with paranoia become very angry or feel extreme guilt. The anger may derive from a feeling that they are being wrongly and unjustly persecuted, while the guilt may be fostered by their conviction that they are being singled out for trouble because they are 'bad' people.

Paranoia can be mild, meaning that affected people realize their suspicions may not be justified, or it may be extreme, meaning that affected people are convinced they are right whatever the evidence to the contrary. The disorder can be a symptom of a mental health problem such as **depression** or **schizophrenia**. It can also develop for other reasons – older people or those who are ill may feel they are becoming a burden, while people who are partially deaf can convince themselves that others are keeping their voices low in order to trade secrets about them.

Paranoid personality disorder may be diagnosed when people have suffered paranoia since early adulthood. Paranoid schizophrenia may be diagnosed when a person also hears voices.

CAUSES
A condition as complex as paranoia is unlikely to have a single, simple cause. Often, it is linked to a lack of self-esteem that is rooted in childhood. This will shape the way in which people view the world and the relationships they have with others. Children who are repeatedly told that they live in a wicked world and that others are out to hurt them, say, may develop a paranoid outlook. Some researchers say that people with paranoia tend to jump to conclusions and have difficulty understanding other people's thoughts and feelings. This can interfere with their relationships and cause further paranoia, creating a vicious circle.

Paranoia can also have physical or chemical causes. For example, illnesses such as **dementia** or drugs such as cocaine, cannabis and alcohol can bring on the condition.

TREATMENT
Getting help and treatment is often difficult, because people suffering from paranoia may not accept that there is anything wrong with them. A GP may refer a person with paranoia to a psychiatrist or psychologist for medication or talking therapies, or both.

Medication usually involves anti-psychotic drugs, such as haloperidol. These have a tranquillizing effect. Cognitive behaviour therapy can be effective for paranoia. It involves examining a person's way of thinking for evidence of damaging negative patterns, and seeking to replace these with more positive beliefs. It can also help people to cope with hearing voices. A short stay in an appropriate hospital may be needed if the person is very disturbed or a danger to him or herself or others.

WHAT CAN FAMILY AND FRIENDS DO?
Living with a paranoid person can be distressing, especially if he or she is aggressive or angry. Ask others to help, and look out for a support group for carers or help from social services. Look on the web sites run by charities for information about paranoia. The more you know about the condition, the better you will be able to cope.

Try not to be confrontational and do not dismiss a paranoid person's beliefs. You can empathize with the person's feelings – fear and anxiety, for example – without sharing his or her view of the world.
SEE ALSO *Mental health and problems*

Paraplegia

Paraplegia is the paralysis of the lower body due to spinal-cord damage. It is usually the result of a severe accidental injury. Paraplegia affects both legs and sometimes part or the whole of the trunk. Sexual function and internal organs, such as the bladder and bowel, may also be affected.

SPINAL DAMAGE

The spinal cord carries all the nerve fibres that pass to and from the brain. These transmit both the outbound signals that instruct the muscles to move, and inbound messages about sensation. If the nerve fibres are severed or badly crushed, or if they are withered by disease, then the signals can no longer get through. The result is that the parts of the body controlled by them are paralysed and dead to sensation.

The amount of function lost depends on where the damage is. A break above the middle of the spinal cord may paralyse the entire trunk as well as the legs. A break lower down may paralyse the trunk below the waist and the legs, or the legs alone. A break at the bottom of the spine will affect only the legs.

SYMPTOMS

Although paralysis is the defining feature of paraplegia, the symptoms of the condition vary widely according to the type of damage, as well as the level in the spine at which it occurs.

■ When the internal organs are affected, there is usually loss of bladder and bowel control.

■ Injury to the neck region may paralyse the diaphragm muscle below the lungs, so the person can breathe only with a respirator.

■ Paralysis and loss of sensation can lead to problems, such as kidney and bladder stones, urinary infections, and circulation problems that cause sores and slow healing of injuries.

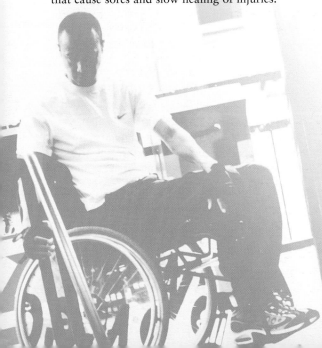

■ When the cord damage occurs high up in the spine, the autonomic nervous system may become hypersensitive and cause profuse sweating, high blood pressure, a slow pulse rate and blackouts. This can be triggered by a variety of factors, including a very full bladder or bowel, or bedsores.

CAUSES

Paraplegia usually occurs as the result of an accident. A person who is conscious throughout the event will probably be aware of suffering a major injury to the back and realize immediately that something catastrophic has occurred. The level of pain is not a good guide to the severity of a spinal injury, because once the damage has been done the affected area of the body stops sending pain signals to the brain. After an accident, the most obvious sign that someone is paralysed is their inability to move or to feel the lower part of the body. Onlookers may notice that the person is lying in a peculiar twisted position and apparently making no attempt to alter it.

Two out of three of those paralysed by spinal-cord damage are young men between the ages of 19 and 35. The main causes are:

■ motor accidents (70 per cent);

■ falls (8 per cent);

■ sporting accidents – especially in sports such as diving, horse-riding, shooting and mountain-climbing (10 per cent);

■ a disease such as a tumour on the spine or a severe spinal infection (12 per cent).

TREATMENT

Medical care of spinal-cord injuries improved greatly in the second half of the 20th century. During the Second World War, injury to the spinal cord was usually fatal. Post-war advances in emergency care and rehabilitation allowed many patients to survive, but methods for reducing the extent of injury were virtually unknown. Significant advances in recent years, including an effective steroid drug therapy for acute spinal-cord injury and better imaging techniques for diagnosing spinal damage, have improved the recovery rates of patients with spinal-cord injuries.

But the most important advance has been the recognition that, in most cases, spinal-cord damage continues to occur after the initial injury. This damage occurs in a variety of ways. The crushing of the spinal cord causes the immune system to release a cascade of chemicals that affect the nerve cells. Some of these chemicals poison the injured cells, effectively killing them off. Others trigger a process which causes cells to self-destruct. The injury may also block the chemicals that healthy cells need in order to survive. Medical

The people most likely to sustain an injury to the spinal cord are young men who risk injury by doing competitive sports or driving too fast.

understanding of these processes is improving all the time, and with this understanding comes the hope of new treatments that will minimize and perhaps even reverse the damage. At the moment, however, there is no cure for severe spinal injury.

Immediate care

If someone is severely injured in an accident and spinal damage is suspected, it is crucial to avoid moving the person unless there is danger of imminent death – for example, if the person is in a burning car. Call for an ambulance, and keep the patient still and warm while waiting for it to arrive. Check for vital signs and start cardiopulmonary resuscitation if needed.

Hospital care

When a patient with a spinal-cord injury arrives in hospital, the priority is the diagnosis and the relief of cord compression. Techniques such as magnetic resonance imaging (MRI) and CT scanning are used to pinpoint the site of injury and to see precisely what needs to be done to prevent further injury from broken or misaligned vertebrae.

■ **Drug treatment** Methylprednisolone is a steroid that has been shown to reduce the secondary damage caused by the body's own defences following injury to the spinal cord. It reduces inflammation near the site of the injury and suppresses the activation of immune cells that appear to contribute to nerve cell damage. The steroid drug may also block the formation of free radicals – charged, highly energetic molecules that can disrupt the membranes of cells that were not initially injured. Preventing this damage helps to spare some nerve fibres that would otherwise be lost, improving the patient's chances of recovery. Studies of the drug show that it is most beneficial when given within three hours of a spinal-cord injury occurring, and when treatment is continued for up to two days.

■ **Surgery** If the spinal cord is compressed, surgery may be undertaken to remove bone splinters or other tissue that is pressing on the nerves. However, the use of surgery is controversial – in some cases surgical intervention has actually worsened the patient's condition. In other cases, however, early surgery allows earlier movement and earlier physical therapy, which are important for preventing complications and regaining as much function as possible.

■ **Spinal stabilization** If an operation is carried out, a metal plate, screws or similar devices may be put in place to prevent further compression or twisting of the spinal cord. Where surgery is not performed, patients may be put in traction. This usually involves placing the

patient in a frame that allows him or her to be hoisted upright. Lifting the injured person into an upright position helps to relieve pressure on the affected area and minimize further damage.

COMPLICATIONS

If the paralysis resulted from an accident, the injured person is likely to be suffering from other peripheral damage. But paralysed areas of the body are usually insensitive to pain as well as to touch, which can cause problems. The victim may be unaware that a foot, say, is injured or has become infected in some way. It is therefore important that affected areas are not left lying still for too long and any sores are treated with antibiotics to prevent infection.

LONG-TERM CARE

Rehabilitation therapy for patients with spinal-cord injuries takes many forms, depending on the site and extent of injury and the age and general medical health of the patient. Almost all patients with spinal-cord injuries can achieve a partial return of function. Physical therapy can keep the muscles and joints flexible, and can help to reduce the risk of blood clots.

Psychological rehabilitation

The sudden onset of paraplegia after an accident usually has a massive psychological impact as well as causing profound lifestyle changes. The mobility of sufferers is, of course, hugely reduced and – for a while at least – this forces them to depend heavily on other people for help with even the simplest tasks. Sometimes, injured people have to give up their existing jobs and look for work better suited to their reduced mobility. Sexual activity is also impaired.

The speed and extent to which people who have suffered spinal-cord injury adapt psychologically to their state depends largely on their own and other people's attitudes. Patients and carers should be encouraged to take an optimistic outlook, and to concentrate on making the most of the affected person's existing abilities rather than dwelling on what he or she has lost.

OUTLOOK

Fifty years ago, 70 per cent of people with severe spinal-cord injuries died within days of the accident. Today, however, the life expectancy of people with such injuries – providing they survive and get treatment within the first few hours – is about 90 per cent of the average lifespan.

The major dangers of injury are secondary complications such as kidney failure, caused by untreated infections. These tend to occur because people with paraplegia cannot tell when their bladder is full and are unable to empty it normally, so urine may collect in the bladder

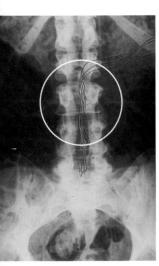

▲ **Nerve stimulator**
A person paralysed from the waist down may be able to use a spinal nerve stimulator, implanted under the skin near the base of the ribs, to restore bladder, bowel and sexual function. An external remote control is used to trigger the stimulator and send signals down wires (shown green) in the spinal canal, stimulating the nerves there.

and become infected. It is therefore most important that people with bladder dysfunction are aware of the potential dangers and take antibiotics at the first sign of infection.

Experimental cell transplantation

Specialized cells called Schwann cells are responsible for producing myelin, the sheath surrounding the fibres that carry electrical impulses from a nerve cell to its target. Myelin increases the speed of nerve cell impulses and is necessary for the normal functioning of most nerve cells in the brain and spinal cord.

Researchers are experimenting with implanting Schwann cells into damaged spinal tissue in the hope that such cells may act as a bridge, supplying the nourishing chemical factors that encourage regeneration, and allowing the normal functioning of undamaged or regenerated fibres. The procedure involves:
■ removing a small amount of nerve tissue from the network of nerves outside the patient's brain and spinal cord – from a nerve in the ankle, say;
■ isolating Schwann cells from the nerve tissue;
■ growing the Schwann cells in culture dishes in an incubator;
■ implanting the cultured Schwann cells into the site of spinal-cord injury.

It is too early to tell whether the treatment works, and it is not yet widely available.

SEE ALSO *Disability; Quadraplegia*

Parasites and parasitic diseases

A parasite is an organism that lives on or inside another living organism and cannot survive alone. It feeds off nutrients taken from its host. This usually damages the host in some way, causing a disease or – in extreme cases – death.

Human parasites live in the intestines or blood, or in the skin. They include worms, insects such as lice, mites and ticks, fungi and micro-organisms such as bacteria and protozoa (a simple single-celled organism). The diseases they cause are widespread throughout the world, but are most common in warm and tropical climates.

Some parasites are on the increase. For example, there is a rising incidence of bedbugs in the UK, USA and Australia. It is believed that they are carried in luggage when people travel.

Poor hygiene and carelessness are the main reasons why people pick up a parasitic disease, particularly in the developed world. Parasites are often ingested in contaminated food and drink. Washing your hands with soap and water, particularly before preparing a meal,

is one of the best measures to take to prevent their spread. Some parasites, however, can enter the body via wounds and insect bites.

Abdominal pain, nausea, diarrhoea, watery stools, flatulence, weight loss and occasionally fever are the most common symptoms of parasitic diseases. A number of antiparisitic drugs have been developed – and as scientists unravel the structure of the enzymes that allow parasites to attack our immune systems, the diseases they cause will become easier to treat.

Acanthamoeba infection

Acanthamoebas are microscopic creatures found in dust, soil and fresh water. They often live in air-conditioning and heating units. Several species infect human beings, particularly people with weakened immune systems. They can enter the skin through a cut, or be inhaled. People who wear contact lenses may also pick them up by using a non-sterile solution, such as ordinary tap water, to store and clean their lenses.

SYMPTOMS

Symptoms take the form of eye infections and skin lesions, and vary widely in severity.

TREATMENT

Eye infections are healed with a combination of anti-amoebic and antifungal eyedrops. Skin infections are treated with antiseptic ointment.

Complementary therapies

The herbal remedies blackwalnut hull, cloves and wormwood are sometimes helpful.

PREVENTION

Use commercial contact-lens cleaning solution to avoid eye infections.

COMPLICATIONS

A serious infection of the whole body, called granulomatous amoebic encephalitis, may develop, causing hallucinations, headaches, confusion and seizures. It often results in death. **Ulcers** may develop on the corneas of the eyes, in which case surgery may be necessary.

OUTLOOK

Eye and skin infections usually heal well. The infection cannot be spread from person to person.

Amoebiasis

Amoebiasis is caused by the microscopic parasite *Entamoeba histolytica*. It is found mainly in the developing world, and results from poor sanitation. It is spread by swallowing anything that has touched the stool of an infected person, and sometimes by anal sex.

SYMPTOMS

Only one in ten people infected with the parasite become ill. Symptoms take the form of loose stools and stomach cramps, but can be very mild.

TREATMENT

Usually antibiotics are used to kill the parasite.

Complementary therapies

Quassia is a useful herbal remedy for easing the symptoms.

PREVENTION

Wash hands with soap and water before eating or touching the face.

■ Cook all food thoroughly.

■ Drink only bottled or filtered water when travelling in the developing world.

COMPLICATIONS

Diagnosis can be difficult as some other parasites look similar.

■ Hepatic amoebiasis can result if the liver is infected. Signs include fever and pain in the abdomen below the ribs.

■ A severe form of amoebiasis called amoebic dysentery may develop. It causes chills and severe diarrhoea and can last for a few weeks.

OUTLOOK

The outlook is good as this disease is treatable and medication seems to have few side effects.

Cryptosporidiosis

The parasite *Cryptosporidium parvum* lives in the intestines of both human beings and animals. It is passed on by contact with infected stools, usually from contaminated water. It is one of the most common water-borne diseases in the Western world. Cryptosporidiosis, often known simply as crypto, can be very contagious and outbreaks are common in childcare settings. People whose immune systems are weakened or damaged in some way – such as AIDS patients – are particularly vulnerable.

SYMPTOMS

Symptoms appear two to ten days after infection and usually last for up to two weeks. An affected person will often feel better and then worse again throughout the duration of the infection. Symptoms include:

■ diarrhoea;

■ loose and watery stools;

■ abdominal pain;

■ low fever.

TREATMENT

An otherwise healthy person will recover without treatment, as long as plenty of water is given to avoid dehydration.

For people with AIDS, anti-retroviral therapy to boost the immune system assists recovery.

PREVENTION

■ Always wash your hands thoroughly with soap and water after using the toilet or changing a nappy.

■ Toddlers should wear clothing over nappies to avoid leakage of faeces and prevent any spread of the disease.

■ Avoid exposure to faeces during sex.

■ Do not swim – even in chlorinated pools – during and for two weeks after an infection.

COMPLICATIONS

■ Severe symptoms are most likely among those with immune-system problems, small children and pregnant women.

■ In extremely severe cases, the disease can be life-threatening.

OUTLOOK

Most people recover completely.

Fascioliasis

A type of flatworm, the liver fluke – *Fasciola hepatica* – is a parasite of sheep. It can be passed on, via their droppings, when humans eat watercress collected from streams near grazing areas. It is fairly rare in the UK, but common in Eastern Europe and the Far East.

SYMPTOMS

There are often no symptoms, but those affected may develop fever and the liver may become enlarged and tender. The severity of an individual's symptoms depends on the number of flukes present.

TREATMENT

A stool sample will be examined for signs of the fluke eggs. Treatment is with the drug bithionol, which kills the worms.

PREVENTION

■ It is important to check that any watercress eaten is from a safe source, which all farmed watercress in the UK should be.

■ Watercress used uncooked in salads should be washed thoroughly before being eaten.

COMPLICATIONS

Flukes can make their way from the liver into the bile duct causing inflammation and obstruction that can lead to **jaundice**.

OUTLOOK

Most people make a complete recovery.

Giardiasis

Giardiasis is an intestinal disease caused by the single-celled *Giardia lamblia*, which attaches itself to the lining of the small intestine. It is contracted either through sexual contact or by drinking contaminated water.

SYMPTOMS

There are often none, but some people have:

■ cramping abdominal pain;

■ flatulence;

■ diarrhoea, which can last for a week or more.

TREATMENT

A stool sample will be microscopically examined for signs of the parasite. If the diagnosis is confirmed, a single dose of Fasigyn is usually very effective at treating the illness. Flagyl is also sometimes used.

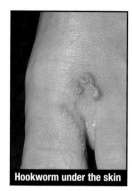

Hookworm under the skin

▲ **Skin parasite**

When hookworm larvae – picked up by walking barefoot on contaminated soil or sand – penetrate the skin, they burrow around randomly, causing extreme irritation.

More than 2 billion people throughout the world are infected with parasitic worms.

COMPLICATIONS

Flukes can make their way from the liver into the bile duct, causing inflammation and obstruction that can lead to **jaundice**.

PREVENTION

■ Avoid consuming contaminated water, ice, fruits and salad.
■ Ensure stringent hygiene by washing your hands thoroughly.

OUTLOOK

Most people recover completely.

Hookworms

The hookworm is one of the most common types of roundworm. It is spread through human faeces in insanitary conditions. The parasite is widespread in tropical countries, where hookworm eggs are often found in the soil, and can enter the human body in contaminated food or through the skin. If people walk barefoot on soil that contains any hookworm larvae, some of them may enter the body by piercing the skin. The larvae then migrate in the bloodstream to the lungs and windpipe, from where they can be swallowed and pass into the intestine. Once in the digestive system, the larvae mature and eventually produce eggs that will appear in the affected person's stools.

SYMPTOMS

If worms enter via the skin, an itchy rash may be the only symptom initially. As the infestation progresses, others develop, including:
■ diarrhoea;
■ abdominal pain and cramps;
■ nausea;
■ intense itching at site of entry.
   If a person is affected by dog or cat hookworm, an itchy red rash is the only symptom, as this type of hookworm stays under the skin and does not enter the bloodstream.

TREATMENT

Treatment with the drug albendazole is effective within one to three days, but is rarely given in countries where re-infection is likely.

Complementary therapies

Homeopathic remedies such as Spigelia anthelmia (spigelia) are sometimes used.

PREVENTION

The infection can be prevented by good hygiene, taking care with what you eat and by avoiding walking barefoot.

COMPLICATIONS

When the worms suck blood from the intestine wall, the affected person may suffer a low iron count and develop **anaemia**.

OUTLOOK

An otherwise healthy person will recover completely with appropriate treatment.

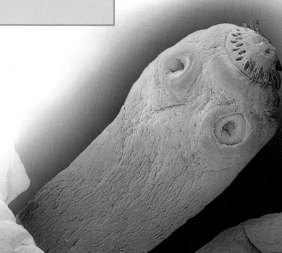

▶ **Head of a tapeworm**
Suckers and a crown of tiny hooks at the top of a tapeworm's head allow it to attach itself to its host's intestine and feed off semi-digested food found there.

Threadworms

Threadworms – also known as pinworms – are the most common type of roundworm parasite. They are widespread throughout the Western world. Threadworms infect large numbers of children and are often found in schools and daycare centres. Their eggs enter the body when swallowed in contaminated food, or off dirty fingers. The adults that develop live in the colon and rectum.

SYMPTOMS

Symptoms can be mild, but usually include:
- itching of the anus or vagina;
- small worms seen occasionally on a child's bottom or in stools.

TREATMENT

Cream is given to relieve the itching, and drugs such as mebendazole are used to destroy the parasite. Homeopathic and herbal remedies such as Artemisacina (cina) and Quassia amara (quassia) can help.

PREVENTION

- Wash hands regularly, especially before eating.
- Take frequent baths or showers.
- Avoid scratching the infected site.

OUTLOOK

The infection is always treatable.

Lice

Lice are tiny wingless creatures that feed by piercing the skin and sucking up blood. There are three species, head lice, body lice and crab lice – which are also known as pubic lice. Head and crab lice lay eggs that are known as nits and attach to hair, while body lice lay their eggs on clothing. An infestation can cause an intensely irritating itch. (See **Lice.**)

Lyme disease

Also known as borrelia or borreliosis, Lyme disease is caused by bacteria that are transmitted to human beings by tick bites. Changes in climate have been blamed for the recent increase in the number of cases occurring in the UK. (See **Lyme disease.**)

Malaria

Malaria is caused by a parasite that infects red blood cells. It is transmitted to human beings by mosquito bites. The disease originates in the tropical areas of Africa, Asia and Central and South America, but over a thousand cases are reported every year in the UK, brought in by returning travellers. (See **Malaria.**)

▼ Bloodsucker
The parasitic worm that causes schistosomiasis attaches itself by a large suction pad to blood vessels in the bladder and intestines of its host. It feeds on nutrients in the blood.

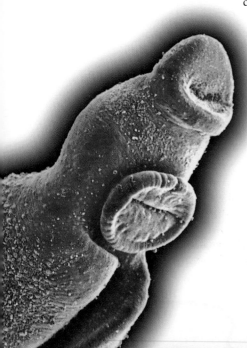

Scabies

Commonly known as mange mites, *Sarcoptes scabies* can burrow under the skin and live there, causing the infection scabies. The mites are transmitted from person to person by close contact or by infected bedding.

SYMPTOMS

In an initial infestation, symptoms are rare for the first month. In subsequent infections, they appear within four days. Symptoms include:
- severe itching that worsens at night;
- rash in the creases between the fingers, behind the elbows and knees, under the breasts, around the penis, and between the shoulder blades.

TREATMENT

Clothes and bedding should be washed thoroughly in hot water two days before any treatment begins.
- Lotions such as permethrin are applied to all areas of the body, then washed off up to 24 hours later. Anyone who is in close contact with the affected person should also be treated, and all bedding and clothing washed.

Complementary therapies

The herbal remedy Rumex crispus (yellow dock) can sometimes be helpful.

PREVENTION

Good hygiene can prevent infection.

COMPLICATIONS

A more severe variety of scabies called Norwegian scabies is characterized by thick crusts on the skin and is common in people with immune system problems. Secondary bacterial infections can occur.

OUTLOOK

Treatment if highly effective, if clothes and bedding are kept scrupulously clean.

Schistosomiasis

Two hundred million people worldwide, mainly in the tropics, are infected with the flatworm *Schistosoma mansoni*. It lives in the intestines and bladder, causing schistosomiasis, which is also known as bilharziasis. The worm's eggs are passed in the victim's urine and faeces into freshwater rivers and lakes, and the disease is contracted when the larvae penetrate the skin of someone swimming in the infected water. These larvae develop into adults, which settle in the new victim's intestines or bladder.

SYMPTOMS

Initially, there may be no sign of infection, although there may be itchy skin and a rash. After a month, an affected person may experience a fever and chills, a cough and aching muscles.

TREATMENT

Treatment may include antibiotics and drugs such as praziquantel, which kill the worms.

PREVENTION

■ Do not swim in freshwater rivers or pools in countries where the parasite is common. Caution should be maintained in Southern and sub-Saharan Africa, South America, the Caribbean, the Middle East, southern China and Southeast Asia.

■ Drink bottled water only when travelling in any of the countries in the regions mentioned above – check that the seal of the bottle is still intact before drinking.

COMPLICATIONS

Repeated infections over a number of years can result in liver, lung, intestinal and bladder damage. This is due to the parasitic worms growing inside the blood vessels and producing eggs which then travel to the intestines and bladder. The body reacts to the eggs.

OUTLOOK

The infection can be difficult to treat.

Toxoplasmosis

Toxoplasmosis is caused by the micro-organism *Toxoplasma gondii*. It can be transmitted to human beings in undercooked meat, and after contact with cat faeces – a typical example is when someone cleans out a litter tray and does not wash his or her hands thoroughly before eating or preparing food.

SYMPTOMS

There may be no symptoms, although an infected person may experience:

■ mild flu-like symptoms;

■ slightly enlarged lymph nodes.

TREATMENT

A blood sample is taken and tested for evidence of the disease. Antibiotics may be given to people with poor immunity, but often no treatment is necessary.

PREVENTION

Avoid eating raw or undercooked meat and handling cat litter, especially if you are pregnant or have immunity problems.

COMPLICATIONS

Toxoplasmosis can sometimes cause serious damage in people with impaired immunity, and if contracted by a pregnant woman may lead to malformation of the fetus and even stillbirth.

OUTLOOK

Most people recover fully.

Trichomonas infection

The *Trichomonas vaginalis* parasite is found throughout the world and causes one of the most common **sexually transmitted diseases**. It is most prevalent in sexually active women under the age of 35 but can also be transmitted to men.

SYMPTOMS

The infection can be symptom-free, but some people experience:

■ in women – a foul-smelling discharge, which can froth from the vagina;

■ in men – a discharge from the urethra;

■ pain during sexual intercourse;

■ a strong urge to urinate.

TREATMENT

Antibiotics are the usual treatment.

PREVENTION

Using a latex condom during sex should provide protection from this infection.

COMPLICATIONS

Re-infection can occur if a partner is not treated at the same time as the affected person.

OUTLOOK

The outlook is good if treatment is prompt.

SEE ALSO *Infectious diseases; Travel and tropical diseases*

Paratyphoid

Although very similar to **typhoid fever**, paratyphoid is generally much less severe. It is an infectious disease caused by the bacterium *Salmonella paratyphi*. The symptoms include fever, tiredness, loss of appetite, constipation, diarrhoea, headache, rose-coloured spots on the chest area and an enlarged spleen and liver. The incubation period is about one to three weeks and symptoms generally last for about a week.

Paratyphoid is related to hygiene and sanitary conditions. It is common in countries where there is unsafe drinking water, where sewage disposal is inadequate, and where flooding occurs. Paratyphoid bacteria are passed in the faeces and urine of infected people. You can also become infected after eating food or drinking beverages that have been handled, and therefore contaminated, by an infected person, or by drinking water contaminated by sewage containing the bacteria. In some countries, shellfish from sewage-contaminated beds can be a source of infection. Once the bacterium enters the body, it multiplies and spreads from the intestines into the bloodstream.

TREATMENT

Treatment with antibiotics is highly effective.

PREVENTION

Since paratyphoid is often transmitted by contaminated water, it is advisable to drink only bottled water when in less industrialized countries; always check that the seal is intact before drinking. Good hygiene and sanitation prevent the spread of paratyphoid.

Parkinson's disease

Parkinson's disease is a slowly progressive disease of the nervous system. The classic sign is a slow tremor, but symptoms vary. In some sufferers there may be little outward sign of the disease for many years.

The cause of Parkinson's disease is unknown and the condition is very rare in people under the age of 40. Symptoms are usually noticed when people are in their 60s or 70s. Around 120,000 people in the UK have Parkinson's disease and every year 10,000 new patients are diagnosed with the condition.

The first visible symptom of Parkinson's disease is often an involuntary shaking or tremor on one side of the body. Typically it starts in the fingers or hand. The tremor may progress to the legs, jaw, tongue and forehead, and is usually worse when the person is resting and better during movement. Which parts of the body are affected – and how badly they shake – varies from person to person. About one-quarter of people with Parkinson's disease do not have a tremor at all.

As the condition slowly progresses, movement may become jerky and the limbs rigid. People tend to shuffle when they walk and cannot swing their arms as they move along. They take small, quick steps, and then run to prevent themselves from falling. Some people find it difficult to speak clearly, others cannot write legibly. If facial muscles are affected, it may become hard to smile, frown or use the normal body language that we all take for granted. This can make people with Parkinson's disease feel frustrated, misunderstood and, in some cases, depressed. People who have had Parkinson's disease for many years may also experience some memory loss and confused thinking.

CAUSES

Parkinson's disease affects a part of the brain called the substantia nigra, located in the basal ganglia in the cerebrum (see **Brain and nervous system**). The substantia nigra produces a chemical messenger called dopamine that is responsible for passing messages from one nerve cell to another. Dopamine and another chemical, acetylcholine, control the movement of the body.

In Parkinson's disease, the cells that produce dopamine deteriorate and so there is an increasing loss of dopamine. When the levels of dopamine fall to 80 per cent of what they should be, the balance between dopamine and acetylcholine is upset and messages from the brain to some parts of the body are interrupted or travel very slowly. It is this failure of the body's communication system that causes the symptoms of Parkinson's disease.

DIAGNOSIS

Parkinson's disease is usually diagnosed by a specialist in neurological diseases, largely on the basis of observable symptoms and a physical examination. For example, gently manipulating a limb of someone with Parkinson's disease is likely to make it go rigid. Scans and other tests help to rule out other illnesses, particularly in elderly people who may have movement problems or be suffering from **depression** or **dementia**.

Parkinsonism

Symptoms similar to those of Parkinson's disease sometimes occur in people as a secondary effect of other disorders, following exposure to toxins or in reaction to some drugs – as a side effect of some antipsychotic agents, for example. In these cases, the sufferers are said to have Parkinsonism rather than Parkinson's disease. A person with Parkinsonism will be troubled by tremor, jerkiness, rigidity and other movement problems.

LIVING WITH PARKINSON'S DISEASE

If you have been diagnosed with Parkinson's disease, your GP, hospital specialist and other health workers will be an invaluable source of help and advice. They will be able to put you in touch with local services and volunteer support groups. These vary from area to area, but most offer help and information for sufferers and their family or carer as well as opportunities for social gatherings and outings.

It is quite common to feel anxiety and depression when you are first diagnosed. But if you can keep a positive and practical outlook, this will help you to make the most of the pleasures and opportunities of life.

As Parkinson's disease progresses, it may become more difficult to cope with everyday living. Simple tasks may require more effort and take much longer than previously, but persistence is worthwhile. Keeping the following advice in mind may help.

- Take things steadily. Planning your activities will enable you to avoid rushing.
- Accept help, but only with the tasks that are really difficult.
- Take all medicines you have been prescribed as directed and let your doctor know how well they are working.
- Do any exercises that have been recommended by your physiotherapist and try not to be discouraged if they seem difficult at first.
- Remember – the more you do, the longer you will be able to do more.

CARING FOR SOMEONE WITH PARKINSON'S

If you are looking after a parent, other relative or friend with Parkinson's disease, encourage him or her to do as much as possible for him or herself for as long as possible. For advice and support, keep in touch with the person's GP and health workers, and contact the Parkinson's Disease Society and other self-help groups.

Help for carers

Looking after someone with a long-term, disabling condition such as Parkinson's disease is very demanding. Many carers find it helpful to talk with other people in the same situation or with a counsellor or therapist. It is important to have a day off from time to time – don't feel guilty about taking advantage of respite care schemes for people with chronic conditions. Staff from the hospital or social services department should be able to explain what is available in your area.

TREATMENT

There is no cure for Parkinson's disease, but a great deal can be done to relieve symptoms, particularly in the early stages. Drug treatment falls into two categories: drugs that mimic dopamine and drugs that reduce the rate of loss of natural dopamine. Other treatments include surgery and physical therapies.

Levodopa

For many years, the aim of Parkinson's disease treatment has been to replace the dopamine that is missing in the brain. This has largely been done with a drug called levodopa – a synthetic chemical that is converted into dopamine when it gets into the brain. Levodopa is most effective at relieving the rigidity and slow movements associated with the disease, though it can also reduce the tremor. Initially, levodopa treatment can help someone newly diagnosed with Parkinson's disease to move almost normally.

The main drawback of levodopa is its side effects, which include nausea, low blood pressure, involuntary movements and restlessness. Taking a second drug – usually carbidopa – to block levodopa's activity outside the brain may help

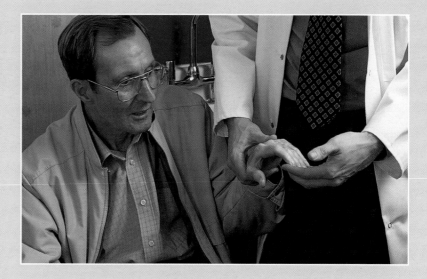

▲ **Parkinson's diagnosis**
A doctor checks the fingers of a man for the slow movement and response that is recognized as a sign of Parkinson's disease.

to reduce the nausea and drops in blood pressure when you stand. But abnormal involuntary movements, including facial tics and other muscle spasms, are common side effects of levodopa that cannot be avoided or blocked. People may be unwilling to put up with these, which will limit the dose of levadopa that can be used. After two to five years of treatment with levodopa, more than half of those with Parkinson's disease experience fluctuations in their response to the drug – the so-called 'on-off' effect.

Within a single day symptoms can fluctuate enormously. One minute, they are well controlled and someone with Parkinson's disease can get dressed and eat normally. The next minute, the person can barely move and is helpless. The longer levodopa treatment continues, the shorter the beneficial effects after each dose.

As a result of these problems, many doctors prefer to avoid using levodopa in the early stages of Parkinson's disease, especially in younger people, and hold it in reserve for when other drugs stop working.

Selegiline and other drugs

Several drugs are now available that either boost the activity of a person's own dopamine or mimic that of the nerve transmitter.

Selegiline blocks the activity of an enzyme called monoamine oxidase B, which breaks down dopamine in the brain. It is used on its own in the early stages of Parkinson's disease or, later on, combined with levodopa. There is some evidence that selegiline delays the need for levodopa.

The antiviral drug amantadine is also thought to enhance the availability of dopamine, but by a different and, as yet, uncertain mechanism. Entacapone is used in combination with levodopa to prolong its duration of action by inhibiting one of the enzymes that break down dopamine.

Another option in the treatment of Parkinson's disease is to improve the balance between

If you have Parkinson's disease, keep as healthy and active as possible, with plenty of exercise, fresh air and a balanced diet.

dopamine and other nerve transmitters, for example, by blocking the activity of acetylcholine with anticholinergic drugs such as benztropine. These drugs are useful for treating tremor in the early stages of Parkinson's disease. Some anticholinergic agents, such as amitriptyline, also have antidepressant effects.

Dopamine receptor agonists

Oral dopamine-like drugs known as dopamine receptor agonists stimulate receptors in the brain. Like selegiline, they are used on their own or together with levodopa to improve its effectiveness. These drugs have similar side effects to levodopa, including nausea, vomiting, drowsiness, hallucinations and confusion, and doses have to be carefully tailored to individual needs. Anti-emetic agents, such as domperidone, can be useful in blocking the nausea and vomiting associated with dopamine agonists.

Some dopamine agonists, such as apomorphine and lisuride, are given as injections under the skin. Apomorphine injections may be used to help people during sudden 'off' periods. The drug is also used as a continuous infusion for those with severe and frequent movement fluctuations, so that the dose of levodopa can be reduced and, with it, abnormal movement.

Non-drug treatments

Drug treatment of Parkinson's disease should be used as part of a coordinated plan to minimize the disability associated with the condition, and treatment should include appropriate use of **physiotherapy**, **speech therapy** and **occupational therapy**.

People vary enormously in how their disease progresses and how they cope with it. So it is important to review your drug and non-drug treatments at regular intervals, or as soon as there is a change in your responses or ability to cope.

Physiotherapists can advise on an exercise programme, massage and other techniques to relax overactive muscles and reduce spasms. Exercise will not stop the progression of Parkinson's disease, but it can strengthen and relax the muscles whose overactivity and rigidity are common features of the condition. Exercises can also help people to walk more smoothly and improve their balance so they become less prone to falling over.

For those with speech and swallowing problems, speech therapists can recommend exercises to help them to communicate more effectively. Occupational therapists assess what aids and adaptations to the home and elsewhere could help people with Parkinson's disease to cope more effectively with their disabilities. This may mean putting up railings and banisters to make moving about easier, or installing labour-saving devices for cooking, washing and cleaning.

Recent research has uncovered new information about dopamine receptors in the brain that could revolutionize the use of drugs for Parkinson's disease.

As depression is a common symptom of Parkinson's disease, some people benefit from counselling or other psychological therapies. It may be easier to discuss emotions of anger, frustration and unhappiness with a trained counsellor than with friends or family.

Complementary therapies

Some people with Parkinson's disease find that stress-relieving therapies are helpful. It is widely accepted that stress and tiredness can aggravate symptoms, so techniques such as visualization and therapies such as aromatherapy, which help people to relax, are likely to be helpful.

If you have Parkinson's disease, choose a diet that is low in fat and refined sugar and high in fibre-rich fruit and vegetables. A high-protein diet can interfere with the absorption of levodopa, so some doctors recommend restricting protein consumption to the evening meal. Hopes that antioxidant treatment, such as vitamin E, might delay the progression of Parkinson's disease have not been supported by research.

Surgery

Before the introduction of levodopa in the 1960s, surgery was quite often used to try to relieve the symptoms of Parkinson's disease. A thin probe was inserted into the brain through a hole in the skull. For example, in an operation called pallidotomy, surgeons carefully destroyed overactive nerve cells in an effort to reduce tremors and abnormal movements.

With the success of levodopa, surgery was used less often. But when doctors realized that levodopa became less effective with time, they began to reconsider whether surgery might still be an effective way of treating Parkinson's disease. The beneficial effects of pallidotomy have recently been confirmed in studies showing improvements in movements and tremor for about five years.

A further option is to operate on a part of the brain called the thalamus. Either an electrode can be implanted in the thalamus and stimulated from outside, or part of the thalamus can be destroyed. Both approaches have been shown to relieve tremor in Parkinson's disease. But technical difficulties and cost have limited the use of implants, and further surgical destruction of cells may be needed if people go on to develop other movement problems.

A more controversial treatment has been fetal brain cell transplants to try to replace the damaged brain cells in the basal ganglia. Transplants were first attempted in the late 1980s and promising results were reported in a handful of cases. However, there have been doubts over the long-term effectiveness of these and subsequent transplants, and ethical concerns about the use of fetal tissue have limited this type of surgery in many countries.

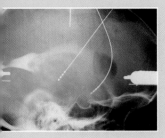

◄ Electrode implant
One surgical method of treating Parkinson's disease is to implant an electrode in the brain. The electrode is then activated remotely to destroy the overactive nerve cells that are responsible for tremor and other symptoms.

In one placebo-controlled trial in the USA, embryonic brain cell transplants were performed on 40 people with severe Parkinson's disease. In patients aged under 60, the procedure resulted in some improvements in movement that lasted at least 12 months after surgery. Older patients did not improve. Brain scans of the people who had had the transplants showed their dopamine activity had increased by at least 20 per cent. But there were ethical concerns about performing 'sham' operations on members of the placebo group (who had all given full consent) as these involved a general **anaesthetic** and making a hole in the skull.

OUTLOOK

Parkinson's disease is not fatal. Current drug, surgical and other treatments ensure that people who develop the disease can expect to live for much of their normal lifespan. The disease does not have a regulated pattern of progression and it is not possible for doctors to predict how quickly the symptoms of the disease will affect the sufferer. In some people, the condition can cause disabling deterioration within 5–10 years, while others remain physically very able for 15 or even 20 years.

THE FUTURE

Parkinson's disease is one of many conditions that it is hoped may ultimately benefit from stem cell transplants. These are the multipurpose cells that develop into a variety of different cells needed for the brain, heart, kidney and other organs. Intensive research is underway in many institutions around the world to find out more about the triggers that make stem cells develop into one type of tissue or another.

At present, embryos are the best sources of stem cells for research. But, as scientists learn more about how to switch stem cells on and off, they hope to be able to avoid the ethical concerns of using embryonic tissue by harvesting and manipulating adult stem cells.

In this way, they may one day be able to replace the damaged nerves of the substantia nigra with fresh, healthy, dopamine-producing cells and so give back normal control over their movements to people with Parkinson's disease.

SEE ALSO *Brain and nervous system*

Patch test

A patch test is the application of a suspect substance to the skin in order to determine whether it is a cause of contact **dermatitis** or **eczema**. Either of these conditions can be the result of a sensitivity to a particular substance that the body has encountered in the past. A patch test can help to identify the substance that causes the dermatitis or eczema. Once this has been done, avoiding the trigger substance will go a long way towards curing the problem.

People can be sensitive to a wide range of substances used in everyday life. They include soap, detergents, cosmetics, plants, fabric such as wool, and the fur of pets. People can also develop reactions to substances, such as particular brands of make-up or soap, that have been used without any symptoms for long periods of time.

Patch testing can be especially useful for people who have become sensitive to a constituent of creams or bath emollients that they may be using to treat other conditions, such as non-allergic eczema. Common culprits are lanolin and the preservatives in steroid creams, which can antagonize the effect of the steroid.

WHAT'S INVOLVED

Patch testing is carried out by a dermatologist. A sample of the substance to be tested is placed on a small piece of fabric (usually cotton), which is attached to the skin of the inner forearm or the back with waterproof tape. The tape is left in place for 48 hours, but it can be removed earlier if the site becomes uncomfortable. After 48 hours, the site is inspected when the tape is removed, and again one hour later when the marks left by the tape have faded. Further changes are also noted over the following three days. Several suspect substances are usually tested at the same time, using different patches.

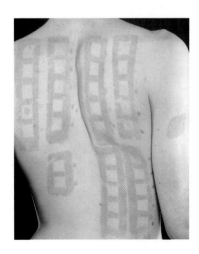

◄ Patch test positive
Raised red marks on the skin are caused by the waterproof tape that has held the patch tests in place. They will fade within an hour. The red spots on the mid-upper right and lower left back indicate allergy to the substances tested there.

AFTER THE TEST
The appearance of an itchy rash or raised blemish at the test site suggests an allergic or hypersensitive reaction to the substance being tested. Patch tests are a useful tool, but they are not foolproof. A negative result does not rule out a substance as a cause of the problem. This is because the immune system has many ways of reacting to a sensitive substance, and the patch test only investigates one of those ways.
SEE ALSO *Allergy*

Pelvis and disorders

The pelvis is a girdle of bones that supports the spine and connects the upper body to the lower limbs. It also protects the organs found in the space within it, which is known as the pelvic cavity. These organs are different in men and in women. The shape of the pelvis is also different between the sexes (see box, opposite).

A girdle of bones
The pelvis consists of the two hip bones and, behind them, the triangular sacrum and the coccyx, a small bone at the base of the spinal column.

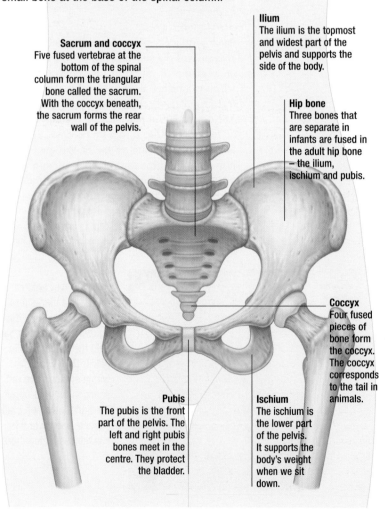

Sacrum and coccyx
Five fused vertebrae at the bottom of the spinal column form the triangular bone called the sacrum. With the coccyx beneath, the sacrum forms the rear wall of the pelvis.

Ilium
The ilium is the topmost and widest part of the pelvis and supports the side of the body.

Hip bone
Three bones that are separate in infants are fused in the adult hip bone – the ilium, ischium and pubis.

Coccyx
Four fused pieces of bone form the coccyx. The coccyx corresponds to the tail in animals.

Pubis
The pubis is the front part of the pelvis. The left and right pubis bones meet in the centre. They protect the bladder.

Ischium
The ischium is the lower part of the pelvis. It supports the body's weight when we sit down.

The pelvis is wider at the top, which is called the pelvic inlet, than at the bottom, the pelvic outlet. Occasionally, the outlet is too narrow in women to allow the birth of a child – a Caesarean section is then necessary for delivery.

The bladder and rectum – and in women, the womb – are normally prevented from sinking out of the pelvis by a system of muscles and ligaments known as the pelvic floor.

Pelvic injury
An injury to the pelvis may result in damage to the organs in the pelvic cavity or to the blood supply in that part of the body. A fall or heavy collision can cause a fracture of the pelvic bones, which can have serious consequences.

In particular, pelvic injuries to men may cause problems with sexual function. Difficulties in having and maintaining an erection quite commonly result from pelvic injuries – research in the USA shows that one-third of men who suffered a fracture of the pelvis or damage to the pelvic blood supply subsequently suffered erection problems.

Pelvic injuries in women may cause damage to the womb, ovaries or Fallopian tubes and may impair fertility.

Pelvic tumours
Tumours in the pelvis, both cancerous and non-cancerous, can become quite large before they cause symptoms. These often result from pressure on neighbouring organs.

Possible symptoms of a pelvic tumour include frequently needing to urinate or having difficulty urinating, swelling of the abdomen, vague pain in the abdomen, tiredness and weight loss.

Common pelvic tumours include tumours of the ovaries and fibroids in the womb. These may need surgical treatment. An **ultrasound** scan, **laparoscopy** or **laparotomy** may be necessary to make an exact diagnosis.

Most pelvic tumours can be successfully treated, but those caused by ovarian cancer are more difficult to eradicate.

Prolapse
A prolapse is the forward or downward displacement of part of the body. Some of the most common types are the displacement of the uterus, bladder or rectum in women. These occur when the muscles and ligaments of the pelvic floor have been weakened.

Women often notice a lump coming down from the vagina. Other symptoms include urinary incontinence, a dragging pain in the pelvis and experiencing difficulty in opening the bowels.

The pelvic floor may be weakened by childbirth, the menopause, previous surgery such as a hysterectomy, obesity or a long-term increase in pressure within the abdomen – caused, for example, by a large tumour, constipation or coughing.

Treatment options include regular exercises to strengthen the pelvic floor muscles or inserting rings into the vagina to support its walls. Doctors will also treat any aggravating factors, such as a cough, constipation and obesity.

Most women are able to strengthen their pelvic floor muscles and the prolapse is corrected. But repair operations, which are usually carried out via the vagina, are sometimes necessary.

Pelvic inflammatory disease

In pelvic inflammatory disease (PID), the Fallopian tubes, ovaries and surrounding structures have become infected and inflamed. Without early treatment, the disease may cause permanent damage to the pelvic organs, which can lead to infertility and sometimes persistent pain. Pelvic inflammatory disease is a major cause of infertility worldwide. In the UK, about 100,000 women develop the condition each year.

Some women with pelvic inflammatory disease have no symptoms, while others suffer pain or discomfort in the lower abdomen, experience pain during sexual intercourse, have an abnormal vaginal discharge or develop a high fever.

Pelvic inflammatory disease is usually a result of a sexually transmitted infection. About 50 per cent of infections are caused by chlamydia. In many cases, the cause of PID is not identified.

Antibiotics are used to treat acute pelvic inflammatory disease. Sexual partners should be screened and treated if necessary. Chronic pelvic inflammatory disease often fails to respond to even prolonged courses of antibiotics and a hysterectomy is sometimes necessary to relieve symptoms. About 20 per cent of women with pelvic inflammatory disease become infertile and about 20 per cent develop long-term pain in the pelvis. Around 10 per cent of those who conceive have a tubal pregnancy (see page 470).

Endometriosis

Endometriosis is a non-cancerous condition in which tissue similar to the lining (endometrium) of the womb forms at other sites, usually in the pelvis. It affects about 1.5 million women in the UK.

Sometimes endometriosis causes no symptoms at all. Alternatively, it may result in severe

Factfile

Differences between the male and female pelvis

A woman's pelvis is shaped differently to a man's, in order to facilitate the birth of children. The organs within the pelvis are different in men and women, too.

In women, the two ilia bones at the top of the hip are less deep and farther apart than in men. This is why women have wider hips. The sacrum is usually less curved than in men and the outlet at the bottom of the pelvis is wider. This maximizes the width of the birth canal. In women, the protruberances on the ischia bones are smaller and do not project so far into the pelvic cavity. The pelvic cavity contains the bladder, bowel and reproductive organs. In women, this includes the uterus, Fallopian tubes and ovaries. In men, it contains the prostate gland and the seminal vesicles, glands behind the bladder.

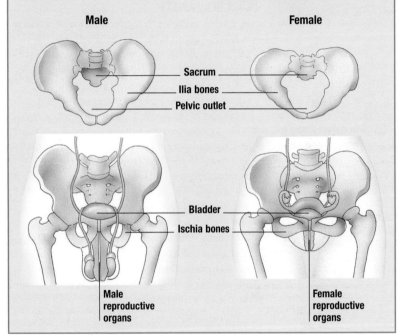

Male   Female

Sacrum
Ilia bones
Pelvic outlet

Bladder
Ischia bones

Male reproductive organs

Female reproductive organs

prolonged period pain or pain during sexual intercourse, particularly with deep penetration. Other possible symptoms are infertility, pressure in the rectum and blood in the urine.

The exact cause of endometriosis is unknown. One possibility is that, during a period, cells from the lining of the womb pass back along the Fallopian tubes into the pelvis and implant themselves on the surface of pelvic organs such as the uterus and ovaries. They then proliferate and undergo changes similar to those that occur each month in the womb lining. This leads to internal bleeding, which causes inflammation and adhesions. Endometriosis often runs in families and is increasing in frequency as women have fewer pregnancies and therefore more periods. Taking the Pill appears to have a protective effect.

Treatment may consist of medication to reduce oestrogen levels, such as the contraceptive pill (taken continuously) or

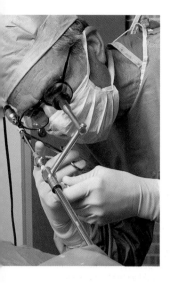

▲ **Laparoscopy**
A doctor has inserted a laparoscope – a tube fitted with light and a magnifying lens – into a woman's pelvis to determine whether or not she has endometriosis. If she has the condition, he will see blood blisters and cysts on the pelvic organs.

progestogens, such as dydrogesterone, medroxyprogesterone, danazol or gestrinone. Alternatively, a doctor may prescribe a preparation that acts like GNRH (the gonadotrophin-releasing hormone that helps to stimulate ovulation) by nasal spray or injection.

Surgery by **laser** or **diathermy** (heat) treatment to remove the displaced tissue is sometimes successful. In severe cases of endometriosis, a hysterectomy with removal of the ovaries and Fallopian tubes may be the best way to relieve symptoms. Rates of recovery vary, but endometriosis will improve with **menopause**.

Tubal pregnancy

In a tubal pregnancy, the fetus starts to develop in the Fallopian tube. This may rupture the tube and cause life-threatening internal bleeding. In recent years, the incidence of tubal pregnancies has increased as the incidence of pelvic inflammatory disease has increased. About one in 200 pregnancies develop outside the uterus.

The symptoms of a tubal pregnancy are those of a normal pregnancy plus pelvic pain, usually on one side only. Sometimes women with a tubal pregnancy collapse suddenly.

A woman who has previously had a pelvic inflammatory disease, particularly if connected to chlamydia, is more likely to have a tubal pregnancy. Other factors that increase the likelihood are using a progestogen-only pill, an IUD (intrauterine contraceptive device) or undergoing in vitro fertilization (IVF) or gamete intra-Fallopian transfer (GIFT).

Women with a suspected tubal pregnancy will need to be admitted to hospital for investigation. Women who have collapsed may need immediate surgery as delay can be fatal. A ruptured Fallopian tube is usually removed. If the tube is intact, it may be possible to remove the fetal sac and preserve the tube. Many women who have a tubal pregnancy later go on to have a successful pregnancy.

SEE ALSO *Ovaries and disorders; Pregnancy and problems; Reproductive system; Uterus and problems*

Pemphigoid

Pemphigoid is an autoimmune disease in which the body produces antibodies that attack a skin protein responsible for holding cells together. It is similar to another blistering condition, pemphigus vulgaris, but different proteins are targeted and the blisters are deeper. Diagnosis is made by biopsy, which shows a splitting of the skin through the layer known as the basement membrane. The condition can be treated with corticosteroids and immunosuppressive drugs, which usually have to be taken for at least two to three years.

Bullous pemphigoid is a form of the condition that mainly affects people over the age of 60. Multiple large blisters form, which are very tense and may have a red or bloodstained base. They are often intensely itchy.

SEE ALSO *Skin and disorders*

Penis and disorders

The penis is the male sexual organ. It contains the urethra, the tube through which urine and semen are discharged. The penis consists mainly of spongy erectile tissue full of blood vessels. When a man is sexually excited, the erectile tissue fills with blood which, because the veins are then so tight, cannot drain out again and so produces an erection.

WHAT CAN GO WRONG
Conditions that commonly affect the penis include disorders involving sexual function and a man's ability to achieve and maintain an erection; problems with the foreskin; certain sexually transmitted diseases; urination problems; congenital disorders; and, more rarely, cancer. Blood in the urine should be reported to your GP promptly as it may indicate a problem such as a kidney, prostate or bladder disorder or infection. Blood in the sperm is usually an isolated incident, although a second occurrence should be reported. A blockage of the urethra can result from inserting objects into the end of the penis. If an object is not retrievable with the use of forceps, it may need to be removed under anaesthetic.

Sexual function problems
Erectile dysfunction or impotence is a condition in which a man is unable to produce or maintain an erection adequate for his chosen sexual activity. When a man ejaculates before or immediately following sexual penetration, this is referred to as premature ejaculation.

The inability to ejaculate at all, known as retarded ejaculation, may be the sign of an underlying medical condition. However, if a man can ejaculate through masturbation, the cause is more likely to be either tiredness or psychological inhibition.

Priapism is a potentially dangerous condition in which the penis becomes erect for long periods in the absence of sexual arousal.

In Peyronie's disease, thick, hard scars develop inside the penis, causing it to bend when erect and making sexual intercourse awkward or impossible. Peyronie's disease can be painful and, as the plaques restrict blood flow, can make it difficult to achieve erections. Worrying about this problem may cause **impotence**. Men who suspect that they may have Peyronie's disease should consult their doctor promptly.

Peyronie's disease is known to affect 80,000 men in the UK, usually those aged over 40. But the real incidence could be much higher, since embarrassment may stop some men from seeking help. It is thought that it may affect up to one per cent of the older male population. The cause is unclear, although it may be the result of damage to the penis or internal bleeding. The disease is not sexually transmitted. Usually Peyronie's heals itself – a doctor may recommend drug treatment in the form of painkillers or other drugs – but in about one in ten cases surgery will be advised.

Problems with the foreskin

The foreskin can be affected by a number of complaints. Phimosis, a condition in which the foreskin is too tight and cannot be drawn back, is the main medical reason for **circumcision** in young boys. The common initial tightness of the infant foreskin should not be mistaken for phimosis, and action to correct the condition is best delayed because full retractability of the foreskin can be expected in almost all boys by their early teens.

Poor personal hygiene can lead to **balanitis**, in which the foreskin becomes inflamed, and to a buildup of smegma, a smelly white substance that can accumulate under the foreskin of an unwashed penis. It is formed from the secretions of the sebaceous glands in the penis glans.

Sexually transmitted diseases

Whenever you have sex without using a condom with a partner whose medical history you cannot be sure about, you risk contracting a **sexually transmitted disease**. Possible symptoms of a sexually transmitted disease include:

■ an unusual discharge from the penis;

■ pain or a burning feeling when urinating or having sex;

■ urinating more often than usual;

■ rashes, itchiness, **warts**, sores, soreness, blisters or pain in the genital area.

People who suspect that they have contracted a sexually transmitted disease (for example, if a partner has one) should consult a GP or visit a sexually transmitted disease clinic or genito-urinary medicine (GUM) clinic, even if symptoms have not appeared.

Congenital disorders

The penis can be affected by a number of congenital disorders. Hermaphroditism is a very rare congenital problem in which a baby has both male and female sex organs. With pseudohermaphroditism, a baby has only one

The structure of the penis

The penis consists of three cylinders of spongy erectile tissue, which fill with blood during sexual excitement. This causes the penis to become erect.

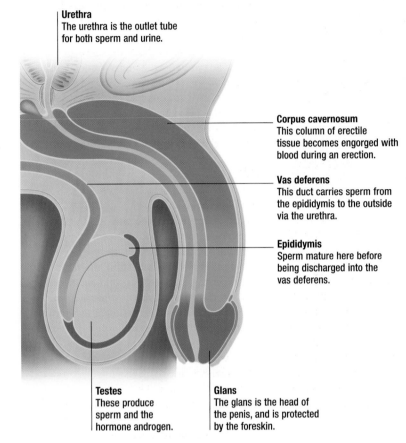

Urethra
The urethra is the outlet tube for both sperm and urine.

Corpus cavernosum
This column of erectile tissue becomes engorged with blood during an erection.

Vas deferens
This duct carries sperm from the epididymis to the outside via the urethra.

Epididymis
Sperm mature here before being discharged into the vas deferens.

Testes
These produce sperm and the hormone androgen.

Glans
The glans is the head of the penis, and is protected by the foreskin.

set of genitals, but these may more closely resemble those of the opposite sex – for example, in a boy the penis may be very small and resemble a clitoris.

Hypospadias is a congenital problem in which the opening of the urethra appears in the wrong place – generally on the underside of the head of the penis, but in more severe cases closer to the scrotum. Surgery is usually performed before a boy is two years old to straighten the penis and create an artificial urethra from other skin. Normal urination and, later, sexual intercourse are both then possible.

Penile cancer

There are probably fewer than 400 cases of penile **cancer** a year in the UK, making it one of the rarest cancers. Keeping the penis clean reduces the risk still further. Symptoms include a red, velvet-like patch, ulcer or other growth on the penis. If cancer of the penis is diagnosed early in its development, the condition can usually be successfully treated by using **radiotherapy**; otherwise surgery is needed.

SEE ALSO *Prostate and disorders; Reproductive system; Urinary system*

Peritonitis

Peritonitis is inflammation of the peritoneum, the membrane that lines the abdominal cavity. The infection is usually caused by bacteria, which enter the cavity through a perforation in the stomach or intestine. This may be caused by **appendicitis**, **diverticular disease**, a peptic ulcer or a ruptured gallbladder. Other, rarer, causes include an injury in which the abdominal wall is pierced, an infection that spreads through the bloodstream (**septicaemia**), an infection that spreads from the female genital tract or accidental contamination during surgery.

The symptoms of peritonitis include acute abdominal distension and pain (this is not always present), a high fever, vomiting, shock and **dehydration**.

Peritonitis is diagnosed primarily by physical examination, but **endoscopy** and **X-rays** may also be used. Immediate treatment is essential: antibiotics combat the infection, an intravenous infusion counteracts dehydration and surgery is generally required to identify and treat the cause of the problem. If treatment is prompt, the outlook is usually good.

Pharyngitis

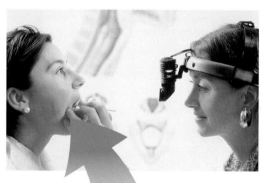

▲ **Sore throat**
An examination of a patient with a sore throat may pinpoint infected tonsils (white patches) as the cause of pain.

Pharyngitis, or an inflammation of the pharynx, is the most common cause of sore throats. Pharyngitis is generally caused by a virus, such as the influenza virus or the common cold virus. Some cases arise from infection with bacteria such as *Streptococcus* or *Haemophilus influenzae*. When pharyngitis is caused by *Streptococcus*, it is known as 'strep throat', a condition that can sometimes lead to complications such as rheumatic fever and kidney problems if left untreated. Pharyngitis is most common in winter, and is often passed round between people in the same household.

SYMPTOMS

- Sore throat.
- In viral pharyngitis, runny nose.
- In strep throat, fever, headache, swollen lymph nodes in the neck.
- In severe cases of pharyngitis, swallowing difficulties and, more rarely, breathing problems.

DURATION

The symptoms of viral pharyngitis should ease gradually over the course of one week. Someone who has bacterial pharyngitis can expect the symptoms to subside within two to three days of starting a course of antibiotic treatment. For the treatment to be successful it is important to complete the course of antibiotics.

TREATMENT

A physical examination of the pharynx is usually sufficient to diagnose most cases of pharyngitis. If strep throat is suspected your GP may take throat swabs for analysis. The treatment of pharyngitis depends on the underlying cause. Antibiotics should be given for bacterial cases, including strep throat. Antibiotics and antiseptic lozenges should not be used to treat viral pharyngitis: they upset the natural balance of microbes which may lead to chronic infection.

What you can do

A viral infection usually clears up on its own, but gargling with warm salt water, taking painkillers such as aspirin, and drinking plenty of fluids will help to relieve symptoms.

When to consult a doctor

Seek medical attention if:
- a sore throat does not clear up in several days;
- you have a fever, swollen glands in the neck or a rash;
- breathing difficulties develop.

COMPLICATIONS

Almost all patients with viral or bacterial pharyngitis recover completely and rapidly, without developing any complications. However, if streptococcal sore throat is not treated with antibiotics, the bacteria can remain in the pharynx. It may go on to cause further complications such as **otitis media** (ear infection), sinusitis, rheumatic fever or glomerulonephritis (kidney inflammation).

Phenylketonuria

Phenylketonuria, often referred to as PKU, is an inherited metabolic disorder in which the body cannot break down proteins properly. If it is not treated, harmful substances build up in the blood and can cause brain damage.

Since the 1960s, all newborn babies have been tested for phenylketonuria using a blood test called the Guthrie test six to ten days after birth. About one in 10,000 children is found to be affected, and the condition is more common among white and Asian babies than among those of Afro-Caribbean descent.

Following a special protein-sensitive diet ensures that the affected child develops normally. But adults born before the 1960s, who were untested and untreated, may have developed learning difficulties.

SYMPTOMS

- **Eczema**-like rash.
- Musty odour.
- Short stature, flat feet and small head.
- Infants often have blue eyes and fairer skin and hair than other family members.

CAUSES

In this inherited disorder, the enzyme that breaks down the amino acid phenylalanine is defective. Excess phenylalanine builds up in the blood, and results in damage to the nervous system.

DURATION

The inability to convert phenylalanine is lifelong, but early treatment prevents brain damage.

TREATMENT

If the Guthrie test is positive, your doctor will arrange for further tests to be carried out to determine how severe the phenylketonuria is in your child. Regular monitoring of blood levels ensures that measures can be taken to keep phenylalanine levels within safe limits. These measures include:

- a special milk substitute for babies;
- a low-phenylalanine diet: no meat, fish, cheese and eggs (rich in protein and therefore phenylalanine) and small, measured amounts of foods containing some protein, such as potato, milk and cereals. Fruit and vegetables, sugar and fats may be eaten freely;
- a special protein substitute mixture from which the phenylalanine has been removed;
- vitamin and mineral supplements.

What you can do

Follow your doctor's dietary advice.

COMPLICATIONS

Women with severe phenylketonuria may give birth to babies with brain damage or have a miscarriage or stillbirth. This risk is reduced if the woman eats a low-phenylalanine diet before conception.

PREVENTION

Phenylketonuria cannot be prevented, although early diagnosis and treatment can head off most complications. If both parents have the condition, there is a 50:50 chance that any child will have phenylketonuria. A Guthrie test in the first week of life ensures early treatment.

OUTLOOK

If the diet is strictly followed from infancy, the child will develop normally. It may be advisable to continue with the diet in adulthood and annual reviews are usually recommended by your doctor. If planning to start a family, phenylketonuric women and their partners should see clinical and dietetic experts before trying to conceive.

Phlebitis

Phlebitis is an inflammation of a vein wall and its lining. The vein becomes red, hot, sore and hard, and the person may feel unwell.

Phlebitis commonly occurs in surface varicose veins. It may be linked to an increase in blood clotting, as occurs in pregnant women or those taking the combined contraceptive pill. The vein may then contain a blood clot (thrombophlebitis). Phlebitis may also be the result of infection, injury, underlying disease or toxic chemicals (including medical or recreational drugs injected intravenously). The problem may be recurrent.

Treatment involves addressing the underlying cause, where necessary, plus rest, elevation of the affected part, antibiotics and anti-inflammatory drugs. In severe cases the vein may be permanently damaged.

SEE ALSO *Veins and disorders*

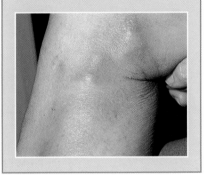

Phlebitis

Phlebitis most commonly occurs in the lower legs, as a complication of varicose veins.

Rashes, peeling, redness, swelling and permanent darkening may occur. There may also be blistering with serious infection. In the most severe cases, so much tissue may be involved that amputation is necessary.

Phobia

A phobia is an intense fear of an object or situation that would not trouble most people. Some phobias are mild and do not affect day-to-day life very much; others are so severe that people are confined to their home, find it impossible to hold down a job and have no social contact of any sort.

Phobias are common, and probably affect around 10 million people in the UK. People can have phobias about any object or any situation. Some people may fear going outside the home (**agoraphobia**) or enclosed spaces (**claustrophobia**). Others may be afraid of illness, of social situations or they may have a specific phobia involving insects, animals or birds.

SYMPTOMS

People with phobias suffer distressing symptoms of anxiety and panic when confronted with the phobic object or situation. These include:

- rapid heartbeat and sweating;
- churning stomach and nausea;
- dizziness and muddled thinking;
- dry mouth and shortness of breath;
- trembling and jelly legs.

These feeling pass, but afterwards the affected person may feel depressed and embarrassed.

TREATMENT

There is no single treatment for phobias – different treatments work for different people and there are several possibilities available. If a phobia is restricting your freedom, your GP may refer you to a counsellor or psychologist for behavioural or cognitive therapy. Medication such as tranquillisers and antidepressants may be helpful in the short term for the relief of anxiety and depression but these may be detrimental in the long term.

What you can do

Many people develop coping strategies and self-help techniques on their own but there are programmes that provide a structured approach to coping with a phobia and a wide range of self-help groups that offer support. Organizations such as the National Phobics Society (see page 652) can provide information on local groups.

Physiotherapy

Physiotherapy (known as physical therapy in the USA) is a form of treatment that uses physical measures rather then drugs or surgery in the treatment of disease or disability. Qualified physiotherapists in the UK have completed a degree course and are known as Members of the Chartered Society of Physiotherapists (MCSP). In order to work in the NHS they must register with the Council for Professions Supplementary to Medicine.

Every hospital and Primary Care Trust has a physiotherapy department – patients are seen on the wards, as out-patients or in the community.

WHAT'S INVOLVED

Physiotherapy treatments are tailored to the needs of the individual, and play a major role in the rehabilitation of patients after an illness, accident or operation.

Exercises

Exercises are used to treat various conditions. There are three types.

■ Passive exercises – the physiotherapist, rather than the patient, moves the joints to ease joint congestion and prevent stiffness.

■ Active exercises – the patient is taught a series of graduated exercises that are performed under the supervision of the physiotherapist.

■ Isometric exercise – the patient tenses a muscle repeatedly without moving it – for example, you might tense your calf muscle while holding your leg quite still.

These exercises are used when movement causes a patient pain or when a joint is immobilized, for example, by plaster.

Electrical treatments

Electrical treatment, also known as **diathermy**, uses short-wave electricity to produce heat within the tissues. It is used to relieve the pain of stiff, arthritic joints and muscle spasms.

Transcutaneous electrical nerve stimulation (TENS) is a method of electrical stimulation that is used for the relief of pain – for chronic back pain, for example, or following an amputation.

Ultrasound

Ultrasound uses very high frequency soundwaves, which are inaudible to the human ear, to treat acute soft tissue injuries by stimulating the healing processes. It is frequently used for sports injuries.

Heat and cold treatments

Heat treatment is given to ease muscle spasm, to relieve pain and improve circulation, by heat lamps or hot pads. Diathermy is also a form of heat treatment. Cold treatment involves applying ice packs or cold sprays to reduce pain and inflammation and relieve congestion and bruising. It is especially beneficial immediately after an injury because it helps to reduce swelling and promote healing.

Hydrotherapy and massage

In hydrotherapy, exercises are performed in water, which supports the body's weight. Massage is used to relax the patient, reduce tissue swelling, ease muscle spasm and to break down tense muscular nodules (trigger points).

Pica

People with pica eat or have cravings for bizarre substances that have no food value. Non-foods that may be craved and consumed include laundry starch, clay, earth, ice, paint, plaster, hair and gravel. Consuming these substances commonly results in abdominal pain.

Pica is common in children between the ages of one and six years. The term should not, however, be applied to infants and children who are aged up to about 18 months old and 'put everything in their mouth' – this is normal and a baby's way of assessing texture. Pica often occurs in pregnancy, and also in mentally handicapped and psychotic patients.

CAUSES

Pica is caused by an instinctive need to replace minerals absent in the diet. For example, people have been known to eat clay for its iron content, particularly during pregnancy, when iron-deficiency **anaemia** is common (see **Pregnancy and problems**).

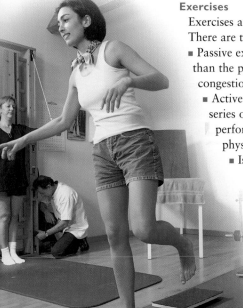

▼ **Balance exercises**
The hospital physiotherapist has devised a series of exercises that involve standing one-legged on a movable block to help a young woman rebuild strength and confidence after an operation.

Psychological factors can also lead to pica. The triggers are not well understood, but can be related to poor housing, low income or emotional deprivation. Pica is more likely to occur in people with a family history of pica, poor nutrition, or in those who live in poverty.

PREVENTION

- Remove commonly consumed items from the reach of children.
- Ensure that the diet is well-balanced and contains adequate minerals.
- Ensure that the person has emotional support.

Pituitary gland and disorders

The pituitary is a pea-sized organ at the base of the brain. It is the most important of the endocrine glands, whose job is to manufacture hormones and pass them into the bloodstream for distribution to the organs and tissues. The release of pituitary hormones is regulated by an adjoining part of the brain called the hypothalamus. The pituitary is egg-shaped, and sits in a hollow in the base of the skull.

Disorders of the pituitary gland are relatively rare. They may be caused by underproduction or overproduction of one or more of the pituitary hormones, resulting in changes in the organs and tissues usually controlled by that hormone.

Hypopituitarism

A shortage of pituitary hormones, called hypopituitarism, may result from impaired blood supply, head injury, ageing, a pituitary tumour or **radiotherapy** for a pituitary tumour. In some cases, the cause is unknown.

If a doctor suspects you may have hypopituitarism, blood tests and other specialized tests designed to detect hormone deficiencies will be asked for. You will also be sent for an **X-ray** and a CT scan or magnetic resonance imaging (MRI) scan to investigate whether there is a problem with the pituitary.

SYMPTOMS

Symptoms of hypopituitarism may develop gradually. They include:

- retarded growth, tiredness and weakness;
- reduced body hair, poor libido and **impotence** in men, and lack of menstruation (amenorrhoea), painful intercourse and hot flushes in women;
- in young people, delayed onset of puberty;
- weight gain, lack of energy, constipation, sensitivity to cold, and dry skin;
- pallor, weight loss, low blood pressure, dizziness and tiredness;
- thirst and production of excessive urine.

Occasionally, symptoms develop suddenly and dramatically. They include headache, collapse, hypothermia, low blood glucose and abnormally low blood pressure. In such cases, emergency treatment is needed.

TREATMENT

Treatment usually consists of replacing the missing hormones in the target glands affected, or in some cases involves directly replacing pituitary hormones. When the shortage of hormones is caused by a tumour, the tumour must be treated by surgery, drugs or radiotherapy, and the missing hormone or hormones replaced.

Pituitary dwarfism

Growth hormone deficiency – also called pituitary dwarfism, panhypopituitarism or proportionate short stature – is caused by underproduction of growth hormone or by failure of the body to respond to growth hormone. The physical proportions of children affected by this condition are normal, but the children fail to grow. Growth hormone deficiency is distinct from genetic dwarfism (disproportionate short stature), in which body proportions are abnormal.

It may be a result of a pituitary tumour or treatment for childhood cancer; occasionally, it can be hereditary. The condition may first become obvious when a baby or toddler fails to grow normally (see **Growth and disorders**). The child's growth curve, which is plotted on a height and weight chart by a community nurse or health visitor, is either flat or below normal.

Pituitary dwarfism may be linked to shortages of other pituitary hormones. The rate of growth, rather than short stature alone, gives the clearest indication of growth hormone deficiency. For example, children with a hormone deficiency but tall parents might start out as tall for their age, and their short stature may only become obvious over a period of time.

Tests conducted to establish whether a child is suffering from pituitary dwarfism include **X-rays**, measurements of growth hormone and other hormone levels in the blood, and CT or MRI scans of the head. Early diagnosis is important so that hormone replacement therapy can begin as soon as possible.

SYMPTOMS

In some cases, children may have physical defects of the face and skull. A small number of babies born with cleft lip or cleft palate are found to have reduced levels of growth hormone (see **Cleft palate and hare lip**).

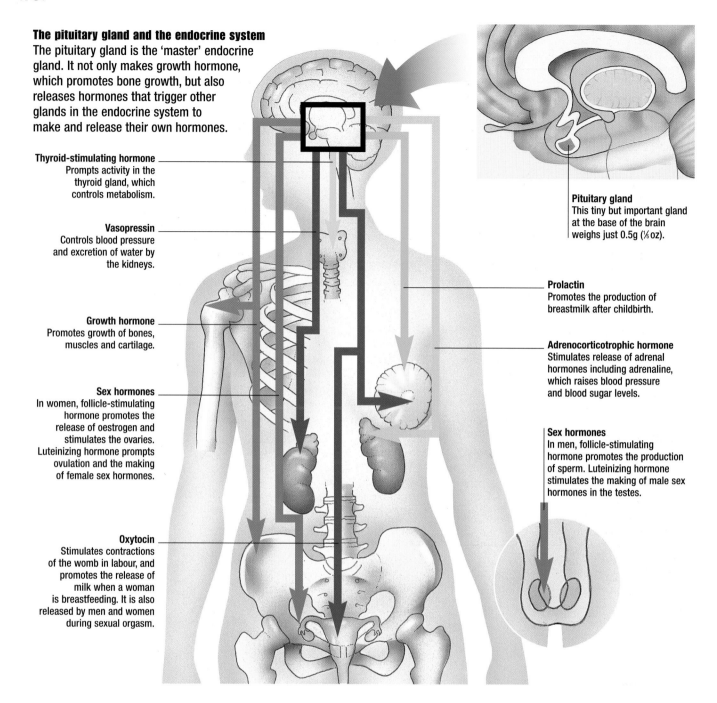

The pituitary gland and the endocrine system
The pituitary gland is the 'master' endocrine gland. It not only makes growth hormone, which promotes bone growth, but also releases hormones that trigger other glands in the endocrine system to make and release their own hormones.

Thyroid-stimulating hormone
Prompts activity in the thyroid gland, which controls metabolism.

Vasopressin
Controls blood pressure and excretion of water by the kidneys.

Growth hormone
Promotes growth of bones, muscles and cartilage.

Sex hormones
In women, follicle-stimulating hormone promotes the release of oestrogen and stimulates the ovaries. Luteinizing hormone prompts ovulation and the making of female sex hormones.

Oxytocin
Stimulates contractions of the womb in labour, and promotes the release of milk when a woman is breastfeeding. It is also released by men and women during sexual orgasm.

Pituitary gland
This tiny but important gland at the base of the brain weighs just 0.5g (⅕oz).

Prolactin
Promotes the production of breastmilk after childbirth.

Adrenocorticotrophic hormone
Stimulates release of adrenal hormones including adrenaline, which raises blood pressure and blood sugar levels.

Sex hormones
In men, follicle-stimulating hormone promotes the production of sperm. Luteinizing hormone stimulates the making of male sex hormones in the testes.

More common symptoms of growth hormone deficiency in children include:
- absent or slow growth;
- short stature;
- delayed or absent sexual development at puberty;
- headaches;
- excessive thirst, and production of larger than usual amounts of urine.

TREATMENT
The earlier treatment is started, the more likely children are to reach their full growth potential. Treatment involves regular injections of growth and other hormones; these can be given at home by a parent.

The long-term benefits and potential effects of growth hormone replacement are still being debated by doctors. Most children who have been treated with growth hormone do show improved levels of growth, although the effectiveness of the treatment may diminish over time.

Left untreated, a child with insufficient levels of growth hormone may have delayed sexual development at puberty and will be short in stature as an adult. In the past, some cases of **CJD** (Creutzfeldt-Jakob disease) were caused by taking human growth hormone. The growth hormone used today, known as recombinant human growth hormone (rhGH), is synthetically produced, but has the same structure as the normal human hormone. There is no risk of CJD with this treatment.

Growth hormone deficiency in adults

Until recently, deficiency of growth hormone in adulthood was dismissed as being unimportant. However, research has shown that adults lacking growth hormone have higher cholesterol levels, a higher risk of heart disease and an increased risk of dying early.

Other symptoms of low growth hormone levels include:
- obesity;
- loss of strength and stamina;
- chronic fatigue;
- anxiety;
- depression;
- a raised risk of sustaining fractures;
- debilitating attacks of fatigue, leading to a decreased ability to exercise.

Causes may be a tumour or treatment for a tumour, or problems with blood supply to the pituitary such as a **stroke**. Treatment is by means of injections of growth hormone.

Graves' disease

Graves' disease is the most common cause of hyperthyroidism, in which the body produces antibodies that attack the **thyroid**, instead of the thyroid-stimulating hormone made by the pituitary gland. This causes overproduction of thyroid hormone from the thyroid gland and, in response, the pituitary gland shuts down production of the hormone.

The symptoms of Graves' disease are over activity, sweating, trembling hands, loss of weight, bulging eyes, emotional disturbance and swelling of the thyroid gland in the neck. If the condition is left untreated, it can lead to eye infections, raising of body temperature, heart failure and nervous breakdown.

SEE ALSO *Growth and disorders*

Pityriasis rosacea

Pityriasis rosacea is a common skin rash caused by a mild viral infection. At first a large, round 'herald' patch appears on the trunk. This is followed a week or so later by a widespread rash of flat, scaly, round or oval patches on the trunk and upper arms. The patches are dark pink or copper-coloured and can last for six to eight weeks. They sometimes itch.

No treatment is necessary, although the topical application of calamine lotion or taking antihistamines will relieve the itching.

SEE ALSO *Skin and disorders*

Plague

The word 'plague' is used to describe any epidemic disease with a high death rate. More specifically, it refers to a serious infectious disease of rats, caused by the bacterium *Yersinis pestis*. This is transmitted to human beings by blood-sucking rat fleas. It is spread from person to person mainly through infected droplets expelled during coughing and sneezing. The plague was the cause of the Black Death, which killed more than half of Europe's population in the 14th century. Today, rat-borne epidemics still occur but are mostly confined to parts of Africa, South America and Southeast Asia. There are between one and two thousand cases a year worldwide, but the last case reported in Europe was soon after the Second World War. Outbreaks occur both in rural communities and in cities, in areas where housing conditions and sanitation are poor; they are usually associated with infected rats and rat fleas that live in the home.

BUBONIC PLAGUE

Bubonic plague, the more common form of the disease, has an incubation period of two to six days. Early symptoms are headache, nausea, vomiting and aching joints. Sufferers develop buboes – painful swellings of the lymph nodes in the armpits and groin – and a fever. After about a week, the buboes may burst and discharge pus, and then heal. Otherwise, subcutaneous (under the skin) bleeding may occur. This produces black patches, and can lead to ulcers that may prove fatal.

PNEUMONIC PLAGUE

Pneumonic plague, in which bacteria enter the lungs, can occur as a complication of bubonic plague. It is also transmitted by coughing and sneezing. The skin of a pneumonic plague victim turns purplish and the patient becomes exhausted. Left untreated, most pneumonic plague victims will die.

TREATMENT

Both forms of plague respond to antibiotics, especially streptomycin; prompt treatment reduces the risk of death to around 5 per cent.

PREVENTION

A vaccine is available for people at high risk. The injection gives protection for six months.

Plantar fasciitis

Plantar fasciitis is an inflammation that occurs where the plantar fascia (connective tissue layer) in the sole of the foot joins the heel bone (calcaneus). This causes pain mainly under the heel. Sometimes a small bony protuberance forms on this part of the heel bone and produces a calcaneal spur. The pain from this may be eased by special padded insoles, **physiotherapy** and sometimes corticosteroid injections.

Pleurisy

Pleurisy is an infection of the two-layered membrane (the pleura) that envelops the lungs and facilitates breathing. The outer layer of the pleural sac lines the ribcage and the inner layer encloses each lung. As the lungs expand and contract in breathing, the two layers glide across each other. If either layer of the pleura becomes inflamed from infection, they rub together causing pain.

Since the advent of antibiotics, pleurisy is rare; most people make a full recovery.

SYMPTOMS
- One-sided chest pain, which starts suddenly and is likely to be severe.
- Pain when breathing. Deep breathing or coughing makes the pain worse.
- Sometimes, a fever, and pain in the neck, shoulder or abdomen.

CAUSES
- Other infections, such as **tuberculosis** or **pneumonia**.
- Chest injury, or small pneumothorax – in which air enters the pleural cavity.
- Occasionally no cause can be found.

TREATMENT
The treatment of pleurisy depends on the underlying cause. You will be prescribed painkillers, and if the cause is an infection, antibiotics.

When to consult a doctor
You should see a doctor if you develop any of the above symptoms, especially if they are associated with difficulty in breathing.

What a doctor may do
The doctor will base a diagnosis on the description of your symptoms. He or she will also want to listen to your chest. You may be referred for a chest **X-ray**, and the hospital specialist may then wish to draw off a sample of pleural fluid to confirm the cause.

PREVENTION
Prevention is mainly by prompt treatment of chest infections, such as pneumonia or tuberculosis.

COMPLICATIONS
Pleurisy can lead to pleural effusion, in which fluid collects between the layers of the pleura. This fluid squashes the lung beneath it, making it very hard to breathe.

SEE ALSO *Lungs and disorders*

Pneumonia

'Pneumonia' is a general term for an acute inflammation of the lungs – specifically the air sacs (alveoli). The many types of pneumonia are all caused by infection with one of three micro-organisms: bacteria, viruses and mycoplasma.

In the UK, 150,000 people develop pneumonia each year – most cases are bacterial. Thanks to effective antibiotics, the vast majority of people recover. But the condition can be fatal – in the UK, 3000 people aged between 15 and 55 die from pneumonia each year, and the disease causes up to a quarter of all deaths in elderly people. Pneumonias caused by mycoplasma are rarely life-threatening, but can take a long time to clear up; viral pneumonia is less serious than the other forms.

Pneumonia is the third most common infection acquired by patients staying in hospital – one to two per cent of all post-operative patients and 25 per cent of those in intensive care pick up the infection. The death rate from hospital-acquired pneumonia is much greater than that from pneumonia caught in day-to-day life. About two-thirds of people who acquire pneumonia in hospital and half of those who develop it while in intensive care survive.

WHO IS AT RISK
Anyone can develop pneumonia, but people who are most at risk are:
- the very young;
- elderly people;
- people with underlying health problems, such as chronic obstructive pulmonary disease, diabetes, heart problems, **AIDS** or **asthma**;
- people with a weak immune system, such as those undergoing **chemotherapy** or **radiotherapy** treatments for cancer or those who have recently had a transplant;
- people in inadequate housing.

In addition, major risk factors include:
- excess alcohol;
- cigarette smoking;
- the infection bronchiectasis, which affects the smallest airways in the lungs;
- obstruction in the airways;
- drug abuse.

SYMPTOMS
The symptoms vary from person to person and also depending on

Symptoms in children

Children may experience extra symptoms. If your child is breathless or has a fever with chest pain, you should see a doctor immediately.

Symptoms in children under 18 months

- Sudden rise in temperature.

- Fast breathing and difficult breathing. Often the distress caused by the infant trying to breathe makes feeding impossible. If breathlessness leads to a blueish tinge around the lips, the child needs immediate medical attention.

Symptoms in children over 18 months

- Brief cold at first, followed by high temperatures.

- Shaking and chills.

- Possible tummy pains.

- Fast, shallow breathing.

- Drowsiness and delirium.

the cause of the pneumonia. The main symptoms include:

- a cough – this may start off dry, but within a couple of days you will start to bring up mucus. People infected with mycoplasma will probably experience very forceful coughs that produce white phlegm;
- infected mucus (sometime blood-flecked);
- high fever;
- shortness of breath;
- pains in the chest. These are caused by an infection of the sac that contains the lungs and protects them from rubbing against the chest (the pleura). They are usually associated with bacterial forms of pneumonia.

In addition, general symptoms include:
- generally feeling very ill;
- shaking;
- loss of appetite;
- sweating, often profusely;
- headaches;
- aching muscles and joints.

TREATMENT

Pneumonia is a serious disease – the sooner it is diagnosed and treatment started, the better.

When to consult a doctor

If you have the symptoms of pneumonia, especially if they last more than a couple of days, consult your doctor at once. If you have symptoms of pneumonia that come on very quickly, if you become breathless without any exertion, or if you have a pulse rate that is higher than 100 beats per minute, you should have someone drive you immediately to your nearest casualty department. If you are alone, call an ambulance.

What a doctor may do

Most forms of pneumonia are diagnosed from the physical symptoms. In addition, a doctor will probably tap on your chest – the sounds made will help to locate the infection. A chest X-ray may also be taken, as well as a sample of your phlegm, which will be sent for analysis to discover the cause of the pneumonia.

There is no direct treatment for viral pneumonia, but it is generally less severe than pneumonia caused by bacteria or mycoplasma. You may be given painkillers to alleviate chest pain or drugs to reduce fever.

Antibiotics are an effective treatment against bacteria, the most common cause of pneumonia. Antibiotics may also be helpful if you have a pneumonia caused by mycoplasma; although these drugs do not work directly on mycoplasma, they may help to speed up recovery by preventing the development of any secondary infection.

The doctor will also ask about your recent movements to determine where you may have

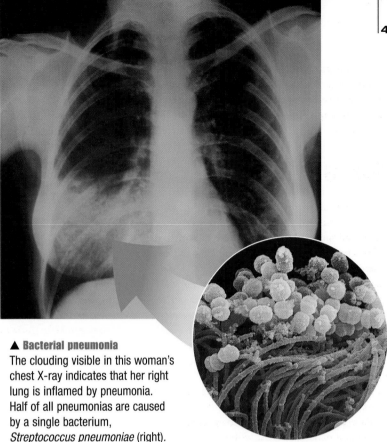

▲ **Bacterial pneumonia**
The clouding visible in this woman's chest X-ray indicates that her right lung is inflamed by pneumonia. Half of all pneumonias are caused by a single bacterium, *Streptococcus pneumoniae* (right).

caught pneumonia. For example, it is significant if you have been travelling abroad – in Spain, 30 per cent of *Streptococcus pneumoniae* bacteria are resistant to the usual antibiotics.

If there is no noticeable improvement within 48 hours of starting treatment, contact your doctor again – the treatment will probably have to be changed. If symptoms become more severe, go to casualty immediately.

Severe cases of pneumonia require hospital treatment. In hospital, antibiotics may be given intravenously (direct into the bloodstream) and you may also be given pain relief and oxygen.

What you can do

- Rest in a warm atmosphere.
- Drink plenty of fluids.
- Avoid smoking and smoky atmospheres.

PREVENTION

There is no sure way to prevent all forms of pneumonia. But there are vaccines for the main form of bacterial infection. Since one of the complications of flu is pneumonia, those at risk should have both the vaccine for flu and for bacterial pneumonia (see also **Influenza**).

COMPLICATIONS

Most people make a full recovery from pneumonia, but complications can include: pleural effusion (liquid in the sac enclosing the lungs), which can lead to **pleurisy**; lung abscess (in less than one per cent of people); blood poisoning; and scarring of the lungs (fibrosis).

SEE ALSO *Chest pain, Lungs and disorders; Respiratory infections*

Pneumothorax

In pneumothorax, air enters the pleura, a two-layered sac that encloses the lungs. This causes the lung to collapse, partially or completely.

Pneumothorax is quite rare, but the people most at risk are tall, thin men aged between 15 and 30, and those over 55. Smokers, those with a family history of the condition and anyone with an underlying lung disease such as **emphysema** are particularly at risk of developing pneumothorax. More men than women are affected, by a ratio of six to one.

SYMPTOMS

- Breathlessness, which may be severe.
- Pain, usually on one side of the chest, that comes on very quickly. It can start during sleep.
- Pain may also occur at the base of the neck.

Some young, fit people may experience only a slight feeling of breathlessness and slight chest discomfort.

CAUSES

A pneumothorax can occur spontaneously, with no apparent cause, or because of an injury such as a broken rib puncturing the pleura. It can also be the result of a small blister that forms on the lung and then ruptures, releasing air into the pleural cavity – this is a common cause in young men. Other lung conditions, such as emphysema, may cause pneumothorax.

TREATMENT

You should consult a doctor immediately if you have the symptoms of pneumothorax. A chest **X-ray** will be needed to confirm diagnosis.

Treatment will depend on the severity of the condition. No treatment is given for a small pneumothorax, which generally heals itself. But if your symptoms get worse, you should seek medical help immediately. For a larger pneumothorax, the air will need to be extracted (aspirated). This is done under local **anaesthetic**.

In cases of severe pneumothorax or if aspiration fails, a chest drain will be necessary. In this procedure, a tube is inserted into the chest, between the layers of the pleura, to release the air. A pump may be used to extract the air more quickly although it can take two days for the air to be removed. A chest drain is carried out under local anaesthetic while in hospital. If this fails to improve the condition, a thoracoscope, a viewing device, may be used to inspect the inner side of each layer of the pleura. Once the hole through which air is seeping is found, it can be sealed up by chemical means. If you have more than one attack of pneumothorax, a more extensive operation may be necessary to stick the two layers of pleura together so that air cannot find its way between them.

What you can do

Avoid smoking or smoky atmospheres. Do not fly until fully recovered – the reduction in pressure in the aircraft could cause another or a more severe collapse.

COMPLICATIONS

The condition recurs in about 50 per cent of patients.

Poliomyelitis

Generally known as polio, poliomyelitis is an infectious viral disease that invades the central nervous system. Polio **immunization** is now widespread and cases of polio are rare.

Infection ranges in severity from a mild illness to a paralytic disease that can result in death. Polio is more common in infants under three years old. Most polio victims experience a mild form of the disease, and paralysis is more common when infection occurs in older people.

The virus is excreted in the faeces of infected people, and so polio often occurs in areas with poor sanitation. But even in modern and hygienic conditions it can strike people who have not acquired immunity during childhood.

SYMPTOMS

After entering the body through the mouth, the virus multiplies in the intestine. In the vast majority of cases, paralysis does not occur. The virus may get no farther than the bloodstream, causing mild flu-like symptoms. If it enters the central nervous system, symptoms will include headache, vomiting and stiff muscles in the neck and back. Many people recover at this stage.

Muscle weakness and paralysis occur if the virus goes on to destroy nerve cells. The limbs, particularly the legs, are most commonly affected, but paralysis can occur in abdominal muscles and those of the back, neck and face. Polio becomes life-threatening if the throat or breathing muscles are paralysed.

TREATMENT

There is no cure for polio, although specific symptoms may be treated.

PREVENTION

The single most effective preventive measure is polio immunization. For those who cannot be given the live oral vaccine – for example, anyone with a weakened immune system – an alternative exists. If not already immunized, travellers to high-risk areas, including parts of Africa and Asia, should be vaccinated.

OUTLOOK

Most people make a full recovery. If nerve cells are destroyed, paralysis is permanent, otherwise muscles may recover after six months or so.

In 2000, there were fewer than 3500 cases of polio reported worldwide.

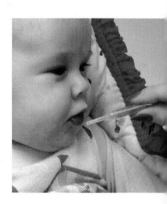

▲ **Polio vaccination**
The vaccine is given by mouth in three doses at four-week intervals. It is recommended for all children and confers long-lasting protection.

Polymyalgia rheumatica

Polymyalgia rheumatica is a disorder causing stiffness and aching in the region of the neck, shoulder and hip. It is common among elderly people, and rarely affects those aged under 50. Twice as many women as men suffer from the condition, which is rare in Asians and black people. It often strikes suddenly – typically with pain and stiffness in the shoulders, hips and thighs, neck and torso.

Up to 80 per cent of people suffering from the condition also have temporal arteritis or giant cell arteritis – a painful inflammation of the arteries in the skull.

SYMPTOMS

Sufferers are often unaware that they have polymyalgia rheumatica and put their symptoms down to old age or vague rheumatism. The symptoms may include:
- severe pain and stiffness in affected muscles, which may be worse in the morning and get gradually better during the day;
- slight fever and feeling unwell;
- depression and weight loss.

Giant cell arteritis also causes headaches and pain in the muscles of the head.

TREATMENT

You should not try to treat the condition at home, because medical advice is essential. See a doctor as soon as possible.

What a doctor may do
- Arrange blood tests for diagnosis.
- Prescribe corticosteroids as appropriate.
- Refer you to a rheumatologist.

What you can do
- Eat a balanced diet.
- Keep as fit and active as possible.
- Report pain or swelling in the scalp immediately, especially if you experience eye problems such as blurred or double vision.

OUTLOOK

If polymyalgia rheumatica is diagnosed and treated at an early stage, the outlook is excellent. The condition is not progressive and can be cured. Corticosteroid treatment often brings about dramatic and rapid improvement, suppressing symptoms until the condition is cured. This usually takes one to two years, but a minority of people may need to continue treatment for up to four years.

Porphyrias

Porphyrias are a group of rare disorders of body chemistry in which the body cannot manufacture the enzymes needed to form the blood pigment haemoglobin. As a result, substances called porphyrins, which are used in the manufacture of haemoglobin, are produced to excess and accumulate in the bloodstream. Porphyrias are usually inherited, but sometimes develop during life.

Excessive production of porphyrins may occur in the liver, when the condition is known as hepatic porphyria, or in the bone marrow, when it is called erythropoietic porphyria. The most common type of the condition, acute intermittent porphyria (AIP), is hereditary and mainly affects adults under the age of 35.

SYMPTOMS

People with porphyria are acutely sensitive to sunlight, which causes blistering skin rashes, and can bring on attacks of the condition. The sensitivity arises because the excess of porphyrins in the blood affects the skin. Attacks of porphyria can also be sparked off by alcohol, by drugs such as some anaesthetics, barbiturates, tranquillizers, contraceptive pills and sedatives, by chemicals and by certain foods. Hormonal changes in pregnancy can also trigger an attack in some individuals.

Some people suffer relatively mild porphyria attacks that consist only of skin rashes and similar problems. In other people attacks are more severe and may bring on pain in the abdomen, vomiting, constipation, weakness, muscle cramps and weakness, high blood pressure and rapid heartbeat. Porphyria can also cause mental disturbances, which may include **hallucinations**, **schizophrenic** behaviour, **depression** and related conditions such as **insomnia** and **anxiety**.

All people who suffer from porphyria will excrete porphyrins in their urine, which turns reddish-purple when left to stand for an hour or so.

PRECAUTIONS

If you have porphyria take the following precautions.
- Don't take a new medicine unless you are absolutely sure it will not provoke an attack. Check with the pharmacist or your GP that over-the-counter products such as dietary supplements are safe for you.
- In general, avoid taking medication unless strictly necessary.

THE FUTURE

Scientists have used spacesuit technology to design a garment that protects children with porphyria from the sun's ultraviolet (UV) rays and other light sources. Meanwhile, the discovery of a faulty gene involved in one common type of porphyria has led to the development of a simple blood test to identify the disease.

SEE ALSO *Liver and disorders*

Postnatal depression

For one out of ten new mothers motherhood is initially spoiled by postnatal depression. Family, friends and doctors can do much to support and comfort the mother and help her through this serious condition.

Postnatal depression should not be confused with the 'baby blues'. Three or four days after giving birth, at least half of all new mothers have a brief period of depression and mood swings. This is thought to be caused by changing hormone levels. Most women get through it with the help of a sympathetic partner or friend and a supportive midwife.

Postnatal depression – also called postpartum depression – is less common than 'baby blues', but is still widespread. It can last for several months, and so naturally has an impact on a new mother's relationship with her baby – and with her partner. For this reason you should seek medical help if you find that you are developing the symptoms described below. Remember that postnatal depression is not your fault: it is an illness that can be cured with the right treatment and support.

▼ New mother's long day
Some women with postnatal depression are fine in the morning, but become more miserable as the day goes on, feeling unable to cope.

SYMPTOMS

Postnatal depression builds up gradually. One of its most striking effects is exhaustion. Even when the mother is getting enough sleep, she feels constantly tired. She may develop obsessions and suffer from sleep disruption not caused by the baby waking. Other symptoms of the disorder include anxiety, tearfulness and despondency, unfounded feelings of rejection, disregard for personal hygiene and grooming, panic attacks and poor concentration.

DIAGNOSIS

The demands of caring for a new baby can make it difficult to identify postnatal depression. Some of the symptoms, such as tiredness and sleep disruption, are normal with a new baby in the house. Your GP should be sympathetic and skilled enough to recognize that you are depressed and not just tired. But you may have to raise the issue with him or her yourself. If you feel that your doctor is not taking your concerns seriously, ask your midwife or health visitor for advice.

To aid diagnosis, your health visitor may ask you to fill in a questionnaire. This enables your depression to be assessed against the Edinburgh Postnatal Depression Scale. Postnatal depression usually lasts for many months, although it is not unusual for it to last even longer. Early diagnosis and treatment can help offset any debilitating effect on the mother and prevent damage to the relationship with the baby.

CAUSES

Postnatal depression has no clearly identifiable cause, but a number of factors appear to increase the risk of depressive illness after childbirth. These include having had a difficult labour, having a child with a handicap or disability, having a preterm baby or one who requires treatment in a special care unit.

The condition is more likely to strike women who have low self-esteem or whose mother also experienced postnatal depression. Women with marital problems or an unsupportive partner are more likely to suffer from the condition. Other causes often associated with depression include moving house, particularly if this involves moving a long way away from family and friends, and giving up a career to care for the baby.

SUPPORT FROM FAMILY AND FRIENDS

Encouragement and support can do much to aid recovery, but family members and friends need to recognize that postnatal depression is a clinical disorder that must be taken seriously. A woman

Case study
Counselling helped young mother

Janet, 27, suffered from postnatal depression following the birth of her first child, Nathan.

Janet became depressed soon after Nathan's birth – but this was not a case of the 'baby blues'. She had difficulty in concentrating, felt worthless and was irritable with all her family. She became tearful for no apparent reason, experienced panic attacks and lost interest in how she looked.

Her depression went on for several weeks before she sought medical advice. When she did contact her GP, she was diagnosed with postnatal depression. She responded well to counselling. This took place at the GP's surgery, using the practice's counsellor. The doctor did not feel that Janet needed to take antidepressants.

Janet's husband and mother shared out domestic responsibilities until Janet was able to cope. Janet has now fully recovered and reports being 'back in charge' of her home. She and Nathan appear to have no further problems.

experiencing depression cannot be jollied along or chivvied into feeling better. However, she does need to be reassured that she will get better and that depression is not a sign of weakness.

If the depressed mother fears being left alone with her child, family members and friends can organize a rota so that she is always with someone she likes and trusts. Give her space when she wants it and allow her to do as much, or as little, as she feels able to do. It can be a great help if someone takes over domestic chores and responsibility for family meals – but not if the mother is unhappy about relinquishing control of household duties.

TREATMENT
In many cases of postnatal depression, counselling may be a very effective treatment, and cognitive therapy, which focuses on coping skills, is often helpful. Antidepressants or tranquillizers may be prescribed. If depression gets worse just before a period, progesterone therapy may help.

The contraceptive pill appears to be linked with depression in some women – if you are taking the Pill and feeling depressed, it is worth considering another form of contraception. If you are suffering from postnatal depression, do not cut short your treatment. You may experience a dramatic improvement after taking antidepressant drugs, but it is important to allow time to make a full recovery. Problems can be avoided by gradually reducing the dose rather

than stopping medication suddenly. If you do stop taking medication and feel the depression returning, go back to your doctor and explain the situation.

WHAT THE MOTHER CAN DO
Accept that it is perfectly natural to worry about caring for a newborn baby and that many women suffer aches and pains after childbirth. You can use relaxation techniques such as deep breathing and meditation to reduce tension and anxiety.

To prevent hypoglycaemia (low blood sugar), which may exacerbate depression, make sure that you eat regular healthy meals. If you are worried about putting on weight, cut down on sweet and starchy foods but eat plenty of fruit and raw vegetables. Vitamin B_6 or a general vitamin supplement may help to relieve your symptoms.

Rest when you can, and don't try to be a superwoman. Find out about local mothers' groups – sharing your experiences and worries can counter feelings of isolation.

ANTENATAL DEPRESSION
Although postnatal depression has been recognized by the medical profession for many years, recent research suggests that depression is actually more common during pregnancy than after childbirth. A study reported in the *British Medical Journal* found that depression is at its lowest point around the 32nd week of pregnancy.

PUERPERAL PSYCHOSIS
One or two women in every 1000 develop an extreme form of depression called puerperal psychosis. It usually appears quickly, often a day or two after the delivery. A woman suffering from puerperal psychosis may completely lose touch with reality and is likely to exhibit bizarre and at times frightening behaviour. Symptoms include hallucinations, feeling very restless, unsettled and unable to sleep, denying that the baby is hers and trying to harm the baby.

If puerperal psychosis is diagnosed, the mother is admitted to a psychiatric unit immediately. In many areas, specialist mother and baby units are available – if at all possible, continued contact between the mother and infant is encouraged. If the condition is diagnosed early, the prognosis is usually good, although recurrent bouts of severe depression are likely to continue, particularly in later pregnancies.

SEE ALSO *Babies and baby care; Birth and problems; Pregnancy and problems*

The key to coping with postnatal depression is to acknowledge that it is a temporary condition and you will get better.

Pregnancy and problems

The nine months of pregnancy can be exciting, scary, nervewracking and uncomfortable. But despite the worries, it should be remembered that in most cases the outcome is the delivery of a normal healthy baby.

Pregnancy is a time of joy, but it places great physical and emotional demands on a prospective mother. It can also be an anxious time – especially as the due day draws near.

THE BEGINNING OF PREGNANCY

For conception to occur naturally, a woman needs to be ovulating – releasing an egg from one of her ovaries – which happens around the middle of each menstrual cycle. And her partner needs to be producing an adequate quantity of sperm.

During the first week or so after menstruation, there is a slow increase in levels of oestrogen and follicle stimulating hormone (FSH). This initiates the growth of an egg within one of the ovaries and prompts changes to the uterine lining, making it thicker and spongy with blood, so that it is ready to receive a fertilized egg. Roughly two weeks after the beginning of a woman's last period, an egg is released from one of her ovaries and 'caught' by the frilled membranes at the end of each Fallopian tube. The cilia, tiny grass-like fronds that line the tubes, gently ease the egg towards the womb and the possibility of fertilization. If sex takes place around the time of ovulation, conception can occur.

There are probably no more than 100 days in a year when a woman of childbearing age is likely to conceive, and fewer days of peak fertility.

Around 300 million sperm are released during sexual intercourse, but only a few hundred ever reach the Fallopian tube that contains an egg. Sperm that do reach an egg release enzymes that slowly soften and break down the protective layer of cells surrounding the egg (corona radiata), until one finally breaks through. The moment a sperm reaches the surface of the egg the two cells – one from the sperm and one from the egg –

merge. This merged cell forms a tough outer surface that repels any remaining sperm.

Pregnancy tests

Some women have an intuitive feeling that they are pregnant even before they have missed a period, although many women have no sign at all. You can test whether you are pregnant with a pregnancy testing kit. Most kits are so sensitive that they can confirm a pregnancy if your period is only one day late. Over-the-counter pregnancy tests work by measuring a hormone called human chorionic gonadotrophin (HCG). Kits consist of a small plastic stick containing a panel that reacts to HCG. This is dipped into a urine sample taken first thing in the morning; if HCG is present, the reactive panel changes colour in a few minutes. If there is no reaction within 15 minutes, pregnancy is unlikely. But home pregnancy tests are not infallible. A false positive result can be caused by hormones administered for fertility treatment, and a recent miscarriage or pregnancy.

Detergent in the container used to collect urine, or a test taken too early, when HCG is still very low, and some drugs including tranquillizers and antihistamines, may give a false negative result.

Keeping healthy

Women often do not realize that they have conceived until around the eighth week of

When is the baby due?

As many women are not sure of the exact date of conception, the length of pregnancy is measured from the first day of their last period.

The date on which the baby is due is calculated by counting 40 weeks, or 280 days, from the first day of a woman's last period – but fewer than 10 per cent of babies arrive on their due date.

For instance, if your last period was on January 1, your estimated date of delivery (EDD) is October 8. The duration of your pregnancy is based on that first date. So two weeks after your next period would have been due, you will be described as being six weeks pregnant – although it is actually only four weeks since you conceived.

pregnancy, when they know they have missed a period. By now, most of the baby's organs are developing, so it is wise to adopt a healthy lifestyle and diet before trying to conceive. It is usually safe to work throughout pregnancy, and many women choose to work right up until the birth.

Keeping fit is an important part of a healthy pregnancy, and low-impact exercise such as swimming, walking and yoga are excellent.

Here are some guidelines that will help you give your baby the best possible start:

■ Take 400mcg folic acid each day for the first three months of pregnancy. This will reduce your baby's risk of neural tube defects such as **spina bifida** and other problems including **cleft palate**. Ideally, you should take folic acid before pregnancy too, so begin a course of tablets as soon as you decide to try for a baby.

■ Make sure that your diet includes plenty of B group vitamins – thiamin, niacin, riboflavin and B_6 – to cut the risk of a low-birthweight baby.

■ Avoid soft and unpasteurized cheeses, raw eggs and raw or undercooked meats; they could carry **salmonella**, **listeria** and other bacterial infections.

■ It is best to avoid alcohol. The safe level is not known, and individual tolerance varies. Alcohol abuse can cause fetal alcohol syndrome, resulting in low birthweight and mental retardation.

■ Don't smoke. Smoking increases the risk of miscarriage and having a low-birthweight baby.

■ Avoid liver and liver pâté: liver is high in retinol, the form of vitamin A found in animal products, which has been linked to birth defects. If you are taking a multivitamin or supplement, look for one that contains vitamin A in the form of beta carotene and has no more than 1250mcg.

■ Avoid touching pregnant livestock; they may carry bacteria that cause miscarriage.

■ Avoid exposure to X-rays and anaesthetic gases.

■ Be wary of toxoplasmosis, a parasitic infection that causes miscarriage and stillbirth. It can be picked up by eating raw or undercooked meat, or from animals.

■ Avoid saunas and extremely high temperatures.

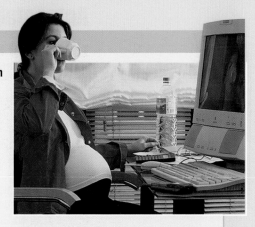

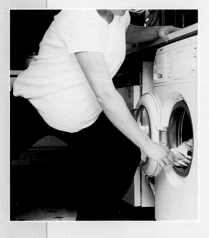

In late pregnancy, you may begin to feel the extra weight the baby is placing on your back. It's important to spend a little time each day making yourself comfortable and ensuring that your spine is properly aligned.

1 If you sit at a desk all day at work, get up and walk around regularly. Straighten your back, tuck in your bottom, drop your shoulders and hold them back, and tighten your tummy muscles to support the weight of the baby.

2 When doing anything at low level – dressing a toddler or loading the washing machine – bend your knees and keep your back as straight as possible.

THE BABY'S UMBILICAL LIFELINE

The fetus is completely dependent on its mother for nourishment and oxygen, both of which pass from mother to baby via the placenta. The placenta is attached to the mother via the uterine wall and to the baby through the umbilical cord. Inside the placenta is a thin membrane, known as the chorion, which allows blood to pass freely in either direction. Every minute, about 600ml (just over a pint) of blood flows from the mother to her baby through the placenta. This carries oxygen and nutrients to the baby and removes waste products, which are then processed and eliminated by the mother's body.

▼ Sleeping position
When the bump gets bigger, try lying on your side with one leg bent and supported with a cushion. Just one or two pillows under your head is best for your spine.

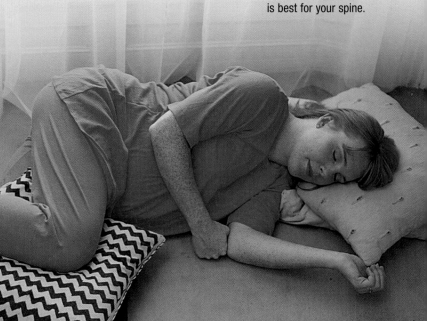

Antenatal care

The health of both mother and baby are monitored throughout pregnancy

Antenatal care is designed to look after both the mother and her unborn child, and to ensure the best possible outcome of the pregnancy.

Once your pregnancy has been confirmed by your GP, arrangements will be made for your care up to and including the birth. There are several options for antenatal care, but if you have chosen a hospital birth you are most likely to receive shared care, which means visiting the hospital two or three times during the pregnancy, and being looked after by your community midwife or GP for the rest of the time. If you want a home birth, you are legally entitled to have one, even if this is your first baby. A GP who does not offer maternity care for a home birth may recommend that you transfer to another doctor.

FIRST ANTENATAL CHECK

The first antenatal check, or booking visit, takes place at around 12 weeks. You may be asked to go to a hospital clinic or your GP's surgery, or your midwife may visit you at home.

■ You will be asked about your medical history and your immediate family's medical history. Questions will include whether you have been pregnant before, and whether you smoke or drink.

■ Your blood pressure will be checked, and you may be weighed and your height measured.

■ You will have a blood test to determine your blood group and iron levels, to find out whether you are Rhesus positive or negative (see box, page 488), and to see if you are immune to rubella. Most hospitals offer to test your blood for HIV, but this will not be done without your consent.

■ You will be asked for a urine sample, which is tested for signs of protein or sugar or any urinary infection. Sugar in the urine may indicate **diabetes** brought on by pregnancy. This can be confirmed or ruled out by doing a glucose intolerance test in which your blood is tested before and after fasting and then drinking a measure of glucose.

■ The midwife or doctor may ask to feel your abdomen to get an idea of the size of your uterus. Occasionally, but very rarely, you will be asked permission for an internal examination.

ULTRASOUND SCREENING

Often, the first ultrasound scan takes place at the 12 week appointment. Ultrasound uses soundwaves to build up an image of the baby,

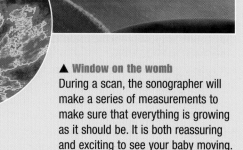

▲ **Window on the womb**
During a scan, the sonographer will make a series of measurements to make sure that everything is growing as it should be. It is both reassuring and exciting to see your baby moving.

which can be seen on a monitor by parents and health professionals. It is usually performed externally, using a gel to conduct waves between the abdomen and a hand-held probe. If the image is unclear, or the sonographer thinks that there may be a hidden twin, the scan may be performed via a vaginal probe. This is completely painless and poses no known risk to the pregnancy.

The first scan will confirm how many weeks pregnant you are, how many babies there are, whether your baby's heart is beating, and whether there are any major problems with how your baby's body and limbs have developed. It can also check the position of the placenta and the condition of the mother's cervix.

Some hospitals can also offer what is known as a nuchal translucency scan. This measures a thin layer of fluid between two folds of skin at the back of your baby's neck, and the result predicts the risk of your being pregnant with a baby with Down's syndrome. If you appear to be at risk, you will be offered amniocentesis or chorionic villus sampling (see below).

Most pregnant women have two scans. The second scan is carried out at about 20 weeks to check your baby's spine, arms, legs, hands and feet, and the heart and other internal organs.

Further scans are likely if there are any other risk factors or complications. A late scan may be recommended to assess your baby's birthweight and to check that your pelvis is large enough to allow a vaginal delivery.

PRENATAL TESTING

You will be offered various antenatal tests that are used to ascertain the health of your baby – but these tests are not compulsory. There are two types of test: screening tests predict your chances of having a baby with a particular condition; diagnostic tests confirm one way or the other whether your baby has such a condition. Diagnostic tests carry a slight risk of miscarriage.

Blood tests

A blood test can be carried out at 16 to 18 weeks to screen for Down's syndrome and spina bifida. If your blood test shows that the risk of your baby having Down's syndrome is higher than that predicted for your age, you may want to have a diagnostic test, such as an amniocentesis, to find out. Other blood tests are used to detect inherited blood disorders such as thalassaemia and sickle cell anaemia.

Amniocentesis

Amniocentesis is a diagnostic test that involves taking a small sample of amniotic fluid (the fluid that surrounds the baby in the womb) and analysing it for Down's syndrome or other chromosomal abnormalities. It is routinely offered to mothers aged 35 and over, and is carried out at 16 weeks. The results may take up to four weeks.

Chorionic villus sampling

Chorionic villus sampling (CVS) is another diagnostic test. It too provides information on chromosome abnormalities such as Down's syndrome, single-gene conditions including **cystic fibrosis** and **haemophilia** and some blood disorders. It can be carried out at around 12 weeks and the results are available within a week.

BECOMING A FATHER

It may have taken two of you to conceive a child, but finding out that your partner is pregnant can still come as a shock – even if this is followed by delight, excitement or perhaps disbelief.

The focus of any pregnancy is on the mother. But while she is preoccupied with her changing shape and what's going on inside, you are also preparing, psychologically, for fatherhood.

Try to remember that, although your partner is going through huge, and often uncomfortable, physical changes, her pregnancy isn't an illness. Your support and involvement will make a real difference to how she copes: try to be there for any scans or prenatal testing, and feel the baby move through her abdomen.

Today, it is almost a foregone conclusion that a father will be there for the birth, but this is not compulsory. While some fathers are overwhelmed by the sense of awe and joy at the birth of their child, others feel very awkward or cannot bear to see their partner in pain. It is essential that you talk through these issues, and come to a decision with which you both feel happy.

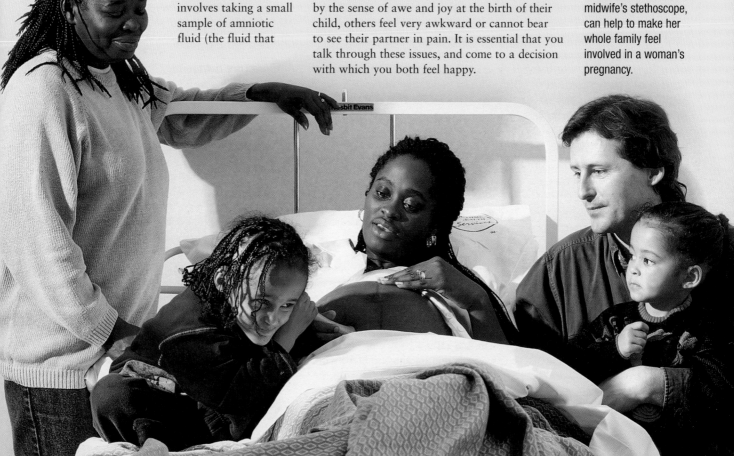

▼ **A family affair**
Feeling the baby kick, or listening to it through the midwife's stethoscope, can help to make her whole family feel involved in a woman's pregnancy.

Problems during pregnancy

The majority of established pregnancies are free of serious problems, but sometimes things go wrong.

Most parents embark on a pregnancy full of optimism and looking forward to a new addition to the family, so it can be particularly devastating when things do not turn out as expected.

It is thought that at least one in five pregnancies ends in **miscarriage** – the loss of a pregnancy at any time in the first 28 weeks. Almost all miscarriages occur in the first 12 weeks, sometimes before a woman knows she is pregnant when there may be a late, heavy 'period'. Early miscarriage can be caused by a number of factors, including maternal illness – especially with a high temperature – and fetal abnormality. Sometimes a fertilized egg implants in a Fallopian tube rather than the uterine wall. This is known as an **ectopic pregnancy**, and it always ends in miscarriage or termination. Late miscarriages are rare; one cause is an incompetent cervix, in which the neck of the uterus is weakened and does not close properly.

Antenatal checks usually pick up other common problems such as maternal **anaemia**, placenta praevia and pre-eclampsia.

■ Anaemia is common in pregnant women because increased blood volume increases the body's need for iron. The baby also builds up its reserves by taking iron from its mother.

■ Placenta praevia, or a low-lying placenta, can cause bleeding during pregnancy and may obstruct the birth canal. This usually necessitates delivery by Caesarean section.

■ Pre-eclampsia is a dangerous complication of pregnancy. Symptoms are high blood pressure, swelling and protein in the urine. The only cure is delivery of the baby, but early treatment can prolong a pregnancy and lessen complications for both mother and baby. (See also **Eclampsia**).

WHEN A BABY DIES IN THE WOMB

In rare cases a baby dies in the womb, and parents are faced with the tragic prospect of giving birth to a baby that they know is dead.

Sometimes a routine scan shows that the heart is no longer beating; sometimes a woman becomes aware that she hasn't felt the baby moving for a while. It may just be keeping still, but if you notice a lack of movement, contact your midwife or hospital so that they can check the heartbeat. Other women simply no longer 'feel' pregnant.

If doctors confirm that your baby has died, you can wait for labour to start naturally, you can have labour induced, or you can have a Caesarean delivery. Whatever route you decide on, the experience is devastating, and you will both need time to come to terms with your loss.

FETAL ABNORMALITY

If an antenatal check suggests that there may be a serious problem with your baby, you will be offered further tests. Results can take days, or even weeks, to come through, and waiting is a time of great anxiety. If a serious abnormality is found, you will be offered a termination of the pregnancy. But you do not have to have any tests: for some couples, whatever may be wrong with their baby a termination is unthinkable.

It is heartbreaking to have to choose whether to end the life of a fetus who would be born with severe disabilities. Some couples decide that they do not want a termination; others feel unable to cope with raising a severely disabled child. Most hospitals offer counselling to help you work through this difficult decision.

PREMATURE BIRTH

A baby born before 37 weeks is said to be premature. Babies born as early as 26 weeks can survive, though the risk of handicap and serious health problems is high. Those born after 32 weeks generally do well. Premature delivery may be induced if the baby is not growing, or if the mother is at risk because of complications such as pre-eclampsia. It may also occur naturally if there is a rupture in the amniotic sac that encloses the fetus. Since their lungs and liver may not be fully developed, premature babies are at risk of jaundice and breathing difficulties. Very early arrivals may also have to be fed by tube.

In most cases, the reason for premature birth is not known, and it cannot be prevented.
SEE ALSO **Birth and problems**

Rhesus incompatibility

The Rhesus factor is a term used for certain proteins in the blood. Most people have these proteins and are described as Rhesus positive. But the 15 per cent who do not have them are Rhesus negative.

If a mother is Rhesus negative and her baby is Rhesus positive, they have what is known as Rhesus incompatibility. This means that, if some of the baby's red blood cells leak into the mother's system, her body may produce antibodies to the Rhesus factor in the baby's blood – a condition called sensitization. These antibodies can destroy the red blood cells in her unborn baby or in the next Rhesus-positive baby she carries.

A blood test taken early in pregnancy identifies mothers who are Rhesus negative. Once diagnosed, Rhesus incompatibility can usually be treated. Further blood tests are taken at 28 and 34 weeks to check for antibodies. To prevent the mother becoming sensitized and making Rhesus antibodies, she is given an injection to destroy fetal red blood cells whenever there is a risk of her baby's blood reaching her own body. Risks include tests such as amniocentesis, any miscarriage, and the birth itself.

Pregnancy, termination of

Termination of pregnancy, or elective abortion, is the removal of an embryo or fetus from the uterus at a stage of pregnancy when it would not be capable of independent survival, that is up to the 24th week of pregnancy.

Elective abortion has been legal in England, Scotland and Wales since 1967, and about 185,000 terminations are performed every year. Before 1967, abortions did take place, but they were often performed illegally by people who had little or no medical training and at great risk to the women involved.

Abortions are permitted in Northern Ireland only in cases in which there is a risk of serious fetal abnormality, but the law is ambiguous and in practice very few terminations are performed. Abortion is illegal in the Republic of Ireland. Every year around 1500 women from Northern Ireland and more than 6000 from the Republic have terminations on the British mainland.

Under NHS rules, a GP is obliged to offer support and advice to any woman who is seeking an abortion. If religious views prevent a GP from writing a referral for termination, the GP is obliged to refer you to another doctor who will provide this service. Contact your local health authority if your doctor refuses to refer you for an abortion, or to another doctor who will. Terminations are also available through family planning clinics and charities such as Marie Stopes International and the Brook Advisory Centres.

LEGAL POSITION

Termination is permitted up to 24 weeks of the pregnancy if two doctors agree that any of the following applies:
- the woman's life is at risk if the pregnancy continues;
- the baby is likely to have a serious handicap;
- continuing the pregnancy poses a serious risk to the physical or mental health of the woman;
- continuing the pregnancy poses a serious risk to the physical or mental health of her family.

Most terminations are carried out for the two latter 'social' reasons.

DECISION MAKING

Deciding whether or not to have an abortion is a deeply personal matter, and one that is rarely taken lightly. If you are considering termination, it is crucial to think through all the issues involved, and if possible to discuss them with the father. You may wish to make use of any counselling offered. Factors that may influence your decision include:
- your relationship with the father;
- your ability to provide for a baby;
- other children;
- your age, and the likelihood of your being able to conceive in the future;
- religious beliefs;
- the accuracy of any tests that indicate fetal abnormality;
- your ability to cope if the child were born with some form of handicap.

COUNSELLING

If you are considering an abortion, you need to feel absolutely sure about going ahead, because any doubt can lead to subsequent feelings of guilt and emotional distress. Hospitals and clinics offer counselling, and online counselling and information is also available from the Marie Stopes International web site. But it is not mandatory to have counselling before an abortion. Some women have thought through all the issues before they seek advice and do not feel the need to discuss their decision.

WHAT'S INVOLVED

The first step is to confirm that conception has taken place and calculate the length of the pregnancy. If this is not clear, an **ultrasound** scan may be done to confirm your dates. You will be asked about your medical history and the reasons why you want a termination. Blood samples and vaginal swabs are taken to check your blood type and ensure that no infection, such as chlamydia, is present.

If a doctor agrees that a termination is appropriate, the doctor will sign an HSA1 form authorizing the procedure. You will then be referred to a second doctor, usually a gynaecologist, who may repeat some of the tests and go over the same questions relating to your decision to have a termination. If the second doctor agrees, and signs the HSA1 form, the termination can go ahead. At some clinics, it is possible to complete this procedure in one day.

TYPES OF TERMINATION

The type of termination depends on the length of the pregnancy and the place where the procedure is being carried out. The options are a medical termination, a surgical termination or a late termination. The stage of pregnancy up to which a medical or surgical procedure is offered varies between health authorities and individual clinics, but a medical termination is not usually carried out beyond nine weeks.

Medical termination

Early in the pregnancy, it may be possible to have a medical abortion. This involves three visits to the clinic or hospital. On the first, you will be given a drug called mifepristone, which disrupts the pregnancy. This is a synthetic hormone that blocks progesterone, another hormone that supports the fetus. Bleeding and pain may occur, but unless this is more severe than period pain there is no need for concern.

If you are considering an abortion, it is important to seek advice as soon as possible. Later terminations can sometimes carry an increased risk of complications.

Two days after taking the mifepristone, you will return to the hospital or clinic for a pessary containing prostaglandin to be inserted into the vagina. This activates uterine contractions. The lining of the womb is broken down and the fetus is expelled. Since the pregnancy is at such an early stage, the main physical effects are similar to those of a heavy period, although side effects may include headaches, nausea and diarrhoea. If contractions fail to expel the pregnancy, it will be necessary to have a D&C (dilation and curettage, which removes the lining of the womb) under general **anaesthetic**. Bleeding may continue for a week to ten days. A follow-up visit is usually arranged to ensure that the entire pregnancy has been expelled and there are no further complications.

Surgical termination
From nine or ten weeks, a surgical termination is performed. This is done under local **anaesthetic** or a light general anaesthetic. An hour or so before the operation, a pessary of prostaglandin may be inserted into the vagina to soften and open the cervix.

Your legs will be placed in stirrups and a thin syringe or tube will be inserted into the uterus and the pregnancy gently suctioned out. The lining of the womb is scraped away to ensure that all of the pregnancy has been removed. If any remains, there is a risk of infection; antibiotics may be given to prevent infection.

Late termination
After about 14 weeks, there are two methods of terminating the pregnancy. It can be done surgically, by removing sections of the fetus under a general anaesthetic. Alternatively, from 13 or 14 weeks up to 24 weeks, a late medical termination can be performed by administering prostaglandin to induce contractions and expel the fetus. Prostaglandin can be given as a pessary, by intravenous drip, injection into the abdomen, or as a combination of these. The experience is similar to going into early labour, and pain relief is offered to ease contractions.

SEE ALSO *Pregnancy and problems*

Presbyopia

Presbyopia is the gradual decline with age in the eye's ability to focus on near objects. The lens loses its elasticity and ability to increase its curvature, so that by middle age it can be difficult to perform close tasks or read at normal distance without wearing reading glasses. General poor health or certain drugs may hasten the effects of presbyopia.

SEE ALSO *Eye and problems*

Presenile dementia

Presenile dementia is the chronic deterioration of the intellect. It affects intellectual functions such as thinking, reasoning and memory skills. It occurs in middle-aged people but can also affect young adults. Presenile dementia may be the result of a genetic disorder (such as **Huntington's disease**), infection (such as **CJD** or **HIV**), disease affecting the blood vessels (such as vascular dementia), a brain tumour, or a complication of a neurodegenerative condition such as **Parkinson's disease**.

SYMPTOMS
Poor memory, language problems, clumsiness, confusion, rigid muscles, paralysis, failure to recognize objects, anxiety, fear, **delusions** and **paranoia** may occur at different stages of dementia. In the later stages, people may no longer recognize family members and may be unable to do anything for themselves.

TREATMENT
Treatment is generally geared to enabling people to lead lives as near to normal for as long as possible. It may take the form of practical help in the home, providing meals and assistance with personal and domestic hygiene, and emotional support for both the person with dementia and his or her carers.

Tranquillizers and antidepressant drugs may relieve symptoms such as aggression, irritability, restlessness and depression.

Complementary therapies
Some essential oils, such as that of rosemary, and herbs such as ginkgo biloba and lecithin are said to help memory. Relaxation techniques, aromatherapy and **massage** may be soothing.

Music and art therapies can help to relieve frustration and tension by enabling people to express themselves when they are unable to take part in normal day-to-day conversations.

PREVENTION
Dementia related to poor blood supply to the brain (vascular dementia) may be prevented by reducing risk factors such as high **blood pressure** and **smoking**.

COMPLICATIONS
As dementia progresses, people can no longer manage their own affairs. It is therefore important that those affected by dementia and their carers seek legal advice before any major problems arise. In many cases, it is likely that residential care will be the safest option.

OUTLOOK
Research is rapidly uncovering more about the type of brain damage that leads to presenile dementia, bringing with it the possibility of more effective treatments.

SEE ALSO *Alzheimer's disease; Dementia*

Priapism

Priapism is a condition in which the penis becomes erect in the absence of sexual arousal, and remains so for long periods.

An erection results from an increased flow of blood to the spongy tissue in the penis. Priapism occurs when the increased blood supply fails to drain. The condition is painful and potentially dangerous. It requires prompt treatment to avoid the risk of permanent damage to the penis and **impotence**.

Any man whose erection continues for four hours or more should see a doctor. Priapism is treated with medication and, if necessary, minor surgery. In some cases, priapism might indicate another medical problem such as a reaction to a drug, damaged nerves or blood vessels, a blood disease or tumour.

SEE ALSO *Penis and disorders*

Prickly heat

Prickly heat is a common and irritating skin rash, which is linked with excessive sweating. The medical name, miliaria rubra, means 'red millet seeds', and describes the many tiny, itchy spots that appear in affected areas such as at the chest, waist, armpits and groin.

The exact cause is unknown, but it may be linked with a buildup of unevaporated sweat in hot, humid conditions, which causes the skin to become soggy and the sweat glands to become blocked. Sweat is believed to leak from the glands into the surrounding tissues, triggering inflammation and an irritating prickly sensation. In some cases, salt crystals form in the sweat gland ducts, and small, fluid-filled blisters appear. Antihistamine tablets or creams help to reduce itching. In some cases, heat rash is complicated by fungal skin infections, in which case an antifungal cream is needed.

SEE ALSO *Skin and disorders*

Proctitis

Proctitis is the inflammation of the rectum. The most common cause is a **sexually transmitted disease**, such as gonorrhoea, especially in gay men. It can also be caused by diseases such as ulcerative colitis and **Crohn's disease**, bacterial infection, **allergies**, and rectal injury. It can sometimes be a side effect of **radiotherapy** or antibiotics.

Symptoms include soreness of the rectum and anus, rectal bleeding and discharge (blood and mucus), left-sided abdominal pain, a feeling of rectal fullness, and constipation. The diagnosis is made by viewing the rectum through the anus using either a rigid proctoscope or flexible sigmoidoscope (see **Endoscopy**). The cause of inflammation may also be determined by taking a **biopsy** of a small piece of rectal tissue.

Treatment is of the underlying cause and is usually successful. Antibiotics are given to combat infections, and corticosteroid drugs are used (as suppositories or enemas) in the case of gastro-intestinal disorders. Without treatment proctitis can lead to severe bleeding, **anaemia** and **fistulas** – openings that occur between the anal canal and the surface of the skin.

SEE ALSO *Rectum and disorders*

Prostate and problems

The prostate is a gland found just below the bladder and against the rectum in men. The urethra runs through the middle of it (see **Urinary system**).

The role of the prostate is not fully understood. One of its functions is to secrete some of the fluids that, with sperm, make up the semen. It also contracts during orgasm, which may heighten sensation. The prostate gland is the size of a pea in an infant and normally increases to the size of a walnut in a young adult male. It naturally becomes larger from middle-age onwards and can, in extreme cases, reach the size of an orange.

WHAT CAN GO WRONG

Possible problems include an enlarged prostate, prostatitis and prostate cancer. The symptoms of these disorders are sometimes very similar, making the specific problem hard to diagnose. Seek medical advice if you:
■ are urinating more often than three to four times a day and once at night;
■ feel pain on urination;
■ have a weak or intermittent flow of urine;
■ have a flow of urine, which is very slow to start and finishes with a trickle;
■ have a sensation that you haven't finished urinating when the urine flow has actually stopped;
■ urinate when you don't intend to.

Enlarged prostate

The natural enlargement of the prostate is thought to be linked to the action of the sex hormone testosterone in men as they mature. As the prostate enlarges, it presses upon the urethra, impeding the flow of urine. This condition becomes a problem for four out of five men by the age of 80 or so. Doctors often refer to it as benign (or non-cancerous)

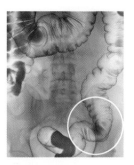

▲ **Proctitis X-ray**
A barium enema inserted into the rectum makes it and the adjoining colon clearly visible on X-rays. Proctitis is indicated by signs of granularity in the rectum wall (circled).

Factfile

A healthy prostate

Implementing some simple steps into your daily routine from a young age can help you to stop prostate cancer developing later in life.

If you want to maintain a healthy prostate gland, the usual lifestyle tips apply: don't smoke, do eat plenty of fruit and vegetables, and eat fewer foods with high levels of saturated fat. Drinking too much alcohol has a direct effect on the prostate, making you urinate more. Although regular urination is good for the prostate, it is better done naturally than as a result of too much alcohol (see **Alcohol and abuse**). Keeping your body weight down may ease pressure on the bladder. Foods that are rich in vitamin B$_6$, zinc and

selenium appear to be good for the prostate. Zinc is found in shellfish, seeds (including pine, sunflower and pumpkin seeds), yoghurt, beans and lean meat. Fatty acids from linseeds and oily fish such as sardines and salmon may also be helpful. Some studies suggest that eating tomatoes a couple of times a week may help to reduce the risk of prostate cancer. Lycopene, an antioxidant found in cooked tomato products such as tomato sauce, may be responsible for the lowered risk.

prostatic hyperplasia. An enlarged prostate can force the bladder muscles to work harder, which in time may cause it to swell and misfunction.

SYMPTOMS

The most obvious symptoms are in changes to urination.

- Difficulty when beginning to urinate.
- A weak or intermittent flow of urine.
- Increased frequency of urination.
- Occasionally, mild incontinence.

DIAGNOSIS

A doctor will diagnose an enlarged prostate through a combination of rectal examination – using a finger – and an **ultrasound** scan. Blood tests are carried out to check for poor kidney function. Any man with the symptoms of an enlarged prostate is advised to consult his doctor so that he can have treatment if necessary and so that more serious causes can be excluded.

TREATMENT

Treatment for an enlarged prostate itself is not always necessary. If it is, drugs that relax the muscle in the prostate or inhibit the production of the form of testosterone that seems to cause it to grow are available. Side effects may include decreased libido and impotence. Surgical options range from a simple procedure to release pressure on the urethra to a prostatectomy (removal of part of the prostate) in more serious cases of enlargement.

Prostatitis

Prostatitis is the inflammation of the prostate caused by a bacterial infection that is sometimes **sexually transmitted**. Symptoms are more acute than in an enlarged prostate. Urination is very frequent and painful. There may also be fever, pain in the lower back and genitals, pain during bowel movements and a discharge from the penis, sometimes including blood. The method of diagnosis is similar to that for an enlarged prostate; with blood and urine tests to reveal any infection. Treatment is with antibiotics.

Prostatitis can recur in some individuals. This is called chronic bacterial prostatitis. Although an enlarged prostate is most common in men over 50, prostatitis more commonly affects younger men.

Prostate enlargement and the bladder

The prostate sits below the bladder. If enlarged, it impairs urination by obstructing the neck of the bladder, which may in turn damage the kidneys.

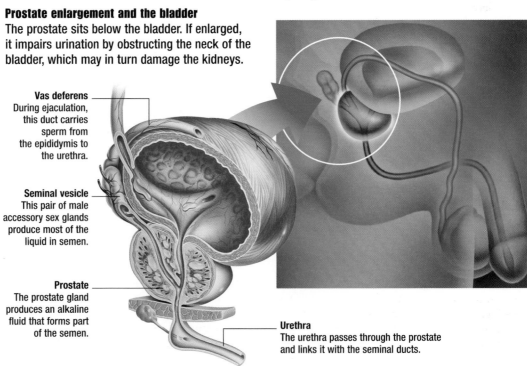

Vas deferens
During ejaculation, this duct carries sperm from the epididymis to the urethra.

Seminal vesicle
This pair of male accessory sex glands produce most of the liquid in semen.

Prostate
The prostate gland produces an alkaline fluid that forms part of the semen.

Urethra
The urethra passes through the prostate and links it with the seminal ducts.

Prostate cancer

Cancer of the prostate is the second most common **cancer** in men after testicular cancer. Its initial symptoms are often similar to those of an enlarged prostate, which is why men experiencing urination problems are advised to visit their GP promptly. Other symptoms – which may sometimes be the only symptoms – include blood in the urine, pain in the lower back and unexplained weight loss.

Prostate cancer affects one in 13 men in England and Wales, but is rare before the age of 45. Some doctors would like to see a screening programme in which the prostates of older men are routinely checked.

DIAGNOSIS

The diagnostic procedure for prostate cancer is similar to that for an enlarged prostate. Several blood tests are made, including the measurement of prostate-specific antigen (PSA), an enzyme produced by the prostate. If high levels of the enzyme are present, this may indicate cancer (see also **PSA test**). A **biopsy** may be taken to confirm the diagnosis.

If an elderly man has a small, slow-growing, non-aggressive cancer that does not affect his life expectancy, he and his doctor may decide that regular monitoring is the best course of action – with no treatment given unless his health deteriorates.

TREATMENT

If treatment is thought to be necessary, its nature will depend on how advanced the cancer is. Prostate cancer can be treated in many ways. Options include surgery, **radiotherapy**, **chemotherapy** and hormonal therapy designed to reduce levels of testosterone.

OUTLOOK

More than 90 per cent of men with prostate cancer can expect to live at least five years after the initial diagnosis. According to the American Cancer Society, 67 per cent of men diagnosed with prostate cancer survive for at least 10 years and 52 per cent survive for 15 years. As many men who get prostate cancer are already elderly, they are more likely to die from other causes than from the cancer.

Prosthesis

A prosthesis is an artificial replacement of a missing or non-functioning body part.

Amputated limbs and worn joints can be replaced with artificial limbs and individual joints. Advances in bionics have revolutionized limb prostheses and their ability to replicate normal human actions; legs are now available with joints at the knee and ankle so that they can mimic normal walking. Artificial arms can be fitted with elbow joints and wrists capable of rotation, while springs controlled by shoulder movements can manipulate artificial hands. Small artificial joints, such as knuckles and toe joints, are now also available.

In the vascular system, early mechanical heart valves have largely been replaced by those made from animal or human tissue. Pacemakers are used to produce and maintain a normal heartbeat, and grafts replace blocked coronary arteries. Flexible, self-expanding metal springs (stents) can be implanted to overcome blockages in arteries in various parts of the body.

Penile prostheses are flexible rods that are implanted into the penis as a cure for impotence.

Hearing aids and cochlear implants are now able to improve hearing.

Breast implants, artificial eyes and dentures are forms of cosmetic prostheses, which are used to improve appearance rather than function. Prostheses can also be used to correct facial deformities resulting from birth defects or injury.

OUTLOOK

Nerve prostheses – fine tubes filled with mouse nerve cells – are being investigated as a means of replacing damaged nerves.

PSA test

The PSA test is a way of testing for prostate cancer and other prostate conditions in their early stages. Prostate cancer may grow for many years before causing any symptoms. In older men, a prostate tumour may never cause any problems and can safely be left untreated.

The PSA (prostate specific antigen) blood test can contribute to earlier diagnosis of the condition. PSA is a 'marker' protein, which is made by the prostate gland. Normally, a small amount of PSA enters the blood, and research has shown that raised levels are often linked to prostate gland problems that may, or may not, develop into cancer. But PSA levels also rise with age, and elevated PSA is often found in cases where the prostate is enlarged but not cancerous.

It is not yet clear how useful the PSA test really is on its own. Normal levels do not necessarily exclude cancer, while raised levels may lead to men who do not have cancer being investigated unnecessarily.

Some doctors may give a PSA test and a rectal examination to all men over 50 if they ask for one. Men over 50 should certainly have one if they have symptoms of prostate disease (for example, an enlarged prostate gland causing difficulty urinating), or a family history of prostate cancer. But at present offering the test to healthy men is not thought to be useful. If the PSA test can be made more sensitive and specific, this position could change.

SEE ALSO **Prostate and problems**

Psittacosis

Psittacosis, also known as ornithosis and parrot disease, is a disease caught by inhaling dried secretions from birds. Birds most likely to be carrying the disease are pets (such as parrots, parakeets, macaws) and poultry (turkeys, ducks).

Psittacosis is very rare. In the USA, for example, only 50 cases a year are reported. Bird breeders, pet shop owners, vets and poultry farm workers are most at risk of infection.

SYMPTOMS

Following a 6–19-day incubation period, symptoms can include fever, chills, headaches, severe muscle ache and a dry cough.

TREATMENT

Psittacosis responds to antibiotics.

COMPLICATIONS

Psittacosis can lead to inflammation of the heart, nervous disorders and severe pneumonia. Occasionally it can be fatal.

SEE ALSO **Zoonoses**

Psoriasis

Psoriasis is a long-term inflammatory disease of the skin that affects one in 50 people in the UK. Symptoms usually appear between the ages of 10 and 30, although the condition can occur at any age. Psoriasis occurs when new skin cells in parts of the body are produced too quickly and push up to the surface rapidly, forming raised, red patches covered with fine, silvery scales or thick, white plaques. Psoriasis flares up from time to time, causing attacks of varying severity.

TYPES OF PSORIASIS

There are several types of psoriasis. Discoid or 'plaque' psoriasis is the most common, affecting nine out of ten sufferers. Patches appear on the trunk and limbs, especially on the elbows, knees, hands, around the navel, over the lower back and on the scalp; the nails may show pitting, thickening or lifting from the nail bed.

In guttate psoriasis, small patches develop over a wide area to resemble drops of paint; it occurs most frequently in children, often after a viral infection such as influenza or **glandular fever**, or a sore throat due to the streptococcus bacteria (see **Throat and problems**).

Napkin psoriasis develops in the nappy area of an infant, causing a bright red, weeping rash or the more typical plaques. Children who are affected do not seem to have a higher risk of psoriasis in later life.

Scalp psoriasis causes redness and flaking, and a buildup of plaques, often around the hairline. Another form, flexural psoriasis, produces well-defined, red areas in skin folds such as the armpits, groin and under the breasts; there is little or no scaling. In pustular psoriasis, small, deep-seated pustules form, usually affecting only the palms and soles. Occasionally, the pustules become more widespread with fever and a high white blood cell count (leukocytosis) that requires hospital admission.

The rarest and most serious form is erythrodermic psoriasis, in which widespread redness of the skin occurs, without scaling. This is due to an abnormal dilation of blood vessels under the skin, which leads to a rapid heat loss and disruption in the fluid balance of the body. It is potentially life-threatening and needs urgent treatment.

Up to one in five people with psoriasis also develop inflamed joints, a condition known as psoriatic arthritis, which needs drug treatment.

TREATMENT

Psoriasis is treated mainly with creams or ointments that moisturize the skin or reduce the rate at which new skin cells are produced. Older treatments, such as coal-tar extracts and dithranol, are effective, but can stain skin or clothing. Newer treatments, such as tazarotene gel and calcipotriol ointment or cream, are less messy to use. Phototherapy using ultraviolet-B light may be recommended.

Complementary therapies

Some sufferers visit the Dead Sea in Israel – the combination of sunlight and mineral-rich mud and sea water is known to be helpful for treating psoriasis. **Acupuncture** may also help.

OUTLOOK

Treatment can relieve the symptoms of psoriasis, but it can take time to find the best treatment for each individual.

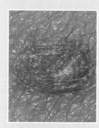
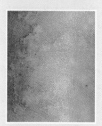
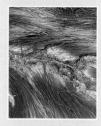
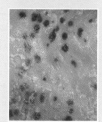

Psychiatric disorders

The mind is as susceptible to illness as any other organ of the body. Most people will have to grapple with a mental health problem at some point in their lives, but too many of us are reluctant to ask for help. This is a mistake, because most mental illness is eminently treatable.

Psychiatric or mental illness is notoriously difficult to define. A mental illness is not like a physical illness such as a cancer, which can be diagnosed in irrefutably objective ways. An oncologist can spot a malignant tumour and do something about it without having to worry about the cultural background or the personality of the sufferer. A psychiatric doctor, on the other hand, has to take into account the norms of the society in which the patient lives when deciding whether or not he or she is ill and, if so, what treatment is most suitable.

After all, every one of us at some time exhibits symptoms that may be considered abnormal: prolonged sadness, a sense of disappointment in oneself, irritability, impulsiveness and aggression. These traits can be signs of illness – or they can be core personality traits. Some people, for example, are naturally melancholy – that does not mean to say that they are suffering from clinical depression.

Patterns of behaviour become a mental health issue when they begin to change drastically from what is normal for that individual, or if they go way beyond what is acceptable to society. Even then, no one – not even a trained professional – can say definitively or objectively when a pattern of eccentric or unsocial behaviour crosses the boundary that takes it into the realm of mental disorder. Madness and sanity – to use two popular terms – are concepts that depend on your point of view.

Psychosomatic illness

The term 'psychosomatic' is used to describe symptoms that arise as a result of psychological or stress-related factors. This does not mean that symptoms are imaginary or 'all in the mind'.

Doctors recognize that after an event such as a bereavement, for example, a person might develop high blood pressure or even have a heart attack. In another person, the same situation might lead to a peptic **ulcer**. A third individual, just as grief-stricken, might not get sick at all.

Treatment for psychosomatic illness will take account of this unpredictable psychological element: symptoms can disappear once the person knows that there is no underlying physical illness.

THE VARIETIES OF MENTAL DISORDER
Although there are difficult philosophical issues involved in the definition of psychiatric illness, it is nevertheless possible for doctors to classify mental disorders, and to use those categories as a diagnostic tool. There are three groups of psychiatric disorder, and they are usually classified under the headings neuroses, psychoses and mental deficiency.

Neuroses
Neuroses are illnesses in which normal thoughts and feelings are exaggerated to the point where

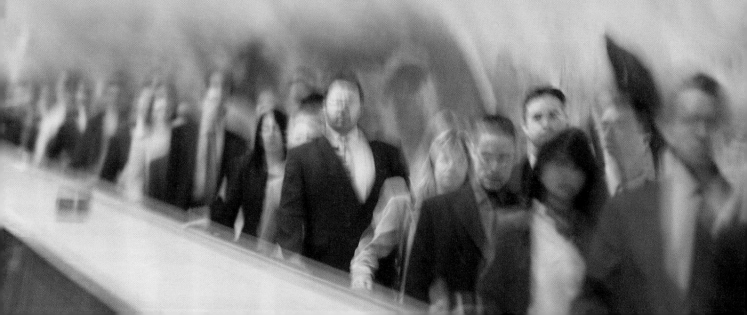

▼ **Troubled mind**
Psychiatric illness can strike anyone at any time, but it is often triggered by traumatic events such as divorce and bereavement.

Factfile

How to get psychiatric help

It is difficult to know where to start when you are looking for help for a mental health problem. A good first step is to visit your GP, who will know what is available on the NHS in your area.

Your doctor can refer you to a psychiatrist, to a psychotherapist or to another practitioner on the NHS. But choice may be limited, and there may be a waiting list.

If you decide to pay for treatment, you will have to do some research – although your GP may be able to make some useful recommendations. The range of fees can be surprising: some therapists offer a sliding scale according to your income; others have hourly rates that rival those of solicitors and barristers. You must also bear in mind that the approach of a psychological therapist will depend on the school and tradition in which he or she has been trained: a Jungian psychoanalyst, for example, will treat you very differently from a cognitive behaviour therapist.

The biggest factor in successful therapy is finding a practitioner who suits you. It is also important to choose someone who belongs to a reputable professional body with a code of ethics and practice. Anyone can advertise as a therapist, so do not merely pick a name from the local paper.

Before going for therapy or analysis, or before seeing a psychiatrist, write down your goals. Ask yourself what problems you want to deal with, how active you want to be in the treatment, and how much time and money you have to invest in it. If you are willing to explore your past and you feel your problems are long term and recurring, then psychotherapy or psychoanalysis may be appropriate. If you are experiencing psychotic symptoms that are disrupting your life, it may be best to see a psychiatrist. If you are having problems because of a bereavement or recent loss, and do not want to delve into your past too much, brief counselling might be the best option.

they interfere with the sufferer's everyday life. **Anxiety** is by far the most common form of neurosis – the other most prevalent forms are **depression** and the many varieties of **phobia**. What all these disorders have in common is that the sufferer is aware of the condition and its effects. Neuroses might also be said to include such conditions as **anorexia nervosa**, which could be described as an 'eating phobia'. Anorexia also has some of the characteristics of obsessive-compulsive behaviour (see **Obsessions and compulsions**).

Psychoses

A person suffering from a psychosis, unlike someone with neurosis, is unaware of the condition. A psychotic is out of touch with reality, and unable to function within the parameters of society. The illness is obvious to everyone else – often painfully so – but psychotics themselves have no idea that they are behaving abnormally. One might say that 'psychosis' is the medical term for madness.

Psychosis covers such serious conditions as **manic depression** and the various forms of **schizophrenia**. Schizophrenics become irrational and delusional: they hear voices and see visions, entertain bizarre beliefs and thoughts of persecution, and speak in unreal or disturbing ways. Psychotics can sometimes be violent. For this reason, and because they are unaware of their condition, some psychotics may require compulsory admission to hospital.

Mental deficiency

The term mental deficiency covers a group of conditions generally termed mental disability. They are not illnesses so much as conditions. In other words, the difference between mental illness and mental deficiency is that illnesses are usually temporary and treatable and have an entirely psychological root. Mental disability, on the other hand, is usually permanent, and often has a physical cause: infection of the baby in the womb, brain damage during birth, or genetic abnormalities such as Down's syndrome. Mental deficiency is usually diagnosed in childhood.

WHO IS AT RISK?

Anyone can succumb to a psychiatric or mental illness, but some groups appear to be more vulnerable because of their social position, personal circumstances or heredity. Those who are statistically more likely to have a mental illness include members of large, low-income families, the unemployed, those who lack a close friend or confidant, people who have suffered a prolonged serious illness, and alcoholics. Mental illness can also be triggered by extreme stress and loneliness, and by life-changing events such as marriage, divorce or bereavement.

Situations that can cause mental illness often contribute to the reluctance of a sufferer to seek help. People with depression, say, often feel embarrassed that they are not coping; others feel that to take the problem to the doctor is 'giving in'. It is important to bear in mind that mental illness is no more the fault of the sufferer than a broken arm. If you feel that you need help with a psychiatric problem, go to your GP – who will take you seriously and be sympathetic (see box, above left).

SEE ALSO *Psychosis*

Psychosis

'Psychosis' is a term used for a severe mental disorder in which someone cannot tell the difference between what is real and what is imaginary. This can cause delusions in which the person hears voices or sees things that are not there (see **Hallucinations**).

People can develop psychotic symptoms for various reasons – they might be very depressed, physically ill, or misusing drugs or alcohol. Most people recover fully, but for some, the symptoms persist, or go away and then return. Some people develop psychotic symptoms as part of another illness such as **schizophrenia, postnatal depression** or **manic depression**.

Doctors do not know what causes psychosis. It is probably the result of several influences, including genes, family background, suppressed feelings and chemical changes in the brain.

SYMPTOMS

Various behavioural signs might indicate that someone is psychotic.

■ Hallucinations: hearing or seeing things that others do not.

■ **Delusions:** believing him or herself to be a celebrity, or that people are sending messages.

■ **Paranoia:** believing that others are stealing from or threatening him or her in some way.

■ Extreme mood swings or one dominant mood.

■ Changed behaviour: the person withdraws socially or becomes aggressive.

TREATMENT

It is important that symptoms of psychosis are recognized and treated early on. But getting help or treatment may be difficult because people with psychotic symptoms may not accept that there is anything wrong. The affected person should see his or her GP. The GP may be able to help directly, or refer the patient to a psychiatrist or other practitioner.

The main treatment for psychosis is drug-based. Anti-psychotic drugs include strong tranquillizers such as haloperidol and chlorpromazine. These have a calming effect and can control disturbing thoughts and hallucinations. While medication is needed in a crisis, talking treatments, such as counselling or psychotherapy, can help at other times when people have some insight into their situation.

Compulsory admission to hospital

Sometimes people become seriously ill but cannot recognize that they need help. People who are a danger to themselves or to others can be admitted to hospital against their will in the UK. This is done under a section of the *Mental Health Act 1983* – hence the term 'sectioning'. This type of hospital admission is unusual: about one in 15 of all patients in psychiatric units are there against their will; the rest are voluntary patients.

HOW OTHERS CAN HELP

Psychotic symptoms are difficult for carers, family and friends to cope with, as well as for the person him or herself. There may be marked changes in a person's behaviour, such as aggression, which can be hard to deal with. The way that others help and respond to the situation can aid the person's recovery.

■ Be sensitive and reassuring. The person may be frightened and need someone to open up to.

■ Try not to be judgmental – the person needs support and acceptance; try to understand why he or she is behaving in a particular way.

■ Encourage the person to seek help – find out about support groups where the person can share his or her feelings and experiences with others.

■ Be sure to get some help and support for yourself – from other family members, support groups or carers groups.

SEE ALSO *Mental health and problems; Psychiatric disorders*

Pyelonephritis

Pyelonephritis is a kidney infection, which has often travelled up from the lower urinary tract as a complication of untreated **cystitis**. It may come on quickly (acute) or cause long-term repeated problems (chronic).

SEE ALSO *Kidneys and disorders*

Pyloric stenosis

Pyloric stenosis is a narrowing of the pylorus, the lower part of the stomach that leads to the pyloric sphincter. It mainly occurs in infants. Within weeks of birth, muscles around the pylorus thicken, stopping the passage of food into the small intestine. The cause is unknown, but genetic factors may play a role. In the UK, it affects about one in 4000 newborns, being four times more likely in boys. It occasionally occurs in adults as a result of a gastric tumour or scarring from a gastric ulcer.

Symptoms include spitting, often followed by projectile vomiting within 30 minutes of eating, weight loss, **dehydration** and diarrhoea. A **barium investigation** or an **ultrasound** scan may be used to confirm the diagnosis.

Treatment is by surgery. Vomiting may occur during feeding after the operation, but this quickly subsides. Recurrence is very rare.

SEE ALSO *Digestive system; Stomach and disorders*

Q fever

Q fever is an acute, infectious disease, with severe, influenza-like symptoms. It is caused by *Coxiella burnetii*, a bacterium harboured by farm animals, such as sheep, cattle and goats. Q fever can be present in the urine, faeces, milk and flesh of infected animals, and is transmitted to human beings by inhaling infected particles, drinking contaminated milk, or by ticks.

After an incubation period of about 20 days, symptoms develop, including a cough, high fever, headache and muscle and chest pain. Q fever is diagnosed with a blood test; treatment with antibiotics is usually effective.

Two in every three patients will then recover, but some develop a form of **pneumonia** in the second week, and others may develop **hepatitis**. In 1 or 2 per cent of cases Q fever is fatal.

Quadraplegia

Quadraplegia is the paralysis of all four limbs. It is usually caused by a severe injury to the spinal cord in the neck. The spinal cord contains nerve cells and bundles of long nerve fibres running through the centre of the vertebrae of the spinal column. The nerve fibres carry signals to and from the brain. If they are severed or badly crushed, the signals cannot get through and the body parts that are served by the damaged nerves become paralysed.

The nerve fibres that lie higher up the spinal cord control movement and feeling in the upper limbs and the torso, and those that lie lower down control the lower limbs and the internal organs. If the entire bundle of spinal cord nerve fibres is damaged at a high level, all parts of the body beneath the injury area will be affected.

SEE ALSO *Disability; Paraplegia*

Quarantine

'Quarantine' is the term used to describe the period of time for which a person or animal recently exposed to a serious infectious disease is kept in isolation. The aim of quarantine is to stop the spread of disease, and quarantine may be applied whether or not the people or animals concerned display any symptoms of the infection to which they might have been exposed.

Nowadays, it is extremely rare for a person to be placed in quarantine because of the greatly reduced incidence of many serious infections and the extensive use of immunization.

Quinsy

Quinsy is an abscess that forms in the area around the tonsils – and is probably the most common complication of tonsillitis. Today, thanks to the availability of antibiotics to treat tonsillitis, quinsy is far less common than it used to be. It occurs more frequently in adults than in children.

SYMPTOMS
Symptoms include:
- very severe sore throat;
- swallowing difficulty and earache;
- tender glands in the jaw and throat;
- facial swelling;
- headache;
- drooling;
- fever;
- chills.

TREATMENT
The symptoms are far more severe than they would be with a simple case of tonsillitis, and medical aid should be sought immediately if quinsy is suspected. An examination of the pharynx will reveal redness and swelling of the tonsils and the surrounding area, while the uvula (the central flap of tissue that hangs down at the back of the throat) will usually have been displaced to one side by the abscess.

Admission to hospital may be necessary so that the patient can be given antibiotics by injection. Meanwhile, the abscess usually needs to be drained. This procedure can be carried out by a GP, who will spray the affected area with a local **anaesthetic** and then puncture the abscess with a scalpel. The patient should feel immediate relief if the diagnosis is correct. When a child is being treated, this is usually done under a general **anaesthetic**.

As a preventive measure, doctors may consider removing the tonsils of a patient who has suffered from repeated bouts of tonsillitis.

COMPLICATIONS
In the majority of cases quinsy responds to prompt treatment, but complications do sometimes occur. These might include:
- **cellulitis** of the jaw, neck or chest;
- **pneumonia**;
- pericarditis – an inflammation of the membrane surrounding the heart;
- pleural effusion – fluid around the lungs;
- airway obstruction.

You should always call a doctor if someone has had tonsillitis and the symptoms start to become worse, especially if that person develops a persistent fever, a cough, breathing difficulties or a pain in the chest.

SEE ALSO *Tonsils and disorders*

Rabies

Rabies is an acute viral infection that mainly affects animals in Asia, Africa and Central and South America. It is rare in Europe and North America. Although best known as a disease that makes dogs sick and mad, it can affect all warm-blooded creatures, including human beings. It is also known as hydrophobia.

A rabid animal such as a dog can transmit the infection to people by a bite or even just a lick over a small cut in the skin, which is why all dogs in many northern European countries are routinely vaccinated against the disease.

CAUSE

The virus that causes rabies is called the lyssa virus. After a bite, the virus travels from the wound along the nerve pathways of the muscles into the central nervous system. It replicates quickly and spreads into many parts of the brain. The brain becomes inflamed, often resulting in delirium, and many functions of the central nervous system are affected. The virus spreads via the nervous system to many tissues of the body, including the skin, mucous membranes and salivary glands.

SYMPTOMS

Symptoms may progressively include:
- fever;
- vomiting;
- loss of appetite;
- headache;
- copious salivation and weeping;
- paralysis;
- spasms in the throat, making swallowing difficult;
- a terror of water;
- anxiety and hyperactivity (it is in this phase that animals become mad and bite);
- uncontrolled movement, confusion and delirium.

Once symptoms appear, the disease can no longer be cured – rabies in human beings is almost always fatal. But it can be prevented with a vaccine, and anyone who has been bitten can be treated with a vaccine before symptoms develop. Immunization should be given within two days of the bite for rabies to be prevented.

PREVENTION

When in developing countries, avoid stray dogs. Vaccination against the rabies virus requires three injections: two that are given with an interval of one week between them, and one that is given three weeks later. Vaccination provides protection for three years and is recommended for people living in areas where there is a regular incidence of rabies and for travellers planning to spend time in areas with no immediate access to preventive treatment.

After a rabid bite, you will need treatment with a rabies vaccine whether or not you received pre-travel rabies vaccination.

SEE ALSO *Immunization, Travel and tropical diseases*

Radiation sickness

Radiation sickness is the effects on the body of high doses of ionizing radiation – from **radiotherapy**, a nuclear accident, or fall-out from a hydrogen bomb. Radiation is measured in units called Grays (Gy).

SYMPTOMS

The effects of radiation vary according to the degree of exposure. The radiation received during radiotherapy treatment for breast cancer, for example, is targeted at a particular area of the body in a carefully calculated and controlled dose. It may therefore cause only mild symptoms, such as a general feeling of ill health, nausea and vomiting, diarrhoea and loss of appetite.

Complications can include anaemia and serious infections caused by damage to the bone marrow and the immune system.

The exposure to radiation during a nuclear accident produces wider-scale damage to the body's cells. The immediate symptoms are severe vomiting and disorientation. In time, an affected person may develop major infections and cancers such as **leukaemia**, thyroid cancer, skin cancer, and bone cancer (see **Cancer**).

TREATMENT

- The affected person needs to be isolated from the risk of infection until the immune system recovers, and any infections contracted must be treated with antibiotics.
- In severe cases, a bone marrow transplant is needed to speed recovery and reduce infection and anaemia.

OUTLOOK

Symptoms from radiotherapy usually disappear when treatment ends, although some of the effects may last for a couple of months after the end of treatment. Progress is monitored by regular appointments with a doctor. These checks will probably become less frequent as time passes.

Research into the effects on health of nuclear accidents such as the one that occurred in Chernobyl in 1986 has proved inconclusive. However, some studies have linked exposure to such high doses of radiation with an increased risk of developing certain cancers such as thyroid cancer, and with congenital abnormalities in the next generation.

SEE ALSO *Anaemia*

Radiotherapy

Radiotherapy is a treatment that is primarily used for **cancer** and involves the use of high-energy beams of radiation. These beams are very precisely directed at the cancer cells to kill them. Cancer cells are particularly sensitive to radiotherapy and so are killed more easily than normal cells, which recover fairly quickly.

Radiotherapy is targeted at the areas of the body where the cancer cells are, and the beams are often given from several angles, all focused on the same spot to reduce any damage to surrounding tissues.

Treatment must be carefully planned, both to calculate the correct dose needed to treat the cancer and also to minimize any harm to other organs. The radiotherapist is likely to practise putting you in the correct position for treatment and extra scans of the tumour may be taken. Sometimes a plastic mould is made of the part of your body needing treatment in order to hold it exactly in place while the radiotherapy is given. This is usually done for areas that are difficult to pinpoint such as the head and neck. You may have a single treatment or a course of treatments at regular intervals over several weeks, depending on why radiotherapy has been recommended for you.

SIDE EFFECTS

The treatment is completed in a matter of minutes and is quite painless. However, the following side effects may occur and can be uncomfortable and even distressing.

- Tiredness.
- Nausea, vomiting and diarrhoea.
- Redness and irritation of the skin in the area being treated.
- Stiffness in the joints and muscles in the area treated.
- Hair loss and reduced sweating in the area treated (usually temporary).
- Cough and shortness of breath.
- Urinary discomfort.

COPING WITH RADIOTHERAPY

People react differently to radiotherapy treatment. Some general measures will help you to cope with the particular effects you are experiencing, and help you to feel as comfortable as possible.

- Treat your skin very gently. Take showers rather than baths, use unperfumed soap and avoid chemicals on the skin (baby powder is a good mild deodorant).
- Wear soft, comfortable clothing.
- Protect your skin from sun or cold winds.
- Eat as well as possible – your body will need nutrients to recover and repair itself.

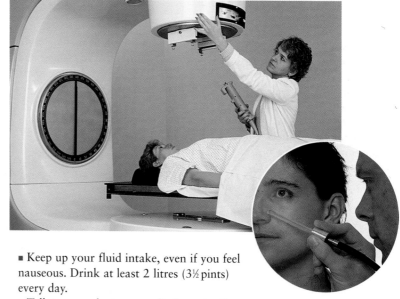

- Keep up your fluid intake, even if you feel nauseous. Drink at least 2 litres (3½ pints) every day.
- Talk to your doctor or radiotherapist if you are having any problems: side effects can be minimized, for example, the symptoms of nausea and be reduced with drug treatment.
- Go out for a short stroll every day.
- Drink cranberry juice to relieve urinary discomfort.

▲ **Radiotherapy**
Radiotherapy is often used to treat cancers affecting the face. This is because removal of tumours by surgery is problematic in difficult sites such as the nose, eyes and ears.

Raynaud's syndrome

Raynaud's syndrome is a condition that includes Raynaud's disease and Raynaud's phenomenon. Both of these cause spasms, usually in the arteries of the fingers and toes but also in the ears and nose when they are subjected to cold.

Raynaud's disease affects up to one person in 10 in the UK, two-thirds of whom are female. One per cent of those with Raynaud's also have Raynaud's phenomenon, in which the symptoms are due to an underlying disease. Raynaud's phenomenon is commonly caused by scleroderma, a connective tissue disorder.

SYMPTOMS

Cold or stress triggers spasm in small arteries (arterioles), usually in the fingers. The fingers change colour – they are pale at first, changing to blue and then red. There may be numbness and sometimes pain. This may last for minutes or hours, and is usually relieved by rewarming.

If there is an underlying cause, the circulation may be poor, leading to skin changes, ulceration or even **gangrene**.

TREATMENT

Although self-help measures can help to relieve the symptoms, medical attention is advisable.

When to consult a doctor

Seek medical advice if you have any of the symptoms above.

Raynaud's syndrome can be hereditary, although in such cases the condition is usually mild.

What a doctor may do
- Check for underlying causes.
- Advise warm or artificially heated clothing.
- Prescribe vasodilator drugs, such as nifedipine.
- Suggest surgery to cut the nerves that control the arterioles (in extreme cases only).

What you can do
- Buy and wear thermal gloves, hats and socks.
- Stop smoking (nicotine constricts arterioles).

Complementary therapies
Take fish oil or evening primrose oil supplements.

Referred pain

Referred pain occurs when a disorder in one part of the body can be felt as a pain in another area of the body. Typical examples are angina (heart pain) which is felt in the wrists, neck, jaw, or ear lobes; and ureteric colic (spasm of the ureters associated with kidney stones), which is felt in the testicles or the labia.

Refractive surgery

More and more people are having surgery to correct refractive errors in the eye such as **myopia, hypermetropia** or **astigmatism**. The **cornea** is reshaped to allow light to be refocused upon the retina without the need for correction with glasses or contact lenses. Radial incisions made in the cornea cause the eyeball to shrink as the wounds heal, thereby reducing its length and correcting myopia.

WHAT'S INVOLVED
The advent of **lasers** has allowed more precise treatment of a wider range of refractive errors. Photorefractive keratectomy involves scraping away the the epithelium, which is the front layer of the cornea, burning away tissue from the exposed surface and then allowing the epithelium to regrow.

More popular nowadays is laser in-situ keratomileusis, more popularly known as LASIK. A liftable flap of cornea is created, allowing exposed tissue to be removed by laser; and the flap is then replaced. It takes only 20 minutes to treat both eyes by this method, which is less painful and has a quicker recovery time. There is, however, a risk of long-term complications due to flap dislodgement.

Some high street opticians offer this treatment in specialist laser eye clinics. Although in theory anyone with a thick enough cornea is treatable, the best results are on people with low- to medium-prescription myopia, and those with only mild hypermetropia or astigmatism.

AFTER THE TREATMENT
Successful treatment may remove the need for optical correction, although anyone with **presbyopia** will still require reading glasses. Regular **eye tests** are recommended to detect any post-operative effects; these may include glare or haze around lights. It is important to avoid excessive rubbing of or trauma to the eye, especially after LASIK.

Reiter's syndrome

Reiter's syndrome is an inflammatory disease that affects the urethra (**urethritis**), both eyes (**conjunctivitis**), and one or more of the joints (**arthritis**).

Reiter's syndrome is the most common cause of arthritis in young men, and usually affects one or two joints – generally the knees or ankles. The affected joints become hot, swollen, stiff and painful, and there may be a fever and a general feeling of being unwell. The tendons, ligaments and the soles of the feet may become inflamed and a skin rash is also common.

The condition is most common in those who have recently had a new sexual partner followed by urethral inflammation and discharge (see **non-specific urethritis**).

Treatment of Reiter's syndrome is with painkillers and anti-inflammatory drugs. Anti-inflammatory eyedrops may be prescribed for the conjunctivitis. The NSU – which may be due to chlamydia – is treated with antibiotics.

Most first attacks clear up within two to six months, but recovery may be delayed for as long as a year. In about one in three cases, especially after further episodes of NSU, the arthritis flares up again.

Relapsing fever

Relapsing fever is, as its name suggests, characterized by recurrent fever. The illness is caused by a bacterial infection transmitted to human beings by lice or ticks. It occurs in most parts of the world, although not in the UK.

A week or so after being bitten by an infected tick, the victim develops a fever, accompanied by headache, muscle and joint pain, nausea and vomiting. The symptoms last two to nine days. If the illness is left untreated, there may be up to ten subsequent, progressively milder relapses, but treatment with antibiotics is effective.

To prevent relapsing fever and other diseases, ticks should be removed promptly and carefully, using tweezers.

AMNIOTIC FLUID

The amniotic fluid is a buoyant liquid that lets the growing baby move within the womb. It is contained inside the membrane that forms a sac around the embryo and, later, the fetus. The fluid, which stops the amnion (membrane) from sticking to the fetus, is produced by both the fetus and the placenta. Being surrounded by liquid helps the baby to grow uniformly, and allows its bones and muscles to develop. Breathing amniotic fluid in and out while in the womb helps a baby's lungs to prepare for breathing air after birth.

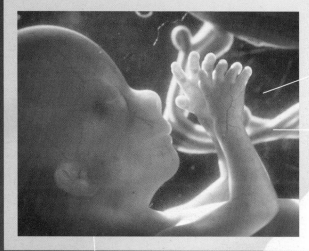

Amniotic fluid

Umbilical cord

12 weeks old

When a baby nears full term, it becomes harder to move in the confined watery world of the uterus. Most babies now assume a head-down position ready for birth.

Amniotic fluid

Umbilical cord

Fetus

Fetal head

THE MOMENT OF FERTILIZATION

The instant at which the head of a sperm breaks through the surface of the egg is the moment of fertilization. The nuclei of both egg and sperm cells fuse, forming a zygote, and the tail and body of the sperm drop off. The surface of the egg then becomes impenetrable to other sperm.

Millions of sperm are released at ejaculation, and swim instinctively for their goal – the egg in the Fallopian tube. Those that make it to the egg release special enzymes that dissolve its outer layer.

Surface of egg

Head of sperm

Reproductive system

A human life begins when a sperm cell from the male partner fertilizes an egg from the female partner and becomes an embryo. Fertilization takes place in one of the woman's Fallopian tubes, the fertilized egg is then transported along the tube to the uterus for implantation, and pregnancy is established.

But in order for conception to happen, both partners have to be biologically fit for reproduction. This means that their hormones need to be functioning properly: both female ovulation and male sperm production depend on specific hormone activity taking place. Both partners' reproductive organs have to be in good working order, too. For example, a woman's egg must be able to travel unhampered along an unblocked Fallopian tube in order to be fertilized, and the man needs to produce millions of healthy sperm – even though only one will eventually penetrate the egg. The uterus must be ready to nurture a pregnancy, which means that the womb lining must be receptive to an embryo embedding itself in it. Once this has happened, a complex chain of hormone production will need to take place in order to keep the pregnancy going. All of these vital components are more likely to occur in people whose general levels of health are good. However, with today's demanding lifestyles and often inadequate diets it is not surprising that many couples have

THE BEST TIMING

Conception can only occur if you make love near the time of ovulation.

To give sperm the best chance of reaching the egg, they need to be deposited near to or on the cervix, which means deep vaginal penetration. An egg is released 14 days before the first day of a woman's next expected period and can survive for up to 24 hours. Sperm can live for two to four days inside a woman's body and will be most numerous if a man makes love every other day. So, for maximum fertility, you should have sex every other day from day 11 to 16 of the menstrual cycle.

The miracle of conception

Once a sperm has succeeded in fertilizing an egg, a complex chain of events has to take place to result in pregnancy.

During a normal menstrual cycle, an egg – or ovum – is released from one of a woman's ovaries about 14 days before her next menstrual period. This is called ovulation. The egg is swept into the fronded funnel-like end of the nearby Fallopian tube. Here, fertilization may occur, but if the egg is not fertilized, it breaks down to be passed with the woman's next menstrual period.

If a sperm succeeds in penetrating the egg, it begins to grow into an embryo through a series of cell divisions. (If more than one egg is released and fertilized, a multiple pregnancy occurs.) The fertilized egg divides repeatedly as it moves along the Fallopian tube, entering the uterus about five days after conception. On arrival, the egg – now called a blastocyst – embeds itself into the spongy uterine wall. Here, it continues its rapid development, and divides into various layers of cells that will develop into specialized parts of a baby's body, such as the skeleton or organs: it is now known as an embryo.

At the same time, the placenta, the organ that will nourish the growing baby by linking it to the mother's circulation via the umbilical cord, begins to form at the site of implantation. The amniotic fluid that surrounds and protects the baby throughout pregnancy is also forming inside an encircling membrane. By the end of the first week, the embryo is about a millimetre long – roughly the size of a pinhead.

A woman is now medically described as three weeks pregnant because doctors measure the term from the first day of the last menstrual period. This stage is the peak time for **miscarriage**. It is thought that as many as one in four pregnancies ends in miscarriage – often before the women knows that she has conceived.

THE LIFE-CYCLE OF SPERM

From puberty onwards, at least 1000 sperm a minute are manufactured in the testicles. Each sperm is tadpole-shaped, about 0.05mm long, and takes some 10 weeks to mature. The last couple of weeks of its life are spent in the epididymis. A masterpiece of engineering, the epididymis is a microscopically narrow 6m (20ft) long tube folded into a space 5cm (2in) in length.

On average, sperm swim at 150mm (6in) a second and reach the cervix within two minutes of ejaculation, and the Fallopian tubes in another five minutes. This is a lot easier during the most fertile part of the menstrual cycle (when the egg is released) because there is plenty of fertile mucus around for the sperm to live on. During infertile periods of the cycle, the mucus is thicker and harder for the sperm to negotiate.

The average ejaculation contains 200–300 million sperm, but it only takes one to fertilize the egg – and only about 40 super-fit sperm get anywhere near the end of the race.

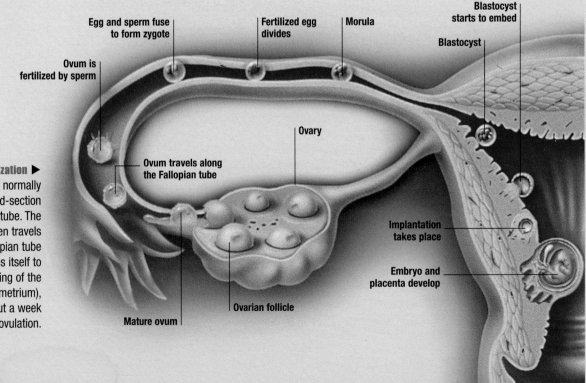

Egg and sperm fuse to form zygote

Fertilized egg divides

Morula

Blastocyst starts to embed

Blastocyst

Ovum is fertilized by sperm

Ovary

Fertilization ▶
Fertilization normally occurs in the mid-section of a Fallopian tube. The egg (ovum) then travels down the Fallopian tube and attaches itself to the spongy lining of the womb (endometrium), about a week after ovulation.

Ovum travels along the Fallopian tube

Implantation takes place

Embryo and placenta develop

Ovarian follicle

Mature ovum

Disorders of the reproductive system

Around one in five couples in the UK has difficulty in conceiving, and the figure is rising.

Some women become pregnant after just one act of intercourse, but for most couples having regular intercourse, it takes about three to six months for the woman to conceive. If you have been having regular unprotected intercourse for 18 months without conceiving, you may have a problem and should seek medical advice. In many cases, the cause is minor and easily treated.

However, a woman who wishes to conceive but whose periods are irregular should see her doctor promptly. And a woman over 35 who is trying for a baby but has not conceived within 6 months should also be referred for tests.

An estimated one in seven Britons will at some time in their lives consult their doctor on infertility. In about 50 per cent of cases, the problem lies with the woman, in about 30 per cent of cases it lies with the man, and in the remainder it is shared between both partners.

MALE REPRODUCTIVE PROBLEMS

Statistics vary, but it is thought that around 30 per cent of men are sub-fertile and at least one man in fifty is totally infertile. Scientific debate continues to dispute the evidence that suggests male fertility is falling as a result of modern living. What is undeniable is that the most common male problem is poor-quality sperm or a low sperm count – and sperm counts do appear to be falling in much of the Western world.

Environmental changes – such as pollutants from pesticides and industry in our air and water – can have a major impact on sperm counts. And just a slight increase in body temperature can impede sperm production. So men who spend a great deal of time driving, or sitting behind a desk (with their testicles kept too warm) may also be at risk of lowered sperm counts. The advice given is to cut down excess alcohol, stop smoking and to wear loose, cool underpants and trousers. It is still undecided as to the exact cause of falling sperm counts but, globally, overpopulation remains a greater threat than declining fertility.

Poor sperm function

Sperms' effectiveness is not only a question of numbers but also of their ability to swim – known medically as motility – and appearance. Even in fertile men, most sperm are either deformed, unable to swim properly, or both. As a rule of thumb, a 'normal' sperm sample should contain at least 20 million sperm per millilitre, at least half of which are motile (though fertility is still possible with lower levels).

FEMALE REPRODUCTIVE PROBLEMS

The female reproductive system is vulnerable to infection from sexually transmitted diseases, many of which can be unnoticed and damage a woman's fertility. In polycystic ovary syndrome, hormonal imbalance may prevent ovulation. A woman who suffers from increasingly painful periods or experiences pain during intercourse may have a pelvic infection or a condition called **endometriosis**. In either case, she should see a doctor. Any woman who has suffered from a severe pelvic infection in the past, or who has had a burst appendix or a miscarriage might have a problem with her Fallopian tubes or her womb.

Blocked Fallopian tubes

The Fallopian tubes collect eggs released by the ovaries and pass them to the uterus by means of muscular contractions of their walls and the sweeping action of the fine hairs (cilia) that line the tubes. The Fallopian tubes are very thin, so any damage to them by infection or inflammation is likely to cause a blockage – a major cause of female infertility and also of **ectopic pregnancy**.

Hormone imbalances

The hormones progesterone, oestrogen, prolactin, luteinizing hormone, and follicle stimulating hormone all play a key role in a woman's reproductive cycle. If any of these hormones are too low or too high, this can hinder conception. An imbalance may, for example, trigger the physical signs of ovulation but not actually stimulate the ovary to release an egg. And if there are fewer than 10 days between ovulation and menstruation, this will prevent a pregnancy.

UNEXPLAINED INFERTILITY

Many couples decide against starting a family until the woman is over 30. If they encounter problems in conceiving a baby, doctors will be conscious of the need not to waste time. Whenever possible, tests will lead to a diagnosis of the problem, and hopefully, a solution. But for many couples, no matter how rigorous the tests, doctors are unable to pinpoint a cause and will describe the problem as 'unexplained infertility'.

Fortunately, many infertility problems can be overcome using in vitro fertilization (IVF) and assisted reproductive technologies. These have helped several thousand infertile couples to have children. Nevertheless, as many as one in ten couples will still be unable to have children.

SEE ALSO *Infertility; Ovaries and disorders; Testicles and disorders; Uterus and problems*

Male disorders

Impotence
The inability to achieve or maintain an erection.

Cryptorchidism
A testis is not in its normal position in the scrotum. Usually, it is in the abdomen or groin instead.

Hypogonadism
Low levels of hormones cause lack of testicular function.

Retrograde ejaculation
Semen shoot into the bladder instead of out of the penis.

Azoospermia
No sperm in the semen – possibly due to a blockage.

Respiratory infection

Respiratory infections are one of the most common reasons for people to see their GP. They are split into two types:

- upper respiratory infections;
- lower respiratory infections.

The airways from the nose to the bottom of the neck are known as the upper respiratory tract, while the airways in the chest are known as the lower respiratory tract. (See also **Respiratory system**.)

Infections of the lower respiratory tract are usually much more serious than upper ones. People most at risk from respiratory infections of all types include:

- young children;
- elderly people;
- smokers;
- people with underlying medical conditions;
- people whose immune systems may be weakened, for example, after an operation.

SYMPTOMS

It can be difficult to distinguish an upper respiratory infection from the more serious lower respiratory infections as some symptoms such as coughing, headache and fever can be common to both.

Symptoms specific to upper respiratory infections include:

- sneezing and runny nose, also sinus pain;
- sore throat and loss of voice;
- headache;
- ear ache;
- fever.

Symptoms specific to lower respiratory infections include:

- coughing and producing mucus;
- wheezing and breathlessness;
- fever and fatigue.

TREATMENT

Treatment depends very much on the cause. There are no effective treatments for infections caused by viruses, which account for most of the upper respiratory infections, although treatments are given to ease the symptoms. These are available from a pharmacist and may include syrup to soothe a sore throat or paracetamol to treat fever and headaches. Most upper respiratory infections are relatively mild and clear up by themselves.

Antibiotics are the main treatment for bacterial infections, such as pneumonia.

When to consult a doctor

You should see a doctor urgently for any of the following symptoms:

- breathlessness without exertion;
- blue-tinged skin, especially around the lips;
- coughing up blood, or infected mucus. This

Infections of the airways

Upper airway infections are not usually the same as those that affect the lower airways, but upper airway infections may develop into a more serious disorder lower down.

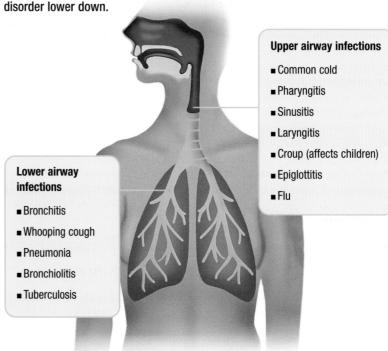

Upper airway infections

- Common cold
- Pharyngitis
- Sinusitis
- Laryngitis
- Croup (affects children)
- Epiglottitis
- Flu

Lower airway infections

- Bronchitis
- Whooping cough
- Pneumonia
- Bronchiolitis
- Tuberculosis

may be coloured green or yellow and have an unpleasant smell;

- high fevers;
- wheezing or persistent coughing.

Complementary therapies

Echinacea helps to prevent colds but there is no evidence that it helps other respiratory infections.

Respiratory system

SEE PAGE 508

Restless leg syndrome

Restless leg syndrome is also known as Ekbom's syndrome. It is a deep and uncomfortable sensation of restlessness, usually in the legs, although it sometimes involves the whole body. It tends to occur at night and is relieved only by moving or walking. If persistent, it therefore leads to problems with sleeping.

The cause of restless leg syndrome is generally unknown, but it may occasionally be associated with **diabetes, anaemia,** or a defect in the region of the brain known as the basal ganglia.

There is no specific medical treatment for the condition. Drugs such as anticonvulsants can bring relief and may be prescribed in cases where the symptoms are severe.

Retinoblastoma

Retinoblastoma is a rare malignant tumour of the retina that affects one in 20,000 children, usually within the first three years of life. One of the reasons why a light is shone into the eyes of newborn babies is to check for signs of retinoblastoma. A white pupil may indicate a large tumour or, more commonly, a congenital **cataract**. If retinoblastoma is present, it is usually necessary to remove the eye surgically, although if both eyes are affected, more conservative treatment such as **radiotherapy** may be tried first, in an attempt to save at least one eye.

SEE ALSO *Eye and problems*

Rheumatic fever

Rheumatic fever is a disease that leads to the inflammation of many tissues of the body, especially those of the heart, joints, brain or skin. It carries a serious risk of permanent heart damage (rheumatic heart disease).

Rheumatic fever generally occurs in children aged 5–15 and young adults, although it is now very rare in developed countries. The resulting rheumatic heart disease can last for life.

SYMPTOMS

Symptoms of rheumatic fever vary greatly from person to person, but usually include fever, pain, inflammation and swelling of the joints, a rash and nodules beneath the skin.

CAUSES

The precursor to rheumatic fever is always a throat infection caused by certain strains of streptococcal bacteria. These bacteria are believed to bring about an autoimmune response that makes the body attack its own tissues.

TREATMENT

Penicillin or other antibiotics may be prescribed to prevent acute rheumatic fever developing from a streptococcal throat infection. Bed rest is usually advised, and aspirin can be taken to relieve joint pain.

Once diagnosed with rheumatic fever, people are usually given monthly or daily antibiotic treatment continuously, perhaps for life.

COMPLICATIONS

Damage to the heart valves can occur, with the result that a valve fails to open or close completely. The effects of this may not be noticeable immediately, but eventually damaged valves can cause serious problems, such as congestive heart failure. The nervous system can also be affected, causing irregular, uncontrolled jerky movements.

OUTLOOK

People who have had an attack of rheumatic fever are more prone to further attacks and to the risk of heart damage.

Rheumatoid arthritis

Rheumatoid arthritis is a progressive form of arthritis that attacks the joints, causing pain, inflammation and swelling. It typically affects the fingers, wrists, knees, hips, shoulders and neck, although any joints may become affected.

Starting in the synovial lining of the joints, rheumatoid arthritis can go on to damage the surrounding bones. So it is essential to start treatment as early as possible. An **autoimmune disease**, which has no cure, rheumatoid arthritis affects more than 600,000 people in the UK.

SEE ALSO *Arthritis*

Rhinitis

Rhinitis is an inflammation of the mucous membranes lining the nose. It generally leads to congestion, a runny nose, sneezing, redness and irritation. The most common cause of rhinitis is the common **cold**; the second most common cause is **allergy**. With an allergy, the nasal lining becomes oversensitive to substances such as pollen, animal dander, feathers and house-dust mites, as well as foods such as wheat, eggs and milk. Where pollen is the cause, rhinitis is seasonal and is commonly known as **hay fever**.

Rhinitis is usually treated with steroids, antihistamines and sodium cromoglicate nasal sprays. Rhinitis may also be caused by overuse of nasal decongestants (rhinitis medicamentosa).

Rhinopyma

In rhinopyma, the nose takes on a bulbous, ruddy appearance. The skin also thickens and has more oil glands than usual.

The cause is unknown, but it is thought to be a form of **rosacea**, a condition where there is an abnormal degree of flushing of the skin. Rhinopyma is almost never seen in women, and in men occurs mainly in the over-40s. It is often wrongly linked with excessive alcohol consumption; in fact, it can occur in men who do not drink at all. It can be corrected by **laser surgery**, but may recur.

Cilia

Cilia are microscopic hair-like fronds that line the tiny airways – the bronchioles – in the lungs. Mucus in the lungs trap bacteria and foreign bodies, and the cilia waft it up to the throat, where it is then coughed up or swallowed.

Respiratory system

The respiratory system consists of all the organs of the body that contribute to breathing. They include the nose, mouth, throat, trachea (windpipe) and the bronchi. All these are passages that lead into the lungs.

In the lungs, the oxygen in air is passed into the bloodstream. At the same time, carbon dioxide is passed back out of the blood and into the lungs to be exhaled. This process, called gaseous exchange, takes place in millions of alveoli, the tiny air sacs in the depths of the lungs that are fine enough to allow the passage of oxygen through their membranous walls and into the blood.

The passageways of the respiratory system do more than direct air to the lungs; they also filter out unwanted foreign bodies such as germs (bacteria and viruses) and dust. This means that they are in the front line of the body's never-ending battle against infection. The nose and throat stop diseases before they can reach the vital lungs but often succumb to infection in the process. This is why colds, runny noses and sore throats are so common.

LUNGS: THE RESPIRATORY ORGANS

The job of the respiratory system is to provide the oxygen that allows us to burn the fuel stored in the body. The lungs make up one of the largest organs in the body. Each day the body draws 10,000 litres of air from the atmosphere, delivers it to the lungs, and then expels the waste products with the outward breath. The lungs are surrounded by the ribcage, which forms a protective casing around them. Beneath the lungs is the diaphragm, a dome-shaped muscle that works with the lungs as they inhale and exhale air.

BREATHING

Breathing is a two-stage process: inhalation, or breathing in, and exhalation – breathing out. It is made possible by the action of the diaphragm. As the diaphragm flattens out, it causes the chest to be lifted up and outwards. This expands the lungs, creating a partial vacuum, and air rushes in to balance the pressure. The diaphragm then relaxes upwards and the ribcage contracts, increasing the pressure within the chest and forcing air out of the lungs.

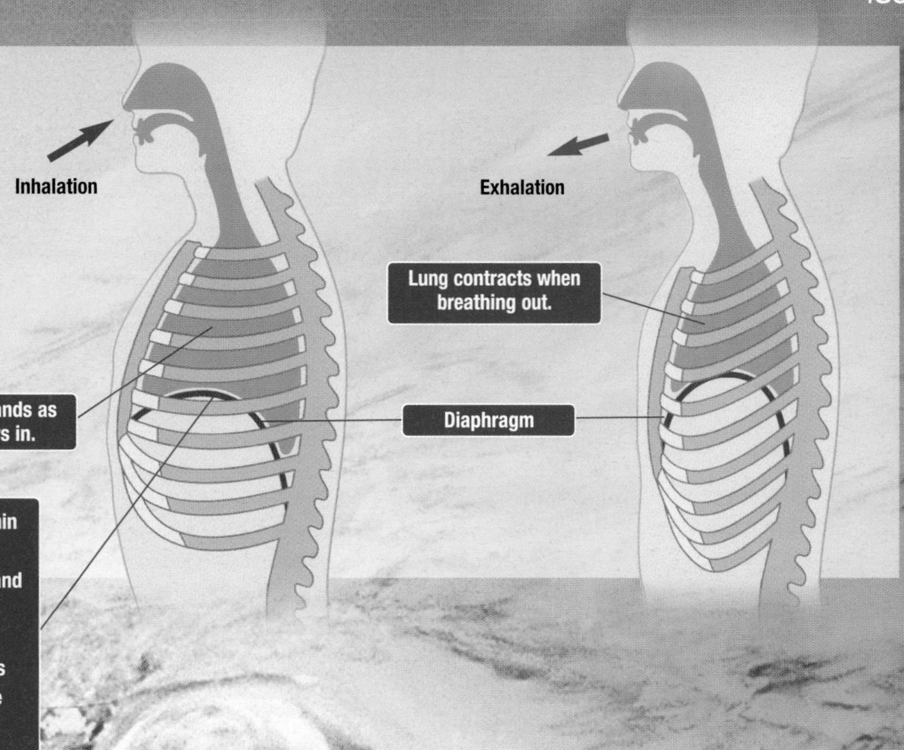

Inhalation

Exhalation

Lung contracts when breathing out.

Lung expands as air flows in.

Diaphragm

Diaphragm

The diaphragm is a thin sheet of muscle that separates the upper and lower body organs. It is attached to the lower ribs at the sides and to the breastbone at the front and back.

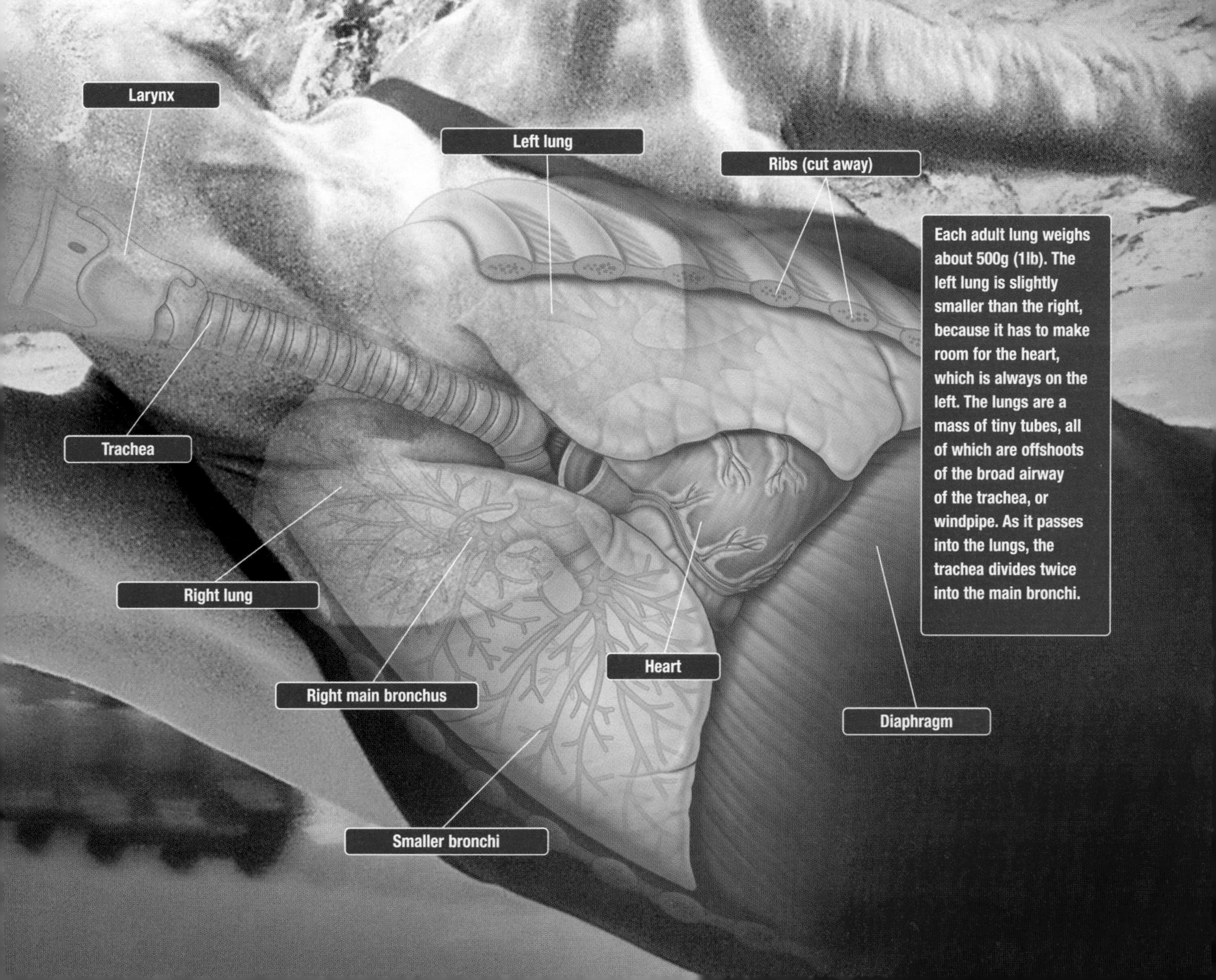

Larynx

Left lung

Ribs (cut away)

Each adult lung weighs about 500g (1lb). The left lung is slightly smaller than the right, because it has to make room for the heart, which is always on the left. The lungs are a mass of tiny tubes, all of which are offshoots of the broad airway of the trachea, or windpipe. As it passes into the lungs, the trachea divides twice into the main bronchi.

Trachea

Right lung

Heart

Right main bronchus

Diaphragm

Smaller bronchi

How the lungs work

The lungs are responsible for exchanging carbon dioxide –
a gas that the body has to get rid of – for the oxygen it needs.

If our respiratory centres send extra impulses to the diaphragm, they cause unwanted contractions – or hiccups. Unborn babies hiccup because their respiratory centres begin working before birth.

Each of our lungs is like an incredibly complex honeycomb or sponge forming a mass of tiny tubes. The airways in the lungs are the largest area of the body exposed to the external environment. If they were spread out flat, they would cover the area of two tennis courts. Connecting the lungs to the outside world is the windpipe, which divides twice into the main bronchi. Each of these tubes divides another 15 to 25 times into smaller and narrower airways, collectively known as the bronchial tree. The smallest airways are known as the bronchioles. These connect with the tiny grape-like air sacs, the alveoli (of which there are between 150 and 400 million). Each alveolus is a kind of dead end in the branching network of passages that riddle the lungs. But the walls of the alveoli are thin enough to allow oxygen molecules to pass through into the bloodstream. Here the oxygen is picked up by a chemical called haemoglobin.

The gas exchange
This magnified illustration of a bronchiole shows how the lungs keep the body's cells supplied with oxygen and get rid of the waste carbon dioxide.

The haemoglobin in the blood is like a string of barges on the fast-flowing river of the body's circulation. It carries the oxygen molecules downstream and deposits them where they are needed to assist the burning of energy in cells. At the same time, waste carbon dioxide crosses from the capillaries back into the alveoli, ready to be exhaled. This exchange of gases occurs very rapidly, in fractions of a second. The carbon dioxide leaves the alveoli when we exhale.

EFFICIENT BREATHING
We breathe more when we use our muscles because muscles need oxygen to work. The oxygen gets to the muscles from the air we breathe via our bloodstream.

People often become out of breath when they exercise. Aerobic exercise – such as running, cycling or dancing – needs oxygen to produce energy. It involves many of the large muscles in the body, including the heart.

A person's ability to exercise depends on how efficiently his or her cardiovascular system supplies the muscles with oxygen. The heart plays a major role in this, pumping blood to the lungs and through the body. But if the body's demand for oxygen is not met because there is not enough oxygen-rich blood pumping around, the lungs will respond by gasping for more air. All muscles, including the heart, need to be overloaded to an extent in order to develop. The fitter your heart becomes, the less breathless you will feel.

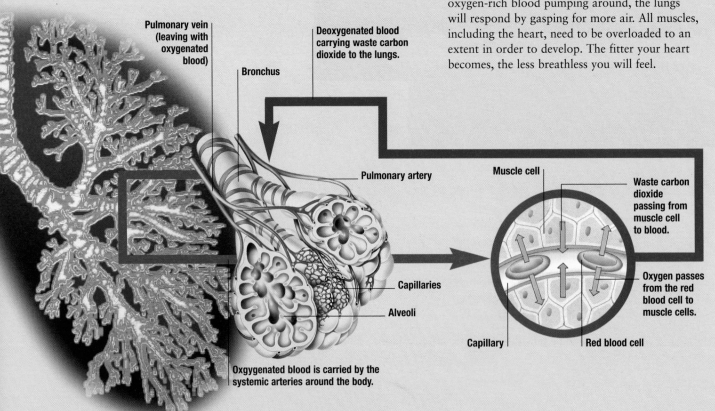

Pulmonary vein (leaving with oxygenated blood)

Bronchus

Deoxygenated blood carrying waste carbon dioxide to the lungs.

Pulmonary artery

Capillaries

Alveoli

Muscle cell

Waste carbon dioxide passing from muscle cell to blood.

Oxygen passes from the red blood cell to muscle cells.

Capillary

Red blood cell

Oxygenated blood is carried by the systemic arteries around the body.

What can go wrong

The delicate lungs are exposed to the external environment, which makes them susceptible to irritation and infection.

Respiratory problems are one of the most common reasons that we visit our GPs. Dust, pollen, fungal spores, bacteria, viruses and airborne pollutants can all damage the lungs. The respiratory system has several forms of defence to stop invaders from entering and to expel those that do gain access. Defences include:
■ nose hairs that filter the air;
■ the epiglottis: a flap of cartilage that covers over the trachea during swallowing, stopping food and drink being 'breathed' (aspirated) into the lungs;
■ the airways becoming smaller when foreign objects are detected, making it more difficult for them to penetrate any deeper into the lungs.

A foreign body that makes its way past these defences can be removed by several methods.
■ It can be coughed up.
■ It can be passed up the airways, which are constantly being cleared, by tiny hairs, called cilia, that line the airways and waft unwanted material up to the mouth. It is then swallowed.
■ It can be ingested by special cells in the alveoli, which then move unwanted matter as mucus to the bronchioles to be cleared by the cilia.

The immune system is activated if bacteria and viruses get through these physical defences, particularly if they get into the lining of the lungs or airways. The immune system consists of a complex chain of cells that recognize foreign invaders and call up attack cells to destroy foreign cells, while other specialist cells come along to mop up dead particles.

RESPIRATORY DISORDERS

Despite the sophisticated defence mechanisms of the respiratory system, problems do occur. Our lungs achieve their peak performance when we are between the ages of 15 and 25. There follows a gradual but relentless decline as our respiratory system becomes less efficient, so that problems increase with age.

Many illnesses, such as colds and **influenza**, are confined to the upper tract. Most clear up within a few days and require simple home treatment.

Problems affecting the lower respiratory tract are more serious. They include bacterial and viral infections, such as **pneumonia** and **tuberculosis**; disorders of the airways such as **asthma**, bronchitis and chronic obstructive pulmonary disease (COPD); occupational lung disease caused by such substances as asbestos and cancer, which can also affect parts of the upper respiratory tract.

Symptoms of respiratory disorders

The main symptoms of something having gone wrong include: breathlessness (fighting for breath), a persistent cough, odd breathing sounds, including wheezing, pain when trying to breathe, difficulty breathing when lying down, and a blueish tinge to the skin – this is an important sign to look out for in babies.

All problems with the chest and respiratory system should be taken seriously, and it is always best to err on the side of caution and see your doctor if you are at all worried.

Some symptoms are serious and should be treated as an emergency. They are:
■ intense chest pains;
■ severe breathlessness (especially if you have not exerted yourself);
■ coughing up blood;
■ lips or fingers that have turned blue.

Who is at risk

Anyone can develop a respiratory problem, but those most at risk are babies; elderly people; people with other underlying diseases; and smokers or people that live or work in a smoky environment.

Treating respiratory problems

Over-the-counter drugs are used to relieve the symptoms of viral infections – such as coughs, headaches and stuffy noses. For short-term respiratory infections they can be a great help. But they should not be used long term since they could be suppressing the body's natural defences. A cough, for example, is the body's way of clearing mucus. Always describe your symptoms to your pharmacist and ask advice on which over-the-counter drugs are best for you. If symptoms persist you should see your doctor.

Different drugs are prescribed for different respiratory conditions, but the main ones are:
■ antibiotics – for infections caused by bacteria, such as pneumonia and tuberculosis;
■ bronchodilators – which widen the bronchi and are especially effective in asthma, but are also used in chronic obstructive pulmonary disease;
■ **chemotherapy** – a course of toxic drugs used to treat some types of lung cancer;
■ corticosteroids – which help to prevent inflammation in the lung and are used in a range of conditions including asthma, COPD and sarcoidosis.

SEE ALSO *Capillaries and disorders; Chest pain; Heart and circulatory system; Lungs and disorders; Respiratory infection*

Other disorders

Asthma causes the bronchial tubes to overreact to certain environmental triggers. This reaction narrows the tubes causing breathing to become difficult.

Bronchitis is an inflammation of the lining of the bronchial tubes. This affects breathing, making it harder than normal for air to pass in and out of the lungs.

Cystic fibrosis is an inherited disease that causes the body to produce a mucus that is thick and sticky. This mucus clogs the lungs, making breathing very difficult.

Rickets

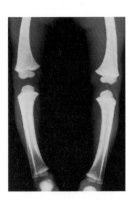

▲ **Bent bones**
One of the most distinctive symptoms of rickets is a bowing of the long bones in the legs.

Rickets is a disease of childhood in which growing bones fail to harden. Instead, they become soft and malformed. Typically, the long bones in the legs become bowed. Rickets is caused by a lack of vitamin D – resulting from a poor diet or lack of exposure to sunlight, or both.

The body requires vitamin D in order to absorb calcium and phosphorus, which are essential for building strong, healthy bones. Dietary sources of the vitamin include oily fish, such as salmon, herring and tuna, and fortified breakfast cereals. But, with enough exposure to sunlight, the body can make all the vitamin D it needs.

The adult counterpart of rickets is known as osteomalacia. Elderly people who are housebound or confined to a nursing home and rarely exposed to sunlight are particularly at risk of vitamin-D deficiency. Some people with intestinal problems such as **Crohn's disease** and coeliac disease may also become short of vitamin D.

SYMPTOMS

Children with rickets suffer bone pains and visible enlargement of the bones at joints, such as the wrists, knees and ankles. Other symptoms include bow legs and knock-knees. In adults with osteomalacia, muscle weakness and fractures can occur.

TREATMENT

Consult a doctor as soon as you suspect rickets or osteomalacia: if bones in the wrists, knees or ankles swell and are painful, or if you notice any apparent deformity, such as bow legs.

What a doctor may do
- Arrange diagnostic blood tests.
- Arrange **X-rays** of the affected bones in a child.
- Arrange a bone-density scan in an adult.
- Advise regular daily doses of vitamin D and calcium.
- Administer a single injection of 7.5mg or 15mg of ergocalciferol (vitamin D). Its effect can last for up to a year. Ergocalciferol is the optimum treatment for a vitamin-D deficiency caused by intestinal problems.

What you can do
- Take vitamin D and calcium supplements.
- Eat plenty of foods that contain vitamin D: fatty fish such as salmon and sardines; breakfast cereals, dairy products and margarines fortified with vitamin D.
- Spend plenty of time outside in the sunlight: 15 minutes' midday sunlight on your face, hands and arms three times a week enables the body to make all the vitamin D it needs.

OUTLOOK

If rickets is diagnosed early, and the vitamin-D deficiency is corrected before damage and deformity occurs, the prospect of full recovery is excellent. But, since the condition is rare in the UK, many doctors are unfamiliar with the symptoms and diagnosis may not be made before permanent damage has been done.

Ringworm

Ringworm is the popular name for certain types of fungal infections of the skin, feet, groin, scalp and nails – collectively known as tineal infections. In the medical names, the term 'tinea' is followed by the Latin word for the affected area of the body. For example, tinea cruris affects the groin and tinea pedis affects the feet.

A tineal infection is often characterized by ring-shaped, reddened skin or blistery patches on the skin.

CAUSES

Most infections are caused by a group of fungi called the dermatophytes. They can be acquired from another person – by sharing towels or from the floors of communal areas such as showers or changing rooms – or from household objects such as carpets, or from an animal or from soil.

SYMPTOMS

The symptoms of tinea vary according to the site of the fungal infection.
- The most common type, tinea pedis (**athlete's foot**), causes cracking and itching between the toes.
- Tinea corporis (ringworm of the body) is characterized by circular itchy patches with a prominent edge.
- Tinea cruris (jock itch), which is more common in males, produces a reddened, itchy area spreading from the genitals over the inside of the thigh.
- Tinea capitis (ringworm of the scalp) causes one or several round, itchy patches of hair loss.
- Tinea unguium (ringworm of the nails) is often accompanied by scaling of the soles or palms. The nails become thick and turn white or yellow.

TREATMENT

Seek medical advice if you suspect that you have tinea. Most types of infection can be diagnosed from their appearance.

In most cases, treatment is with antifungal drugs in the form of skin creams, lotions or ointments. For widespread infections, or those affecting the hair or nails, an antifungal drug in tablet form may be prescribed. The treatment may be continued for some time after symptoms have subsided to eradicate the fungi and prevent symptoms recurring.

Complementary therapies

Zinc taken for three to six months may help to ward off fungal infections affecting the nails.

Rosacea

Rosacea is an inflammatory skin condition affecting around 1 per cent of people in the UK. It is most common in fair-skinned women aged between 30 and 50, and some estimates suggest that as many as one in ten women are mildly affected. But rosacea can occur in both sexes, and at any age.

The cause of rosacea is unknown, although it is thought to be due to abnormal sensitivity of blood capillaries, which readily dilate. It has also been linked with overuse of corticosteroid creams, and to infection of sebaceous glands with the skin mite *Demodex folliculorum*.

SYMPTOMS

Rosacea starts with temporary facial flushing – especially after drinking alcohol, eating spicy foods, consuming hot drinks or entering a warm room. If the condition is allowed to progress, the skin becomes permanently red from the development of fine, dilated capillaries, and pustules appear.

In severe cases, there is a persistent eruption of acne-like pimples on the forehead and cheeks, with redness, puffiness and prominent blood vessels. The eyes may be affected, which can cause **conjunctivitis** and inflammation of the eyelids (**blepharitis**). In some people – especially older men – the skin on the nose becomes thickened and red due to enlargement of sebaceous glands (**rhinopyma**).

Symptoms tend to recur over five to ten years, after which they may subside.

TREATMENT

Medical treatment usually involves antibiotics, such as oral tetracyclines or metronidazole gel. Repeat courses are often needed. In resistant cases, oral metronidazole or oral isotretinoin (a derivative of vitamin A used in hospitals to treat severe acne) may be recommended.

Laser surgery is often successful in reducing dilation and redness of blood vessels.

What you can do

■ Avoid factors that may trigger flare-ups of rosacea. These include stress, hot liquids, spicy foods, alcohol, vigorous exercise, heat and exposure to sunlight – use a non-greasy high-protection cream (SPF 15 or higher) or apply a product that reflects and blocks out ultraviolet rays with titanium dioxide or zinc oxide.

Although women are three times more likely than men to develop rosacea, men who are affected tend to have more severe symptoms.

■ It may also help to exclude tea, chocolate, cheese, yeast extract, eggs, citrus fruits and wheat from your diet.

■ People who have rosacea often lack A and B-group vitamins, especially vitamins B_2, B_3 and B_6, so rosacea may respond to supplements of vitamin B complex. But try to ensure that these contain vitamin B_3 in the form of nicotinamide rather than niacin, as niacin can itself cause flushing.

■ Applying tea tree oil or aloe vera may help.

■ Use skincare products designed for use in rosacea, which contain vitamin K.

SEE ALSO *Skin and disorders*

Roseola infantum

Roseola infantum is a common infection, mainly affecting children between six months and three years old. It is caused by a herpes virus transmitted through the respiratory tract.

The main symptom is a high fever, which comes on abruptly, often accompanied by irritability. The temperature may rise to 40°C (104°F). When the fever subsides, after about three to four days, a pink raised rash appears on the trunk, often spreading quickly to the neck, face and limbs. This usually lasts for a day or two. Other symptoms may include a sore throat and enlarged lymph nodes in the neck.

Occasionally a child may have a fit (**febrile convulsion**) during the fever, but the illness has no serious long-term effects. The only treatment is to try to keep the child cool – for example, by keeping the room temperature quite low – and to make sure that the child drinks plenty of fluids.

Roundworms

The term 'roundworms' refers to any of a large group of worms known as nematodes, which have long, cylindrical bodies. Some species live independently; others as parasites in plants, animals and human beings.

Worms can sometimes inhabit human intestines without causing any symptoms. Problems caused by roundworms invading the human intestine include threadworm, which mainly affects children, toxocariasis, trichinosis, whipworm and ascariasis.

Roundworm diseases are much more common in tropical countries. Most types of roundworm infestation are effectively treated with anthelmintic drugs such as mebendazole.

SEE ALSO *Parasites and parasitic diseases; Travel and tropical diseases*

RSI

RSI (repetitive strain injury), is more accurately termed 'work-related upper limb disorder'. It encompasses hand-and-arm problems brought on by frequent and repeated movements, and affects workers in many occupations – from shift workers on a conveyor belt to keyboard operators and musicians. It is the cause of many people taking time off work because of pain or, at worst, disablement. In many cases, no abnormality of muscles, tendons or nerves can be found, but sometimes the problem can be attributed to tenosynovitis, an inflammation of the tendon sheath that is usually due to overuse.

RSI may not be based solely on the strain of physically repetitive tasks, but may also be linked to psychological factors. A study in 2001 showed that those under stress at work were the most likely to suffer from the condition.

SYMPTOMS
Symptoms of repetitive strain injury include cramp, heaviness and weakness in a limb, pins and needles, a dull ache and excruciating pain.

CAUSES
Symptoms can be produced by any action that is forced or awkward, that involves a heavy weight or is repeated many times in rapid succession. Workers who develop upper limb disorders are most likely to be performing tasks that require repetitive finger, hand or arm movements – such as squeezing, pounding or hammering; or pushing, pulling, lifting or reaching movements.

TREATMENT
Seek medical advice as soon as you notice a persistent problem. Also notify your employer, who has a duty to ensure your welfare.

What a doctor may do
■ Assess the problem and its connection with your job.
■ Write to your employers about possible time off work or changes to your work pattern.
■ Prescribe stronger analgesic and anti-inflammatory drugs.
■ Apply a bandage or splint.
■ If your symptoms persist, despite trying all other remedies, refer you to a rheumatologist.

What you can do
■ Take paracetamol, preferably about an hour before starting the action that brings on the pain.
■ If there is swelling as well as pain, ibuprofen may help.
■ Warmth can help – for example, a hot-water bottle on the affected area.

OUTLOOK
Only in very few rare cases does RSI lead to any permanent damage of the joints.

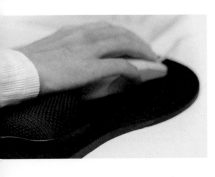

▼ **Mouse control**
Sit upright and close to your desk, so you don't have to sit with your mouse arm stretched.

Rubella

Also known as German measles, rubella is a mild but highly contagious viral infection that mainly affects children. It is characterized by enlarged lymph nodes in the neck area and a rash of tiny, pinkish red spots. It is only serious when it affects women in early pregnancy, because there is a risk of the virus infecting the fetus, causing severe birth defects. However, **immunization** programmes have greatly reduced the incidence of rubella in the developed world.

SYMPTOMS
Symptoms appear after an incubation period of two to three weeks, and include: headache; light fever; sore throat; painful swelling in the neck and a rash of small, flat or slightly raised, pinkish-red spots, which usually starts on the face, spreads all over the body, and then disappears after about a week.

TREATMENT
Rubella requires no special treatment except a few days' rest in bed. But it is important to remember that you can spread the disease by close contact with others.

If you have rubella, you are infectious from a week before the rash appears right up to five days after it has disappeared. You must therefore avoid contact with anyone to whom rubella could cause serious harm – that is, women in the early stages of a pregnancy or those who are trying to conceive, since they may already be pregnant without knowing it.

PREVENTION
You can catch rubella only once in your life – one attack usually confers immunity. Because of the risks to pregnant women, it is an advantage for girls to acquire immunity before puberty. But it may be difficult to know for sure if you have had rubella, since many people who suffer a mild attack do not even notice the disease. Therefore, to prevent problems during a possible future pregnancy, a vaccine against rubella is recommended for adolescent girls who may be uncertain as to whether or not they have gained immunity in childhood. Women who are planning a pregnancy can be tested to see if they have acquired immunity and, if not, can be vaccinated before they attempt to conceive; it is advisable not to become pregnant until three months after having the vaccination.

In the UK, most young children are now offered the **MMR vaccine** (measles, mumps and rubella) to protect them from rubella.

COMPLICATIONS
If a woman is infected with rubella in the early stages of a pregnancy, particularly in the first three months, there is a risk that the fetus will develop abnormally.

Salivary glands and disorders

Saliva is the fluid produced by the salivary glands that drain into the mouth, and by the mucous membrane lining the mouth itself. Saliva helps to lubricate food, aiding chewing and swallowing, and contains an enzyme, amylase, which breaks down starch and so starts the process of digestion even before food reaches the stomach. Saliva also helps to keep the mouth moist and, because it is alkaline, stops the environment of the mouth from becoming too acidic. A healthy flow of saliva helps to prevent tooth decay.

Most saliva is produced from three pairs of glands that drain by ducts into the mouth.
■ The parotid glands – the largest of the salivary glands – are situated over the top end of the upper jaw, just in front of and below the ears. Their ducts open into the inner surface of the cheeks near the upper teeth.
■ The submandibular glands lie beside the jaw bone, below the parotid glands. Saliva from them flows out into the mouth via a pair of ducts that open underneath the tongue.
■ The sublingual glands – the smallest salivary glands – are located in the floor of the mouth

The salivary glands
The salivary glands are not only crucial to the health of the mouth, teeth and gums, but play a vital role in kick-starting digestion and hence in the fuelling of all the organs of the body.

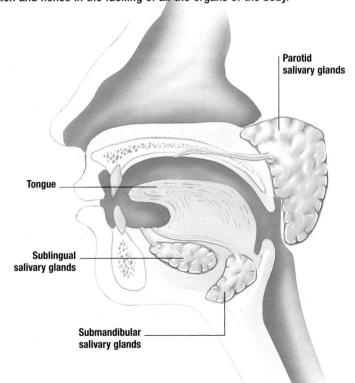

Parotid salivary glands

Tongue

Sublingual salivary glands

Submandibular salivary glands

underneath the tongue on each side. Each one has about 20 ducts, which open directly into the floor of the mouth above.

In addition, there are many tiny glands, producing small quantities of saliva, in the lining of the mouth and in the lips and cheeks.

A small amount of saliva is being produced continuously in order to keep the mouth wet and clean, but when stimulated by food the flow increases dramatically.

INFECTION

Since the mouth is open to the atmosphere, it is impossible to keep it free of germs. This means that if anything reduces the body's natural defences, the salivary glands will become vulnerable to infection. Infection can also spread from other areas of the body, including the nearby lymph nodes during a sore throat or from a dental **abscess**. Increasing fluid intake may help to increase the flow of saliva and so clear the infection, but it may be necessary to treat it with antibiotics.

Infections of the salivary glands can cause them to swell up and become painful, and may be linked to a host of other problems, such as the formation of salivary stones and general difficulties with the production and flow of saliva (see below).

Mumps

Mumps, known medically as infectious parotitis, is the most common infection of the salivary glands. It is due to a virus and its most noticeable feature is swelling of the parotid glands. The person remains infectious until the swelling has completely gone down. Symptoms also include fever, headache and vomiting.

The infection occasionally spreads to other organs, including the testicles, and may impair fertility. Mumps was once very common in children, but has become less so since the introduction of the **MMR vaccine**. It is less common but more severe in adults.

DRY MOUTH

A lower than normal flow of saliva, known to doctors as xerostomia, can lead to a variety of unpleasant side effects including:
■ speech problems;
■ difficulty swallowing;
■ sore throat;
■ **gum disease**;
■ tooth decay.
Causes include:
■ **dehydration**;
■ connective tissue diseases, such as **lupus**;
■ rheumatoid **arthritis**;
■ diabetes;
■ **alcohol** abuse;
■ damage to the salivary glands by surgery or **radiotherapy**.

- various medicines, including diuretics and antidepressants;
- Sjögren's syndrome (see below).

A saliva substitute can help, but often the best way to maintain a healthy flow of saliva is to drink plenty of fluids, preferably water. Patients also need to take meticulous care with dental hygiene and diet, especially avoiding sugar.

Sjögren's syndrome

A common cause of a dry mouth, especially in women, is Sjögren's syndrome, an **autoimmune disease** of the lacrimal (tear-producing) and salivary glands. It causes dry eyes as well as a dry mouth, sometimes with other symptoms such as fatigue and joint pain, and may be associated with conditions such as rheumatoid arthritis or lupus.

TOO MUCH SALIVA

Excessive production of saliva is known as ptyalism or sialorrhoea. It may occur with any irritation in the mouth, or may be a symptom of infection, such as **rabies**, or of poisoning (with mercury, organophosphate insecticides or the toxins found in poisonous mushrooms) or occasionally of nervous system disorders.

SALIVARY STONES

Salivary stones, or calculi, may form in susceptible people, particularly when their saliva becomes very concentrated because of dehydration. They are most often found in the duct of a submandibular gland, and sometimes in the parotid, and they obstruct the flow of saliva. Symptoms therefore tend to occur while eating, when the gland is producing an increased flow of saliva that cannot drain normally into the mouth. They include:

- pain;
- swelling;
- reduced saliva flow.

Sometimes the blockage leads to infection, and worsening of symptoms.

Treatment is with surgery to remove the stone or with lithotripsy, in which a special machine sends out shockwaves that shatter the stone. The pieces then pass harmlessly out into the mouth. Patients are likely to be advised to increase their fluid intake to prevent recurrences.

TUMOURS

Tumours of the salivary glands may be benign or cancerous and usually start with painless enlargement on one side – although there are many other causes of salivary gland swelling. Malignant tumours can spread rapidly and may become painful and interfere with movement of the face, or affect the facial nerves, causing a droop on one side. They require urgent medical treatment, usually by surgery. Radiation treatment may be recommended afterwards.

Medical terms

Amylase
An enzyme contained in saliva that helps to break down starch in food.

Calculus
A stone, usually formed from calcium deposits, within some biological tissue such as the salivary glands.

Enzyme
A substance that speeds up a biological reaction without being itself affected by it.

Gland
A bodily organ that produces and secretes particular fluids, such as saliva or hormones.

Salivation
The process by which saliva is secreted from the salivary glands into the mouth.

Causes of salivary gland problems

Many factors may cause the swelling and malfunction of the salivary glands.

- Infections, including mumps, and other viral infections, bacterial infection, cat-scratch fever, tuberculosis, abscess in the parotid gland.
- Salivary stones.
- Reduced saliva flow.
- Excessive saliva flow.
- Nutritional deficiencies.
- Bulimia.
- Alcoholism.
- Diabetes.
- Hypothyroidism.
- Various medicines.
- Cysts.
- Benign tumours.
- Cancerous tumours, including secondary tumours that have spread from elsewhere in the body.
- After effects of radiation treatment.
- Lymphoma.
- Sarcoidosis.

WHEN TO CONSULT A DOCTOR

It is advisable to seek medical advice if any of the following occur.

- You develop any lumps or swelling around your mouth, jaw, cheek or neck.
- The lymph glands in your neck become swollen.
- Your face droops or you cannot properly close the eyelid on one side.
- Part of your face becomes numb.
- You develop persistent pain in the face, chin, neck or ear.

Investigations for salivary gland problems

Sometimes special investigations will be needed to confirm diagnosis of a problem. If your doctor suspects your symptoms are caused by a salivary stone, probing and dilating the duct under local anaesthetic may help to locate it, and can sometimes help small stones to pass. Stones may also show up on ordinary dental X-ray or on X-rays taken after a radio-opaque solution, which shows up on X-rays, has been introduced into the salivary duct.

In cases where the symptoms are not clear-cut, a computed tomography (CT) or magnetic resonance imaging (MRI) scan of the glands may be taken, sometimes with a biopsy.

SEE ALSO *Digestive system; Lymphatic system; Mouth and disorders; Teeth and problems*

Salmonella

The bacteria salmonella live in human and animal intestines and cause various diseases. One species of salmonella causes **typhoid fever**; another **paratyphoid**; and others commonly cause food poisoning and **gastroenteritis**.

Common sources of salmonella food poisoning are raw or lightly cooked eggs, undercooked poultry, and cooked foods or salads that have been left at room temperature for several hours. Food poisoning can be serious. Those particularly at risk include pregnant women, young children and sick and elderly people, who may have weak immune systems.

The salmonella bacteria attack the stomach and intestines. In serious cases, the bacteria may enter the lymph tract, which carries water and protein to the blood, and the blood itself.

SYMPTOMS

The following may occur within 8–36 hours:
- diarrhoea;
- headache;
- abdominal pain;
- nausea and vomiting;
- fever;
- blood in faeces.

TREATMENT

If symptoms are mild, drink plenty of fluids to avoid **dehydration**. Rehydration solution, available from pharmacies, may also be helpful.

When to consult a doctor

See a doctor if any of the following occur:
- diarrhoea continues for more than 24 hours;
- diarrhoea is frequent and intense;
- severe stomach cramps;
- blood in faeces;
- fever of 38°C (100°F) or higher;
- signs of **jaundice** – a yellowish discoloration of the skin or eyes. This may indicate problems with the liver or the bile ducts;
- signs of dehydration – a dry tongue or mouth, increased thirst, dry chapped skin, dark urine, a reduction in or lack of urine and weakness.

What a doctor may do

In severe cases, antibiotics may be given. Diarrhoea and vomiting can drain the body of fluids, salts and minerals, so rehydration therapy – in which fluids and salts are given intravenously – may be needed. Hospital treatment may be necessary, especially for babies and elderly people.

PREVENTION

Good hygiene and preparing and cooking food correctly minimizes the risk of food poisoning.
- Make sure that all foods, especially poultry and minced meat, are thoroughly cooked.
- Always wash your hands with soap after going to the toilet and before preparing food.
- Always wash your hands when you switch from preparing one type of food to another – for example, from vegetables to meat.
- Wash kitchen utensils properly with soap and water before using with another type of food.
- Use different cutting boards and knives for preparing different foods.
- Wash dishcloths in water over 60°C (140°F).
- In most eggs, salmonella exists only on the shell, so always crack a raw egg with a knife, and never on a bowl containing other foods.

SEE ALSO *Food poisoning*

Salpingitis

Salpingitis is an inflammation of one or both of the Fallopian tubes, usually caused by a bacterial infection, such as **chlamydia**, acquired during sexual intercourse. Acute salpingitis can cause fever and pain in the lower abdomen, but sometimes no symptoms result. Antibiotic treatment is needed. Scarring of the tubes after salpingitis is a major cause of infertility.

SEE ALSO *Reproductive system*

SARS virus

Severe acute respiratory syndrome (SARS) first appeared in 2003. Scientists now know that the SARS agent is a new type of coronavirus, an infectious virus family that causes various diseases including the common cold.

SARS is spread by close contact with airborne droplets, produced when an infected person coughs or sneezes. From a small outbreak in Southern China, SARS spread rapidly around the world. Fears of a global epidemic prompted international quarantine and isolation measures to prevent the spread of the virus. In July 2003 – when SARS had affected 8400 people in 32 countries – the World Health Organization (WHO) reported that the spread of SARS had been contained. However, the possibility of further outbreaks remains.

SYMPTOMS

SARS initially causes flu-like symptoms – cough, fever, headache and muscle pains. These develop rapidly and may cause severe breathing difficulties and **pneumonia**.

TREATMENT

Patients usually require hospital treatment and may need a ventilator to help them breathe.

OUTLOOK

Around one in ten of those affected dies; nearly one in two of those are over the age of 65. There is no specific treatment, but efforts are being made to develop a vaccine.

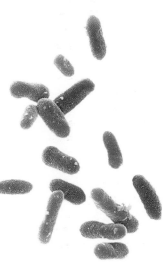

▼ **Salmonella bacteria**
In 2001, salmonella bacteria accounted for about 17,000 reported cases of food poisoning in England and Wales.

Scabies

Scabies is a **skin** infestation of the tiny parasitic mite *Sarcoptes scabiei*, which burrows into the skin. The mite deposits faeces, which trigger an allergic-type reaction and produce an intensely itchy rash of fine raised lines.

TREATMENT

■ Antiscabies lotions containing malathion and permethrin can be bought over the counter. Apply to cover all skin from the neck down, sparing the head and face unless advised otherwise. Pay particular attention to the webs of fingers and toes, and brush lotion under the ends of nails. Usually, only one application is needed but all members of the household should be treated to avoid reinfection.

■ Don't wash your hands after applying lotion or it will need to be reapplied. And be sure to use clean bed linen and clothes after treatment so you don't reinfect yourself from these sources.

■ Using tea tree soaps and lotions on your skin may help to reduce the risk of reinfection.

■ Taking oral antihistamines that will aid sleep may help to reduce itching.

OUTLOOK

Itching and scaliness may last for two or three weeks after treatment because the mites' faeces will still be present in the skin.

SEE ALSO *Skin and disorders*

Scarlet fever

Scarlet fever is a highly infectious disease that most commonly affects children and is caused by a strain of streptococcal bacteria.

SYMPTOMS

These occur three to four days after exposure, and include: sore throat; fever; headache; and a rash, which develops on the body (but not usually on the face). The child often appears scarlet, hence the name. The rash, caused by a toxin released by the bacteria, is initially a mass of tiny red spots on the neck and upper body. It then spreads rapidly. The face is flushed except round the mouth, and a white coating with red spots may develop on the tongue. After a few days, this coating comes off to reveal a bright red appearance. Soon afterwards, the fever subsides and the rash fades. Often the skin peels.

TREATMENT

See a doctor if you or a child have any of the symptoms listed above.

What a doctor may do

Diagnosis is confirmed from the symptoms and by examining your throat and, if necessary, by taking a swab. Treatment is with antibiotics, which shorten the course of the disease.

COMPLICATIONS

If not treated promptly, there is a very slight risk of **rheumatic fever** or an inflammation of the filtering units in the kidneys.

Scars and scarring

Scars are formed as a part of the body's natural healing process. A wound, ulcer or other area of damage is initially plugged by a blood clot. This becomes infiltrated with scavenger cells and a network of supporting fibrous material. Small superficial areas of minimal damage will usually heal without scarring, as the tissues are able to regenerate. But if damage is more extensive, such as through the full thickness of skin, fibrous tissue is replaced by scar tissue – collagen – that shrinks and forms a pale scar.

If the sides of the wound are well-aligned and close together, the scar forms a thin white line – a process referred to as primary healing. If the edges of the wound are separated or there has been extensive tissue loss, healing is slower and is known as secondary healing. The exposed tissue starts to expand to form pink granulation tissue. Skin at the sides of the wound slowly grows inwards to cover the defect, and by the time healing is complete, the granulation tissues have formed a tough, wide scar.

Scars produce a mark that has a different colour and texture to the surrounding skin. Initially, scar tissue looks dark red or pink, but eventually it shrinks and forms a paler scar.

PROMOTING HEALING

To encourage a scar to heal, you should increase your intake of vitamin C, which is needed for the formation of collagen, and essential fatty acids, which help to improve tissue suppleness. Vitamin E tablets are sometimes recommended and vitamin E cream may be helpful to soften new scar tissue, but sensitization is common, so stop using it if redness or irritation occurs.

KELOIDS

Some people form keloid scars that are harder, more irregular and thicker than usual. These are due to an overactive healing response in which there is excess laying down of collagen fibres. The tendency to produce keloids runs in families, and they are most common over the sternum and shoulders. Keloids are initially raised and itchy, but most start to flatten and stop itching after a few months.

STRETCHMARKS

Stretchmarks, known medically as striae, are visible linear scars caused by stretching and damage to the collagen fibres in the lower skin layers. They occur when body shape increases rapidly, such as during puberty and pregnancy.

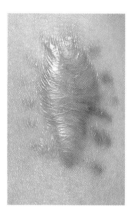

▲ **Tough scar**
Keloid scars consist of a tough mass of collagen that forms as a result of a defective healing process.

Schizophrenia

In the UK, about 1 in 100 men and women are diagnosed with schizophrenia at some point in their lives – usually as young adults. It is probably the most misunderstood of all mental illnesses.

Many people believe that schizophrenia means a split or multiple personality. This is in fact a very rare condition, called dissociative disorder (which is a personality disorder). In schizophrenia, it is the person's thoughts and feelings – not their personality – which are split or fragmented.

The experience of schizophrenia is different for each person, but it usually involves a dramatic disturbance in thoughts and feelings, resulting in behaviour that seems odd to other people. Some people hear voices, others see things that are not there, or feel they are under threat or being persecuted in some way. Schizophrenia is the most common of the psychotic illnesses, in which a person cannot tell the difference between what is real and what is imaginary.

Some people have only one psychotic episode in their lifetime and some people recover completely from schizophrenia. Others recover partly, but have occasional episodes or relapses. About one-third of those diagnosed with schizophrenia live with the condition over a period of years and need regular medical care.

Schizophrenia exists in all cultures and countries, but is treated differently. Hearing voices, for example, has a spiritual meaning in some cultures or religions.

A person who has schizophrenia is no more violent than the rest of the population, despite some media stories. The small number of violent crimes committed by people with mental illness has remained at the same low level for ten years. Recent research has found that people who drink alcohol or take drugs are twice as likely to commit a violent crime as someone with schizophrenia.

CAUSES

Although the cause of schizophrenia is unknown, scientists have identified certain risk factors.

Schizophrenia appears to run in families, but the risk of getting it if a family member is affected is still relatively small. Stressful life events can also be a contributing factor – schizophrenia may be triggered by the death of a loved one, for example, or losing a job, or by ongoing pressures such as poverty, homelessness or discrimination. Family life may also have a role to play in the

development of schizophrenia. Early childhood experiences, such as sexual or physical abuse, affect people in different ways, and may be significant in some cases.

A combination of factors is usually responsible. For example, genetic make-up may make a person more vulnerable to schizophrenia, but stressful events or specific life experiences might trigger the start of symptoms.

SYMPTOMS

The symptoms of schizophrenia vary between individuals, but people with the condition may experience some of the following.

■ Hearing voices or seeing, feeling or even smelling things that are not there (see **Hallucination**).

■ Strange beliefs or thoughts: you may think that you have special powers or that somebody is trying to control you (see **Delusions**).

Partners, relatives and friends

A diagnosis of schizophrenia in a family member or friend can be devastating. Thinking carefully about your reactions to them can be helpful.

Do

✔ Listen to, accept and support the person.

✔ Focus on the person's feelings – he or she may feel frightened and alone.

✔ Let the person know that you accept that he or she hears voices or interprets things in a particular way.

✔ Encourage the person to get help and support.

✔ Look after and get support for yourself.

Don't

✘ Blame the person, or say 'pull yourself together'.

✘ Blame yourself.

✘ Dismiss the person's delusions, but don't agree with them either.

✘ Take over, but consult the person and listen to any views about what sort of help he or she wants.

Self-help

Dealing with your schizophrenia

If you have schizophrenia, your needs and feelings may change over time. But here is a checklist of things you can do to help yourself.

■ Learn to recognize early signs that you are becoming unwell and get help early.

■ Try to reduce stress or worry in your life: identify what makes you feel unwell or particularly stressed and avoid these 'triggers'.

■ Contact a self-help or support group for advice on practical issues, such as medication and your rights.

■ Try talking therapies such as psychotherapy as well as or instead of medication. But never stop taking medication without first discussing this with your doctor.

■ Take up new activities: art, drama or music can help, as can yoga and relaxation techniques.

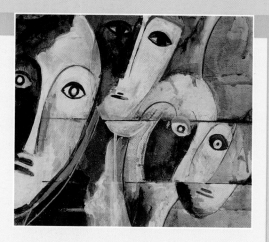

▲ Unforgiving witness
Some schizophrenics are tormented by the idea that their every move is being watched or controlled. Painting can be a therapeutic expression of these anxieties.

■ Thoughts jumping between different topics.
■ Feeling apathetic, depressed and unable to concentrate.
■ No longer enjoying social activities that you used to like; wanting to avoid people or be protected from them.

TREATMENT

If you suspect that you have symptoms of schizophrenia, the first step is to contact your GP or the health professional in charge of your care. If you are concerned that a relative or friend may have symptoms, encourage the person to go for help and offer to accompany him or her. Getting help early on may prevent schizophrenia from developing.

Your GP is likely to refer you to a psychiatrist who will assess you and arrange treatment. This will usually be in the community, but you may be offered short-term hospital care if it is deemed appropriate.

In extreme circumstances, a person who is unwilling to seek help and is a danger to him or herself or to others, may be compulsorily admitted to hospital in the UK under the *Mental Health Act 1983*. This is called sectioning.

Medication

People with schizophrenia are usually given antipsychotic medication to deal with psychotic symptoms. Older antipsychotics, such as haloperidol, reduce hallucinations and delusions in many people, but cause unpleasant side effects such as muscle spasms. Newer antipsychotics, such as clozapine, have fewer side effects. But like all tranquillizers, antipsychotics have some sedative effect.

These drugs can take between one and three months to work, and you may need to try several before you find one that suits you. Check that you are on the lowest possible dose, to minimize side effects. About one-third of people with schizophrenia do not take their antipsychotics because of unpleasant side effects.

Talking therapies

Many people with schizophrenia and their families want to talk about their feelings and experiences and get support in coping with the illness. Talking therapies, such as counselling and psychotherapy, can be used alongside drug treatment. Cognitive behaviour therapy can help with symptoms of schizophrenia, such as delusions and hallucinations. It aims to challenge and test negative thoughts.

Talking therapies are available on the NHS in some areas; ask your GP to refer you. Some voluntary groups, such as Mind or Relate, offer low-cost or free counselling, or you can go privately.

Other treatments

New treatments are being researched, and those showing positive results include:
■ oestrogen supplements (for women);
■ fish oils (found in sardines, pilchards and supplements);
■ vitamin E and vitamin B_6 supplements (for some side effects of antipsychotics).

Sciatica

Sciatica is a pain in one side of the back, often radiating into the buttock, thigh or leg. It commonly occurs following an awkward or straining movement, such as lifting a heavy object. Sciatica usually starts suddenly, with an excruciating pain in the lower back, often accompanied by spasms or 'locking', in which even the slightest movement exacerbates the pain.

CAUSES

The cause of sciatica is pressure on one of the two sciatic nerves – two major nerves that emanate from nerve roots in the lower part of the spinal cord and run down the back of the thigh. The pressure may be due to swelling around an injured muscle or a prolapse of one of the intervertebral discs. Women can sometimes develop sciatica in late pregnancy, because changes in their posture may put pressure on a sciatic nerve. The pain is usually felt in only one leg, and tends to worsen with coughing or straining. It is relieved by resting horizontally.

TREATMENT

The initial treatment is rest, the application of heat or cold compresses to the affected area, and the taking of analgesics or anti-inflammatory drugs. It is advisable to start moving about again as soon as possible, even if this necessitates the use of painkillers.

Physiotherapy, especially learning lifting techniques, is essential to avoid a recurrence.

If the pain comes on gradually and persists, further investigations may be needed to exclude causes such as **arthritis**, tumours or **tuberculosis**, which can have similar symptoms. Investigations include blood tests, X-rays and MRI (magnetic resonance imaging) scanning.

PREVENTION

Sciatica is a common work-related condition, but your employer is under a legal obligation to minimize any physical risk to you. Preventive measures include rotating tasks so that repetitive lifting is avoided, using mechanical lifting devices where possible, and improving the ergonomics of workstations.
SEE ALSO **Back and back pain**

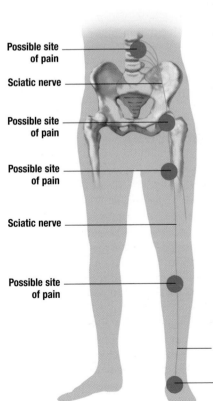

▼ **Sciatic pain**
The pain felt during an attack of sciatica begins when a spinal nerve root is compressed. The pain then moves sharply down the back and outer side of the thigh, leg and foot.

Possible site of pain

Sciatic nerve

Possible site of pain

Possible site of pain

Sciatic nerve

Possible site of pain

Sciatic nerve

Possible site of pain

Scoliosis

Scoliosis is an unnatural curve of the spine to either the left or right, so that it takes on an S- or C-shape when viewed from behind. It can be present at birth or can develop when one leg is shorter than the other. Unlike poor posture, these curves cannot be corrected simply by teaching someone to stand up straight.

It is important that any indication of scoliosis is detected early, to make sure the curve does not progress. Most spine curves in children with scoliosis remain small and will need only regular checks so that signs of progression can be spotted as soon as possible. If a curve does progress, an orthopaedic brace can be used to prevent it from worsening. If a scoliotic curve is severe or if treatment with a brace does not control the curve, surgery may be necessary. In cases such as these, surgery has proved to be highly effective.
SEE ALSO **Spine and disorders**

Seasonal affective disorder

Seasonal affective disorder, commonly known as SAD, is a type of depression that affects people in the winter months. Most of us feel energetic and cheerful when the sun is shining and subdued and less active in the winter months. But seasonal affective disorder is more severe than this. Some people are unable to hold down a job in winter because of lethargy, tiredness and poor concentration; relationships often break down because the sufferer becomes irritable and unloving. Some people cannot function at all in winter without treatment.

Between October and April, 1–3 per cent of the UK population have symptoms of seasonal affective disorder, and a further 20 per cent have a milder version known popularly as the 'winter blues'. It can begin at any age, but is most common between the ages of 18 and 30. Symptoms disappear in spring, either suddenly (with a bout of hyperactivity) or gradually.

Seasonal affective disorder is caused by lack of light. In winter, there are fewer hours of daylight and the light is much less intense. This can mean that insufficient light gets to a part of the brain called the hypothalamus, which controls the important bodily functions of sleep, appetite, temperature, sex drive, mood and activity. For people with SAD these functions slow down and become reduced.

SYMPTOMS

People with seasonal affective disorder often have a low immune system in the winter and get regular colds, infections and other illnesses.

To be diagnosed with the disorder you must have had three years of winter symptoms, including some of the following:

- sleepiness during the day or oversleeping;
- lack of energy for normal routine;
- overeating and putting on weight;
- feeling low; sometimes helplessness and despair;
- unwillingness to see people or to socialize;
- anxiety, tension and irritability;
- lack of interest in sex or physical contact.

TREATMENT

Light therapy is one successful option; others include antidepressant drugs and supplements.

Light treatment

Bright light treatment helps 85 per cent of people diagnosed with seasonal affective disorder. It means spending up to four hours a day exposed to very bright light, or 'full-spectrum' light – which mimics natural sunlight and is ten times the intensity of domestic lighting. Light boxes that produce this light can be bought commercially.

Antidepressant drugs

Newer antidepressants, such as Lustral and Prozac, can help people with severe seasonal affective disorder, and can be combined with light treatment.

Complementary therapies

The medicinal herb St John's wort (*Hypericum perforatum*) is now a popular treatment for depression, and may also help people with seasonal affective disorder. It should not be taken with conventional antidepressants.

What you can do

- Make the most of any available daylight: go for a walk at midday in winter; decorate your home in light colours.
- Simplify your life in winter; leave big upheavals until the summer.
- Take a holiday in January or February.

SEE ALSO *Depression*

Seizure

A seizure is defined as disturbed activity in the brain due to conditions such as epilepsy, infection, fever, low or high blood sugar, head injury, brain haemorrhage or cancer. Alcohol and drug abuse can also cause seizures

A seizure can last for a few seconds or continue until medical treatment is given.

SYMPTOMS

The symptoms depend on the type of seizure. They range from numbness and tingling and muscle spasms to more generalized, rhythmic movements of the limbs. There may be partial or full loss of consciousness.

TREATMENT

Anyone experiencing a seizure for the first time should seek urgent medical help to identify the cause and prescribe treatment.

What a doctor will do

If you are taken to hospital as an emergency you will probably undergo a range of tests.

If epilepsy or brain injury is suspected, referral to a nerve specialist is usually recommended. A detailed examination will be conducted, often including an EEG (electroencephalogram) of electrical activity in the brain, and a brain scan (magnetic resonance imaging or MRI) is usually recommended. If a brain tumour is suspected, you will be referred to a cancer specialist.

Treatment of seizures depends on the cause:
- epilepsy is usually treated with drugs or, in some cases, surgery;
- febrile seizures are treated by reducing fever and supporting body systems as necessary;
- central nervous system (CNS) infections, such as meningitis, falciparum malaria and rabies, are treated with anti-microbial therapy and organ support;
- brain haemorrhages and brain tumours may require surgery.

COMPLICATIONS

Severe, prolonged or recurrent seizures can cause brain damage.

PREVENTION

Vaccines are available against some forms of meningitis and rabies; and epileptic seizures may be prevented by regular medication. To prevent alcohol and drug-induced seizures, seek professional support to help reduce your intake and then give up altogether.

SEE ALSO *Brain and nervous system; Epilepsy; FIRST AID; Fits*

Senile dementia

Senile dementia is a term used to describe the confusion and gradual lessening of intellectual ability in some older people. While most people's memories deteriorate as they get older, dementia is not an inevitable part of ageing. In senile dementia, a person gradually becomes less able to learn, pay attention, exercise judgment, think clearly, and remember recent events. In the UK, one in 20 people over the age of 65 have some degree of dementia; over the age of 80 the figure rises to about one in five.

The most common cause of **dementia** is **Alzheimer's disease**, in which parts of the brain degenerate. Another common cause is a **stroke** or series of strokes that damages the blood vessels leading to the brain and reduces the oxygen supply. Less common causes of

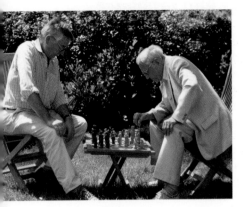

▲ Mental exercise
Short-term memory loss does not stop you from remembering skills learnt in the past. Research has shown that using your brain helps to slow down the rate of deterioration.

dementia include **Parkinson's disease, AIDS, CJD** and Pick's disease, which is similar to Alzheimer's disease.

SYMPTOMS
The first signs are often so slight as to be hardly noticeable. They include lapses in memory, mood swings, and difficulty in finding the right words. As time goes on mood swings may become more obvious and worsening memory can lead to confusion and depression or anger. However, the person affected may, in moments of lucidity, have some insight into his or her condition.

TREATMENT
There is no cure for dementia, but a range of drug treatments may reduce symptoms and delay the deterioration of mental function.

Septicaemia

Septicaemia is more commonly known as blood poisoning. It occurs when bacteria escape from the site of an infection into the bloodstream and multiply. People most at risk of septicaemia are those whose natural resistance is weakened by an immunodeficiency disorder like AIDS, or by immunosuppressant drugs. People with severe burns, or who have widespread cancer, leukaemia or diabetes are also at risk. Drug addicts who share contaminated needles commonly get blood poisoning, too.

SYMPTOMS
Symptoms include a high temperature and shivering, a headache, rapid breathing and sometimes a rash. It is vital to get a person with these symptoms to hospital. Urgent treatment is vital, as otherwise there is the possibility that it will lead to septic shock, which is often fatal.

Septic shock
When bacteria multiply rapidly in the bloodstream, they produce powerful poisons, or toxins, that severely damage the blood vessels, allowing fluid from the bloodstream to escape into surrounding tissue. When so much fluid is lost from the blood that normal circulation cannot be maintained, the blood pressure plummets and the person goes into shock.

Symptoms include a weak but rapid pulse and pale, cold clammy skin. When the blood supply fails to reach all parts of the body, the result is multiple organ failure.

TREATMENT
Both septicaemia and septic shock need urgent medical attention. Septicaemia is treated with intravenous antibiotics combined with glucose

or saline, or both. Doctors will also try to identify and treat the original source of the infection. As long as septicaemia does not progress to septic shock, most patients recover.

Septic shock is a medical emergency. It is treated with large doses of antibiotics and rapid fluid transfusions to replace the blood lost. It is fatal in about 60 per cent of cases.

Serum sickness

Serum sickness is an illness that follows about eight days after a vaccine containing animal serum is given to someone who has previously had contact with, and been sensitized to, the serum. Symptoms include fever, swollen glands, widespread **nettle rash** and painful swollen joints. Such vaccines are rarely used today.
SEE ALSO *Allergies; Immunization*

Sexually transmitted diseases

Sexually transmitted diseases – commonly known as STDs – are infections caused by micro-organisms passed on from person to person during intimate sexual contact.

Practising safer sex by using a barrier method of contraception, such as the male condom, helps to reduce the risk of contracting a sexually transmitted disease, but does not remove the risk altogether.

SYMPTOMS
Telltale symptoms may include: an unusual or unpleasant genital odour; soreness; itching; a rash; lumps; and ulcers. In addition, women may notice an increased vaginal discharge, and men may develop a penile discharge that stains their underwear, and experience pain when urinating.

Certain infections (see below) can cause more serious health problems: chlamydia, for example, can cause infertility.

If you suspect you may have an STD, do not ignore it. Any unusual symptoms should be checked by your doctor or, if you prefer anonymity, at a hospital clinic. These clinics are usually known as GUM clinics, short for genito-urinary medicine, and will give free, confidential advice and treatment. You do not even have to give your real name.

Many sexually transmitted diseases do not have any obvious symptoms, but if you think you could be at risk – through having had unprotected sex, for example – you should make an appointment for a check-up at a GUM clinic. If you are found to have an infection, any recent sexual partner must also be treated.

INFECTIONS

Commonly encountered STDs are listed below.

■ **Trichomoniasis** is caused by a tiny parasite. Commonly known as 'trich', it causes a green, frothy vaginal discharge. There may be no symptoms in men, or there may be urethritis, which causes stinging on urination and a discharge from the penis. Trich is treated with antibiotics, and partners should be treated, too.

■ **Genital warts** are among the commonest sexually transmitted infections. They are caused by the human papillomavirus. White or pinkish lumps may appear on the skin of the genitals one to three months after contact with an infected person, or the infection may be symptom-free. Visible warts can be removed using laser treatment, liquid nitrogen or a painted-on lotion. The wart virus lies dormant in skin cells, so recurrences and transmission to others are common. Some strains encourage cancer of the cervix, so women may be offered more frequent smear tests.

■ **Genital herpes** is caused by the Herpes simplex virus. Many people remain symptomless, but it can produce a flu-like illness plus a crop of painful ulcerating blisters around the genitals. Treatment with the antiviral drug acyclovir can hasten healing. Recurrences are common.

■ **Chlamydia** is one of the most common sexually transmitted diseases. It often has no symptoms, but can cause infertility. Men may have penile discharge and **urethritis**; women may have pelvic discomfort on intercourse and bleeding between periods. It is treated with antibiotics.

■ **Gonorrhoea** is a bacterial infection. It may cause no symptoms, or mild urinary discomfort, or severe urethral pain plus a heavy pus-stained discharge. It can spread to infect the prostate and testicles in men or to cause pelvic inflammatory disease in women. Gonorrhoea is treated with a single dose of antibiotics.

■ **Syphilis** is a bacterial infection. A painless, shallow ulcer appears at the site of infection. If untreated, the disease progresses to secondary syphilis, causing a flu-like illness and skin sores. It then lies dormant for anything from 3–40 years when the final debilitating, and sometimes fatal, stage of syphilis develops. Syphilis is generally treated with penicillin injections.

■ **Non-specific urethritis (NSU)** describes a discharge from the penis, often accompanied by pain on urination, before the cause has been diagnosed. Chlamydia is frequently the culprit.

■ **Hepatitis B and HIV** can be passed on sexually. A vaccine can protect against hepatitis B.

Of the 25 sexually transmitted diseases that are known, eight have no obvious symptoms, most can be treated, but four are incurable.

Shoulder and problems

The shoulder is made up of two bones, the clavicle – this is more commonly known as the collarbone – and the scapula or shoulder blade. These two bones project from the trunk of the body forming a framework from which our arms hang. The main joint in the shoulder links the bone of the upper arm (humerus) to the shoulder blade.

The collarbone is a slender arc of bone that forms a bridge from the top of the sternum, in the ribcage, to the shoulder socket at the end of the shoulder blade. It is the only bone in the shoulder that is connected directly to the ribcage. The collarbone supports the weight of the entire arm. If someone has a broken shoulder, this usually means that the collarbone is broken. If the collarbone is snapped right through, the entire shoulder droops.

The shoulder blade is a roughly triangular, large flat bone. It is not connected to the ribcage but is held in place by muscles. At the end farthest from the ribcage is the shoulder socket into which the bone of the upper arm fits. This is a ball-and-socket joint, which means that the spherical end of one bone fits into the hollow of another.

The shoulder socket is saucer-shaped and shallow and the bones are held in place by ligaments. This makes the joint very flexible but, because the ligaments that surround it are looser then those of the hip joint, say, the joint is weak and can be dislocated quite easily.

The shoulder muscles

An arrangement of muscles allows movement of the arms, neck and head (see **Muscular system**). One group, known collectively as the rotator cuff muscles, helps to stabilize the shoulder joint and is involved in moving the arm. Another muscle, the trapezius, turns the head and bends the neck backwards; this muscle, along with several others, also raises the shoulder blade and the arm behind the back. The main chest muscle – the pectoralis major – forms the front of the armpit, and is mostly used for arm movement. The deltoid muscle forms a cushion on top of the shoulder. It raises the arm up out to the side, and helps with all shoulder movements. The biceps and triceps muscles of the upper arm also help with certain shoulder movements.

WHAT CAN GO WRONG

The complex of joints and muscles in the shoulder can sometimes run into problems.

Arthritis

The shoulder is rarely affected by osteoarthritis because it is not a weight-bearing joint. However, rheumatoid arthritis can affect both shoulders simultaneously and cause severe disability. Occasionally, a child may develop arthritis in the shoulder if the upper end of the humerus is affected by osteomyelitis.

Painful arc syndrome

Inflammation of one of the so-called rotator cuff muscles (the supraspinatus) can cause this condition. This weak, vulnerable muscle is easily strained by unaccustomed repetitive actions or by a sudden wrench or a blow. The muscle tenses, and its tendon becomes pinched between the end of the shoulder blade and the head of the humerus, causing pain.

Any action that involves lifting the arm can cause a severe pain to shoot down from the shoulder. (To see whether the cause of this type of shooting pain is painful arc syndrome, lift your arm straight out to your side and up to your head. If it is painful arc syndrome, the pain will start when the angle of your armpit is 60° and fade after it reaches 120°.) Without treatment, a calcified deposit can form in the tendon, increasing the inflammation and pain – which can be so severe that the arm becomes virtually immobile.

Physiotherapy, including ultrasound, traction and mobilizing exercises, can help mild cases. In more serious cases hydrocortisone injections

around the tendon may be given and the arm rested. Occasionally, doctors will operate to remove the calcified deposit.

Rotator cuff tear

The rotator cuff muscles can be torn by a fall or a sudden strain. This is more likely in elderly people whose tendons have been weakened and made vulnerable by age. Depending on which muscles are affected, the symptoms may be similar to those for painful arc syndrome (see above), but worse. When several muscles tear and the joint itself is affected, there is pain at the tip of the shoulder and down the arm, and it is excruciatingly painful – if not impossible – to raise the arm.

If such an injury affects a younger person, the tear can be repaired surgically. This is followed by several months of physiotherapy. But it is rarely possible to repair damage in older people, whose treatment will involve exercises.

Dislocation

Dislocation of the shoulder joint is common because the joint is relatively weak. It usually happens as a result of a violent wrenching movement or a fall. However, some people are born with extremely loose ligaments, and their shoulders can dislocate without any injury.

Once a shoulder has dislocated, it may do so again. This is because the spherical head of the humerus is usually dented by the injury, and this makes it likely to slip out of its socket.

After the joint has been clicked back into place and the surrounding tissues have healed, a course of physiotherapy can help to strengthen the muscles, tendons and ligaments and so increase the stability of the joint. But if a shoulder repeatedly becomes dislocated, physiotherapy is unlikely to help and an operation may be needed to stabilize the joint.

This may involve surgically tightening the cavity to stop the ball from popping out of the socket so easily, or grafting on a piece of bone to increase the depth of the socket, or operating on the muscles so as to limit the amount the arm can rotate outwards, thereby lessening the likelihood of dislocating the shoulder.

Fractures

Fracture of the shoulder blade is very rare, but both the collarbone and humerus are prone to cracking or breaking as a result of a direct blow, accident or fall (see **Fractures**).

Bursitis

A bursa is a sac that contains a joint's lubricating fluid. If the bursa that lies over the shoulder joint becomes inflamed it causes tenderness and pain (see **bursitis**). It can result from overuse or dislocation; it may also be caused by disease.

The bones and joints of the shoulder

The shoulder socket gets its strength from the shoulder blade, the collarbone and the muscles that support them. The bones of the arm and shoulder have rough areas on their surfaces where muscles are attached. When muscles tense, this pulls the bone and moves the limb.

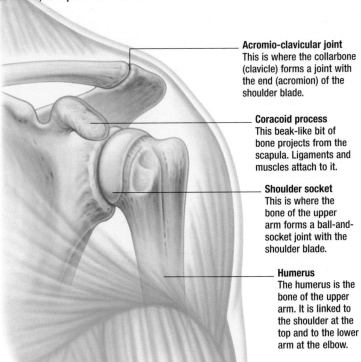

Acromio-clavicular joint
This is where the collarbone (clavicle) forms a joint with the end (acromion) of the shoulder blade.

Coracoid process
This beak-like bit of bone projects from the scapula. Ligaments and muscles attach to it.

Shoulder socket
This is where the bone of the upper arm forms a ball-and-socket joint with the shoulder blade.

Humerus
The humerus is the bone of the upper arm. It is linked to the shoulder at the top and to the lower arm at the elbow.

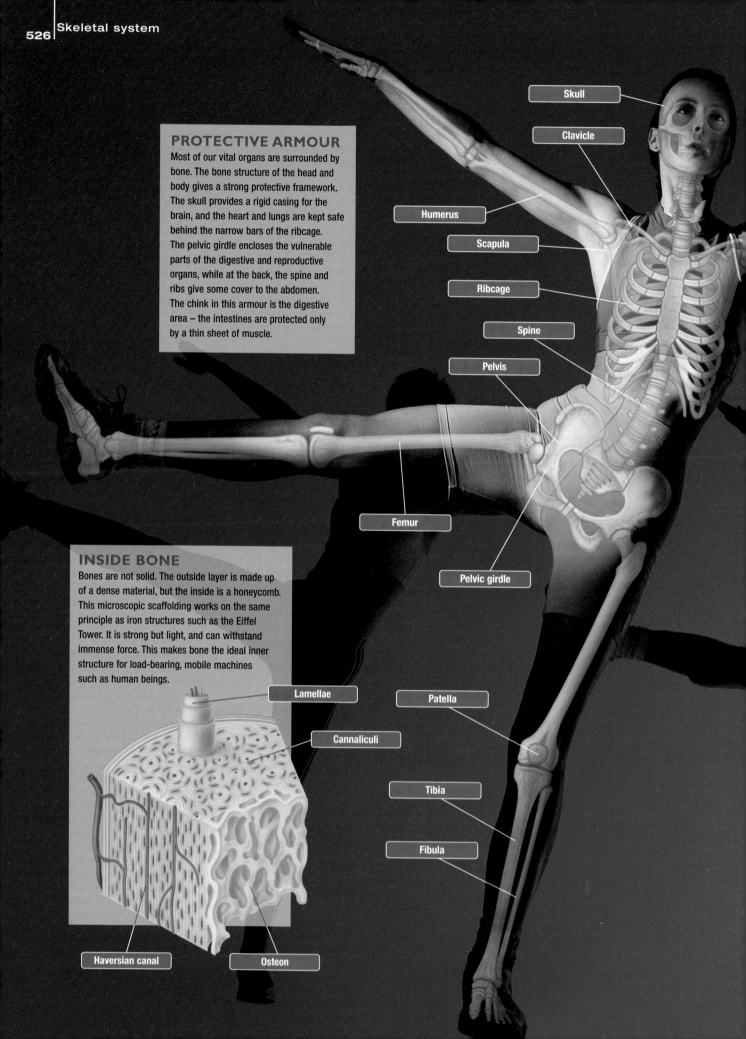

PROTECTIVE ARMOUR

Most of our vital organs are surrounded by bone. The bone structure of the head and body gives a strong protective framework. The skull provides a rigid casing for the brain, and the heart and lungs are kept safe behind the narrow bars of the ribcage. The pelvic girdle encloses the vulnerable parts of the digestive and reproductive organs, while at the back, the spine and ribs give some cover to the abdomen. The chink in this armour is the digestive area – the intestines are protected only by a thin sheet of muscle.

INSIDE BONE

Bones are not solid. The outside layer is made up of a dense material, but the inside is a honeycomb. This microscopic scaffolding works on the same principle as iron structures such as the Eiffel Tower. It is strong but light, and can withstand immense force. This makes bone the ideal inner structure for load-bearing, mobile machines such as human beings.

Skull

Clavicle

Humerus

Scapula

Ribcage

Spine

Pelvis

Pelvic girdle

Femur

Patella

Tibia

Fibula

Lamellae

Cannaliculi

Haversian canal

Osteon

Radius

Carpals

Ulna

Metacarpals

The sponge-like matrix, found at the centre of our bones, is a honeycomb structure that is much lighter than compact bone. The struts are arranged along the lines of greatest pressure, giving our bones great strength.

Skeletal system

The skeleton is a superb piece of biological engineering. It is the tough but delicately wrought framework that allows us to stand upright, change position, and manipulate objects. The skeleton also forms a protective barrier around vital organs such as the brain and heart: it is our internal armour. Bones, working with muscles, act as levers that allow us to move from place to place and to lift and carry heavy objects.

The skeleton is not rigid, because part of its function is shock absorption. Every time a sprinter takes a stride, for example, the force through each foot is equivalent to 20 times the body weight. Some of this force is absorbed by the bones' collagen, a tough rubbery substance that provides resilience, or 'bounce'. The skeleton is strong enough to support this burden, but light enough to allow ease of movement. And all the time, the bones take the constant strain of muscle flexion, which tugs at them like the taut rigging on a ship's mast.

The skeleton is the manufacturing centre for our red blood cells, nearly all of which are made within the marrow of bones. And the skeleton is a storehouse for calcium, which not only gives the skeleton its structural strength, but is essential to many body functions such as blood clotting, muscle contraction and nerve conduction.

THE BODY'S FRAMEWORK

The skeleton accounts for one fifth of our body weight. There are 206 bones in the body. The largest of them is the thigh bone, and the smallest is the stapes in the inner ear. The precise shape and size of the bones vary from person to person: tall people have much longer leg bones and larger vertebrae than those who are short.

There are also some small but significant differences between the skeletons of men and women. The female pelvis, for example, is shallower and wider than in men, to allow for childbearing.

How bones develop and grow

Bones are living tissue with a complex physical structure. They are subject to growth and disease just like the soft organs of the body.

We tend to think of bone as being hard, rigid and static. In fact, it is an active living material that is continuously being renewed. It has rich blood and nerve supplies, which is why injuries to bones bleed a lot and are painful.

The two main structural components to bone are minerals and collagen. The mineral element, which provides strength, is a complex salt that contains calcium, phosphorous, magnesium and other trace minerals. Collagen, a complex protein also found in cartilage, provides shock absorption and resilience. Together they make a strong structure with the mechanical ability to withstand high forces. The tensile strength of bone is greater than that of steel, but it is lighter than aluminium.

WHAT IS BONE?

Bone can be of two types: compact or spongy. Compact bone is dense and looks solid to the naked eye. It is actually made up of rod-like elements called Haversian systems. These consist of a central canal containing blood and lymph vessels and nerves, surrounded by concentric sheets of bone. Between these are gaps (lacunae) containing lymphatic fluid and bone cells (osteocytes). The Haversian systems give compact bone a tubular structure, which provides greater strength than it would have if it were solid. Compact bone tissue is generally found at the ends and near the outside of the bone – the parts that are most vulnerable to injury.

The central part of our bones is made up of spongy bone. This has larger Haversian canals than compact bone and fewer concentric sheets, giving a honeycomb structure. Spongy bone is light but extremely strong – and it acts as scaffolding for the bone's outer layers. The spaces in the 'honeycomb' are filled with bone marrow, which manufactures blood cells.

Bones are covered by a fibrous membrane to which the various tendons and ligaments are attached. But on the articular surfaces of our synovial joints, this membrane is replaced by a form of cartilage called hyaline. This is smooth and virtually friction-free, and aids movement.

Bone renewal

Bone tissue, like all tissue, is subject to a constant process of renewal. In a healthy body, a continual turnover of calcium ensures the body's supplies are kept in balance. Turnover can be rapid. It has been said that calcium absorbed from milk drunk at breakfast could be part of a bone by lunch, and excreted in the urine in the evening.

The essential building blocks of strong and healthy bone come from a healthy diet. Calcium is particularly important, but to absorb the calcium and phosphorus needed for bone formation, the body requires vitamin D. When the skin is exposed to sunlight, the body can make sufficient vitamin D, but people confined indoors must obtain it from food sources.

A vitamin D deficiency causes lower leg bones to bend – a condition known as **rickets**. Additional intakes of calcium and vitamins are recommended during pregnancy and breastfeeding, because a baby's need for nutrients before it is born, and for breast milk afterwards, can deplete the mother's calcium stores.

HOW DOES BONE DEVELOP?

The skeleton begins to form in the womb, soon after conception. Within the fetus there is a buildup of columns of cartilage, the precursor of bone. By the seventh week after conception these proto-bones can be seen on an **ultrasound** scan. It is about this time that ossification begins, that is, the process whereby cartilage is replaced by hard deposits of calcium and so transformed into genuine bone.

In the centre of long bones – such as those in the leg – there is a specialized growing region where cells called osteoblasts gather to make new bone. This is the point from which growing bones lengthen and strengthen, and it is also the main centre of ossification. Meanwhile, at the bone ends, there are other centres of ossification known as epiphyses. In the epiphyses, the growth happens at the epiphyseal plate. This is found between the end of the straight part of long bones and the more rounded end pieces, and is clearly visible on children's X-rays.

The growing frame

The skull consists of several separate bones, which eventually fuse together. Initially, in the womb, the skull is a strong membrane, but by birth this has largely been converted into hard bone. At birth the separate plates of the skull are not fused together into a hard casing. This means that the head is still pliable enough to squeeze through the birth canal and flexible enough to accommodate the rapid growth of the brain in the first weeks and months of life. The fontanelles, the membrane-covered gaps in a baby's skull, do not close until a child is over a year old. All the bones in the body continue to grow until the age of 18 in boys and 16 in girls.

▼ **Longhand**
Bones and joints do not become fully formed until early adulthood.

2½ years

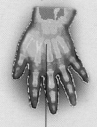

In early childhood bone formation occurs only in the middle of long bones.

6½ years

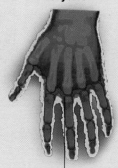

Spaces narrow as cartilage becomes bone.

19 years

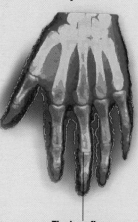

The long finger bones have fully formed and plates have closed up.

What can go wrong

Problems with the bones and joints are among the most common causes of poor health and disability, especially among elderly people.

Despite their inner strength, bones can break and they are also susceptible to various diseases, including cancer. With advancing age, more calcium is removed from the bones than is replaced and they become less dense, or 'lighter', making them weak and more prone to fractures.

BONE FRACTURES

A **fracture**, or break, occurs if excessive stress is put on a bone. This is often as a result of an awkward fall. Anyone can be affected, but fractures are much more likely to occur if the bone has already been weakened by osteoporosis (see below).

All fractures require medical attention. The initial treatment is usually to correct any displacement of bone by realigning the bone ends. Depending on the severity of the break and the displacement, this may have to be done in an operating theatre. The affected part will usually have to be immobilized until the break is healed. This may be done internally, using plates and screws to hold the bone pieces in place. An external plaster cast or fibreglass splint may also be applied to ensure that the body part maintains the correct position until the bone has healed.

Healing time varies, depending on the severity of the fracture, the part of the body affected and the age of the patient. All body healing is quicker in children and at its slowest in older people.

The three most common fractures are:

Colles fracture: this is a fracture of the lower end of the radius bone, just above the wrist. It is usually caused by the person falling onto an outstretched hand. It is particularly common in older people, especially if the bones are weakened. The wrist may be pushed back over the broken bone, giving it a forked appearance. Treatment is to immobilize the bone in a plaster cast or splint, after correcting any deformity.

Pottes fracture: this is a fracture of the ankle caused by the foot being forced outwards at the ankle joint. The lower part of the tibia, known as the shinbone, is cracked and can easily be displaced. Sometimes the bottom end of the fibula is also broken and the ankle joint may be dislocated. Treatment is to correct any deformity using internal splints and screws as necessary and then immobilize the lower leg by cast.

Fractured hip: this is a very serious fracture that occurs as the result of a fall. It most commonly affects elderly people with osteoporosis. There is often major internal bleeding after a hip fracture.

The treatment is surgical, and may involve either fixing the hip joint with a plate and screw, or replacing the broken part of the hip joint with an artificial joint.

BONE DISEASES

Bones can be affected by several disorders as well as by nutritional and hormonal factors.

Osteomalacia is a metabolic disease that can occur at any age. It results in the bone having a lower mineral content than normal. This causes it to soften and become vulnerable to fractures.

Osteoporosis is a common condition in which the natural processes of bone regeneration are disrupted. The holes in spongy bone become larger, making the bone much more fragile.

Osteomyelitis is an infection of bone, which causes severe pain as well as swelling of the surrounding tissues. It usually occurs after a fracture or hip replacement operation but it can also be the result of the *Staphylococcus aureus* bacteria entering the bloodstream and infecting the bone tissue.

Paget's disease is a rare metabolic bone disorder in which there is increased and irregular formation of bone. Over time, the deformed new bone becomes larger and weaker than normal bone, making it prone to fracture.

Bone tumours are rare but they do occur either as a primary tumour or secondary deposit from a primary tumour that has occurred elsewhere in the body (see **Cancer**).

Bone conditions affecting the young

Some bone disorders are congenital, meaning that children are born with them. They include achondroplasia, a genetic disorder causing defective bone growth and short stature.

Children can also suffer from bone disorders that occur during development. **Perthes' disease** affects the hip in children aged 3–11 causing pain in the groin and sometimes the knee. Pain in the knee or hip joints in children should always be assessed by a medical professional, who will usually arrange for X-rays to be taken.

Osgood Schlatter disease commonly affects teenagers, usually following sporting activities that involve a lot of jumping. It is a painful inflammation of the area where the tendon from the kneecap (patella) attaches to the shinbone (tibia). The condition generally heals itself within 12–24 months.

SEE ALSO *Bone and problems; Bone marrow and disorders*

Skin and disorders

Tough and resilient, the skin is the body's first line of defence. It provides a protective barrier against infection and a waterproof layer that prevents excessive loss or absorption of moisture.

Men have thicker skin than women and, because of the effect of testosterone, are less prone to dry skin.

The skin is the largest human organ, with a surface area of up to 2 square metres (22 square feet). It continually regenerates itself during life, though this process slows down as we age. The skin can be damaged in many ways, from cuts and deeper wounds to sunburn. We can all benefit from looking after our skin.

As well as protecting the body, skin also helps to regulate body temperature by varying the amount of heat lost. When blood vessels near the surface of the body dilate, more heat is lost, and when these blood vessels contract and tiny hairs on the surface of the body become erect, body heat is conserved. The skin also contains a number of different sensory nerve endings that can detect light touch, sustained pressure, cold, warmth or pain. Pain receptors are stimulated when tissues are damaged, and release chemicals that trigger irritation and inflammation.

THE FOUR LAYERS OF SKIN
The skin cells form four main layers:
- an outer layer called the epidermis;
- beneath it, the basal cell layer;
- an inner layer, the dermis;
- an underlying fatty layer.

Skin cells in the outer epidermal layer contain a strong structural protein known as keratin. New cells are made by division of cells in the basal layer and slowly move towards the body surface, pushed up by the production of new cells beneath. They gradually become flattened and hardened ('cornified') before finally dying to produce a tough, waterproof outer layer for the body that is continually worn away and replaced.

The inner dermis is made up of living cells and contains structural collagen and elastin fibres, nerves, blood vessels, sense receptors, sebaceous glands, sweat glands and hair follicles.

SWEAT GLANDS
Sweat cools the body as evaporation draws energy away from the skin surface. The average person produces around 1 litre (1¾ pints) of perspiration per day – more in hot conditions or when exercising vigorously.

We each have around three million sweat glands. There are two main types.
- Eccrine glands are found on all skin (except for the eyelids) but are concentrated on the palms of the hands and soles of the feet. They secrete water and salts directly onto the skin's surface.
- Apocrine glands only become active at puberty. They are found on hair-bearing skin, mainly on the armpits, groin, nipples and scalp. They produce modified sweat (containing proteins, fats and sugars) into hair follicles rather than onto the skin surface. This sweat is initially odourless, but once it is broken down by skin bacteria, it produces body odour.

Sweating problems
Excessive sweating occurs when the metabolic thermostat is set too high, leading to overactivity of the nerves that regulate the sweat glands. Excess sweating affects an estimated one in 100 people. The condition is usually due to overactive sweat glands but, in rare cases, is associated with a skin disease – eccrine angiomatous hamartoma.

The structure of skin
Skin is made up of two layers – the surface layer, the epidermis, and the underlying dermis. Every minute of the day we lose about 30,000 to 40,000 dead skin cells from the surface layer of our skin.

Epidermis

Hair

Basal cell layer

Sweat gland

Hair follicle

Dermis

Fatty layer

SKIN DAMAGE

The skin is one of the first places to show signs of illness or the effects of an unhealthy lifestyle, including dryness, itching, flakiness and increased susceptability to skin infections. Other common types of skin damage include friction blisters (see **FIRST AID**), corns (see **Foot and problems**), **ulcers** and chapping.

Chapping

Frequent washing with soap and water, and especially contact with the chemicals in some washing-up liquids and other cleaning fluids, can damage the horny top layer of skin, causing excessive scaling known as chapping.

To ease chapping, dry hands carefully after washing and use an unperfumed hand cream. Use waterproof gloves when washing dishes and clothes, or using bleaches and cleaning chemicals.

Burns

Skin heated to more than 49°C (120°F) will burn. **Burns** are classified as first-degree, second-degree and third-degree, with third-degree being the most serious. When second or third-degree burns cover more than 10 per cent of the body, the effects often trigger clinical shock, where the pulse speeds up and the blood pressure falls. Burns can also result from contact with chemicals and electricity. All but the most superficial burns should be checked by a doctor.

Keloid scars

A keloid scar is a thickened area of scar tissue that forms due to an overactive production of collagen in some skin wounds (see **Collagen diseases**). This is most common over the breastbone and shoulders. Keloids cannot simply be cut out as they often re-form as the cut heals.

Applying an adhesive silicone gel sheet improves the appearance of keloids in 90 per cent of cases – even where scars are 20 years old – although results are better on recent scars.

Stretchmarks

Stretchmarks are a common problem, due to crease-like breaks in the lower layers of skin as a result of thinning and stretching.

The usual cause of stretchmarks is gaining weight quickly, as can happen at puberty or during pregnancy. You cannot prevent or remove stretchmarks, although they do eventually fade.

INFLAMMATORY SKIN DISEASES

Inflammatory skin diseases usually cause redness, swelling and itching and include:
- **dermatitis** – a term covering many types of skin rashes, sometimes caused by an allergy;
- **eczema** – itchy, scaly skin that may blister;
- **psoriasis** – thickened red patches of skin with white scales. It tends to run in families;
- **seborrhoea** – a form of dermatitis that produces an itchy, scaly rash on the scalp. **Cradle cap** is a form of seborrhoeic dermatitis that commonly affects newborn infants;
- Lichen planus – a skin disease with intensely itchy, raised, purple sores, often on the lower legs and inside the wrists, but can occur anywhere.

Skin infections

The skin is vulnerable to bacterial infections that can cause problems such as:
- **boil** – an inflamed pus-filled spot;
- **abscess** – an accumulation of pus;
- **impetigo** – a very contagious infection, causing crusty blisters, often near the nose and mouth;
- **cellulitis** – a hot, tender reddened area of skin.
Viral infections that affect the skin include:
- **wart** – a horny, non-malignant growth;
- Molluscum contagiosum – a harmless but contagious infection that forms multiple, shiny, pearly white lumps on the skin;
- **herpes** – cold sores;
- shingles – a painful recurrence of chickenpox;
- pityriasis rosea – a mild, pink rash in young adults that affects the trunk, arms and thighs. It clears up in 6 to 8 weeks without treatment;
Fungal infections can result in:
- **ringworm** – itchy ring-shaped lesions;
- **athlete's foot** – intensely itchy areas, usually between the toes.

Some conditions such as **acne vulgaris** and **acne rosacea** are also associated with skin infections that have triggered an inflammatory skin reaction. Flare-ups of eczema can also result from an increase on the skin of the bacterium *Staphylococcus aureus*.

THE SKIN AND SUNLIGHT

The skin protects the body from the ultraviolet radiation in sunlight. However, this radiation also damages the skin and interferes with normal cell division. There are two forms of ultraviolet rays:
- UVA rays, which do not burn, but are responsible for photosensitivity reactions. These rays also accelerate the skin's ageing process.
- UVB rays, which cause sunburn and long-term changes in the skin responsible for ageing and skin cancer.

Skin that is exposed to the sun in the long term eventually loses elasticity and becomes thickened, and wrinkled with a coarse, leathery texture.

Vitamin D

Vitamin D is one of the few vitamins that can be made in the body. It is produced by the action of UVB rays in sunlight on the skin. Blood levels of vitamin D are naturally higher in the summer and lower in winter, so when the sun comes out in the winter months it is important to spend as much time as possible outdoors.

Skin pigmentation

The basal cell layer of the epidermis contains pigment cells known as melanocytes. These make

Types of skin cancer

Skin cancer affects around 50,000 Britons every year and kills more than two per cent of them. Tell your doctor about any sores that do not heal.

Malignant melanoma begins in the skin's pigmentation system – the layer that tans in summer. Melanomas usually start in moles but can appear in areas of normal-looking skin.

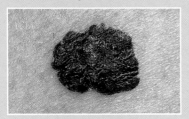

Basal cell carcinoma is often seen on the face or neck. Also known as rodent ulcer, it begins in the basal cell layer of the epidermis. It is not one of the most dangerous cancers but it must still be treated to stop it spreading.

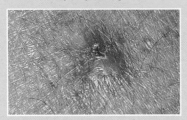

Squamous cell carcinoma often starts like a patch of eczema on the face or neck. It is less common than basal cell carcinoma and grows faster – especially when located near the eyes, ears or mouth.

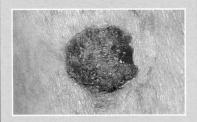

the brown tanning pigment melanin. We each have around 2 billion melanocytes. Exposure to sunlight causes melanocytes to inject granules of melanin pigment into surrounding cells. This protects the cell nucleus and shield chromosomes from the damaging effects of UV light.

Moles, freckles and skin blemishes

■ Freckles occur when pigment cells produce melanin more quickly than melanocytes on surrounding non-freckled skin. Freckles often fade in winter, although exposure to the sun will tend to bring them out again.

■ A mole is a brown skin mark, known as a pigmented naevus, produced when overactive melanocytes inject too much pigment into the adjacent cells.

■ Other common blemishes include cherry spots, chloasma, spider naevus and **birthmarks**.

■ Skin can also lose pigmentation in patches, known as **vitiligo**.

SKIN CANCER

More than 90 per cent of all skin cancers are due to exposure to the sun – often during childhood. Skin cancer is now the second most common cancer in the UK.

There are three main types of skin **cancer**: malignant melanoma, basal cell carcinoma and squamous cell carcinoma. Malignant melanoma is the most serious and is potentially fatal. It is a tumour of melanocytes. Malignant melanoma can be triggered by UV exposure built up over years. The two other most common forms of skin cancer, basal cell carcinoma and squamous cell carcinoma, are also linked with sun damage.

Malignant melanoma

Malignant melanomas and other forms of skin cancer are most common on areas of skin exposed to the sun such as the backs of the hands, nape of the neck and face. But they can occur anywhere on the body. Melanomas on the back are difficult to spot. Use a long mirror or ask your partner or a family member to check your back regularly.

If a mole starts to itch, grow, weep, become scaly or change in other ways, it may be a sign that it will develop into a skin cancer. Many skin cancers have a high cure rate if caught in the early stages, so never ignore the problem.

Basal cell carcinoma

Basal cell carcinoma initially forms a pearly skin growth, and usually appears on the face or back of the hands. It progresses slowly to form a small, painless lump that eventually develops a raised edge with a central depression. If left untreated, the lump will ulcerate – this is known as a rodent ulcer – and it may bleed, but it will not heal. It rarely spreads or causes death but should always be treated to prevent ulceration and disfigurement of the area affected.

Squamous cell carcinoma

Squamous cell carcinoma initially forms an area of thickened, scaly skin that makes a hard, painless lump with an irregular edge and a reddish hue. This slowly enlarges and eventually ulcerates. Squamous cell carcinoma can spread throughout the body, so early detection and treatment are important.

SKIN TREATMENTS

Treatment of skin problems depends on the condition. Dry skin conditions are soothed and moisturized with emollient creams; infections are treated with antibiotic creams, ointments or tablets. Wounds are protected with dressings and sometimes need skin grafts. Laser therapy can be used to get rid of birthmarks. Steroid creams may be used to treat conditions such as psoriasis: these creams should be used sparingly, exactly as prescribed; prolonged and excessive use can lead to thinning of the skin, especially on the face.

Skin grafting

Skin grafting is used to cover large defects in the skin such as burns, ulcers, injuries, or areas where tumours have been cut out. A donor site is selected from elsewhere on the body – often the thigh or back – and skin is taken for grafting onto the affected area.

Laser therapy

Laser therapy uses laser light energy of varying wavelengths to cut tissues during surgery, to seal them and prevent bleeding, or more superficially to treat certain skin problems. For example, laser pulses can be used to destroy the small dilated capillaries that cause facial redness in rosacea: each laser pulse lasts only a few thousandths of a second so heat does not build up in the skin. Red birthmarks, moles and tattoos can be treated in a similar way.

SEE ALSO *Cancer; Cosmetic and plastic surgery; Dermatitis; Eczema; Scars and scarring*

Smoking

Although we all know that smoking is bad for our health, it is a habit that is extremely hard to kick. But the good news is that from the moment you put out that last cigarette, your body starts to recover.

In western Europe, tobacco kills one person every minute – 500,000 each year. In the UK alone, 120,000 people die from tobacco-related illness each year, making smoking the leading single cause of avoidable ill health and premature death. Tobacco smoke contains more than 4000 chemicals, but it is the quantity and toxicity of the chemicals that is so damaging to health. They include tar, gases like carbon monoxide and, most importantly, the addictive drug nicotine.

Lung **cancer** is the cancer most strongly associated with smoking, and tobacco is responsible for 85–90 per cent of cases of lung cancer in developed countries. In fact, smoking is a factor in a third of *all* types of cancer.

Each year in the UK, tobacco smoking accounts for 26,000 deaths from coronary heart disease (see **Heart and circulatory system**). Compared to a non-smoker, a cigarette smoker is two or three times more at risk of having a heart attack. Inhaling smoke dramatically affects the heart and blood vessels: within one minute, the heart rate begins to rise, increasing by up to 30 per cent in the first ten minutes. Blood pressure rises, as blood vessels constrict and force the heart to work harder to deliver oxygen to the rest of the body. Simultaneously, carbon monoxide exerts a negative effect on the heart by reducing the blood's ability to carry oxygen. With raised fibrinogen levels and platelet counts that make the blood more sticky (see **Blood and disorders**), smokers are also at increased risk of developing arterial disease, peripheral vascular disease (blocked blood vessels in legs or feet that can eventually lead to tissue death and amputation) and **stroke**. Heavy smokers have two to four times the risk of a stroke.

Smoking is now known to be implicated in about two dozen causes of death, including:
- several forms of cancer;
- myeloid leukaemia;
- tuberculosis;
- pneumonia;
- chronic bronchitis and emphysema;
- heart disease;
- myocardial degeneration;
- arteriosclerosis;
- cerebral thrombosis;

- brain haemorrhage;
- stroke;
- aortic **aneurysm**;
- stomach and duodenal ulcers;

In addition, smokers face an increased risk of many other conditions, including osteoporosis and infertility, and suffer from more severe symptoms of asthma.

WOMEN AND SMOKING

In the UK, smoking is responsible for about a quarter of female deaths in middle age. This figure will soar over the next 25 years, reflecting the increase in smoking by women in the latter part of the 20th century.

QUITTING

Surveys show that at least 70 per cent of adult smokers want to stop smoking. Ask your doctor for help. He or she may recommend nicotine replacement therapy, at least in the short term. This comes in the form of chewing gum, skin patches, tablets, nasal sprays or inhalers. Alternatively, a drug called buproprian desensitizes the brain's nicotine receptors. The effectiveness of these aids is clinically proven, and both are available on prescription through the NHS. Acupuncture, hypnosis and support groups can also help.

Withdrawal symptoms

Giving up smoking can cause unpleasant withdrawal symptoms, but these will fade in time. It is quite normal to feel lightheaded for a couple of days, and you may find yourself waking at night for no apparent reason during the first week. People often feel irritable or aggressive, depressed and restless and find it hard to concentrate. But these feelings will subside, though it may take a month or so. Increased appetite, however, is a longer-lived side effect, and the chances are you will put on weight. But the health benefits of quitting far outweigh the disadvantages of a few excess pounds.

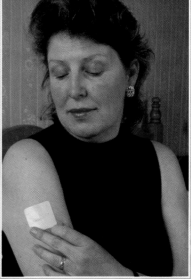

▼ Nicotine patch
The slow release of nicotine is intended to reduce withdrawal symptoms and enable the smoker to quit.

Speech disorders

Speech disorders are not uncommon. About two-and-a-half million people in the UK have a speech or language problem, and in a third of stroke cases there is a persisting speech and language difficulty.

The words 'speech' and 'language' are often used interchangeably, but they are not the same thing. Language is a mental ability to understand the complex symbols and rules behind words and grammar; speech is the physical production of language. The mechanics of talking require the coordinated movement of the tongue, lips, cheeks, throat and upper body muscles to produce verbal sounds. In contrast, language depends on the ability of the brain to link the sounds of words with their meanings (understanding) and to translate thoughts into words that can then be formed into sentences.

SPEECH DEVELOPMENT
Children learn to speak by interacting with their parents and through play. Their instinctive thirst for language – to understand and be understood – begins almost as soon as they are born.

- Year one: most babies begin to babble – make speech-like sounds – in the first year of life, and start to show an understanding of some of the words that are said to them.
- Year two: most children can say several words clearly by the time they are two years old, and can attempt to pronounce the strongest syllable of many others.
- Year three: by the time they reach the age of three, children should be able to speak in two- to three-word sentences; they should also be able to follow simple instructions and repeat words they have heard and used in conversation.
- Year four: most four-year-olds are able to follow an instruction that consists of two or three steps, recognize and identify practically all common objects and pictures, and understand most of what is said to them.

Common speech development problems

If your child has any of the problems described below, you may be able to find a solution to the problem by taking the recommended action.

PROBLEM	POSSIBLE CAUSE	ACTION
Your active and healthy two-year-old makes no effort to speak. He or she understands you and communicates non-verbally.	Slower than normal rate of speech development.	Read and speak with him or her one-to-one, giving plenty of opportunities to reply.
Your child responds to your voice only when he or she can see your face.	Hearing problem.	Ask your doctor to conduct a hearing test.
Your child hesitates, stammers, repeats syllables or confuses word order.	Possible cause: normal period of non-fluency.	Speak clearly and read to your child. Don't overcorrect him or her or finish sentences. This stage usually passes quickly.
Your school-age child lisps or consistently mispronounces consonants.	Possible cause: lisp or other speech impediment.	If the impediment is marked, ask your doctor to recommend a speech therapist for an evaluation.
Your school-age child stutters or hesitates and grimaces when trying to get words out.	Possible cause: stammering.	Consult your doctor about speech therapy.

- Year five: average five-year-olds have mastered the basic rules of grammar and have a vocabulary sufficient to express abstract ideas (that allows them to talk, for example, of events in the future as well as what is happening right now). Mispronunciation of words remains common.

THE ORIGIN OF SPEECH DISORDERS

People with speech disorders may have an underlying impairment in their language skills or they may have perfect language skills but are unable to produce coherent speech sounds. If any part of the complex process of interpreting language and making sounds is disrupted, a speech disorder may occur.

If the problem arises at the start of the process – in the brain – the disorder may take the form of aphasia, the inability to understand or 'find' words. If it occurs later in the process – when the signals from the brain are translated into muscle movements – it will manifest itself as a speech impediment such as stammering, a lisp, or slow, indistinct speech.

CAUSES OF SPEECH DISORDERS

Speech disorders have a very wide range of possible causes. These include hearing impairment, neurological abnormalities, cleft palate, vocal cord paralysis and throat cancer.

Hearing impairment

More than half of all speech disorders are thought to be associated with hearing abnormalities. Children naturally repeat what they hear, so a child who is hard of hearing will not develop normal speech without special help.

Neurological abnormalities

Speech disorders may be the result of neurological problems in the brain or in the nerves supplying the larynx, mouth and jaw.

- **Autism.** Children with severe autism rarely speak. This failure is thought to be due to lack of function in the frontal lobes of the brain, where ideas are generated and turned into language-based thought. Less severely autistic children may speak, but they tend to use very concrete language such as simple nouns rather than abstract sentences.
- **Cerebral palsy** is often associated with speech by problems in the part of the brain that processes speech or by weakness in the mouth and jaw muscles, which affects the production of sounds.
- **Dyspraxia** – inability to control fine movements – may prevent a child from making the subtle mouth and tongue movements required to articulate words.
- **Strokes** affecting the language centres of the brain may prevent language understanding or articulation (aphasia). If Wernicke's area is

Factfile

Speech areas in the brain

Language involves the integration of several areas of the brain. In a brain that's working normally it all happens in an instant without you even 'thinking' about it.

Wernicke's area takes incoming speech and links the sounds to memories of the objects to which it refers. Broca's area takes these symbols and translates them into sounds. Signals from Broca's area travel to the muscles controlling the vocal cords, the mouth and throat that produce speech. The movements are coordinated by a third area of the brain, the cerebellum, not indicated in the diagram on the right.

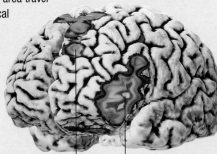

Wernicke's area | Broca's area

affected, stroke victims may speak fluently but nonsensically, whereas a stroke in Broca's area may leave understanding intact but prevent sufferers from 'finding' the words they require and from forming them into sentences.

Cleft palate

A person with a **cleft palate** is unable to move the mouth in the way required to produce normal speech sounds. Most children born with the condition are operated on in early infancy, and such surgery – combined with treatment to correct any problems in the development of the teeth – usually solves the problem. However, cleft palate surgery sometimes causes impaired hearing, and as a consequence of this many children who have undergone such surgery may need speech therapy. Providing therapy is given early, there is no reason why a child should not grow up to have normal speech.

Laryngeal dystonia

Also known as spasmodic dysphonia, this condition involves involuntary movements of one or more muscles of the larynx, or voice box. The muscles may cause the vocal cords to open suddenly, stopping the air that flows over them from vibrating and resulting in a weak, breathy or whispery voice. Alternatively, the cords may stiffen and cut off the flow of air, causing the voice to sound strained or strangled. The disorder usually occurs in middle age, and it tends to run in families. It is sometimes treated by small injections of botulinum toxin (botox) in the larynx, which partially paralyses the muscles.

Stammering

About one per cent of adults and four per cent of children stammer. Stammering, also known as stuttering, can manifest itself in several different ways and lead to a variety of communication problems.

The cause of stammering is unknown, although recent brain-imaging studies suggest that it may occur as a result of the two hemispheres of the brain 'competing' for dominance – almost as though two people were trying to speak at the same time. Stammering usually starts between the ages of two and five, but most children grow out of it. Boys are five times more likely to have a stammer than girls. People generally do not stammer when they sing, whisper or cannot hear their own voice.

The degree to which people stammer varies widely. Some people who stammer have more natural control over their speech than others. And the degree of stammering depends on the particular situation, the difficulty of the words they need to speak, and how they feel, in general, at a particular moment. People who stammer report having 'good days' and 'bad days'.

Vocal cord paralysis

When one or both of the vocal cords or vocal folds fail to open or close properly vocal cord paralysis results. People with the condition experience abnormal voice changes, changes in voice quality and discomfort from vocal straining. Surgery and voice therapy are among the methods used to treat vocal cord paralysis. In some cases, the voice returns without treatment and so doctors often delay corrective surgery for at least a year to give the voice time to recover spontaneously.

Cancer of the throat

Treatment for throat cancer may involve a laryngectomy, that is, surgical removal of the voice box. Instead of breathing through the mouth, people who have undergone laryngectomy breathe through an opening in the neck called a stoma. After the operation, they have to learn to speak in an entirely different way in order to communicate with others. There are three ways in which this can be done.

■ Electro-laryngeal speech involves using a small hand-held device rather like an electric shaver that is placed against the neck. The device produces a vibration in the throat similar to the vibration of the lost vocal cords. Learning to use the device takes practice, but many people achieve very good results, although the voice produced in this way has a mechanical sound to it.

■ Oesophageal speech is produced by a person using the walls of the oesophagus (the muscular tube that leads to the stomach), rather than the vocal cords, to produce the controlled vibrations that make voice sounds. It is relatively easy to learn, and requires no devices or additional surgery. However, the voice tends to sound rough,

and it is difficult to produce sentences that are more than a few words long.

■ Tracheo-oesophageal speech is similar to oesophageal speech, but involves surgery to divert air into the oesophagus in order to produce more standard speech sounds.

SPEECH THERAPY

Speech and language therapists are trained to help with all types of speech and language disorders. They also help people experiencing swallowing problems.

The first appointment will usually involve taking a case history and carrying out an assessment of the client. This can take different forms depending on the client's age and particular problem. The diversity of the clients includes:

■ children with learning difficulties, speech or language delay;

■ people who stammer;

■ people who have progressive neurological conditions such as **multiple sclerosis, Parkinson's disease** and **motor neurone disease;**

■ people with voice disorders.

Speech therapy for children

Games are often employed with young children. A speech and language therapist may observe how a young child plays, as this indicates the child's level of language skills. The therapist will assess whether a child has understood what has been said to him or her, whether the child uses single words or words joined together and how the words are pronounced. The speech therapist will also check the mouth and palate for any physical abnormalities, as well as observing whether the child has any difficulties in eating or drinking.

After the assessment, the speech and language therapist will devise a treatment plan for the child which, where indicated, may involve individual or group sessions at the health clinic, school or home. Speech and language therapists who work with adults may see clients in hospital, day centres or at home.

SEE ALSO *Deafness; Learning difficulties*

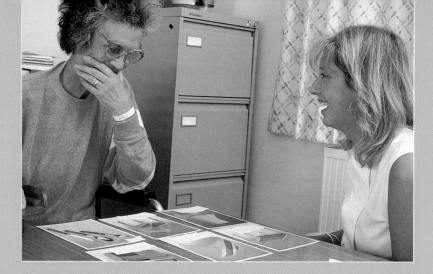

▲ **After a stroke**
A speech therapist uses pictures of familiar objects to help a woman who has aphasia after a stroke in the left side of her brain.

Spina bifida

Spina bifida is a birth defect characterized by incomplete closure of the spinal column. The term usually refers to myelomeningocele, the most severe form of the condition, in which a portion of the spinal cord protrudes from the back. The protrusion may occur anywhere along the spinal cord, but is most common in the lower back. The bulging nervous tissue may either be covered by skin or fully exposed.

Until recently, about one child in 1000 in the UK was born with spina bifida, but the incidence has fallen rapidly since it was found that folic acid supplements taken in pregnancy protect against the disorder.

DIAGNOSIS

The spinal cord normally closes within a few weeks of conception, so diagnosis is often made before birth by **ultrasound** or maternal blood tests. In other cases, spina bifida is not spotted until the child is born, when malformation of the spinal column makes the condition obvious. Most children with spina bifida also have **hydrocephalus**, an accumulation of fluid on the brain, which may cause the head to be swollen or misshapen.

TREATMENT

Surgery is generally performed within the first few days of life to close the opening. Its purpose is to protect the exposed cord from infection and to prevent further damage; it cannot put right damage that has already been done. If hydrocephalus is present, doctors will drain the excess fluid from the baby's skull; this should be done as quickly as possible after birth because buildup of fluid on the brain can cause mental retardation.

PROGNOSIS

The protrusion of the spinal cord damages it and causes permanent paralysis in the area of the body below the site. This means that the child cannot walk normally, and may be very weak in the hips and lower back, making sitting and balancing difficult. The degree of **disability** depends on where the protrusion occurs – the higher up the spine the more body area is affected by paralysis – and the amount of tissue that is exposed.

Depending on the degree of disability, the child may need a walking aid or a wheelchair. However, **physiotherapy** can help with mobility and promote a feeling of independence. Bladder and bowel control are likely to be affected, but can be relieved with the appropriate use of a catheter and laxatives.

CAUSES AND PREVENTION

Folic acid, one of the 'B' group of vitamins, is essential for normal neural development in

Types of spina bifida

There are three types of spina bifida: spina bifida occulta, meningocele and myelomeningocele.

Spina bifida occulta

This is the most common and least serious form. There is an opening in one or more of the vertebrae without apparent damage to the spinal cord. Research suggests that nearly 40 per cent of adults have the condition without being aware of it.

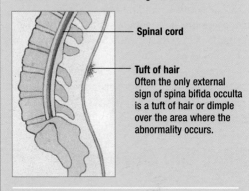

Spinal cord

Tuft of hair
Often the only external sign of spina bifida occulta is a tuft of hair or dimple over the area where the abnormality occurs.

Meningocele

This is where the protective covering around the spinal cord, but not the spinal cord itself, has pushed through an opening in the vertebrae. The problem can be easily repaired by surgery.

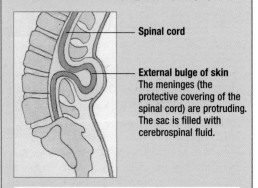

Spinal cord

External bulge of skin
The meninges (the protective covering of the spinal cord) are protruding. The sac is filled with cerebrospinal fluid.

Myelomeningocele

This is the most serious form of spina bifida, where the spinal cord is malformed and protrudes through a gap in the vertebrae. It results in severe disability.

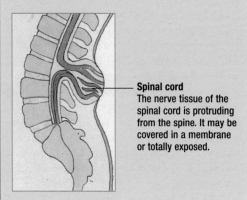

Spinal cord
The nerve tissue of the spinal cord is protruding from the spine. It may be covered in a membrane or totally exposed.

fetuses. Folic acid depletion in pregnant women is thought to be the major cause of spina bifida and other neural tube deficits. The vitamin is found in a wide range of foods, including green leafy vegetables, eggs, cereals and some fruits. Many women do not normally eat enough of these foods to ensure that, if they become pregnant, the fetus has a sufficient supply of folic acid. Pregnant women are therefore advised to take daily folic acid supplements of 0.4 mg. The most crucial period of neural development is the first few weeks after conception, so a woman should ideally take supplements whenever there is a chance of her becoming pregnant.

Parents of a child who has spina bifida should seek advice and support from their GP if they intend to have more children.

SEE ALSO *Pregnancy and problems*

Spine and disorders

The spine is a bony column running from the skull to the pelvis. It is made up of 33 bones called vertebrae. Each vertebra has a main body, a central canal that carries the spinal cord, and three bony protrusions to which ligaments and muscles are attached, one on either side and one that points backwards – the spinous process. Each vertebra is connected to its neighbour by a joint called a facet joint; these joints both strengthen the spine and allow it to move.

A BONY COLUMN OF VERTEBRAE

There are five groups of vertebrae: the cervical, thoracic, lumbar and sacral vertebrae and the coccyx. Each group has different characteristics. The seven cervical vertebrae, in the neck, are comparatively small and delicate. They have an extra canal on either side that carries blood vessels supplying blood to the brain. The twelve thoracic vertebrae, in the chest region, are similar to the cervical vertebrae but a little bigger. They have extra joints – called the costo-vertebral joints – to which the ribs are attached on either side. The five lumbar vertebrae, in the lower back, are thick and sturdy because they bear the greatest weight. The five sacral vertebrae, in the pelvis, are fused together and form the sacrum. This bony triangle is thick at the top and pointed at the bottom. It forms a joint with the pelvic bone called the sacro-iliac joint. At the base of the spine, the final group of four vertebrae are also fused together. These form a residual tailbone known as the coccyx.

Between each pair of vertebrae is a disc of cartilage with a jelly-like middle. These discs act as cushions, protecting the vertebrae by absorbing impact when we jump or run.

Spine and cross-section of a vertebra

Below is a cross-section of a cervical vertebra (from the neck). All vertebrae in the spine are jointed, making the spine strong and flexible.

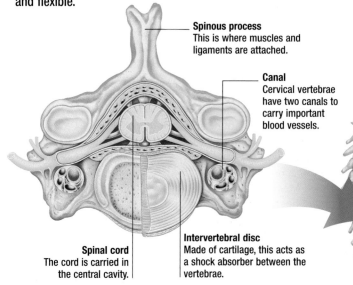

Spinous process
This is where muscles and ligaments are attached.

Canal
Cervical vertebrae have two canals to carry important blood vessels.

Spinal cord
The cord is carried in the central cavity.

Intervertebral disc
Made of cartilage, this acts as a shock absorber between the vertebrae.

Spine
The spine provides main skeletal support and protects the spinal cord.

What the spine does

The spine supports the head and body in an upright position and provides attachment sites for the ribs, ligaments and muscles of the back. It protects the delicate spinal cord from damage. The spine is also a reservoir for calcium and other minerals, while the main bodies of the vertebrae store the bone marrow that makes blood cells.

WHAT CAN GO WRONG

The vast majority of spinal problems are the result of soft-tissue damage, such as muscle strains and ligament sprains caused by poor posture, weak muscles, incorrect lifting techniques, osteoarthritis or **osteoporosis**. Osteoarthritis affects the joints in the spines of most people over 60. Osteoporosis, which causes a thinning and softening of bone, affects the spines of older women, in particular, and can cause the vertebrae to fracture.

The small percentage of other problems that affect the spine include conditions present at birth such as **spina bifida** and **scoliosis**, inflammatory diseases such as **ankylosing spondylitis**, fractures and bruising, slipped disc, facet joint injuries, stenosis and **cancers**.

Fractures and bruising

Various different types of fracture can affect the bones that form the spine.

■ A major **fracture** of the spine is rare unless it occurs as a result of an accident, such as a fall from a height, being struck by a heavy object or a car crash. But, if a vertebra is fractured, it can cause catastrophic injury to the spinal cord and nerves, leading to complete paralysis of the body below the site of the damage. Anyone who suspects that they have damaged their back in an accident should lie completely still until the emergency services arrive.

■ A minor 'avulsion' fracture happens when the tip of one of the vertebral bony protrusions is cracked or torn off. This usually occurs as a result of a sudden, violent muscular action. There is a sudden sharp pain at the affected vertebra, which returns if the same muscle is used again. The only treatment is to rest the area until it has healed and to take painkillers.

■ A small 'microfracture' can occur in a vertebral body or a facet joint. It is usually caused either by a minor accident, overuse of one area of the spine, or by lifting a heavy weight incorrectly. Most microfractures heal without treatment, but the area should be rested or supported during the healing process.

■ Crush fractures, in which the body of a vertebra collapses, are caused by a violent accident, such as a heavy object falling on the back, or result from osteoporosis.

■ Spondylolysis is a condition where there is a small crack in the arch round the spinal canal in a lumbar vertebra. It can occur as a result of injuries, especially a fall onto the buttocks, or through overuse in, for example, long-distance running. A susceptibility to this problem seems to run in families. A spondylolysis may go undetected and cause no problems, but sometimes it develops into a more serious condition called spondylolithesis, in which the crack in the arch widens and breaks right through. The vertebra is then poorly connected to its neighbour and slips, usually forward, out of alignment. The problem is more common in women than men and can also be a complication of osteoarthritis of the lumbar spine in elderly people.

■ A fall on the 'tailbone', or coccyx (see **Coccyx and problems**), can cause painful local bruising and occasionally a small crack in the bone. This problem, called coccydinia, can cause severe discomfort for several months, especially when sitting, but there is no specific treatment, other than to take painkillers while it heals.

Slipped disc

A slipped disc is more correctly known as a prolapsed disc. It happens when the outer shell of one of the cartilage discs that cushion the vertebrae is damaged in any way, allowing the inner jelly to protrude or leak out. The outer shell can crack as a result of a sudden, awkward movement such as bending and twisting. Often this does not cause any symptoms, but sometimes the prolapsed disc squashes nerves or ligaments outside the vertebra or puts pressure on the spinal cord inside it. In about half of cases, a prolapsed disc

clears up on its own within a few days, but if the pain is severe and the surrounding muscles go into spasm, recovery may take up to six weeks. Only about one case in twenty needs medical or surgical treatment.

Facet joint injury

The facet joints on either side of each vertebra connect it to its neighbours and limit the amount of movement possible between individual vertebra, giving the spine stability. These small joints are very vulnerable to damage. If a joint becomes inflamed, it can press on the surrounding tissues, causing pain in the area and **referred pain** in the buttock and leg (though there is no numbness or pins and needles). The facet joints can be injured by:

■ sudden, awkward movement;

■ dryness and shrinkage of intervertebral discs, allowing bone surfaces to grind together;

■ the onset of osteoarthritis, which causes joint inflammation.

Central canal stenosis

The spinal canal is normally wide enough not to compress the spinal cord inside it. But the cord is very sensitive to pressure, and even a small reduction in the diameter of the canal – known as stenosis – can cause severe pain, numbness, pins and needles, muscle weakness and bladder and bowel problems. There are three main causes of a central canal stenosis.

■ Congenital malformation of the canal: this is a condition present at birth in which the canal is either smaller than normal or not the usual circular shape. The spinal cord fits so snugly in the canal that the tiniest variation in the canal's size can damage nerves.

■ A prolapsed disc pushing into the spinal canal: this problem is more likely to affect people under 40, since the disc loses its fluid with age and is less likely to prolapse.

■ Osteoarthritic changes: bony outgrowths may grow into the spinal canal, reducing its diameter. This problem mainly affects the lumbar spine area in elderly people.

Cancers

Several cancers may affect the spine. A tumour may originate in the spine or, more commonly, it may be secondary, which means that the original cancer started elsewhere in the body and has spread to the spine. Some back cancers affect the bones, some the lining of the spinal cord or nerves and some the soft tissues nearby.

The signs and symptoms of spinal tumours depend on the type of tumour and its site. The pain of most bone cancers is worse at night.

SEE ALSO *Back and back pain*

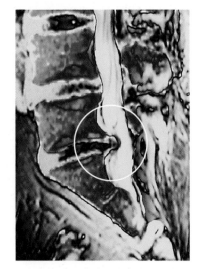

▲ **Slipped disc**
A magnetic resonance image shows a slipped disc (dark blue) that is protruding into the spinal cord (light beige).

Spleen and disorders

The spleen is a fist-sized, dark purple, bean-shaped organ that lies in the upper left part of the abdomen, behind the lower ribs and just under the diaphragm. It plays an important part in a person's immune system. The spleen is part of the **lymphatic system** and, like the lymph nodes, it contains lymphocytes that make antibodies. These antibodies weaken or kill bacteria, viruses and other organisms that cause infection.

Blood is brought to the spleen by a large artery called the splenic artery. If blood passing through the spleen contains any damaged or worn-out red blood cells, white blood cells called phagocytes in the spleen will engulf and destroy those cells and clear them from the bloodstream. This ensures that the red blood cells in circulation are kept healthy. The spleen also manufactures new infection-fighting white blood cells, and helps to regulate the number of red blood cells circulating in the body.

AN EMERGENCY BACK-UP

In the fetus, the spleen produces red blood cells. After birth, red blood cells are normally formed in the bone marrow, but the spleen continues to contain a small number of immature red blood cells. In times of great need, these cells are able to divide and replace any of the blood cells that are missing. This can occur, for example, in certain severe types of anaemia or if the bone marrow becomes diseased and stops producing red blood cells.

Despite the importance of the spleen's various functions, it is not an essential organ. This means that people can survive without their spleen if, for any reason, it has to be surgically removed. In this case, the organ's function will largely be taken over by other parts of the immune system and the liver.

WHAT CAN GO WRONG

The spleen is usually so small that it cannot be felt by a doctor pressing on the abdomen. However, it can enlarge to several times its normal size and become firmer, in which case it can be felt under the ribs on the left side. Many conditions can cause this to happen, including various viral infections, blood diseases and cancers. One of the most common causes of an enlarged spleen, especially in adolescents, is **glandular fever** (infectious mononucleosis), usually caused by the Epstein-Barr virus. This can be dangerous because an enlarged spleen is easily ruptured – in a rugby tackle, for example – and could cause a life-threatening loss of blood. For this reason, anyone with an enlarged spleen must avoid contact sports.

Even if the spleen is not enlarged, it can be ruptured by a fall, an industrial injury or a serious car crash. The large size of the artery supplying the spleen means that the danger from rupture is severe internal bleeding. Even relatively minor damage to a normal spleen can cause an internal haemorrhage requiring emergency treatment. And if the spleen is already enlarged for any reason, it is far more vulnerable to injury.

The medical term for an enlarged spleen is splenomegaly. It can be caused by any of the following conditions.

- Infections, such as septicaemia, glandular fever, tuberculosis, brucellosis, and certain tropical diseases, including malaria and sleeping sickness.
- Blood diseases, such as leukaemia (especially chronic myeloid leukaemia) and certain types of anaemia in which the red cells are abnormal,

A sophisticated filter

The spleen is the body's main blood filter. It removes the waste products generated by the constant breakdown of red blood cells. It also manufactures new antibodies and lymphocytes that help the body to fight infection.

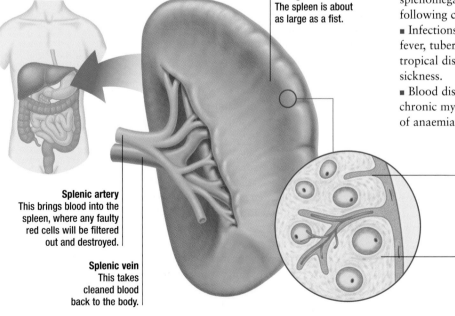

Enlarged view
The spleen is about as large as a fist.

Splenic artery
This brings blood into the spleen, where any faulty red cells will be filtered out and destroyed.

Splenic vein
This takes cleaned blood back to the body.

Outer casing
Many fibrous bands run into the spleen from the casing to form a kind of sponge.

Lymph tissue
This mass of pulpy material is mostly made up of lymphocytes and red blood cells.

and are destroyed prematurely by the spleen, as occurs in haemolytic anaemia (see **Blood and disorders**).

■ Diseases of the bone marrow, such as myelofibrosis, in which the marrow fails and the spleen has to start producing blood cells, or myeloproliferative disease, in which the bone marrow becomes overactive so that the spleen has to destroy more blood cells than usual (see **Bone marrow and disorders**).

■ Inflammatory diseases including rheumatoid arthritis, sarcoidosis and systemic lupus erythematosis.

■ Other conditions, including **cirrhosis of the liver** and syphilis.

Hypersplenism

When the spleen becomes grossly enlarged it may lead to hypersplenism, which can cause the following symptoms.

■ Pallor, tiredness and shortness of breath, if the spleen's indiscriminate destruction of red blood cells has caused anaemia.

■ Abnormal bleeding, usually into the skin, which will appear as bruises or tiny red spots, but also elsewhere, such as in the kidneys, resulting in blood in the urine. This happens because the enlarged spleen destroys too many platelets, thereby disrupting the blood-clotting mechanism.

■ Increased susceptibility to infection, if there are insufficient white cells to fight it.

REMOVAL OF THE SPLEEN

Surgical removal of the spleen is called splenectomy. It is most frequently performed as an emergency operation after an injury to the spleen has resulted in internal haemorrhage. If the outer casing of the spleen has been damaged, bleeding is usually severe because the spleen is an organ with a plentiful supply of blood. Since the spleen is difficult to repair surgically, the only way to stop the bleeding is to seal off the artery that supplies the organ and to remove the spleen itself.

The spleen may also be removed when it has become enlarged as a result of a tumour. The most likely cancers to affect the spleen are Hodgkin's disease, lymphosarcoma and other malignant lymphomas. Splenectomy may also be recommended when:

■ an underlying condition results in hypersplenism;

■ there is bleeding under the skin, (of the type idiopathic thromocytopenic purpura) because the spleen has removed too many platelets;

■ a person suffers from a type of anaemia in which the red cells are an abnormal shape and are too rapidly removed by the spleen.

A splenectomy is a major operation and usually means staying in hospital for a week to 10 days, although some surgeons are now able to remove the spleen using **keyhole surgery**. Since the spleen plays such an important role in removing infection-causing bacteria from the bloodstream, patients who have had a splenectomy are very vulnerable to infection. So, before the operation, vaccinations are given to protect patients from the most harmful of these organisms: *Streptococcus pneumoniae*, which causes pneumonia among other infections, and HiB, which can cause serious lung infection and bacterial meningitis. Most people will then also need to take lifelong antibiotics and should keep a 'medic alert' card or bracelet with them at all times.

SEE ALSO *Lymphatic system*

Spots

A spot is a small, discoloured mark or lump on the skin. When raised, and due to infection, it may be referred to as a pimple. The term for a number of spots appearing together is a rash.

The medical name for a small, discoloured area that feels the same as the surrounding skin – a freckle, for example – is a macule. A spot that feels different from the surrounding skin is a papule. A rash that both looks and feels different from the surrounding skin is called a maculopapular rash. A spot that forms a fluid-filled swelling may be known as a vesicle, blister or cyst, depending on its size and solidity. Milia, small keratin cysts, popularly known as whiteheads, are a common type of white papule that forms on the face.

Seek medical advice if you have any persistent skin blemish.

Sterilization

Sterilization is a permanent and often non-reversible surgical procedure that results in **infertility** – the inability to reproduce. People choose to be sterilized for many reasons. For those who do not wish to have children, it is a convenient method of contraception; others may opt for sterilization because there is a high risk that a child would be affected by a serious hereditary disorder.

FEMALE STERILIZATION

Female sterilization is performed under general anaesthetic and involves clipping or cutting the Fallopian tubes (known as tubal occlusion) so that an egg cannot reach the uterus. One in 200 women in the UK becomes pregnant some time after a tubal occlusion, and if this happens there is an increased risk of ectopic pregnancy.

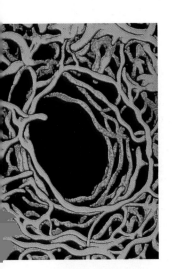

▲ **A fibrous framework**
This coloured electron micrograph of a section of spleen shows its fibrous, almost spongy texture.

Reversal of the procedure does not always work and may not be available on the NHS.

A **hysterectomy**, the surgical removal of the uterus, also results in sterilization. It may be performed to treat cancer of the womb or some other serious gynaecological problem.

MALE STERILIZATION

The procedure for male sterilization is known as a vasectomy. A small section of the vas deferens, the tube that carries sperm from the testes to the penis, is removed. This has no effect on the sexual drive or on the ejaculation of semen. Traces of sperm may be present for up to 16 weeks after the operation and an alternative form of contraception should be used until a sperm count confirms that the vasectomy is working. Reversal of the procedure does not always work and may not be available on the NHS.

SEE ALSO *Contraception; Reproductive system; Uterus and problems*

Stomach and disorders

The stomach is a large, muscular sac situated in the upper left abdomen and separated from the left lung and the heart by the diaphragm. It is divided into two parts: the body (corpus) and the antrum. The gullet (oesophagus) opens into the corpus, the larger part, but is separated from it by a circular band of muscle called the cardiac sphincter. The antrum is the area of stomach closest to the duodenum, separated from it by the pyloric sphincter. Both sphincters act as one-way valves, ensuring that food passes only in one direction.

The stomach lining contains glands that secrete acidic gastric juices and mucus. The mucus is alkaline, and forms a protective barrier that prevents the stomach lining from being damaged by these juices.

FUNCTIONS OF THE STOMACH

The stomach acts as a reservoir for food and can contain up to 1.5 litres (2½–3 pints) of it at any one time. This storage facility means that we can eat just a few times a day rather than every half hour or so.

As food enters the corpus the glands in the mucous membrane secrete: hydrochloric acid; a precursor chemical called pepsinogen; and a protein called intrinsic factor, required for the absorption of vitamin B_{12} in the small intestine. The hydrochloric acid breaks down foods that are not soluble in water, disinfects the contents of the stomach by destroying bacteria and other micro-organisms and changes pepsinogen into the stomach enzyme pepsin (which breaks down proteins). The antrum of the stomach releases

Stomach muscles and lining
Contractions of the stomach's muscular walls churn and thoroughly mix any food arriving there with the strong digestive juices secreted by its lining.

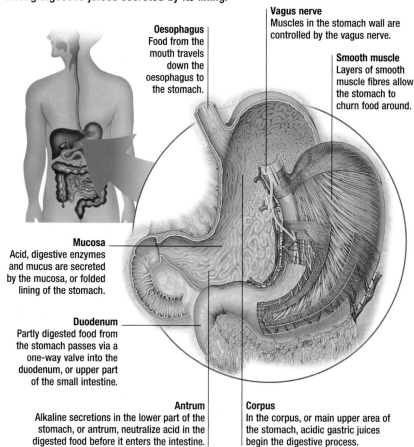

Vagus nerve
Muscles in the stomach wall are controlled by the vagus nerve.

Oesophagus
Food from the mouth travels down the oesophagus to the stomach.

Smooth muscle
Layers of smooth muscle fibres allow the stomach to churn food around.

Mucosa
Acid, digestive enzymes and mucus are secreted by the mucosa, or folded lining of the stomach.

Duodenum
Partly digested food from the stomach passes via a one-way valve into the duodenum, or upper part of the small intestine.

Antrum
Alkaline secretions in the lower part of the stomach, or antrum, neutralize acid in the digested food before it enters the intestine.

Corpus
In the corpus, or main upper area of the stomach, acidic gastric juices begin the digestive process.

mucus, dilute sodium bicarbonate (so that the acidic juices are modified before they enter the duodenum) and a hormone called gastrin.

The release of pepsin stimulates the muscles of the stomach wall to contract weakly in a wave pattern (peristalsis). This mixes the food thoroughly with the gastric juices, the final mixture being known as chyme. Stronger peristaltic contractions then pulp the chyme and push it down to the pyloric sphincter. The pyloric sphincter opens with each contraction and allows a small part of chyme through.

WHAT CAN GO WRONG

The complex process of digestion can be affected by imbalances in the gastric juices.

Overproduction of gastric juices

If the stomach produces too much gastric juice, the lining of the stomach can become inflamed (**gastritis**). The condition can be acute, chronic or atrophic (resulting in the loss of the stomach's secretory glands).

Underproduction of gastric juices

Too little gastric juice results in a susceptibility to bacterial infections, such as **salmonella** and shigellosis (see **Dysentery**).

Overproduction of gastrin

If the stomach releases too much of the hormone gastrin it can result in a duodenal **ulcer**, **heartburn**, diarrhoea and steatorrhea (undigested fat in the stools). Causes include a certain type of tumour (a gastrinoma) that secretes gastrin, and a high-protein diet that stimulates gastrin production.

Underproduction of gastrin

Too little gastrin may result from too much fat or too much acid in the chyme. The stomach muscles will be less effective and the time food spends in the stomach will be increased.

Gastric ulcer

Gastric ulcers are a common condition in late middle-age (see **Ulcer**).

Cancer of the stomach

Stomach cancer is the sixth most common cancer among adults in the UK. Worldwide, there are marked geographical differences in incidence: high in Japan, for example, but low in the USA. The UK incidence is higher than that of the USA: more than 10,000 people are diagnosed with the disease each year. Eight out of ten of these are aged over 60 and more men than women are affected. Overall, the incidence of stomach cancer has fallen since the 1930s, but the incidence of cancer near the cardiac sphincter has increased. More than 90 per cent of stomach cancers start in the glands that produce mucus and gastric juices. Several risk factors have been identified.

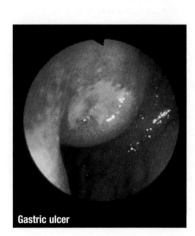
Gastric ulcer

■ Diet: pickled, smoked, barbecued, salty and preserved foods that contain nitrites increase the risk of stomach cancer.
■ Bacteria: *Helicobacter pylori*, a common bacterium that affects many people and is associated with gastric ulcers, is thought to increase the risk three-fold, but it also seems to have a protective effect against cancer around the cardiac sphincter. An infection can be cured by a course of antibiotics.
■ Blood group A: there is a statistical link between having this blood group and a higher risk of stomach cancer. This indicates that there may be a genetic predisposition to the disease.
■ Certain medical conditions: pernicious **anaemia** and atrophic **gastritis**, which both cause less acid to be produced in the stomach. This may allow more bacteria to survive and it is thought that the nitrite chemicals the bacteria release may cause cancer. Past surgery for a gastric ulcer is also a risk factor. It is thought that this may be because bile juices from the duodenum tend to regurgitate after some types of surgery and irritate the lining of the stomach.

■ Smoking and drinking alcohol: both have been linked to stomach cancer – drinking beer, in particular, increases the risk. Tobacco and alcohol both contain nitrites and other chemicals that irritate the lining of the stomach.

The symptoms of stomach cancer include:
■ indigestion;
■ stomach acidity and belching;
■ feeling full after eating a small amount, and so losing weight;
■ vomiting, difficulty in swallowing and pain;
■ anaemia and blood in the stools, as a result of bleeding from the tumour;
■ a high risk of a **deep vein thrombosis** (DVT).

In all but the most advanced stages, treatment is **gastrectomy** – removal of the stomach – followed by **chemotherapy**. If the cancer has spread and is at an advanced stage then treatment is palliative and aimed at relieving symptoms.

SEE ALSO *Cancer; Digestive system; Oesophagus and disorders*

Stones in the urinary tract

Stones (known as calculi) can form anywhere in the urinary tract, and may occur in the kidneys, ureters or bladder. About three out of four stones are made up of calcium oxalate and calcium phosphate. Some urinary stones result from chronic urinary tract infection or metabolic abnormalities, such as **gout** or hyperparathyroidism (a disorder of the parathyroid gland), but in many cases, there is no obvious cause. Kidney stones can cause severe pain (renal colic) and blood in the urine, while bladder stones can cause urinary difficulties and a complete blockage of urinary outflow.

SEE ALSO *Urinary system*

Strains

Strains arise after overuse or overstretching of muscles, often a result of sporting activity. The term is sometimes used in the same sense as sprains. Symptoms are pain and swelling, and treatment is with a cold compress or ice-pack to discourage further swelling. Firm bandaging achieves a similar effect, and raising the injured part above the level of the heart also helps.

This should be followed by painkillers, if necessary, and resting the affected part to allow healing to occur. A poultice may also help to ease symptoms. To prevent stiffness, gentle movement and exercises should be started as soon as the immediate symptoms subside.

Stress

Brief episodes of stress can raise our energy levels and improve performance. But high levels of stress on a regular basis can damage our physical and mental health and lead to life-threatening diseases.

Stress is something we all encounter at some time in our lives, no matter what our circumstances. It is an unavoidable part of being alive. When we are faced with change, or threatened or challenged in any way, we come under stress. How we respond varies from person to person. A situation that one person finds intolerable may be stimulating and exciting to another. Too little stimulation, resulting in boredom, can also cause problems, which is why some people may feel more stressed after they have retired from work than when they were doing a highly demanding job.

'FIGHT OR FLIGHT' RESPONSE

Stress affects us not only mentally but can bring about physical changes too. In fact, our bodies' response to stress clearly illustrates the way in which our mental health can be directly linked to physical problems.

Animals respond to danger by turning to face the fight or fleeing. This is called the 'fight or flight' response. Human beings share this automatic bodily reaction, and we respond to emotional stress as if it were a physical threat. You may only be having an argument with a colleague at work, but you are physically ready for a life-or-death struggle with a lion. Your muscles grow tense, ready for action, your heart beats faster, your blood pressure goes up, you breathe faster and sweat more, and your mouth becomes dry. These physical reactions are caused by the release of adrenaline and other hormones into the bloodstream.

The reason why different people react differently to stress is because the intensity of the hormone response varies from person to person, according to lifestyle and genetic make-up. Your personality affects how stressful you judge a situation to be and how you deal with it. A troubled childhood may make you more vulnerable to stress, while being in a supportive relationship or family situation is thought to give some protection from stress.

STRESS TRIGGERS

In modern life, stress is most likely to be caused by worries concerning your job, finances, health, personal life or surroundings that make you feel under constant pressure. Generally speaking, stress arises from events that create a sense of anxiety, uncertainty or loss.

In addition, a feeling of being out of control frequently accompanies such events. If you feel in control of your life, you will often still function well despite being subjected to a constant flow of highly demanding situations.

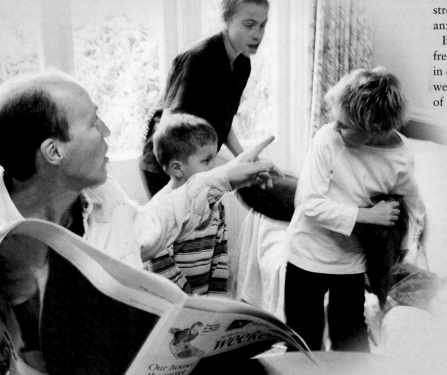

◀ **Family strife**
When a person is feeling the effects of stress even the day-to-day games among siblings can seem almost intolerable.

Stressful life events

A number of common life events have been graded according to the amount of stress they tend to generate. The extent of stress caused by any particular event varies considerably from person to person.

VERY HIGH STRESS FACTORS	MODERATE STRESS FACTORS
Death of partner or close family member	Large mortgage
Divorce or separation	More arguments than usual with partner
Imprisonment	Changed responsibilities at work
Personal injury or illness	Problems with boss
Getting married	Son or daughter leaving home
Loss of a job	Outstanding personal achievement

HIGH STRESS FACTORS	LOW STRESS FACTORS
Death of close friend	Change in work hours or conditions
Moving to a new home	Change in sleeping habits
Marital reconciliation	Holiday
Sexual problems	Christmas
Pregnancy and having a baby	
Retirement	
Change in finances	

RESPONDING TO STRESS

Experiencing a certain amount of stress can result in a surge of energy that will help you to achieve your goals in life. Without it, you may not be alert enough to perform well or to make appropriate changes should any difficulties or obstacles arise.

However, problems tend to occur when you are constantly reacting to stressful situations without taking, or feeling you are able to take, any action to counter their effects.

When someone is under too much stress for too long, it can threaten their health and well-being. The resulting continual rise in levels of adrenaline can lead to the development of certain illnesses. These may be relatively minor such as insomnia, backache or headaches, but stress has also been identified as as contributory factor in several potentially life-threatening conditions, including high blood pressure and heart disease.

Some people have a good awareness of their stress levels – even if they succumb to stress easily, they know how to recognize its symptoms and to deal with them effectively – while others fail to recognize their condition or try to cope by ignoring it. It is common for people affected by stress to turn to alcohol, cigarettes, tranquillizers or other drugs as a way of dealing with the problem. But such responses can eventually cause physical, emotional and behavioural problems, which can also affect their health and peace of mind. These problems can have an impact on relationships at home and in the workplace.

SIGNS OF STRESS

Stress shows itself in various ways. If you are under stress, you may notice a number of the following physical, emotional or behavioural signs.

Physical signs
- Breathlessness or palpitations.
- Muscle cramps, aches or spasms.
- Constipation or diarrhoea.
- Headaches, migraines or backache.
- Skin problems such as eczema or acne.
- Tiredness or insomnia.
- Panic attacks.
- Asthma.
- Frequent colds.

Emotional signs
- Irritability or impatience.
- Depression.
- Anxiety and fear.
- Tearfulness.
- Anger or aggression.
- Mood swings.
- Inability to express or feel emotion.

Behavioural signs
- Difficulty concentrating.
- Problems making decisions.
- Eating, smoking or drinking more.
- Emotional outbursts.
- Never finishing anything.
- Losing sense of humour.
- Withdrawing from social activities.

COMBATING STRESS

The key to managing stress is to know your personal tolerance for stressful situations and to try to live within these limits. You can keep stress under control if you learn to recognize the signs of it in yourself and take action to counteract it. There is plenty you can do to deal with stress or reduce the stress in your life. But you should always remember that lasting change will not come overnight. It will take persistence. It may even be necessary to make big changes in your lifestyle in order to reduce your stress levels.

The best stress treatments are those that help you to manage stress yourself, which involve specific relaxation exercises, which you can use when you are alone. You will need to seek professional help for other treatments, such as medication, talking therapy or **complementary therapies**. Your first point of contact should be your GP, who may treat you personally or refer you to a counsellor or other practitioner.

Active relaxation therapy
One type of relaxation therapy involves a combination of controlled deep breathing and muscle relaxation, often using progressive muscle relaxation – in which you tense and release muscles.

Meditation

Most relaxation involves some form of meditation – where the mind and body are still and you take 'time out' from your surroundings. It involves sitting in a comfortable position, with closed eyes, and steering your attention away from your racing thoughts. Staring at a candle flame, visualizing a peaceful place, concentrating on a symbol or repeating a particular sound (mantra) may help to focus your attention. The aim is to reach a state of 'being' with no movement or sensation.

Meditation can change the heart rate and breathing, helping to reduce stress. As thoughts slow down, tension in the body drops and feelings of calm, peace and detachment can fill the mind and the body.

It is possible to learn meditation from a book or tape, or from a teacher. But, if full meditation is not for you, then 10–20 minutes each day of quiet reflection may help to alleviate your stress levels. You could use the time to listen to music and try to think of pleasant things – or of nothing at all.

Exercise

Exercise helps to release physical tension and the mental effects of stress. It uses up the adrenaline and other hormones that the body produces under stress, and relaxes the muscles. It improves strength, stamina and resilience, and heart and blood circulation also benefit. For some people, an exercise session is an ideal way to throw themselves into an activity and forget about whatever is troubling them. For other people, a run or swim might provide an opportunity to focus on and resolve a problem.

Physical activity also makes you feel better. This is because it releases mood-improving chemicals, known as endorphins, into your bloodstream. These can raise your level of self-esteem, reduce any feelings of anxiety or depression, and help you to sleep better. An aerobic exercise, such as walking, cycling or swimming, performed for 20–30 minutes three times a week, is a good antidote to stress. Yoga is another exercise option, and one that many people turn to for stress relief. It is a workout for the body and mind that can be used safely by most people. But any activity is helpful. You do not have to take up a competitive sport; simply become more active as part of your daily routine. Try walking to the shops rather than driving there; use the stairs rather than the lift; take a walk during your lunch break; get off the bus a few stops before home and walk the rest of the way. But always remember to build up your activity gradually: too much too quickly could make you feel even more stressed.

Talking things over

Talking about your feelings to your friends and family is important when you are under stress. But if you want to get to the bottom of recurring problems, such as failed relationships, or if you simply want to understand your situation better, it may be helpful to see a qualified counsellor, psychotherapist or psychologist. You can go to one privately – the British Association of Counsellors and Psychotherapists has a list of practitioners – or you could ask your GP to refer you for talking therapy on the NHS. Some GPs run stress clinics of their own, where a combination of practical advice and talking therapy is available. Contact your local health authority to find out which GPs offer this service.

Medicines for stress

Some GPs prescribe tranquillizers, such as Valium, for stress and anxiety. These drugs will not help you to deal with the cause of your stress, but they can help you to get through a crisis. Since tranquillizers are addictive, you should be given a low dose for a few days only.

Complementary therapies

Massage can help to relax your body and give you a feeling of emotional well-being. It offers relief from stress, anxiety and headaches, with special benefits for alleviating tension in the neck, back and shoulders. You can visit a massage therapist for a full massage. Alternatively, you can perform a home massage: lie down, close your eyes gently and massage your face and head for about 15 minutes. This will help to relieve a headache or just make you feel better after a stressful day.

Aromatherapy massage (with essential oils) or reflexology (foot massage) can also help you to relax. Aromatherapy is also ideal for self-help treatment – add a few drops of a relaxing oil such as lavender to a warm bath or use it in a burner to scent a room. The herbal remedies valerian and passiflora are included in many over-the-counter stress treatments because they have sedative properties.

The **Alexander technique** is helpful too, especially for stress-related conditions such as anxiety, breathing disorders and back, neck and joint pain.

SEE ALSO *Anxiety; Depression; Panic attacks*

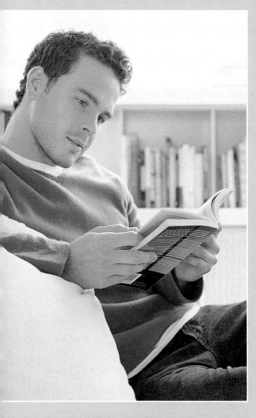

▲ **Be good to yourself**
Set aside time to do something you enjoy such as reading, listening to music or gardening.

Stroke

A stroke disrupts the blood supply to the brain and is the greatest single cause of severe disability in the UK. But in many cases, the brain's adaptability allows damaged cells to recover some of their function.

Of those who survive a stroke around 50 per cent are left with severe disability, but better drugs and intensive rehabilitation therapies are improving the outlook for people who have a stroke. Scientists are also discovering that we can do a lot to reduce the risk of stroke, with a healthier lifestyle and regular checkups.

WHAT IS A STROKE?

A stroke occurs when the flow of blood to part of the brain is disrupted. When this is due to a blockage of one of the arteries that supply the brain with blood, it is called an ischaemic stroke. Arteries can become blocked when the inner lining of the blood vessel is damaged, allowing a blood clot to form around the diseased area. As other cells clump around the blood clot in an effort to patch up the damage, the blood vessel becomes progressively narrower until little or no blood can get through.

Less often, a stroke occurs when an artery bursts and blood leaks into nearby brain tissues. This is called a haemorrhagic stroke. If the bleed occurs beneath the arachnoid membrane (one of three layers of tissue protecting the brain) it is called a subarachnoid haemorrhage.

Starved of blood or swamped in it, nerve cells quickly start to die. Dying cells release chemicals that destroy neighbouring cells in a cascade effect, leading to varying amounts of brain damage.

Every year, in the UK, about 1000 people under 30 years old have a stroke.

SYMPTOMS

The symptoms of a stroke depend on which part of the brain is affected. They include:
- muscle weakness or paralysis, numbness or pins and needles on one side of the body;
- speech difficulties (slurring or problems finding the right word);
- double vision or loss of vision on one side;
- confusion;
- dizziness;
- headache and vomiting;
- drowsiness or unconsciousness.

Because of the way nerve pathways from the brain to the spinal cord are 'wired', weakness and paralysis usually occur on the opposite side of the body to the side of the brain where the stroke has occurred. Persistent speech problems are most common following a stroke in the left side of the brain, where the language centre is generally found.

Anyone who experiences one or more symptoms of a stroke should see a doctor immediately. If the symptoms are severe, call for an ambulance.

INVESTIGATIONS

If a stroke is suspected, hospital tests will be needed. These will include:
- a physical examination and checks for weakness, numbness and other symptoms;
- blood tests;
- an ECG (electrocardiogram) to monitor heart rhythm, and a brain scan;
- a CT (computed tomography) scan, to distinguish between an ischaemic stroke caused by a blocked artery and a haemorrhagic stroke due to a burst blood vessel. This is very important, as the treatment of an ischaemic stroke is different from that used in the case of a haemorrhagic stroke.

Some hospitals do magnetic resonance imaging (MRI) rather than CT scans. While CT uses X-rays to produce pictures of the brain and its blood vessels, MRI uses magnetism. MRI can produce more detailed pictures and may pick up signs of a bleed for a longer period after a haemorrhage than is possible with a CT scan.

MEDICAL TREATMENT

Before deciding on a suitable course of treatment for someone who has suffered a stroke, a doctor will order tests to determine whether their stroke was ischaemic or haemorrhagic. Only then can the appropriate treatment be started.

Drug treatments

If the scan confirms an ischaemic stroke, initial treatment is likely to involve taking anti-clotting drugs to reduce the risk of blood clots forming in any blood vessels to the brain or other parts of the body. Aspirin is the most commonly used anti-clotting drug because it prevents the particles (platelets) that form the core of a clot from sticking together.

But two other agents, dipyridamole and clopidogrel, which reduce the risk of clots in

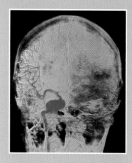

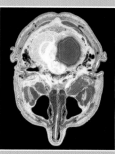

▲ **Causes of Stroke**
Top: If an aneurysm occurs in arteries supplying the brain, its rupture results in a stroke.
Bottom: A less common cause of stroke is an internal bleed due to a burst artery.

slightly different ways, may be used instead of, or in addition to, aspirin.

Warfarin, another anti-clotting agent, is often used to treat people who have a stroke due to a blood clot that formed in their heart and moved to a blood vessel in the brain. Such clots usually arise in the heart as a result of an abnormal heart rhythm (atrial fibrillation). Anyone taking warfarin needs regular blood tests to make sure that their blood does not become too thin.

Clearly, anti-clotting drugs are not suitable for someone whose stroke is due to a haemorrhage in their brain since this could make the bleeding worse. Hence the importance of having a brain scan as soon as possible after a stroke to distinguish between an ischaemic and a haemorrhagic stroke.

Many people who suffer a stroke have high **blood pressure**. Once their condition has stabilized, they are likely to be prescribed drugs to reduce their blood pressure. Latest research suggests that even people with relatively normal blood pressure may also benefit from lowering it after a stroke.

High **cholesterol** is another problem linked to strokes, and some people will also be given drugs to reduce their cholesterol levels.

Other treatments

Further tests carried out within a few days or weeks after a stroke may show that other treatments are needed. These tests include an **ultrasound** scan of the heart (echocardiogram) to check for disease, or an ultrasound scan of the carotid arteries in the neck. These are the main blood vessels that supply the brain with blood and, if they are partially blocked, an operation may be needed to clear away the blockage.

The operation is called a carotid endarterectomy, and it may be recommended for people who have a 70–90 per cent blockage in one or both of their carotid arteries. If the blockage is less than this, surgery is not worthwhile, and if the arteries are completely blocked, then surgery is not an option.

During a carotid endarterectomy, the surgeon makes an incision in the neck and opens the carotid artery at the point where it is partially blocked. The obstruction is carefully scraped out and, if necessary, synthetic tubing is inserted into the artery to replace the damaged tissue. The procedure may sound dramatic but patients are soon up and about and can go home within a few days. In some cases the operation is performed under local rather than general anaesthetic.

LIVING WITH A STROKE

The brain is remarkably adaptable, and in the months and years following a stroke many of the damaged cells recover some of their function. At the same time, other areas of the brain take over the functions performed by cells that have died. Recovery time for stroke patients is very variable, but most people have a surge of recovery in the early weeks following a stroke. A slower period of continued recovery may then take a year to 18 months or more.

Most people need some form of rehabilitation therapy after a stroke to help them to overcome or cope with the effects that the stroke has had on their daily lives. Rehabilitation therapy aims to encourage and enhance the recovery process and should be tailored to each individual's problems (for example, movement, speech, bladder, bowel, vision, emotions). Rehabilitation should start as soon as possible as it can greatly improve recovery from a stroke, as well as reduce the effects of disability.

Rehabilitation helps people to relearn skills and abilities that have been lost as a result of a stroke. It may also teach new skills to overcome certain disabilities or new ways of adapting to some limitations caused by the stroke. Rehabilitation is designed to help people to live as independently as possible – managing their cooking, shopping and getting around inside and outside the home – it will also guide them towards any social, emotional and practical support they may need.

Rehabilitation is most successful when it is carried out by a team of different specialists working together. These are likely to include doctors, nurses, physiotherapists, occupational therapists, speech and language therapists, dietitians, continence advisers, counsellors and social workers.

The first step is to assess how much disability has occurred and work out goals and targets for treatment, according to the person's physical and emotional needs, home situation, social and leisure interests and priorities. For example, one person's priority might be to continue managing his or her garden; while others might want to be able to continue cooking, painting or taking part in a drama group or choir.

Physiotherapy

Physiotherapy uses specific exercises, techniques and massage to keep muscles and joints working. Ideally, a course of physiotherapy should begin as soon as possible (within one or two days) after a stroke and continue for as long as it is useful. The aims can range from preventing muscle spasms in someone who is chair or bed-bound to enabling them to get back on their feet. Other stroke patients may need to relearn how to sit, stand, walk and perform other everyday activities. Movements are built up gradually and may take several months to achieve. The exercises need to be practised as often as possible.

After a stroke it is natural for patients to try to use the unaffected side of their body to keep moving about independently. A physiotherapist will discourage this over-compensation with the unaffected side of the body, and encourage the patient to use both sides of their body to regain balance and movement.

Physiotherapy usually begins at the earliest opportunity in hospital, with the patient returning for sessions as an outpatient following discharge. If someone has a mild stroke that does not require hospital treatment, a physiotherapist will visit them at home to advise the patient and their carer on safe ways to move about at home, get dressed and use the bathroom.

Occupational therapy

Occupational therapy is aimed at finding practical solutions to problems with washing, dressing, eating, bathing, walking up stairs or other everyday activities. It may involve learning new skills or techniques or adapting the home to make life easier.

Speech therapy

The aim of speech therapy is to help someone with speech problems after a stroke to communicate more effectively. This may include helping people to form the sounds of speech, to use clues and cues to find words, or to use gestures, word and picture charts, writing, drawing or computers.

Other forms of support

Other therapists may be called upon to provide rehabilitation, but this will depend on the type of disability. In addition to the confusion and troubled thinking that many people experience after a stroke, some become anxious or depressed about what has happened to them. This is a perfectly natural reaction. Talking to family and friends may help, but counselling and other forms of psychological support may also be worthwhile.

Much of the improvement that occurs after a stroke happens quite quickly in the weeks or months after the event. But people continue to get better for a long time after a stroke, especially if they can learn or relearn skills and techniques to overcome their disabilities. Although much of the formal rehabilitation occurs in the immediate weeks after a stroke, it is never too late to ask for further assessment and help months or even years after a stroke.

PREVENTION

There is much that you can do to reduce your risk of having a stroke.

■ Don't smoke: smoking doubles the risk of the arterial damage that can lead to blockages, transient ischaemic attack and stroke. Quitting can halve your risk of a stroke – whatever your age or however long you have smoked.

Stroke warning

While a stroke occurs suddenly for many people, others have a warning that they are at risk.

This warning takes the form of a 'mini-stroke' or transient ischaemic attack (TIA). The symptoms are similar to those of a stroke (weakness, tingling, blurred vision, slurred speech, confusion), but they only last from a few minutes up to 24 hours. The cause of a TIA is nearly always the same as that of an ischaemic stroke – an obstruction in an artery that supplies the brain with blood. But the blockage moves so that the blood supply is restored before any damage is done to the brain.

This type of warning should not be ignored. It requires the same tests and investigations as a full stroke and, if a TIA is confirmed, similar treatment. Without treatment, someone who suffers a TIA has a 10 per cent chance of having a stroke within the following 12 months and a 5 per cent chance after that. It is therefore important for an affected person to be assessed for anti-clotting drugs and for treatment with drugs to lower blood pressure and cholesterol. If the carotid arteries are sufficiently narrowed, a carotid endarterectomy may also be recommended.

■ Be more physically active: this helps to lower blood pressure and control weight, both of which are important factors in reducing the risk of suffering a stroke.

■ Drink alcohol in moderation: excessive consumption is linked to stroke. Stick to 2–3 units per day for women and 3–4 for men, but don't save them up for a binge. Binge drinking is particularly bad for you.

■ Eat a healthy diet: aim to eat at least five portions of fruit and vegetables a day and keep the fat (especially animal fat) and salt content of your diet as low as possible.

■ Avoid being overweight: this increases your risk of stroke, heart attack and many other diseases.

People with high blood pressure are at increased risk of a stroke, so it is important to have a regular checkup. For adults whose pressure has previously been normal, that means at least once every five years, although women taking the contraceptive pill or who are pregnant, and those on some medicines, need checks more often.

If you have had a high or borderline reading in the past but don't currently need medicines, your blood pressure should be measured at least once a year. Anyone already taking medicines to control their blood pressure will need a check at least twice a year.

SEE ALSO *Brain and nervous system*

Sudden infant death syndrome

'Cot death' is the sudden, unexpected death of a baby for no obvious reason. It is one of the most shocking and distressing events that parents ever have to cope with. There are several things you can do to reduce significantly the risk to your baby.

Sudden infant death syndrome, or cot death, is every parent's nightmare. No one knows why some babies die suddenly and for no apparent reason. If your baby has died, some of your anger and grief may be to do with not being able to understand why it happened. Researchers believe that, rather than there being one single cause, there is likely to be a combination of factors that can affect a baby at this vulnerable stage of development.

The Foundation for the Study of Infant Deaths (FSID) was founded in 1971. It funds most of the research into cot death in England and Wales, and it is partly due to this work that there has been a dramatic decline in the rate of cot death in the UK. Nevertheless, cot death is still the most common cause of death in babies aged under one.

IF YOUR BABY HAS DIED

Different parents deal with losing a baby in different ways. Some find their family and friends help them through this traumatic period. But what many parents want is to talk to someone who has been through the same thing. If you would like to talk to someone, the FSID helpline can help (see **Contacts**). The charity has a network of volunteer befrienders across the UK who are there to listen, support and, if you wish, share their own experiences with you.

During the hours, days and weeks after a baby's death, parents find themselves wanting answers to all sorts of questions: 'Why our baby?' for example, or 'Did he suffer any pain?', or 'Will it happen again?'. And if you have other children, you will need to help them to deal with the loss of their baby brother or sister, too. Midwives, doctors, counsellors and various support organizations can all help you to find the answers you need. The important thing is to talk, and to allow yourselves to grieve.

People often feel they should not talk to the bereaved parents about their baby for fear this will bring on another wave of grief. But most parents say it hurts if their baby is not mentioned, almost as though he or she had never existed. So it is worth trying to remember happy times, to look at photographs, and to talk about things that made this baby so uniquely lovable.

In the UK the rate of SIDS has fallen by 70 per cent in the past decade, but there are still seven cot deaths each week.

Reduce the risk of cot death

The Foundation for the Study of Infant Deaths lists nine key steps to cut the risk of cot death.

- Place your baby on his or her back to sleep.
- Give up smoking in pregnancy – fathers, too.
- Do not smoke yourself or let anyone else smoke in the same room as your baby.
- Do not let your baby get too hot.
- Keep the baby's head uncovered – place your baby with his or her feet to the foot of the cot, to prevent him or her from wriggling down under the covers.
- Keep the baby's cot in your bedroom for the first six months.
- Avoid falling asleep on the sofa with your baby.
- If your baby is unwell, get medical advice promptly.
- It's best not to share a bed with your baby if you smoke, have been drinking, take medication or drugs that make you drowsy, or if you are overtired.

RESEARCH FINDINGS

Letting a baby get too hot increases the risk of cot death – the abdomen of a baby who is too warm feels hot to the touch. Even if your baby is asleep, always take off outdoor clothes once you get indoors or into a warm car, bus or train.

A baby's room should be 16–20°C (61–68°F). If the weather or the room is very warm, a vest and nappy may be all the baby needs. Don't put the cot near a radiator or in direct sunlight.

Research has shown that it is best not to use a second-hand mattress, and also that there is no risk of SIDS from fire-retardant materials used in some cot mattresses. Keep the mattress aired and clean. Sheets and blankets are safer than quilts; if your baby comes into your bed, use blankets rather than a duvet, and watch those pillows.

SEE ALSO *Babies and baby care*

Surgery and surgical techniques

Having an operation is a major event in anyone's life, but understanding what is involved can help reduce any anxiety and disruption, and can help to make the experience less stressful for everyone involved. If an operation has to be performed as an emergency procedure, however, this may not be possible.

Surgery is a branch of medicine that uses operations to treat a wide range of injuries, deformities or diseases. Developments in the technology and equipment used in surgery have lead to major advances in surgical techniques and improvements in patient care.

BEFORE THE OPERATION

Doctors and nurses often arrange to see the patient a few weeks before their operation is due to take place. This meeting is called a pre-operative assessment, and it gives medical staff the opportunity to carry out routine tests, such as blood tests and **X-rays**. Such tests vary, depending on the operation to be performed and the patient's general health. The meeting also allows the person having the operation to ask any questions. You should be given information about your operation with the complications outlined.

Most people need to take some time off work after an operation; it may take anything from a few days to several weeks for you to recover, depending on the procedure. People who smoke often take longer to recover from an operation and also have a higher risk of chest infections after a general anaesthetic. It is advised that you stop **smoking** two weeks before any operation.

GOING INTO HOSPITAL

Do not wear any make-up or nail varnish on the day of the operation, and don't bring any valuables or jewellery into the hospital because of the security risk. Wedding rings, however, can be left on and covered with tape for the operation.

The anaesthetist will ask if you have any crowns or dentures. If you have dentures, these will need to be removed to stop them interfering with your breathing. If you have crowns, they might be damaged if the anaesthetist needs to use a breathing tube; knowing where they are will mean that they can be avoided.

You will not be allowed to eat or drink anything for at least six hours before surgery, although you may be permitted a sip of water. This is because food or drink in the stomach may make a patient sick while under anaesthetic and if vomit enters the lungs, it will not be coughed up because the coughing reflex is suppressed by the

anaesthetic. This can cause serious lung damage. A card saying 'nil by mouth' will probably be hung on your bed to alert staff.

THE CONSENT PROCESS

Everyone undergoing a surgical procedure is required to sign a consent form to indicate that they wish the operation to proceed. This states that the person has received information about the operation and understands both the procedure and the main risks associated with the operation.

The consent form has to be signed by the person undergoing the operation, except under special circumstances, and your signature will be witnessed. Children usually have their consent form signed by their parent or guardian. If a patient is unable to give his or her consent – they may be unconscious or have a mental illness, for example – then the doctors looking after the patient can perform procedures or operations that are 'in the patient's best interests'. A relative or next of kin does not have to sign the consent form, but is usually involved or informed.

DAY SURGERY

Day surgery means that a person is admitted to hospital, undergoes a surgical procedure and goes home, all in the same day. Not all operations are suitable for day surgery; it is usually restricted to uncomplicated and relatively short operations: hernia repair and varicose vein removal are two common examples. Day surgery has become more usual over recent years because it is usually more convenient for the person having the operation, and is more efficient for the hospital.

Day cases can be carried out under either general or local anaesthetic. If a general anaesthetic is required, you will be asked not to eat or drink for six hours beforehand.

Many small operations can be performed under a local anaesthetic in either a GP's surgery or at the out-patient department by surgeons at the hospital. GPs have different levels of training and experience in performing operations but most will do simple procedures, often in designated clinics.

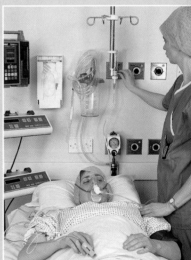

▲ Recovery room
Recovery from a general anaesthetic, following surgery, may be assisted in several ways: an adjustable oxygen supply helps to maintain breathing while the patient comes round; an intravenous drip corrects the balance of fluids in the body, and a meter on the finger monitors the pulse rate.

These include the removal of small skin growths such as moles, skin tags and cysts, and cryosurgery (freezing) of warts and verrucas.

MAJOR SURGERY

Major operations require patients to be in hospital for several days and cannot be performed as day surgery. They are usually carried out under general anaesthetic. The patient is generally admitted to hospital the day before the operation. The length of the hospital stay for major operations varies widely; your surgeon can let you know roughly how long your stay will be.

Pain after the operation

Post-operative pain is likely to be worse if the scar is large and the operation is a major one, but even small scars can be very sore. The anaesthetic takes several hours to wear off, and as it wears off the pain will probably get worse. However, there is no need to suffer undue pain after an operation as there are many effective painkillers available. Pain relief can be given in the form of a drip, injection, suppository or tablet.

After an operation, a patient may have a number of tubes attached. These are not as alarming as they look. A drip may be used to administer painkillers, antibiotics or fluids, and there may be a surgical drain in the wound itself. This is often a soft flexible plastic tube that allows air to be released, or fluids to drain away.

THE RISK OF CLOTTING

People who undergo major operations have an increased risk of developing **deep vein thrombosis**, a potentially dangerous complication in which a clot forms in a vein in the leg. A piece of the clot can then break off and travel through the veins to the lungs, where it can lodge causing a pulmonary embolism, a very serious complication. People undergoing surgery have a higher risk of developing clots, partly because of immobility during the operation and because they spend a period of time in bed afterwards.

Other risk factors for clots include taking certain medication (such as HRT), being a smoker, being overweight, or having a condition that makes blood clot more easily – **lupus**, for example. Some run in families, so it is important to tell your doctor if you have any relatives who have had clots in their legs or lungs.

Reducing the risk of clots

People are now less likely to develop a post-operative clot than in the past. Many people now receive injections of heparin before their operation; this thins the blood slightly, making it less likely to clot in the body. In addition, operations are usually quicker, with shorter recovery periods than before, so people spend far less time in bed afterwards. Many people are also given surgical stockings to wear or their legs are encased in inflatable

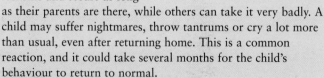

Children and surgery

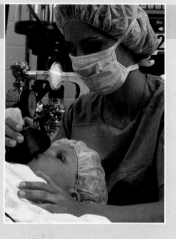

Children can find it difficult to cope with strange surroundings, unfamiliar people and different routines, and having an operation can be a frightening and bewildering experience.

There are many ways of making a child's stay in hospital a less traumatic experience, especially if the surgery is planned in advance rather than as an emergency operation. If the parents and child are well informed and relaxed about a hospital stay, then it is more likely the child will recover quickly, thereby reducing the length of hospital stay.

Where possible, children should visit the ward with their parents before being admitted. This gives them an opportunity to meet some of the staff and get to know the ward layout. Often, children are given a theatre hat and mask to take home so that they can become more familiar with theatre uniforms. There are also good books available on preparing for an operation or a hospital stay, which can help parents to explain to children what will happen. It is also worth involving children in the process of packing a bag or suitcase to take to hospital. Include some favourite toys and books so that they have some familiar items.

There is usually a parents' room for parents to stay in while their child is in hospital. It is worth enquiring about this in advance, preferably at the first visit, to ensure that it will be available. Parents are usually encouraged to stay with children until they are taken to the theatre for the operation, and may accompany them to the anaesthetic room.

Children react differently to being in hospital. Some feel safe and secure as long as their parents are there, while others can take it very badly. A child may suffer nightmares, throw tantrums or cry a lot more than usual, even after returning home. This is a common reaction, and it could take several months for the child's behaviour to return to normal.

Children who are frightened often behave badly, so it is important that they feel supported and comforted. It is useful for parents and the hospital staff to explain what children should expect and what is going to happen at all stages of the hospital stay, so that they remain informed and feel prepared.

leg cuffs during an operation; these both stimulate the flow of blood through the leg veins.

OTHER COMMON COMPLICATIONS

There are risks involved with every operation and these vary enormously with their frequency and severity. There is always a small risk of the scar becoming infected, for example, which usually responds to a short course of antibiotics. It is important to understand the likelihood of complications of an operation before signing the consent form. Surgeons will always be able to answer questions regarding complications and risks of the operation they are about to perform.

Confusion after an operation

Some elderly people become confused for short periods of time after an operation, which can be distressing both for the patient and for visiting relatives. The reasons vary, but unfamiliar surroundings, and the effects of dehydration, infection, pain and the side effects of medication can all cause an elderly person to become confused. Usually such confusion is short-lived and does not lead to further problems.

SURGICAL STITCHES

There are two different types of stitches used by surgeons: absorbable stitches, which the body breaks down, causing them to 'dissolve' over a period of time, and non-absorbable, which need to be removed. When and where the stitches are removed will depend on the operation and the type of material used in the stitches; often the practice nurse in the GP's surgery removes non-absorbable stitches. The procedure is straightforward and painless – people are often surprised at how quick it is.

Staples are used in some operations, particularly major ones such as a Caesarean section, as they are quick and easy for the surgeon to insert and are easily removed with a special instrument.

SURGICAL TECHNIQUES

In open surgery, a surgeon opens the body and uses his or her hands and instruments to operate. This is the most invasive form of surgery, and has long recovery times. There is a strong trend away from open surgery and towards improved techniques of minimally invasive surgery, which generally minimizes the risk to patients and speeds up recovery.

New technology and innovations in equipment mean that surgery is developing all the time. Advances that are likely to have a growing impact over the next decade include the use of virtual reality and robots in surgery. The newest techniques often result in quicker, less traumatic operations with faster recovery times.

Keyhole surgery

Keyhole surgery, or endoscopy, is minimally invasive surgery carried out through natural body openings or small artificial incisions – the 'keyholes' that give rise to the term keyhole surgery. A fine tube with a lens or an electronic chip on the end is used in combination with several long, thin, rigid instruments and a high definition TV monitor. Images are shown on screens in the operating room and the surgeon uses these to navigate to the site of the operation. Some common gynaecological operations are carried out using keyhole surgery, and it is becoming increasingly widely used for such commonly performed operations as those to remove the gallbladder or to treat knee cartilage problems.

New operations that use keyhole surgery continue to be devised and introduced.

Virtual reality and surgery

Virtual reality in surgery uses interactive computer technologies to help plan, simulate and perform surgical procedures. It is now being applied in all three major areas of surgery: open surgery, endoscopic surgery and radiosurgery.

Virtual reality gives a surgeon three-dimensional views of areas within a patient. It can be used pre-operatively to plan an operation, allowing doctors to determine an approach to surgery that will involve minimum damage to the patient. In a breast reconstruction operation, for example, the procedure might be rehearsed and the predicted end result shown three-dimensionally. This helps and reassures the woman as she can see the end results on a computer screen before the operation is performed. But this technique is not offered routinely, and is still in the early stages of development.

Virtual reality simulation is becoming a valuable training tool. It can be used in routine training, or to focus on particularly difficult cases and new surgical techniques. Surgeons are able to learn operative procedures away from the operating theatre using real patient data combined with anatomical information from a human 'atlas'.

WHAT HAPPENS AFTERWARDS?

Often patients are seen by their surgeon in an out-patient clinic several weeks after their operation to ensure that they are recovering fully and any scars are healing. However, not all patients need to be seen again by the surgeon – for more minor operations, patients are discharged and advised to consult their GP if any problems arise.

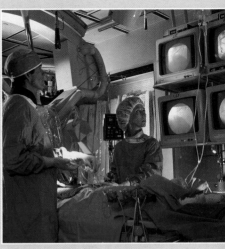

▲ **Inner vision**
On monitors the surgical team can follow the progress of a catheter in a coronary angioplasty operation. It is guided through the patient's blood vessels until it reaches the heart.

Tears and problems

Tears are the fluid constantly secreted by the lachrymal glands in the eye to keep the front of the eyeball lubricated and clean. They drain away through small openings at the inner corner of the eye into two tubes, then empty into the back of the nose via a larger tube (the nasolacrimal duct). A blockage at any point prevents drainage, resulting in a persistently watery eye.

A watery eye can also be due to excess tear formation rather than an obstruction. To discover if this is the case, your optometrist or doctor will carry out a simple, painless test to establish whether or not dye inserted into the tears reaches the nose. There is no treatment for excess tear formation, which is a nuisance but not medically worrying.

An obstruction may be congenital and persist from birth, although the tear drainage in one in ten newborns is often not fully developed for weeks. Alternatively, it may be acquired as a result of injury, infection, ageing or the presence of a foreign body.

Treatment is rarely necessary, because the obstruction will generally resolve itself. But persistent blockage may require the insertion of a sterile tube into the duct, or surgery to reopen the duct.

SEE ALSO *Eye and problems*

Teeth and problems

Modern dental care is centred firmly around conservative care and prevention of disease. By taking care of our teeth and maintaining a sensible diet, most of us can now expect to keep our teeth throughout our lives.

The mouth contains many kinds of bacteria, only a few of which are harmful. Some bacteria form a sticky film (plaque) on the teeth. In the presence of sugary foods, snacks and drinks, the bacteria in plaque produce acid that attacks teeth, resulting in decay. Plaque is also the main cause of gum disease.

Good brushing technique, regular flossing and avoiding frequent snacks of sweet, sugary foods or drinks can substantially reduce the need for dental treatment. Good brushing involves moving the brush in small circular movements on all the surfaces of every tooth, upper and lower, for about two minutes twice a day. A dentist or dental hygienist can advise you further on brushing and diet. A dentist may also warn you against smoking, which exacerbates gum disease as well as staining the teeth and causing **halitosis.**

You should see a dentist at least once a year for a check-up. He or she will be able to identify early signs of decay as well as other problems such as gum disease.

WHAT CAN GO WRONG

Various disorders can affect the teeth, and most people suffer from decay at some point in their lives. But prompt treatment can minimize the damage and prevent further problems.

Decay

Tooth decay – also known as dental caries – is the most common of all human diseases. Decay occurs when the acid produced by bacteria in plaque comes into contact with the protective enamel of the teeth. It is easily treated, but if left unchecked, the decay will reach the soft dentine, then the pulp of the tooth, which contains the nerves and blood vessels. If the decay progresses and the pulp becomes infected, the tooth may die.

Early signs of decay can be picked up by a dentist during a check-up, either by examining your mouth or by the use of **X-rays**. Otherwise, toothache is often the first sign, but by then the damage to the tooth has already begun and prompt treatment is essential. Severe pain is likely if the decay reaches the pulp or if an abscess forms (see below).

Treatment for decay will depend on how far it has spread. Usually the area of decay is removed by drilling and the cavity filled to prevent further decay. Silver fillings are made of amalgam, which is a mixture of mercury, silver, tin and sometimes copper. Apart from hypersensitivity in some people, no health problems are thought to be caused by amalgam use. But, as a precaution, pregnant women are advised to avoid having amalgam fillings placed or removed. An alternative filling is made from a composite quartz resin. Some people prefer the appearance of this white-coloured filling.

Drilling and filling a tooth is a simple procedure usually performed under local anaesthetic. If the cavity is large, however, the dentist may recommend a crown. This is placed over the tooth after preparation to help to protect the remaining tooth. If the pulp has been affected and died, an abscess may form within the tooth. You will need to take antibiotics to destroy the infection. Once the infection has cleared up, root canal treatment may be necessary to save the tooth. This is quite a complicated procedure, which may involve several visits. The dentist drills into the top of the tooth, removing the nerve and pulp and replacing them with an inert material designed to stop further infection. A filling is used to restore the tooth to its former shape, and a crown may be used to strengthen the tooth.

Structure of a tooth

A tooth consists of a layer of enamel covering the dentine, which in turn covers the pulp with its nerve fibres and blood vessels. The gums help to protect the roots of the tooth, which are connected to the bone by the peridontal ligament.

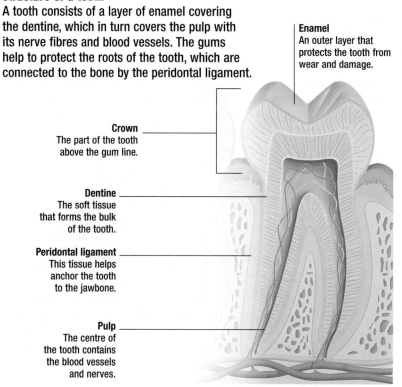

Enamel
An outer layer that protects the tooth from wear and damage.

Crown
The part of the tooth above the gum line.

Dentine
The soft tissue that forms the bulk of the tooth.

Peridontal ligament
This tissue helps anchor the tooth to the jawbone.

Pulp
The centre of the tooth contains the blood vessels and nerves.

Researchers in the UK and USA are currently developing vaccines that attack dental caries. It is hoped that vaccinating all children will eliminate decay in the future.

Root decay

Decay usually occurs between the teeth and on the biting surfaces. But if your gums recede due to gum disease, you risk developing decay on the root surface of the tooth, near the gums. People on medication that reduces the flow of saliva, such as drugs for heart problems, blood pressure and depression, are particularly at risk. This is because saliva neutralizes acids in the mouth and so protects the teeth from decay.

If you have root decay, your dentist may coat your teeth with a varnish to inhibit further decay. If the decay is more advanced, a filling will be necessary. Good oral hygiene and a sensible diet will help to prevent root decay.

Abscess

A dental **abscess** is a collection of pus in or around the root of the tooth. It forms when the pulp at the centre of the tooth has died as a result of decay or an injury such as a blow to the mouth. It is characterized by pain, particularly on biting, and the tooth may feel raised in its socket. If left untreated, there may be local and facial swelling and severe pain. The swelling may burst, releasing the pus.

Antibiotics are usually prescribed to treat infection, and root canal treatment is carried out to remove the inflamed nerve and pulp.

Occasionally, root fillings are not successful and the infection lingers at the tip of the root. In these cases, an apicetomy is performed. This is a surgical procedure in which an incision is made in the gum so that the end of the root can be cleaned and trimmed.

Erosion

Dental erosion is the loss of tooth enamel caused by acid attack from food and drink. It usually shows up as hollows in the teeth and a general wearing away of the tooth surface and biting edges. Eventually, the dentine may be exposed, giving the tooth a darker yellow appearance and leading to some sensitivity and, in extreme cases, pain and the death of the tooth.

Erosion may affect any surface of the tooth. It is caused by frequent exposure to acid, and the most likely sufferers are children who regularly drink fizzy drinks or concentrated fruit juices. Half of all children in the UK show some signs of tooth erosion. The front teeth and their visible surfaces are most affected.

Another cause of erosion is the eating disorder **bulimia nervosa**. The teeth are damaged by acid in vomit. Typically, the inner surfaces of the front teeth are most affected. The reflux of gastric acid into the mouth of people suffering from a hiatus **hernia** can also cause erosion.

Everyone is at risk of erosion and the best defence is to brush your teeth twice a day with fluoride toothpaste, and to floss daily. But don't brush your teeth straight after a meal as acids in the mouth, whatever the cause, make the enamel soft. Sweet fizzy drinks should be avoided; at the very least, drink them through a straw to minimize contact with the teeth.

Chipped, cracked or missing teeth

Injuries to the teeth range from minor damage, such as chipped enamel, to the loss of an entire tooth. If a crack or chip in the enamel leaves the dentine exposed, the tooth may become sensitive to hot or cold food and drink, or pain may be felt on biting.

Depending on the damage, the tooth may be smoothed or, in more severe cases, may require a veneer, filling or crown. In the case of a bad fracture, a root filling may be necessary and, in the worst cases, the tooth may have to be extracted. If a tooth is knocked out fully, you may be able to put it straight back in its socket. Avoid touching the root while doing this. If it is not possible to replace the tooth in the socket, your dentist may be able to do so. You should keep the tooth in milk or in your cheek so that it stays moist until you can get to the dentist. The tooth may then require a splint to keep it stable until it has re-attached to the bone.

Impacted teeth

Extreme pain can result when a tooth (most commonly a wisdom tooth) has no room to erupt and becomes 'impacted'. If there is an infection, antibiotics may be required and it is likely that the tooth will have to be extracted.

Irregular, misaligned or protruding teeth

Most people have some teeth that are not ideally positioned. If misaligned or protruding teeth affect the way that you speak or chew your food, or if they are difficult to clean, your dentist can refer you to an orthodontist.

An orthodontist can also help if you wish to improve the appearance of your teeth. Treatment usually involves wearing a brace for several months or even years. Some teeth may need to be removed from an overcrowded mouth. Your dentist may also recommend veneers, thin porcelain replacement surfaces, to improve the appearance.

Discoloured teeth

Teeth can become discoloured or stained due to poor oral hygiene, smoking or drinking large amounts of coffee or tea. When teeth die, they may become yellowish-brown.

Sometimes children's teeth have a yellow appearance. This can be due to the child being given the antibiotic tetracycline when the tooth was being formed. Fluorosis, caused by excess amounts of fluoride, can cause mottling.

If your teeth are discoloured, there are various techniques that can be used to whiten them. Professional bleaching is the most common. Your dentist applies a whitening product to your teeth, using a specially made tray that fits into your mouth like a gum-shield. You will need to continue the treatment at home, applying the whitening product at home for up to four weeks, for 30 minutes to one hour each time.

Laser whitening is a speedier option in which a light or laser is shone on the teeth to activate the whitening product. The light speeds up the chemical reaction of the whitening product and the colour change can be achieved within an hour.

If your teeth are discoloured by nicotine or caffeine stains, your dentist may advise regular polishing. Children's teeth can be cleaned by a dentist or hygienist, but they should be treated cosmetically only when the child is older.

Sensitive teeth

Gum disease can cause your gums to recede, leaving them sensitive to hot and cold. Elderly people are particularly susceptible to receding gums. This is due to the changed bacterial flora in the mouth and reduced flow of saliva that occur with age. Your dentist may be able to coat any sensitive areas with fluoride varnish. You may also need to use a toothpaste designed for sensitive teeth, and to avoid food and drink which is very hot or cold.

SEE ALSO *Dentists and dentistry; Gums and disorders*

Temperature

A normal healthy body temperature is considered to be 37°C, although this varies slightly from person to person. It also fluctuates depending on the time of day or (in women) the day of the menstrual cycle.

Body temperature is controlled by a complex system (thermoregulation). The overall temperature control centre is located within the hypothalamus, a part of the brain that deals with automatic functions of the body.

Active heat generation within the body occurs in the liver, as part of its breakdown of food substances, and as a result of muscle activity. Heat loss occurs directly through the skin and increases when the environmental temperature is lower than the temperature of the skin. Another cause for increased heat loss is moisture evaporation from the skin, which itself is increased by air movement and decreased humidity. A certain amount of heat is also lost through urine, faeces and exhaled breath.

The most common cause of raised body temperature is infection – viral or bacterial. This is the body's reaction to chemicals released by its activated immune system that is fighting the infection. Other causes include: heatstroke, which arises after exposure to too much sun, and an environmental temperature that is too high for the body's cooling mechanism to cope with; severe thyrotoxicosis (overactive thyroid gland); a reaction to stimulant drugs (amphetamine, Ecstasy and cocaine); and, rarely, a reaction to anaesthetic agents which can also increase temperature.

Excessively low body temperature is known as **hypothermia**. It can be brought on by dressing inadequately in a freezing environment and may occur with walkers in mountain regions. Physical inactivity, malnutrition and self-neglect commonly contribute to hypothermia in the elderly. Neglect may also be the case when infants suffer from hypothermia.

People that are immersed in cold water – usually accidentally – can quickly succumb to hypothermia. Low body temperature is also a feature of severe hypothyroidism (underactive **thyroid** gland).

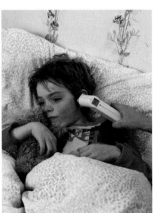

▲ **Taking a temperature**
The boy's flushed face indicates a fever but the tympanic thermometer (in the ear) confirms it.

Tendons and disorders

Tendons, or sinews, are strong, flexible bundles of tissue attaching muscle to bone. They are made of a fibrous protein called collagen. A muscle is connected at each end by tendons to one or more bones. When the muscle contracts, the tendons transmit to the bones the power of the whole muscle, producing movement (see **Muscular system**). Tendons are inelastic, however, and can be ruptured by an excessive force such as the sudden flex of a muscle.

Tendons can be very long. For example, the complex tendons that move the fingers and toes run from the muscles in the forearms and shins to the tips of the fingers and toes.

Bands of fibrous ligaments called retinacula hold down the tendons at the wrists and ankles to prevent them from 'bowing' out. Some tendons are also joined to bands of connective tissue called fascia, or to the ligaments that link bones together at the **joints**.

In some places, such as the back of the wrist and around the ankles, tendons are enclosed by a double-layer of sheath made from synovial membrane. This secretes synovial fluid, which helps to minimize friction within the tendon.

WHAT CAN GO WRONG

Tendons are much tougher than muscles and less likely to be damaged. Indeed, the most common site of muscle injury is neither the tendon nor the muscle 'belly', but the fibrous join between the two. But, if tendons are injured, they take longer to heal than muscle because they have a poorer blood supply. The tendons of the shoulder and arm are the ones most often injured or ruptured.

As well as injury, tendons can be damaged by disease. Certain disorders that affect the body's connective tissues, such as rheumatoid **arthritis**, weaken the tendons; and long-term steroid therapy (for asthma, for example) is particularly damaging to tendons, making them thinner, weaker and more prone to rupture.

Otherwise, most tendon injuries are caused either by a single severe incident – most likely to occur during sport or exercise – or by repeated minor damage, known as repetitive strain injury or chronic overuse syndrome.

Surgical repair of a tendon is not easy because the two ends move apart as the muscle goes into spasm. If the ends cannot be brought together a tendon graft may be needed, whereby a tendon is taken from another part of the body, often the foot. There may also be damage to other tissues (nerve damage is particularly serious) or complications resulting in scarring that will prevent free movement of the tendon.

After surgery, the damaged part is immobilized in a splint to allow the tendon to heal. The process of rehabilitation that follows tendon surgery can take several weeks or even months.

UPPER LIMB INJURIES

Conditions affecting the upper limbs include tennis elbow, golfer's elbow, tenosynovitis of the wrist, thumb or finger, and rupture or tear of the finger tendons (see also **Ganglion**).

Tennis elbow and golfer's elbow

Elbows are particularly vulnerable to repetitive strain injury. The flexing muscles of the wrist and fingers come from the forearm, where they are linked by a common tendon to the funny bone (see **Elbow and problems**). Continued repeated gripping activity can cause inflammation around the tendon on the funny bone, resulting in pain on the inside of the elbow and the inner forearm. This is called golfer's elbow, although playing golf is only one of its many causes.

The bony prominence on the outside of the arm has a tendon where many of the finger and wrist extensor muscles pull; this can become inflamed, in a condition called tennis elbow.

Tennis elbow and golfer's elbow are difficult to treat. The first step is to rest from the activity that caused the problem. Other options include various kinds of physiotherapy, stretching and hydrocortisone injections. Surgery may be performed in persistent cases.

Muscle control

Tendons are strong bands of fibrous tissue that connect muscles to bone and enable movement. When a tendon is damaged the muscle cannot function and movement is severely restricted.

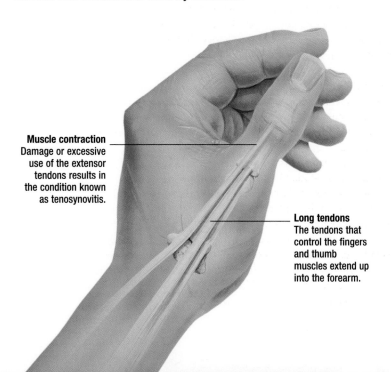

Muscle contraction
Damage or excessive use of the extensor tendons results in the condition known as tenosynovitis.

Long tendons
The tendons that control the fingers and thumb muscles extend up into the forearm.

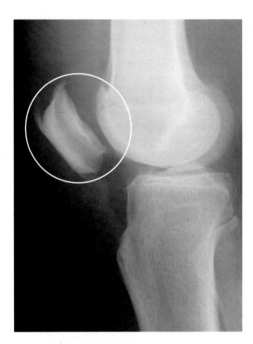

▲ **Ruptured patella tendon**
X-ray of a ruptured patella tendon resulting from a sports injury. Normally, the tendon holds the patella (circled) close to the thigh bone.

Tenosynovitis of the wrist, thumb or finger

The sheath around a tendon can become inflamed and hardened, restricting movement and causing considerable pain. This condition is called tenosynovitis. It can occur in any tendon, but the most common site is around the wrist.

If it affects the tendons that straighten the thumb, the problem is know as de Quervain tendinitis; if it affects a finger, it is called finger extensor tendinitis. These conditions are caused by repetitive strain injuries and result in pain in the wrist and arm; they may be associated with overuse of computer keyboards.

When tenosynovitis in a long finger flexor causes the tendon to become 'locked' in the sheath, the condition is called trigger finger. The finger suddenly releases in a snappy, jerky movement. It may be caused by overuse of round-handled tools.

Rupture or tear of the finger tendons

All finger tendons are close to the surface of the skin, making them especially vulnerable to being wholly or partly severed. Accidents with sharp tools are the most common cause. Falling through a glass pane with an outstretched hand is a common cause of cut wrist tendons.

All such injuries need immediate and specialized treatment because the impairment of even a single hand tendon can severely restrict the function of the hand as a whole.

Total or partial tendon rupture is very rare above the elbows, but it sometimes occurs around the shoulder. The rotator cuff muscles connect the shoulder blade to the upper arm and stabilize the shoulder joint when lifting the arm. A sudden stretch of any muscle while the fibres are strongly contracting can cause a tendon or muscle tear. The result is pain around the shoulder, and probably an inability to lift the arm out to the side. The extent of pain and disability depends on which muscle or tendon is injured – and how badly.

Repetitive strain injury

Repetitive strain injury, or chronic repetitive trauma, is more common than partial or complete tendon rupture. An injury develops gradually over weeks, months or even years as a result of repeated stress on a particular body part. During work, sport or leisure activities, similar movements repeated without rest over a long period can inflame a tendon, or its sheath, and cause pain and impair movement. The condition can sometimes suddenly worsen, leaving the affected limb completely disabled.

The tendons of the rotator cuff muscles are prone to inflammation caused by any unaccustomed, repeated activity of the arm in the shoulder joint. As there is very limited space in the region just above the shoulder, any inflammation causes tendons to be pinched, resulting in severe pain. Sometimes a calcium nodule forms in the tendon, leading to pain and stiffness in the shoulder. Extreme pain can 'freeze' the shoulder joint, so that even when the inflammation has resolved, the joint is stiff.

LOWER LIMB INJURIES

The most common tendon-related conditions affecting the lower limbs are Achilles tendon rupture and hamstring or quadriceps injuries.

Achilles tendon rupture

The Achilles tendon runs from the powerful calf muscle to the heel bone. Injury is caused by a sudden stretch of the calf muscle, when jumping, for example. Injury to the muscle fibres is more likely than a torn tendon, but the symptom of both is a severe pain in the calf (as though hit by a brick) and an inability to walk. A torn tendon may require surgery.

The Achilles tendon is also particularly prone to chronic inflammation due to repetitive injury, such as that caused by long-distance running, especially when wearing shoes that dig in behind the heel. The tendon sheath becomes inflamed and needs rest, physiotherapy and possibly local steroid injection. In some cases surgery may be needed.

Hamstring injuries

The hamstring tendons behind the knee attach the hamstring muscles at the back of the thigh to the tibia and fibula in the lower half of the leg. The hamstring muscles are responsible for bending the knee and acceleration.

Injuries to the hamstring tendons are common among football players, sprinters and squash players. Inflammation caused by overuse (tendinitis) or pulling muscle fibres is more common than tears in the tendon. A carefully paced warm-up and stretch before taking part in sports reduces the risk of injury.

Quadriceps injuries

We use our quadriceps muscles, or 'quads', to straighten our knees – when going upstairs, for example. These important anti-gravity muscles at the front of the thighs are put to the test in almost every sport. The powerful patella tendon links the quadriceps to a point just below the knee joint. The kneecap (patella) is a round bone within this tendon.

The short section of tendon below the patella is prone to inflammation (patellar tendinitis). This can be caused by doing a lot of jumping. But kneeling for a long time can also precipitate tendon (or bursa) problems. Very rarely, the patella tendon can rupture.

TENS

Transcutaneous electronic nerve stimulation (TENS), is a form of pain relief that uses small electrical currents to block the pain of, for example, **osteoporosis**, rheumatoid **arthritis**, **sciatica** and other muscle and joint problems. It is also used to reduce the pain of contractions during labour. Medical opinion is divided over the efficacy of TENS.

HOW TENS WORKS

It is thought that the electrical currents disrupt the pain signals sent by nerve endings to the brain, while stimulating the production of endorphins, the painkilling opiates that occur naturally in the body. This then brings pain relief to the part of the body to which the electrical currents are applied.

USING A TENS MACHINE

TENS units can be hired or bought from some hospitals and pharmacists and from specialist companies. The unit consists of four adhesive pads linked to a small hand-held control that regulates the type of current and its intensity. Initially, the current may feel like little more than a tingling sensation, but as it is increased it may feel more like a mild electric shock.

As a device to help labour pains, TENS is most effective when used from the early stages. Pads should be placed on the woman's back, according to the instructions, when contractions begin. Correct positioning of the pads, directly above key nerve junctions, is crucial.

Testicles and disorders

The two testicles manufacture sperm and testosterone, the male sex hormone. They are located in the scrotum, a sac of skin hanging below the **penis**, where the temperature is slightly below that of the rest of the body. This is essential because successful production of sperm requires a temperature about 3°C lower than normal body temperature.

Sperm are produced at a rate of about 1000 per second, and new sperm mature in the epididymis, which can be felt as a small bump at the top of each testicle. From here they travel up the vas deferens just before ejaculation (see also **Reproductive system**).

Testes

The testes, the male reproductive glands, are well supplied by blood capillaries, nerves and lymph vessels. They are packed with sperm-producing tubules.

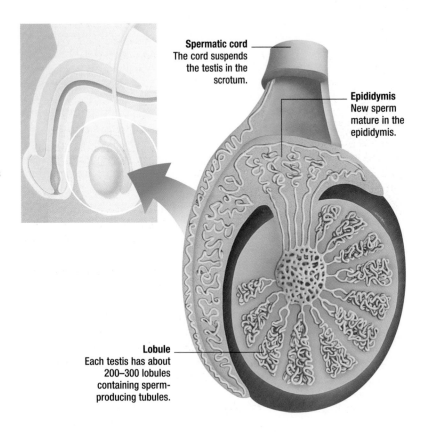

Spermatic cord
The cord suspends the testis in the scrotum.

Epididymis
New sperm mature in the epididymis.

Lobule
Each testis has about 200–300 lobules containing sperm-producing tubules.

WHAT CAN GO WRONG

A baby's testicles should descend from his body at birth; if they do not, problems can occur (see **Cryptorchidism**). It is common for a testicle to disappear temporarily into the abdomen in response to worry, cold or tight clothing. Such an event is not a health hazard. If the cause of its disappearance is removed, the testicle will again descend.

There are a number of common problems related to the testicles.

■ A swollen epididymis is usually caused by an infection; this is called **orchitis**, and is most common in teenagers. The characteristic symptom of orchitis is a burning pain in the scrotum. It is diagnosed through a urine test and treated with antibiotics and applying ice.

■ **Hydrocele** is swelling of the scrotum caused by excess fluid. Although the condition is usually harmless, it may be advisable for comfort's sake to have the fluid drained.

■ Itching in the area of the testicles, sometimes called jock itch, is caused by the fungus responsible for **athlete's foot**. To counteract jock itch, use an unperfumed soap, dry yourself thoroughly and wear loose cotton underpants (rather than pants made from synthetic material). If the condition persists, ask your GP or pharmacist about creams that will heal the condition.

■ A lumpy or swollen testicle may, rarely, be a sign of **cancer**. It is more likely to be caused by orchitis or perhaps an epididymal **cyst**. Seek medical advice without delay. A lump on the skin of the scrotum tissue may be a boil, a cyst or, rarely, scrotal skin cancer (usually caused by repeated exposure to carcinogenic chemicals such as oil and tar).

■ If swelling comes on quickly or is very painful, seek medical help immediately. The spermatic cord around the vas deferens may become twisted and within a few hours could cut off the the blood supply, causing permanent damage. This is called torsion of the testicle and is most common in teenagers.

■ The usually harmless development of varicose veins around a testicle is called a varicocele. Surgery may be offered if the problem appears to be affecting the sperm count.

■ Occasionally, an injury resulting from a blow to the testicles may require treatment. Don't let embarrassment keep you from consulting a doctor.

Testicular cancer

Testicular cancer is the most common form of cancer in men under 40. It is still rare (only 1600 cases a year in the UK), but rates have nearly doubled since 1980, possibly due to environmental factors, including rising levels of oestrogen in cow's milk. Survival rates for men with testicular cancer are over 90 per cent if the disease is caught early.

SYMPTOMS

The main symptom of testicular cancer is a lump, although sometimes there may also be feelings of heaviness, pain or swelling.

CAUSES

If you wear close-fitting underpants or tight trousers, your testicles are kept at higher temperatures than if you wear looser garments. Higher temperatures do not cause testicular cancer, but may encourage cells that already have a cancerous tendency to develop into full-blown cancer. You are at greater risk of testicular cancer if:

■ someone else in your family has had it;

■ you had an undescended testicle (see **cryptorchidism**) or an early puberty;

■ you take little exercise.

PREVENTION

Men can identify early signs of cancer by regularly examing their testicles. After a warm bath or shower, roll each testicle gently between

the thumb and the tips of the fingers. The slight lump at the top is the epididymis. Any other lumps, especially any that feel particularly firm, should be reported to a doctor, even if they cause no pain.

TREATMENT

If testicular cancer is suspected after blood tests and an ultrasound scan, the testicle is likely to be surgically removed (orchidectomy). Other tests and X-rays are performed to see if the cancer has spread. If it has, **radiotherapy** or drugs are required and, occasionally, further surgery.

OUTLOOK

The outlook for someone with testicular cancer is excellent if the disease is caught early enough. Provided that the other testicle is not affected by the cancer or the treatment, fertility is also unaffected.

SEE ALSO *Cancer*

Tetanus

Tetanus is a severe infectious disease that affects the central nervous system. It is commonly known as lockjaw, because the main early sign of infection is a spasm of the chewing muscles that makes it very difficult to open the mouth.

Tetanus is caused by the bacterium *Clostridium tetani*. Infection occurs when spores of the bacterium contaminate a wound. The bacteria then multiply and produce a toxin that acts on the nerves controlling muscle activity, causing spasmodic contractions.

In the UK there are fewer than 20 cases of tetanus each year. These occur in non-immunized people. Most cases arise in developing countries. There are an estimated half a million cases of tetanus worldwide each year, but with modern methods of treatment the mortality rate has been cut from 60 per cent to about 20 per cent.

SYMPTOMS

■ Stiffness of the jaw (known medically as trismus), making it hard to open the mouth.

■ The jaw spasm spreads to the muscles of the face and neck, producing a facial expression known medically as the risus sardonicus.

■ Stiffness of the abdominal and back muscles.

■ Fast pulse rate.

■ Fever.

■ Profuse sweating.

■ Eventually, painful muscle spasms develop, which can affect the larynx or chest wall, causing asphyxia.

TREATMENT

As soon as the diagnosis is suspected, tetanus is treated with tetanus antitoxin and antibiotics.

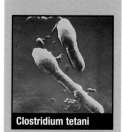

When to see a doctor

See a doctor as soon as symptoms appear.

What a doctor will do

The doctor will make a diagnosis from the symptoms. The patient will be admitted to hospital for a course of tetanus antitoxin injections and antibiotics or metronidazole. In severe cases, where respiratory muscles are affected, a tracheotomy (insertion of a breathing tube into the windpipe) may be needed. A ventilator may also be needed to help the patient to breathe. With prompt treatment most patients make a full recovery.

PREVENTION

Tetanus is easily prevented by **immunization**, and everyone should be protected. It is given routinely in the UK during childhood. Thereafter, booster shots are recommended every 10 years. You should also have a booster if you injure yourself with a dirty implement, such as a muddy garden fork, and before travelling to tropical countries.

Thalassaemia

Thalassaemia is a genetic disorder afflicting people from Mediterranean countries or of Mediterranean origin. It is caused by an abnormality in haemoglobin, the red blood pigment that carries oxygen from the lungs to the cells. This abnormality causes the red blood cells, or erythrocytes, to break down too easily.

BETA THALASSAEMIA

Beta thalassaemia major is a form of the disorder that affects children from the age of one year. Its symptoms are profound **anaemia**, poor growth, breathlessness, tiredness after minor exertion, repeated infections and yellow skin – known medically as jaundice. The spleen is also enlarged. These symptoms are caused by the anaemia and the resulting impairment of the blood's ability to carry oxygen around the body. A further visible sign of the disorder in children is a bulging skull. This happens as a result of the body producing red blood cells in the bone marrow of the skull.

The worst-affected children need regular blood transfusions in order to survive beyond early childhood. However, multiple transfusions themselves eventually cause iron overload, which can damage many parts of the body, including the liver, but in most cases, the heart. The disorder has been successfully treated with bone marrow transplantation, but this is not routinely offered because it carries major risks.

Milder forms cause no symptoms, and no treatment is needed, though sufferers may be more vulnerable to infections and gallstones.

ALPHA THALASSAEMIA

Alpha thalassaemia has a different genetic cause from beta thalassaemia. The worst-affected babies die in the womb or soon after birth, or else the child remains severely anaemic. The course and treatment are otherwise similar to beta thalassaemia.

OUTLOOK

Genetic identification and counselling are vital in controlling the spread of thalassaemia. Prenatal diagnostic techniques such as chorionic villus sampling and amniocentesis can detect whether a fetus is affected by thalassaemia.

Thermography

Thermography is a non-invasive scanning technique based on detection of temperature differences on the surface of the skin. This reveals variations in the underlying blood supply, indicating problems such as inflammation or a tumour.

In one type of thermography, a camera picks up infrared radiation emitted by the skin and displays the temperature variation as an image. In another type, temperature-sensitive liquid crystals are applied to the skin; these change colour according to the skin temperature.

Many medical conditions lead to changes in skin temperature, and thermography alone is not specific enough for use as a diagnostic tool. Hopes that thermography could be an alternative technique for detecting early breast cancer have not, so far, been fulfilled.

▼ **Thermographic image** Thermography is a screening procedure that may be used, along with other investigations, to check breast tissue for early active tumours.

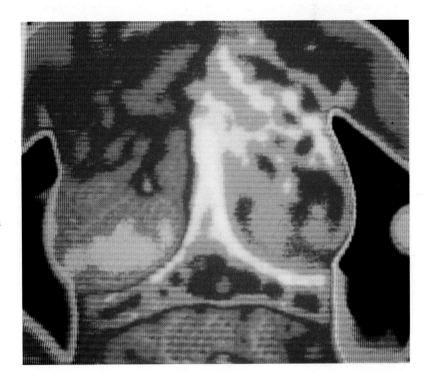

Throat and problems

The throat, also known as the pharynx, is a funnel-shaped muscular tube that runs from the back of the nose and mouth down to the upper section of the **oesophagus** and the top of the larynx. Sometimes the word 'throat' is also used to refer to the front of the neck from the jaw to the collarbone.

The throat is made up of three continuous sections: these are divided into the nasopharynx (upper section), the oropharynx (middle section) and the laryngopharynx (lower section).

The nasopharynx connects the nasal cavity to the area around the soft palate, while the oropharynx runs from the nasopharynx to below the tongue. The laryngopharynx, which joins the oesophagus, is found behind and to each side of the larynx.

During swallowing, the nasopharynx is sealed off by the soft palate, which prevents food from entering it. The oropharynx is a passage for both air and food. Only food passes through the laryngopharynx.

The throat also plays an important role in speech. Being muscular, it can change shape and so helps the formation of vowel sounds. It also acts as a resonant cavity that aids the quality and volume of sounds produced by the larynx.

The pharynx

The pharynx forms part of both the digestive system and the respiratory system. It contains the gullet (oesophagus) which carries food to the stomach and the windpipe (trachea), which is the airway to the lungs.

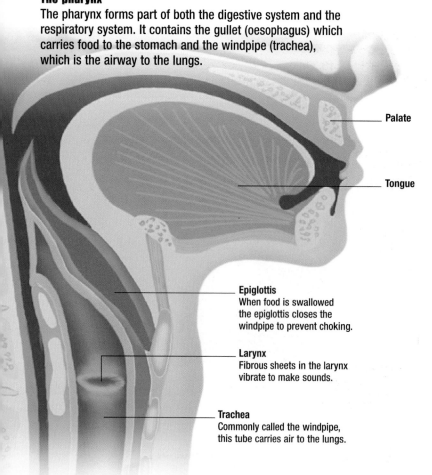

Palate

Tongue

Epiglottis
When food is swallowed the epiglottis closes the windpipe to prevent choking.

Larynx
Fibrous sheets in the larynx vibrate to make sounds.

Trachea
Commonly called the windpipe, this tube carries air to the lungs.

WHAT CAN GO WRONG

The most common problems affecting the throat are soreness, pain, hoarseness and lumps. Causes include infections, injury or a tumour. Swallowing difficulties, especially in men over 50, may be caused by a pharyngeal pouch. The sensation of a lump in the throat can have a physical or psychological origin.

Throat infections

Pharyngitis, the most common cause of a sore throat, is generally caused by a viral or sometimes a bacterial or fungal infection. Laryngitis (see **Larynx and disorders**), signalled by hoarseness and loss of voice, is another common cause of a sore throat. It is usually due to a viral infection but can also be part of an allergic reaction to a drug or other substance. Tonsillitis (see **Tonsils and disorders**), **influenza**, the common **cold, bronchitis, quinsy** and **glandular fever** are other infections that often have sore throat as a predominant symptom, frequently accompanied by fever, a cough, swallowing difficulties and a runny nose.

A severe sore throat with white patches on the tonsils may indicate strep throat – a bacterial infection that requires medical attention and probably a course of antibiotic treatment. But most sore throats clear up of their own accord.

Injury

A foreign body, such as a fish bone or chicken bone, may become lodged in the throat, causing pain and choking. A pricking sensation or pain on every swallow is common, and distinguishes an injury from an infection (which usually causes a more gradual onset of sore throat). Accidental swallowing of a caustic substance such as bleach will cause intense pain and swelling of the mucous membrane lining the throat and needs emergency treatment.

More chronic damage to the mucous membrane lining the throat may be caused by gastro-oesophageal reflux, heavy smoking or alcohol abuse. This can set the scene for the development of a throat cancer in later life.

Cancer

Throat **cancer** is relatively rare in the West, accounting for less than one per cent of cases of cancer. The condition is almost always related to smoking and heavy alcohol consumption; those who use both tobacco and alcohol have about a 15-fold greater risk of developing throat cancer than those who abstain from both. It is more common among men and its incidence rises with age.

A malignant tumour in the oropharynx often causes swallowing problems, sore throat and earache. Bloodstained phlegm may be coughed up. Sometimes a lump can be felt in the neck. Symptoms of a tumour in the laryngopharynx include hoarseness, increased difficulty in swallowing and a sensation of incomplete swallowing.

Throat tumours can be treated by surgery or radiotherapy, or both. Surgery is difficult in the nasopharynx, so radiotherapy is usually preferred. The outlook is variable, depending upon the location of the malignancy and the stage at which it is detected.

Pharyngeal pouch

A pharyngeal pouch is a sac-like protrusion from the top of the oesophagus, where it meets the pharynx, caused by failure of the sphincter muscle at the oesophageal entrance to relax during swallowing. The condition is most common in men over the age of 50. Once formed, the pouch enlarges and food becomes trapped in it, causing swallowing difficulty, throat irritation, bad breath and regurgitation.

Endoscopic surgery (where a flexible tube with a light source and a lens is passed into the throat enabling the surgeon to get a close-up view) is used to staple off a pharyngeal pouch; at the same time, the sphincter muscle is cut to relax it and thereby prevent recurrence of the condition.

A lump in the throat

The sensation of a lump in the throat, perhaps accompanied by swallowing difficulty, has a variety of possible causes, including chronic sinusitis, a gastric **ulcer**, smoking and psychological stress. If you are worried about a lump in the throat, seek medical advice. A doctor will probably arrange for you to have a barium X-ray or an endoscopy to investigate the cause of the problem.

Where the cause is psychological, affected individuals may have a strong feeling of interference with swallowing or breathing, which can lead to panic attacks. They may also worry that they have cancer – especially if they have just lost someone close to them from the disease. Breathing techniques, relaxation and psychotherapy may be helpful in alleviating the condition.

WHEN TO SEE A DOCTOR

Problems affecting the throat have many possible causes. For instance, a lump in the neck may be caused by anything from a harmless cyst or glandular fever to lymphoma or other forms of cancer. See a doctor if you have any of the following symptoms:

- a persistent lump in the throat;
- a lump in the neck;
- difficulty in swallowing;
- unexplained hoarseness – especially if present for more than three weeks.

Thyroid gland and disorders

The thyroid is a small, butterfly-shaped gland situated just below the larynx, which is in the front of the neck. It consists of two lobes joined by a bridge of tissue called the isthmus.

Thyroid hormone (TH) is produced by the thyroid gland and has a wide range of functions (see chart, page 564). In fact, with the exception of the brain, spleen, testes, uterus and the thyroid itself, TH affects virtually every cell in the body.

Thyroid hormone actually consists of two hormones, thyroxine (T4), and triiodothyronine (T3). T4 is the major hormone secreted by the thyroid, while T3 is mainly synthesized in other tissues from T4. The formation of T3 and T4 is controlled by thyroid-stimulating hormone, which is produced by the pituitary gland.

WHAT CAN GO WRONG

The thyroid may either produce too little or too much thyroid hormone. Both under- and overactivity can produce severe disturbances of the metabolism.

Hypothyroidism

Underactivity of the thyroid is referred to as hypothyroidism or **myxoedema**. The symptoms of hypothyroidism include:

- fatigue;
- energy loss;

Thyroid gland

The structures of the neck are closely linked – with the parathyroid glands at the back of the thyroid and the front of the trachea passing through it.

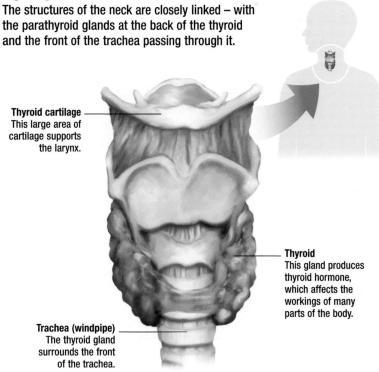

Thyroid cartilage
This large area of cartilage supports the larynx.

Thyroid
This gland produces thyroid hormone, which affects the workings of many parts of the body.

Trachea (windpipe)
The thyroid gland surrounds the front of the trachea.

- weight gain;
- intolerance of cold;
- dry skin and hair;
- menorrhagia (abnormally heavy bleeding during menstruation);
- **constipation;**
- slowed thinking.

Hypothyroidism is commonly the result of Hashimoto's thyroiditis, a condition in which the immune system attacks the thyroid cells. It is often accompanied by a swelling of the neck due to enlargement of the thyroid gland (see **goitre**). The condition may also occur after radioactive iodine therapy (used to treat thyroid problems) or surgery to treat hyperthyroidism. Temporary underactivity of the gland may also occur following childbirth when it may be mistaken for **postnatal depression**. The condition may also be present from birth.

In babies and children, severe hypothyroidism is called cretinism. The child has a short, disproportionate body, a thick tongue and neck, and mental retardation. A heel prick test at birth (see **Birth and problems**) for thyroid hormone, and early treatment, has virtually eliminated this condition in the UK.

Hypothyroidism is diagnosed by means of thyroid function tests, although sometimes these do not produce a clear result. Treatment involves thyroid replacement therapy – taking thyroid hormone in the form of a pill or tablet. This normally continues for the rest of the person's life.

Hyperthyroidism

Hyperthyroidism is experienced when too much thyroid hormone is produced. Symptoms of the condition include:

- a higher than normal metabolic rate (see **Metabolism and disorders**);
- restlessness;
- feeling hot and sweaty;
- rapid, irregular heartbeat or palpitations;
- nervousness, shaking and irritability;
- weight loss;
- fatigue;
- more frequent bowel motions;
- shorter or lighter menstrual periods.

The most common, and mystifying, form of hyperthyroidism is Graves' disease, an **autoimmune disease** in which the body turns against itself. It is more common in women and those with a family history of the condition,

What thyroid hormone does

Thyroid hormone plays an important role in many of the body's systems. As well as those listed below, it affects bone growth, the function of the gastro-intestinal tract, the reproductive system and the skin.

BODY SYSTEM	EFFECTS	WHAT CAN GO WRONG
Metabolism	Regulates metabolism by promoting oxygen consumption and heat production.	Too little leads to a lower basal metabolic rate (BMR), low temperature, intolerance of cold, appetite loss and weight gain; too much causes raised BMR, higher temperature, heat intolerance, appetite increase and weight loss.
Carbohydrate, fat and protein metabolism	Helps the body metabolize glucose and fats and to synthesize protein; enhances the liver's secretion of cholesterol.	Too little causes decreased glucose metabolism, raised cholesterol, decreased synthesis of protein and swelling; too much leads to increased metabolism of glucose and fat, weight loss and muscle wasting.
Nervous system	Vital for the development of the nervous system in the fetus and needed for normal function in adults.	Too little in a fetus or baby leads to poor brain development or retardation. In adults, too little causes depression, forgetfulness, slowed thinking and listlessness; too much causes irritability, restlessness, insomnia and personality changes.
Heart	Needed for normal heart function.	Too little causes reduced efficiency of heart, low heart rate and lowered blood pressure; too much leads to rapid heart rate, high blood pressure and heart failure.
Muscles	Needed for normal muscular development.	Too little causes sluggish muscle action, cramps and muscle pain; too much leads to muscle wasting and weakness.

and the incidence increases with age. There may be painless swelling of the thyroid and a painless goitre. Left untreated, there is a higher risk of heart disease and the bone disease **osteoporosis**. There may also be an increased risk of **dementia** or **Alzheimer's disease**. Some people with Graves' disease develop Graves' ophthalmopathy, which causes eye symptoms such as staring, bulging eyes (exophthalmos) and retraction of the lids. There may also be pain, excess production of tears, irritation, photophobia (an abnormal intolerance of light) and muscle weakness leading to double vision.

Diagnosis of hyperthyroidism involves blood tests and thyroid function tests, which track the uptake of radioactive iodine in the thyroid gland. A thyroid scan may be performed to detect other thyroid conditions that could be causing symptoms.

Treatment is by means of radioactive iodine to destroy the thyroid, and thyroid replacement therapy. Medications that slow the thyroid can also be given, but these are not always effective and may cause serious side effects. Surgical removal of part of the thyroid is occasionally used as a treatment.

Thyroid nodules

These are fairly common and normally harmless, but about 4 per cent are cancerous. A doctor usually does a **biopsy** to rule out the possibility of cancer. Treatment with thyroid hormone to decrease the size of the nodule may be recommended if the nodule is benign. If it is cancerous, or is so large as to interfere with swallowing or breathing, it may need to be surgically removed.

OUTLOOK

There is a great debate about how mild degrees of thyroid problems should be treated, and whether routine thyroid screening should be introduced to identify people with abnormal levels of thyroid hormones. Mild cases of hypothyroidism are common in older women and may affect as many as one in ten people.

Symptoms are less severe than those of severe hypothyroidism, but they can still be debilitating. The condition has been linked with other disorders including **migraine**, mood swings, **panic attacks**, premenstrual syndrome, heart disease, eating disorders, **obesity**, **chronic fatigue syndrome** and **allergy**, as well as ageing.

Mild hyperthyroidism is less common but has been linked to an increased incidence of **atrial fibrillation**, a type of abnormal heartbeat found in older people.

SEE ALSO *Pituitary gland and disorders*

TIA

TIA, or transient ischaemic attack, is also known as a 'mini-stroke' because it causes similar symptoms to those of a **stroke**. Weakness, numbness, tingling, blurred vision, slurred speech and confusion may all occur, and last from a few minutes up to 24 hours.

TIAs are caused by a temporary blockage of an artery to the brain. They should always be investigated as they indicate a high risk of subsequent stroke.

SEE ALSO *Brain and nervous system*

Tinnitus

Tinnitus is a ringing, buzzing or whistling sound in the ears, which is not caused by an exterior source. The noise may be continuous or it may come and go. It can vary from a low roar to a high-pitched whine, in one or both ears.

CAUSES

Tinnitus can be one of the symptoms of an ear infection (see **Ear and problems**). It will subside once the infection has been eradicated.

The chronic form arises from damage to the endings of the acoustic nerve in the inner ear. The damage may be caused by:
- the ageing process, which causes a certain degree of nerve impairment;
- exposure to loud noises;
- **otosclerosis** – a disorder of the middle ear;
- **allergy**;
- high **blood pressure**;
- **diabetes**;
- **thyroid problems**;
- medications such as aspirin, antibiotics or sedatives.

PREVENTION

The following measures may help to reduce the likelihood of getting tinnitus.
- Avoid exposure to loud sounds and noise.
- Keep your blood pressure under control.
- Decrease your salt intake.
- Avoid stimulants such as tea, coffee, cocoa, and tobacco.
- Exercise regularly, to improve the circulation.
- Avoid fatigue.

TREATMENT

There is no specific treatment for tinnitus. If the underlying cause can be detected, treating this may reduce or eliminate the noises.

What you can do

If tinnitus is interfering with your life, try to find some way of distracting yourself from the sound. Relaxation techniques may be helpful, as might introducing a competing low-level sound, such as a ticking clock or a white-noise device.

Tongue and problems

The tongue is a large flap of muscular tissue attached to the floor of the mouth. It has three main functions:

- providing taste sensation;
- manipulating food while chewing;
- aiding speech production.

The body of the tongue joins its root at the back, where muscles attach it to bones in the throat (pharynx). It is covered with mucous membrane, like that lining the mouth. On its top surface are little mounds called papillae, around which the taste buds are arranged in grooves. A fold of membrane (the frenulum linguae) connects the middle of the base of the tongue with the floor of the mouth.

TASTE BUDS

The taste buds – which are also found in the soft palate, epiglottis and pharynx – detect four basic tastes. Bitter and sour tastes are tasted towards the back of the tongue, sweet tastes are felt at the tip, and saltiness is detected at the front sides.

Loss of taste

Our sense of taste is closely allied to our sense of smell – which is why we often cannot taste food properly during a cold.

Other causes of loss of taste include:

- ageing;
- smoking;
- nasal polyps;
- prolonged use of decongestants;
- rarely, a nerve lesion or brain tumour.

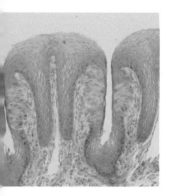

▲ Taste buds
The surface of the tongue has tiny grooves called papillae, which contain about 10,000 taste buds in total. They have sensory cells that detect sweet, salty, sour and bitter flavours.

Sophisticated senses
Our taste buds – on the tongue, soft palate and other areas near the mouth – work with olfactory receptors to help us to distinguish subtle flavours.

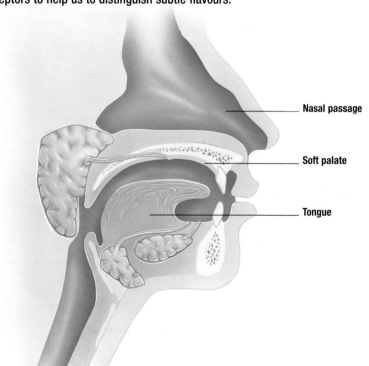

Nasal passage

Soft palate

Tongue

See a doctor if you lose your sense of taste suddenly and without obvious cause, or if the loss persists for more than two weeks after an infection. You should also seek medical advice if your loss of taste is accompanied by loss of smell in one nostril only.

THE TONGUE'S APPEARANCE

A thin coating of yellowish 'fur' on the surface of the tongue is very common and is not necessarily a sign of illness. The furring worsens in **dehydration**, fever and when saliva flow is reduced. It can also occur in kidney disease.

The tongue's coating may turn black after drinking red wine, smoking heavily or taking antibiotics. Sometimes – particularly after taking a course of antibiotics – this indicates a fungal infection that may need treatment. Otherwise, gentle scraping with a toothbrush will clean it quite safely. Many Eastern cultures have a long tradition of cleaning the tongue as well as the teeth.

Complementary therapies

The tongue is widely used for diagnosis in traditional **Chinese medicine**. Practitioners believe that the different areas on the tongue reveal the workings of different bodily organs and systems.

SEE ALSO *Nose and problems; Salivary glands and disorders; Mouth and disorders*

Tonsils and disorders

The tonsils are a pair of oval-shaped tissue masses visible on either side of the back of the throat. They are part of the lymphatic system, which helps to protect the body from infection. The function of the tonsils is to trap micro-organisms entering the body through the nose and mouth. They seem to be at their most active between the ages of four and ten years – with the result that many children experience problems at this stage.

The most common problem affecting the tonsils is infection by one of a range of viruses or bacteria. Infection, or tonsillitis, is mainly a childhood condition, although adults may also be affected by it.

SYMPTOMS

The symptoms of tonsillitis include:

- sore throat;
- difficulty in swallowing;
- fever;
- general malaise;
- swollen glands in the neck;
- tonsil enlargement.

The symptoms of tonsillitis are similar to those of **glandular fever**, but a doctor can readily distinguish the two conditions by examining the tonsils and throat. If a more serious condition is suspected, a throat swab may be taken for analysis to give an accurate diagnosis. In tonsillitis, there are frequently white and inflamed patches on the tonsils, while in glandular fever the tonsils are covered with a thick white or grey fluid.

TREATMENT

In milder cases of tonsillitis, bed rest, painkillers and plenty of fluids may be all that is needed by way of treatment. More severe cases require antibiotic treatment – intravenously if the patient's throat is so sore that he or she cannot swallow a tablet properly.

Surgical treatment

Tonsillitis tends to recur, and in some cases removal of the tonsils (tonsillectomy) is the only long-term solution. But the operation is now performed less frequently than it was 20 or 30 years ago. While there is no evidence that removal of the tonsils has any serious adverse effect upon the immune system, doctors no longer recommend this as a routine procedure for children.

Tonsillectomy is usually considered if there have been five or more bouts of infection in a year, or three or more annual bouts for two consecutive years. A child or young adult who has missed a substantial amount of education through tonsillitis would also be a prime candidate, regardless of the number of attacks. Enlarged tonsils causing sleep apnoea – episodes of breathing cessation linked with snoring – are usually removed. A tonsillectomy is also performed if there is any suspicion of a malignant tumour.

In a tonsillectomy, the tonsils are eased away from the throat with forceps and then cut out. **Diathermy** – a form of heat treatment – is used to reduce bleeding, the main complication of this operation. More recently, laser tonsillectomy and radio-frequency removal of tonsillar tissue has been used in an attempt to reduce post-operative bleeding.

The pharynx has a rich nerve supply, so many people experience pain after the operation. Bleeding that occurs five to ten days after the operation is normally due to infection.

As far as eating after surgery is concerned, the modern view is that the person's diet should return to normal as soon as possible, as it is believed that chewing speeds recovery and helps to prevent post-operative infection.

COMPLICATIONS

Nowadays, complications of tonsillitis are rare. But **quinsy**, which is an abscess of the tissue on the side of the tonsils, may sometimes occur.

SEE ALSO *Lymphatic system; Throat and disorders*

Toxaemia

Toxaemia is a type of blood poisoning caused by the release of poisons (toxins) from a severe localized bacterial infection, such as a lung or bowel abscess. Symptoms include high fever, shaking, low blood pressure, confusion and abnormal blood clotting. Treatment involves antibiotics, a high intake of fluids and, in extreme cases, blood transfusion.

Toxic shock syndrome

Toxic shock syndrome (TSS) is a rare but life-threatening condition. It is usually due to an infection with the bacterium *Staphylococcus aureus*, which produces a poison (toxin). Other bacteria, such as *Escherichia coli* (E. coli), can also cause TSS.

Some cases of TSS have been associated with tampon use during menstruation, possibly as a result of the tampon becoming contaminated during insertion by staphylococci bacteria on the hands and skin. TSS can also occur after surgical operations and as a result of infections acquired in hospital, insect bites, burns, childbirth and the use of barrier contraceptives.

SYMPTOMS

- Sudden severe fever.
- A widespread red rash that later peels.
- Vomiting and diarrhoea.
- Severe muscle pains.
- Shock.

TREATMENT

Patients with toxic shock syndrome require immediate intensive care with intravenous fluids and antibiotics. Kidney and liver failure may occur. TSS is fatal in about 10 per cent of cases.

TAMPON USE

To reduce the risk of toxic shock syndrome:
- wash your hands before inserting a tampon;
- change tampons at least every 4–6 hours during the daytime;
- wear an external pad at night;
- if you have an abnormal vaginal discharge, avoid wearing a tampon and seek medical advice immediately.

SEE ALSO *Contraception; Menstruation*

Toxocariasis

Toxocariasis is a disease that primarily affects children, who become infested with the larvae of *Toxocara canis*, a roundworm that lives in the intestines of dogs. It occurs when they ingest *Toxocara* eggs, which can be present on hands or in food contaminated with the faeces of infected domestic pets. Symptoms are mild fever and malaise, which soon clear up.

Dogs that live with children should be dewormed monthly until the dog is six months old and annually thereafter. Do not allow children to play or crawl in areas where dogs may have been. Wash your hands after handling or cleaning up after your dog. Teach your children to wash their hands after handling animals, particularly before touching food.

Transplants

A transplant is the transfer of healthy living cells, tissues or organs from a donor to a recipient. Examples include heart, lung and liver transplants. Transferring an organ from one person into another involves complex procedures to avoid rejection. This is because the body's immune system recognizes a transplanted organ as foreign and so attacks it. Although doctors had perfected the necessary skills and techniques to perform the surgery, the transplanted organs would always be rejected by the recipients' bodies.

The development of transplant surgery, in which a diseased organ is replaced with a healthy one, was one of the most profound medical breakthroughs of the last century, and now saves thousands of lives every year.

RETRIEVING SUITABLE ORGANS

All internal organs except kidneys have to come from someone whose heart is still beating. This is because organs need a good supply of oxygenated blood in order to function properly. As soon as they lose their supply of oxygenated blood they begin to deteriorate and die. Although kidneys can be retrieved within one hour of heart-death, and there are developments to extend this period to four hours, beating-heart kidney retrieval is the preferred method. Most beating-heart donors are people who have consented to their organs being used after death. Before the organ can be removed, two experienced doctors who are not involved with the transplant unit must declare the donor brain dead. Breathing and heartbeat are maintained artificially until the organs can be retrieved.

The other type of beating-heart donor is a relative, partner or friend who has consented to donate an organ while still alive. Segments of liver and lung can be donated in this way, as well as one kidney. Cystic fibrosis patients can end up in the unusual position of being able to donate their hearts. A person with cystic fibrosis often requires a heart-lung combination transplant, so leaving a healthy heart that can be transferred to another recipient.

THE PROBLEMS OF REJECTION

When a patient receives a new organ, the immune system recognizes that the organ is not a natural part of the body and attacks it and this leads to rejection of the organ. Various methods have been used to minimize rejection.

■ Donors are selected with a similar genetic make-up to the recipient. Identical twins offer the ideal solution; close relatives (parent, sister, brother, half sister/brother, first cousin, uncle, aunt, nephew or niece) are the next best thing.

■ Medication is given to prevent the immune system from attacking the transplanted organ.

Travel and tropical diseases

SEE OPPOSITE

Trigeminal neuralgia

Trigeminal neuralgia, also known as tic douloureux, causes spasms of severe, stabbing facial pain. It affects areas of the face supplied by the trigeminal, or fifth, cranial nerve, which transmits sensations of touch, heat, cold and pain from the face, mouth, nose and teeth, it also controls chewing movements of the jaw.

SYMPTOMS

Pain affects one or more branches of the trigeminal nerve and is usually short-lived, lasting 5 to 30 seconds, but may recur several times a day and be extremely painful. It is sometimes accompanied by a spasm of the muscles of the face, and tears.

CAUSES

The cause remains uncertain, but it may be due to pressure from blood vessels where the nerve enters the brain. Occasionally it is found in association with other neurological conditions, including multiple sclerosis.

TREATMENT

Anticonvulsant drugs such as carbamazepine, originally developed to treat epilepsy, are one form of treatment. Common side effects include drowsiness, nausea, dizziness and muscular weakness – but many sufferers feel that these are worth enduring to be rid of the pain. If drug treatment is not effective, various forms of surgery can be performed to block pain impulses from the nerve, although this may leave the face numb, and treatment may need to be repeated after a few years if pain recurs.

OUTLOOK

Remissions lasting weeks or months do occur, particularly early on, but rarely last. Without treatment, attacks become more frequent with age. Most people gain relief with treatment.

Travel and tropical diseases

Travelling around the world has never been easier or cheaper. But it almost always brings with it some risks to health. By taking a few simple precautions, you can minimize your exposure to travel-related health hazards.

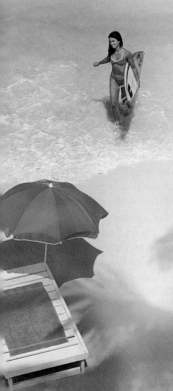

Foreign travel is increasing year by year – and many travellers are venturing to places where unfamiliar climates and environments may pose dangers to their health. For example, of the 43 million British residents who travelled abroad in 1998, more than 4 million visited tropical and east European countries, where the risk of communicable diseases is higher than it is in the West. To meet the needs of the growing number of people exposed to travel-related health hazards, a new branch of medicine – travel medicine – has evolved. As well as training specialist doctors how to manage travel-related illnesses, travel medicine educates travellers to assess their health needs and take precautions and preventive measures, such as immunization.

PREPARATION

Preventing illness, the key to good travel health, demands preparation. If you frequently travel, internationally, you can take action that will stand you in good stead for future trips.

■ Check your immunization status: diseases such as polio, tetanus, mumps and rubella are widespread in many countries. All can affect children and adults. Tuberculosis is re-emerging in the West, and travellers often pick up influenza. Have the shots or boosters as soon as you can, well before your next trip. If you have to travel at short notice you should still see a doctor. Some protection is better that none.

■ Exercise: two or three times a week. Sitting immobile on a long journey strains the back and may encourage deep vein thrombosis (DVT). Regular exercise keeps the back flexible, boosts the circulation, discouraging the formation of blood clots and strengthening resistance to stress.

■ Ask your doctor for a blood test. One person in 20 may have a Factor V Leiden blood-clotting abnormality that predisposes them to DVT. If the result is positive, take special care to protect yourself against developing DVT.

■ If you travel by air regularly, work out a strategy for overcoming **jet lag,** or your health will be permanently affected.

■ Consult travel books and leaflets to make sure you are aware of any specific risks.

TROPICAL DISEASES

Tropical diseases are those prevalent in the regions between the Tropic of Cancer and the Tropic of Capricorn – latitudes 23.5°N and 23.5°S. Since the onset of global warming, however, average summer temperatures in temperate regions are increasing, and summer seasons are lasting longer. There is concern that climate change may therefore extend the habitats of disease-causing organisms such as the Anopheles mosquito, which thrives only in hot, humid conditions, into the temperate zones, and so widen the geographical distribution of malaria and other infectious tropical diseases.

Diseases such as **plague, diphtheria, typhoid fever** and **typhus** were once epidemic as far north as Scandinavia; they have since been controlled by public health and immunization programmes, but outbreaks still occur in poorer tropical countries. **Tuberculosis** is rife in China, India and Pakistan, parts of Southeast Asia, the Philippines and southern Africa, and is now re-emerging in temperate-zone cities from which it was once eradicated, such as London and New York. Some tropical diseases are declining, notably leprosy (Hansen's disease). This illness has a low infection rate and is treated easily and cheaply. It occurs worldwide, and no vaccine is available, but the risk of contracting it is minimal and no preventive measures are necessary.

Many people are unaware that the greatest disease hazard facing travellers to most tropical countries today is malaria. There is no vaccine for this disabling illness, which affects 3–5 million people and causes 1–2 million deaths every year. Preventive measures could be life-saving.

Most travellers are aware of newly identified diseases – for example, Lassa, Ebola and Marburg fevers, which occur in tropical Africa – for which no vaccines are available. Awareness is high that AIDS has reached epidemic proportions in central African countries and is close to becoming epidemic in some Asian countries, but many travellers do not realize that other **sexually transmitted diseases** (STDs) are far more widespread. Lymphogranuloma venereum and chancroid – both characterized by sores around the genitals – are STDs specific to the Tropics.

Travel immunization chart

Most of the major infectious diseases are widespread in tropical areas, but always check with a specialist travel clinic which vaccinations you need for the area(s) you intend to visit.

DISEASE	SYMPTOMS	VACCINATION	BOOSTER
Cholera	Gut infection	Single-dose oral or injection	After 6–9 months
Diphtheria	Suffocating throat infection	Injection	After 10 years
Flu	Respiratory virus	Injection	Annual
Hepatitis A	Liver disease	2 shots 6 months apart	After 10 years
Hepatitis B	Liver disease often spread by needles or blood	3 shots over 6 months	After 5 years
Japanese encephalitis	Viral brain inflammation	3 injections over 1 month	After 3–5 years
Measles	Virus with fever and rash	Injection (part of MMR)	After 3–5 years
Meningococcal meningitis (Hib)	Bacterial infection causing inflammation of the brain	3 shots 4 weeks apart	After 3–5 years
Mumps	Glandular virus	Injection (part of MMR)	After 3–5 years
Plague	Respiratory or all-encompassing with boils	Injection	Every 6 months for those at risk of exposure
Polio	Paralysing infection	Oral	After 3–5 years
Rabies	Nervous system disease with fits and delirium	2 injections 4 weeks apart	Annual for those at risk of being bitten by animals
Rubella	Rash and mild fever	Injection (part of MMR)	After 3–5 years
Tetanus	Nervous system disease in which jaw seizes up	Injection	After 10 years
Tuberculosis	Lung disease	Injection	After 10–15 years
Typhoid	Digestive tract infection with fever and headache	Injection	After 3 years
Whooping cough	Respiratory with cough	Injection	After 3–5 years
Yellow fever	Infection affecting liver with severe headache	Injection	After 10 years

POOR SANITATION AND POOR HYGIENE

Many tropical diseases are spread by consuming food or drinking water contaminated through poor personal hygiene of those infected, especially after going to the lavatory. The following are the most common.

■ **Cholera**: has been spreading through Africa and South America for some years.

■ **Diarrhoea** and **dysentery**: found worldwide, including the UK. (See also **E. coli; Food poisoning; Giardiasis; Salmonella**.)

■ **Hepatitis A**: distribution is worldwide, with a high incidence in Central and South America, Africa, the Middle East and across Asia.

■ **Typhoid fever** and the **paratyphoids**: found worldwide, including recent occurrences in the UK; common in countries with poor sewage systems and where human excreta is used to fertilize the land.

Prevention

Be scrupulous about personal hygiene and what you consume. Drink only boiled water, milk and other drinks. Some organisms that cause traveller's diarrhoea are resistant to all chemical methods of water decontamination. Do not drink aerated water, or drinks cooled by ice cubes, or eat frozen products such as ice cream.

Do not eat shellfish, uncooked or partially cooked vegetables, cooled rice or unpeeled fruit. Eat only well-cooked food that has been freshly prepared. Do not eat food that may have been left standing or contaminated by flies.

Wash hands frequently with bactericidal soap, especially after using the lavatory and before eating. This will reduce the risk of contaminating food and passing on infection. Never put your fingers in your mouth or rub your eyes with unwashed hands.

PARASITE INFECTIONS

Many infections by protozoa, such as *Giardia lamblia*, *Cryptosporidium*, *Entamoeba histolytica* and worms can be transmitted through the consumption of contaminated food and water after poor hygiene (see above), but they may also be picked up by swimming in infested waters and by walking with bare feet. The following are the most widespread.

- Filarial diseases occur when biting flies transmit microscopic worms into the bloodstream. They occur in Central America, the Caribbean, north and northeast regions of South America, East and Southeast Asia, and include loiasis and onchocerciasis (river blindness) of West and Central Africa.
- Fluke infestations may be caused by schistosome worms, which live in freshwater lakes, rivers and streams and penetrate the skin rapidly. They occur in northern and eastern regions of South America, West, Central and East Africa, parts of the Middle East, and East and Southeast Asia. Liver flukes are widespread and a problem in East Asia, where infection occurs after eating raw or lightly cooked fish, beef and pork.
- Guinea worms, *Dracunculus medinensis*, are transmitted by drinking water containing tiny Cyclops water fleas. The worms infest the tissues beneath the skin. They occur in tropical Africa, South America and South Asia.
- Roundworm infestation – by threadworms, hookworms, *Ascaris lumbricoides*, *Trichinella spiralis* and other nematodes that live in the bowel. These are a hazard in all tropical and temperate regions and are usually transmitted by the contamination of food by infected faeces. It is possible for hookworm larvae to enter the feet from the soil.
- Tapeworms enter the gut via infected pork, beef or fish. They can occur worldwide.

Prevention

There are no vaccines against parasitic infections. To prevent infection and passing on any disease you may have contracted, attend scrupulously to personal hygiene, and wash your hands and scrub your nails with bactericidal soap after using the lavatory and before eating. Never put your fingers in your mouth. Wear shoes indoors and out; change clothes frequently; wash clothes in hot water and iron them if possible. Do not swim in freshwater lakes or rivers. Never eat raw or undercooked vegetables (especially watercress and water chestnuts), beef, pork or fish.

INSECT-BORNE DISEASES

Many infectious diseases are transmitted by insects. Discover which disease-causing insects inhabit the area you intend to visit, and what precautions are required to prevent infection.

Use insecticides and insect repellents, take other precautions at times of the day when they are active, and cover the body – including the neck, arms, legs and feet.

Protect yourself from mosquito bites

Preventing mosquito bites is one of the most important things you can do to protect yourself from diseases such as malaria and dengue fever when travelling in tropical countries.

Deet (diethyl-meta-toluamide), the active ingredient in most insect-repellent sprays and creams, has been linked with occasional severe reactions – so apply insect repellent sparingly to exposed skin.

The more deet a repellent contains, the longer it will protect you from mosquito bites – so a higher percentage of deet in a repellent does not mean that your protection will be better, simply that it will last longer.

Before you use an insecticide or insect repellent, carefully read the manufacturer's directions for use. Repellents can irritate the eyes and mouth, so don't apply them to children's hands. Mosquitoes can bite through thin clothing, so spray clothes with repellents containing either permethrin or deet. Repellents containing permethrin should not be used on bare skin.

Peak mosquito biting times are at dawn, dusk and in the early evening, so it may be worth trying to stay indoors at these times. Whenever you are outdoors you should wear long-sleeved shirts and long trousers. Cover any pram, buggy or baby-carrier with mosquito netting.

TREATING TROPICAL DISEASES

Be aware of unusual symptoms while travelling or living in tropical areas and see a doctor urgently if any arise. Many tropical diseases clear up quickly if treated promptly with the right medication, but can be serious if left untreated. If you experience any symptoms of tropical disease, remember that local doctors are more likely to recognize these than your GP at home. However, some tropical diseases can occur long after the initial infection, and some can recur years after the first outbreak.

If you have any worrying symptoms on your return home – even if they occur several months later – visit a clinic that specializes in travel medicine, or a hospital for tropical diseases.

West Nile virus

West Nile virus is commonly found in Africa, West Asia and the Middle East. However, in 1999, the disease spread to the USA.

West Nile virus is spread by the bite of an infected mosquito, and can infect people, horses, many types of bird and some other animals. Most people who become infected with West Nile virus have no symptoms or only mild ones. However, in rare cases, the infection can cause West Nile encephalitis or West Nile meningitis – severe and sometimes fatal illnesses. Symptoms of severe infection can include headache, fever, stiff neck, disorientation, coma, tremors, convulsions, muscle weakness and paralysis. It is estimated that one in 150 people infected with the West Nile virus will develop a more severe form of the disease.

Tuberculosis

Tuberculosis, often called TB, is an infectious disease affecting both people and animals. It damages the lungs, reducing the area available for the exchange of gases and making it hard to breathe. Left untreated, the victim may die through lack of ventilation and exhaustion.

Tuberculosis, which used to be known as consumption, caused some 25 per cent of all deaths in Europe during the 17th and 18th centuries. The death toll began to fall with improved health and hygiene in the early 20th century, and was further reduced with the development of penicillin and other antibiotics. But the disease is still common in areas where people are badly nourished, in poor health and living in overcrowded conditions. About 3 million people a year die from the disease, mainly in less developed countries.

In the UK, the incidence of tuberculosis is rising, especially among alcoholics and people with weakened immune systems such as those who are **HIV**-positive. The resurgence of TB worldwide may in part be due to the emergence of drug-resistant strains.

There is a difference between being infected with tuberculosis and having the disease. Many people infected with tuberculosis bacteria do not develop the disease, because their immune system protects them. But the infection can remain dormant for years, and then strike if the immune system is weakened.

SYMPTOMS

Symptoms of tuberculosis include:
- a chronic or persistent cough;
- bringing up phlegm that may contain blood;
- severe fatigue;
- lack of appetite and weight loss;
- fever and night sweats.

TREATMENT

Tuberculosis is treated with antibiotics that must be taken for several months.

When to consult a doctor

See a doctor if coughing and bringing up phlegm persists for more than three weeks.

What a doctor may do

A GP will refer anyone suspected of having tuberculosis for a chest **X-ray** and may send a sample of phlegm for analysis. Bacteria from the phlegm can be tested; the results take up to six weeks to come through. A tuberculin skin test may be carried out: if this is positive, the patient has either been inoculated or exposed to the infection.

Early treatment of tuberculosis with a combination of antibiotics means that most people recover completely. The patient may become non-infectious quite quickly, but

a complete cure often necessitates drug treatment for about nine months.

PREVENTION

Prevention of tuberculosis largely depends on good hygiene and nutrition. In the UK, most teenagers are routinely inoculated with the **BCG vaccine** at school; this gives them lifelong immunity to tuberculosis infection. Inoculation is also recommended for anyone travelling to areas where the disease is prevalent.

SEE ALSO *Immunization*

Tularaemia

Tularaemia is an infectious disease that affects wild animals such as rabbits and squirrels, and which can be passed to human beings. It does not occur in the UK but exists in parts of Europe and the USA. Anyone who handles a diseased animal abroad might be at risk.

The disease-causing bacterium enters the skin through a cut, or via flea or tick bites. Flu-like symptoms are followed by an **ulcer** at the site of infection. Swollen glands and bouts of fever can occur over several weeks. The disease is treated with antibiotics.

Turner's syndrome

Turner's syndrome is a chromosomal disorder that it is found only in women. Those affected are much shorter than average; they do not develop breasts and usually lack ovaries. Other minor abnormalities affect appearance but not intelligence. It is possible to diagnose Turner's syndrome by prenatal chromosome analysis. If an affected girl is treated with growth hormone from infancy, she may reach normal height.

SEE ALSO *Chromosomal disorders*

Typhoid fever

Typhoid fever is a highly infectious disease. It affects 16 million people, and kills some 600,000, each year worldwide. It is caused by the *Salmonella typhi* bacterium infecting the gastro-intestinal tract. Typhoid fever is not a tropical disease – it is related to hygiene and sanitary conditions rather than the climate itself. It is found mainly in countries where water or food supplies are liable to faecal contamination, such as much of Asia, Africa, Central and South America. Many of those infected on holiday pick up the disease in the Far East. Typhoid is caught by eating food or drinking water contaminated with the faeces

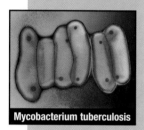

Mycobacterium tuberculosis

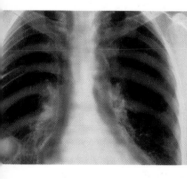

▲ **Tuberculosis X-ray**
If someone has TB, an X-ray will reveal characteristic shadows on the lungs.

or urine of someone who has the disease, or who is carrying it without symptoms.

SYMPTOMS

A person who has typhoid fever will show signs of illness between one and three weeks after exposure to the bacterium. Symptoms include:
- severe headache;
- sustained high fever, of 39–40°C (102–104°F);
- loss of appetite;
- constipation, which soon gives way to a soup-like diarrhoea;
- a rash on the chest and abdomen.

DURATION

If typhoid is left to run its course, the feverish phase can last for four or five weeks. Then the temperature falls and a slow recovery begins.

TREATMENT

Someone with typhoid fever will be admitted to hospital for treatment to replace lost fluids and salts, and antibiotic drugs to kill the bacteria.

PREVENTION

Travellers to areas where food and water are likely to be contaminated can be vaccinated against typhoid. The jab is available at GPs' surgeries and private travel clinics, and should be administered at least two weeks before you travel. It is effective for three years.

If you are visiting a country with poor sanitation, drink only boiled or bottled water and be careful about food sources and hygiene.

SEE ALSO *Travel and tropical diseases*

Typhus

Typhus is completely unrelated to typhoid fever. The term is used to describe infections caused by rickettsiae – micro-organisms similar to bacteria – which are spread by insects. Epidemic typhus is spread by body lice, endemic typhus is transmitted to people by rat-borne fleas, and other forms are spread by ticks.

Historically, typhus epidemics occurred in crowded, insanitary conditions, often during wars and at times of famine. Today, infection is rare, and confined to parts of tropical Africa and South America. A vaccination is available.

SYMPTOMS

Typhus symptoms include:
- headache;
- back and limb pain;
- coughing;
- constipation;
- high fever and delirium;
- a widespread rash, like that of **measles**.

TREATMENT

Different types of typhus are diagnosed using blood tests, and all are treated with antibiotics. Without treatment, the infection can be fatal.

Ulcer

An ulcer is an inflamed, often painful break in the skin or in the mucous membranes that line the body's cavities. There are several different kinds of ulcer, from the small ulcers that appear in the mouth to more serious ulcers in the stomach and duodenum. A pressure sore is an ulcer that forms in areas of the body put under pressure by a person's own body weight. Pressure sores usually develop when the person is immobilized and are particularly common in elderly people who are bedridden.

Peptic ulcers

Peptic ulcers occur in the stomach (where they are called gastric ulcers) and in the first part of the intestine (duodenal ulcers). They affect one in 10 men and one in 20 women in the UK.

More than 80 per cent of peptic ulcers develop as a result of *Helicobacter pylori* bacteria in the gut. Other causes include excess stomach acid secretion; this can be related to stress, smoking and the long-term use of certain medication, especially aspirin, ibuprofen and other non-steroidal anti-inflammatory drugs (NSAIDs).

SYMPTOMS

Peptic ulcers, whether in the stomach or duodenum, often cause severe abdominal pain.
- **Duodenal ulcers** These can cause a gnawing, burning pain in the upper abdomen and excessive salivation. The problem is worse at night and is relieved either by eating, or by drinking milk. However, about half of all duodenal ulcers have no symptoms.
- **Gastric ulcers** The pain is also in the upper abdomen but is usually made worse by eating. This in turn is likely to lead to weight loss.

TREATMENT

The treatment of ulcers has changed in recent years. In the past, surgery was often necessary, but with modern drugs ulcers can be cured within a few weeks. People with ulcers should:
- avoid foods that make the pain worse;
- avoid drinking alcohol;
- stop smoking, since smoking increases the likelihood of relapse for duodenal ulcers, and slows down the healing of gastric ulcers.

If tests for *Helicobacter pylori* are positive, then the bacterium must be eradicated with what is known as 'triple therapy', so that the ulcer can heal. Triple therapy involves taking high doses of three different drugs for a short period – usually a week. One is a powerful acid-reducing drug, known as a proton-pump inhibitor, and two are different types of antibiotics. Usually a week of treatment is enough to kill all the bacteria. But sometimes it is necessary to continue taking acid-inhibiting drugs for a few weeks to allow the wound to heal fully.

An ulcer caused by taking aspirin or other NSAIDs is treated with acid-reducing drugs. The patient must stop taking the drug that caused the ulcer. Once the ulcer has healed, the patient may be able to resume taking aspirin or NSAIDs, but if there are complications, such as bleeding or perforated ulcers, then treatment with the culprit drug should never be resumed.

COMPLICATIONS

Peptic ulcers can cause:

■ blood leakage – if slow, this can cause **anaemia** in the long term and, if fast, it may cause a life-threatening haemorrhage;

■ perforation of the gut, a surgical emergency;

■ **pyloric stenosis**, in which narrowing of the outlet of the stomach causes projectile vomiting;

■ duodenal ulcer can perforate the pancreas causing pancreatitis, a serious illness (see **Pancreas and disorders**).

PREVENTION

■ Drink alcohol within sensible limits.

■ Cut down on salt and salty foods.

■ Do not eat very spicy foods.

■ Keep down your intake of caffeine.

■ Don't smoke.

OUTLOOK

Most peptic ulcers are cured within a few weeks if diagnosed and treated promptly.

Mouth ulcers

Mouth ulcers are a common problem. They are usually short-lived and minor. By far the most common cause is superficial damage from biting the inside of the mouth, or a scald from hot food or drink. Thrush infection of the mouth is widespread in babies and elderly people. Viral infections such as **glandular fever** or **hand, foot and mouth disease** can cause ulcers in children.

Occasionally mouth ulcers signify other illness, such as inflammatory **bowel** disease, mouth **cancer**, **leukaemia**, and rare infections and **autoimmune diseases**. So seek medical advice if the ulcers are very painful or extensive.

SYMPTOMS

Ulcers may occur singly or in crops, and cause whiteish areas inside the mouth or on the tongue. They are sore to the touch. Ulcers that are infected cause bad breath.

TREATMENT

Most ulcers get better without any treatment in a week to ten days. Because no one is sure what causes most mouth ulcers, no specific treatment has been developed. Mouthwashes and pastilles may help to ease the pain and speed up healing – ask your pharmacist for advice.

Complementary therapies

Some people find the homeopathic remedies Arsenicum album (arsen alb) or Cantharis vesicatoria (cantharis) helpful.

PREVENTION

Good oral hygiene will help to prevent ulcers. Keep your mouth clean and visit the dentist regularly. If you wear dentures, make sure they fit properly and keep them scrupulously clean. Smoking can damage the delicate tissues of the mouth so, if you are a smoker, it is worth trying to give up. There is little evidence that changing your diet has any effect on mouth ulcers.

Leg ulcers

Leg ulcers are the most common type of skin ulcer. Ulcers that do not heal are described as chronic; they mainly affect elderly people or people with **diabetes**. About 70 per cent of all leg ulcers are venous ulcers, which develop as a result of poor blood circulation. The other main type of leg ulcer is an arterial ulcer, caused by poor blood flow through the arteries.

SYMPTOMS

Leg ulcers look and feel different depending on whether they are arterial or venous ulcers.

■ **Venous leg ulcers** The leg becomes swollen and the skin around the ulcer is dry, itchy and may look brownish. The ulcer is usually painless and appears raw and weeping.

■ **Arterial ulcers** The feet and legs often feel cold and may look whiteish or blueish and shiny. The ulcers can be painful, especially when the legs are at rest and raised. If the person sits on the edge of the bed with the feet on the floor, gravity increases blood flow into the legs and this helps to ease the pain. Cramp-like pains in the legs when walking are known medically as **claudication**. The pain usually goes away if the patient stands still for a few minutes.

CAUSES

■ Venous leg ulcers can develop from old leg ulcers, or they may be due to a bone **fracture** or other injury, a blood clot in the deep veins (**deep vein thrombosis**), surgery, doing a job that involves a lot of sitting or standing, inflammation in the veins (**phlebitis**), **pregnancy** and **obesity**.

■ Arterial leg ulcers can be caused by arterial disease, which is associated with smoking, high blood pressure or diabetes (see also **Arteries and disorders**).

TREATMENT

Treatment depends on what caused the ulcer or what is stopping it from healing. Once these factors are dealt with, the ulcer should heal by itself. Meanwhile, the wound needs cleansing and dressing regularly. The most effective form of dressing is compression bandaging, but this

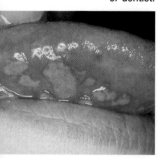

▼ Mouth ulcers
Mouth ulcers rarely need medical advice, but recurrent ulcers may signify an underlying problem and should be checked by a doctor or dentist.

cannot be used if the patient has arterial disease, because compression can reduce the blood supply to the leg below the bandage.

Patients with venous leg ulcers should sit with their feet up. Patients with arterial ulcers may be offered surgery or, alternatively, balloon **angioplasty**, a procedure that relieves narrowing and obstruction of the arteries.

Sometimes an ulcer is closed using a skin graft: skin is taken from elsewhere on the patient's body and placed over the ulcer (see **Cosmetic and plastic surgery**).

PREVENTION

To prevent both arterial and venous leg ulcers:
- stop smoking;
- lose weight if you are overweight;
- take exercise to improve the blood circulation in your legs. You can even exercise while sitting down: move your feet around in circles, then up and down;
- look after your feet: keep them warm and make sure shoes fit properly, and visit a chiropodist regularly;
- check your legs and feet regularly for sores or changes in colour;
- if you are diabetic, make sure your diabetes is well controlled by following diet, monitoring procedures and any treatment recommended by your doctor.

You can also help to prevent venous leg ulcers by sitting with your feet up whenever possible and avoiding crossing your legs – which impairs blood circulation. If you have to stand or sit a lot at work, vary your position and walk about whenever you can.

OUTLOOK

Leg ulcers often recur in elderly patients and often do not completely heal, necessitating years of treatment.

Ultrasound

Ultrasound scanning uses high-frequency soundwaves to generate a detailed image of the internal organs. Although ultrasound is used to investigate any soft tissue, such as the heart, liver or kidneys, it is most widely used during pregnancy to check the baby in the womb.

WHAT'S INVOLVED

An ultrasound scan is painless and, in the case of pregnancy, usually lasts about 15 minutes. Clear gel is poured onto the abdomen and a hand-held unit is moved across the stomach. Signals relayed to a monitor are translated into a detailed black-and-white image of the baby.

Most women are offered at least two scans during the course of their pregnancy. The first, at around 12 weeks, confirms dates and looks for signs of **Down's syndrome**. The scan also checks other anatomical details such as the position of the cervix, amniotic sac or placenta. A second scan is carried out at 18–20 weeks to make sure there are no fetal abnormalities.

Further scans may also be carried out:
- as a guide during tests such as amniocentesis and CVS (chorionic villus sampling);
- when there is concern about a baby's growth;
- to check that a woman's pelvis is large enough to allow vaginal delivery;
- to investigate vaginal bleeding;
- to check if the cervix is opening too early (cervical incompetence);
- to check the amount of amniotic fluid surrounding the baby.

IS ULTRASOUND SAFE?

Most doctors believe that ultrasound scans are completely safe. However, unnecessary scans are avoided because it is thought best not to subject a fetus to prolonged exposure. Small studies that linked scans with low birthweight and hearing problems have been discounted.

SEE ALSO *Pregnancy and problems*

Ultraviolet radiation

Ultraviolet radiation, or UVR, is invisible light, the most common source of which is sunlight. Underexposure to ultraviolet radiation causes vitamin D deficiency. It is common in dark-skinned people living in climates where days are short in winter because the melanin in dark skins screens out UVR.

Overexposure commonly affects light-skinned people and people living in areas no longer protected by the ozone layer, which absorbs UVR. Overexposure causes:
- sunburn, particularly in light-skinned people;
- drying and wrinkling of the skin;
- damage to skin cells; this can lead to **cancers** of the skin;
- damage to the eye, including **cataracts**.

SEE ALSO *Skin and disorders*

Urethritis

Urethritis is an inflammation of the urethra. It is caused by infection either from micro-organisms such as **candida**, normally found in the bowel or on the skin, or from **sexually transmitted diseases** such as **chlamydia**. It can also result from chemical irritation or allergy – for example, to bubble-bath or spermicides. Urethritis should be investigated at a genito-urinary medicine (GUM) clinic.

SEE ALSO *Urinary system*

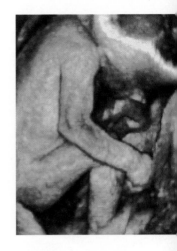

▲ **Ultrasound**
Ultrasound scans can be seen as a 3D image and reveal small details, such as the gender of an unborn baby.

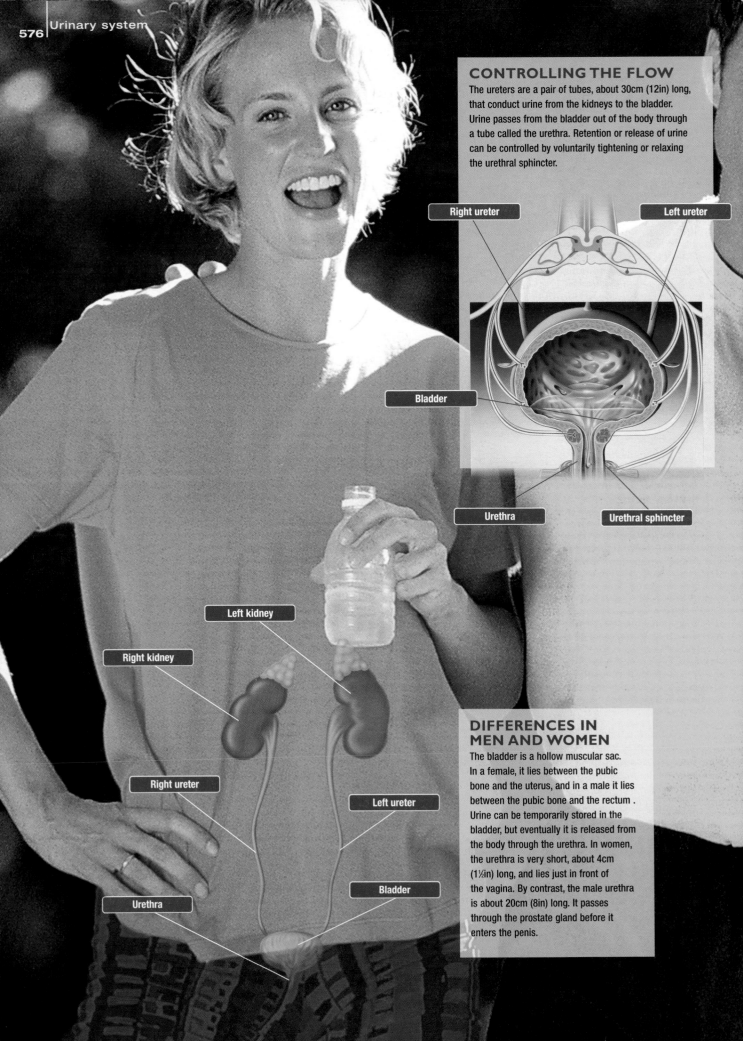

CONTROLLING THE FLOW

The ureters are a pair of tubes, about 30cm (12in) long, that conduct urine from the kidneys to the bladder. Urine passes from the bladder out of the body through a tube called the urethra. Retention or release of urine can be controlled by voluntarily tightening or relaxing the urethral sphincter.

Right ureter

Left ureter

Bladder

Urethra

Urethral sphincter

Left kidney

Right kidney

Right ureter

Left ureter

Bladder

Urethra

DIFFERENCES IN MEN AND WOMEN

The bladder is a hollow muscular sac. In a female, it lies between the pubic bone and the uterus, and in a male it lies between the pubic bone and the rectum . Urine can be temporarily stored in the bladder, but eventually it is released from the body through the urethra. In women, the urethra is very short, about 4cm (1½in) long, and lies just in front of the vagina. By contrast, the male urethra is about 20cm (8in) long. It passes through the prostate gland before it enters the penis.

MICROSCOPIC FILTERS

Each kidney has about one million tiny tubules called nephrons, which filter waste products from the blood and reabsorb useful substances. A nephron consists of a tangled knot of blood capillaries (a glomerulus), surrounded by a cup-shaped capsule (Bowman's capsule). Blood reaches the glomerulus under high pressure, forcing waste materials, glucose, salts and other substances through the capillary walls into the Bowman's capsule, where further filtration begins.

A kidney glomerulus is made up of a tight knot of tiny blood vessels. It filters the blood that is constantly being delivered through a branch of the renal artery.

Capillaries in a glomerulus

Branch of the renal artery

Urinary system

A FILTER FOR THE BLOOD

The urinary system consists of the kidneys, ureters, bladder and urethra. The function of the kidneys is to maintain the health of the blood by filtering out unwanted substances and by maintaining the water, salts and acids in the body at a constant level. All the body's blood passes through the kidneys many times each day, so it is kept constantly purified. The kidneys produce a waste-carrying solution – urine – that passes through the ureters to the bladder and is expelled from the body through the urethra.

The urinary system is constantly at work, filtering and expelling the body's liquid waste products and regulating the volume and composition of body fluids.

The kidneys filter 1.3 litres (more than 2 pints) of blood every minute, a vital process that stops the body being poisoned by its own waste. In temperate climes, the body produces and expels up to 2.5 litres (4½ pints) of urine in the course of a single day and night.

The kidneys are bean-shaped organs that lie just under the ribcage at the back of the abdomen, one on each side. The right kidney is located below the liver, so it is a little lower than the left one. Each kidney is about the size of a computer mouse or a child's fist. The kidneys are connected to the body's main artery and vein – the aorta and interior vena cava – by short, wide arteries and veins. Blood enters the kidneys under high pressure. Here, it is filtered, and useful substances are reabsorbed into the bloodstream. The filtered fluid – filtrate – then travels down the renal tubule where the levels of water, salts and acidic substances are adjusted to ensure that the body's needs are met. The resulting fluid is urine, which contains unwanted substances and excess water that can be excreted from the body.

How the urinary system works

The principal function of the urinary excretory system is to dispose of urea, a waste product produced by the liver as it breaks down protein.

Four elements make up the urinary system: the kidneys, the ureters, the bladder and the urethra. The kidneys filter excess fluid and wastes from blood to form urine, which is carried from the kidneys to the bladder in two thin tubes, one from each kidney, called ureters. The bladder stores urine until it can be expelled from the body via another tube, the urethra.

Urine consists of around 95 per cent water plus water-soluble waste substances produced by the body's metabolism. When blood delivers nutrients to cells, chemical reactions occur to break down those nutrients. Some of the waste (such as urea, made in the liver during the metabolism of protein) is the result of these chemical reactions. Some are salts, such as sodium and potassium chloride, that are surplus to requirements. The main tasks of the kidneys are:

- excreting wastes;
- regulating body fluid volume and composition;
- producing some hormones;
- metabolizing vitamin D and some proteins.

Depending on an individual's age and sex, the kidneys filter up to 170–180 litres (300–320 pints) of fluid per day. This high volume is necessary because wastes such as urea are present in the blood in low concentrations.

The kidneys also balance the volume of fluids and minerals in the body – this balance is called homeostasis. The body takes in water when we drink, and when we eat foods such as fruits and vegetables. Water leaves the body in several ways: it comes out of the urethra as urine, out of the skin as sweat, and out of the

mouth and nose when we breathe. There is also water in stools.

When there is too little fluid in the body, the brain communicates with the kidneys via a hormone that tells them to retain fluid and at the same time tells you that you are thirsty. When you have a drink, the hormone level falls and the kidneys release more fluids.

Urine flows from the kidney to the bladder through the ureters. The ends of the ureters do not allow urine to flow back from the bladder to the kidneys. The ureters contract in a rhythmic, pulse-like way up to five times per minute, each contraction squirting urine from the kidneys through the ureteral openings into the bladder. The highly elastic bladder can stretch to hold more than half a litre (1 pint) of fluid. The urine is passed from the bladder to the outside of the body through the urethra.

URINE

Urine is produced from excess fluid and soluble substances that are filtered through the kidneys. Around 60–80 per cent of the filtered substances are reabsorbed into the bloodstream; the rest are wastes and are expelled as urine. The volume of urine passed each day depends on an individual's fluid intake.

Urine has a faint smell that becomes stronger when it becomes more concentrated. Women may notice that the odour of their urine varies according to the time of their menstrual cycle. Eating certain foods such as asparagus can cause a strong unpleasant urine odour, as can the presence of a bacterial urinary tract infection.

The colour of urine varies depending on how much water you drink – it can range from a pale straw colour to dark orange. Urine may look:

- cloudy if there is a urinary tract infection;
- dark brown in people who have jaundice, owing to the presence of the pigment bilirubin (see **Liver and disorders**);
- smoky or pink-red if stained with blood (see **Kidneys and disorders**);
- red in someone who has eaten beetroot;
- orange in someone who has been taking the antibiotic drug rifampicin;
- green in people who have had certain treatments – for example, injections of fluorescein (to check for abnormalities in the eye) turns urine a dark yellowish-green until the dye is excreted;
- bright yellow in people who have taken dietary supplements containing vitamin B_2 (riboflavin).

▼ **Nephrons at work**
Every minute, more than a litre (2 pints) of blood is pumped through the kidneys. This blood is cleaned by filters called nephrons. There are more than a million nephrons inside each kidney. Blood enters the kidney through the renal artery and, once filtered, leaves via the renal vein.

Bowman's capsule
Glomerulus
Branch from renal artery
Capillaries
Collection duct for urine
Renal vein
Renal artery

What can go wrong

A problem in the urinary tract may be indicated by the production of too much or too little urine, pain on passing urine and incontinence.

Disorders of the urinary system are common. Half of all women, for example, suffer at least one attack of the bladder infection cystitis. Another widespread problem is the development of stones, or crystallized waste, in the bladder or kidneys. More serious diseases, such as diabetes and cancer, can also affect the urinary organs.

Symptoms include changes to urine frequency or colour (see page 578), a loss of control, or pain on passing urine. Pain in the abdomen or lower back can also be a sign that something is wrong.

URINE PRODUCTION PROBLEMS

Sometimes a person produces too much or too little urine. The production of excess urine is known as polyuria. Causes include:
■ diabetes, in which glucose spills over into the urine when its concentration in blood reaches a certain level known as the renal threshold;
■ raised blood calcium levels;
■ reduced blood potassium levels;
■ rarely, a condition known as diabetes insipidus;
■ polydipsia – a compulsion to drink fluids.

Producing a low volume of urine – less than 300ml (½ a pint) per day – is known as oliguria. It is usually caused by kidney diseases or obstruction, but other causes include low blood pressure or loss of blood, for example, in someone who is seriously ill with shock.

FREQUENT OR PAINFUL URINATION

The frequent passing of urine is often triggered by infections such as cystitis or **urethritis** that can make urination excruciatingly painful.

Pain on passing urine is known medically as dysuria. Other causes include genital herpes (see **Sexually transmitted diseases**), candidiasis, or a bladder or kidney stone. Mild discomfort may be caused by passing very concentrated urine or by an allergy – for example, to bath additives.

If frequent urination is painless, it may be caused by anxiety. Other causes include diabetes, stones in the bladder, an enlarged **prostate** or, rarely, a bladder tumour or kidney failure.

URINARY RETENTION

Urinary retention is an inability to empty the bladder completely. The bladder may empty only partially, leaving a quantity of urine that sometimes becomes stagnant and infected. Complete urinary retention is a surgical emergency, since urine will continue to build up in the bladder, causing extreme pain.

Urinary retention is usually due to a urinary outflow obstruction. A blockage may result from a urethral stricture (see below), a bladder stone, blood clot or tumour (see **Bladder and problems**).

In men, urinary retention is commonly caused by an enlarged prostate gland. Much more rarely, it may be caused by a swollen, tight foreskin (phimosis). Rarely, urine retention in women can be caused by pressure from an enlarged uterus (in **pregnancy** or as a result of **fibroids**). Other possible causes include disorders of the nervous system, such as **multiple sclerosis**, and drugs that act on the bladder.

Treatment involves inserting a catheter into the urethra to drain retained urine. If this is not possible – for example, when there is severe narrowing of the urethra as it passes through an enlarged prostate gland – the catheter may have to be inserted into the bladder through the abdominal wall above the pelvic bone. In most cases, the problem corrects itself. But sometimes a catheter may need to stay in place permanently.

Urethral stricture

An abnormal narrowing of part of the urethra – called a urethral stricture – may cause problems in passing urine. A stricture may be present from birth or it can be caused by shrinkage of scar tissue in the urethral walls following injury, or an untreated infection such as **urethritis**.

The use of antibiotics to treat urinary tract infections has made urethral stricture less common. Treatment may involve the dilation of the urethra using a slim probe, cutting the scar tissue using a device called a urethrotome, or reconstructive surgery.

URINARY INCONTINENCE

The involuntary loss of urine may be due to an overactive bladder, weakness of the pelvic floor muscles or a disease of the nervous system.

Pelvic floor exercises, done little and often, help to strengthen the muscles supporting the bladder neck. A simple exercise involves pulling up the front and back passages tightly as if trying to stop the bowels and bladder from opening. Hold tight for a count of four and repeat five times, every hour. Pull in the pelvic floor muscles before coughing, sneezing or lifting.

SEE ALSO *Bladder and disorders; Incontinence; Kidneys and disorders; Liver and disorders; Prostate and problems*

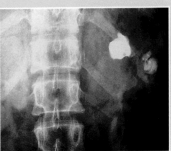

▲ **Kidney stone**
An X-ray reveals the presence of a kidney stone (shown in white, upper right). The stone may cause severe pain, especially when it passes down the urinary tract.

Other disorders

Vesicoureteral reflux is a condition in which urine abnormally flows backwards from the bladder into the ureters. It may even reach the kidneys, causing damage through infection and scarring.

Kidney stones, also called calculi, result from the buildup of crystallized salts and minerals, such as calcium, in the urinary tract.

Nephritis is an inflammation of the kidney. It may be caused by infection, an autoimmune disease (such as lupus), or occur for unknown reasons.

Uterus and problems

The uterus, commonly known as the womb, is a muscular organ that forms part of the female reproductive system. It allows an embryo to be implanted in its inner wall and nourishes the growing fetus with its mother's blood. It lies in the pelvis just behind the bladder. In adult women, the non-pregnant womb is about 8cm (3in) long and about 5cm (2in) wide.

The womb looks like a pear with the narrow end pointing downwards. This part is the cervix, which opens into the vagina; the upper part or body of the uterus opens into the Fallopian tubes. Both the cervix and the body of the uterus can be affected by health problems.

RETROVERTED UTERUS

In most women, the womb is tilted forward or anteverted; in about a quarter of women it is upright or tilted back or retroverted. This is perfectly normal and does not affect a woman's ability to conceive or bear a child.

Sometimes, however, a pelvic cyst or tumour or some other condition alters the position and size of the uterus (see **Pelvis and disorders**).

PERIOD PROBLEMS

Menstruation is the shedding of the lining of the uterus. It happens throughout a woman's fertile life, beginning in adolescence and ending at menopause. Abnormal menstrual bleeding is one of the most common disorders affecting women. It can be caused by a variety of factors, from hormonal disturbances to abnormalities of the uterus, such as fibroids (see **Menstruation**).

CERVICAL CANCER

Cervical **cancer** affects about one per cent of women in the UK and kills about four women in every 1000. It is most common among women in their early 30s and in those over 60.

The disease has a precancerous stage in which there are no symptoms, but the changes can be detected on a cervical smear. Treating the precancerous stage can prevent cancer (see **Cervix and disorders**).

Cervical smear tests

The aim of a cervical smear is to prevent cancer. A smear test looks for changes in the cells of the cervix that may indicate a risk of cancer developing. Precancerous changes occur around the entrance to the cervical canal, where cells lining the uterus meet those lining the vagina.

CERVICAL EROSION

Now known medically as cervical ectropion, cervical erosion is a harmless but common cause of increased vaginal discharge, or of mild bleeding after sexual intercourse or if the cervix is touched (see **Cervix and disorders**).

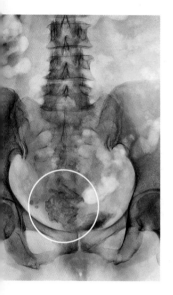

▲ **Fibroid**
A coloured pelvic X-ray of a calcified fibroid (lower centre) in the womb of a 65-year-old woman. A fibroid is a benign tumour of fibrous and muscular tissue.

POLYPS AND FIBROIDS

Polyps are mucous membrane growths that can develop from the lining of the uterus – the endometrium. Signs of polyps include painful periods, heavy periods, bleeding between periods and postmenopausal bleeding. Polyps are easily removed, and should be sent for microscopic examination to make sure they are non-cancerous. They can recur.

A fibroid is a non-cancerous growth within the uterine wall made up mostly of muscle tissue. A fibroid may be pea-sized or as large as a melon (see **Fibroids, uterine**).

UTERINE CANCER

Cancer of the uterus usually develops in the endometrium – the lining of the uterus. It is often preceded by abnormal overgrowth of the endometrium – known as hyperplasia. The disease tends to affect women after the menopause.

The most common symptom of uterine cancer is postmenopausal bleeding or a bloodstained vaginal discharge. In younger women, heavy periods or bleeding between periods may be warning signs. Diagnosis involves taking a biopsy of the uterine lining for investigation. Uterine cancer cannot be detected with a cervical smear. Women at increased risk for uterine cancer include those who:
- are clinically obese;
- have had no children;
- have a late menopause;
- are on hormonal treatment for breast cancer, for example, tamoxifen;
- are on oestrogen replacement therapy without progestogen: an excess of oestrogen in the body increases the risk of uterine cancer especially if progesterone levels are low (see **Hormone replacement therapy**).

Cancer of the uterus is treated by a full hysterectomy to remove the womb, Fallopian tubes and ovaries. If the cancer has spread, a course of radiotherapy might be needed. If uterine cancer is caught and treated early, the chance of survival for five years or longer is more than 80 per cent.

AFTER THE MENOPAUSE

Giving birth, and the normal ageing process, weaken the pelvic floor – a term used to describe the muscles and ligaments that support the uterus and vagina. This can result in a uterine prolapse, a condition rarely seen before the menopause. In a prolapse, the uterus descends from its normal position into the vagina; in the most severe cases the uterus protrudes out of the vagina. A surgical repair or a hysterectomy may be recommended.

SEE ALSO *Cervical smear test; Hysterectomy; Infertility; Reproductive system*

Vagina, vulva and disorders

The vagina is a sheath-like muscular tube that forms the lower part of the female reproductive tract and connects the cervix to the exterior of the body. It receives the penis during sexual intercourse, and widens and elongates to form the birth canal during childbirth. The vagina is normally about 10cm (4in) long, but is capable of considerable extension when a woman is sexually aroused.

The vulva is the female external genitalia. It is made up of two pairs of fleshy folds called the labia, which surround the opening of the vagina and the urethra, and extend forward to the clitoris. (See **Reproductive system**.)

Disorders of the vagina and vulva are very common. If you are concerned about an abnormal discharge, irritation, swelling or any other symptom affecting the vagina or vulva, seek medical advice – even if this means overcoming some initial embarrassment.

VAGINAL DISCHARGES

A clear or white discharge from the vagina is normal in adult women. No discharge should occur until puberty, and after the menopause discharge is much reduced.

A discharge is abnormal if it is unpleasantly smelly, itchy, greenish-yellow or bloodstained. Abnormal vaginal discharges are frequently associated with infection and inflammation in the vagina, known as vaginitis.

COMMON VAGINAL INFECTIONS

Most common vaginal infections are sexually transmitted. The exceptions are candida, or thrush, and bacterial vaginosis, which is not necessarily sexually transmitted.

If an infection could have been acquired during sexual intercourse, you should attend a GUM (genito-urinary medicine) clinic with the special facilities needed to make a diagnosis. (See also **Sexually transmitted diseases**.)

Candida

Candida, or thrush, is recognized by a white discharge that sometimes resembles cottage cheese. The vagina and vulva may be red, swollen, cracked, and very itchy. It may be painful to urinate or have intercourse.

Bacterial vaginosis

Bacterial vaginosis is caused by overgrowth of *Gardnerella vaginalis* and other bacteria. There may be unpleasant discharge with a fishy odour, but there are often no symptoms except for mild irritation. Treatment is with oral metronidazole or clindamycin vaginal cream.

VULVOVAGINITIS

Inflammation of both the vagina and the vulva is called vulvovaginitis. Apart from infection, possible causes of vulvovaginitis include irritation by chemicals, for example, those found in perfumed toiletries, contraceptive agents and disinfectants; an item such as a tampon or contraceptive device mistakenly left in the vagina; an abnormal opening (fistula) between the vagina and bladder or rectum, caused by injury, surgery or a tumour. Lack of oestrogen – atrophic ('senile') vaginitis is common in postmenopausal women; the vaginal walls become thin and inflamed, and bacterial infections occur (see **Vulvitis**).

VULVAL SKIN DISORDERS

The vulval skin is very sensitive to friction from clothing, antiseptics, detergents, perfumes and anaesthetic or antihistamine creams. Any of these may lead to itching, which can be severe. With prolonged itching, areas of the vulva may become leathery and thickened. Mauve or white patches of skin sometimes appear.

Steroid creams often relieve the itching. If any abnormal tissue remains, a doctor may remove a small portion for examination to make an exact diagnosis. Itchy conditions can be precancerous, particularly in older women.

VULVAL TUMOURS

Non-cancerous lumps – for example, sebaceous cysts, Bartholin's cysts and varicose veins – often appear in the vulva. Treatment depends on the nature of the tumour.

Cancer of the vulva is rare, and chiefly affects women over the age of 60. The initial symptom may be itching, a painless lump or a scaly raised area of skin. Treatment involves surgical excision of the vulva or **radiotherapy**.

SEE ALSO *Sexually transmitted diseases*

Female genitalia and personal hygiene

Keeping the area around the vagina and vulva clean and dry is important to avoid the spread of bacteria from the neighbouring anus or urethra.

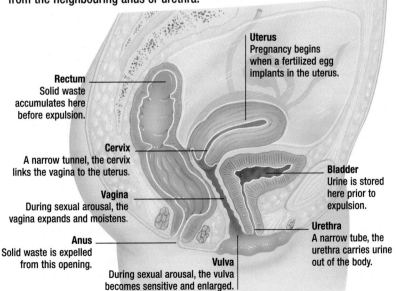

Rectum
Solid waste accumulates here before expulsion.

Cervix
A narrow tunnel, the cervix links the vagina to the uterus.

Vagina
During sexual arousal, the vagina expands and moistens.

Anus
Solid waste is expelled from this opening.

Uterus
Pregnancy begins when a fertilized egg implants in the uterus.

Bladder
Urine is stored here prior to expulsion.

Urethra
A narrow tube, the urethra carries urine out of the body.

Vulva
During sexual arousal, the vulva becomes sensitive and enlarged.

Veins and disorders

The veins act as a collecting system carrying blood from capillaries throughout the body and returning it to the heart. There are three main sets of veins.

■ The pulmonary veins bring oxygenated blood back from the lungs to the left side of the heart.

■ The systemic veins bring deoxygenated blood back from the muscles, body organs and skin to the right side of the heart.

■ The portal vein takes blood containing absorbed nutrients from the intestine to the liver (which removes the nutrients and returns the blood to the systemic veins).

Veins often run alongside the arteries, but, unlike arteries, they join together to make larger veins. The jugular veins from the head and neck meet the veins returning from the arms to form the superior vena cava. The veins from the abdomen and lower half of the body eventually drain into the inferior vena cava.

HOW VEINS WORK

Blood flow in veins is smoother and slower than in arteries. This is because veins are wider and the blood is not under pressure from the force of the heart. Vein walls are thin and contain little muscle, but a series of one-way valves ensures that blood can only flow forward. Damage to the valves allows blood to leak backwards, and makes varicose veins worse.

The pressure of blood in the veins is very low, so the body relies on the pumping action of muscles to help squeeze the blood back to the heart. In the legs there are two connecting sets of veins, superficial (under the skin) and deep (in the muscles). The calf muscles compress these veins during walking, pushing the blood up against the force of gravity.

Breathing also affects the flow by increasing and decreasing the pressure in the chest.

HOW VEINS ARE EXAMINED

There are two principal methods.

■ **Ultrasound** is used to examine peripheral veins for blood flow and the presence of clots.

■ Central venous catheterization (a tube passed into the superior vena cava) measures pressure and volume in life-threatening conditions and can also deliver nutrients or medicines directly into the circulation.

WHAT CAN GO WRONG

Any sudden pain and swelling in the leg should receive urgent medical attention.

Varicose veins

Leg veins become twisted and raised, producing itching, aching, swelling, skin changes or ulcers. Treatment includes support stockings, injection therapy and surgery.

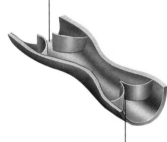

Valves open
When muscles contract valves open and allow blood to return to the heart.

Valves close
When the muscles relax, the valves close to prevent the blood from flowing backwards.

▲ **Cross-section of a vein**
Blood is pumped around the body by breathing and movement. This flow is maintained by hundreds of small valves in a vein. The valves open and close as activity is reduced or increased.

Thrombophlebitis

In certain circumstances veins may become inflamed (red, hot, sore and hard) or develop blood clots (see **Phlebitis**).

Blood clot (thrombosis)

Blood clots may form in veins for many reasons. They may cause damage in the surrounding area, or may travel to the lungs (see **Deep vein thrombosis**).

Spider veins (telangiectases)

These are actually fine dilated capillaries (see **Capillaries and problems**).

Vertigo

Vertigo is usually a symptom of ear infection or, less commonly, a disturbance in the brain. The term is often mistakenly used to mean a fear of heights. The most common causes of vertigo are viral infection of the balance organs and nerves, and middle ear infection; these are usually temporary and symptoms settle within a few days. **Ménière's disease**, postural vertigo (due to a change in position) and poor blood flow to part of the brain are also common. Ménière's disease may cause symptoms to recur for years; these will eventually cease, but at the price of total hearing loss in the affected ear.

SYMPTOMS

Vertigo affects both vision and sense of balance. It usually begins suddenly, and can quickly become acute. Symptoms include:

■ lightheadedness;

■ nausea;

■ ringing or continuous sound in the ear;

■ a disruption to balance that makes standing very difficult; affected people feel that the room they are in is spinning, or that they are spinning within it.

TREATMENT

Once vertigo is diagnosed, the underlying cause should be treated by a doctor. Treatment may include a phenothiazine drug (such as prochlorperazine). Phenothiazines are fast-acting and useful in the early stages of vertigo; cinnarizine and betahistine are useful for longer-term control in Ménière's disease. Ménière's may also be helped by relaxation exercises.

COMPLICATIONS

Acute vertigo is severe and disabling. Complications include:

■ falling over, with risk of injury;

■ increased risk of accidents, from driving, for example;

■ in the longer term, depression.

SEE ALSO *Ear and problems*

Viral infections

Viruses are responsible for many illnesses of varying severity. Some, including the common cold and gastroenteritis, cause temporary illness; others, such as hepatitis and HIV, can be resistant to medication.

A virus is a minute particle that can only replicate itself within living cells. Research has shown that viruses are able to evolve into more virulent strains by altering their genetic material, something particularly true of the flu virus, which changes continuously. This is why people catch colds and flu year after year rather than acquiring immunity to them – and also why developing a successful vaccine is difficult. Unlike bacterial infections such as tonsillitis, virus infections do not respond to antibiotic treatments, although such treatments may be useful in the case of a weakened immune system and secondary bacterial infection.

Traditionally, vaccination against viruses has focused on using the protein that coats the virus surface to create a 'memory' in the body's immune system. This enables antibodies to identify and fight the invading virus.

However, mutating viruses such as **HIV** (human immunodeficiency virus) may differ from country to country. There can even be different strains of HIV within the same person. This has made a strain-specific vaccine impossible to produce. HIV vaccines being tested at the start of the 21st century aim to block the virus from growing in the body rather than bolstering immunity.

Viruses can have long-term effects on the immune system, even when the viral infection seems to have passed. One post-viral illness is **chronic fatigue syndrome**, which may be diagnosed when a person feels fatigued for longer than six months and no other medical condition can be identified. Similar symptoms are caused by **glandular fever** and **Hodgkin's disease**.

VIRAL INFECTIONS

Viruses are divided into families and include papillomaviruses (**warts**), herpes viruses (**chickenpox**, shingles, **genital herpes** and Epstein-Barr virus), orthomyxoviruses (flu), corona viruses (common cold) and retroviruses (**HIV/AIDS**). Many viral infections such as colds, **cold sores** and **conjunctivitis** are common and the infection is usually short term. The affected person recovers with little or no long-term effect. Other viruses, such as **hepatitis**, can become chronic, continuing for months or years.

Children fall prey to numerous viral infections. **Croup**, for example, is an acute inflammation and obstruction of the respiratory tract in young children. **Hand, foot and mouth disease** is common in small children, causing a mild fever and a general feeling of being unwell. Other common childhood diseases caused by viruses include **measles**, **mumps** and **rubella**, for which there is a combined vaccine (**MMR**). Vaccinations against the **poliomyelitis** (polio) and **meningitis** viruses (meningococcal C and HiB) are also part of childhood **immunization** programmes.

Some viruses are restricted to certain areas of the world. The **Ebola virus**, for example, has been reported in several African countries including Gabon and Sudan, and **yellow fever** is most common in the jungle areas of Africa and South America (see **Travel and tropical diseases**).

VACCINES

Many vaccines contain live, attenuated (less virulent) viruses. For example, the measles vaccine contains live, attenuated measles virus. This allows the human body to gain immunity to the virus without usually becoming ill. The measles vaccine is available as a single injection or combined with live, attenuated mumps or rubella vaccine, or both (see **MMR**).

Some vaccines can cause muscle pain or minor symptoms of the virus, and there is a very small risk that the vaccine will be fatal. Always ask your doctor about risks and complications.

Booster vaccines are often required every few years to maintain immunity to a virus.

ANTIVIRAL DRUGS

A variety of antiviral drugs is available. For example, interferon is used to treat hepatitis. Interferons are a family of small protein molecules that are produced by cells in the body when attacked by a virus. They are not yet fully understood and work in a complicated way. They boost the immune system and attack infected and cancerous cells. These drugs can be harmful and may damage the liver.

SEE ALSO *Cold, common; Herpes; Infectious diseases; Rabies*

Currently 34.3 million people are infected with HIV worldwide. No vaccine is yet available.

Von Recklinghausen's disease

Also known as neurofibromatosis (NF), Von Recklinghausen's disease is an inherited disorder affecting between one in 2500 and one in 3300 live births. The disorder was first recognized by the German pathologist F. D. von Recklinghausen in 1882. Neurofibromatosis causes numerous benign tumours, which can occur in various organs of the body.

Symptoms vary greatly, and in many cases coffee-coloured patches of skin may be the only symptom. An estimated 95 per cent of cases are undetected. Those who are severely affected suffer from thousands of small growths, which may occur in the brain, spinal cord, eyes, liver, stomach, kidneys or intestines. About 50 per cent of people with NF also have learning disabilities.

A more severe form of the disease, known as NF2, occurs in one in 50,000 live births and causes multiple tumours of the spinal and cranial nerves. This can often lead to deafness and paralysis. The gene that must be defective to cause NF2 has been identified, and prenatal and diagnostic tests are now available.

Neurofibromatosis can lead to isolation for many affected individuals, as other people may react negatively to their disfigurement and have unfounded fears that the disorder is contagious.

TREATMENT
There is no treatment for the disease, but small cutaneous or subcutaneous neurofibromas can be removed if they are painful.

Vulvitis

Inflammation of the vulva, the outer part of the female reproductive system, is known as vulvitis. The usual symptoms are soreness and itching, and sometimes a discharge. Causes include bacterial, viral, and fungal infections, chemical irritation (from detergents, perfumes or spermicides, for example), allergies, psoriasis, eczema, menopause and precancerous and cancerous conditions.

TREATMENT
Treatment depends on the cause. A swab will be taken from the vagina to check for infection, which may be treated with antibiotics. If no infection is found, it is advisable to stop using any products that may be causing the irritation. Hormonal creams may be prescribed if vulvitis occurs during the menopause.

SEE ALSO *Reproductive system; Vagina, vulva and disorders*

Warts

Warts are caused by infection with a skin virus, human papillomavirus (HPV). They usually affect the hands, elbows, face, knees and scalp but may also appear on the genitals. Those on the soles of the feet become flattened by the weight of the body to form painful verrucas. Warts are benign but highly contagious, and often appear in crops, especially in children.

Half of sufferers find that their warts disappear within a year without treatment. But they can be treated earlier by freezing (cryosurgery), painting with wart-dissolving liquids, or burning off under local anaesthetic.

If you develop **genital warts**, always seek medical advice from a doctor or a genito-urinary medicine clinic (see **Sexually transmitted diseases**).

Weil's disease

Also known as leptospirosis, Weil's disease is an infection caused by the *Leptospira* bacteria. It occurs in dogs, rats and other mammals and is transmitted to human beings through exposure to water contaminated with the urine of infected animals.

Symptoms include fever, headache, vomiting, abdominal pain and diarrhoea, muscle aches, eye inflammation and skin rash. The disease may also affect the kidneys and liver. Treatment with antibiotics is effective.

Whiplash injury

Whiplash injury occurs when the neck is jerked forward and backwards forcefully. It happens most commonly in vehicle crashes involving sudden braking, but can also happen in the course of strenuous activities, such as diving. Whiplash effect can damage the soft tissues and the nerves in and around the spinal column, as well as the bones of the neck.

SYMPTOMS
These may appear immediately, or may start a day or two after the accident.
- Headache.
- Pain and stiffness in the neck.
- Weakness or heaviness in the arms.
- Pins and needles in the shoulders and arms.

TREATMENT
Self-help measures can bring relief, but medical attention may be required in some cases.
When to consult a doctor
- If you have periods of memory loss or unconsciousness.

- If you have severe pain in the back of the head.
- If you experience pins and needles or heaviness in the arms.

What a doctor may do

- Make a diagnosis based on your description of the injury and symptoms.
- Arrange an X-ray to check for broken bones.
- Prescribe anti-inflammatory drugs.
- Suggest wearing a collar to support the neck.

What you can do

As often as possible in the 24 hours after the injury, lie on a bed, your head supported by a pillow, and apply a towel-wrapped ice pack or bag of frozen peas to your neck for 20 minutes. This will help to reduce inflammation.

Rest and taking paracetamol for pain relief can also help.

Complementary and other therapies

Physiotherapy or **chiropractic** with appropriate manipulation and exercises may help.

OUTLOOK

Complete recovery is to be expected, but may take several months.

Self-help

Exercises to relieve whiplash

You may be able to relieve your whiplash symptoms with regular practice of these simple exercises.

1 Stand against a door or wall, head facing forward. Move your eyes towards two, four, eight and ten o'clock positions. Repeat five times. This eye movement gently exercises the deep muscles in the back of the head.

2 Use a beach ball or soft ball to exercise head and neck muscles. Place the ball between a wall and your forehead. Slowly move the ball against the wall in circles or figures of eight. Repeat, with the ball between the back of your head and the wall.

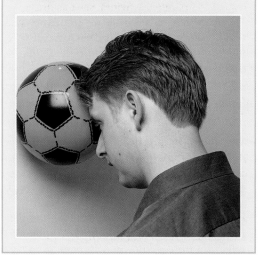

Whooping cough

Whooping cough, also known as pertussis, is a serious inflammation of the lungs that makes it very difficult to clear mucus. The mucus forms into plugs that are moved only by bouts of severe coughing – followed by a sucking in of air that makes a 'whooping' noise.

Children under the age of one account for a quarter of all cases; a further half occur in children under five. It usually lasts eight weeks, followed by an often-lengthy convalescence period (up to three months).

Whooping cough is a very contagious bacterial infection. It is spread by droplets of infected moisture from sneezing or coughing.

SYMPTOMS

There is a gap of 3–21 days between infection and symptoms. Consult a doctor if there are symptoms. Whooping cough has three stages.

- Catarrhal stage – about two weeks. Symptoms of the common cold.
- Paroxysmal stage – one to six weeks. Bouts of severe coughing that end in a whooping noise or vomiting. About 15 coughing attacks take place every 24 hours, during which facial redness, bulging eyes and possibly a blue tongue and lips may occur. Often children are too tired to hold themselves up during such coughing fits.
- Convalescence stage – up to three months. Coughing gradually reduces.

In infants under one there may be no 'whooping' noise, but there may be periods where breathing stops (apnoea). If these last for more than 20 seconds, call an ambulance.

TREATMENT

Antibiotics are the main treatment. Depending on the severity of the infection, hospitalization may be required (especially for children under the age of one).

COMPLICATIONS

The vast majority of cases recover with no further complications. But one in ten people develop pneumonia, and a smaller number go on to develop a widening of the bronchi or their branches, forming pockets where infections can occur (bronchiectasis).

PREVENTION

The main protection against whooping cough is vaccination. Since 1958, when a comprehensive vaccination programme was introduced in the UK, the number of cases has dropped from a high of 400 people per 100,000 to 20 per 100,000. There has been some controversy over the safety of the vaccine, however, although the risk of not being vaccinated is much greater than any theoretical danger from the vaccine.

Vaccinated children can still get whooping cough, but only as a mild cough.

Medical terms

Lower respiratory tract
The airways including the lower part of the trachea downwards (bronchi, bronchioles and alveoli).

Mucus
A viscous fluid produced by the mucous membranes. Also referred to as sputum or phlegm.

Pertussis
Another name for whooping cough, caused by *Bordetella pertussis* bacterium.

Pneumonia
Infection of the part of the lung where breathing actually takes place (the alveoli).

Wrist and problems

The wrist is a complex joint that allows the hand to bend forward and backwards at the joint with the lower arm. The wrist (carpus) is made up of eight small interlocking bones, known as the carpals. Four of the carpals work with the two bones of the lower forearm (radius and ulna), while the others work with the five bones in the palm of the hand (metacarpals).

The wrist also contains a number of tendons running from the fingers and thumb to the forearm, which are held close to the wrist by

The structure of the wrist
The wrist consists of eight carpal bones divided equally in two rows. It also contains a number of tendons, joining the hand to the forearm.

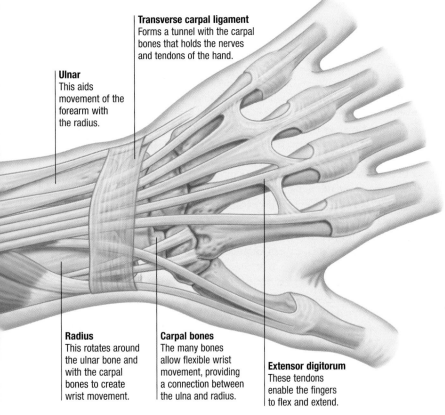

Ulnar
This aids movement of the forearm with the radius.

Transverse carpal ligament
Forms a tunnel with the carpal bones that holds the nerves and tendons of the hand.

Radius
This rotates around the ulnar bone and with the carpal bones to create wrist movement.

Carpal bones
The many bones allow flexible wrist movement, providing a connection between the ulna and radius.

Extensor digitorum
These tendons enable the fingers to flex and extend.

strap-like ligaments. The radial artery, which can be felt on the inner side of the wrist on the same side as the thumb, is often used to assess a patient's pulse rate.

PROBLEMS AFFECTING THE WRIST
Problems involving the wrist can affect hand movements and may interfere with a person's occupation, as well as causing discomfort.

Fractures
A Colles' fracture occurs when the lower end of the radius is broken. This typically occurs when falling onto the outstretched hand. The hand and wrist below the fracture are displaced backwards. It is common in elderly people, particularly in postmenopausal women whose bones have been weakened by **osteoporosis**. Treatment involves reducing the fracture to restore normal alignment of the wrist, and encasing the lower arm in plaster while it heals. The scaphoid bone can also be fractured by a fall onto the outstretched hand. This type of fracture usually occurs in younger people, whose radius is strong enough to resist a Colles' fracture. As a fracture of the scaphoid reduces its blood supply, this injury often fails to heal properly and surgery may be needed to pin it together.

Carpal tunnel syndrome
The carpal tunnel is a narrow opening into the hand made up of the wrist bones on the bottom and the carpal ligament on the top. This connects the base of the thumb and little finger. The median nerve passes through this space, and carpal tunnel syndrome (CTS) occurs when the nerve becomes pinched. This causes painful tingling in the hand, wrist and forearm. In severe cases, numbness, weakness and muscle wasting may occur. Symptoms classically affect the thumb, index and middle finger and the inner side of the ring finger. Carpal tunnel syndrome is diagnosed by looking at symptoms, and by tapping over the median nerve, which causes tingling. Nerve conduction studies may be performed to confirm the diagnosis.

Treatment may include painkillers, and wearing wrist splints at night – those that hold the wrist at a neutral angle seem to relieve pain more effectively than those that hold the wrist in an upwards, bent position. Steroid injections or surgery to free the trapped nerve by cutting the ligament may be suggested.

Wrist drop
Wrist drop is caused by damage to the radial nerve and produces an inability to straighten the hand and bring it up into alignment with the forearm. Damage may be caused by pressure in the armpit (from prolonged use of a crutch, for example) or from a fracture of the humerus. Treatment is with splinting, or occasionally by fusing the wrist bones.

Writer's cramp

Writer's cramp is a condition characterized by difficulty with writing, or an inability to write, due to spasm of muscles in the forearm. It also affects other fine hand functions, such as playing an instrument. The cause is unknown and treatment (with acupuncture, splints or magnetic therapy) is often unhelpful. Rest may bring some relief, but the condition may be permanent.

X-rays

An X-ray is an examination commonly used to investigate the skeleton, the chest, the teeth, blood vessels and the digestive system.

Since their discovery in 1895 by the German scientist Wilhelm Roentgen, X-rays have become a vital diagnostic tool in a wide range of medical conditions. Most of us will have had an X-ray examination at some time during our lives, whether to diagnose a fractured bone, check for dental decay or as a routine screening test, such as a mammogram to detect the early signs of breast cancer.

HOW X-RAYS WORK

X-rays are a form of radiation known simply as X-radiation. This is produced by the impact of an electron beam upon a heavy metal target. The radiation is absorbed to a differing extent by body tissues, depending upon their density; bone, for example, absorbs X-radiation well because it is dense, while skin, fat, blood and the air inside hollow organs absorb X-radiation relatively poorly. The X-rays emerging from the body after exposure are recorded on a special film, creating an image of the exposed part. Dense tissue, such as bone, casts a shadow, and looks dark, whereas the soft tissues form a lighter contrast. When the image is developed onto film these contrasts are seen in reverse – that is, the images of the bones are white, and those of the soft tissues are dark. With modern imaging techniques, very high quality pictures of the body can be generated.

WHAT'S INVOLVED

Most X-ray examinations are entirely painless but a few specialized procedures may cause some discomfort. With the exception of dental X-rays, X-rays are normally carried out in hospital by a radiographic technician.

You will be asked to expose just the area of the body being investigated, while the technician positions the X-ray machine. The X-ray film is usually inserted into a flat cassette, which is placed in contact with the relevant body area. Next, the technician leaves the room – to avoid undue exposure to radiation – and then presses an exposure button to take the X-ray. The whole procedure is normally over in a few minutes.

A doctor called a radiologist interprets the X-ray image. Some problems, such as bone fractures, are immediately evident, while tumours may take more time to assess.

SPECIALIZED X-RAYS

The hollow or fluid-filled parts of the body, such as the bladder or digestive tract, do not show up well on an X-ray film on their own. New techniques have been developed that can detail all the body tissues and this has led to the development of a number of specialized X-ray examinations.

Contrast X-rays

To achieve a clear image, a fluid that is opaque to X-rays is introduced into the relevant part of the body. The X-ray cannot pass through the contrast medium and this produces an image similar to that of bone density. There are various forms of contrast X-ray.

■ **Barium X-rays** These are used to examine various parts of the digestive tract. To highlight the soft tissue of the digestive tract, a solution of barium sulphate mixed with water is used as a contrast medium. In the single-contrast technique, barium alone is used. This creates an outline image of the entire part being examined. In the double-contrast technique, both barium and air are used, to create images of the surface of the digestive tract.

To examine the oesophagus, stomach or small intestine, the patient swallows the barium. If the large intestine is being imaged, the barium is introduced into the rectum, via a catheter, as an enema.

Although barium X-rays have now largely been replaced by **endoscopy**, they are still a useful alternative in some circumstances, particularly when a patient has swallowing difficulties or rectal bleeding.

■ **Urography** This is used to examine the urinary system and involves the injection of a fluid

▼ **Viewing X-rays** X-ray images are similar to photographic negatives. The detail of the image can be seen very clearly when viewed against a lightbox.

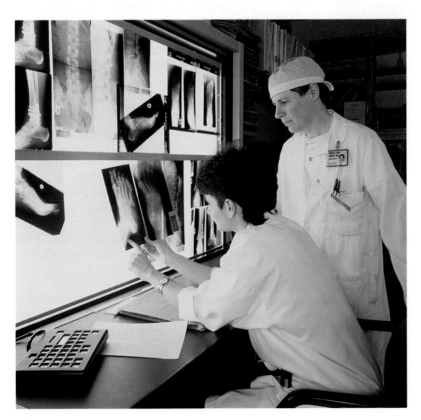

Viewing X-rays

X-rays reduce the need for investigative surgery.
The type of X-ray used for diagnosis depends on the
injury or disorder involved and the information needed.

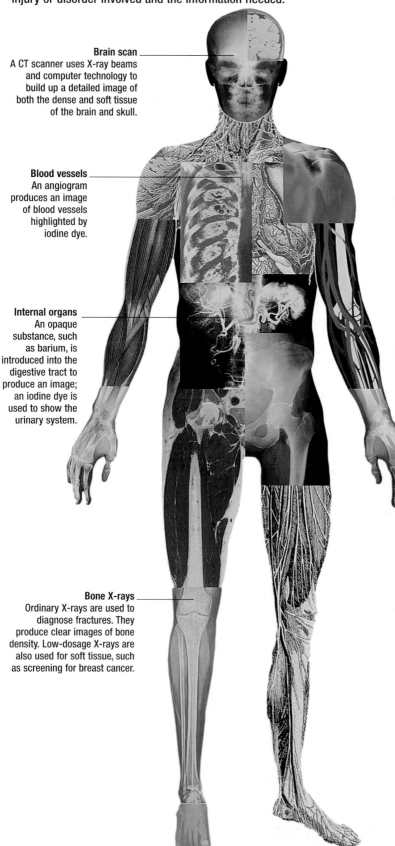

Brain scan
A CT scanner uses X-ray beams
and computer technology to
build up a detailed image of
both the dense and soft tissue
of the brain and skull.

Blood vessels
An angiogram
produces an image
of blood vessels
highlighted by
iodine dye.

Internal organs
An opaque
substance, such
as barium, is
introduced into the
digestive tract to
produce an image;
an iodine dye is
used to show the
urinary system.

Bone X-rays
Ordinary X-rays are used to
diagnose fractures. They
produce clear images of bone
density. Low-dosage X-rays are
also used for soft tissue, such
as screening for breast cancer.

containing iodine as the contrast medium. This
is usually injected into a vein in the arm, but
it may be introduced directly into the bladder
via a catheter. As the iodine passes through the
kidneys, ureters and bladder, an X-ray image
of the urinary system can be taken. Urography
is used to look for obstructions in the urinary
system, such as kidney stones, as well as for
kidney disease.

■ Angiography Angiography produces an image
of the blood vessels. The contrast medium
is introduced via a catheter in the groin, elbow
or the carotid artery in the neck. Angiography
is being increasingly used in the diagnosis
of **coronary artery disease,** since it can detect
any narrowing or blockages of the arteries.

CT scans

A major development in X-ray examination has
been CT or computed tomography scanning.
To create a whole image, a series of X-rays is
taken. These show 'slices' through the body
which are then built up into an accurate three-
dimensional image with a computer. CT scans
are used to diagnose tumours and in the
investigation of **strokes** and head injuries.
They are increasingly replacing contrast X-rays.

Mammography

Mammography is an X-ray examination of the
breasts. It is used to investigate breast lumps
and as a screening test for the early signs
of cancer because it can detect breast lumps
that are too small to be found by physical
examination. To take a mammography
image, the breast is compressed between the
X-ray plate (below the breast) and
a plastic cover (above). X-rays may be
taken from several angles to get a more
complete picture. The procedure is very safe,
using only very low-dosage X-rays, but it may
cause some discomfort, especially among
younger women whose breast tissue is more
dense. An alternative method is to X-ray the
breast from the side.

THE RISK TO THE PATIENT

X-radiation has the potential to damage tissue
– that is why it is used to destroy tumours
in **radiotherapy.** Modern X-ray machines
deliver the minimum possible dose of radiation,
and the benefits of the examination generally
far outweigh any health risk involved. However,
X-rays are usually avoided if there is any
possibility of pregnancy; a patient's reproductive
organs can be protected with a lead shield
during abdominal X-ray exams. Because of the
risk of cumulative damage from X-ray exams
over a lifetime, children's feet are no longer
X-rayed routinely to check growth and
development. Your dentist will usually also
restrict X-ray examination for small areas
of decay to every second visit.

Yaws

Yaws is an infectious tropical disease caused by the presence of a spirochaete, a spiral-shaped bacterium similar to the one that causes syphilis, in the skin and underlying tissues. The infection is almost always acquired in childhood and causes ulceration and tissue destruction.

The spirochaetes enter through small abrasions in the skin. After initial symptoms of fever, pain and itching, a single highly infectious itchy growth appears at the site of infection. Scratching spreads the infection, causing more crusty growths to appear elsewhere on the skin. Left untreated, these may eventually develop into deep **ulcers.**

Treatment with penicillin or other antibiotics is effective. Without drugs, the growths may heal slowly over about six months.
SEE ALSO *Travel and tropical diseases*

Yeast infections

Certain yeasts can cause infections of the skin or mucous membranes. The most common is *Candida albicans*, which causes **candida** or thrush, also known as candidiasis. It most commonly affects the vagina and mouth (oral thrush), but also occurs in other areas. This form of candida is common in the very young and the elderly. Vaginal thrush is a common, often recurrent problem for women.

The fungus that causes candidiasis is normally present in the vagina and the mouth. It is also found in skin folds, for example, under women's breasts, in the groin and in the area around the anal orifice. Its growth is kept under control by the bacteria usually present in these organs. However, if the body's resistance is lowered, for example, through a metabolic disorder such as **diabetes** or an immunodeficiency disorder, or if the natural balance of yeast microbes is upset by a course of antibiotics – candida or another type of yeast may proliferate, resulting in infection.

SYMPTOMS

Symptoms can be localized, as in vaginal or oral thrush, or generalized. They include:
- red, very itchy patches on the skin;
- a degree of scaling on the patches;
- in vaginal thrush, a thick white vaginal discharge, and itching.

TREATMENT

If you suspect you may have candidiasis, you should consult a doctor to obtain a diagnosis.
What a doctor may do
A doctor will prescribe antifungal medication against yeast fungus. This is usually in the form of a cream or ointment. The medication may be given in tablet or injection form for more serious conditions, such as generalized candidiasis, which affects the whole body.
Complementary therapies
Berberine-containing plants, such as garlic and goldenseal, have shown natural antibiotic activity against yeast, including *Candida*. Caprylic acid, a naturally occurring fatty acid, has also been reported as an effective antifungal compound in treating *Candida*.

PREVENTION
- Wash regularly.
- Dry skin thoroughly after washing.
- Do not share towels.
- Avoid wearing trainers.

OUTLOOK
In most cases, the infection disappears after antifungal treatment. But since the condition tends to recur, preventive measures are advised.

Yellow fever

Yellow fever is an infectious disease that occurs in tropical and subtropical Africa and South America. It is caused by a virus spread between human beings by the *Aedes aegypti* mosquito. The virus causes degeneration of the liver and kidney tissues. Three to six days after infection, symptoms appear. These include high fever and **jaundice** – the disease is given the name yellow fever because of the yellowing of the skin. In severe cases, the disease may lead to low blood pressure and kidney failure. Treatment is usually designed to maintain the level of red blood cells in the blood. The disease is fatal in about 10 per cent of cases, but recovery from an attack gives lifelong immunity. Yellow fever can be prevented by **immunization** and control of mosquitoes.

Zoonoses

Zoonoses are animal diseases that can infect people. Many zoonoses, including **anthrax,** from cattle, are parasitic diseases and are not infectious among people. Zoonoses include **toxocariasis** and **rabies** from dogs; **psittacosis** from birds such as parrots; toxoplasmosis or cat-scratch fever; **brucellosis** from cows, goats, sheep and pigs; leptospirosis from rats and mice; and **bubonic plague** from rat fleas.
SEE ALSO *Parasites and parasitic diseases*

FIRST

You could be faced with a medical emergency at any time. You could be the first person at the scene of a traffic accident or be present when a health crisis occurs at home, and your actions in those first few minutes may be vital. Knowing just a few simple techniques will equip you to offer basic first aid to treat and relieve minor injuries – and may help you to save a life. Read these pages now and you will be ready to give effective help while waiting for professional medical assistance.

AID

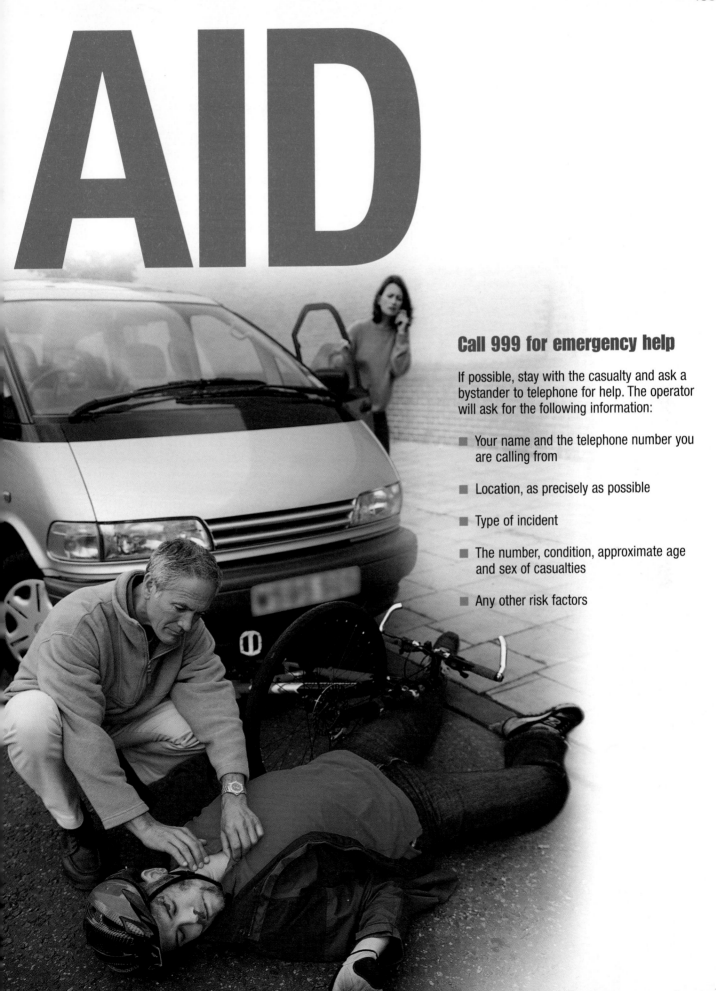

Call 999 for emergency help

If possible, stay with the casualty and ask a bystander to telephone for help. The operator will ask for the following information:

- Your name and the telephone number you are calling from

- Location, as precisely as possible

- Type of incident

- The number, condition, approximate age and sex of casualties

- Any other risk factors

What to do at the accident scene

✚ CALL FOR AN AMBULANCE AS SOON AS POSSIBLE.

✚ STAY CALM AND ASSESS THE SITUATION.

✚ MAKE SURE THE SCENE IS SAFE BEFORE YOU OFFER YOUR HELP.

Priorities in an emergency

1 Call for help Wherever possible ask someone else to call the emergency services, and to come back to confirm that he or she has done so.

2 Assess the situation Make sure that you are not putting yourself in danger – you will be no help to the victim if you get run over and become a casualty, too. Be alert to less obvious potential dangers, such as smoke and gas or petrol leakage.

3 Make the scene safe for others If you are at the scene of a road accident and in a separate vehicle, switch on your hazard warning lights to warn other vehicles and, if possible, ask someone to warn approaching traffic. Turn off the ignition and check the handbrake of all vehicles involved in the accident.

4 Assess the victims If there are multiple victims, you will need to decide who is the most seriously injured and treat those with life-threatening conditions first.

5 Start treatment If the victim is unconscious, follow the ABC procedure (see page 594). If the victim is not breathing, he or she must be resuscitated immediately in order to maintain heartbeat and breathing (see pages 596-7). Action may also be required in order to stem major bleeding (see pages 606-8).

Knowing just a few simple techniques may help you to save a life.

Observation notes

Note observations at 10 minute intervals while waiting for medical help.

Follow this list of tests. Pass your notes to the doctor or paramedic, or send them to the hospital with the casualty.

Eyes
This is a useful gauge for reaction while checking other responses
■ Open spontaneously
■ Open in response to voice
■ Open in response to stimulus such as pinching
■ No response

Speech
Speak clearly to the victim and listen carefully for a response
■ Answers questions coherently
■ Answers questions but confused
■ Answers but words cannot be understood
■ No response

Movement
Give verbal instructions for movement or apply physical stimulus such as pinching the skin
■ Follows verbal instructions to move (a hand or foot)
■ Can point to site of injury or pain
■ Responds to physical stimulus
■ No response

Pulse
Check an adult or child's pulse at the wrist or neck; check on the inner arm of a baby. Count the number of beats a minute and note the type
■ Strong or weak
■ Regular or irregular

Breathing
Count the number of breaths a minute and note the type
■ Quiet or noisy
■ Easy or difficult

First-aid kit

Every home and car should be equipped with a well-stocked first-aid kit, which is checked regularly – supplies should be replenished when they are used or become out of date.

You can buy first-aid kits from most pharmacists, or you can make up your own, provided that you keep it in a container with a well-fitting lid, that is both clean and watertight. A first-aid kit should be clearly marked and kept in a clean dry place where it is readily accessible and where anyone can find it easily in an emergency.

Basic contents

- adhesive dressings (plasters)
- sterile dressings
- bandages in various sizes, including triangular bandages
- dressing tape
- disposable latex gloves
- safety pins or bandage clips
- eye pads
- scissors
- antiseptic cream or spray
- cotton gauze swabs
- cotton wool for padding (not to be placed directly on a wound)
- notebook and pencil
- tweezers

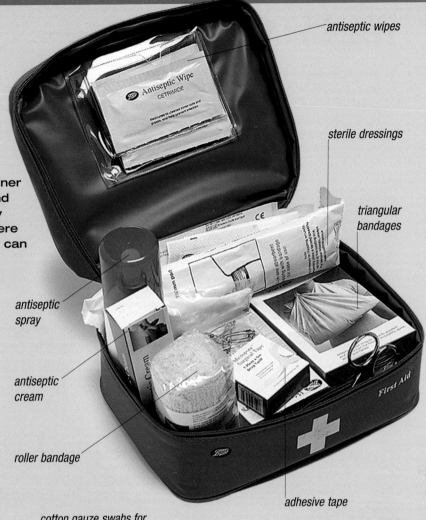

antiseptic wipes

sterile dressings

triangular bandages

antiseptic spray

antiseptic cream

roller bandage

adhesive tape

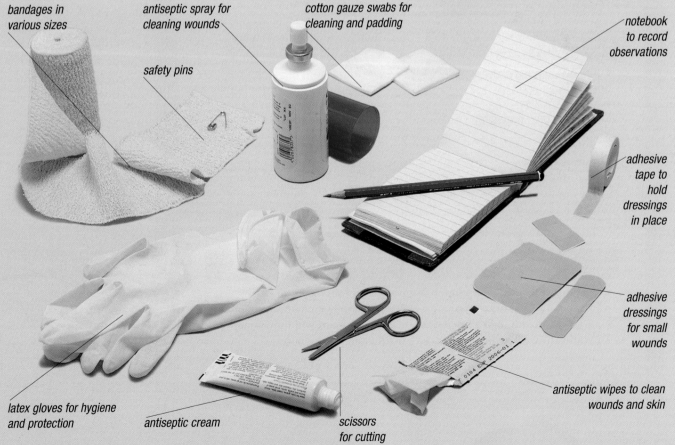

bandages in various sizes

antiseptic spray for cleaning wounds

safety pins

cotton gauze swabs for cleaning and padding

notebook to record observations

adhesive tape to hold dressings in place

adhesive dressings for small wounds

antiseptic wipes to clean wounds and skin

latex gloves for hygiene and protection

antiseptic cream

scissors for cutting bandages

The ABC of First Aid

In a life-threatening emergency, the strict priorities are to:
• Make the area safe if necessary
• Observe the ABC of first aid according to the basic life-support chart (see below)
• Treat for severe bleeding (see pages 606-8)

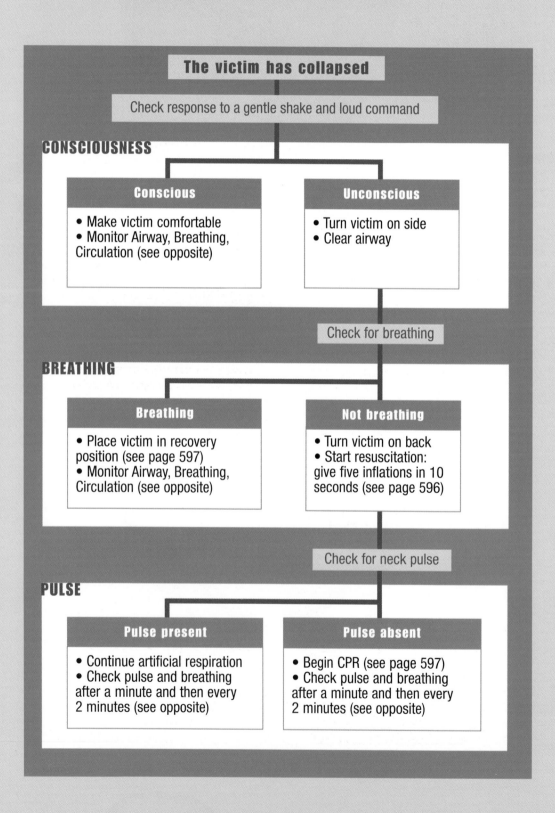

The victim has collapsed

Check response to a gentle shake and loud command

CONSCIOUSNESS

Conscious
• Make victim comfortable
• Monitor Airway, Breathing, Circulation (see opposite)

Unconscious
• Turn victim on side
• Clear airway

Check for breathing

BREATHING

Breathing
• Place victim in recovery position (see page 597)
• Monitor Airway, Breathing, Circulation (see opposite)

Not breathing
• Turn victim on back
• Start resuscitation: give five inflations in 10 seconds (see page 596)

Check for neck pulse

PULSE

Pulse present
• Continue artificial respiration
• Check pulse and breathing after a minute and then every 2 minutes (see opposite)

Pulse absent
• Begin CPR (see page 597)
• Check pulse and breathing after a minute and then every 2 minutes (see opposite)

AIRWAY In an emergency, first check for any obstruction of the airway and then position the person to keep the airway open. The recovery position is the only safe position for an unconscious person. **RECOVERY POSITION, SEE PAGE 597**

BREATHING If the victim is not breathing, artificial respiration is given mouth to mouth to ventilate the lungs and provide vital oxygen to tissues. **RESUSCITATION, SEE PAGE 596**

CIRCULATION If there is no pulse, the victim's heart is not beating. There will be no circulation of blood, no breathing and he or she will die unless CPR, cardiopulmonary resuscitation, is given. **CPR, SEE PAGE 597**

Airway check

When a person is unconscious, he or she cannot cough or swallow. Any food, fluid, vomit or blood can cause a fatal blockage of the airway, which leads from the mouth and nose to the lungs. The tongue can also cause a blockage by flopping backwards in the mouth.

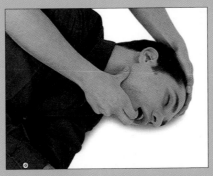

1 Look inside the mouth and if necessary use two fingers to check for anything that could block the airway. Remove any obvious obstructions but DO NOT try to probe the back of the throat. Leave any dentures in place unless they are broken.

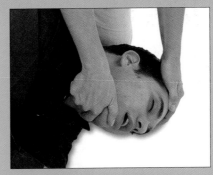

2 Gently tilt back the head and bring the chin forwards by supporting the jaw. This will keep the airway open and prevent the tongue from blocking it. Ensure that the face is inclined slightly downwards to aid the drainage of any fluids.

Breathing check

Look for rising movements of the chest or abdomen, listen for breathing sounds and feel for air coming from the victim's mouth or nose. Be alert for very shallow breathing and keep looking, listening and feeling for up to 10 seconds.

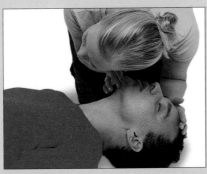

1 Hold the airway open and lean down with your face close to the casualty's mouth. Look along the chest for movement while listening for sounds of breathing and feeling for the movement of breath against your cheek.

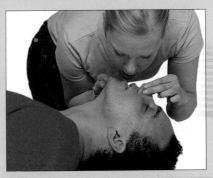

2 Be alert for very shallow breathing, but if you are sure breathing is absent, give five quick breaths of artificial respiration (see page 596) and follow with a pulse check (below).

Pulse check

It does not matter where on the body you take a pulse, but the carotid artery in the neck is the easiest to find when a victim is unconscious. If in any doubt about the presence of a carotid pulse, it is easy to compare the location and sensation with the pulse in your own neck. A healthy adult pulse rate is between 60 and 80 beats a minute. It is faster in children.

For an adult or child
The pulse in the carotid artery is the easiest to find. It can be felt on the neck, on either side of the windpipe. Feel for the pulse for up to 10 seconds. If the pulse is absent, begin CPR (see page 597) at once.

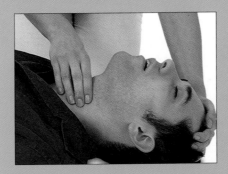

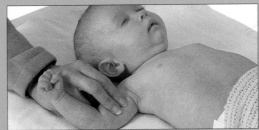

For a baby
If the pulse in the neck is hard to find, use the pulse in the inside of the upper arm. With your first and middle fingers feel for the pulse in the groove between the two upper arm muscles.

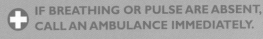
IF BREATHING OR PULSE ARE ABSENT, CALL AN AMBULANCE IMMEDIATELY.

Resuscitation

BREATHING AND PULSE CHECKS

- Breathing and pulse checks should be made every 2 minutes during resuscitation to see whether the heart and breathing have restarted

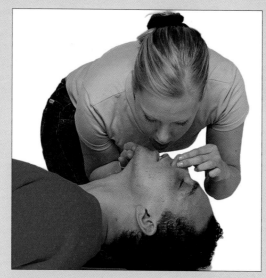

1 Kneel beside the victim and tilt the head back gently to keep the airway open. Place two fingers under the chin to support the jaw in this position. Pinch the victim's nose with your thumb and first finger. Take a deep breath and seal your lips around the victim's mouth. Blow into the victim's airway for about 2 seconds – watch for the chest to rise.

2 Draw back for about 4 seconds turning your head to the side to watch the chest falling. Give a repeat inflation and then check the pulse (see page 595). If you find a pulse, continue to breathe for the victim, checking the pulse after every ten breaths. If there is no pulse, start CPR (cardiopulmonary resuscitation, see opposite).

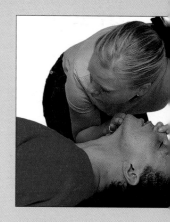

For a baby or child

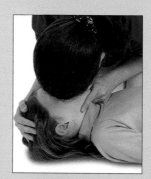

Use the same pattern of inflations for a child as for an adult, but use shorter breaths and pause as soon as the chest rises. For a baby or infant, seal your lips around the mouth and the nose before inflating the chest, and stop breathing out as soon as the baby's chest rises.

Cardiac compression

ACTION TO TAKE IF SOMEONE'S HEART STOPS

If no pulse is present, and therefore there is no circulation of blood around the body, the tissues are likely to die of oxygen starvation within 3 to 4 minutes.

- **External cardiac compression** should begin along with mouth-to-mouth respiration (see above) as soon as the pulse is discovered to be absent. These two techniques together are known as CPR (cardiopulmonary resuscitation, see opposite).

Push vertically downwards with your arms straight.

Grasp your lower hand with the fingers of your upper one.

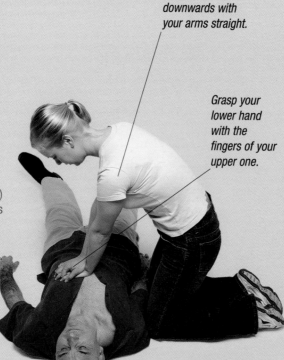

1 Kneel beside the victim and if necessary roll him or her onto the back. Find the lower end of the ribcage and run your first two fingers inwards until you find the bottom of the breastbone. Place your index finger at this point as a marker. Place the heel of your other hand on the breastbone just above this finger and maintain this position.

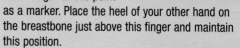

2 Move the other hand on top of the first and interlace your fingers. Lean forwards with your shoulders over the victim. Keeping your arms straight, push down, aiming to press the lower breastbone down by about a third of the depth of the chest. Release the pressure without removing your hands. Repeat 15 times at a rate of 100 thrusts a minute (almost two a second), then give mouth-to-mouth respiration (see above).

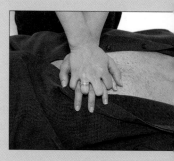

CPR Cardiopulmonary resuscitation

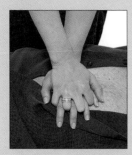

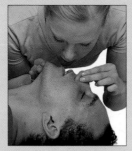

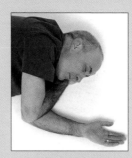

1 Start with a steady series of 15 cardiac compressions (see below left). Follow this with two breaths of mouth-to-mouth respiration (see top left). Repeat this cycle, giving two breaths after each 15 cardiac compressions, until help arrives. If there are two rescuers, one can give the compressions and the other the mouth-to-mouth respiration.

2 After one full minute of CPR, hold the victim's head in the open airway position (see page 595) and recheck for a neck pulse (see page 595). If the pulse is present, do not continue with compressions. Check breathing and if necessary carry on with respiration until normal breathing returns or medical help arrives.

3 If the victim regains a pulse and is breathing unassisted but remains unconscious, place him or her in the recovery position (see below). Check pulse and breathing regularly until help arrives, and be prepared to start CPR again if necessary.

CPR for babies and children

Use adult CPR techniques on children aged over eight years, unless they are particularly small for their age. For babies and children, you need to give gentler chest thrusts and very gentle breaths.

For a baby

Give breaths by sealing your lips around the baby's mouth and nose. Place two fingers one finger's width below an imaginary line between the baby's nipples. Give chest compressions with the fingers only, at a rate of five compressions to one breath.

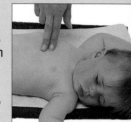

For a child (age 1–7)

Use one hand only to compress the chest and perform cycles of five chest compressions to one breath. Monitor pulse and breathing between each cycle, as for adults.

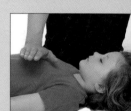

Recovery position

The recovery position is the safest position in which to place an unconscious casualty. It protects from further injury by stopping the victim from rolling over, and ensures that the airway stays open and fluids – blood, saliva or vomit – can drain away without risk of choking.

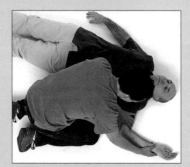

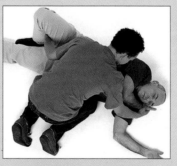

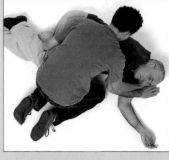

1 Kneel at the side of the victim, straighten the legs and place the arm nearest to you at a right angle to the body, with the forearm at a right angle to the upper arm.

2 Place the victim's other arm across the chest and support the cheek on the back of the hand. Bend the opposite knee upwards and roll the victim towards you.

3 Support and protect the victim's head while rolling over. Keep the upper knee bent to prevent the victim from rolling too far onto his or her front.

4 Tilt the victim's head back to keep the airway open, keeping it supported by the back of the victim's hand. Check pulse and breathing regularly until medical help arrives.

Bend one leg to prevent the victim rolling.

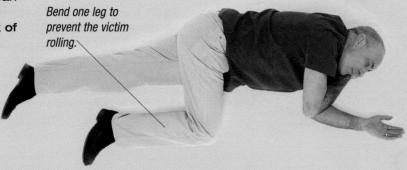

Abdominal injury

The abdominal cavity contains the stomach, liver, spleen, intestines, kidneys and some major blood vessels. Damage may occur without any obvious external wounds. It is vital to assess the patient carefully in order to detect internal injuries which may lead to life-threatening collapse.

1 Help the victim to lie down in the most comfortable position possible. If a wound cuts across the abdomen, ease a cushion or rolled-up clothing under the knees to avoid straining the injury. Do not raise the knees if the wound runs up and down the abdomen.

For wounds across the abdomen, place a soft support under the knees.

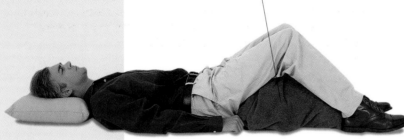

2 Loosen any tight clothing. If the wound is small, apply a sterile dressing fixed with a wide stretch-cotton bandage or wrap a towel around the abdomen.

Use a clean towel if there is no dressing to hand.

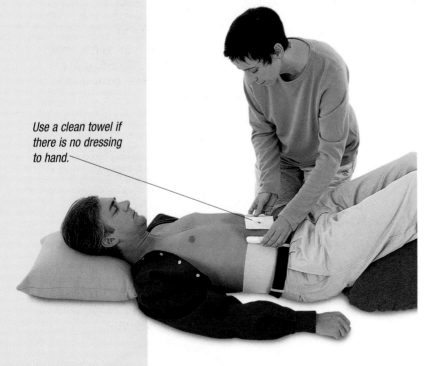

Use a damp dressing over the first dressing to keep it from drying out.

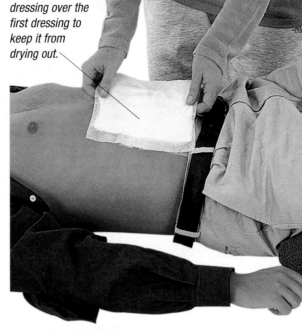

3 If internal organs are visible through the wound, do not touch or try to put them back in place. Cover the wound with plastic film or a plastic bag to prevent the intestine from drying out, or use a sterile, non-stick dressing moistened with a damp dressing or towel on top. If blood seeps through, cover with another dressing.

➕ **IF THE VICTIM COUGHS, SNEEZES OR VOMITS, APPLY LIGHT PRESSURE WITH YOUR PALMS ON TOP OF THE DRESSING TO PREVENT THE ABDOMINAL CONTENTS FROM PROTRUDING.**

4 Cover the victim lightly with a blanket or clothing to maintain the body temperature. If the victim is lying on a hot, cold or wet surface, ease a blanket, clothing or even newspapers under them. Take care to avoid any movement of the abdominal area.

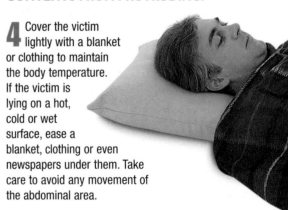

5 While waiting for the ambulance, check the victim's airway, breathing and pulse every few minutes and monitor for signs of shock such as rapid and shallow breathing and weakening pulse (see page 633). Be prepared to give CPR (cardiopulmonary resuscitation, see page 597) if necessary. If the wound is covered and secure, place an unconscious victim in the recovery position (see page 597).

Allergic reaction

**WHAT TO
LOOK FOR:**

- Skin rash, redness or blotchiness
- Intense itching
- Abdominal pain, nausea or vomiting
- Breathing difficulty or wheezing
- Puffiness around the eyes
- Swelling, especially around the face

➕ **CALL AN
AMBULANCE
IMMEDIATELY.**

Almost anything can trigger an allergic reaction, but common causes are food, drugs or medicine and insect stings. An allergic reaction can vary from an annoying but relatively harmless skin rash, to severe and life-threatening collaspe, known as anaphylactic shock.

Localized allergic reaction

Signs of less severe, localized allergic reactions include:

- Swelling of a body part (other than the face)
- Redness or heat under the skin
- Skin rash, itching or blistering
- Sneezing, runny eyes or nose

Offer first-aid treatment for symptoms where possible. Advise the victim to seek medical advice if there is a history of allergic reaction or symptoms do not improve.

Anaphylactic shock

Develops rapidly when an allergic reaction causes swelling and constriction of the airway. Signs include:

- Spreading skin reaction
- Swelling of the face
- Anxiety or panic
- Difficulty in breathing
- Rapid pulse
- Collapse

1 Help the victim to sit up in the most comfortable position to aid breathing.

2 Ask about previous allergic reactions. If the victim is aware of a severe allergy and carries emergency adrenaline (an Epi-Pen syringe), help him to use it.

3 If the victim becomes unconscious, open the airway and check pulse and breathing (see page 595). If necessary, be prepared to start resuscitation (see page 596). Place the victim in the recovery position (see page 597).

Ankle and foot injury

**WHAT TO
LOOK FOR:**

- Pain in and around the injured area
- Swelling around the joint
- An open wound
- Inability to walk or to put weight on the foot
- Feeling faint or giddy
- Numbness in the foot or toes
- Loss of power and movement at the ankle joint threatening collapse

The most common ankle injury is caused by twisting the joint or from impact when jumping or falling from a height. The injury may be a sprain or fracture (broken bone), but it can be difficult to be sure without an X-ray. To avoid the risk of further damage, treat all severe ankle injuries as possible fractures and advise the victim to seek medical advice as soon as possible.

➕ **IF PAIN
PERSISTS AND
YOU SUSPECT A
FRACTURE, TAKE
THE VICTIM TO
HOSPITAL. DO NOT
GIVE ANY FOOD
OR DRINK AS AN
ANAESTHETIC MAY
BE NEEDED.**

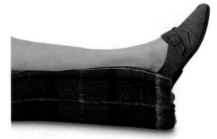

1 Help the victim to sit or lie down, avoiding moving or touching the injured joint. Carefully raise and support the injured leg in the most comfortable position for the victim.

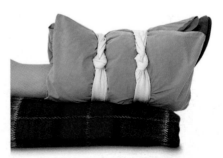

2 Carefully pad around the ankle using a soft pillow or light blanket held in place with two or three bandages. Reduce any swelling by applying an ice pack or cold compress (see page 605).

Arm and elbow injury

WHAT TO LOOK FOR:
- Pain in and around the injured area, often increased by movement
- Swelling
- Feeling cold and shivery
- Feeling faint and giddy
- Numbness in the extremities
- Loss of power and function in the joint

✚ **IF THE PULSE CANNOT BE FELT TAKE THE VICTIM TO HOSPITAL FOR URGENT ASSESSMENT.**

Arm injuries include dislocations of the elbow joint and fractures of one or more bones. An X-ray is often needed to confirm the diagnosis, and any serious injury should be treated as a fracture until medical advice has been obtained.

Forearm

1 Gently support the arm and place a rolled newspaper under the forearm as a temporary splint. Secure it with a sling (see page 604), keeping the fingers slightly higher than the elbow.

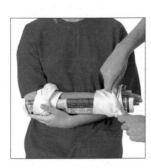

2 Check the pulse and colour of the fingertips every few minutes. If necessary, remove the bandages and splint and reposition them.

Elbow

Rest the injured arm on a soft support.

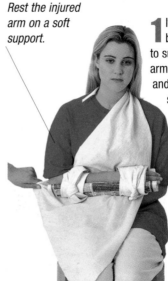

1 If the elbow can bend, ask the victim to support the injured arm across the chest and place it in an arm sling (see page 604), with soft padding between the arm and the chest. Check the pulse and if necessary gently straighten the elbow until the pulse can be felt. Take the victim to hospital.

2 If the elbow cannot bend, call an ambulance. Do not try to move the injured limb and do not bandage the arm unless it is necessary to move the victim to safety. Ask the victim to lie down and place padding around the elbow to support it. Keep checking the pulse until the ambulance arrives.

Asthmatic attack

WHAT TO LOOK FOR:
- Difficulty in breathing
- Wheezing, especially when breathing out
- Coughing, especially at night
- Difficulty in talking
- Blue lips
- Anxiety

✚ **BE PREPARED TO START RESUSCITATION IF THE VICTIM STOPS BREATHING (SEE PAGE 596).**

During an asthma attack, the airways are narrowed, restricting breathing. The muscles go into spasm, the mucous membrane lining swells and thick, sticky mucus is produced. Attacks may be triggered by allergy, cold, exercise or infection, although often no trigger can be identified.

✚ **CALL AN AMBULANCE IF:**

- **THERE IS NO IMPROVEMENT AFTER 5–10 MINUTES.**
- **THE ATTACK IS GETTING WORSE DESPITE MEDICATION.**
- **THE VICTIM IS BECOMING EXHAUSTED.**
- **THE VICTIM COLLAPSES, STOPS BREATHING OR FALLS UNCONSCIOUS.**

1 Help the victim into a comfortable position – sitting and leaning forwards on the arms often helps to reduce breathing effort. Ask the victim to breathe slowly and deeply, and offer frequent reassurance.

2 Help the victim to use a reliever inhaler if available, preferably through a 'spacer' device if the victim is a child. If the attack eases, another dose can be taken after 5 to 10 minutes.

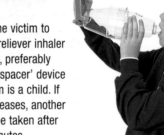

Asthma medication

Most asthmatics carry a 'reliever' inhaler to use at the first sign of an attack. Inhalers usually have a blue cap and should ease symptoms within 5 to 10 minutes. A plastic 'spacer' may make it easier to breathe in the medicine.

Back injury

**WHAT TO
LOOK FOR:**
- Back pain,
  sometimes radiating
  down the outer leg
- Any signs of recent
  injury
- Drowsiness or loss of
  consciousness

✚ **CALL AN
AMBULANCE
AT ONCE IF
THE INJURY IS
ASSOCIATED
WITH AN IMPACT
OR SEVERE FALL,
AND THE VICTIM
IS CONSCIOUS.
AVOID ANY
MOVEMENT OF
THE HEAD, NECK
OR BACK.**

Back muscles can be injured by heavy lifting, a severe fall or sudden twisting. The lower back is most commonly injured and the victim may also suffer painful muscle spasm.

More rarely, the spine itself may be injured after a heavy fall or impact. If the pain is severe or accompanied by any of the symptoms listed on the left, seek urgent medical advice.

✚ **CALL AN AMBULANCE IF THERE IS:**

- **RESTRICTED MOVEMENT IN THE
  LOWER LIMBS.**
- **LOSS OF SENSATION, TINGLING
  OR BURNING IN THE LEGS.**
- **HEADACHE.**
- **STIFF NECK.**
- **BLURRED OR DOUBLE VISION.**
- **BLOODSTAINED URINE (FROM
  INTERNAL BLEEDING).**

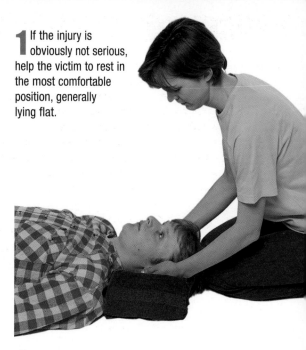

1 If the injury is obviously not serious, help the victim to rest in the most comfortable position, generally lying flat.

2 If there is soreness of the lower back after carrying a heavy load or after a sudden twisting movement, the victim should rest for up to an hour. This will help to ease the muscle spasm.

Bandages

Applying bandages and dressings is an important part of first aid. Sterile dressings come in various sizes and are made either with an absorbent surface for use on major wounds and to control bleeding, or with a non-adherent surface for use on burns or a weeping graze. Adhesive dressings are used for minor wounds and should be changed daily because the adhesive softens the skin and can delay healing. Roller bandages have many uses: to apply pressure, to control bleeding, support an injury and secure dressings on a wound.

Roller bandages

*Sterile wound dressings
and bandages*

*Adhesive
dressings*

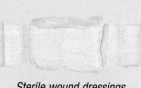

*Sterile combined
dressing*

*Safety
pins*

*Sterile non-adherent
dry dressings*

*Adhesive
tape*

Triangular bandage

Cotton gauze swab

Bandaging triangular

USING A TRIANGULAR BANDAGE:

- Use to make a sling, tie a splint to a limb, or to create a comfortable protective covering
- Secure dressings on a wound, but remember that the bandage will not supply enough pressure on its own to control bleeding
- Use to support an injured elbow with the arm partly bent, if this is possible

Hand injury

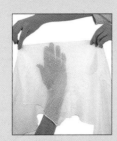

1 With the hand on an open triangular bandage – held upright or laid on a flat surface – bring the point over the injury so that the hand is covered.

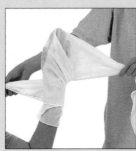

2 Cross the ends around the wrist, pulling the bandage around the hand. Make one full turn around the wrist.

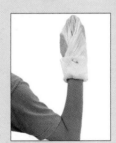

3 Tie the ends over the point, using a secure knot. Tuck the bandage ends around the wrist. Bring the point up over the knot and secure with a safety pin.

Foot injury

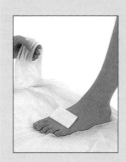

1 Place the foot on the open triangular bandage, with toes pointing towards the point.

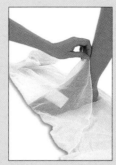

2 Bring the point up as far as the ankle, covering the dressing and the whole foot.

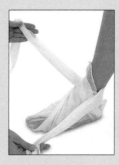

3 Cross the ends around the ankle to secure the point. Tie a secure knot in the front. Bring the point down over the knot and pin to fix in position.

Head injury

1 Fold a narrow hem inwards along the long edge of the bandage to make a firm edge.

2 Place the hem around the forehead of the victim, with the point hanging down towards the back and the ends away from the head.

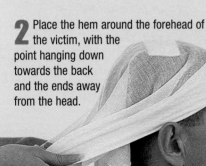

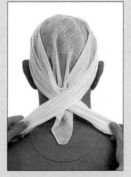

3 Carry the ends over the point, cross them, and return them around the head and back to the forehead.

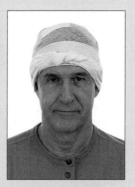

4 Tie the ends with a secure knot, being careful not to tie too tightly and create excessive pressure.

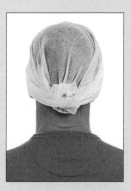

5 Lift the point at the back of the head to cover the crossed ends, tuck it in and use a safety pin to secure.

Knee injury

1 Cover the bent knee with the open triangular bandage, the point upwards and the base under the knee. Cross the ends behind the knee and bring them up around the thigh.

2 Tie the ends above the knee in front, using a secure knot. Bring the point down over the knot and fasten it with a safety pin.

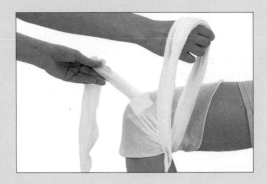

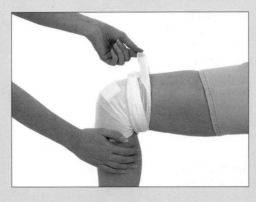

Elbow injury

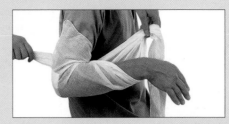

1 Place the bandage over the elbow with the point upwards and the base below the elbow on the outside of the lower arm. Cross the ends behind the elbow, bring to the outside upper arm and tie with a secure knot.

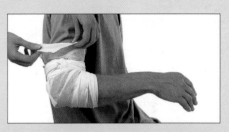

2 Tuck the ends of the bandage away, bring the point down over the knot and pin.

Bandaging roller & tubular

USING A ROLLER BANDAGE:
- Position yourself facing the victim, on the injured side
- Place the bandage end against the skin, with the roll on top
- Unroll only a short length of bandage at a time
- Apply the bandage from the inner side of the body and work outwards
- Start the turns below the injury or wound, and work upwards
- When bandaging, cover two-thirds of each previous turn to hold the bandage firmly in place

Roller bandages

Roller bandages have four main uses: to support an injury, apply pressure, control bleeding and secure a dressing. Widths vary from 2.5cm (1in) for fingers to 15cm (6in) for the trunk.

1 Start the bandage below the injury applying one or two turns in order to hold it in place.

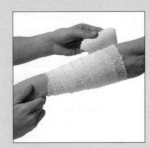

2 Wind the bandage with a series of overlapping spiral turns around and up the limb.

3 Finish with a straight turn and fix the end with a safety pin or adhesive tape. Check that the skin colour above and below the bandage is the same on both limbs. A change of colour indicates the bandage is too tight and should be loosened.

Tubular gauze

Tubular gauze is a seamless, tube-shaped bandage, which is useful for bandaging fingers and toes. It comes with an applicator.

1 Cut a piece of gauze three times longer than the injured finger, and push the whole cut length onto the applicator. Slide the applicator gently over the finger.

2 Hold the end of the gauze firmly onto the base of the finger and gently pull back the applicator, leaving a gauze layer on the finger. Twist the applicator twice, then gently push it back over the finger.

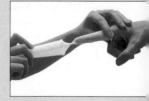

3 With a second layer of gauze in place, withdraw the empty applicator. Fix the gauze in place at the base of the finger or toe with small sections of adhesive tape. Do not encircle the finger with the tape, as this could cut off the blood supply.

Bandaging slings

Elevation sling

An elevation sling is used to keep the hand and fingers in a raised position and also to provide support for a chest injury or fractured collarbone.

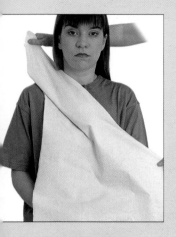

1 Ask the victim to support the injured arm across the chest, with the fingertips touching the opposite shoulder. Hold a triangular bandage over the injured arm, with the longest side over the uninjured side of the body and the point of the triangle over the elbow on the injured side. Wrap the top end of the bandage around the upper hand.

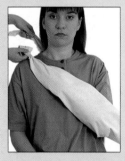

2 Tuck the bandage under the injured arm. Take the lower end up the back to the shoulder. Secure the fingers inside the sling by twisting the end gently before tying the ends at the shoulder.

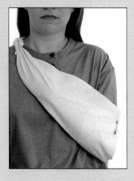

3 At the elbow, ease the loose fabric backwards and tuck the point into the sling, or use a safety pin to secure it. Insert the pin with the point facing downwards for safety. Check the colour of the fingers. If there is any change of colour, a sign of possible impaired circulation, remove the sling and loosen any bandages.

Arm sling

An arm sling is designed to support the lower arm, hand and fingers across the chest. It is used for various injuries to the upper or lower arm and wrist, including some fractures.

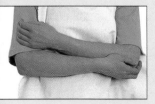 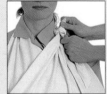 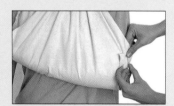

1 Ask the victim to support the injured arm as shown above. Hold the longest side of the sling down the uninjured side of the body, with the top end around the back of the neck.

2 Bring the lower end of bandage up to support the forearm and tie it securely to the other end. The knot should sit in the hollow above the collarbone on the injured side.

3 Bring the point forwards, over the elbow, and fasten it to the front of the sling with a safety pin. Make sure the point faces downwards in case the pin becomes unfastened. Check that hand and wrist are supported in a position that is slightly higher than the elbow.

Collar-and-cuff sling

A collar-and-cuff sling is used to support an upper arm injury or collarbone fracture, or when the hand and fingers need to be raised. It is also used when an elevation sling would be too uncomfortable for the victim.

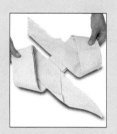

1 Begin by making a 'clove hitch'. Fold a triangular bandage into a narrow strip and make two loops: one pointing upwards and one downwards.

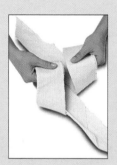

2 Fold both loops into the middle, so that they form a secure and firm support for the arm.

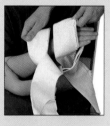

3 Place the injured arm against the chest and in a raised position, with the fingers pointing towards the opposite shoulder. Slip the two loops gently over the hand and place them so that the arm is comfortable and there is no pressure on an injured area.

4 Tie the long ends of the bandage behind the casualty's neck and allow the sling to take the full weight of the arm.

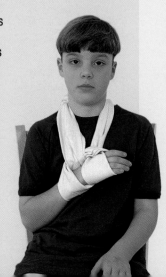

Bites and stings animal & insect

WHAT TO LOOK FOR:

- Bleeding from a wound made by a bite
- Teeth marks anywhere that the skin is broken
- Pain, swelling or soreness
- A sting remaining in the skin
- Difficulty in breathing
- Spreading redness and swelling of the skin
- Wheezing or gasping for air
- Rapid pulse

Bites

As well as causing wounds to the skin and deeper tissues, there is a high risk of infection from both animal and human bites unless prompt medical treatment is given. A tetanus injection and antibiotics may be prescribed.

Small animal wound

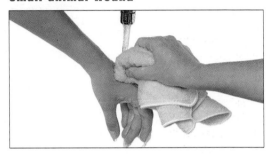

1 Wash the area which has been bitten as thoroughly as possible, using an antiseptic wash or soap and warm water.

2 Dry the area with a clean towel or blot it dry with clean tissues. Apply a sterile adhesive dressing over the entire area of the wound.

✚ **SEEK URGENT MEDICAL HELP IF AN ANIMAL OR HUMAN BITE HAS BROKEN THE SKIN.**

Large animal wound

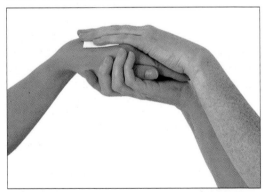

1 Where there is obvious skin damage and some bleeding, apply pressure with your hand or fingers over a sterile or clean dressing. Raise the affected part if possible.

2 When the bleeding is under control, apply a bandage to maintain pressure and keep the dressing in place. Always roll bandages from the inside of the limb outwards.

Stings

Insect stings may be painful but are usually not serious. A few people are allergic to stings and may develop breathing difficulties with a dramatic fall in blood pressure (anaphylactic shock). Emergency treatment is vital.

✚ **CALL AN AMBULANCE IMMEDIATELY IF THERE ARE SIGNS OF ALLERGY, IF BREATHING DIFFICULTIES DEVELOP, OR IF THE VICTIM HAS MULTIPLE STINGS OR STINGS NEAR THE MOUTH.**

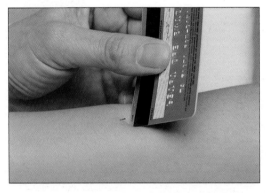

1 If the sting is still in the skin, scrape it out with a fingernail or hard object, such as the corner of a credit card. Do not remove it with tweezers, because this may squeeze more poison into the skin.

2 To relieve pain, prepare a cold compress or an ice pack. Soak a cloth in very cold water and then wring it out, or make an icepack by placing ice cubes in a plastic bag and covering with a damp cloth.

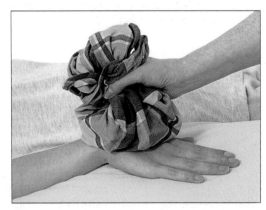

3 Apply the ice pack or cold compress to the site of the sting. An ice pack should not be applied for more than 10 minutes every hour, but can be reapplied hourly to relieve pain if needed.

Bleeding internal

WHAT TO LOOK FOR:

- Violent injury
- Pain or tenderness
- Bleeding from orifices
- Increasing thirst
- Pattern bruising at the site of injury
- Cold, clammy and pale skin
- Weak and increasingly rapid pulse
- Confusion or irritability
- Collapse or unconsciousness

✚ CALL AN AMBULANCE AS SOON AS POSSIBLE. THE VICTIM MAY SUDDENLY COLLAPSE OR BECOME UNCONSCIOUS.

Internal bleeding means loss of blood into the skull, chest or abdomen. It may follow an injury or be the result of a medical condition, and always requires urgent medical attention. You should suspect internal bleeding if signs of shock develop (see page 633) after an injury with no visible bleeding, or if there is bleeding or fluid loss from body orifices (see table below).

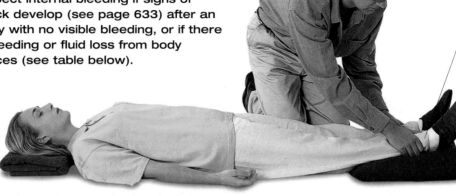

Raise the victim's legs slightly to help to reduce shock symptoms.

1 Help the victim to lie down in the most comfortable position. The victim will choose the position which eases the pain and you should try to provide support with pillows or blankets. Generally, a conscious victim will feel better with the legs raised slightly and this will also help to reduce the symptoms of shock.

2 Cover the victim lightly with clothing or a blanket. If you are outdoors, ease some fabric, such as a blanket, clothing or even newspapers, under the victim to reduce heat loss from a cold surface. Try to keep the victim still to avoid further internal blood loss.

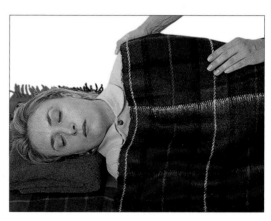

3 Reassure the victim frequently. Keep checking pulse and breathing and monitor for signs of shock (see page 633). Be prepared to start resuscitation if necessary (see page 596). Place an unconscious victim in the recovery position (see page 597).

Visible signs of internal bleeding		
Body part	**Injury**	**Result**
Ear	• Fractured skull • Damage to ear canal or eardrum	Blood or clear fluid
Nose	• Fractured skull • Damage to nose	Blood or clear fluid
Mouth	Fractured jaw or damage to mouth	Fresh blood
Lung	Lung or upper airway injury	Bright red frothy blood, coughed up
Stomach	Stomach or duodenal ulcer	Red or dark brown material, like coffee grounds, vomited up
Bowel	Damage to intestines	Fresh blood or black tarry stools
Vagina	Miscarriage Injury to womb or vagina	Fresh or dark blood
Urethra	Damaged kidney, ureter or bladder	Red or smoky urine; blood or clots in urine

Bleeding wounds

➕ **APPLY PRESSURE TO THE WOUND AS QUICKLY AS POSSIBLE TO REDUCE BLOOD LOSS.**

➕ **PLACE A CLEAN CLOTH OR DRESSING OVER THE WOUND TO AVOID CONTACT WITH ANOTHER PERSON'S BLOOD.**

With a small cut, instinct usually takes over and the victim applies firm pressure over his own wound to stop the bleeding and ease the pain. Raising the injured part further eases the pain by reducing pressure in the cut blood vessels. The first-aid treatment required for severe or deep wounds is exactly the same.

1 As long as there are no protruding objects, apply direct pressure over the wound, using a sterile dressing or clean pad. If you do not have one, a bulky pad can be made from tissues. Ideally, the victim should apply the pressure, as he or she will know how hard to press.

Bandage the dressing firmly, but not too tightly.

2 Raise the injured part above the level of the victim's heart to reduce blood flow to the wound. Ask the victim to lie down.

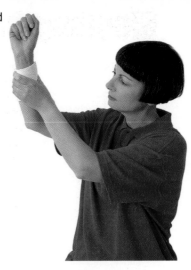

3 Fix the dressing in place with a clean bandage. If blood seeps through, leave the first dressing in place and apply another bandage on top.

4 Check fingertip colour to make sure that the bandage is not too tight. If the skin on the injured side looks blue, white or mottled, loosen the bandage. Keep the wounded area elevated.

➕ **MONITOR FOR ANY SIGNS OF SHOCK (SEE PAGE 633). FOR ALL BUT THE SMALLEST WOUNDS, SEEK MEDICAL ADVICE.**

➕ **CALL AN AMBULANCE IMMEDIATELY IF THE INJURY IS SEVERE, BLEEDING CONTINUES, OR SHOCK DEVELOPS.**

Foreign objects in wounds

Any foreign object embedded in a wound should be left in place until medical help arrives, so that it can be expertly removed without the risk of causing further damage. Seek medical advice as soon as possible.

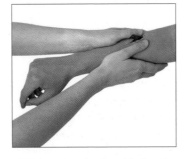

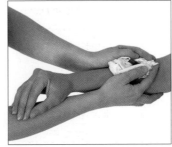

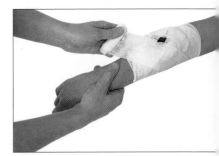

1 If there is a foreign object such as a fragment of glass or metal, or a large splinter in the wound, apply pressure equally on both sides of the object to stop bleeding.

2 Build up padding either around, or on both sides of the wound. DO NOT try to remove the foreign object, because this could make any bleeding worse.

3 Keep the padding in place and apply pressure to the wound with a bandage wrapped in a figure-of-eight (criss-cross) around the protruding object.

Bleeding wounds

Deep cuts

A deep cut may not appear to be large, but blood vessels, nerves, tendons, ligaments and muscles may have been damaged. If the wound was caused by a long blade, assume there is internal damage. Most deep wounds need prompt control of bleeding and medical assessment, because of the risk of complications, including tetanus infection.

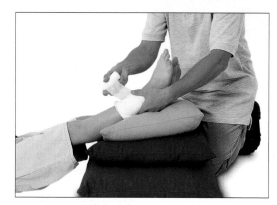

1 Apply firm pressure over the wound with a sterile dressing to control bleeding. Depending on the location of the injury, either the victim or the first aider can do this. If a sterile dressing is not available, folded tissues may be used.

Ensure that bleeding is controlled before preparing to bandage the wound.

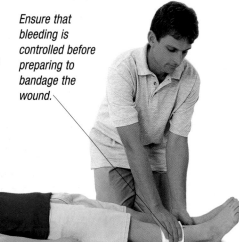

2 Ask the victim to lie down. Raise an injured limb above the level of the heart to reduce blood flow to the part. If an object is protruding from the wound, pad around it before applying a dressing (see page 607). Secure the dressing with a bandage.

3 If blood seeps through the dressing, place another one on top. For leg wounds, compare the colour of the toes on both feet and loosen the bandage if the toes on the injured leg start to swell or become discoloured. Treat for shock as necessary.

✚ **CALL AN AMBULANCE AS SOON AS POSSIBLE.**

Surface cuts

Small surface cuts are common. If there is very little bleeding they can usually be treated without any specialist care. However, if the cut is on the face, there is a risk of scarring, and if it is on a hand or is deep or gaping, there is a risk of injury to deeper tissues. In these cases, medical advice should be sought.

1 Control any bleeding by applying firm pressure over the wound. The victim should hold either a sterile dressing or one or two folded tissues firmly over the wound. Raise the injured part as high as possible to reduce blood flow to the area.

Raise the injured part to control bleeding.

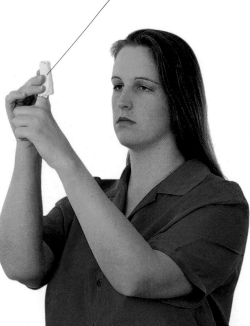

✚ **IF BLEEDING CONTINUES, SEEK MEDICAL ADVICE PROMPTLY.**
• **IF THE WOUND HAS NOT PARTIALLY HEALED WITHIN 24 HOURS, SEEK MEDICAL ADVICE.**

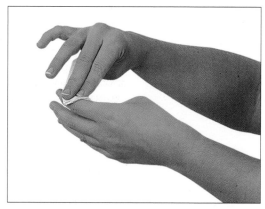

2 Clean the wound with an antiseptic solution or soap and warm water. Use a gauze or cotton swab and wipe away from the wound to avoid soiling it with any skin bacteria. Use several swabs if necessary, using each one once only.

3 Apply an adhesive dressing. Advise the victim to remove the dressing at night to allow the wound to dry. A new adhesive dressing should only be applied if the wound is moist and appears to need protection.

Blisters

WHAT TO LOOK FOR:

- Severe pain, or no pain but loss of sensation
- Hot, sensitive skin
- Black or red skin which may be blistered
- Swelling
- Clear fluid weeping from the skin

➕ **NEVER BURST A BLISTER AS THIS CAN CAUSE INFECTION.**

Blisters form as a result of allergic reaction, infection, friction or heat. Fluid leaks into a damaged or infected area under the skin's surface, creating a protective cushion which allows new skin to form below the blister. If there is a risk that a blister could be damaged by friction, it should be protected by a dressing.

Identifying types of blister

Cause	Symptom	Action
Injury	Injury is visible and with obvious cause, such as friction, heat, chemical burns or insect bites. Blisters are usually more than 5mm (¼ in) in diameter.	Do not burst a blister; cover it with a dry dressing. Seek medical advice promptly if redness spreads out from the blister and pain increases, as infection is possible.
Cold sore (herpes simplex) 	A crop of blisters in one area, usually on or around the mouth and less than 5mm (¼ in) in diameter. Blisters are preceded by skin tingling and pain.	Apply an antiviral cream as soon as possible. Seek medical advice urgently if the rash spreads beyond the original outbreak.
Shingles (herpes zoster)	Blisters are usually less than 5mm (¼ in) in diameter. They always occur on one side of the body, spreading out in a band around the trunk or down a limb.	Seek medical advice urgently as shingles is contagious: avoid contact with adults who have not had chickenpox, especially pregnant women, until the last blister has burst and scabbed over.
Eczema	Blisters are often more than 5mm (¼ in) in diameter, and may be painful. Commonly appear on hands, palms or soles of feet.	Seek medical advice as soon as possible, urgently if the skin is very painful – this is unusual and may indicate that the skin is infected.

Bruises

WHAT TO LOOK FOR:

- Pain, swelling or a bluish discoloration at the site of an injury
- Pressure building up beneath the skin

Bruises are caused by a blunt blow to the skin, which breaks the tiny blood vessels, or capillaries, close to the surface, so that blood seeps into the tissues. Sometimes there is a more serious underlying injury. The colour of a bruise gradually changes as the blood is reabsorbed into the body.

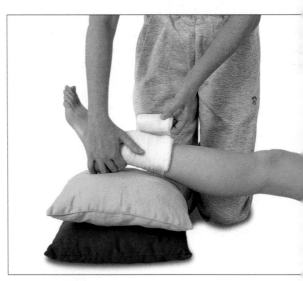

A blow to the area around the eye will often result in dramatic swelling and severe bruising, known as a black eye. A cold compress applied hourly for 10 minutes will reduce the swelling. Seek medical advice if vision is affected in any way.

If the injury is only a few minutes old, first reduce the spread of bleeding into the tissues by raising the affected part and applying an ice pack or cold compress (see page 605). This helps to lessen any later pain and swelling. After 10 minutes of firm pressure, treat any associated injuries, such as a sprain (see page 634).

Burns and scalds

WHAT TO LOOK FOR:

- Severe pain or no pain (see right)
- Black or red skin which may be blistered
- Swelling
- Clear fluid weeping from the skin
- Cold, clammy skin
- Nausea or vomiting

➕ **SEEK MEDICAL HELP FOR ALL BUT THE MOST MINOR BURN. IF THE BURN IS DEEP OR COVERS AN AREA GREATER THAN THE SIZE OF THE VICTIM'S OWN PALM, CALL AN AMBULANCE.**

➕ **DO NOT BURST ANY BLISTERS THAT FORM AFTER A BURN OR SCALD.**

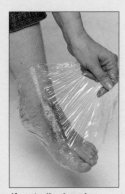

If a sterile dressing is not available, use plastic film or a plastic bag.

Burns are caused by contact with a heat source such as hot metal, or by corrosive chemicals, friction, radiation or electricity. Scalds are caused by steam or hot liquid.

The amount of pain felt is not a true guide to the severity of the injury. Superficial and partial-thickness burns (involving only the skin) tend to be more painful than full-thickness burns, in which the underlying tissues are damaged and nerve endings destroyed.

1 Cool the burn or scald at once with cold running water from the nearest tap. In an emergency, any cold, non-flammable fluid can be used. Continue cooling with cold water for at least 10 minutes, even if the burn has stopped hurting. Do not apply any lotion, ointment or oil to a burn or scald.

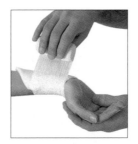

2 Remove any jewellery from the burned area in case of swelling. Cover the burn with a clean, non-stick dressing to reduce the risk of infection.

3 Do not try to remove clothing or debris stuck to the burn, since this could increase the risk of infection. Cut around any attached material and cover the burned area. If a sterile dressing is not available, use a clean plastic bag, plastic film, or any clean, non-fluffy material.

Raise the legs on a blanket or pillow.

Treatment of burns and scalds

Chemical burn

First, make the area safe. Flood the burnt part with water for at least 20 minutes (longer than for a heat burn). Meanwhile, call an ambulance and monitor breathing – be prepared to resuscitate the victim if necessary (see page 596). Gently remove any contaminated clothing. Household chemicals, insecticides and weedkillers can be highly toxic if absorbed through the skin as well as causing chemical burns, so be alert to signs of poisoning, such as nausea, headache or dizziness.

Send details of the chemical involved with the victim to hospital.

Electrical burn

Electricity, including a lightning strike, leaves burns both where the current entered and where it left the body. There is also a high risk of cardiac arrest. Make sure that the power source is safe before approaching the victim. Call an ambulance immediately, then treat burn injuries by cooling while waiting for help. If cardiac arrest occurs, give CPR (cardiopulmonary resuscitation, see page 597) until the ambulance arrives.

Burns to the airway

Burns to the face, or inhalation of smoke in a fire, can be very dangerous. The victim may suffer pain and extensive swelling of the lining of the mouth and throat, resulting in the narrowing or closure of the upper airway. This can be life-threatening. Call an ambulance at once if you know the victim has inhaled smoke or if you notice soot or damaged skin around the mouth or nose, swelling of the mouth or tongue, or breathing difficulties. Observe the victim closely in case resuscitation is needed.

4 Make the victim comfortable, while waiting for help. Keep monitoring their pulse and breathing and check for signs of shock (see page 633). Be prepared to resuscitate if necessary. Avoid giving any food or drink, unless the burn is very small, in case an anaesthetic may be needed. Monitor the victim's breathing, especially after smoke inhalation, and be prepared to give CPR (see page 597) if necessary.

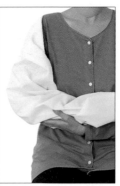

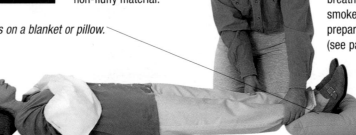

Chest injuries

WHAT TO LOOK FOR:

- Difficulty breathing, with shallow and gasping breaths
- Chest pain
- Bright red, frothy blood coughed up
- Blueness of tongue and lips
- Sucking noise as air enters the chest cavity with each breath
- Bloodstained fluid bubbling around the wound

✚ **CALL FOR AN AMBULANCE AS SOON AS POSSIBLE.**

An injury to the chest can cause internal bleeding or lung damage, which may be life-threatening.

1 Immediately help the victim into a resting, half-sitting position, with support where required. The victim should lean towards the injured side.

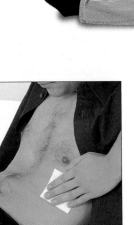

2 Check for a penetrating wound. If one is found, place a thick, sterile dressing or pad of clean tissues over the wound and press down gently but firmly with the palm of your hand. This should stop any bleeding and restrict the entry of air into the chest cavity.

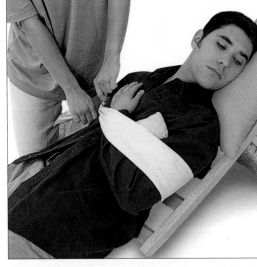

3 Seal the dressing on three sides with adhesive tape, leaving one edge open. This allows air to escape, but not enter.

4 Place some padding over the dressing, between the arm and chest wall. Then apply a broad bandage around the chest and over the arm on the injured side to provide support to the injured area.

5 Monitor breathing and pulse while waiting for the ambulance. If the victim becomes unconscious, be prepared to give CPR (cardiopulmonary resuscitation, see page 597). Place the victim in the recovery position but with the injured side downwards. This allows the uninjured lung to work efficiently.

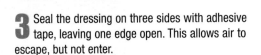

An up-ended chair is a useful support.

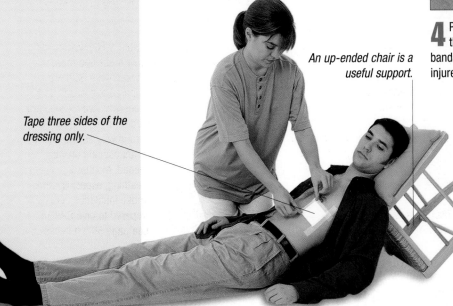

Tape three sides of the dressing only.

Childbirth

➕ CALL FOR MEDICAL ASSISTANCE AS SOON AS POSSIBLE.

When a baby arrives unexpectedly but after a normal pregnancy, he or she will usually be born naturally, without any complications. Labour has three stages: first, the birth canal stretches and the uterus contracts every few minutes in preparation for pushing the baby out – this may last for several hours, with contractions gradually increasing in frequency and intensity; second, the baby is born; third, the placenta (afterbirth) is delivered. There is usually plenty of time to arrange assistance. If not, stay calm and listen to the mother's wishes. Never try to delay the birth, and interfere as little as possible – the baby will usually be expelled naturally. DO NOT pull on the head and shoulders as they emerge.

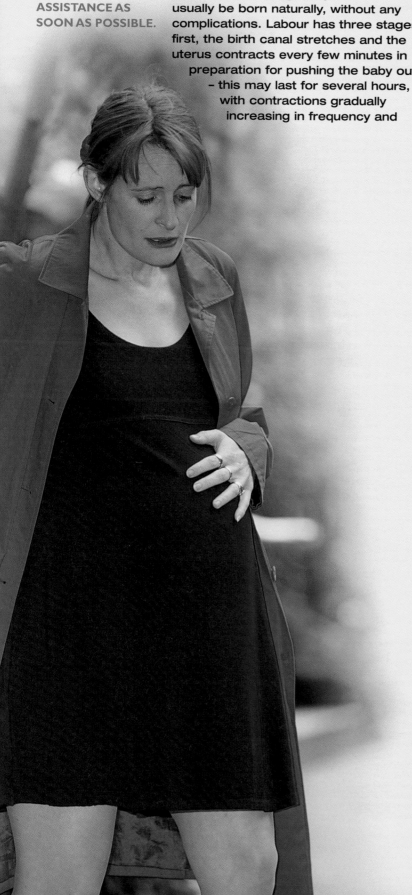

1 Help the mother to assume whatever position is most comfortable for her. Provide support if she wishes with pillows or rolled-up clothing. Place clean towels or old cotton sheeting under her for the birth.

2 Wash your hands and scrub under the nails thoroughly, if there is time, and wear plastic gloves if available.

3 Encourage the mother to rest between contractions. When the birth is imminent, the widest part of the baby's head will become visible. At this stage, ask the mother to stop pushing, and take fast, short breaths instead.

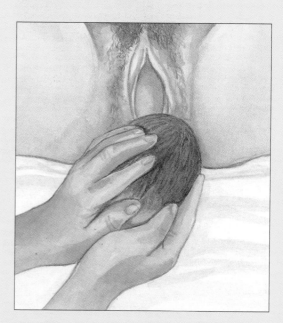

4 When the baby's head appears, support it lightly on your hands until the next contraction comes and expels the body. The head will rotate slightly on your hands as the shoulders turn sideways ready to be born. Do not interfere with the natural movement of the baby because any resistance can be harmful.

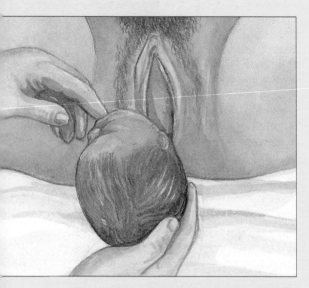

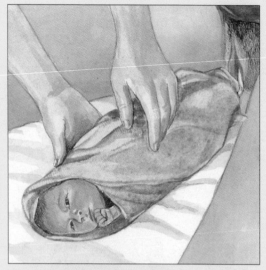

5 If there is any membrane covering the face, gently remove it to enable the baby to breathe. Check to see if a loop of cord is around the baby's neck. If so, carefully slip it over the head to avoid it tightening around the neck as the baby is born.

7 When the baby slips out of the birth canal, lift it away carefully – it will be slippery. Gently pass the baby to the mother and place it on her abdomen. Cover the baby in a towel or blanket, keeping the head covered to conserve heat. Keep the head low so that fluid and mucus can drain from the mouth. DO NOT pull on or cut the umbilical cord.

8 A short time after the birth, the placenta (afterbirth) will be expelled. This will happen naturally with the mother's contractions – DO NOT pull on the cord. Wrap the placenta in a plastic bag, but leave it still attached to the baby. The midwife will want to examine it, to ensure that there are no fragments left inside the mother, which could be dangerous. Leave it to the midwife to cut the cord.

9 It is normal for the mother to bleed a little after the birth. If available, supply warm water and towels and help her to clean herself up. Provide a sanitary towel if available.

✚ **IF BLEEDING IS SEVERE, WATCH FOR SIGNS OF SHOCK (SEE PAGE 633) AND CALL AN AMBULANCE, IF ONE IS NOT ALREADY ON ITS WAY.**

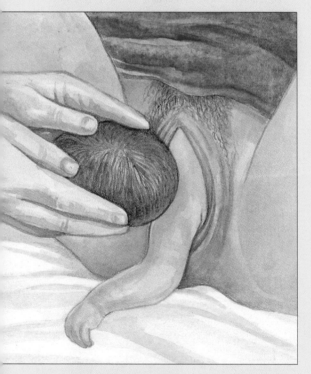

6 At the start of the next contraction, the shoulders will appear, one at a time. Do not attempt to pull on the baby but let the mother's contractions do the work naturally.

IF THE BABY DOES NOT BREATHE ON ITS OWN, IMMEDIATELY CHECK THE AIRWAY (SEE PAGE 594) AND BE PREPARED TO CARRY OUT RESUSCITATION (SEE PAGE 596). DO NOT SMACK THE BABY.

Choking adult

WHAT TO LOOK FOR:

- Difficulty in breathing (shortness of breath)
- Difficulty in speaking
- Clutching the throat
- Distress
- Noisy breathing, wheezing or a high-pitched 'crowing' noise
- Congested facial skin with bluish lips
- Later, collapse and unconsciousness

✚ **CHOKING CAN CAUSE DEATH WITHIN MINUTES – TREAT IT AS AN EMERGENCY.**

In a choking emergency, it is vital to act fast to clear the airway. If there is total obstruction of the airway, the victim will quickly collapse, but even a partial blockage, when the victim will be coughing (and therefore still breathing), should be treated as an emergency.

If the victim is conscious

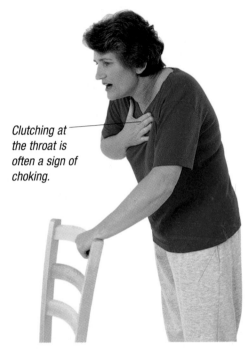

Clutching at the throat is often a sign of choking.

1 Be reassuring and encourage coughing. DO NOT slap the person on the back – this can push objects farther down the airway. Don't let a choking person rush from the room in embarrassment.

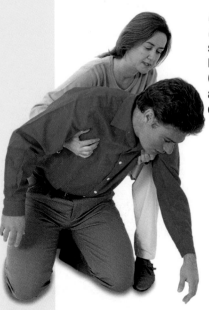

2 Help the person to bend forwards so that the head is lower than the chest. Check inside the mouth and remove any obvious obstruction.

3 If this fails, perform the Heimlich or abdominal thrust manoeuvre. Stand behind the person and place one clenched fist, thumb inwards, just below the breastbone. Grasp this fist with your other hand and pull sharply upwards and inwards. The object should shoot out as air is forced violently outwards. Repeat up to five times if necessary, then check inside the mouth again.

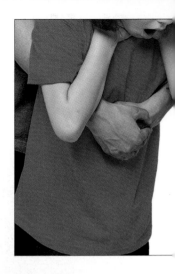

✚ **NEVER PRACTISE THE HEIMLICH MANOEUVRE ON ANYONE WHO ISN'T CHOKING – THERE IS A RISK OF DAMAGE TO THE INTERNAL ORGANS.**

If the victim becomes unconscious

1 Call an ambulance as a first priority or ask someone else to do this.

2 Attempt to clear any obstruction from the person's mouth.

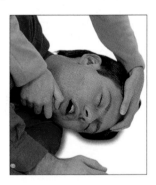

3 Give abdominal thrusts by rolling the victim onto the back and kneeling astride him or her. Place the heel of one hand midway between the navel and breastbone, cover it with the other hand and keep your elbows straight (as for CPR). Press sharply upwards and inwards several times. Check the mouth again.

4 If the airway is apparently clear and breathing is still absent, begin resuscitation (see page 596) in an attempt to blow air past the obstruction.

5 Check for breathing and circulation. Start CPR (cardiopulmonary resuscitation, see page 597), if necessary. Repeat abdominal thrusts between each CPR cycle if necessary.

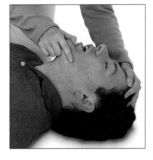
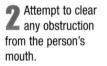

Choking child

Toddlers and older children

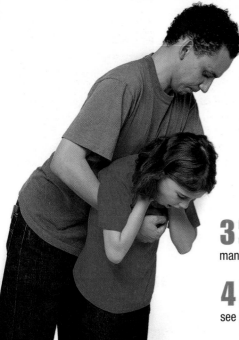

1 Encourage the child to bend forwards and cough, to clear any obstructions from the mouth.

2 Stand behind the child and place a clenched fist against the lower breastbone. Grasp with the other hand and give up to five chest thrusts by pulling sharply upwards and inwards. Check the mouth.

3 If this fails, move your fist down to the upper abdomen and perform the Heimlich manoeuvre, as for adults (see opposite page).

4 If the child lapses into unconsciousness, start CPR (cardiopulmonary resuscitation, see page 597).

For a baby

➕ **DO NOT USE ABDOMINAL THRUSTS ON A BABY.**

1 Lay the baby face down over your forearm with the head lower than the chest.

2 Give up to five sharp back slaps between the shoulder blades to dislodge any obstruction.

3 Check the mouth and remove any obvious obstruction.

4 If this fails, place the baby face upwards and put two fingertips onto the lower part of the breastbone, just below the nipples. Press vigorously up to five times and check the mouth again.

Collarbone fracture

WHAT TO LOOK FOR:

- Pain and tenderness at or around the site of the injury
- Pain increased by even slight movement
- The victim supporting the weight of the arm at the elbow
- Head tilted to the injured side to ease the pain
- Injured shoulder joint a little lower than the uninjured side
- Obvious swelling or deformity over the injury site
- Nausea or vomiting

The collarbone, which runs between the shoulder blade and breastbone, is usually broken by a blow to the shoulder or by a fall onto an outstretched hand.

1 Ask the victim to sit down and support the injured limb at the elbow with the other hand. The injured shoulder often droops lower than the uninjured side because the shoulder joint has lost the support of the collarbone.

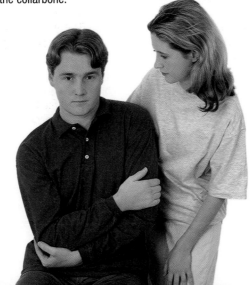

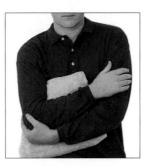

2 Gently ease soft padding – such as a folded towel or sweater – between the arm and chest wall to provide extra support.

3 Support the injured arm with an elevation sling (see page 604).

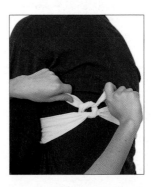

4 Apply a broad bandage around the body, fastening the arm against the chest. Tie off using a secure knot on the uninjured side of the body.

➕ **SEEK MEDICAL ADVICE PROMPTLY IF A FRACTURE IS SUSPECTED.**

Concussion

Concussion

WHAT TO LOOK FOR:

- Headache
- Nausea or vomiting
- Tiredness
- Blurred or double vision
- Temporary loss of consciousness
- Confusion or disorientation
- Irritability
- Loss of hand-to-eye coordination
- Short-term memory loss of events before the accident

Concussion is a head injury which can follow a blow to the head or jaw, or result from a heavy fall onto the head, feet or buttocks. The jarring that occurs causes the brain to be shaken around inside the skull, causing internal bruising, swelling and sometimes bleeding. Sometimes, a brief loss of consciousness occurs with concussion.

1 Check the victim's response to simple instructions such as, 'Squeeze my hand. Now let it go'. If the victim fails to respond promptly, turn them onto their side immediately because they may lose consciousness.

Place a victim who is unconscious, or in danger of becoming so, into the recovery position (see page 597).

2 If the victim is fully conscious, help them into a comfortable position, preferably with the head slightly raised. Check for any injuries, including wounds, bumps or bruises. If a wound is found, stop any bleeding promptly with direct pressure, elevation and rest for the injured part.

3 If there is a bump or bruise on the head, prepare a cold compress (see page 605) and encourage the victim to hold it in place so that you can check their ability to coordinate the task. Observe the victim closely for any deterioration, including sleepiness, irritability or headache.

➕ **CALL FOR AN AMBULANCE, AND WATCH FOR ANY CHANGE IN THE VICTIM'S CONDITION WHILE YOU WAIT.**

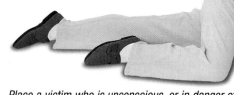

Convulsion, febrile

WHAT TO LOOK FOR:

- Flushed, ill appearance
- High temperature of 38°C (100°F) or more
- Skin hot to the touch with bluish lips
- Twitching or jerking movements of the trunk and limbs
- Unconsciousness: no response to voice or to touch

Child convulsions, resulting from a fever, usually occur before the age of five years and are not related to epilepsy. During a convulsion, the body will twitch and jerk. These movements are caused by an overheated brain, which results from a high temperature or the start of an infection. The convulsion usually lasts no more than 2 minutes, often less. Doctors no longer recommend active cooling of a feverish child because this makes the fever recur.

1 Remove all clothing, including any bedclothes, to allow the child to cool down naturally, but do not sponge with water or fan the child's skin.

2 Do not attempt to restrain the child, but make the area around him safe to avoid him sustaining an injury. Move furniture away or place clothing or blankets against heavy items to cushion them.

3 When the convulsions have stopped, check the child's pulse and breathing and cover him or her with a light sheet or a thin blanket. Repeat the pulse checks every 10–15 minutes, until the child has recovered fully.

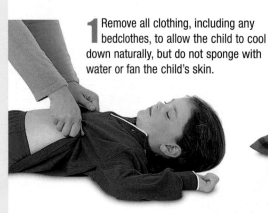

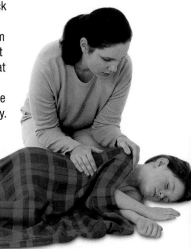

Cramp

WHAT TO LOOK FOR:

- Waking at night due to muscle spasm
- Painful spasm in a muscle that has been over-used

Keeping a limb in one position for a long time can slow the circulation to major muscles in one area of the body, causing a tight muscle mass in the affected area and cramp. In hot weather, cramps occur when the victim has failed to maintain an adequate fluid intake. A cramp may also occur in cold conditions or following heavy exercise.

Lower leg

Help the victim to lie down and slowly straighten the affected leg while gently pressing down on the knee with your other hand. Hold the foot under the heel and use the other hand to gently push the toes upwards. When the spasm eases, gently massage the affected muscles until the area feels relaxed.

Gently stretching the foot helps to relieve lower leg cramp.

Hand

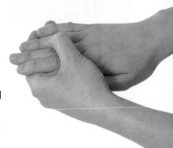

Ask the victim to straighten and massage the affected fingers until the muscles relax. Warmth can be comforting when the spasm eases, especially in cold weather.

Foot

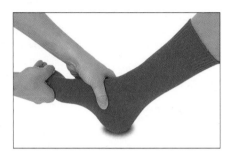

Ask the victim to stand with the affected foot firmly on the floor. If the toes are in severe spasm, gently try to straighten them with your hand. In cold weather, advise the victim to put on some warm socks.

Croup

WHAT TO LOOK FOR:

- A barking or crowing sound with each intake of breath
- Frequent spasms of coughing that cause breathlessness
- Exhaustion from frequent coughing
- Deteriorating skin colour with bluish lips and fingertips
- High temperature of 38°C (100°F) or more
- Attempts to sit upright to ease breathing

Croup is a breathing disorder that affects babies and small children. The attacks often occur at night and are caused by an infection which leads to swelling of the upper respiratory tract.

1 Help the child to breathe more effectively by propping him or her upright with a pile of pillows. Give plenty of reassurance.

Reassure the child – croup is a very frightening condition.

2 Create a steamy atmosphere to help to relieve the inflammation and swelling in the upper respiratory tract. Take the child into the bathroom and run the hot-water tap for some time. Keep the child a safe distance from the water.

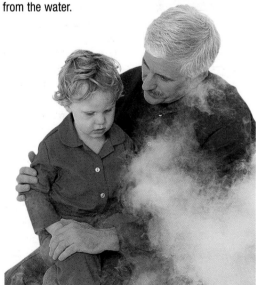

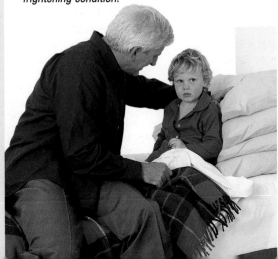

➕ **IF BREATHING DOES NOT IMPROVE RAPIDLY, SEEK MEDICAL HELP PROMPTLY.**

Crush injury

**WHAT TO
LOOK FOR:**

- Signs of a crushing force on the trunk or a limb
- Swelling and bruising of the crushed tissues
- Pale, cold and clammy skin
- Tingling or numbness in the affected area
- Feeling cold, faint, dizzy and nauseous
- Severe pain

Crush injuries are usually very serious, leading to extensive soft tissue and bone damage. Toxins build up around the injury so that if the crushing force is suddenly removed there is a risk of serious complications from kidney failure.

1 If the casualty has been crushed for less than 10 minutes, remove the crushing force, if possible. While waiting for an ambulance, treat any wounds or fractures, and watch for signs of shock (see page 633).

2 If the victim has been crushed for more than 10 minutes, DO NOT attempt to remove the crushing force. Doing so may release toxins around the body. Offer reassurance and make the victim as comfortable as possible while waiting for help.

✚ **CALL AN AMBULANCE AS SOON AS POSSIBLE. WHILE WAITING, NOTE ANY CHANGES IN THE VICTIM'S CONDITION.**

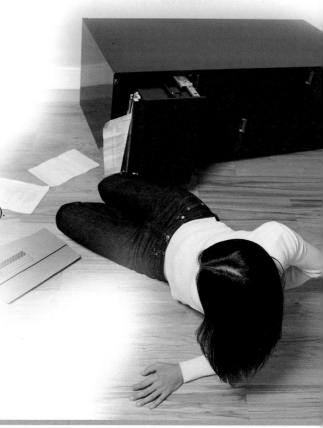

Cuts, grazes and splinters

**WHAT TO
LOOK FOR:**

- Pain at the site of injury
- Profuse bleeding
- A splinter in a wound
- Broken skin
- Numbness of the skin
- Deep cuts on a hand or the face
- Difficulty in moving part of a limb or a digit

✚ **IF BLEEDING FROM A CUT CONTINUES, SEEK MEDICAL ADVICE PROMPTLY.**

Minor wounds are very common. A cut may not appear serious, but if it is deep or gaping, underlying structures may have been damaged. Cuts on the face may lead to scarring, and cuts on the fingers or hands can cause muscle or tendon damage. Seek prompt medical assessment if you are in any doubt.

Cuts

Make sure your hands are clean, and clean the wound with running water or antiseptic. Apply firm pressure to stop any bleeding. Elevate the wound if bleeding continues. When bleeding stops, apply a sterile dressing, secured with a bandage if necessary.

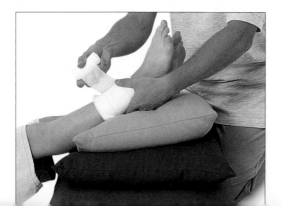

Grazes

1 Control any bleeding by applying firm pressure over the wound using a sterile dressing or tissues and the palm of your hand. Raise the injured part as high as possible to reduce blood flow to the area.

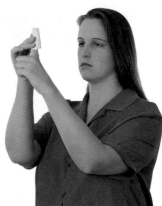

2 Clean the wound thoroughly with an antiseptic or soap and warm water. Use a gauze or cotton swab and wipe away from the wound to avoid soiling it with skin bacteria.

✚ **SEEK MEDICAL ADVICE IF THE WOUND HAS NOT PARTIALLY HEALED WITHIN 24 HOURS.**

Splinters

Splinters are very common. Ensure the area is clean, then remove the splinter with tweezers. If unsuccessful, or if the splinter breaks off, seek medical advice.

Diabetic complications

WHAT TO LOOK FOR:

LOW BLOOD SUGAR
- Feeling faint, giddy and weak with trembling limbs
- Shaking or trembling
- Confusion or strange behaviour in a known diabetic
- Pale skin and sweating
- Shallow breathing with a rapid pulse

HIGH BLOOD SUGAR
- Unconsciousness
- Dry skin and rapid pulse
- Difficult or noisy breathing
- Smell of pear drops or nail-varnish remover on the breath

High-energy foods quickly boost the blood sugar levels in a hypoglycaemic attack.

Diabetes occurs when the body cannot control the level of blood sugar properly, because of a lack of the hormone insulin. Even with treatment, blood sugar levels can become imbalanced, causing problems.

Low blood sugar

The most common emergency for a diabetic is low blood sugar, known medically as hypoglycaemia. Unconsciousness can occur rapidly without emergency treatment. If low blood sugar is suspected, give a conscious victim a sweet drink or sugar lumps to suck, followed by high-energy food such as chocolate, cake, biscuits or a sandwich to raise the blood sugar level.

High blood sugar

If the victim is suffering from too much sugar, known as hyperglycaemia, deterioration is slower and there is usually plenty of time to call an ambulance. Place an unconscious victim in the recovery position (see page 597), ensuring that the airway is kept clear. Call an ambulance at once. If necessary, give the person CPR (see page 597).

Place an unconscious victim in the recovery position until an ambulance arrives.

Dislocation

WHAT TO LOOK FOR:

- An inability to move the injured part
- Severe pain in and around the joint, increased by movement
- Some loss of sensation
- Obvious deformity and swelling around the joint
- Bruising

✚ **DO NOT TRY TO REPLACE THE DISLOCATED BONES. THIS MAY CAUSE FURTHER DAMAGE AND COMPLICATIONS.**

A dislocation occurs when a severe twist or wrench displaces a bone from its normal position in a joint. There may also be bone fracture and damage to nearby blood vessels and nerves which can cause serious complications. Help the victim to find a position in which the injured area can be supported and made comfortable.

✚ **TREAT ALL DISLOCATIONS AS FRACTURES UNTIL A DIAGNOSIS IS MADE.**

Finger

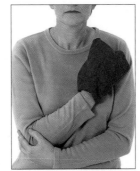

For a dislocated finger, use soft padding to support the injury. Wrap a bandage lightly in place unless this is more painful. Do not apply firm pressure because of the risk of further damage to nerves and blood vessels.

Shoulder

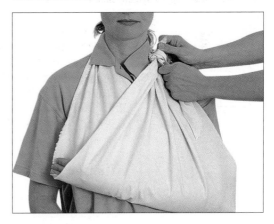

For a dislocated shoulder, place the arm across the chest and support it using a triangular bandage as a sling (see page 604). Pillows or blankets are also useful for supporting a dislocated shoulder, hip or elbow joint.

✚ **SEEK MEDICAL ADVICE URGENTLY, BECAUSE THERE IS OFTEN A RISK OF COMPLICATIONS. CALL AN AMBULANCE AS SOON AS POSSIBLE IF THE VICTIM IS IN SEVERE PAIN.**

Drowning

WHAT TO LOOK FOR:

- Anyone struggling in the water
- A victim is lying or floating face-down in the water
- In a rescued person, mottled blue or white skin colour, noisy breathing or no breathing at all and an inability to speak

⊕ **ANYONE RESCUED FROM WATER MUST BE ASSESSED BY A DOCTOR.**

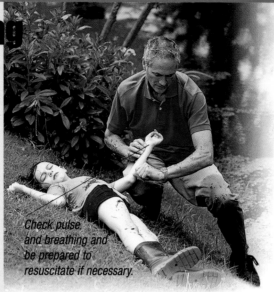

Check pulse and breathing and be prepared to resuscitate if necessary.

Drowning is a common cause of accidental death, especially in children. Summon help immediately – prompt rescue followed by efficient cardiopulmonary resuscitation can save lives. Unless you are a very strong swimmer, you should not enter the water yourself, since this can place your own life at risk.

1 Whenever possible, throw the victim a flotation device or rope, or hold out a pole or tree branch. Unless you are a trained lifesaver, or the victim is unconscious, do not enter the water.

2 If you must go into the water, wade rather than swim if possible. Attempt deep-water rescue only if you are a strong swimmer. Carry an unconscious victim with the head low, to reduce the chance of choking.

3 If the victim is unconscious, check the pulse and be prepared to start cardiopulmonary resuscitation (see page 597). If not, place the victim in the recovery position (see page 597) and continue to check pulse and breathing while awaiting help.

4 Anyone who has been in water for more than a few minutes is at risk of hypothermia (see page 629). Remove wet clothing and cover with towels, blankets or dry clothing to warm the victim as soon as possible. If the victim regains consciousness, give hot drinks while awaiting help.

⊕ **CALL FOR AN AMBULANCE AS SOON AS POSSIBLE, UNLESS THE VICTIM APPEARS TO BE FULLY RECOVERED.**

Ear problems

WHAT TO LOOK FOR:

- Sharp pain
- Bleeding from the ear
- Clear or straw-coloured fluid draining from the ear canal
- Hearing loss
- Persistent earache with fever
- Foreign body wedged in the ear canal

The ears can be damaged by blows to the head, sudden loud noises, pressure waves from an explosion or foreign bodies inserted into the ear canal. Earache is most often due to infection, and commonly occurs during or after a cold or other respiratory infection.

An insect lodged in the ear canal can usually be removed by flooding the ear with water.

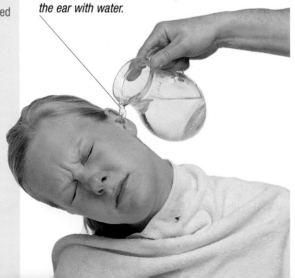

Does the victim have any:

- Bleeding or fluid draining from the ear canal?
- Severe pain in the ear?

NO →

Has the victim experienced:

- Sudden loss of hearing?
- Ringing in the ears?
- Dizziness?
- Foreign body stuck in the ear canal?

 YES

 YES

SEEK MEDICAL ADVICE URGENTLY

MAKE AN APPOINTMENT WITH A DOCTOR

⊕ **IF THERE IS NO IMPROVEMENT WITHIN 24 HOURS, SEEK MEDICAL ADVICE PROMPTLY.**

Electric shock

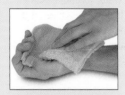
*If the skin has been
burned, flood with cold
water for at least 10
minutes, then apply a
cold compress (see
page 605).*

Low-voltage electric shock

Electrical accidents can occur when
equipment or household appliances
have a fault, such as a damaged flex,
or when they are used in an unsafe
manner, such as handling an appliance
with wet hands.

1 Never touch the
victim until you are
certain that contact with
the electric current has
been broken, or you
could be electrocuted
yourself. Switch off the
power, at the mains if
possible, then disconnect
the appliance from the
power point.

2 If you cannot switch
the current off, stand
on some insulating
material – wood, rubber,
plastic or thick paper. Use
a wooden pole, not a
metal one, to push the
current source clear.
Alternatively, pull the
victim away by a loop of
rope if you can, or by
tugging on clothing.

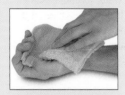 **DO NOT TOUCH THE VICTIM UNTIL
THE CURRENT HAS BEEN
DISCONNECTED.**

3 If the victim is unconscious, start CPR
(cardiopulmonary resuscitation, see page 597)
if necessary. If the victim is breathing and has a pulse,
look for burns on the skin where the electricity entered
the body and where it went to earth. Cool any burns
with cold water (see page 610). Once the victim is
breathing, place him or her in the recovery position
(see page 597).

*Use something wooden,
such as a broom handle
or chair leg, to break the
electrical contact.*

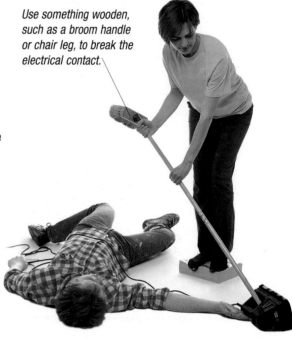

High-voltage electric shock

Power lines and
overhead high-
tension cables
have such a high
voltage current
that contact is
usually fatal.
The current can
arc or jump over
a considerable
distance and can
cause injury to a
person from as
far away as
18m (20 yd).
Wood and other
insulators are no
protection.

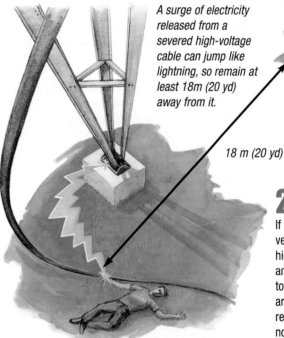

*A surge of electricity
released from a
severed high-voltage
cable can jump like
lightning, so remain at
least 18m (20 yd)
away from it.*

18 m (20 yd)

1 Call the local electricity supply authority for help,
and keep bystanders well clear of the accident
until the power has been turned off.

2 Shout reassurance to
a conscious victim.
If people are inside a
vehicle in contact with a
high-tension cable after
an accident, urge them
to stay in place – they
are safe as long as they
remain in the vehicle. Do
not attempt first aid until
the area is declared safe
– any ill-judged rescue
attempt may be fatal for
both victim and rescuer.

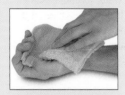

Eye injury

WHAT TO LOOK FOR:

- Intense pain
- A wound or foreign body in or near the eye
- The eye appears bloodshot
- Inability to open the affected eye
- Blood or fluid leaking from the eyeball
- Impaired vision
- Itching and watering of the eye
- Swelling around the eye

Any eye injury is potentially serious. Direct blows, chemical splashes, intense heat and foreign bodies may all cause complications, including scarring, infection and reduced vision. Ensure the victim receives rapid medical attention.

Foreign body

1 Tell the victim not to rub the eye. With the victim facing the light, stand behind and gently separate the eyelids. If you see a foreign body on the white of the eye, flush it out with water or lift it off with the corner of a damp handkerchief or tissue.

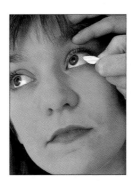

2 If the object is on the coloured part of the eye or is firmly stuck or embedded in the eye, DO NOT attempt to remove it. Cover the eye with a sterile pad secured by adhesive tape and seek urgent medical help.

Chemicals

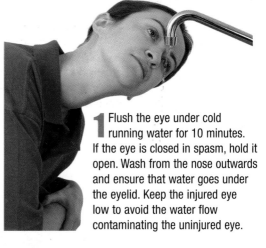

1 Flush the eye under cold running water for 10 minutes. If the eye is closed in spasm, hold it open. Wash from the nose outwards and ensure that water goes under the eyelid. Keep the injured eye low to avoid the water flow contaminating the uninjured eye.

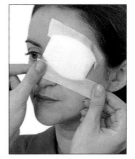

2 Apply a sterile eye pad or dressing secured with lightweight adhesive tape. Take or send a sample of the chemical that entered the eye to hospital with the victim.

Facial injury

WHAT TO LOOK FOR:

- Pain in the injured area
- An inability to speak, chew or swallow
- Swelling and deformity of the injured area
- Bleeding inside the mouth
- Missing or loose teeth
- Dribbling, if the jaw is fractured

Injuries to the face should always be medically assessed to reduce the risks of serious complications or permanent disability. If the nose or mouth is involved, the airway may be obstructed by bleeding. Blindness or a serious head injury can arise from a blow to the cheek or forehead. Injuries that result in loss of consciousness can cause obstruction of the airway by the tongue and inhalation of blood or saliva.

IF THE INJURIES INVOLVE THE EYES OR EYE SOCKETS, THE CHEEKBONE, MOUTH, NOSE OR JAW, CALL AN AMBULANCE AS SOON AS POSSIBLE.

1 If the victim is unconscious, check pulse and breathing and be prepared to start cardiopulmonary resuscitation (see page 597). If there is an injury to the mouth or jaw, ensure that the airway is kept open (see page 595). Place an unconscious victim into the recovery position (see page 597).

2 Help a conscious victim into the most comfortable position – generally sitting with the head forwards. Stop any bleeding with a pad over the wound and apply a cold compress if there is any swelling. Gently support the injured area and arrange immediate transport to hospital.

CALL FOR AN AMBULANCE AT ONCE IF THERE IS CLEAR, STRAW-COLOURED FLUID LEAKING FROM THE EARS OR NOSE – THE VICTIM MAY HAVE A SKULL FRACTURE (SEE PAGE 625).

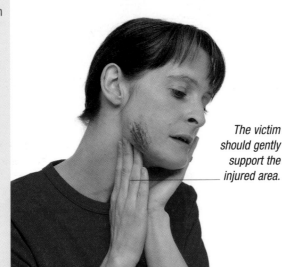

The victim should gently support the injured area.

Fainting

- Feeling dizzy, faint or lightheaded
- Nausea
- Collapse
- Pale, moist skin
- Restlessness and anxiety
- Slow, sighing breaths
- A very slow pulse

Fainting is common. It can occur if there is a temporary loss of normal blood supply to the brain. Once the victim is lying down, the blood returns to the brain and the person regains consciousness.

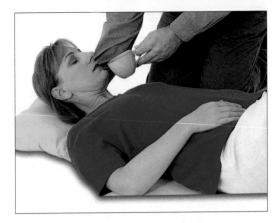

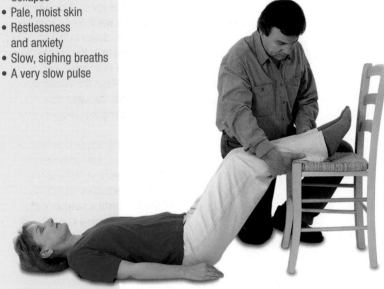

1 Try to anticipate the faint and catch the victim, easing him or her to the ground and protecting the head. Raise the legs to restore the circulation. Loosen any tight clothing at the neck and waist and ensure there is plenty of fresh air. Stay with the victim until he or she recovers, then give small sips of cool water.

2 When the person feels ready to get up, allow him or her a few minutes to adjust to the change of position. If the victim fails to respond to the spoken voice or touch at any time, move him or her promptly into the recovery position to ensure a clear airway (see page 597).

Fits

- Meaningless sounds being made by the victim
- Loss of coordination with staggering and poor balance
- Restlessness and confusion
- Loss of consciousness with a fall to the floor
- Twitching and jerking of some or all limbs with the head tossing from side to side
- Clenching of the teeth with foaming saliva visible
- Loss of bladder and bowel control

Epilepsy is a brain condition in which the victim may have fits. Flashing lights, video games or loud noise can trigger a fit. Some fits follow head injury, poisoning or, in infants, a high temperature (see page 616). In some forms of fits there is no collapse, just a brief disturbance of consciousness, as if the brain has temporarily 'switched off'.

1 Make the area safe to avoid injury while the victim is moving violently on the floor. Move furniture away or place clothing or blankets against heavy items.

➕ **DO NOT ATTEMPT TO RESTRAIN OR MOVE THE VICTIM DURING A FIT.**

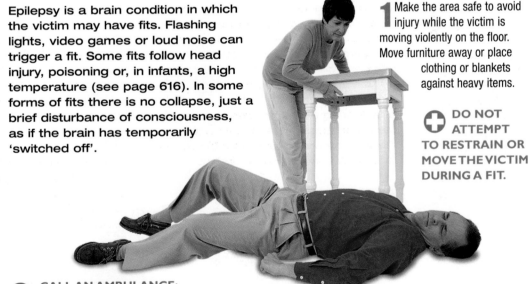

➕ **CALL AN AMBULANCE: IF THE VICTIM:**
- **HAS SUSTAINED INJURIES;**
- **IS HAVING A FIRST FIT;**
- **IS UNCONSCIOUS FOR MORE THAN 10 MINUTES;**
- **HAS A FURTHER FIT.**

2 When the jerking movements stop, quickly roll the victim onto his or her side and check that the airway is clear (see page 595). The victim is likely to fall asleep at this stage so allow him or her to lie quietly until fully recovered.

Gas and smoke inhalation

WHAT TO LOOK FOR:

- Breathing difficulty or breathing failure
- Confusion, listlessness, or 'drunken' behaviour
- Abnormal colour, including pale, bluish or cherry-pink skin
- Burns or soot around the mouth and nose

Carbon monoxide from exhaust fumes or faulty heating appliances is the gas most likely to be inhaled accidentally. This can lead to serious illness, or even death. In most cases, victims of a fire will have inhaled smoke, which may include poisonous fumes given off by burning synthetic fabrics and wall coverings.

1 Do not put yourself in danger. Unless there is a fire, ventilate an enclosed space by opening any doors and windows before entering. If the victim is conscious, help him or her out of the contaminated area into fresh air.

➕ **DO NOT ENTER A CONFINED SPACE FILLED WITH GAS OR SMOKE WITHOUT PROPER SAFETY EQUIPMENT. WAIT FOR THE EMERGENCY SERVICES.**

2 Lift or drag an unconscious victim into the fresh air. Check the airway (see page 595) and begin CPR (cardiopulmonary resuscitation, see page 597) if necessary. Once breathing is regular, place the victim in the recovery position (see page 597).

3 If the victim is conscious, monitor pulse and breathing until the ambulance arrives. Treat any other injuries, such as burns.

➕ **SEND SOMEONE TO CALL AN AMBULANCE AS SOON AS POSSIBLE. MEDICAL ASSESSMENT IS VITAL, BECAUSE SERIOUS COMPLICATIONS CAN RESULT FROM THE INHALATION OF A TOXIC SUBSTANCE.**

Gunshot wounds

WHAT TO LOOK FOR:

- Pain
- Bleeding
- Entry and exit wounds
- Faintness
- Nausea
- Collapse
- Pale, cold and clammy skin
- Rapid breathing and a rapid, weak pulse

Bullet wounds can cause serious internal injuries and infection. Often there is only a small wound at the entry point, but a large exit wound with extensive tissue damage. If the bullet lodges inside the body, there may be only a small entry wound, but massive internal damage is likely.

➕ **CALL AN AMBULANCE IMMEDIATELY.**

1 Check the victim's response to simple instructions. If the victim fails to respond promptly, check the airway (see page 595) and give CPR (cardiopulmonary resuscitation, see page 597) if needed. Place an unconscious victim in the recovery position (page 597).

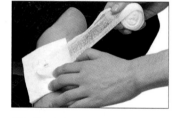

2 Check for entry and exit wounds and apply firm pressure to control any bleeding: if the wound is open and deep, use several large, sterile, bulky pads.

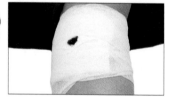

3 If there is a broken bone with the wound, avoid moving the injured part. Apply pressure on either side of the wound and build up padding around it. Hold the padding in position with a bandage that is applied in a criss-cross formation (see page 607).

Head injury

WHAT TO LOOK FOR:

- Headache
- Nausea or vomiting
- Blurred or double vision
- Numbness, tingling or loss of power in the limbs
- Total or partial loss of consciousness
- Loss of short-term memory
- Loss of hand-to-eye coordination
- Signs of weakness or paralysis down one side
- Unequal size of the pupils
- Noisy breathing, flushed face and a strong, slow pulse

✚ **ALL HEAD INJURIES – EVEN THOSE THAT APPEAR TO BE MINOR WITH NO ABNORMAL SYMPTOMS OR SIGNS – SHOULD BE CHECKED BY A DOCTOR BECAUSE OF THE RISK OF COMPLICATIONS.**

Any head injury is potentially serious and some are life-threatening. Seek prompt medical care. While waiting for an ambulance to arrive, observe the victim closely. This is essential to give early warning of any complications that might lead to permanent brain damage.

✚ **CALL FOR AN AMBULANCE AS SOON AS POSSIBLE. STAY WITH THE VICTIM UNTIL IT ARRIVES.**

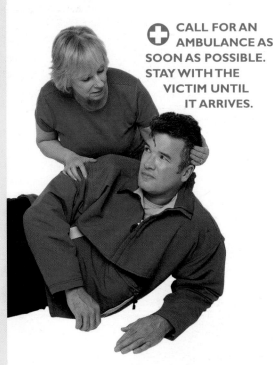

1 Check the victim's response to simple instructions such as, 'Squeeze my hand. Now let it go.' If the victim fails to respond promptly, check the airway and quickly place him or her into the recovery position (see page 597). Be prepared to give CPR (cardiopulmonary resuscitation, see page 597) if necessary.

2 If a victim who has been unconscious wakes up within a few minutes, maintain very close observation in case they lose consciousness again.

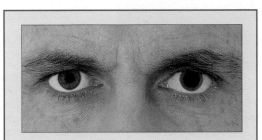

The pupils may be different sizes, with one more dilated or constricted than the other.

✚ **NOTE DOWN YOUR OBSERVATIONS OF THE VICTIM SINCE THE INCIDENT AND PASS THEM ON TO THE AMBULANCE CREW WHEN THEY ARRIVE.**

Ask the victim to hold the dressing in place to assess his coordination.

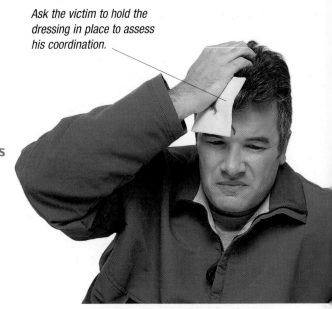

3 Help a conscious victim into a comfortable position and keep a close watch while treating any superficial injuries. Check for any warning signs of serious injury, including loss of short-term memory and poor hand-to-eye coordination.

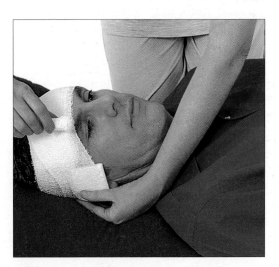

4 Check for head wounds. Control any bleeding by covering the wound with a sterile dressing and applying pressure with the palm of your hand. If any fluid is draining from one ear, apply a sterile pad secured with a roller bandage (see page 603). DO NOT pack the ear canal. Ask the victim to tilt the head towards the injured side.

5 Check the victim at frequent intervals and note any changes in his or her conscious state and coordination.

Heart attack

**WHAT TO
LOOK FOR:**

- Severe chest pain: this may be tight, crushing or vice-like; it may occur in the centre of the chest or around the chest; it may go up the jaw and down one arm (especially the left)
- Breathlessness
- Nausea
- Sudden giddiness or faintness
- Pale, greyish skin with a cold and clammy feel
- Rapid, weak pulse
- Shivering and anxiety
- Collapse

A heart attack is often due to a blood clot causing a blockage in one of the coronary arteries, which supplies blood to the heart muscle. If urgent medical treatment is obtained, the victim may make a full recovery.

➕ **HELP THE VICTIM TO TAKE ANY PRESCRIBED MEDICATION FOR CHEST PAIN. IF PAIN PERSISTS, GIVE ONE 300MG ASPIRIN TABLET.**

1 Help the victim into a position of rest, preferably sitting or half-reclining with the head and shoulders supported.

2 If collapse occurs, check that the airway is clear and open (see page 595). Be ready to give CPR (cardiopulmonary resuscitation, see page 597) if needed. Place the victim in the recovery position (see page 597).

Quickly place an unconscious victim in the recovery position.

➕ **CALL AN AMBULANCE AT ONCE AND STATE THAT THE VICTIM MAY HAVE HAD A HEART ATTACK.**

Help the victim to rest.

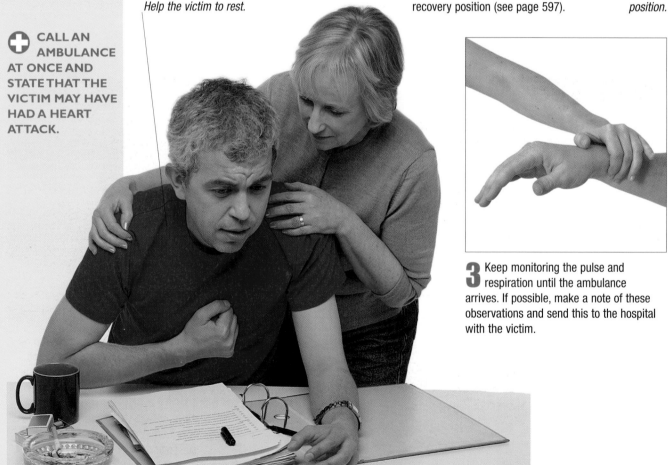

3 Keep monitoring the pulse and respiration until the ambulance arrives. If possible, make a note of these observations and send this to the hospital with the victim.

Heat exhaustion

WHAT TO LOOK FOR:

- Exhaustion and thirst
- Headache, nausea and dizzy spells
- Cramps
- Profuse sweating
- Cool, moist and pale skin
- A rapid and weak pulse
- Confusion

Heat exhaustion is the most common form of heat-related illness. It develops gradually as the body's heat-regulating mechanism is overloaded, resulting in excessive fluid and salt loss from the body through perspiration.

Raise both legs to improve the circulation.

1 Call for an ambulance as soon as possible. Then help the victim to lie down in a shaded place. Loosen any tight clothing at the neck and waist and raise both legs.

If there is no cool breeze, fan the victim.

2 If the victim is conscious, give him or her plenty of liquid to drink. Give water, sweet fluids or a weak salt solution of 1 teaspoon of salt dissolved in 1 litre (1¾ pints) of water.

➕ **SEEK URGENT MEDICAL ADVICE TO AVOID THE ONSET OF HEAT STROKE. NOTE ANY CHANGE IN THE VICTIM'S CONDITION AND RECORD ANY SIGNS OF DETERIORATION.**

3 If the victim becomes unconscious, check the airway is clear and open (see page 595) and be prepared to resuscitate if necessary (see page 597). Place the victim in the recovery position (see page 597).

Heat stroke

WHAT TO LOOK FOR:

- Headache and dizzy spells
- A high temperature with a red, hot and dry skin
- Restlessness and confusion
- A strong, bounding pulse
- Deteriorating level of response

Heat stroke is due to failure of the body's temperature control, resulting in dangerous overheating. Sweating – the body's natural cooling system – ceases, and the body temperature may rise to 40°C (104°F) or more. Heat stroke develops rapidly and requires prompt treatment by rapid cooling.

If the victim's temperature is over 38°C (100°F), cover him or her with a wet sheet, and fan them.

1 Move the victim to a cool place. Remove as much outer clothing as possible.

Help to cool the body by removing the victim's outer clothing.

2 If the victim is fully conscious, give frequent sips of cool water. Wrap the victim in a cold, wet sheet or towel, and keep it wet until the temperature falls to 38°C (100°F). The wet cloth can then be replaced with a dry one. Monitor until help arrives, and be prepared to restart active cooling if the person's temperature rises again.

➕ **CALL AN AMBULANCE IMMEDIATELY.**

3 If the victim becomes unconscious, check that the airway is clear (see page 595). Be ready to start CPR (cardiopulmonary resuscitation, see page 597) immediately. Place the victim in the recovery position (see page 597).

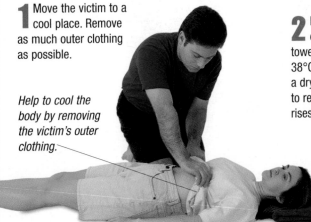

Hip and pelvis injury

WHAT TO LOOK FOR:

- An injured leg with the knee and foot turned outwards
- Severe pain at the site of injury
- Inability to walk
- Nausea, giddiness or faintness
- Paleness, with cold and clammy skin
- A swollen and bruised hip joint

Hip injuries occur most commonly in elderly people after a fall, particularly in women with osteoporosis. The area around the hip will be tender and swollen with blood which has leaked from damaged blood vessels. The victim needs very gentle handling with the minimum of movement to avoid further blood loss and the risk of severe shock.

2 Cover the victim lightly with a blanket to reduce heat loss. If they are lying on a cold or wet surface, gently slide a blanket or cloth under the head, body and uninjured leg, but DO NOT move the injured limb.

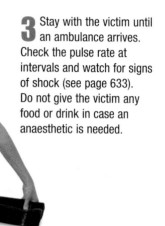

3 Stay with the victim until an ambulance arrives. Check the pulse rate at intervals and watch for signs of shock (see page 633). Do not give the victim any food or drink in case an anaesthetic is needed.

1 Reassure the victim that he or she will not be moved until an ambulance arrives. Try to provide some support for the injured limb by placing a folded blanket or rolled-up clothing gently alongside the leg. DO NOT raise the leg.

Place the support alongside the leg, to run from about mid-thigh to ankle.

✚ **CALL AN AMBULANCE AS SOON AS POSSIBLE.**

Hyperventilation

WHAT TO LOOK FOR:

- Unnaturally fast breathing
- Claw-like finger spasms or shaking
- A choking feeling or an inability to breathe properly
- Tightness in the chest
- Extreme fear and apprehension
- Screaming, shouting or crying
- Tingling and spasm in toes and fingers
- Dizziness, trembling or cramps

✚ **IF A VICTIM IS HAVING DIFFICULTY BREATHING, CALL AN AMBULANCE.**

Hyperventilation or overbreathing is usually due to fear, anxiety or panic. Breathing becomes extremely rapid, causing a temporary imbalance of oxygen and carbon dioxide in the body. Although the situation may appear to be serious, recovery is usually rapid once breathing stabilizes. It is important to remember that some serious medical conditions can cause similar rapid and shallow breathing. If symptoms persist, seek medical attention.

1 Stay calm and speak kindly but firmly. Remove the victim from any source of distress, and keep onlookers away. Reassure the victim that the symptoms will disappear once breathing returns to normal.

2 Encourage the victim to breathe more slowly by counting and deliberately setting a slower rate, telling the victim to breathe on your count. Continue this until breathing is slow and regular. DO NOT use a paper bag for rebreathing – this causes serious complications in some people.

✚ **DO NOT TRY TO RESTRAIN THE VICTIM. DO NOT SLAP THE VICTIM'S FACE OR THROW WATER OVER HIM OR HER.**

Count out loud with the victim.

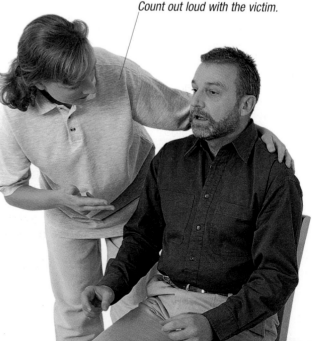

Hypothermia

WHAT TO LOOK FOR:

- Feeling very cold and shivery
- Numbness of the face, fingers and toes
- Apathy or confusion
- Lethargy
- Cold, dry skin
- Failing consciousness
- Slow, shallow breathing
- A slow pulse that becomes irregular

Hypothermia is a medical emergency that occurs when the body cannot produce enough heat to stay warm. If a victim of severe hypothermia is not given prompt first aid and medical care, the heart may cease to function normally and death can occur.

1 If indoors, an elderly victim should only be rewarmed gradually, using layers of blankets, as a sudden change in temperature can be dangerous. Give sips of warm (not hot) liquid, and high-energy foods such as chocolate. Put the victim to bed until help arrives.

A sleeping bag is ideal for raising the body temperature.

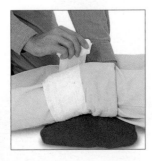

Give sips of warm liquid.

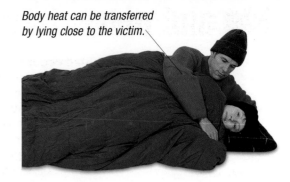

Body heat can be transferred by lying close to the victim.

2 If the victim is out in the open, find or improvise some shelter. If possible remove any wet clothing and cover the victim with dry clothes or blankets. If not, use extra clothing or blankets. Cover the victim's head and place fabric or newspapers underneath to insulate from cold ground. Lie beside the victim and use your own body heat to transfer warmth.

3 Move an unconscious victim into the recovery position (see page 597) and be prepared to start CPR (cardiopulmonary resuscitation, see page 597), if necessary.

✚ **CALL AN AMBULANCE AS SOON AS POSSIBLE.**

Leg and knee injury

WHAT TO LOOK FOR:

- A recent blow or twisting injury to the knee or leg
- Pain in and around the joint or injury site
- 'Locking' of the knee joint, or pain on trying to move or straighten the leg
- Swelling of the knee
- Deformity of the knee or limb
- An injured leg turned or rolled outwards
- Loss of power and function in the affected limb
- Nausea, vomiting or dizziness
- Pale, cold and clammy skin

Knees can be injured in many ways – road accidents, sports activities or a heavy fall at home or work. In such accidents the kneecap is often injured, and occasionally the hinge joint beneath is hurt as well.

Knee injury

1 Help the victim to lie down, steadying and supporting the injured limb. DO NOT attempt to straighten or bend the knee. Place padding or rolled-up clothing under the joint for support.

2 Hold the padding in place with a roller bandage (see page 603). Do not give the victim any food or drink in case an anaesthetic is needed to treat the injury. Call an ambulance or arrange transport to hospital.

Leg injury

1 Help the victim to lie down while supporting the injured limb. If it is positioned at an awkward angle, gently place the leg in the direction of the foot – stop if this causes pain. Place padding along the inside of the injured leg. Position the other leg alongside.

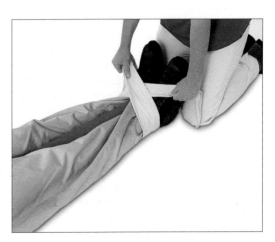

2 Slide bandages above and below the knees to splint the legs together, then bandage the ankles together using a criss-cross pattern. Maintain a firm pull until the knot is secure. If this adds to the pain, stop at once and support the limb as it lies.

Muscle injury

WHAT TO LOOK FOR:

- Pain at the injury site
- Swelling of the injured area
- Pressure beneath the skin
- Reduced function of the injured part
- Tissues that feel hard to the touch
- Bluish discoloration around the injury site

There are many muscles, tendons and ligaments in the leg, and these are easily damaged. Deep bleeding can fill the tissue spaces with blood and may be felt as a hard or cork-like sensation.

✚ **AFTER FIRST-AID TREATMENT, SEEK MEDICAL ADVICE TO AVOID LONG-TERM DISABILITY AND COMPLICATIONS.**

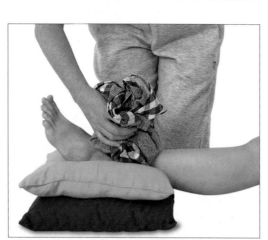

1 If the injury has only just occurred, first stop any further bleeding into the tissues by raising the limb on cushions or rolled-up clothing and applying an ice pack or cold compress (see page 605).

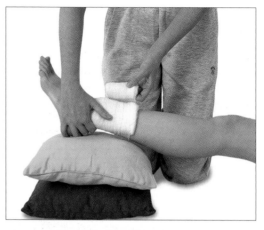

2 Apply firm pressure to the injured area with padding or bandages. This will help to reduce pain and swelling and to lessen later bruising. Advise the victim to rest the muscle and seek medical attention.

Nosebleed

WHAT TO LOOK FOR:

- Bleeding from the nose
- Blood trickling down the back of the throat
- Pain
- Difficulty breathing through the nose

There are many small blood vessels close to the surface in the nose which may be damaged by an impact or by sneezing, picking or blowing the nose. Nosebleeds are rarely serious.

2 Keep the nostrils pinched for at least 10 minutes to allow a firm clot to form. If bleeding continues when the pressure is removed, reapply the pressure for a further 10 minutes. If bleeeding still continues, seek urgent medical attention.

3 When the bleeding has stopped, give the victim a moist tissue to clean around the nose but not inside the nostrils. To avoid repeat nosebleeds, advise the victim not to take strenuous exercise and not to blow the nose for several hours.

1 Sit the victim down with the head tilted forwards. Ask him or her to pinch both nostrils together and breathe through the mouth. Do not plug the nose with a dressing or cotton wool.

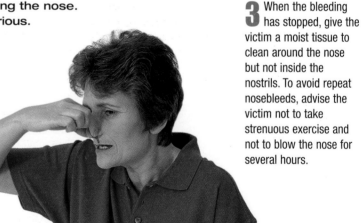

Nose injury or fracture

- Bleeding from the nose
- Clear nasal discharge
- Blood or fluid trickling down the back of the throat
- Pain
- Difficulty breathing through the nose
- Obvious deformity of the nose
- Swelling or bruising

If the skull is fractured after a head injury (see page 625), a bloodstained watery fluid may drain from the nose and be mistaken for a nosebleed. If this is a possibility, seek urgent medical advice.

2 Arrange for the victim to go to hospital for medical attention as soon as possible. Do not give the person any food or drink in case an anaesthetic is necessary.

1 Immediately apply a cold compress (see page 605) to the bridge of the nose to reduce swelling. If necessary, treat any nosebleed (below left).

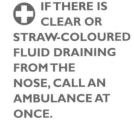

✚ **IF THERE IS CLEAR OR STRAW-COLOURED FLUID DRAINING FROM THE NOSE, CALL AN AMBULANCE AT ONCE.**

Ask the victim to hold a cold compress across the bridge of his or her nose.

Overdose

- Slurred speech
- Staggering or loss of coordination
- Dilation or constriction of the pupils of the eyes
- Vomiting
- Confusion or delirium
- Hallucinations
- Slow, shallow breathing
- Total or partial loss of consciousness

A drug overdose may be deliberate or accidental, and may involve prescription drugs, over-the-counter medicines, illegal street drugs or inhaled solvents such as glue or lighter fuel. The signs vary considerably, depending on what type of drug has been taken.

1 If the victim is unconscious or semi-conscious, check the airway (see page 595) and be prepared to start resuscitation (see page 596). Place the victim into the recovery position (see page 597).

2 If the victim is conscious, be prepared for angry or violent behaviour. Try to persuade the victim to go to hospital. Be ready to start resuscitation if there is a sudden deterioration in the victim's condition.

✚ **CALL FOR AN AMBULANCE AS SOON AS POSSIBLE. DO NOT LEAVE THE VICTIM UNTIL THE AMBULANCE ARRIVES.**

First check the victim's condition. If breathing, but unconscious or semi-conscious, place him or her in the recovery position.

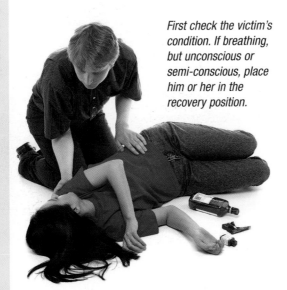

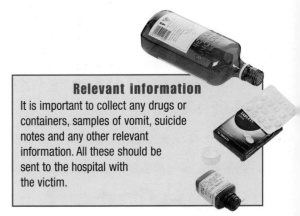

Relevant information

It is important to collect any drugs or containers, samples of vomit, suicide notes and any other relevant information. All these should be sent to the hospital with the victim.

Poison inhaled & swallowed

WHAT TO LOOK FOR:

POISON INHALED
- Breathing difficulty or breathing failure
- Listlessness, confusion or 'drunken' behaviour
- Abnormal colour, including pale, cherry-pink or bluish skin
- Area of redness, blisters or a rash
- Distress

POISON SWALLOWED
- A used container; berries
- Nausea
- Abdominal cramps
- Vomiting
- Seizures or convulsions
- Burns around the mouth and nose
- Drowsiness or loss of consciousness
- Confusion or hallucinations
- Diarrhoea

Emergency procedures

If a victim becomes unconscious after swallowing or inhaling poison, check the airway (see page 595) and be ready to begin CPR (cardiopulmonary resuscitation, see page 597). Place in the recovery position (see page 597) until help arrives.

Inhaled poisons

There are many substances around the home from which poisonous fumes can be inhaled accidentally. In a fire, smoke from burning plastics and synthetic furnishings is likely to contain toxic vapours. Carbon monoxide from faulty heating appliances can also cause severe poisoning.

If the victim is conscious, help them out of the contaminated area into fresh air. Drag an unconscious victim away by the feet or shoulders. Keep the victim under close observation outside until the ambulance arrives.

✚ **SEND SOMEONE TO CALL AN AMBULANCE AS SOON AS POSSIBLE.**

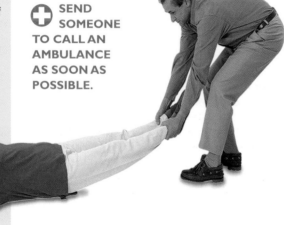

Swallowed poisons

Poison is most often taken by mouth, especially by young children. If a poison has been swallowed, do not give any food or fluid unless directed to do so, as this can cause complications.

✚ **DO NOT TRY TO INDUCE VOMITING. CALL AN AMBULANCE AT ONCE. SEND ANY SAMPLES OF POISON OR VOMIT TO THE HOSPITAL WITH THE VICTIM.**

1 If the victim is conscious, ask what type of poison has been taken, how much and how long ago. Look around for empty containers, or signs of berries or poisonous plants.

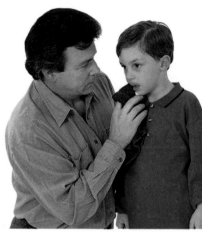

2 If there is any redness on the skin or signs of burning around the mouth or on the lips, wash the area thoroughly with plenty of cold water.

3 If the victim is unconscious, check the airway (see page 595). If necessary, begin CPR (cardiopulmonary resuscitation, see page 597) promptly. Avoid contamination by using a plastic face shield, if available. Place the victim in the recovery position (see page 597) until medical help arrives.

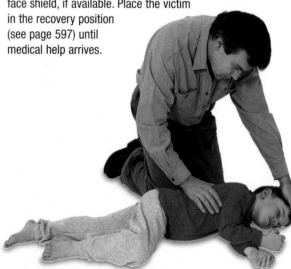

Avoiding accidents

- Keep dangerous substances out of sight and out of reach of children.
- Keep all medications in a locked medicine cabinet.
- Chemicals should be left in their original, correctly labelled containers and should never be mixed or transferred into food or soft drink containers that might be attractive to a child.
- Never mix cleaning products together. Store them in a locked cupboard or on a shelf that is inaccessible to children.
- Keep all medicines and household substances in childproof containers.
- Return out-of-date medicines or those no longer needed to a pharmacy so that they can be disposed of safely.

Severed limb

WHAT TO LOOK FOR:

- A limb or body part is severed
- Bleeding
- Shock

If a limb or digit is severed in an injury, there is a chance that surgery can rejoin the amputated part. However, for this to be successful, immediate care of both the stump and severed part is essential. Controlling the bleeding is the first priority in any emergency care.

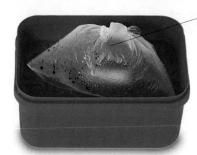

Blow into the plastic bag before tying, to create an air cushion for the severed part.

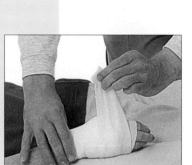

1 Lie the victim down and control bleeding by placing a clean pad over the stump and applying pressure. Do not use a tourniquet. Raise the injured part. When bleeding slows, secure the pad with a bandage, or apply a sterile dressing.

✚ **CALL AN AMBULANCE IMMEDIATELY. REMEMBER TO MENTION THAT AN AMPUTATION IS INVOLVED. SEND THE SEVERED PART TO HOSPITAL WITH THE VICTIM.**

2 Rescue the severed part – in this case, a thumb. Place it in a plastic bag, inflated and tied to create an air cushion. Alternatively, wrap the part in cling film surrounded by gauze or soft fabric. Place the wrapped part in a container filled with crushed ice, or cold water with added ice cubes. Do not allow ice to come into direct contact with the severed part.

3 Treat for shock if necessary. Reassure the victim until the ambulance arrives. If possible, label the container holding the severed part with the victim's name and the time of injury.

4 Check the victim's pulse rate every 10 minutes and note any changes to report to the ambulance staff. Do not give the victim any food or drink as it will probably be necessary to give him an anaesthetic.

Shock

WHAT TO LOOK FOR:

- Pale, cold and clammy skin
- Feeling weak, faint and giddy
- Nausea and vomiting
- Pain (depending on the problem)
- Rapid and shallow breathing
- Yawning or sighing ('air hunger')
- Weak, rapid pulse

Shock happens when the body's circulation system fails, endangering the blood supply to vital organs such as the heart and brain. It can occur after severe injury or illness, including heart attack, infection, allergy or blood loss. It is not the same as psychological shock. Without treatment the blood supply can weaken until the victim falls unconscious and may die.

1 Treat any obvious cause of shock, such as heavy bleeding. Lie the victim down on a blanket (to protect from the cold ground). Raise the legs high and keep the head low. Loosen any tight clothing at the neck, chest and waist.

Raise both the victim's legs to reduce shock.

✚ **CALL FOR AN AMBULANCE AS SOON AS POSSIBLE. AVOID GIVING ANY FOOD OR DRINK IN CASE AN ANAESTHETIC IS NEEDED TO TREAT THE UNDERLYING CONDITION.**

2 Keep the victim warm by covering with coats or blankets. Do not use direct heat, such as hot-water bottles.

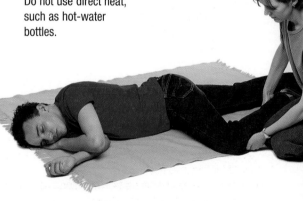

3 Keep checking pulse, breathing and level of response. Be prepared to resuscitate if necessary (see page 596). Turn an unconscious victim into the recovery position (see page 597).

Sprains and strains

**WHAT TO
LOOK FOR:**

SPRAINS
- Sudden pain in and around a joint
- Swelling, with some bruising later
- Nausea, giddiness or fainting
- Pain increased by movement or weight bearing
- Loss of power and function in the joint

STRAINS
- Sudden, sharp pain in the area
- Stiffness and swelling
- Cramp in the injured tissue

➕ **EXCEPT FOR MINOR INJURIES, SEEK MEDICAL ADVICE IN CASE A FRACTURE IS PRESENT.**

An easy way to remember

Treatment of sprains and strains involves the RICE procedure:

Rest the injured part.
Ice or a cold compress should be applied.
Compress the injury.
Elevate the injured part.

Sprains

A sprain occurs when a ligament – a tough band of fibrous tissue connecting bones at a joint – is suddenly overstretched. Provided the ligament has not been torn, gradual healing will occur. The most common places for a sprain are the ankle and wrist. However, as some sprains are associated with other injuries, it can be difficult to tell one from a fracture (broken bone). If in doubt, always seek medical advice.

Rest the injured limb on a soft support.

1 Help the victim into the most comfortable position possible. Avoid moving or touching the injured area more than necessary. Help the victim to steady and support the injured part on a pillow or other soft support. For a back strain, help the victim to lie down on the ground or a firm mattress.

2 Apply an ice pack or cold compress (see page 605) to the injured area to reduce pain, swelling and bruising.

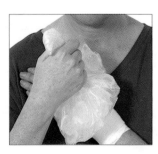

Strains

Strains happen when a muscle is stretched or overworked. They usually occur in the neck, lower back, thigh or calf as a result of a sudden jarring movement.

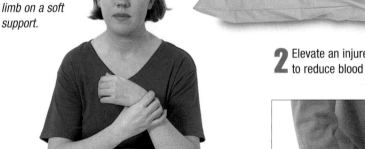

1 If possible, apply gentle pressure to the injured part, using soft padding secured with a bandage. This will also help to control swelling and pain.

2 Elevate an injured limb on a soft pillow or cushion to reduce blood flow and minimize bruising.

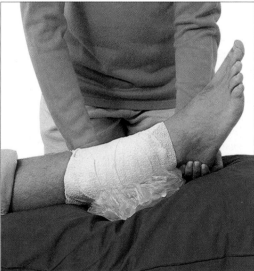

3 Place an ice pack around the bandaged area to bring further relief. Advise the victim to rest and to seek medical attention if symptoms do not improve within 4 to 5 hours.

Stroke

WHAT TO LOOK FOR:

- Weakness or numbness down one side of the body
- Severe headache
- Confusion – which may seem like drunkenness
- Loss of muscle tone in the face muscles
- An inability to speak coherently or slurred speech
- Saliva dribbling from the mouth
- Unequal pupil sizes
- Loss of bladder or bowel control
- Reducing level of consciousness, or unconsciousness

A stroke occurs when a blood vessel in the brain bursts or is blocked by a clot. A part of the brain is then starved of oxygen, resulting in paralysis down one side of the body and loss of the ability to speak. Similar symptoms, from which the victim makes a full recovery within a few minutes, may be a warning sign that someone is at risk of a full-blown stroke and should seek rapid medical advice.

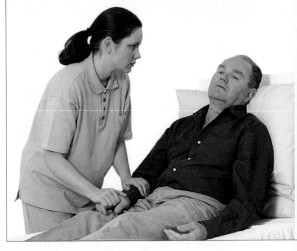

✚ **CALL AN AMBULANCE AT ONCE – TREATMENT WITHIN 2 HOURS MAY AVOID PERMANENT DISABILITY.**

1 If the victim is unconscious, check that the airway is clear (see page 595). Be ready to give CPR (cardiopulmonary resuscitation, see page 597). Turn the victim into the recovery position (see page 597) once breathing and pulse are established.

2 Sit or lie a conscious victim with the head and shoulders slightly raised. Loosen any tight clothing and tilt the head slightly to one side. Use a towel to absorb dribbling.

3 Keep checking pulse, breathing and response level. Reassure the victim that help is on its way. Avoid asking questions if the victim is having difficulty speaking.

4 Remember that the victim may still hear and understand you, even if he cannot respond. Do not give any food or drink because swallowing may be impaired.

Suffocation

WHAT TO LOOK FOR:

- Obvious threat to air supply
- Noisy or difficult breathing
- Blue or grey colour of lips and skin
- Unconsciousness
- Flaring of the nostrils
- Drawing in of the chest wall between the ribs and above the collarbones

Suffocation occurs when oxygen is prevented from entering the airways. It may result from a blockage such as choking (see page 614), smothering, a heavy weight crushing the chest or swelling of the throat. It can also occur when there is not enough oxygen in the air, for example, with fumes (see page 624).

1 Remove any obvious obstruction to breathing, for example, by clearing the airway (see page 595) or moving the victim into fresh air.

2 If the victim is unconscious, open the airway (see page 595). Check for breathing, and start CPR (cardiopulmonary resuscitation, see page 597) if necessary. Once the pulse and breathing are established, place the victim in the recovery position (see page 597).

✚ **CALL AN AMBULANCE IMMEDIATELY IF A VICTIM HAS BEEN UNCONSCIOUS.**

3 If the victim is conscious, check pulse and breathing regularly and call a doctor – even if the victim appears to be fully recovered.

Sunburn

WHAT TO LOOK FOR:

- Pain
- Heat in the burned area
- Redness or tightness of the skin
- Blistered skin
- Skin tender to the touch

Direct exposure to the sun in the middle of the day can cause sunburn after only 20 minutes. Although sunscreen will protect the skin for a short time, it should always be reapplied after swimming. Young children in particular may receive serious and painful burns unless they are closely supervised.

1 Cover the burnt area with loose fabric while helping the victim into a cool or shaded place, preferably indoors. Cool the skin by sponging or soaking in cold water for 10 minutes. Help the victim to change into loose clothes, and to rest without putting pressure on the sunburned area. Encourage the person to take frequent sips of cool water.

2 Apply an after-sun cream, calamine lotion or anaesthetic spray to the painful areas to soothe the skin. If in doubt, seek the advice of a pharmacist.

✚ WHEN THE VICTIM IS UNDER FIVE YEARS OF AGE, OR IS ELDERLY, SEEK PROMPT MEDICAL ADVICE IF HEADACHE, A RAISED TEMPERATURE OR RESTLESSNESS DEVELOP.

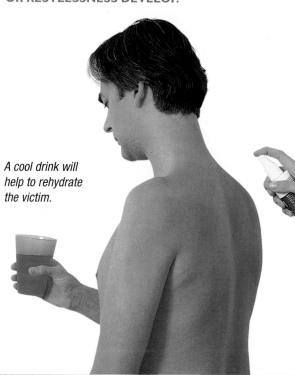

A cool drink will help to rehydrate the victim.

Tooth injury

WHAT TO LOOK FOR:

- Pain
- Bleeding inside the mouth
- Missing or broken tooth
- Irregularity of other teeth

If an adult tooth is chipped or fractured, prompt dental care can often restore or save it. If a tooth is knocked out of the gum, it may be possible to reimplant it successfully. Do not wash the tooth or try to wipe it clean as this can destroy the membrane around its base. Do not try to replace a child's milk tooth.

✚ CONTACT A DENTIST TO ARRANGE AN IMMEDIATE APPOINTMENT.

Ask the victim to bite on a pad held over the replaced tooth, to keep it in place.

1 Help the victim to sit or lie down comfortably with the head tilted forward and towards the injured side. If a tooth has been knocked out, find it and attempt to replace it in the socket as soon as possible.

2 Hold the tooth firmly and carefully position it into the socket. Wrap a gauze pad over the tooth and ask the victim to keep this in place by gripping between upper and lower teeth. Ensure that the victim seeks immediate advice from a dentist or hospital.

3 If the tooth cannot be replaced because of pain or extensive injury, ask the victim to hold it in the mouth, or place it in milk or water, to keep the roots moist until dental care is available. If there is any bleeding, make a firm pad from a rolled tissue or sterile dressing and place it over the socket. Ask the victim to bite firmly on the pad for at least 10 minutes to allow a clot to form.

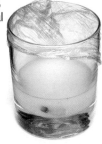

Winding

- Difficulty breathing
- Nausea or vomiting
- Abdominal pain
- Inability to speak

✚ **CALL AN
AMBULANCE
AS SOON AS
POSSIBLE AND
STAY WITH THE
VICTIM UNTIL IT
ARRIVES.**

A blow to the upper part of the abdomen can temporarily affect the solar plexus (a cluster of nerve fibres at the back of the abdominal cavity). Although painful and frightening, the effects of winding pass off quickly. But the victim may feel bruised for a few days.

1 As soon as the victim can move, help him or her into the most comfortable position possible. This is often sitting down or leaning on a table. Loosen clothing at the chest and waist. Keep reassuring the person that the spasm will pass and breathing will become easier. DO NOT attempt to rub the abdomen or 'pump' the legs.

2 Do not give any food or drink to the victim until he or she is fully recovered, or has been assessed by a doctor in case of internal injuries.

3 If the victim becomes unconscious, gently turn him or her onto the side and into the recovery position (see page 597). Clear and open the airway (see page 595). Give CPR (cardiopulmonary resuscitation, see page 597) if necessary.

✚ **ADVISE THE
VICTIM TO
SEEK MEDICAL
ADVICE TO MAKE
SURE THAT
NO LASTING
INTERNAL INJURY
HAS OCCURRED.**

Wrist injury

- Pain around the wrist
- Obvious deformity of the wrist
- Swelling or bruising
- Difficulty in moving the wrist or hand normally
- Fingertips turning blue
- Inability to feel the ends of the fingers

Injuries to the wrist occur frequently, especially after a fall onto an outstretched hand. Sprains of the wrist are common, and it can be hard to distinguish a sprain from a broken bone. A fracture of one of the tiny wrist bones, the scaphoid, may go undetected at first, leading to problems later on.

1 Ask the victim to sit down and gently support the arm and wrist on the injured side. If necessary, treat any open wound.

Rest the injured arm on a soft support such as a cushion.

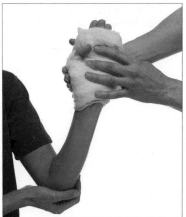

2 Arrange clean, soft padding around the injured area. Place a triangular bandage between the arm and the chest, and tie it up into a sling to support the arm (see page 604).

3 Keep the victim sitting down and arrange transport to hospital.

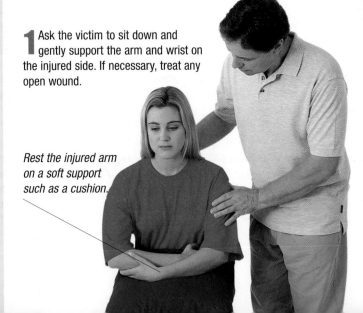

Drugs and their uses

The glossary below lists the main generic drugs and the brand names by which they are most commonly known.

This alphabetical listing includes both branded and generic drugs. Some of them can be bought over the counter; others are only available on prescription. It also explains a number of common pharmacological terms such as 'antibiotic', 'chemotherapy', 'hormone replacement therapy' and 'painkiller'. Words in capital letters indicate cross-references to these general entries.

Where a brand name is given for a drug, it will give the generic name or names for any active ingredient in that drug. Under Actifed, for example, you will see that the active generic drugs contained in this medicine are triprolidine and pseudoephedrine. These each have their own entries in the glossary, informing you that triprolidine is used to treat allergic symptoms such as hay fever and urticaria; and pseudoephedrine is used to relieve general congestion in the airways.

A

ACARBOSE, used to treat non-insulin-dependent diabetes.

ACECLOFENAC, a PAINKILLER used to treat inflammation and pain, particularly that caused by arthritic conditions. It is an NSAID.

ACE INHIBITOR (angiotensin-converting enzyme inhibitor) drugs, used as ANTIHYPERTENSIVE agents and in the treatment of heart failure.

They are widely prescribed, sometimes on their own but often with other medicines such as DIURETIC drugs (for hypertension) or digoxin (for heart failure). They are taken by mouth either as tablets or capsules.

These drugs include captopril and enalapril. They work in a complex way to make the blood vessels dilate. This expansion of the vessels causes blood pressure to fall, which is beneficial to people who suffer from heart failure or hypertension. Some people cannot safely take ace inhibitors: these include those with certain blood vessel conditions and pregnant women. Usually, ace inhibitors have few side effects but they may cause a severe fall in blood pressure, and some people get a persistent cough.

ACICLOVIR, used to treat viral infections such as cold sores that have been caused by the herpes virus.

ACTAL, brand containing alexitol.

ACTIFED, brand containing triprolidine and pseudoephedrine.

ADALAT LA, brand name for nifedipine.

ADVIL, brand of ibuprofen.

ALENDRONIC ACID, used to prevent and treat osteoporosis.

ALEXITOL, an ANTACID.

ALFACALCIDOL, used to treat vitamin D deficiency.

ALFUZOSIN, used to treat urinary retention in men who have benign prostatic hypertrophy.

ALGINIC ACID, a sticky substance added to soothing mouthwashes and indigestion preparations.

ALLOPURINOL, used to prevent attacks of gout.

ALUMINIUM HYDROXIDE, an ANTACID.

ALVERINE, used to relax intestinal muscles and so relieve the pain of irritable bowel syndrome and diverticular disease. It is also used for period pain.

AMILORIDE, a DIURETIC.

AMINOPHYLLINE, used in ASTHMA TREATMENT.

AMIODARONE, used to treat arrhythmias of the heart.

AMITRIPTYLINE, an ANTIDEPRESSANT.

AMLODIPINE, used as an ANTIHYPERTENSIVE and to treat angina. It is a CALCIUM-CHANNEL BLOCKER.

AMOXICILLIN, an ANTIBIOTIC used to treat bacterial infections.

AMPHOTERICIN B, an ANTIBIOTIC used to treat fungal infections.

ANASTROZOLE, used in cancer CHEMOTHERAPY.

ANBESOL, brand containing lignocaine and cetylpyridium.

ANTACID drugs, chemicals that are used to treat indigestion. They work by neutralizing hydrochloric acid in the stomach. This acid, also called gastric acid, is produced by the stomach when food is being digested. However, sometimes too much hydrochloric acid is produced causing stomach pain and other indigestion symptoms. Indigestion is made worse by alcohol and drugs such as aspirin.

Antacids are taken by mouth, and are available over the counter. They can be used for occasional stomach upsets and also heartburn symptoms such as reflux oesophagitis – common in people with hiatus hernia and in pregnant women. Antacids can also relieve the symptoms of peptic ulcers, but ulcers are best treated with prescription ULCER-HEALING DRUGS.

Antacids have side effects. Sodium bicarbonate and calcium carbonate can cause belching and flatulence; aluminium hydroxide can cause constipation; and

magnesium carbonate, magnesium hydroxide and magnesium trisilicate can cause diarrhoea. Some antacids contain a lot of sodium and should not be taken by people who are on a sodium-restricted diet.

ANTIBIOTIC drugs, used to treat infections. Technically speaking, in medical circles, the term 'antibiotic' is restricted to drugs that are made by fungi and used for treating infections. Most antibiotics are used to treat infections caused by bacteria, but some treat infections caused by fungi. It is important to note that no antibiotic is effective against a viral infection so they will not treat a cold or flu.

Antibiotics make up a major proportion of the annual NHS drugs bill. The most-prescribed antibiotics are: amoxicillin, amphotericin, cefaclor, cefadroxil, cefalexin, cefradine, chloramphenicol, clarithromycin, doxycycline, erythromycin, flucloxacillin, fusidic acid, lymecycline, minocycline, mupirocin, neomycin, nystatin, oxytetracycline, phenoxymethylpenicillin and tetracycline.

The majority of antibiotics have few side effects, although some people are allergic to certain ones, such as cephalosporins and penicillins. It is important to tell anyone giving you medication – including your dentist – if you are allergic to any of these.

There is currently a growing problem in treating certain infections because overprescribing has led to the evolution of bacteria that are resistant to a number of common antibiotics.

ANTICOAGULANT drugs, sometimes called blood-thinners because they prevent blood clotting. They are used to stop clots forming in blood vessels and to treat clots that have already formed. Because of this, they are used to treat conditions such as thrombosis and embolism, especially following surgery to prevent deep vein thrombosis.

Many anticoagulants are versions of the blood's own natural anticoagulant, heparin. These must be injected and last for only a short time, so are mainly used in hospitals. Others, including warfarin, can be taken by mouth, and work for longer, so their use is not restricted to hospitals. It is important to get the right dose for each individual, so anyone taking warfarin will need frequent blood tests.

ANTIDEPRESSANT drugs, used to relieve the symptoms of depression. The most recently developed and best-known group includes fluoxetine (Prozac), sertraline (Lustal), paroxetine (Seroxat) and citalopram (Cipramil). These drugs are referred to as selective serotonin reuptake inhibitors (SSRIs). Although they can cause side effects – nausea and stomach upsets are quite common – most people cope well with them.

Other antidepressants include tricyclics such as imipramine, but these have pronounced side effects including sleepiness, sweating, blurred vision and dry mouth.

Monoamine oxidase inhibitors (MAOIs) are not often prescribed now because they can have harmful interactions with constituents of food such as cheese, red wine and yeast extracts, causing a dangerous rise in blood pressure.

The herbal depression remedy St John's Wort should not be taken at the same time as antidepressants prescribed by your doctor because of the risk of serious interactions.

ANTIHISTAMINE drugs, used to treat allergic reactions. When people come into contact with a substance to which they are allergic, a chemical called histamine is released in the body. This causes allergic symptoms such as hay fever, urticaria, the itching of insect bites or stings, and wheezing. Antihistamines prevent histamine causing these effects. They can be taken by mouth, as a nasal spray, or applied to the skin as a cream. Certain antihistamines cause pronounced drowsiness and this can make it unsafe to drive when taking them. Some, such as promethazine, cause so much sedation that they are sold as over-the-counter SLEEP-AID medicines. More modern drugs, such as cetirizine, have a less sedative effect.

ANTIHYPERTENSIVE drugs, used to reduce high blood pressure, and so reduce a person's risk of heart attack, kidney failure and stroke. Several types of drug can be used and they are usually taken by mouth as tablets or capsules. They lower blood pressure either by reducing blood volume or by dilating blood vessels. Often a mild DIURETIC is all that is needed, but other drugs may also be prescribed.

Drugs that might be prescribed include CALCIUM-CHANNEL BLOCKERS such as nifedipine and verapamil; BETA-BLOCKERS such as acebutolol, atenolol, propranolol and timolol; and ACE INHIBITORS such as captopril and enalapril. Side effects depend on the particular antihypertensive drug you are taking. Some may cause dizziness at the start of treatment; beta-blockers can disrupt sleeping patterns and make your hands and feet feel cold; and ACE INHIBITORS can cause an irritating cough.

ANTIPLATELET drugs, used to reduce the stickiness of blood platelets, an important component of blood clots. They can help to prevent clots from forming in the arteries. Dipyridamole and low-dose aspirin are taken as a preventive measure by people who are at risk from blood clots, such as after a heart attack or stroke, or following bypass operations. If you have had a stroke or a heart attack, it may be necessary for you to take antiplatelet drugs for the rest of your life.

ANTIPSYCHOTIC drugs, used to treat schizophrenia and other severe psychiatric disorders. They control symptoms such as hallucinations and disturbed thoughts.

There are many antipsychotic drugs including chlorpromazine, haloperidol, flupentixol, thioridazine, prochlorperazine, sulpiride, olanzapine and risperidone. They work mainly by blocking the action of the neurotransmitter dopamine in the brain. However, this means that they have many unpleasant side effects and sometimes serious adverse effects. Because of this, they are only prescribed by specialists. Antipsychotic drugs, which are administered as long-lasting injection or taken by mouth under supervision, have allowed many people suffering from psychoses to rejoin the community rather than live in institutions.

ANXIETY TREATMENT drugs, used to relieve symptoms of anxiety. They are prescribed for people who do not respond to other therapies such as relaxation or psychotherapy. They are also used for short-term anxiety, such as experienced before surgery or job interviews. The best-known and most widely used are the BENZODIAZEPINE drugs, which include diazepam and lorazepam; and BETA-BLOCKERS, which are good for easing symptoms such as palpitations of the heart, sweating and tremors. Many of these drugs are addictive, so treatment should be carefully monitored and should not be prolonged.

ARTHROTEC, brand of diclofenac.
ASCORBIC ACID, the chemical name for vitamin C. This is sometimes taken in high dosages as an antioxidant and free-radical scavenger. It can also be used to prevent and treat scurvy.

ASPIRIN, used as a PAINKILLER, and to reduce raised body temperature and inflammation such as in arthritis. It is a non-steroidal anti-inflammatory drug (NSAID). Low doses of aspirin may be taken as an ANTIPLATELET drug. Breastfeeding mothers and young children should not usually take aspirin.

ASPRO CLEAR, brand of aspirin.
ASTHMA TREATMENT drugs, used to relieve the symptoms of bronchial asthma or to prevent recurrent attacks. They are also used with other conditions that cause breathing difficulties, sometimes referred to as obstructive airways diseases. In an acute asthma attack, the air passages narrow and become blocked, and drugs called bronchodilators are taken to widen the airways and improve the passage of air. Most are inhaled so that they work quickly and where they are needed – in the lungs – and side effects in the body are minimized. Salbutamol and terbutaline are bronchodilators.

CORTICOSTEROID drugs used to prevent asthma attacks include beclometasone and budenoside. These can be inhaled or taken by mouth.

Anti-inflammatories such as sodium cromoglicate and nedocromil may also be used to treat asthma. Much research has been done to design devices that will deliver the inhaled droplets or particles of drugs into the airways more efficiently, allowing the drug to reach the narrow bronchioles.

ATENOLOL, used as an ANTIHYPERTENSIVE, prescribed for cases of angina and heart arrhythmia.

ATORVASTATIN, a LIPID-REGULATING DRUG.

ATROVENT, a branded asthma drug containing ipratropium.

AZATHIOPRINE, used to reduce tissue rejection in people who have had organ transplants, and to treat autoimmune diseases such as myasthenia gravis and rheumatoid arthritis.

B

BACLOFEN, used to relax muscles that are in spasm, as is sometimes experienced by people with multiple sclerosis.

BAZUKA, brand of salicylic acid.

BECLOFORTE, brand of asthma medication, beclomethasone.

BECLOMETHASONE A, used in asthma treatment and to treat inflammatory conditions of the nose and the skin such as psoriasis and eczema. It is a CORTICOSTEROID.

BECOTIDE, brand of beclomethasone asthma inhaler.

BENDROFLUMETHIAZIDE, a DIURETIC.

BENSERAZIDE, used together with the drug levodopa in treating PARKINSON'S DISEASE.

BENZHEXOL, used to treat PARKINSON'S DISEASE.

BENZOCAINE, a local anaesthetic used on the skin and mouth to relieve pain.

BENZODIAZEPINES, drugs used for many purposes. Diazepam, temazepam, lormetazepam and lorazepam are used as sedatives in ANXIETY TREATMENT. Nitrazepam oxazepam, temazepam and lormetazepam are prescribed as sleeping pills. Benzodiazepines are also used to treat epilepsy and as muscle relaxants. These drugs are quickly addictive so they should only be taken for short periods.

BENZOYL PEROXIDE, used to treat acne and other skin infections such as athlete's foot.

BENZYDAMINE, applied to the skin and mouth as pain relief.

BETA-BLOCKER drugs, used as ANTIHYPERTENSIVES, in MIGRAINE TREATMENT, in angina treatment, ANXIETY TREATMENT, and to treat glaucoma and heart arrhythmias. They are usually taken as tablets, except in glaucoma treatment when eyedrops are used. Those most frequently prescribed are atenolol, betaxolol, carteolol, celiprolol, levobunolol, metoprolol, nebivolol, propranolol, sotalol and timolol.

BETAHISTINE, used to treat Ménière's disease of the ear.

BETAMETHASONE, a CORTICOSTEROID used to treat inflammation.

BETAXOLOL, used as an ANTIHYPERTENSIVE for high blood pressure and to treat glaucoma. It is a BETA-BLOCKER.

BEZAFIBRATE, a LIPID-REGULATING DRUG.

BISACODYL, a laxative.

BISOPROLOL, an ANTIHYPERTENSIVE, also used to treat angina.

BRICANYL, brand of terbutaline.

BRIMONIDINE, used to treat glaucoma.

BROMPHENIRAMINE, used to relieve allergic symptoms such as hay fever and urticaria. It can also be used as a cough medicine. It is an ANTIHISTAMINE.

BUCLIZINE, used to prevent vomiting in MIGRAINE TREATMENT.

BUDESONIDE, used in ASTHMA TREATMENT and other inflammatory conditions such as rhinitis. It is a CORTICOSTEROID.

BUMETANIDE, a DIURETIC.

BUPRENORPHINE, a strong PAINKILLER used to treat moderate to severe pain, such as after surgical procedures.

BUPROPION, used to help people stop smoking.

C

CAFFEINE, a stimulant. It is added to some PAINKILLERS to increase their effect.

CALAMINE, incorporated into some lotions used to soothe itchy skin conditions such as eczema.

CALCIPOTRIOL, used to treat plaque psoriasis.

CALCIUM CARBONATE, an ANTACID. It is also prescribed for high levels of phosphate in the blood.

CALCIUM-CHANNEL BLOCKER drugs, mainly used as ANTIHYPERTENSIVE agents. They work by relaxing blood vessels allowing blood pressure to fall. They are also used in angina treatment, to correct heartbeat irregularities (arrhythmias), to limit brain damage after bleeding in strokes, for treating Raynaud's disease, and after heart attacks. Commonly prescribed calcium-channel blockers include amlodipine, lacidipine, lercanidipine, nifedipine and verapamil.

CALPOL, brand of paracetamol.

CANDESARTAN CILEXETIL, an ANTIHYPERTENSIVE.

CANESTEN, brand containing clotrimazole.

CANESTEN HC, brand containing clotrimazole and hydrocortisone.

CAPSAICIN, rubbed into the skin to relieve pain in underlying muscles and joints.

CAPTOPRIL, an ACE INHIBITOR used as an ANTIHYPERTENSIVE to treat heart failure and in diabetic neuropathy – a complication of diabetes mellitus.

CARBAMAZEPINE, used in EPILEPSY TREATMENT, to relieve the pain of trigeminal neuralgia, in manic depressive illness (bipolar disorder), and in diabetes insipidus and diabetic neuropathy (a complication of diabetes mellitus).

CARBIMAZOLE, used to treat the symptoms of thyrotoxicosis, a condition in which there are excess thyroid hormones in the blood.

CARBOMER, used in artificial tears for dry eyes caused as a result of disease.

CARDURA, brand of doxazosin.

CARTEOLOL, used to treat glaucoma. It is a BETA-BLOCKER.

CEFACLOR, an ANTIBIOTIC used to treat bacterial infections.

CEFADROXIL, an ANTIBIOTIC used to treat bacterial infections.

CEFALEXIN, an ANTIBIOTIC used to treat bacterial infections.

CEFRADINE, an ANTIBIOTIC used to treat bacterial infections.

CELECOXIB, a PAINKILLER used to reduce pain and inflammation in arthritis. It is an NSAID.

CELIPROLOL, used as an ANTIHYPERTENSIVE. It is a BETA-BLOCKER.

CERIVASTATIN, a LIPID-REGULATING DRUG.

CETIRIZINE, used for hay fever and urticaria. It is an ANTIHISTAMINE.

CETYLPYRIDIUM, a skin and mouth antiseptic.

CHEMOTHERAPY, commonly used to mean drug treatment of cancer; the drugs used are also called anticancer drugs. Most anticancer drugs are chemicals that are cytotoxic, meaning that they are poisonous to cancerous cells. They work by preventing new cancerous tissue from growing. Inevitably, this means that production of normal body cells is also affected, which is why there are side effects, some serious. Common side effects of anticancer drugs include nausea, vomiting, temporary hair loss and bone-marrow suppression. Cytotoxic drugs are administered in low doses over a set period. They are often given with other drugs designed to lessen the adverse effects – such as drugs to stop nausea and vomiting – and sometimes in combination with radiotherapy. Treatment is often carried out in hospital. Certain cancers, including some childhood leukaemias, can now be treated successfully and permanently.

Some newer drugs work against cancers that in the past could not be treated. However, these can be very expensive. Taxanes such as paclitaxel and docetaxel are examples; they are used against ovarian and breast cancer. Other drugs used to treat, or even prevent, cancer in people at risk include tamoxifen for breast cancer and OESTROGENS for prostate cancer.

CHLORAMPHENICOL, an ANTIBIOTIC used to treat bacterial infections.

CHLORDIAZEPOXIDE, used in ANXIETY TREATMENT. It is also used to treat acute withdrawal symptoms experienced by alcoholics who are giving up drinking. It is a BENZODIAZEPINE.

CHLORHEXIDINE, used as an antiseptic – for example, as a mouthwash – and as a disinfectant.

CHLORPHENAMINE, used for hay fever and urticaria. It is an ANTIHISTAMINE.

CHLORPROMAZINE, an ANTIPSYCHOTIC drug used to treat schizophrenia. It can also be used to treat anxiety and prevent vomiting.

CHOLINE SALICYLATE, used to relieve pain such as teething pain. Rubbed into the skin, it eases pain in underlying muscles and joints.

CICLOSPORIN, used after organ transplants to stop tissue rejection. It is also used for some other conditions including rheumatoid arthritis and severe dermatitis.

CILEST, brand of contraceptive pill that contains the hormones ethinylestradiol and norgestimate.

CIMETIDINE, an ULCER-HEALING DRUG.

CINNARIZINE, used to prevent vomiting and in the treatment of Raynaud's syndrome.

CIPRAMIL, brand of citalopram.

CIPROFIBRATE, a LIPID-REGULATING DRUG.

CIPROFLOXACIN, an ANTIBIOTIC used to treat bacterial infections.

CITALOPRAM, an ANTIDEPRESSANT.

CITRIC ACID, incorporated into drug preparations including cough-and-cold remedies and laxatives.

CLARITHROMYCIN, an ANTIBIOTIC used to treat bacterial infections.

CLARITYN, branded loratadine.

CLINDAMYCIN, an ANTIBIOTIC used to treat bacterial infections.

CLOBAZAM, a BENZODIAZEPINE used in ANXIETY TREATMENT. It is sometimes used, along with other drugs, in EPILEPSY TREATMENT.

CLOBETASOL, a powerful CORTICOSTEROID drug used to treat severe skin inflammation such as in eczema and psoriasis.

CLONAZEPAM, used in EPILEPSY TREATMENT. It is a BENZODIAZEPINE.

CLONIDINE, mainly used as an ANTIHYPERTENSIVE and in MIGRAINE TREATMENT.

CLOPIDOGREL, used as an ANTIPLATELET drug.

CLORAL BETAINE, a SLEEP-AID drug.

CLOTRIMAZOLE, used to treat fungal infections of the skin.

COAL TAR, used to treat psoriasis and eczema and other skin and scalp conditions such as dandruff.

CO-AMILOFRUSE, the name given to the combined DIURETICS amiloride and frusemide.

CO-AMILOZIDE, the name given to a combination of the DIURETICS amiloride and hydchlorothiazide.

CO-AMOXICLAV, the name given to a combination of the ANTIBIOTIC amoxicillin, and clavulanic acid. It is used for bacterial infections.

CO-BENELDOPA, the name given to a combination of benserazide and levodopa. It is used in PARKINSON'S DISEASE treatment.

CO-CARELDOPA, a combination of carbidopa and levodopa. It is used in treating PARKINSON'S DISEASE.

CO-CODAMOL, a combination of two PAINKILLERS, codeine and paracetamol.

CO-CYPRINDIOL, the name given to a combination of cyproterone and ethinylestradiol, which is used to treat severe acne.

CO-DANTHRUSATE, the name given to the combined laxatives dantron and docusate sodium.

CODEINE, a PAINKILLER. Also used to treat a dry cough and diarrhoea.

CODIS 500, brand containing aspirin and codeine.

CO-DYDRAMOL, the name for a combination of two PAINKILLERS, dihydrocodeine and paracetamol.

CO-FLUAMPICIL, a combination of the ANTIBIOTICS flucloxacillin and ampicillin.

COLCHICINE, used to treat gout.

CO-MAGALDROX, a combination of the ANTACIDS magnesium and aluminium hydroxide.

COMBIVENT, brand containing ipratropium and salbutamol.

CONJUGATED OESTROGEN, an OESTROGEN used in HORMONE REPLACEMENT THERAPY.

CO-PHENOTROPE, the name given to a combination of diphenoxylate and atropine used to treat diarrhoea.

CO-PROXAMOL is the name given to a combination of the two PAINKILLERS dextropropoxyphene and paracetamol.

CORTICOSTEROID drugs, often just called steroids, used on a wide scale to treat many inflammatory and allergic reactions of the skin, airways and elsewhere. They resemble the steroid hormones naturally secreted by the adrenal glands, so some are used to make up for the shortage of hormones in Addison's disease. Commonly prescribed corticosteroids include hydrocortisone, beclomethasone, betamethasone, clobetasol, dexamethasone, fludrocortisone, flumethasone, fluticasone, methylprednisolone, prednisolone and triamcinolone.

The way in which corticosteroids are taken depends on what they are treating. However, because they can cause serious side effects, they are ideally administered close to where they need to act as this reduces potential problems. Many are used in ointments or creams such as for

eczema and psoriasis. Others are inhaled as in ASTHMA TREATMENT and for other lung conditions. Nasal sprays are prescribed for rhinitis, and injections are given into the joints for conditions such as tennis elbow. A weak formulation will usually be tried first, progressing to stronger ones only if necessary. The likely side effects of taking a high-dose or potent corticosteroid over a period of time include frequent infections, water retention, weight gain and a moon-shaped face. When it is time to stop taking high-dose corticosteroid, the dose must be reduced gradually over time. Your doctor will give you a medical alert card explaining this. It should be carried with you at all times.

CO-TENIDONE, a combination of the BETA-BLOCKER atenolol and the DIURETIC chlortalidone. It is used as an ANTIHYPERTENSIVE.

CO-TRIAMTERZIDE, a combination of two DIURETICS, triamterene and hydchlorothiazide.

COVERSYL, brand of perindopril.

COZAAR, brand of losartan.

D

DAKTACORT, brand containing hydrocortisone and miconazole.

DEPO-PROVERA, brand of medroxyprogesterone.

DESLORATADINE, used to treat allergies such as hay fever and urticaria. It is an ANTIHISTAMINE.

DESMOPRESSIN, used to treat diabetes insipidus. It is also used to stop bedwetting.

DEXAMETHASONE, used to treat inflammation. It is a CORTICOSTEROID.

DEXTROMETHORPHAN, used to relieve dry coughs.

DIABETES TREATMENT, of two types. The treatment of Type 1 diabetes – known also as insulin-dependent diabetes mellitus and juvenile-onset diabetes – involves regular injections of insulin. This is because in this type of diabetes the pancreas does not secrete enough of the hormone insulin for the body's needs.

The treatment of Type 2 diabetes – non-insulin-dependent diabetes mellitus or maturity-onset diabetes – involves taking oral hypoglycaemic drugs by mouth. These help the body to store sugar. This treatment is used when the pancreas is still able to produce some insulin. The main oral hypoglycaemics used are glibenclamide, gliclazide, glimepiride, glipizide, tolbutamide and metformin. Researchers are looking for new drugs that work in different ways and suit different people.

DIAMORPHINE, also known as heroin. It is a powerful PAINKILLER used to treat severe pain. It is also given to very ill patients with severe and painful coughing.

DIANETTE, brand of co-cyprindiol.

DIAZEPAM, used as in ANXIETY TREATMENT, in EPILEPSY TREATMENT, and as a SLEEP-AID. It is a BENZODIAZEPINE.

DICLOFENAC, a PAINKILLER, also used to treat inflammation. It is an NSAID.

DICYCLOVERINE, used to relieve painful spasms of the gastro-intestinal tract.

DIDRONEL, brand containing disodium etidronate.

DIETHYLAMINE SALICYLATE, rubbed into the skin to relieve pain in underlying muscles and joints.

DIGOXIN, used to treat heart failure and heart arrhythmias.

DIHYDROCODEINE, a PAINKILLER.

DILTIAZEM, used as an ANTIHYPERTENSIVE and to treat angina.

DIMETICONE (simethicone), used to relieve flatulence.

DIOCALM, brand containing the antidiarrhoeal loperamide.

DIPHENDYDRAMINE, used for allergic conditions. It is also contained in some cough-and-cold remedies, and is used as a SLEEP-AID. It is an ANTIHISTAMINE.

DIPYRIDAMOLE, an ANTIPLATELET DRUG.

DISODIUM ETIDRONATE, used to prevent and treat osteoporosis.

DISPRIN, brand of aspirin.

DISPRIN EXTRA, brand containing aspirin and paracetamol.

DIURETIC drugs, used to reduce excess fluid in the body. They are used in ANTIHYPERTENSIVE TREATMENT, also in acute pulmonary (lung) oedema, congestive heart failure and some liver and kidney disorders. Diuretics act on the kidneys and increase the removal of water and sodium and other mineral salts from the body. They increase urine production and so are often called water tablets.

Various diuretics are used, including amiloride, frusemide and spironolactone. Some deplete potassium from the body, so people taking these must take potassium salts as a supplement. On the whole, diuretics are safe and free from side effects – apart from the frequent need to urinate.

DOCUSATE SODIUM, a laxative. It is also used to soften ear wax.

DOMPERIDONE, used to relieve nausea and vomiting.

DORZOLAMIDE, used to treat glaucoma.

DOSULEPIN (or dothiepin), an ANTIDEPRESSANT.

DOXAZOSIN, an ANTIHYPERTENSIVE. It is also used to treat urinary retention in men with benign prostatic hyperplasia.

DOXYCYCLINE, an ANTIBIOTIC used to treat bacterial infections.

DULCO-LAX, brand of bisacodyl.

E

EFEXOR, brand of venlafaxine.

EFORMOTEROL, used in ASTHMA TREATMENT. It is also known as FORMOTEROL.

ENALAPRIL, used as an ANTIHYPERTENSIVE and to treat heart failure. It is an ACE INHIBITOR.

EPILEPSY TREATMENT, used to prevent the occurrence of epileptic seizures. Specialized drugs are used depending on the type of epilepsy and how severe it is.

Drugs used include sodium valproate, phenytoin, phenobarbital and carbamazepine. Many of these drugs have side effects, and some are not recommended for use in women of childbearing age.

ERGOCALCIFEROL (vitamin D_2), used to make up deficiency of vitamin D.

ERYTHROMYCIN, an ANTIBIOTIC used to treat bacterial infections as an alternative to penicillin.

ESOMEPRAZOLE, an ULCER-HEALING DRUG.

ESTRADIOL, an OESTROGEN used in HORMONE REPLACEMENT THERAPY.

ESTRIOL, an OESTROGEN used to treat menstrual, menopausal and other gynaecological problems.

ETHINYLESTRADIOL, an OESTROGEN used as a constituent of the ORAL CONTRACEPTIVE pill.

ETHOSUXIMIDE, used in EPILEPSY TREATMENT.

ETHYNODIOL, a PROGESTOGEN in the ORAL CONTRACEPTIVE pill.

F

FELBINAC, a PAINKILLER used for the relief of strains and bruises. It is an NSAID.

FELODIPINE, used as an ANTIHYPERTENSIVE and to treat angina. It is a CALCIUM-CHANNEL BLOCKER.

FENOFIBRATE, a LIPID-REGULATING DRUG.

FENOTEROL, used in ASTHMA TREATMENT.

FERROUS GLUCONATE, an iron-rich compound used in iron-deficiency anaemia.

FERROUS SULPHATE, used to treat iron-deficiency anaemia.

FEXOFENADINE, used for hay fever and other allergic conditions. It is an ANTIHISTAMINE.

FINASTERIDE, used to treat benign prostatic hyperplasia.

FLIXONASE and **FLIXOTIDE**, brands of fluticasone.

FLOMAX MR, brand of tamsulosin.

FLUCLOXACILLIN, an ANTIBIOTIC used to treat bacterial infections.

FLUCONAZOLE, used to treat fungal infections.

FLUMETASONE, used to treat inflammatory skin disorders. It is a CORTICOSTEROID.

FLUOXETINE, an ANTIDEPRESSANT.

FLUTICASONE, used to treat inflammatory skin disorders such as eczema. It is also used as an asthma treatment and to prevent hay fever. It is a CORTICOSTEROID.

FLUVASTATIN, a LIPID-REGULATING DRUG.

FOLIC ACID, a vitamin of the B complex. It is taken as a supplement by pregnant women, or women who plan to become pregnant, to help prevent neural tube defects in their babies.

FORMOTEROL, used in ASTHMA TREATMENT. It is also known as EFORMOTEROL.

FUCIBET, brand of betamethasone.

FUCIDIN, brand of fusidic acid.

FUCIDIN H, brand containing hydrocortisone and fusidic acid.

FUCITHALMIC, brand of fusidic acid.

FULL MARKS, preparations of phenothrin against head lice.

FUROSEMIDE, a DIURETIC.

FUSIDIC ACID, an ANTIBIOTIC used to treat bacterial infections.

FYBOGEL, brand of the laxative ispaghula husk.

FYBOGEL MEBEVERINE, brand containing mebeverine and ispaghula husk.

FYBOGEL ORANGE, brand of ispaghula husk, flavoured.

G

GABAPENTIN, used in EPILEPSY TREATMENT.

GAMOLENIC ACID, used to relieve symptoms of breast pain and eczema.

GAVISCON, branded ANTACID preparation that contains alginic acid, sodium bicarbonate and aluminium hydroxide.

GERMOLOIDS, branded preparations containing lignocaine and zinc oxide.

They are used for the relief of haemorrhoids.

GLIBENCLAMIDE, used in DIABETES TREATMENT.

GLICLAZIDE used in DIABETES TREATMENT.

GLIPIZIDE, used in DIABETES TREATMENT.

GLYCEROL, used as a laxative and for treating glaucoma.

GLYCERYL TRINITRATE, used to treat angina.

GOSERELIN, used in INFERTILITY TREATMENT, to treat endometriosis. It is also used in CHEMOTHERAPY for breast and prostate cancers.

H

HALF-INDERAL, brand of generic BETA-BLOCKER, propranolol.

HALOPERIDOL, an ANTIPSYCHOTIC drug that is also used in ANXIETY TREATMENT. It is sometimes used to prevent intractable hiccups and nausea and vomiting.

HEDEX, brand of paracetamol.

HEDEX EXTRA, brand containing paracetamol and caffeine.

HEPARIN, an ANTICOAGULANT.

HEPARINOIDS, drugs with ANTICOAGULANT properties, also used topically to give relief from haemorrhoids, chilblains, varicose veins and bruising.

HIRUDOID, branded heparinoid.

HORMONE REPLACEMENT THERAPY (HRT), used to treat menopausal symptoms. Drugs that act in a similar way to the female sex hormones are given to supplement the diminished production of OESTROGEN hormones by the body, which occurs during the menopause. Conjugated oestrogens, and estradiol (or oestrodiol), are often used. Most women will also be prescribed a PROGESTOGEN, such as levonorgestrel or norethisterone, because there is a small increased risk of uterine cancer if oestrogen is taken alone. Alternatively, a new drug called

tibolone can be used. If you have had a hysterectomy, oestrogen alone will probably be prescribed.

The main purpose of HRT is to alleviate menopausal symptoms such as flushing, night sweats and thinning and drying of the vagina. HRT also reduces postmenopausal osteoporosis and benefits some women by reducing the risk of atherosclerosis, heart attacks and strokes.

However, in other women there is an increased risk of deep vein thrombosis and of pulmonary embolism. There is a slightly increased risk of breast cancer, but a reduced risk of some other cancers.

HRT is usually taken as tablets but may also be applied as vaginal cream, skin gels or skin patches. Sometimes HRT causes side effects such as breast tenderness, nausea, headaches, mood swings and water retention. A doctor will recommend the best type for you, based on your medical history.

HUMAN MIXTARD, brand of insulin.

HYDROCORTISONE, used to treat many types of inflammation, including allergic conditions, skin conditions, inflammatory bowel disease and rheumatic disease. It is a CORTICOSTEROID.

HYDROXOCOBALAMIN, a form of vitamin B_{12} used to treat megaloblastic anaemia.

HYDROXYCHLOROQUINE, used to treat inflammatory disorders such as rheumatoid arthritis and lupus erythematosus.

HYDROXYZINE, used to treat allergic symptoms, and as an ANXIETY TREATMENT. It is an ANTIHISTAMINE.

HYOSCINE, used as a sedative and to prevent travel sickness and symptoms of Ménière's disease of the ear. It is also used in some ophthalmic operations because it paralyses the muscles of the eye.

HYPROMELLOSE, a constituent of artificial tears, is used to treat dry eyes.

I

IBULEVE, brand of pain-relieving cream containing ibuprofen.

IBUPROFEN, a PAINKILLER. It is also used to reduce a high temperature and to treat inflammation. It is an NSAID.

IKOREL, brand of nicorandil.

IMDUR, brand of isosorbide mononitrate, a vasodilator.

IMIGRAN, brand of sumatriptan.

IMIPRAMINE, an ANTIDEPRESSANT.

IMODIUM, brand of loperamide.

IMODIUM PLUS, brand containing loperamide and dimeticone.

INDAPAMIDE, a DIURETIC.

INDERAL, brand of propranolol.

INDOMETACIN (indomethacin), a PAINKILLER used to treat painful inflammatory conditions, such as rheumatic pain, and period pain. It is an NSAID.

INDORAMIN, an ANTIHYPERTENSIVE, also used to treat benign prostatic hypertrophy.

INFACOL, brand of dimeticone.

INFERTILITY TREATMENT drugs, used to help couples who have problems conceiving. The type of treatment depends on the cause of infertility. Sometimes drugs that help a woman to ovulate are used. These include gonadotrophins, goserelin and tamoxifen. A drug regime may also be used as part of assisted conception such as in vitro fertilization (IVF). In cases of male infertility caused by impotence, drugs such as sildenafil – better known as the brand Viagra – may be prescribed.

INNOVACE, brand of enalapril.

INSULIN, used in DIABETES TREATMENT.

IPRATROPIUM, used to treat chronic bronchitis and in ASTHMA TREATMENT for chronic asthma. It is also used to relieve a runny nose in people with rhinitis.

IRBESARTAN, used as an ANTIHYPERTENSIVE. It is an ACE INHIBITOR.

ISOSORBIDE DINITRATE, used to prevent angina attacks.

ISOSORBIDE MONONITRATE, used to prevent and treat angina.

ISPAGHULA HUSK, a laxative used for treating bowel conditions such as irritable bowel syndrome. It is also used as a LIPID-REGULATING DRUG.

ISTIN, brand of amlodipine.

K

KETOCONAZOLE, used to treat serious fungal infections.

KETOPROFEN, a PAINKILLER and anti-inflammatory drug. It is used to treat rheumatic and muscular pain. It is an NSAID.

KWELLS, brand of hyoscine.

L

LACIDIPINE, used as an ANTIHYPERTENSIVE. It is a CALCIUM-CHANNEL BLOCKER.

LACTULOSE, a laxative.

LAMICTAL, brand of lamotrigine.

LAMISIL, brand of terbinafine.

LAMOTRIGINE, used in EPILEPSY TREATMENT.

LANSOPRAZOLE, an ULCER-HEALING DRUG.

LASONIL, branded heparinoid.

LATANOPROST, used to treat glaucoma.

LERCANIDIPINE, an ANTIHYPERTENSIVE. It is a CALCIUM-CHANNEL BLOCKER.

LEVOBUNOLOL, used to treat glaucoma. It is a BETA-BLOCKER.

LEVODOPA, used to treat PARKINSON'S DISEASE.

LEVONORGESTREL, a PROGESTOGEN used in ORAL CONTRACEPTIVE pills, the 'morning-after pill', HORMONE REPLACEMENT THERAPY and intra-uterine devices (IUDs).

LEVOTHYROXINE SODIUM, see thyroxine.

LIGNOCAINE (lidocaine), a local anaesthetic used to relieve pain such as during dental procedures. It is also used to treat heart arrhythmias.

LIPID-REGULATING DRUGS, used to treat people with high levels of certain cholesterol lipids and triglycerides (natural body fats) in the blood. The condition is known medically as hyperlipidaemia. The main drugs used are the statins, which include atorvastatin, cerivastatin, fluvastatin, pravastatin and simvastatin; and the fibrates: bezafibrate, ciprofibrate and fenofibrate. These are all taken by mouth.

Lipid-regulating drugs, along with dietary changes, are used to lower levels of harmful low-density lipoprotein (LDL) cholesterol while raising beneficial high-density lipoprotein (HDL) cholesterol. This can slow down the development of coronary atherosclerosis, a diseased state of the arteries of the heart in which plaques of deposited lipid material cause a narrowing of blood vessels.

Because atherosclerosis contributes to angina pectoris attacks and the formation of the clots that cause heart attacks and strokes, lipid-regulating drugs can be used to help reduce this risk. Lipid-regulating drugs used to be prescribed only for people who had a family history of hyperlipidaemia, or who had very high cholesterol levels. However, large-scale clinical trials have shown that many people, including those with angina or heart failure, as well as those who have really high blood lipids, may benefit. It is likely that these drugs will be used more widely in future to prevent certain cardiovascular diseases.

LIPITOR, brand of atorvastatin.
LIPOSTAT, brand of pravastatin.
LISINOPRIL, used as an ANTIHYPERTENSIVE and to treat heart failure. It is an ACE INHIBITOR.
LITHIUM CARBONATE, used to treat manic depressive illness (bipolar disorder).
LOPERAMIDE, used to treat diarrhoea.
LOPRAZOLAM, used in ANXIETY TREATMENT, in EPILEPSY TREATMENT, and as a SLEEP-AID. It is a BENZODIAZEPINE.
LORATADINE, used to treat allergic conditions such as hay fever and urticaria. It is an ANTIHISTAMINE.
LORAZEPAM, used in ANXIETY TREATMENT, in EPILEPSY TREATMENT, and as a SLEEP-AID and sedative before operations. It is a BENZODIAZEPINE.
LORMETAZEPAM, a SLEEP-AID used to treat insomnia. It is a BENZODIAZEPINE.
LOSARTAN, used as an ANTIHYPERTENSIVE.
LOSEC, brand of omeprazole.
LUSTRAL, brand of sertraline.
LYCLEAR, brand of permethrin.
LYMECYCLINE, an ANTIBIOTIC used to treat bacterial infections.

M

MACROGOL 3350, used in laxative preparations.
MAGNESIUM HYDROXIDE, an ANTACID. It is also used as a laxative.
MAGNESIUM SULPHATE, a laxative.
MAGNESIUM TRISILICATE, an ANTACID.
MALATHION, used to kill head lice and their eggs, and the mites that cause scabies.
MEBENDAZOLE, used to treat worms.
MEBEVERINE, used to treat gastro-intestinal disorders such as irritable bowel syndrome.
MECLOZINE, used to prevent nausea and vomiting such as in travel sickness. It is an ANTIHISTAMINE.
MEDROXYPROGESTERONE ACETATE, a PROGESTOGEN that is a constituent of the ORAL CONTRACEPTIVE pill, HORMONE REPLACEMENT THERAPY and of contraceptive implants. It is also used to boost hormone levels, and is used in CHEMOTHERAPY for some cancers.
MEFENAMIC ACID, used as a PAINKILLER and to treat the inflammation of arthritis. It is also used for period pain and heavy menstrual bleeding. It is an NSAID.
MELOXICAM, used as a PAINKILLER and to treat arthritis inflammation. It is an NSAID.
MEPTAZINOL, a powerful PAINKILLER.
MESALAZINE, used to treat ulcerative colitis.
METFORMIN, used in DIABETES TREATMENT.
METHADONE, best known as a heroin substitute for addicts undergoing detoxification therapy. It is also used as a strong PAINKILLER and to stop coughing in terminally ill people.
METHOCARBAMOL, used to treat muscle spasms.
METHOTREXATE, used in cancer CHEMOTHERAPY, and to treat rheumatoid arthritis and severe psoriasis.
METHYLDOPA, used as an ANTIHYPERTENSIVE.
METHYLPHENIDATE, used to treat attention deficit hyperactivity disorder (ADHD) in children.
METHYLPREDNISOLONE, used to treat inflammation such as in allergic reactions. It is a CORTICOSTEROID.
METOCLOPRAMIDE, used to prevent vomiting.
METOPROLOL, used as an ANTIHYPERTENSIVE, to treat angina and heart arrhythmias, in MIGRAINE TREATMENT and, in the short term, to treat thyrotoxicosis. It is a BETA-BLOCKER.
METRONIDAZOLE, used to treat infections including amoebic dysentery and giardiasis, bacterial infections and worms.
MICONAZOLE, used to treat fungal infections.
MICROGYNON, brand of ORAL CONTRACEPTIVE containing ethinylestradiol and levonorgestrel.
MIGRAINE TREATMENT drugs, used in two ways. Some, such as BETA-BLOCKERS like propranolol, are taken to prevent attacks. Others are taken at the beginning of or during an attack to alleviate symptoms. This type must be rapidly absorbed into the body, so newer drugs such as sumatriptan – marketed under the brand-name Imigran – have been developed that can be self-injected or taken as a nasal spray.

Ordinary PAINKILLERS such as aspirin, codeine and paracetamol, available in quick-absorption formulations, along with drugs to prevent vomiting, such as metoclopramide and domperidone, may be helpful.
MIGRALEVE, brand of migraine medication containing codeine, paracetamol and buclizine.
MINOCYCLINE, an ANTIBIOTIC used to treat bacterial infections such as bacterial meningitis.
MINOXIDIL, best known as a topical treatment for male pattern baldness. It is also used orally as an ANTIHYPERTENSIVE.
MIRTAZAPINE, an ANTIDEPRESSANT.
MOMETASONE, used to treat severe inflammatory skin conditions and allergic rhinitis. It is a CORTICOSTEROID.
MONTELUKAST, used in ASTHMA TREATMENT.
MORNING-AFTER PILL, see ORAL CONTRACEPTIVES.
MORPHINE, a strong PAINKILLER. It is also used to treat dry coughs and diarrhoea.
MOXONIDINE, an ANTIHYPERTENSIVE.
MUPIROCIN, an ANTIBIOTIC used to treat bacterial infections.
MYCIL, branded anti-fungal, tolnaftate.

N

NABUMETONE, a PAINKILLER used particularly for arthritis. It is an NSAID.
NAFTIDROFURYL, used to treat peripheral vascular disease.
NAPROXEN, a PAINKILLER also used to treat inflammation. It is an NSAID.

NARATRIPTAN, used in MIGRAINE TREATMENT.

NEBIVOLOL, used as an ANTIHYPERTENSIVE. It is a BETA-BLOCKER.

NEDOCROMIL, used in ASTHMA TREATMENT to prevent recurrent attacks. It is also used to treat hay fever and other allergic conditions.

NEOMYCIN, an ANTIBIOTIC used to treat bacterial infections.

NICORANDIL, used to prevent and treat angina.

NICORETTE PREPARATIONS, brand of nicotine used to help smokers to give up.

NICOTINE, used in replacement therapy to help smokers to quit.

NICOTINELL PREPARATIONS, brand of nicotine to help smokers to give up.

NIFEDIPINE, used as an ANTIHYPERTENSIVE and to treat angina and Raynaud's disease. It is a CALCIUM-CHANNEL BLOCKER.

NIGHT NURSE PREPARATIONS, brand of cold remedy containing paracetamol, promethazine and dextromethorphan.

NIQUITIN, brand of nicotine to help smokers to give up.

NITRAZEPAM, used as a SLEEP-AID. It is a BENZODIAZEPINE.

NITROFURANTOIN, used to treat bacterial infections.

NIZATIDINE, an ULCER-HEALING DRUG.

NORETHISTERONE, a PROGESTOGEN used in the ORAL CONTRACEPTIVE pill, in HORMONE REPLACEMENT THERAPY and contraceptive implants. It is also used for other gynaecological problems, and in CHEMOTHERAPY.

NSAID (non-steroidal anti-inflammatory drugs), used as anti-inflammatories, analgesics and antipyretics to lower temperature.

NUROFEN, brand of ibuprofen.

NUROFEN COLD AND FLU, brand containing ibuprofen and pseudoephedrine.

NUROFEN PLUS, brand containing ibuprofen and codeine.

NYSTATIN, an ANTIBIOTIC used to treat fungal infections.

O

OESTROGEN, a hormone that is frequently combined with PROGESTOGEN hormones in ORAL CONTRACEPTIVES, HORMONE REPLACEMENT THERAPY and to treat various gynaecological and menstrual problems. Oestrogen is also used to treat certain cancers, such as prostate cancer. Those used include natural oestrogens, estradiol and estriol, and also synthetic versions, including ethinylestradiol and diethylstilbestrol (stilboestrol).

OLANZAPINE, used to treat schizophrenia. It is an ANTIPSYCHOTIC drug.

OMEPRAZOLE, an ULCER-HEALING DRUG.

ORAL CONTRACEPTIVE drugs, taken by women to prevent conception, commonly referred to as the Pill. Most contain both an OESTROGEN and a PROGESTOGEN, and this type of Pill is known as the combined oral contraceptive.

Another type of Pill is the progestogen-only pill; this is safe to use if you are breastfeeding. Contraceptive oestrogens and progestogens can also be given by injection or implant. The so-called 'MORNING-AFTER' pill is an oral contraceptive taken after unprotected sex. All oral contraceptives have side effects, and you need expert advice to find the one best suited to you.

ORIGINAL ANDREWS SALTS, brand containing sodium bicarbonate, magnesium sulphate and citric acid.

ORLISTAT, used to treat obesity.

ORPHENADRINE, used to treat PARKINSON'S DISEASE.

OXAZEPAM, used in ANXIETY TREATMENT and as a SLEEP-AID. It is a BENZODIAZEPINE.

OXITROPIUM, used to treat chronic bronchitis and as an ASTHMA TREATMENT.

OXY PREPARATIONS, brand containing benzoyl peroxide.

OXYBUTYNIN, used for urinary problems such as bedwetting.

OXYTETRACYCLINE, an ANTIBIOTIC used to treat bacterial infections.

P

PAINKILLER drugs, known medically as analgesics. NSAID (non-steroidal anti-inflammatory drugs) such as aspirin and ibuprofen work by reducing the inflammation that is often a cause of pain. These drugs are widely taken to treat arthritic and rheumatic pain, and inflammation and pain in other musculoskeletal disorders. Other NSAIDs include diclofenac, etodolac, felbinac, ketoprofen, indometacin, meloxicam, nabumetone, naproxen, piroxicam and rofecoxib. Most can cause gastro-intestinal upsets ranging from dyspepsia to serious haemorrhage.

Paracetamol is a painkiller. It can also be used to reduce body temperature and can be given to children including babies after immunization.

Narcotic analgesic painkillers can be used to alleviate more intense pain such as that experienced after operations, dental pain and for the severe pain of some cancers. Morphine and diamorphine (heroin) are powerful narcotic analgesics used only for severe pain. Codeine, which has weaker action, is available over the counter only when it is combined with paracetamol. Other narcotic analgesics include buprenorphine, methadone, pentazocine and pethidine. They mimic the actions in the brain of the body's natural analgesics, the encephalins and endorphins. However, most can be addictive and are prescribed with caution.

PANCREATIN, taken to make up a deficiency of pancreatic enzymes in people who have conditions such as cystic fibrosis, or who have had pancreatic surgery.

PANOXYL PREPARATIONS, brand containing benzoyl peroxide.

PANTOPRAZOLE, an ULCER-HEALING DRUG.

PARACETAMOL, a popular PAINKILLER also used to reduce high body temperature.

PARACODOL, brand containing paracetamol and codeine.

PARIET, branded rabeprazole.

PARKINSON'S DISEASE treatment, used to alleviate some of the symptoms of Parkinson's disease. In Parkinson's disease the level of the neurotransmitter dopamine, relative to the level of the neurotransmitter acetylcholine, is reduced.

Drugs are used to try to restore the correct balance. They include levodopa, co-beneldopa, co-careldopa, benzhexol and procyclidine. Specialist medical advice is needed in order to choose the best drug for a given stage of the condition.

PAROXETINE, an ANTIDEPRESSANT.

PEPPERMINT OIL, used to relieve the discomfort of conditions such as irritable bowel syndrome.

PERINDOPRIL, used as an ANTIHYPERTENSIVE and to treat heart failure. It is an ACE INHIBITOR.

PERMETHRIN, used to eradicate lice and their eggs, and the mites that cause scabies.

PETHIDINE, a powerful PAINKILLER often administered to women in labour.

PHENOBARBITAL (or phenobarbitone), a barbiturate used in EPILEPSY TREATMENT.

PHENOTHRIN, used to treat head lice and pubic lice infestations.

PHENOXYMETHYLPENICILLIN (or penicillin V), an ANTIBIOTIC used to treat bacterial infections.

PHENYLPROPANOLAMINE, used to relieve congestion in the airways and nose.

PHENYTOIN, used in EPILEPSY TREATMENT and also for trigeminal neuralgia.

PHOLCODINE, used to treat a dry cough.

PILOCARPINE, used to treat glaucoma.

PINDOLOL, used as an ANTIHYPERTENSIVE. It is a BETA-BLOCKER.

PIRITON PREPARATIONS, brand containing chlorphenamine.

PIROXICAM, a PAINKILLER. It is used to treat pain and inflammation in musculo-skeletal conditions such as arthritis. It is an NSAID.

PIZOTIFEN, used in MIGRAINE TREATMENT.

PLAVIX, brand of clopidogrel.

PLENDIL, brand of felodipine.

POLYVINYL ALCOHOL, used as a constituent of artificial tears to treat dry eyes.

POTASSIUM BICARBONATE, a potassium supplement taken to make up potassium loss from the body, such as after chronic diarrhoea.

PRAVASTATIN, a LIPID-REGULATING DRUG.

PREDNISOLONE, used to treat many inflammatory conditions. It is also used in cancer CHEMOTHERAPY, and for some autoimmune conditions. It is a CORTICOSTEROID.

PREMARIN, brand of conjugated oestrogens.

PRIMIDONE, used in EPILEPSY TREATMENT.

PROCHLORPERAZINE, an ANTIPSYCHOTIC drug for schizophrenia and mania. It is also used to prevent vomiting and as an ANXIETY TREATMENT.

PROCYCLIDINE, used to treat PARKINSON'S DISEASE.

PROGESTOGEN, the natural female progesterone hormone that prepares the lining of the uterus for pregnancy, maintains it throughout pregnancy, and prevents the further release of eggs. Natural progesterones used medically include levonorgestrel, medroxyprogesterone and norethisterone. The hormones are used in ORAL CONTRACEPTIVES,

HORMONE REPLACEMENT THERAPY, and to treat various menstrual and gynaecological problems. Sometimes progestogen is used in the treatment of breast, endometrial and prostate cancers.

PROMETHAZINE, used to treat allergic conditions, travel sickness and as a SLEEP-AID. It is an ANTIHISTAMINE.

PROPRANOLOL, used as an ANTIHYPERTENSIVE, to treat angina, thyrotoxicosis and heart arrhythmias. It is also used as a MIGRAINE TREATMENT and ANXIETY TREATMENT. It is a BETA-BLOCKER.

PROZAC, brand of fluoxetine.

PSEUDOEPHEDRINE, used to relieve congestion in the nose and airways.

PULMICORT, brand of budesonide.

Q

QUINAPRIL, used as an ANTIHYPERTENSIVE and to treat heart failure. It is an ACE INHIBITOR.

QUININE, used to treat malaria and also to relieve night time leg cramps.

QUINODERM PREPARATIONS, brand of benzoyl peroxide.

R

RABEPRAZOLE, an ULCER-HEALING DRUG.

RALOXIFENE, used to prevent and treat osteoporosis.

RAMIPRIL, used as an ANTIHYPERTENSIVE and to treat heart failure. It is an ACE INHIBITOR.

RANITIDINE, an ULCER-HEALING DRUG.

REGAINE, brand of minoxidil.

RESOLVE, brand containing paracetamol, ascorbic acid, sodium bicarbonate, sodium carbonate, potassium bicarbonate and citric acid.

RISEDRONATE, used to prevent and treat osteoporosis.

RISPERIDONE, an ANTIPSYCHOTIC drug.

RIZATRIPTAN, used in MIGRAINE TREATMENT.

ROFECOXIB, a PAINKILLER and anti-inflammatory drug used in arthritis. It is an NSAID.

ROSIGLITAZONE, used in DIABETES TREATMENT.

S

SALBUTAMOL, used in ASTHMA TREATMENT.

SALICYLIC ACID, used on the skin to treat minor infections and conditions such as athlete's foot, and to relieve muscle and joint pain. It is also used to remove warts and calluses.

SALMETEROL, used in ASTHMA TREATMENT.

SEA-LEGS, brand of meclozine.

SENNA, a laxative.

SENOKOT, brand of senna.

SEREVENT, brand of salmeterol.

SEROXAT, brand of paroxetine.

SERTRALINE, an ANTIDEPRESSANT, also used to treat obsessive-compulsive disorders.

SILDENAFIL, used as an impotence treatment.

SILVER SULPHADIAZINE, used to treat bacterial infections, particularly to prevent bedsores and burns becoming infected.

SIMETHICONE (dimeticon), used to relieve flatulence.

SIMVASTATIN, a LIPID-REGULATING DRUG.

SINUTAB, brand containing paracetamol and phenylpropanolamine.

SLEEP-AID DRUGS, known medically as hypnotics. These help to induce sleep and work by acting on the brain. They are used mainly to treat insomnia and to sedate patients who are mentally ill, but they may also be used for the short-term treatment of insomnia due to jet lag, shift work, emotional problems or serious illness.

The best known and most often taken are the BENZODIAZEPINE drugs, such as diazepam and

temazepam. Other drugs that are used include zopiclone, zolpiderm and chloral betaine. Most are available only on prescription, but over-the-counter sleep-aids include promethazine. Some can cause you to feel drowsy the following day.

SODIUM BICARBONATE, an ANTACID.

SODIUM CARBONATE, an ANTACID.

SODIUM CITRATE, used as a laxative and as an enema.

SODIUM CROMOGLICATE, used in ASTHMA TREATMENT and other allergic conditions such as allergic conjunctivitis.

SODIUM FEREDETATE, rich in iron and is used to treat iron-deficiency anaemia or to prevent deficiency. It is also known as SODIUM IRONEDETATE.

SODIUM FUSIDATE, a compound of FUSIDIC ACID, used in the same way.

SODIUM IRONEDETATE, see sodium feredetate.

SODIUM PICOSULPHATE, a laxative.

SODIUM VALPROATE, used in EPILEPSY TREATMENT.

SOLPADEINE, brand containing paracetamol, codeine and caffeine.

SOTALOL, used to treat heart arrhythmias. It is a BETA-BLOCKER.

SPIRONOLACTONE, a DIURETIC.

SULEO-M, brand of malathion.

SULFASALAZINE, used to treat Crohn's disease, ulcerative colitis and rheumatoid arthritis.

SULPIRIDE, used mainly as an ANTIPSYCHOTIC drug for schizophrenia.

SUMATRIPTAN, used in MIGRAINE TREATMENT.

T

TAGAMET 100, brand of the ulcer-healing drug cimetidine.

TAMOXIFEN, used as an INFERTILITY TREATMENT and in cancer CHEMOTHERAPY to prevent or treat breast cancer.

TAMSULOSIN, used to treat urinary retention by men who have benign prostatic hyperplasia.

TEMAZEPAM, used as a SLEEP-AID. It is a BENZODIAZEPINE.

TENORMIN, brand of atenolol.

TERBINAFINE, used to treat fungal infections such as ringworm.

TERBUTALINE, used in ASTHMA TREATMENT.

TETRACYCLINE, an ANTIBIOTIC used to treat bacterial infections.

THEOPHYLLINE, used in ASTHMA TREATMENT.

THIORIDAZINE, an ANTIPSYCHOTIC drug. It is sometimes also used as an ANXIETY TREATMENT to calm elderly people.

THYROXINE, a hormone administered to make up for deficient hormone production by the thyroid gland.

TIBOLONE, used in HORMONE REPLACEMENT THERAPY.

TIMOLOL, used as an ANTIHYPERTENSIVE and to treat angina and glaucoma. It is also used as a MIGRAINE TREATMENT. It is a BETA-BLOCKER.

TOLBUTAMIDE, used in DIABETES TREATMENT.

TOLNAFTATE, used to treat fungal infections such as athlete's foot.

TOLTERODINE, used to treat urinary problems.

TRAMADOL, a strong PAINKILLER.

TRANDOLAPRIL, used as an ANTIHYPERTENSIVE. It is an ACE INHIBITOR.

TRANEXAMIC ACID, used to stem bleeding such as might occur during tooth extraction, or for excessive menstrual bleeding.

TRAZODONE, an ANTIDEPRESSANT.

TRIAMCINOLONE, used to treat inflammatory conditions, especially when caused by allergy. It is a CORTICOSTEROID.

TRIFLUOPERAZINE, an ANTIPSYCHOTIC drug. It is also sometimes used to treat anxiety and severe nausea and vomiting.

TRIMETHOPRIM, used to treat bacterial infections.

TRIMIPRAMINE, an ANTIDEPRESSANT.

TRIPROLIDINE, used to treat allergic symptoms such as hay fever and urticaria. It is an ANTIHISTAMINE.

TRITACE, brand of ramipril.

TYROZETS, brand of lozenge containing benzocaine.

U

ULCER-HEALING DRUGS, used to promote healing of ulcers in the lining of the stomach and small intestine. They are suitable for treating peptic ulcers. Many different types of drug may be used, including so-called H2-antagonist drugs such as ranitidine (known by the brand name Zantac) and cimetidine (branded as Tagamet). The so-called proton-pump inhibitors such as omeprazole (Losec) may also be prescribed. These drugs may be used in conjunction with antibacterial drugs which eliminate the bacterium *Helicobacter pylori* in the stomach. *H. pylori* is known to be one of the main causes of peptic ulcers.

V

VACCINES, used to give immunity against infections and so prevent the vaccinated person from catching that disease. They work by causing a person's own body to create a defence in the form of antibodies. Vaccines can be made from dead microbes, live but weakened microbes, or extracts of the toxins released by the invading microbes. They are usually injected, but some, such as the polio vaccine, are taken by mouth. There are vaccines to treat a wide range of infections, but they are less effective against viruses such as influenza and HIV, that can change rapidly into new forms.

VALSARTAN, used as an ANTIHYPERTENSIVE.

VENLAFAXINE, an ANTIDEPRESSANT.

VENTOLIN, brand of salbutamol.

VERAPAMIL, used as an ANTIHYPERTENSIVE, and to treat angina and heart arrhythmias. It is a CALCIUM-CHANNEL BLOCKER.

VIAGRA, brand of sildenafil.

VIOXX, brand of rofecoxib.

VISCOTEARS, brand of carbomer.

W

WARFARIN, an ANTICOAGULANT.

X

XALATAN, brand of latanoprost.

Z

ZANTAC, brand of ranitidine.

ZANTAC 75, brand of ranitidine.

ZESTRIL, brand of lisinopril.

ZINC OXIDE, used to treat skin conditions such as eczema and nappy rash.

ZIRTEK, brand of cetirizine.

ZOCOR, brand of simvastatin.

ZOLADEX, brand of goserelin.

ZOLMITRIPTAN, drug used in MIGRAINE TREATMENT.

ZOLPIDEM, a SLEEP-AID drug.

ZOPICLONE, a SLEEP-AID drug.

ZOTON, brand of lansoprazole.

ZOVIRAX, brand of aciclovir.

ZYPREXA, brand of olanzapine.

Useful contacts

These organizations can provide practical help and advice for people suffering from a wide range of disorders.

AIDS/HIV

Joint United Nations Programme on HIV/AIDS
www.unaids.org

National AIDS Trust
New City Cloisters, 188–196 Old Street, London EC1V 9FR
Helpline 0800 567 123
www.nat.org.uk

Terrence Higgins Trust
52–54 Gray's Inn Road, London WC1X 8JU
Helpline 0845 122 1200
www.tht.org.uk

ALLERGY

Allergy UK
Deepdene House, 30 Bellegrove Road, Welling, Kent DA16 3PY
Helpline 020 8303 8583
9am–5pm Mon–Fri
www.allergyuk.org
www.allergyfoundation.com

British Society for Allergy, Environmental and Nutritional Medicine
PO Box 7, Knighton, Powys LD8 2WF
Tel: 0906 302 0010
www.bsaenm.org.uk

National Pollen Research Unit
Issues a pollen guide from mid-May to the end of July
www.pollenforecast.org.uk

National Society for Research into Allergy
Box 45, Hinckley, Leeds LE10 1JY
Tel: 01455 250715

ARTHRITIS

Arthritis Care
18 Stephenson Way, London NW1 2HD
Helpline 0808 800 4050
12pm–4pm Mon–Fri
Under 25s helpline 0808 808 2000
10am–2pm Mon–Fri
www.arthritiscare.org.uk

Arthritis Research Campaign
Copeman House, St Mary's Court, St Mary's Gate, Chesterfield, Derbyshire S41 7TD
Helpline 0870 850 5000
Tel: 01246 558033
www.arc.org.uk

CHOICES for families of children with Arthritis
Offers practical support to families of children with chronic arthritis.
PO Box 58, Hove, East Sussex BN3 5WN
www.kidswitharthritis.org

AUTOIMMUNE DISORDERS

Lupus UK
St James House, Eastern Road, Romford, Essex RM1 3NH
Tel: 01708 731251
www.lupusuk.com

Raynaud's and Scleroderma Association
112 Crewe Road, Alsager, Cheshire ST7 2JA
Tel: 01270 872776
www.raynauds.demon.co.uk

BLOOD

Blood Pressure Association
60 Cranmer Terrace, London SW17 0QS
Tel: 020 8772 4994
www.bpassoc.org.uk

National Blood Service
Helpline 08457 711711
www.blood.co.uk

The DASH diet
Diet plan designed to reduce high blood pressure
www.nhlbi.nih.gov

BONE DISORDERS

Anthony Nolan Trust
Holds a register of voluntary bone marrow donors
Tel: 0901 882 2234
www.anthonynolan.com

BackCare
16 Elmtree Road, Middlesex TW11 8ST
Offers information and links to other relevant sites.
Tel: 020 8977 5474
ww.backcare.org.uk
www.coccyx.org

Brittle Bone Society
30 Guthrie Street, Dundee DD1 5BS
Helpline 08000 282459
Tel: 01382 204446
www.brittlebone.org

General Osteopathic Council

Osteopathy House, 176 Tower Bridge Road, London SE1 3LU
Tel: 020 7357 0011
www.osteopathy.org.uk

National Ankylosing Spondylitis Society
PO Box 179, Mayfield, East Sussex TN20 6ZL
Tel: 01435 873527
www.nass.co.uk

National Association for the Relief of Paget's Disease
Tel: 0161 799 4646
www.paget.org.uk

Spinal Injuries Association
76 St James Lane, Muswell Hill, London NW10 3DF
Helpline 0800 980 0501
www.spinal.co.uk

BRAIN AND NERVOUS SYSTEM

Alzheimer's Society
Gordon House, 10 Greencoat Place, London SW1P 1PH
Helpline 0845 300 0336

CJD Support Network
Tel: 01630 673973
www.cjdsupport.net

Headway Brain Injury Association
4 King Edward Court, King Edward Street, Nottingham NG1 1EW
Tel: 0115 924 0800
www.headway.org.uk

Meningitis Trust
Fern House, Bath Road, Stroud, Gloucs GL5 3TJ
24-hour helpline 0845 6000 800
www.meningitis-trust.org.uk

Migraine Action Association
Unit 6, Oakley Hay Lodge Business Park, Great Folds Road, Great Oakley, Northants NN18 9AS
Tel: 01536 461333
www.migraine.org.uk

Motor Neurone Disease Association UK
PO Box 246, Northants NN1 2PR
Helpline 08457 626262
www.mndassociation.org

Multiple Sclerosis Resource Centre

Helpline 0800 783 0518
www.msrc.co.uk

Multiple Sclerosis Society
MS National Centre, 372 Edgware Road, Staples Corner, London NW2 6ND
Helpline 0808 800 8000
www.mssociety.org.uk

Multiple Sclerosis Trust
Spirella Building, Bridge Road, Letchworth, Herts SH6 4ET
Tel: 01462 476700
www.mstrust.org.uk

Neurological Alliance
PO Box 36731, London SW9 6WY
Tel: 020 7793 5907
www.neurologicalalliance.org.uk

Parkinson's Disease Society
215 Vauxhall Bridge Road, London SW1V 1EJ
Helpline 0808 800 0303
9.30am–5.30pm, Mon–Fri
www.parkinsons.org.uk

Scope
PO Box 833, Milton Keynes MK12 5NY
Cerebral palsy helpline 0808 800 3333
www.scope.org.uk

Stroke Association
Stroke House, 240 City Road, London EC1V 2PR
Helpline 0845 303 3100
www.stroke.org.uk

Trigeminal Neuralgia Association
www.tna-support.org

BREATHING AND RESPIRATORY DISORDERS

British Lung Foundation
78 Hatton Garden, London EC1N 8LD
Tel: 020 7831 5831
www.lunguk.org
Breathe Easy Club
Tel: 0207 688 5555

National Asthma Campaign
Providence House, Providence Place, London N1 0NT
Helpline 0845 701 0203
9am–7pm Mon–Fri
www.asthma.org.uk

CANCER

Breast Cancer Care
Kiln House, 210 New Kings Road,
London SW6 4NZ
Helpline 0808 800 6000;10am–5pm
Mon–Fri; 10am–2pm Sat
www.breastcancercare.org.uk

CancerBACUP
3 Bath Place, Rivington Street,
London EC2A 3JR
Tel: 020 7739 2280
Helpline 0808 800 1234 (this
number is staffed by cancer nurses)
www.cancerbacup.org.uk

CancerIndex
A guide to Internet resources
for cancer
www.cancerindex.org

Cancer Research UK
Cancer information service,
PO Box 123, London WC2A 3PX
Tel: 020 7269 3142
email: cancer.info@cancer.org.uk
www.cancerresearchuk.org
www.cancerhelp.org.uk

Hospice Information
Help the Hospices, Hospice House,
34–44 Britannia Street, London
WC1X 9JG
Helpline 0870 9033 903

Leukaemia Care Society
2 Shrubbery Avenue, Worcester
WR1 1QH
Tel: 01905 330003
Helpline 0845 767 3203
www.leukaemiacare.org

Leukaemia Research Fund
43 Great Ormond Street, London
WC1N 3JJ
Tel: 020 7405 0101
www. leukaemiaresearch.org.uk

Lymphoma Association
PO Box 386, Aylesbury, Bucks
HP20 2GA
Tel: 01296 619400
www.lymphoma.org.uk

Macmillan Cancer Relief
89 Albert Embankment,
London SE1 UQ
Tel: 020 7840 7840
Helpline 0845 601 6161
www.macmillan.org.uk

**Sargent Cancer Care for
Children**
Griffin House, 161 Hammersmith
Road, London W6 8SG
Tel: 020 8752 2800
www.sargent.org

The Christie Hospital NHS Trust
Wilmslow Road, Manchester
M20 4BX
Tel: 0161 446 3000
www.christie.nhs.uk

The Royal Marsden NHS Trust
Fulham Road, London SW3 6JJ
Tel: 020 7352 8171
www.royalmarsden.org.uk

CARE OF THE ELDERLY

Age Concern
Astral House, 1268 London Road,
London SW16 4ER
Tel: 020 8765 7200
www.ageconcern.org.uk
www.activeage.org.uk

Counsel and Care
Twyman House, 16 Bonny Street,
London NW1 9PG
Information and advice for seniors
Helpline 0845 300 7585
10am–12.30pm and 2–4pm Mon–Fri
www.counselandcare.org.uk

Help the Aged
207–221 Pentonville Road,
London N1 9UZ
Tel: 020 7278 1114
www.helptheaged.org.uk

CARERS

Carers National Association
20–25 Glasshouse Yard, London
EC1A 4JT
Tel: 020 7490 8818
www.londonhealth.co.uk/
carersnationalassociation.asp

Carers UK
Ruth Pitter House,
20–25 Glasshouse Yard,
London EC1A 4JT
Carers line 0808 808 7777
www.carersonline.org.uk

Extend
22 Maltings Drive,
Wheathampstead, Herts AL4 8QJ
Tel: 01582 832760
www.extend.org.uk

CHILDREN AND CHILDCARE

Action for Sick Children
8 Wakley Street, London
EC1V 7QE
Tel: 020 7843 6444
www.actionforsickchildren.org

ADDISS
PO Box 340, Edgware, Middlesex
HA8 9HL
Tel: 020 8906 9068
www.addiss.co.uk

Anti Bullying Campaign
Tel: 020 7378 1446

**Association of Children's
Hospices**
King's House, 14 Orchard Street,
Bristol BS1 5EH
Tel: 0117 905 5082
www.childhospice.org.uk

Centre for Fun and Families
Advice for parents of children with
behavioural difficulties and
communication problems.
www.funandfamilies.com

ChildLine
Freepost 1111, London N1 0BR
Children's helpline 0800 1111
www.childline.org

Changing Faces
1–2 Junction Mews, London W2 1PN
Help and advice for people suffering
from facial disfigurement
Tel: 020 7706 4232
www.cfaces.demon.co.uk

Child Brain Injury Trust
The Radcliffe Infirmary, Woodstock
Road, Oxford OX2 6HE
Tel: 01865 552467

Child Growth Foundation
2 Mayfield Avenue, London
W4 1PW
Tel: 020 8995 0257
www.heightmatters.org.uk

**Cleft Lip and Palate Association
(CLAPA)**
235–237 Finchley Road, London
NW3 6LS
Tel: 020 7431 0033
www.clapa.com

**Hyperactive Children's Support
Group**
71 Whyke Lane, Chichester,
West Sussex PO19 2LD
Helpline 01243 551313
www.hacsg.org.uk

Kidscape
2 Grosvenor Gardens, London
SW1W 0DH
Tel: 020 7730 3300
www.kidscape.org.uk

**National Family and Parenting
Institute**
Campaigns for a more family-
friendly society and offers
information and advice.
www.nfpi.org

**NSPCC National Child
Protection**
For anyone concerned about the
wellbeing of a child.
Helpline 0800 800 500

Parents Online
Information on health, education
and leisure for parents of primary
school children.
www.parents.org.uk

Parentline Plus
Help and advice for anyone
parenting a child.
Helpline 0808 800 2222
www.parentlineplus.org.uk

Royal College of Psychiatrists
Surviving adolescence factsheet
available online at
www.rcpsych.ac.uk/info/help/adol/
index.htm

COMPLEMENTARY THERAPIES

**Aromatherapy Organizations
Council**
Tel: 0870 7743477
www.apcuk.net

**Ayurvedic Medical
Association UK**
Eastern Clinic, 1079 Garrett Lane,
London SW17 0LN
Tel: 020 8682 3876

British Acupuncture Council
Park House, 63 Jeddo Road,
London W12 9HQ
Tel: 020 8735 0400

**British Complementary Health
Medicine Association**
www.bcma.co.uk

**British Medical Acupuncture
Society**
12 Marbury House, Higher
Whitley, Warrington WA4 4QW
Tel: 01925 730492

**College of Occupational
Therapists**
106–114 Borough High Street,
London SE1 1LB
Tel: 020 7357 6480
www.cot.org.uk

**Institute for Complementary
Medicine (ICM)**
PO Box 194 London SE16 7QZ
Tel: 020 7237 5165
www.icmedicine.co.uk

General Chiropractic Council
44 Wicklow Street, London
WC1X 9HL
Tel: 0845 601 1796
www.gcc-uk.org

**National Institute of Medical
Herbalists**
56 Longbrook Street, Exeter
EX1 6AH
Tel: 01392 426022
www.nimh.org.uk

**Register of Chinese Herbal
Practitioners**
Office G4, Garden Studios, 11–15
Betterton Street, London WC2 9BP
Tel: 020 7470 8740

**Research Council for
Complemetary Medicine**
PO Box 194 London SE16 7QZ
Tel: 020 7935 7499
www.rccm.org.uk

Society of Homeopaths
4a Artizan Road, Northampton
NN1 4HU
The society holds a register of
qualified but non-medical
homeopaths.
Tel: 01604 621400

**Society of Teachers of the
Alexander Technique**
129 Camden Mews, London
NW1 9AH
Tel: 020 7284 3338

**UK Homeopathic Medical
Association**
6 Livingstone Road, Gravesend,
Kent DA12 5DZ
The association holds the register of
medically trained homeopaths.
Tel: 01474 560 336

CONGENITAL DISORDERS

**Association for Spina Bifida and
Hydrocephalus**
42 Park Road, Peterborough
PE1 2UQ
Tel: 01733 555988
www.asbah.org

**Children Living with Inherited
Metabolic Diseases (Climb)**
176 Nantwich Road, Crewe
CW2 6EG
Helpline 0870 7700 326
www.climb.org.uk

Congenital Hyperplasia Group
Golden Gate Lodge, Weston Road,
Crewe CW2 5XN
Tel: 01270 250221

Cystic Fibrosis Trust
11 London Road, Bromley, Kent
BR1 1BY
Helpline 0845 859 1000
www.cftrust.org.uk

Down's Syndrome Association
155 Mitcham Road, London
SW17 9PG
Tel: 020 8682 4001
www.dsa-uk.com

Duchenne Family Support Group
37a Highbury New Park,
London N5 2EN
Tel: 0870 241 1857
www.dfsg.org.uk

Genetic Interest Group
Unit 4D, Leroy House, 436 Essex
Road, London N1 3QP
Tel: 020 7704 3141
www.gig.org.uk

**Grown Up Congenital Heart
Patients Association**
75 Tuddenham Avenue, Ipswich,
Suffolk IP4 2HG
Helpline 0800 854 759
www.guch.demon.co.uk

Marfan Association UK
01252 810472
www.marfan.org.uk

Muscular Dystrophy Campaign
7–11 Prescott Place, London
SW4 6BS
Helpline 020 7720 8055
www.muscular-dystrophy.org

**National Society for
Phenylketonuria**
PO Box 26642, London N14 4ZF
Helpline 0845 603 9136
web.ukonline.co.uk/nspku/

Restricted Growth Association
PO Box 4744, Dorchester DT2 9FA
Tel: 01308 898445
www.rgaonline.org.uk

CONTRACEPTION AND
SEXUAL PROBLEMS

To find your nearest GUM clinic,
look in your phone book under
GUM; contact your nearest general
hospital; or contact NHS Direct
Tel: 0845 4647. www.fpa.org.uk
For advice for young people try
www.playingsafely.co.uk

**British Association for Sexual
and Relationship Therapy**
PO Box 13686, London SW20 9ZH
www.basrt.org.uk

Brook Advisory Service
Confidential contraceptive
counselling
Helpline 0800 018 5023

Sexual Dysfunction Association
Helpline 0870 7743571
Mon–Fri 9am–5pm
www.impotence.org.uk

Marie Stopes Intenational
Offers a wide range of confidential
counselling and treatment
Tel: 020 7574 7400
www.mariestopes.org.uk

COUNSELLING

Relate
Helpline 0845 130 40 10
www.relate.org.uk

National Family Mediation
Alexander House, Telephone
Avenue, Bristol BS1 4BS
Tel: 0117 904 2825
www.nfm.u-net.com

DEATH AND BEREAVEMENT

Cruse Bereavement Care
126 Sheen Road, Richmond, Surry
TW9 1UR
Helpline 0870 167 1677
9.30am–5pm Mon–Fri
www. crusebereavementcare.org.uk

**Foundation for the Study of
Infant Death (FSID)**
Helpline 0870 787 0554 9am–11pm
Mon–Fri; 6pm–11pm weekends.
Answered by trained advisors.
www.sids.org.uk

DIGESTIVE SYSTEM

British Colostomy Association
15 Station Road, Reading, Berks
RG1 1LG
Helpline 0800 328 4257
www.bcass.org.uk

British Liver Trust
Central House, Central Avenue,
Ransomes Europark, Ipswich
IP3 9QG
Tel: 01473 276326
www.britishlivertrust.org.uk

British Thoracic Society
17 Doughty Street, London
WC1N 2PY
Tel: 020 7831 8778
www.brit-thoracic.org.uk

**Children's Liver Disease
Foundation**
36 Great Charles Street,
Birmingham B3 3JY
Tel: 0121 212 3839
www.childliverdisease.org

Coeliac UK
PO Box 220, High Wycombe,
Bucks HP11 2HY
Tel: 01494 437 278
www.coeliac.co.uk

Continence Foundation
307 Hatton Square, 16 Baldwins
Gardens, London EC1N 7RJ
Helpline 020 7831 9831
www.continencefoundation.org.uk

Digestive Disorders Foundation
PO Box 251, Edgware, Middlesex
HA8 6HG
www.digestivedisorders.org.uk

**Irritable Bowel Syndrome
Network**
Northern General Hospital,
Sheffield, Yorkshire S5 7AU
Helpline 01543 492192
www.ibsnetwork.org.uk

**National Association for Colitis
and Crohn's Disease**
4 Beaumont House, Sutton Road,
St Albans, Herts AL1 5HH
Helpline 0845 130 3344
www.nacc.org.uk

DISABILITY

Disability Rights Commission
Freepost MID 02164, Stratford-
upon-Avon CV37 9BR
Helpline 08457 622633
Textphone 08457 622644
www.drc-gb.org

Disabled Living Foundation
380–384 Harrow Road, London
W9 2HU
Helpline 0845 130 9177
Textphone 0870 6039 176
www.dlf.org.uk

Motability
Goodman House, Station
Approach, Harlow, Essex
CM20 2ET
This charity helps disabled people
and their families by providing
vehicles and powered wheelchairs.
Tel: 01279 635999
www.motability.co.uk

**Royal Association for Disability
and Rehabilitation (RADAR)**
12 City Forum, 2500 City Road,
London EC1V 8AF
Tel: 020 7250 3222
www.radar.org.uk

**Royal Hospital for
Neurodisability**
West Hill, Putney, London
SW15 3SW
Tel: 020 8780 4500
www.rhn.org.uk

EATING DISORDERS

British Nutrition Foundation
Tel: 020 7404 6504
www.nutrition.org.uk

Eating Disorders Association
First floor, Wensum House,
103 Prince of Wales Road,
Norwich NR1 1DW
Helpline 01603 621414
Youthline 01603 765050
www.edauk.com

Mind
Granta House, 15–19 Broadway,
London E15 4BQ
Helpline 020 8522 1728 London;
0845 766 0163 outside London
9.15am–5.15pm Mon–Fri
www.mind.org.uk

Overeaters Anonymous
Helpline 07000 784985
www.oagb.org.uk

ENDOCRINE SYSTEM

**Association for Cushing's
Treatment and Help**
Tel: 01628 670389

**British Society for Paediatric
Endocrinology and Diabetes**
www.bsped.org.uk

British Thyroid Foundation
PO Box 97 Clifford Wetherby, West
Yorkshire LS23 6XD
Tel: 0113 392 4600
www.british-thyroidassociation.org

Diabetes UK
Central Office, 10 Parkway,
London NW1 7AA
Tel: 020 7424 1000
www.diabetes.org.uk
Pituitary Foundation
PO Box 1944 Bristol BS99 2UB
Tel: 0870 774 3355
www.pituitary.org.uk

EPILEPSY
Epilepsy Action
New Anstey House, Gate Way
Drive, Yeadon, Leeds LS19 7XY
Freephone helpline 0808 800 5050
9am–4.30pm Mon–Thurs,
9am–4pm Friday
www.epilepsy.org.uk
National Society for Epilepsy
Chesham Lane, Chalfont St Peter,
Buckinghamshire SL9 0RJ
Tel: 01494 601300
www.epilepsynse.org.uk

EYE AND DISORDERS
College of Optometrists
42 Craven Street, London
WC2 5NG
Tel: 020 7839 6000
General Optical Council
Holds a list of optometrists
qualified to undertake eye tests.
41 Harley Street, London W1G 8DJ
Tel: 020 7580 3898
**Guide Dogs for the Blind
Association**
Burghfield Common, Reading
RG7 3YG
Tel: 0870 600 2323
www.gdba.org.uk
**International Glaucoma
Association**
108c Warner Road, London
SE5 9HQ
Tel: 020 7737 3265
www.iga.org.uk
LOOK
National Federation of Families
with Visually Impaired Children,
Queen Alexandra College, Court
Oak Road, Harbourne,
Birmingham B17 9TG
Tel: 0121 428 5038
www.look.graphicbox.co.uk
**Royal National Institute for the
Blind (RNIB)**
105 Judd Street, London WC1H 9NE
Tel: 020 7388 1266
Helpline 0845 766 9999 Mon–Fri
9am–5pm
Talking Book Service 08457 626843
Customer Services 0845 702 3153
minicom 0845 7585691
www.rnib.org.uk

Partially Sighted Society
PO Box 322, Doncaster DN1 2XA
Tel: 01302 323132
**Talking Newspaper Association
of the UK**
Tel: 01435 866102
www.tnauk.org.uk
Macular Disease Society
Darwin House, 13a Bridge Street,
Andover, Hants SP10 1BE
Tel: 0845 241 2041
www.maculardisease.org
The Eyecare Trust
Tel: 01673 857847
www.eyecare-trust.org.uk

FAMILY AND PERSONAL
ADVICE
The Site
Non-patronizing advice for young
people on sex and drugs.
www.thesite.org.uk
EXTEND
Tel: 01582 832760
www.extend.org.uk
NORM-UK
Tel: 01785 814044
www.norm-uk.org

FERTILITY PROBLEMS
**British Infertility Counselling
Association (BICA)**
69 Division Street, Sheffield S1 4GE
Tel: 01342 843880
www.bica.net
CHILD The national infertility
support group
Charter House, 3 St Leonards Road,
Bexhill on Sea, East Sussex
TN40 1JA. Tel: 01424 732361
www.child.org.uk
COTS Childlessness Overcome
Through Surrogacy
Tel: 01549 402 401
Helpline 0844 4140001
**Daisy Network (Premature
Menopause Support Group)**
PO Box 392, High Wycombe,
Bucks HP15 7SH
Tel: 01242 680522 or 01268
473466 evenings only
**Human Fertilisation and
Embryology Authority**
Paxton House, 30 Artillery Lane,
London E1 7LS
Tel: 020 7377 5077
www.hfea.gov.uk
ISSUE
The National Fertility Association,
114 Lichfield Street, Walsall,
West Midlands WS1 1SZ
Tel: 01922 722888
www.issue.co.uk

HAND AND FOOT
**Society of Chiropodists and
Podiatrists**
1 Fellmonger's Path, Tower Bridge
Road, London SE1 3LY
Tel: 020 7234 8620
www.feetforlife.org

HEARING DISORDERS
British Deaf Association
1–3 Worship Street, London
EC2A 2AB
Helpline 0870 770 3300
Textphone 0800 6522 965
www.bda.org.uk
British Tinnitus Association
4th floor, White Building, Fitzalan
Square, Sheffield S1 2AZ
Tel: 0114 279 6600
www.tinnitus.org.uk
Ménière's Society
98 Maybury Road, Woking, Surrey
GU21 5HX
Tel: 01483 740597
www.menieres.co.uk
National Deaf Children's Society
15 Dufferin Street, London
EC1Y 8UR
Helpline 0808 800 8880
www.ndcs.org.uk
**Royal National Institute for
Deaf people (RNID)**
19–23 Featherstone Street, London
EC1Y 8SL
Helpline 0808 808 0123
Textphone 0808 808 9000
www.rnid.org.uk

HEART AND
CIRCULATORY PROBLEMS
Arterial Disease Clinics
Prospect House, 32 Bolton Road,
Atherton, Manchester
Tel: 01942 886644
www.chelationuk.com
British Heart Foundation
14 Fitzhardinge Street, London
W1H 6DH
Tel: 020 7935 0185
www.bhf.org.uk
British Vascular Foundation
Fides House, 10 Chertsey Road,
Woking, Surrey GU21 5AB
www.bvf.org.uk
Cardiomyopathy Association
40 The Metro Centre, Tolpits Lane,
Watford WD1 8SB
Helpline 0800 018 1024
www.cardiomyopathy.org
Heartlink
60 Heatherly Drive, Forrestown,
Mansfield, Nottingham NG19 0PY
Freephone 0500 676670

**Royal Free Hospital, Department
of Vascular Surgery**
www.freevas.demon.co.uk
**UK & Overseas Heart Society
Heartlink**
25 Close Street, Hemsworth,
Pontefract, West Yorkshire WF9 4QP
Freephone 0500 676 670
www.heartlink.org.uk

HOME AND SAFETY
Health and Safety Executive
Helpline 08701 545500
8.30am–5pm Mon–Fri
www.hse.gov.uk
**Royal Society for the Prevention
of Accidents (RoSPA)**
Edgbaston Park, 353 Bristol Road,
Birmingham B5 7ST
Tel: 0121 248 2000

LEARNING DIFFICULTIES
British Dyslexia Association
98 London Road, Reading
RG1 5AU
Tel: 0118 966 2677
www.bda-dyslexia.org.uk
Dyspraxia Foundation
8 West Alley, Hitchin, Herts SG3 1EG
Tel: 01462 454986
www.dyspraxiafoundation.org.uk
**Foundation for People with
Learning Disabilities**
7th floor, 83 Victoria Street,
London SW1H 0HW
Tel: 020 77802 0300
www.learningdisabilities.org.uk

ME
ME Association
4 Top Angel, Buckingham
Industrial Park, Buckingham, Bucks
MK18 1TH
Tel: 01280 816115
www.meassociation.org.uk
Action for ME
PO Box 1302, Wells, Somerset
BA5 1YE
Tel: 01749 670799
www.afme.org.uk
National ME Support Centre
Disablement Services Centre,
Harold Wood Hospital, Romford,
Essex RM3 0BE
Tel: 01708 378050
www.nmec.org.uk
**Association of Young People
with ME (AYME)**
www.ayme.org.uk

MEN'S HEALTH
Male health
www.malehealth.co.uk
Circumcision
Information and Resource Pages
www.cirp.org

MENTAL HEALTH
Alzheimer's Society
Gordon House, 10 Greencoat Place,
London SW1P 1PH
Helpline 0845 300 0336
**Association of Occupational
Therapists in Mental Health**
120 Wilton Road, London
SW1V 1JZ
Tel: 020 7233 8322
Association for Postnatal Illness
145 Dawes Road, London SW6 7EB
Tel: 020 7386 0868
**British Association for
Counselling and Psychotherapy**
BACP House, 35–37 Albert Street,
Rugby CV21 2SG
Tel: 0870 443 5252
www.bac.co.uk
www.counselling.co.uk
British Psychological Society
St Andrew's House, Princess Road
East, Leicester LE1 7DR
Tel: 0116 254 9568
www.bps.org.uk
Depression Alliance
35 Westminster Bridge Road,
London SE1 7JB
Tel: 020 7633 0557
www.depressionalliance.org
**Fellowship of Depressives
Anonymous**
Box FDAI, c/o Self-Help
Nottingham, Ormiston House,
32–36 Pelham Street, Nottingham
NG1 2EG
Tel: 01702 433 3838
Hearing Voices Network
91 Oldham Street, Manchester
M4 1LW
Tel: 0161 834 5768
www.hearing-voices.org.uk
Institute of Family Therapy
43 New Cavendish Street, London
W1M 7RG
Tel: 020 7935 1651
www.instituteoffamilytherapy.co.uk
Manic Depression Fellowship
Castle Works, 21 St George's Road,
London SE1 6ES
Tel: 020 7793 2600
www.mdf.org.uk
Mencap
123 Golden Lane, London EC1Y 0RT
Helpline 020 7696 6020
www.mencap.org.uk

Mind
Granta House, 15–19 Broadway,
London E15 4BQ
Helpline 020 8522 1728 London;
0845 766 0163 outside London
9.15am–5.15pm Mon–Fri
www.mind.org.uk
National Autistic Society
393 City Road, London EC1V 1NG
Helpline 0870 600 8585
www.nas.org.uk
**National Schizophrenia
Fellowship**
28 Castle Street, Kingston-upon-
Thames, Surrey KT1 1SS
National advice line 020 8974 6814
www.nsf.org.uk
Royal College of Psychiatrists
Surviving adolescence factsheet
available online at
www.rcpsych.ac.uk/info/help/adol/
index.htm.
SAD Association
PO Box 989, Steyning, BN44 3HG
Tel: 01903 814842
www.sada.org.uk
Samaritans
The Upper Mill, Kingston Road,
Ewell, Surrey KT17 2AF
Helpline 08457 90 90 90
www.samaritans.org.uk
Stress, Anxiety and Depression
Confidential helpline 01622 717 656
http://stresshelp.tripod.com
**Survivors of Bereavement by
Suicide**
Centre 88, Saner Street, Analaby
Road, Hull, Humberside HU3 2TR
Helpline 01482 826559
www.uk-sobs.org.uk
Wellbeing
27 Sussex Place, London NW1 4SP
Tel: 020 7772 6400
www.wellbeing.org.uk
Young Minds
102–108 Clerkenwell Road,
London EC1M 5SA
Provides advice to anyone
concerned with the mental health of
children or adolescents.
Tel: 020 7336 8445
www.youngminds.org.uk

PAIN MANAGEMENT
Pain Relief Foundation
Clinical Sciences Centre, University
Hospital Aintree, Lower Lane,
Liverpool L9 7AL
Tel: 0151 529 5820
www.painrelieffoundation.org.uk
PainSUPPORT
www.painsupport.co.uk

PHOBIA
First Steps to Freedom
1 Taylor Close, Kenilworth,
Warwickshire CV8 2LW
Tel: 01926 851608
www.first-steps.org
National Phobics Society
Zion Community Resource Centre,
339 Stretford Road, Hulme,
Manchester M15 4ZY
Helpline 0870 770 0456
www.phobics-society.org.uk
No Panic
93 Brands Farm Way, Randley,
Telford, Salop TF3 2JQ
Tel: 0808 808 0545
www.no-panic.co.uk
**PAX (Panic attacks, phobias and
anxiety disorders)**
4 Manor Brook, Blackheath,
London SE3 9AW
Tel: 020 8318 5026
www.panicattacks.co.uk
Triumph over Phobia (TOP UK)
PO Box 1831, Bath BA2 4YW
Tel: 01225 330353
www.triumphoverphobia.com

PREGNANCY
Action on Pre-eclampsia (APEC)
84–88 Pinner Road, Harrow,
Middlesex HA1 4HZ
Tel: 020 8427 4217
www.apec.org.uk
Antenatal Results and Choices
73–75 Charlotte Street, London
W1T 4PN
Helpline 020 7631 0285
www.arc-uk.org
Family Planning Association
2–12 Pentonville Road,
London N1 9FP
Helpline 020 7837 4044
Fetal Alcohol Syndrome Trust
Tel: 0151 284 2900
La Leche League (Great Britain)
PO Box 29, West Bridgeford,
Nottingham NG2 7NP
Tel: 020 7242 1278
www.laleche.org.uk
Maternity Alliance
3rd Floor West, 2–6 Northburgh
Street, London EC1V 0AY
Tel: 020 7490 7639
Info line 020 7490 7638
www.maternityalliance.org.uk
National Childbirth Trust
Alexandra House, Oldham Terrace,
Acton, London W3 6N
Helpline 0870 444 8707
www.nctpregnancyandbabycare.com

SANDS
Stillbirth and Neonatal Death
Society, 28 Portland Place, London
W1B 1LY
Tel: 020 7436 7940

SEXUALLY TRANSMITTED
DISEASES
To find your nearest GUM clinic,
look in your phone book under
GUM; contact your nearest general
hospital; or contact NHS Direct
Tel: 0845 4647. www.fpa.org.uk
For advice for young people try
www.playingsafely.co.uk

Herpes Viruses Association
41 North Road, London N7 9DP
Tel: 020 7609 9061

SKIN AND HAIR
Acne Support Group
PO Box 9, Newquay, Cornwall
TR9 6WG
Helpline 0870 8702263
British Red Cross
Offers advice on camouflage creams
to cover disfiguring skin conditions.
www.redcross.org.uk
Institute of Trichologists
5 Belsford Court, Watnall,
Nottingham NG16 1JW
Tel: 0870 6070602
www.trichologists.org.uk
**Wessex Cancer Trust Melanoma
and Related Cancers of the Skin**
MARCS line 01722 415071
www.wessexcancer.org

SMOKING, ALCOHOL AND
DRUGS
**Action for Smoking and Health
(ASH)**
102 Clifton Street, London
EC2A 4HW
Tel: 020 7739 5902
www.ash.org.uk
ADFAM
A charity for families and friends
of drug users.
Tel: 020 7928 8898
Al-Anon Family Group UK & Eire
61 Great Dover Street, London
SE1 4YF
Tel: 020 7403 0888
www.alanonuk.org.uk
Alcoholics Anonymous (AA)
Helpline 0845 769 7555
www.alcoholics-anonymous.org.uk
Alcohol Concern
Online directory of alcohol
treatment services in the UK.
www.alcoholconcern.org.uk

Advice and Counselling on Alcohol and Drugs ACAD
Charity offering free advice, information and counselling.
www.acad.org.uk

Association of the British Pharmaceutical Industry
www.abpi.org.uk

Cascade
An information service on drugs run by and for young people.
Tel: 0121 788 3436
cascade@cascade.u-net.com

Drinkline
For advice on problem drinking
Helpline 0800 917 8282 9am–11pm Mon–Fri; 6–11pm Sat, Sun

DrugScope
Helpline 0870 7743 682
email: services@drugscope.org.uk
www.drugscope.org.uk

Families anonymous
A support group for the parents of drug users.
Tel: 020 7498 4680

Medicines Control Agency
www.mca.gov.uk

Narcotics Helpline
Tel: 020 7730 0009
www.ukna.org

National Drugs Helpline
For free confidential advice, local services and rehabilitation clinics.
24-hour Freephone 0800 776600
www.ndh.org.uk

NHS Smoking Helpline
0800 169 0 169

Pregnancy Smoking Helpline
0800 169 9 169
www.givingupsmoking.co.uk

Quitline
0800 002200 9am–9pm daily

Re-solv
Helpline 0808 800 2345
www.re-solv.org

SPEECH DISORDERS
Association For All Speech Impaired Children
2nd floor, 50–52 Great Sutton Street, London EC1V 0DJ
Helpline 0845 355 5577
www.afasic.org.uk

British Stammering Association
15 Old Ford Road, London E2 9PJ
Tel: 020 8983 1003
Helpline 0845 603 2001
www.stammer.demon.co.uk

SURGERY
Royal College of Surgeons
35–43 Lincoln's Inn Fields, London WC2A 3PE
Tel: 020 7405 3474

British Association of Aesthetic Plastic Surgeons
Adviceline 020 7405 2234
www.baaps.org.uk

British Association of Plastic Surgeons
www.baps.co.uk

TEETH AND DENTISTRY
British Dental Association
64 Wimpole Street, London W1E 8YS
Tel: 020 7563 4166
www.bda-dentistry.org.uk

British Dental Health Foundation
Smile House, 2 East Union Street, Rugby, Warwickshire CV22 6AJ
Helpline 0845 063 1188
www.dentalhealth.org.uk

British Society for Medical and Dental Hypnosis
28 Dole Parts Gardens, Cookridge, Leeds LS16 7PT
Tel: 07000 560309
www.bsmdh.org

NHS Direct
For a list of NHS dentists
Tel: 0845 4647
www.nhsdirect.nhs.uk

Dental payment plan
www.denplan.co.uk
www.cigna.co.uk

TRANSPLANT
British Organ Donor Society (BODY)
Balsham, Cambridge CB1 6DL
Tel: 01223 893636
www.argonet.co.uk/body

Transplant Support Network
Temple Row Centre, 23 Temple Row, Keighley BD21 2AH
Tel: 01535 692323
Helpline 01535 210101
www.transplantsupportnetwork.org.uk

UK Transplant
Fox Den Road, Stoke Gifford, Bristol BS34 8RR
Tel: 0117 975 7575
www.uktransplant.org

TRAVEL AND HEALTH
Department of Health
Health Advice for Travellers leaflet, available free from post offices or Health Literature Line 0800 555777
www.doh.gov.uk/traveladvice

Foreign and Commonwealth Office
Advice 020 7008 0232
www.fco.gov.uk/travel

Hospital for Tropical Diseases
Mortimer Market, Capper Street, off Tottenham Court Road, London WC1E 6AU
Tel: 020 7387 9300 or 020 7387 4411; Travellers Healthline Advisory Service 09050 567733
www.thehtd.org

Vaccination Awareness Network UK
178 Mansfield Road, Nottingham NG1 3HW
Tel: 0115 948 0829

URINARY SYSTEM
Enuresis Resource and Information Centre (ERIC)
34 Old School House, Britannia Road, Kingswood, Bristol BS15 8DB
Tel: 0117 960 3060
www.eric.org.uk

National Kidney Federation
6 Stanley Street, Worksop, Notts S81 7HX
Tel: 01909 487795
Helpline 0845 601 0209
www.kidney.org.uk

National Kidney Research Fund
Kings Chambers, Priestgate, Peterborough PE1 1FG
Tel: 01733 704650
Helpline 0845 300 1499
www.nkrf.org.uk

British Kidney Patient Association
Borden, Hampshire GU35 9JZ
Tel: 01420 472021

WOMEN'S HEALTH
Breast Cancer Care
Kiln House, 210 New Kings Road, London SW6 4NZ
Tel: 0808 800 6000
www. breastcancercare.org.uk

Daisy Network
Premature Menopause Support Group
Tel: 01242 680 522 or 01628 473 446 evenings only

Hysterectomy Association
60 Redwood House, Charlton Down, Dorchester, Dorset DT2 9HU
Tel: 0871 7811141
www.hysterectomy-association.org.uk

Marie Stopes International
153–157 Cleveland Street, London W1T 6QW
Tel: 020 7574 7400
www.mariestopes.org.uk

National Association for Premenstrual Syndrome NAPS
41 Old Road, East Peckham, Kent TN12 5AP
Helpline 0870 777 2177
www.pms.org.uk

National Endometriosis Society
www.endo.org.uk

OBGYN.Net
www.obgyn.net

Women's Health
www.womens-health.co.uk

Women's Nutritional Advisory Service (WNAS)
PO Box 268, Lewes, East Sussex BN7 1Q1
Tel: 01273 487366
www.wnas.org.uk

Index

Page numbers in bold type identify main entries in the A–Z section of the book.